AF809961

Isidoro Di Carlo
Editor

Difficult Acute Cholecystitis

Treatment and Technical Issues

Springer

Editor
Isidoro Di Carlo
Department of Medical, Surgical Sciences and Advanced Technologies
University of Catania
Catania
Italy

ISBN 978-3-030-62101-8 ISBN 978-3-030-62102-5 (eBook)
https://doi.org/10.1007/978-3-030-62102-5

© Springer Nature Switzerland AG 2021
This work is subject to copyright. All rights are reserved by the Publisher, whether the whole or part of the material is concerned, specifically the rights of translation, reprinting, reuse of illustrations, recitation, broadcasting, reproduction on microfilms or in any other physical way, and transmission or information storage and retrieval, electronic adaptation, computer software, or by similar or dissimilar methodology now known or hereafter developed.
The use of general descriptive names, registered names, trademarks, service marks, etc. in this publication does not imply, even in the absence of a specific statement, that such names are exempt from the relevant protective laws and regulations and therefore free for general use.
The publisher, the authors, and the editors are safe to assume that the advice and information in this book are believed to be true and accurate at the date of publication. Neither the publisher nor the authors or the editors give a warranty, expressed or implied, with respect to the material contained herein or for any errors or omissions that may have been made. The publisher remains neutral with regard to jurisdictional claims in published maps and institutional affiliations.

This Springer imprint is published by the registered company Springer Nature Switzerland AG
The registered company address is: Gewerbestrasse 11, 6330 Cham, Switzerland

Foreword

The book you have in your hands holds all the knowledge that a surgeon should master to perform a cholecystectomy. This intervention is a perfect demonstration of the considerable improvement in the surgical management of patients. The approach and study of all aspects of the pathology, associated with the participation of very high level experts, make this book an essential reference. The choice of authors, all experts and often great teachers, and the choice of chapters allow readers to consolidate their knowledge and, if necessary, to develop it, especially in difficult situations, with confidence. It is Isidoro Di Carlo's success and intelligence to have made these choices and—what a very good idea—not to have hesitated to propose almost seven chapters on the same theme of difficult cholecystectomy! Consecutive reading of these seven chapters certainly brings us more information than many conferences on the subject.

At the time, admittedly distant, of my first years of surgery, a patient operated on for a gallbladder could remain hospitalized for 12 days with, of course, a drainage tube, a gastric tube, and a more or less prolonged postoperative fasting period. So, we could not rely on any morphological examination to know the specific anatomy of the patient, no strategy for the prevention of complications other than "beautiful dissection," and of course no decision algorithm nor guidelines because the surgery was considered an art.

This book shows that we have moved from a culture of gesture and technology to a culture of results and therefore safety. And yet, as rightly says Isidoro Di Carlo, this intervention—a priori and often simple—can be extremely difficult with dire consequences in the event of an error in the surgeon's judgment or strategy.

Finally, the book ends on a high note with the prevention and management of bile duct injuries. The last two chapters insist on the importance of collegiality and the multidisciplinarity of the team, which allows the necessary distance to choose an appropriate attitude, especially during the procedure.

But if you will allow me, former anatomist that I am, I wish to return to three risks of complications that may concern the simplest cholecystectomy and which are explained by anatomical concepts perfectly described or pointed out in this volume, particularly in the remarkable first chapter on anatomy.

Calot's Triangle

We must return to the historical definition of Calot's triangle because some authors have kept this name to define the modern dissection triangle at the risk of misleading a surgeon who would seek to apply it to the latter. As we know today, it is not the exposure of the Calot's triangle that ensures a safe dissection but that of the hepatocystic triangle, allowing a good critical view of safety with its three components (Strasberg): (1) the fibrous and fatty tissue is dissected off the hepatocystic (HC) triangle, (2) at least one third of the gallbladder is dissected from the gallbladder fossa/cystic plate, and (3) only two structures (cystic artery and cystic duct) are seen entering the gallbladder.

The authors of Chap. 15 said "the CVS technique is aimed especially at mobilizing the gallbladder neck from the liver in the appropriate cystic plate to obtain a circumferential identification of the cystic duct and its transition into the gallbladder." But they add: "To establish CVS, two windows need to be created during dissection of Calot's triangle: one window between the cystic artery, cystic duct and gallbladder, and another one between the cystic artery, gallbladder, and liver." Calot's triangle is stricto sensu only the first window. If you add the second window going to the liver, you get the HC triangle.

In 1890, François Calot in his thesis (Fig. 1) very precisely described a triangle.

"The common bile duct forms the right edge of the gastrohepatic omentum and the cystic duct roughly continues its direction. These two channels together describe a curved line with a concavity facing right and forward. The hepatic duct is connected to the union of the two channels, which thus forms, with the artery and the cystic duct, a kind of equilateral triangle." (Fig. 2) "The triangle is not exactly equilateral but rather isosceles, the two upper and lower sides, represented by the artery and the cystic duct being equal and only a little longer than the part of the hepatic duct which enters into the constitution of the triangle."

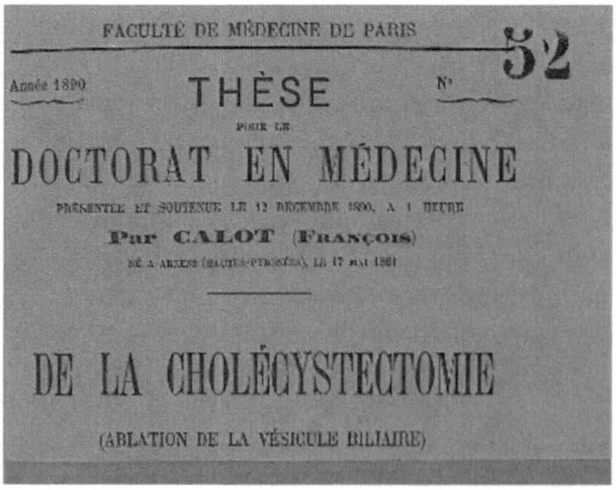
FACULTÉ DE MÉDECINE DE PARIS

Année 1890 THÈSE N° 52

POUR LE

DOCTORAT EN MÉDECINE

PRÉSENTÉE ET SOUTENUE LE 12 DÉCEMBRE 1890, À 1 HEURE

Par CALOT (François)

[illegible]

DE LA CHOLÉCYSTECTOMIE

(ABLATION DE LA VÉSICULE BILIAIRE)

Fig. 1 François Calot's thesis

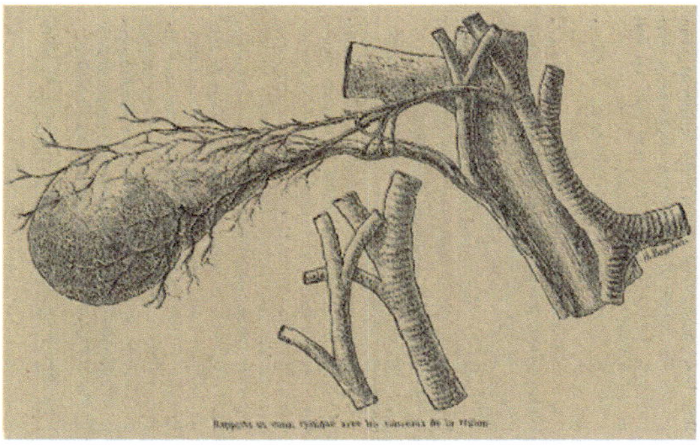

Fig. 2 Calot's triangle: drawing of the area made by Calot himself

Luschka's Duct

Luschka describes subvesical bile ducts in the gallbladder liver bed that may be injured, causing a postoperative bile leak, and specifies in his article that it is rare that this duct drains into the cystic duct (0.07% of cysticohepatic ducts in a series of 2012) and quite exceptional in the gallbladder (cholecystohepatic duct). It is really extremely rare to see a true picture of such a duct, and this is good because the latter is necessarily interrupted during gallbladder release, which requires a ligature or repair if it drains a significant portion of the parenchyma as in the case reported by Maeda in 2020.

There is nothing to add to the description given in the first chapter by Loukas et al.: "In 30% of the population, a small bile duct from segment 5 crosses the gallbladder fossa and is referred to as Luschka's duct. It may drain into the right hepatic duct, the common hepatic duct, or rarely the cystic duct. Since the majority of these accessory ducts are small and insignificant, any additional ducts encountered in the gallbladder fossa could be ligated safely. However, some accessory ducts may drain significant portions of the right hepatic lobe. These cases are defined as aberrant ducts, and studies have emphasized they might need to be protected during surgery."

Anatomical Variations of Pedicle Structures Close to the Cystic Duct

The variations in biliary convergence are reviewed in the very good chapter by Martinez et al. The five anomalies according to Benson and Page are a long cystic duct with low fusion with the common hepatic duct (CHD), abnormally high fusion of cystic duct with CHD, accessory hepatic duct, cystic duct entering right hepatic duct, and finally the cholecystohepatic duct which is, as we have seen, exceptional. These structures must be recognized.

However, some structures, the most dangerous, are missing (Fig. 3). Figure 3a shows a downward slide of the right anterior (or posterior) hepatic duct; Fig. 3b shows a low bifurcation and therefore a cystic duct that empties into the right duct, with the risk of mistaking the left duct for the common bile

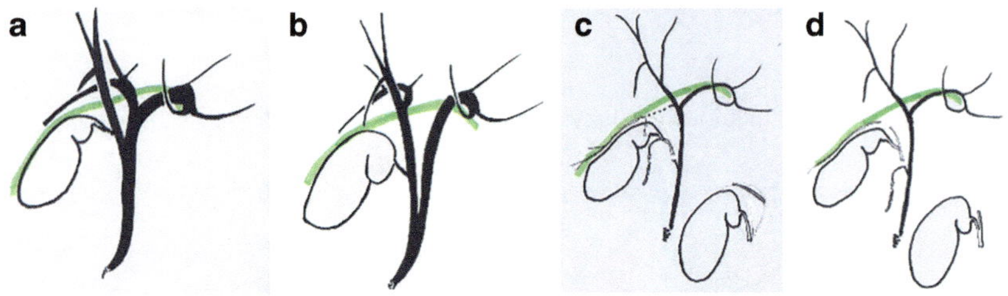

Fig. 3 Anatomical variations of pedicle structures close to the cystic duct

duct (CBD); and finally, Fig. 3c and d show two different connections of a true Luschka's duct, which can drain a more or less important part of the liver and is not protected by the dissection of the Calot's triangle alone.

For the sake of completeness, let us remember that the position of the arteries and especially that of the right hepatic artery can also be a proven risk. In Chap. 11, the authors also perfectly describe risky situations: "One common variation occurs when the right hepatic artery runs within the lower end of the Calot's triangle in a tortuous course referred to as caterpillar or Moynihan's hump. This variation can have an incidence as high as 50%. A Moynihan's hump is clinically relevant as the cystic artery is significantly shorter in these patients. As a result, the right hepatic artery could be misidentified as the cystic artery and could result in erroneous ligation.... In other cases, the right hepatic artery has been found to take another aberrant course in which it passes anterior to the bile duct or even posterior to the portal vein."

We hope that these reminders, which only underline points already mentioned in the various chapters, will at least reduce biliary accidents. These occurrences may seem rare as their incidence is close to 0.3%. However, at 600,000 cholecystectomies per year in the United States, this rate represents 1800 cases each year.

Brice Gayet
Paris Descartes University Medical School
Paris, France

Digestive Surgery Department
Montsouris Institute
Paris, France

Preface

Acute cholecystitis is one of the most common emergencies in the context of acute care surgery. In recent decades, surgical societies and expert groups have produced guidelines that have sought to guide surgical behavior in relation to these diseases. However, despite the advice of many experts, treatment of this disease remains a challenge, especially for the complications that can arise from related surgical procedures. To describe all the tricks that can be used to cure the difficult cases of acute cholecystitis, without complications, represents the main goal of this book. It is important to remember that it is a benign disease, and strong complication cannot be accepted both by surgeons and patients. For this reason in these pages, residents and young surgeons will find all the eminent advice that can be used daily to treat safely all patients affected by this disease.

All the surgeons that have contributed to this textbook are preeminent scientists. With their personal experience, they have contributed to clarify all the aspects of difficult acute cholecystitis. I am indebted to all the authors for their valuable work.

I met during my career skilled surgeons expert in a dedicated field of surgery, but I met only one surgeon who is able to operate all the organs of the abdomen with extraordinary skills both using open and laparoscopic approaches. In my opinion Prof. Brice Gayet is one of the best surgeons of the world, and I am really honored and grateful that he has accepted to write a foreword to this book.

Catania, Italy　　　　Isidoro Di Carlo

Anatomy of the Gallbladder and Biliary Tract

1

Vincent Courant, Michael Montalbano, Anna Zurada, Agnieszka Zurada-Zielińska, Jerzy Gielecki, and Marios Loukas

1.1 Introduction

Cholecystitis accounts for up to 10% of cases of abdominal pain worldwide. For most patients with acute cholecystitis, the preferred treatment is surgical excision of the gallbladder, commonly via laparoscopic cholecystectomy. Other treatment options are open surgery, percutaneous cholecystostomy tube, antibiotics, and supportive therapy. In the U.S alone, around 600,000 people are subjected to cholecystectomy annually [1]. Anatomical variations with clinical significance are found in 20% of laparoscopic cholecystectomies. These mostly include variations in the cystic artery (10%), cystic duct (4%), right hepatic artery (3%), and the gallbladder itself (2%) [2]. Misinterpretation of the exposed anatomy contributes to complications, which occur in 1–6% of laparoscopic cholecystectomy cases. Common iatrogenic injuries are directed toward the biliary tree and surrounding blood vessels, with such injuries possibly causing severe morbidity and life-threatening situations. As a result, it is crucial for surgeons to have a clear understanding of the underlying anatomy, as well as be aware of possible anatomical variations to ensure the best results for their patients.

1.2 Anatomy of the Gallbladder

The gallbladder is a flask-shaped, hollow organ that may vary in size and shape. In adults, the gallbladder usually measures 7–10 cm in length with a capacity of up to 50 mL. The organ is usually found resting on the gallbladder fossa, which is located on the inferior surface and marks the caudal limit of Couinaud segments 4 and 5 (Fig. 1.1), although this location may change between individuals [1]. However, there are cases of intrahepatic gallbladder where the organ lies within the liver parenchyma or under

V. Courant
Department of Anatomical Sciences, St. George's University School of Medicine, St. George's, Grenada

Department of Internal Medicine, Icahn School of Medicine at Mount Sinai/St. Luke's-Roosevelt Hospital Center, New York, NY, USA
e-mail: vcourant@sgu.edu

M. Montalbano
Department of Anatomical Sciences, St. George's University School of Medicine, St. George's, Grenada
e-mail: mmontal1@sgu.edu

A. Zurada
Department of Radiology, Collegium Medicum, School of Medicine, University of Warmia and Mazury, Olsztyn, Poland

A. Zurada-Zielińska · J. Gielecki
Department of Anatomy, University of Warmia and Mazury, Olsztyn, Poland
e-mail: jerzy.gielecki@uwm.edu.pl

M. Loukas (✉)
Department of Anatomical Sciences, St. George's University School of Medicine, St. George's, Grenada

Department of Anatomy, University of Warmia and Mazury, Olsztyn, Poland
e-mail: mloukas@sgu.edu

© Springer Nature Switzerland AG 2021

I. Di Carlo (ed.), *Difficult Acute Cholecystitis*, https://doi.org/10.1007/978-3-030-62102-5_1

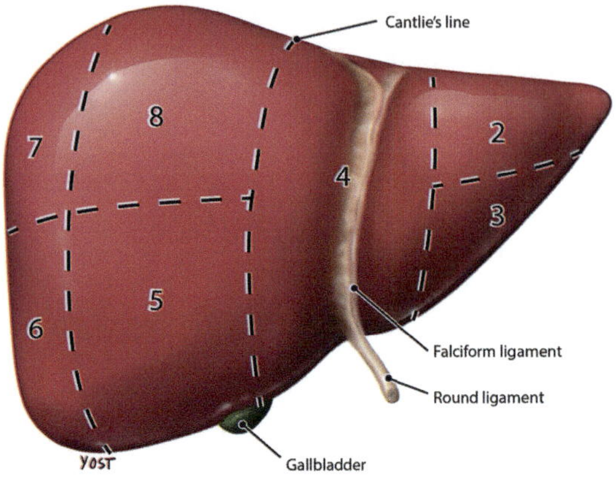

Fig. 1.1 Liver segments and their relation to the gallbladder. (Printed with permission Katie Yost, 2020)

the hepatic capsule at the inferior part of the right lobe. This variation can generate difficulties with dissection as well as heighten the probability of intraoperative hepatic injury. "Floating gallbladders," where the organ hangs freely and is only attached to the cystic mesentery, have also been found [2]. This particular variation may predispose the patient to gallbladder torsion [3]. On rare occasions, additional ectopic locations of the gallbladder have been found to occur at the lesser omentum, falciform ligament, transverse mesocolon, suprahepatic, abdominal wall, retrorenal space, left lower abdomen, and adjacent to the inferior vena cava [2].

The gallbladder is typically separated into three components: the fundus, the body, and the neck.

The neck is defined as the posterosuperior limit of the gallbladder connected to the cystic duct. It is typically 5–7 mm in diameter and takes an S-shaped curve. The neck is located close to the porta hepatis, which is a 5-cm deep fissure extending transversely underneath the left portion of the right hepatic lobe. The porta hepatis is located within the hilum of the liver and contains, from posterior to anterior, the portal vein, the right and left hepatic arteries, as well as the right and left hepatic ducts. A reflection of the peritoneum covering the inferior surface of the liver forms a sleeve around these structures referred to as the hepatoduodenal ligament or free edge of the lesser omentum. A fold of peritoneum connects the hepatoduodenal ligament to the peritoneal layers around the gallbladder, forming the cholecystoduodenal ligament. Of note, on the medial surface of the neck there is a spiral groove that may run along the spiral valves of the cystic duct. The valves are made of several crescentic folds projecting into the lumen of the duct and may be absent in 2% of the population [2].

On the lateral side of the neck, there may be an outpouching referred to as Hartmann's pouch. This expansion is often measured via sonographic imaging to find evidence of dilation or presence of stones. While the pouch may vary in size, a larger Hartmann's pouch can obscure the cystic duct, common hepatic duct, and cystic artery. Similarly, a large stone in a Hartmann's pouch causes an erosion into the bile duct in a condition referred to as Mirizzi's syndrome. These cases can create major difficulties during cholecystectomy.

The body represents the central portion of the gallbladder between the neck and fundus. The body is typically in contact with the liver at the gallbladder fossa, which is usually found anteriorly in relation to the second part of the duodenum and to the right of the transverse colon. The fundus is the most distal part of the gallbladder and forms the anteroinferior margin. It is lateral to the body and often contacts the anterior abdominal wall at the costal margin [4]. The fundus usually folds back on the body of the gallbladder. The gallbladder lumen is widest at the junction of the body and fundus and gets narrower as it travels toward the neck with the most rapidly narrowing segment called the infundibulum.

In some cases, the fundus and body might be separated by an external cleft leading to the formation of a "double" or "bilobed" gallbladder. The second gallbladder is referred to as "accessory" if it drains into a separate cystic duct. An accessory gallbladder may vary in size and may either be separated from its counterpart or contained together within a single peritoneal envelope. The gallbladder might also display a diverticulum along its length, measuring up to 5 cm. In rare cases (0.07%), the gallbladder is entirely absent, with the rest of the biliary tree anatomy remaining normal. In these cases, ultrasound imaging may fail to make the correct diagnosis of absent gallbladder, which can lead to patients undergoing unnecessary surgery [2].

The shape of the gallbladder may also vary. There have been cases of septate gallbladder, which are constituted with the presence of a septum that partly or entirely divides the gallbladder into chambers that are empty via a single cystic duct. The gallbladder might also display a diverticulum along its length, measuring up to 5 cm.

1.3 Biliary Tree

1.3.1 Cystic Duct

The cystic duct is one of the main structures that need to be identified during cholecystectomy. The cystic duct measures from 2 to 4 cm in length and 2 to 3 mm in width. However, size may vary, and a cystic duct larger than 5 mm could be mistaken for the common bile duct. It is also important to note that about 20% of the U.S. population has a cystic duct measuring less than 2 cm, which will make ligations more difficult. The duct commonly travels posteriorly and to the left of the gallbladder neck. The duct usually follows a tortuous course until it meets the common hepatic duct, from the right lateral aspect to form the common bile duct at a variable site ranging from the right hepatic duct to the ampulla of Vater region (Fig. 1.2). Less commonly, the cystic duct may also be S-shaped, curved with acute flexures, or straight.

The cystic duct has been found to exhibit several anatomic variations. The cystic duct junction with the common hepatic duct may occur at a more inferior point in the free margin of the lesser omentum. The cystic duct has also been observed taking different routes as it travels away from the gallbladder. In 75% of cases, the cystic duct joins the common bile duct at an acute angle. It has also been observed to run parallel to the right side of the common hepatic duct in 20% of cases. Rarely, the cystic duct may take a spiral course posterior to the common hepatic duct before entering on its left side (5%) [2].

Since such variations are possible, ligating the cystic duct at its connection with the common bile duct may predispose patients to biliary tree injury. It is helpful to remember that, even with its variations, the cystic duct rarely runs posterior to the duodenum. Therefore, ductal structures that pass behind the duodenum are more likely to be common bile ducts [1]. Another way that may distinguish the two structures is that the cystic duct usually will not have vessels traversing its surface, while the common bile duct does [4].

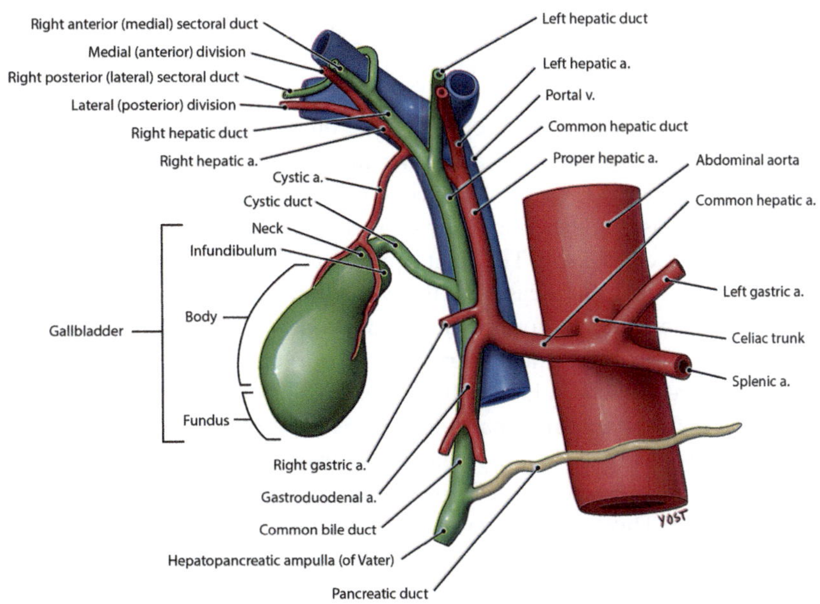

Fig. 1.2 Anatomy of the gallbladder and biliary tree. (Printed with permission Katie Yost, 2020)

The cystic duct may also display aberrant drainage to the left and right hepatic duct, right intrahepatic sectional duct, or drain into the left side of the common hepatic duct. Accessory intrahepatic ducts draining into the cystic duct may also occur. Additionally, the cystic duct may vary numerically as it may be completely absent or present as a double cystic duct, although they are exceedingly rare. As a result, if two ducts are seen entering the gallbladder surgeons should keep a high suspicion that one of the ducts is part of another structure related to the biliary tree [1].

1.3.2 Hepatic Bile Duct

In the liver parenchyma, bile canaliculi fuse to form segmental bile ducts, each draining one hepatic segment. The segmental ducts then combine in a specific pattern to form sectional ducts. Ducts from segments 6 and 7 form the right posterior sectional duct, and ducts from segments 5 and 8 form the right anterior sectional duct. The right hepatic duct arises from the meeting of the right anterior and right posterior sectional ducts at a variable intrahepatic point (Fig. 1.2).

Segments 2 and 3 contribute segmental ducts that coalesce to form the left lateral section duct, which then unites with the duct from segment 4 to form the left hepatic duct. The right and left hepatic ducts meet to form the common hepatic duct near the medial end of the porta hepatis.

The right hepatic duct takes a short vertical course of about 1 cm, while the left hepatic duct travels horizontally for 3 cm along the inferior border of segment 4 (Fig. 1.1). The right hepatic duct system has a higher frequency of variation than the left ductal system. The right hepatic duct may be absent in 15% of cases. In this variation, the common bile duct is formed by a triple confluence from the right anterior, right posterior, and left hepatic ducts. Additionally, a right sectoral duct may join the left hepatic duct in 15% of cases. Occasionally, a right segmental duct may join the common hepatic duct below the normal meeting point. This variation may cause the right segmental duct to be misidentified for the cystic duct during surgery. Consequently, if a structure similar to the cystic duct is to be divided, careful dissection toward the infundibulum should be performed to verify that it is directly connected to the gallbladder [5].

Rarely, the duct from segment 5 or the right posterior sectoral duct drains directly into the cystic duct or the gallbladder itself. Also, infrequently, some branches of the right posterior sectional duct may enter the distal bile duct supraportally and the remaining branches infraportally.

The left intrahepatic ductal system may vary in the arrangement of the segmental duct from segment 5. This segmental duct may drain into the bile ducts from segments 2 or 3, the right anterior sectoral duct, or the common hepatic duct. The bile ducts from segment 1 usually join the origin of the left hepatic duct but may drain into both hepatic ducts.

Finally, there might be multiple accessory hepatic ducts. A more detailed review on accessory ducts will be covered later in this chapter.

1.3.3 Common Bile Duct

The common bile duct is on average between 6 and 8 cm long and travels infero-posteriorly within the right border of the lesser omentum. It travels anterior and to the right of the portal vein, as well as to the right of the hepatic artery. The common bile duct then runs posterior to the first part of the duodenum and to the left of the gastroduodenal artery. It passes posterior to the head of the pancreas, forming its retropancreatic portion. Finally, the common bile duct passes through the sphincter of Oddi to enter the second part of the duodenum at the major papilla, where it may be palpated during surgery [4, 5]. Of note, the pancreatic duct forms a common channel with the common bile duct in 85% of cases; however, the two ducts may enter the duodenum separately. The common bile duct may also vary numerically. In some cases, the common bile duct is completely absent. In this rare variation, the left and right hepatic ducts drain into the gallbladder while the cystic duct directly joins to the duodenum [2]. Conversely, there can be a "double" common bile duct where the ducts run parallel to each other and are separated by a septum.

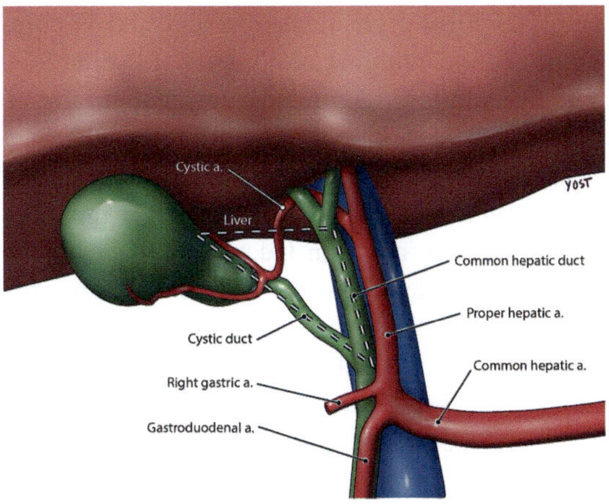

Fig. 1.3 Calot's triangle. (Printed with permission Katie Yost, 2020)

1.3.4 Calot's Triangle

Calot's triangle, or the hepatocystic triangle, was first described in 1891 and represented the triangular space formed by the cystic duct, the common hepatic duct, and the cystic artery [6]. Today, the upper border is now commonly referred to as the inferior edge of hepatic segment 4, while the lateral and medial borders represent the cystic and common hepatic bile ducts, respectively (Fig. 1.3). The triangle usually contains the cystic artery, lymphatics, the cystic lymph node of Lund, small cystic veins, autonomic nerves, and loose connective tissue. Calot's triangle may also contain any accessory hepatic ducts and blood vessels draining into the gallbladder's surrounding anatomy.

This triangular space is clinically important as it is dissected during cholecystectomy to identify and ligate the cystic artery and duct. As a result, it is crucial to be aware of the anatomical structures contained within Calot's triangle to avoid unnecessary damage to the surrounding structure.

1.3.5 Accessory and Aberrant Ducts

The normal biliary anatomy exists in only about 50% of the population [5]. Several accessory ducts are detailed in the biliary drainage system of the liver. The accessory ducts most frequently encountered in a cholecystectomy are those that drain portions of the right lobe, as they remain near the gallbladder. These ducts are usually miniscule and travel through Calot's triangle. Then, they usually join the common hepatic duct where the right and left hepatic ducts merge. In some cases, the cystic duct was found to join an accessory duct prior to its connection with the common hepatic duct. Rarely, a cholecystohepatic duct has been found to join the gallbladder directly. Occasionally, there may be multiple ducts draining segment 4 into the left duct, or the segment 4 duct may join the segment 3 duct before uniting with the segment 2 duct [2].

In 30% of the population, a small bile duct from segment 5 crosses the gallbladder fossa and is referred to as Luschka's duct. It may drain into the right hepatic duct, the common hepatic duct, or rarely the cystic duct [2]. Since the majority of these accessory ducts are small and insignificant, any additional ducts encountered in the gallbladder fossa could be ligated safely [1]. Occasionally, there might also be multiple ducts draining segment 4 into the left hepatic duct, or the segment 4 and 3 ducts may unite before joining the segment 2 duct [2]. However, some accessory ducts may drain significant portions of the right hepatic lobe. These cases are defined as "aberrant" ducts, and studies have emphasized they might need to be protected during surgery [1]. Ligation of these ducts may lead to severe biliary stasis or leak, and the size of the duct can indirectly indicate its functional importance. It is recommended that any injury to a duct over 3 mm in width should be drained into a Roux-en-Y anastomosis. This surgical technique aims at relieving biliary obstruction by creating an anastomosis between the duct and jejunum via choledochojejunostomy. Alternatively, a cholangiogram could be performed through the duct to evaluate the amount of liver drainage and identify whether it is accessory or aberrant.

Detailed classification of iatrogenic bile duct injuries following cholecystectomy needs to include clinically relevant data on every injury pattern since this will influence surgical treatment and outcome [7, 8]. There have been numerous categorizations of common bile duct injury

(BDIs), since Bismuth first introduced them in 1982 [9]. Bismuth classification ranked BDI based on its location in the biliary duct. Since the adaptation of laparoscopic cholecystectomy, more recent classifications have also focused on size, bile leakage, vascular involvement, mechanism of BDI, and severity of injury. A recent classification was introduced by Stewart-Way, whose most common injury type involves the transection and excision of a variable length of the common bile duct and always includes the junction between the common and cystic ducts [10].

1.4 Imaging of the Gallbladder and Biliary Tree

The normal anatomy of the gallbladder may be demonstrated using the imaging techniques that have been developed to examine diseases of the gallbladder. These include oral cholecystography, sonography, scintigraphy, CT scan, and MRI [11]. Right upper quadrant ultrasound is the preferred initial modality when investigating pain that is suggestive of cholecystitis. The normal gallbladder should be visualized in nearly all patients after a 10-h fast. In patients with cholecystitis, imaging may include the presence of stones, distension of the lumen, wall thickening (>3 mm), a positive sonographic Murphy sign, pericholecystic fluid, and a hyperemic wall on color doppler. Detailed information of the biliary anatomy can be obtained by relying on techniques such as magnetic resonance cholangiography or intraoperative cholangiogram. Both of these techniques use a contrast agent that accumulates in the gallbladder and bile duct system. These methods are particularly useful for the diagnosis of biliary tree obstruction by evidence of bile duct dilation and filling defect.

1.5 Vasculature and Lymphatics

1.5.1 Cystic Artery

The arterial supply of the gallbladder arises from the cystic artery. The cystic artery originates from the right hepatic artery and is commonly found within Calot's triangle (Fig. 1.3). The cystic artery then runs anterior to the cystic duct and posterior to the common hepatic duct. As the artery approaches the gallbladder neck, it separates into anterior and posterior branches that ultimately meet on the gallbladder surface. Multiple smaller branches may also supply the hepatic ducts and the superior portion of the common bile duct. Close attention must be made to these vessels during surgery as injury to the artery may lead to severe bleeding.

Additionally, the cystic artery is variable in origin. It could arise from the common hepatic artery, left hepatic artery, and gastroduodenal artery. Rarely, the cystic artery has also been found to originate from the right gastric, celiac, superior pancreaticoduodenal, and superior mesenteric arteries. As seen in these variations, the cystic artery usually crosses the common bile duct anteriorly.

Finally, a double cystic artery has been found to occur in 2–15% of cases. In these cases, the accessory artery has been described arising from the right hepatic artery, common hepatic artery, and left hepatic artery [1, 4]. If the cystic artery branches from the common hepatic or the left hepatic arteries, the cystic artery may cross the bile duct anteriorly, predisposing patients to iatrogenic injury.

1.5.2 Ductal Arteries

The biliary tree is supplied by a network of blood vessels originating from multiple surrounding sources. Blood vessels to the common bile duct run along its entire length. The main contributors to this network of vessels are coming from the retroduodenal branch of the gastroduodenal artery as it nears the upper boundary of the duodenum. Other common sources are the cystic and right hepatic arteries. A retroportal artery has also been found to originate from the celiac or superior mesenteric arteries, the vessel usually runs superior-posteriorly along the portal vein before joining the retroduodenal artery. Rarely, the retroportal artery has also been seen joining the right hepatic artery. The hepatic ducts are supplied by multiple fine blood vessels arising from segmental arteries contained within the Glissonian sheath, which is a layer of connective tissue enveloping the hilar structures inside the liver.

1.5.3 Right Hepatic Artery

The right hepatic artery rises from the bifurcation of the common hepatic artery, usually to the left of the hepatic hilum. The vessel typically courses posterior to the bile duct and anterior to the portal vein until it joins the right pedicle in the Calot's triangle. One common variation occurs when the right hepatic artery runs within the lower end of the Calot's triangle in a tortuous course referred to as "caterpillar" or "Moynihan's" hump. This variation can have an incidence as high as 50% [1]. A Moynihan's hump is clinically relevant as the cystic artery is significantly shorter in these patients. As a result, the right hepatic artery could be misidentified as the cystic artery and could result in erroneous ligation. It is recommended to divide the cystic artery close to the gallbladder wall in order to avoid confusion with other possible blood vessels. In other cases, the right hepatic artery has been found to take another aberrant course in which it passes anterior to the bile duct or even posterior to the portal vein. In addition, an accessory or replaced right hepatic artery from the superior mesenteric artery may occur in approximately 17% of individuals. In these cases, the right hepatic artery courses posterior to the portal vein and the inferior end of the common bile duct.

1.5.4 Venous Drainage

The venous drainage of the gallbladder arises from a system of multiple fine veins. Vessels exiting the superior surface of the body and neck typically enter the liver to join segmental portal veins. The rest of the gallbladder vein system forms small cystic veins that join the intrahepatic drainage either directly or indirectly via veins from the hepatic ducts. Rarely, cystic veins may drain into the right portal branch. There have been only a few reports of clinically significant veins injury involving the portal vein after biliary tree surgery.

1.5.5 Lymphatics

A multitude of lymphatic vessels arises from the plexuses of the gallbladder and cystic duct.

The lymphatic drainage of bile ducts diverges into two pathways. The superior pathway involves lymph nodes along the cystic duct, hepatic artery, and celiac plexus. In contrast, the inferior pathway involves the nodes along the cystic lymph nodes, located superiorly to the cystic duct and embedded within Calot's triangle. This pathway also drains into the anterolateral aspect of the portal vein, the posterior pancreas, and the aortocaval region. Chyle leakage is an extremely rare complication after cholecystectomy.

1.5.6 Nerve Supply

The hepatic plexus innervates the gallbladder and biliary tree. In addition, the common bile duct also receives branches from the pyloric branch of the vagus nerve. Pain sensation arising from these structures is commonly referred to as the epigastric region, while stimulation of the overlying somatic peritoneum will lead to pain in the right upper quadrant. The Murphy's sign is elicited in patients suffering from acute cholecystitis by having the patient hold a deeply inhaled breath while conducting palpation of the right subcostal area. If pain occurs, Murphy's sign is positive. While nerve injury during cholecystectomy is a very rare occurrence, a few cases of unilateral phrenic nerve palsy have been reported in the literature. It has been hypothesized that this might be due to pneumoperitoneum that leads to stretching of the phrenic nerve [12].

1.6 Conclusion

The anatomy of the gallbladder and biliary tract is complex and displays a wide range of variations. Detailed knowledge of the anatomy is needed for surgeons to avoid potential complications and perform a successful procedure.

References

1. Nagral S. Anatomy relevant to cholecystectomy. J Minim Access Surg. 2005;1(2):53–8.
2. Bergman RA, Tubbs RS, Shoja MM, Loukas M. Bergman's comprehensive encyclopedia of human anatomic variation. Hoboken, NJ: Wiley; 2016.
3. Garciavilla PC, Alvarez JF, Uzqueda GV. Diagnosis and laparoscopic approach to gallbladder torsion and cholelithiasis. JSLS. 2010;14(1):147–51.
4. Standring S, editor. Gray's anatomy: the anatomical basis of clinical practice, 40th ed, anniversary ed [Edinburgh]. Philadelphia: Churchill Livingstone/Elsevier; 2008.
5. Fischer JE, Ellison EC, Henke PK, Hochwald SN, Tiao GM. Fischers mastery of surgery. Philadelphia: Wolters Kluwer; 2019.
6. Abdalla S, Pierre S, Ellis H. Calot's triangle. Clin Anat. 2013;26(4):493–501. https://doi.org/10.1002/ca.22170.
7. Chun K. Recent classifications of the common bile duct injury. Korean J Hepatobiliary Pancreat Surg. 2014;18(3):69–72. https://doi.org/10.14701/kjhbps.2014.18.3.69.
8. Bismuth H, Majno PE. Biliary strictures: classification based on the principles of surgical treatment. World J Surg. 2001;25(10):1241–4.
9. Renz BW, Bösch F, Angele MK. Bile duct injury after cholecystectomy: surgical therapy. Visc Med. 2017;33(3):184–90. https://doi.org/10.1159/000471818.
10. Way LW, Stewart L, Gantert W, Liu K, Cm L, Whang K, Hunter JG. Causes and prevention of laparoscopic bile duct injuries: analysis of 252 cases from a human factors and cognitive psychology perspective. Ann Surg. 2003;237(4):460–9.
11. Meilstrup JW. Imaging atlas of the normal gallbladder and its variants. CRC Press; 2018.
12. De U, Maitra D, Mukherjee M. Unusual complications of laparoscopic cholecystectomy: a case series. Int J Case Rep Images. 2012;3(4):5–9.

2 Pathophysiology and Diagnosis of Acute Calculous Cholecystitis

Alberto R. Ferreres

2.1 Introduction

Gallbladder ailments have been affecting humans for thousands of years, as proved by the fact of gallstones found in Egyptian and Chinese mummies. In 1909, an Egyptian mummy was presented to the Museum of the Royal College of Surgeons in London, with a preserved liver and a gallbladder, containing 30 gallstones. The mummy came from Thebes and belonged to a twenty-first dynasty priestess (circa 1500 BC) and was donated by Dr. Elliot Smith, a well-known Egyptologist and anatomist. The gallbladder was described as "large and containing many spherical calculi" (1).

Alexander the Great is believed to have died on July 11,323 BC at age 34 due to peritonitis resulting from the perforation of an acute cholecystitis, fueled by alcohol consumption and abundant intake. In 1867, John Bobbs performed the first cholecystostomy on a 31-year-old lady who survived until the age of 77 in Indianapolis. Fifteen years later, Carl Langenbuch performed in Berlin the first cholecystectomy in a 35-year-old male patient (2).

Acute calculous cholecystitis (ACC) accounts for 3–11% of hospital admissions and carries a mortality of about 0.8% (3). ACC represents more than 90% of all cases of acute cholecystitis, the remaining include acalculous, xanthogranulomatous, and other variations of acute cholecystitis. The gold standard treatment of ACC is laparoscopic cholecystectomy, but its timing (early vs. delayed) is also a matter of discussion.

Although most patients with cholelithiasis remain asymptomatic for long periods, 1 to 4% of those patients per year suffer biliary colics (4, 5). ACC eventually may develop in about 20% of those symptomatic patients if left untreated (6). Nonetheless, most patients with ACC have had previous episodes of biliary colic pain; but for some, ACC may represent the initial episode. In some cases, ACC may coexist with choledocholithiasis, acute cholangitis, or acute biliary pancreatitis. Around 60% of patients with ACC are women; however, ACC develops more frequently in men and tends to be more severe (7). Patients suffering from diabetes are also more prone to develop ACC.

ACC represents the most frequent complication of patients with diagnosis of choledocholithiasis. Gallstone disease incidence is a major world health problem which undoubtedly is expanding. The best method to investigate the real incidence of biliary gallstones is screening ultrasonography, since it is far superior than autopsy findings and clinical diagnosis, which requires biliary symptoms only present in 20% of those individuals with gallstones. The frequency of cholecystectomy, mostly performed in a laparoscopic approach, has a very limited relationship to the prevalence of the disease and

A. R. Ferreres (✉)
Department of Surgery, University of Buenos Aires, Buenos Aires, Argentina

© Springer Nature Switzerland AG 2021
I. Di Carlo (ed.), *Difficult Acute Cholecystitis*, https://doi.org/10.1007/978-3-030-62102-5_2

is more related to the surgeon's driven practice as well as patient access to surgical care (8). In developed countries, 10–15% of white adults carry gallstones. It is estimated that in the USA about 15% of the population are gallstone carriers, with a higher incidence in the Hispanic population than in non-Hispanics. In that country, 6.3 million males and 14.2 million women between 20 and 74 years have gallbladder stones (9). A very high prevalence has been described in American native Indians, such as the Pima group in Arizona. The same applies to original Indian populations in South America. The prevalence of gallstones in the Hispanic population of Latin America (Central and South America) is higher, similarly to native populations in the same areas. In these populations, genetic risk factors lead to lithogenic bile and gallstone early in life (less than 30 years) resulting in gallstone prevalence rates of more than 50% at 50 years of age in both men and women (10). In Europe, the Multicenter Italian Study on Cholelithiasis (MICOL) informed an overall incidence of gallstones of 18.8% in females and 9.5% in males (11). In south east Asia, the prevalence is lower, but usually located in the bile ducts and associated with parasitic infestations (12).

In the West, about 70% of gallstone carriers possess cholesterol gallbladder stones, with a cholesterol content of more than 50%, meanwhile 30% have black pigment gallbladder stones. In eastern Asia, there is a very high incidence of pigment stones lodged in the bile ducts and being responsible for causing severe cholangitis. Nonetheless, in these countries the incidence of cholesterol gallstones has been steadily increasing in the last years, presumably due to the changes in the diet.

Ethnicity is a major determinant of the following facts: cause of the disease, type of stone/s, and location in the biliary tract system. In developed countries, most of the gallstones (around 85%) are predominantly of cholesterol composition, where the remainder 15% are black pigment calculi, due to calcium bilirubinate. Cholesterol and black pigment stones are formed within the gallbladder lumen, but in the first case the starting point is represented by the liver production of supersaturated bile with cholesterol, which tends to precipitate in the gallbladder. The excess secretion of mucin together with an impaired gallbladder motility keep these crystals, aggregating to them other materials and turning them into macroscopic stones (13).

Gallstones may be classified according to their location and composition (Fig. 2.1, see Addenda). The location may be: extrahepatic (choledocholithiasis) where the stones may be present in the

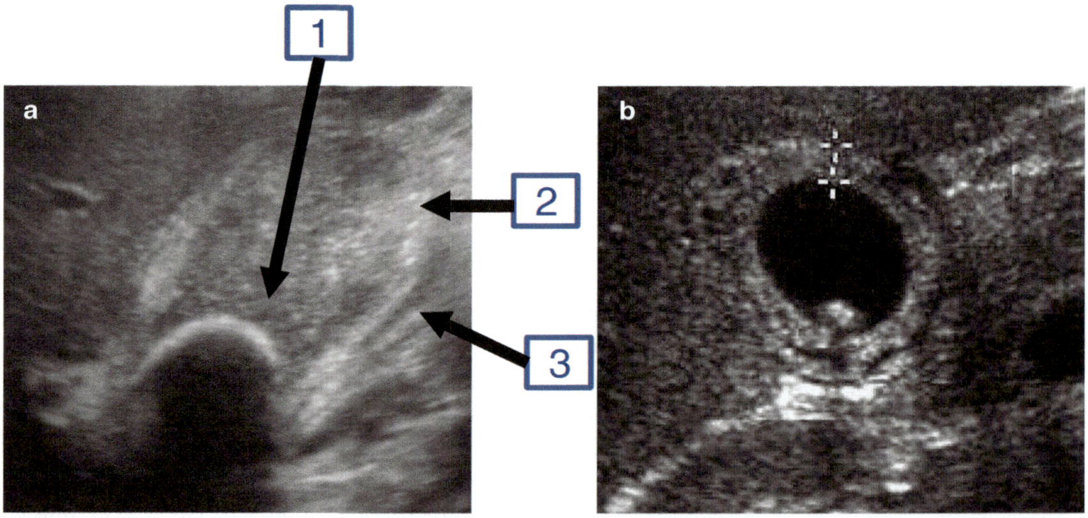

Fig. 2.1 (**a**): 1. Impacted gallstone + sludge. 2. Wall thickening. 3. Pericholecystic fluid. (**b**): Gallbladder wall with thickening of its layers and an impacted gallstone

gallbladder and/or in the common bile duct, or intrahepatic (hepatolithiasis). Stones in the common bile duct may be either primary (originated de novo in that conduct, and usually pigment stones) or secondary, due to migration from the gallbladder and, typically, of cholesterol. Black pigment stones also develop in the gallbladder, but consist of bilirubin polymers (calcium bilirubinate) and are typically associated with advanced age, liver cirrhosis, cystic fibrosis, and hematologic conditions with increased erythrocytes' destruction (sickle cell anemia, chronic hemolytic states).

Bile duct stones may originate in the gallbladder and get there due to migration or otherwise develop primarily in the biliary system. In the Western world, the risk of concomitant common bile duct stones, which migrate from the gallbladder, is estimated in 10–15% and is usually compounded by cholesterol. But choledocholithiasis may develop primarily due to strictures and subsequent inflammation and infection with the appearance of brown pigment stones. In southeastern Asia, pigment stones are predominant, composed by calcium bilirubinate, fatty acids, cholesterol, and mucin (glycoproteins primarily from bacterial biofilms). They tend to aggregate in the common bile duct or in the intrahepatic bile ducts. Infection by bacteria but mostly by parasites (*Clonorchis sinensis*, *opisthorchis species*, and *fasciola hepatica*) as well as stasis represent key factors (8).

Risk factors for gallstone formation are multifactorial (14):

- Constitutional: Represented by age, female gender, genetics, and ethnicity. These are not able to be changed or modified.
- Environmental or exogenous: Include the following factors, which represent modifiable conditions:
  - Dietary factors: Mostly linked with cholesterol gallstone formation, including high carbohydrate/high calories intake, high glycemic upload, low fiber intake.
  - Metabolic aspects: Also linked with cholesterol gallstone formation. Physical inactivity, diabetic or prediabetic conditions, obesity, nonalcoholic fatty disease.
  - Increased enterohepatic bilirubin circulation: Liver cirrhosis, Crohn's disease (both for cholesterol and pigmentary stones), ileal resections, and bariatric procedures (for pigmentary stones).
  - Underlying chronic disease: Cystic fibrosis, spinal cord injuries, some colon conditions are associated with increased risk of gallstones development.
  - Medications: Hormone replacements, octreotide, fibrates, calcineurin antagonists.
  - Alterations in the motility of the gallbladder.

2.2 Pathogenesis of Gallstones

2.2.1 Cholesterol Stones

Bile is a yellow-brown to dark green fluid whose composition is more than 90% water. Bile contains bile salts, cholesterol, and phospholipids as well as little amounts of proteins and inorganic salts. In humans, bile is produced by the liver and stored in a concentrated fashion in the gallbladder. It serves as a surfactant, emulsifying the lipids in the digestive tract. Bile salt anions are hydrophilic on one side and hydrophobic on the other, tending to aggregate around droplets of lipids to form micelles, with the hydrophobic sides towards the fat and the hydrophilic facing outwards.

The organization of cholesterol gallstones is the consequence of a failure in the homeostasis of cholesterol concentration in the bile. The increase in the liver production of biliary cholesterol has been considered the primary pathophysiologic defect in human cholelithogenesis, followed by abnormal secretion rates of bile salts and phospholipids and thus inducing the supersaturation of cholesterol in the gallbladder bile.

There are five primary defects which play a major role in the organization and formation of cholesterol gallstones (Table 2.1, see Addenda):

Table 2.1 Primary defects for cholesterol gallstone formation

Cholesterol gallstones
1. Genetic factors and lith genes
2. Liver cholesterol hypersecretion into bile
3. Alterations in the motility of the gallbladder
4. Rapid phase transitions of cholesterol in bile (with precipitation of cholesterol crystals)
5. Intestinal factors:
• increased absorption of cholesterol
• slow intestinal motility
• dysbiosis

2.2.1.1 Genetic Factors and Lith Genes

A genetic predisposition to gallstone formation seems to be clearly evident (15). The discovery of the lithogenic Lith 1 and Lith 2 genes in mice's chromosomes 2 and 19, respectively associated with quantitative trait locus (QTL) analysis—a powerful genetic study technique—confirmed the genetic role in alterations ending in gallstone formation.

Genome-wide association study (GWAS) has allowed the study in humans, leading to the discovery of two major variants: ABCG5-R50C and ABCG8-D19H, which have been associated with gallstones formation in German, Chilean, Chinese, and Indian populations (16). Nonetheless, less than 25% of the risk of cholesterol gallstones is determined by genetics (17).

2.2.1.2 Liver Cholesterol Hypersecretion into Bile

Although cholesterol secreted into bile recognizes its origin from liver synthesis, reverse cholesterol transport, and chylomicrons, the contribution of each pathway is not yet absolutely clear. Estrogens enhance the formation of cholesterol gallstones by stimulation of the liver synthesis and the production of cholesterol as well as the reduction in the production of bile salts. These mechanisms are the ones responsible for the higher prevalence of stones in females than in males.

2.2.1.3 Alterations in the Motility of the Gallbladder

The emptying of the gallbladder tends to be impaired before gallstones are detected, giving a clinical picture of biliary dyskinesia. This phenomenon is due to the fact of the absorption of large amounts of cholesterol by the epithelial cells of the gallbladder's wall from the supersaturated bile. Cholesterol in excess is transformed to esters and stored in the mucosa and lamina propria, originating changes in the sarcolemmal membranes with further disruption of cholecystokinin I receptors' signaling cascade as well as the alteration of the signal transduction mediated by G proteins (18).

2.2.1.4 Rapid Phase Transitions of Cholesterol in Bile (with Precipitation of Cholesterol Crystals)

The secretion of cholesterol into the bile depends on the balance of the liver's cholesterol input and output. Cholesterol crystal nucleation is considered the first and earliest step in cholesterol gallstone formation and depends on the relative amounts of cholesterol, phospholipids, and bile salts. Although cholesterol solubility in watery solutions is very little, the situation is completely different amidst gallbladder bile. This increase in solubility is due to the incorporation of cholesterol in mixed micelles, together with bile salts and phospholipids, the most representative being phosphatidylcholine.

Supersaturation of the bile occurs when either too much cholesterol or not enough bile salts and phosphatidylcholine molecules are secreted to permit the complete solubilization of micellar cholesterol. The cholesterol in excess may be stored in vesicles or in cholesterol crystals (19). The organization of these crystals is believed to happen from vesicles supersaturated with cholesterol, in the two following stages:

(a) Small unilamellar supersaturated vesicles tend to gather or fuse into larger multilamellar crystals (cholesterol crystal nucleation).
(b) Subsequent phase separation of cholesterol crystals (20).

Wang and Carey studied the cholesterol crystallization pathways and sequences in human gallbladder bile and were able to describe the equilibrium bile salt, phospholipid, and cholesterol ternary phase diagram, which permits to predict the behavior of the three components when present in different proportions (21). Three factors strongly affect the balance of the bile salt–phospholipid–cholesterol ternary phase diagram, with potential alterations of the cholesterol crystallization: the bile concentration, the higher hydrophobicity of bile salts and the type phospholipids, and the composition of their acyl chains.

1. Intestinal factors: are represented by the increased absorption of cholesterol, a slow intestinal motility, and the alterations in gut microbiota.

The small bowel absorbs cholesterol from the diet intake and reabsorbs the cholesterol present in the bile, depending upon the expression of sterol transport proteins (16). Small and large bowel dysbiosis occurs in cholesterol gallstone patients and may be affected by toxins introduced with the food intake.

2.2.2 Pigment Stones

(a) Black pigment stones: Their primary component is calcium bilirubinate, while other components are calcium carbonate and calcium phosphate joined to mucin glycoproteins. In normal conditions, most bilirubin, the breakdown product of hemoglobin, is conjugated in the liver to bilirubin monoglucuronide and subsequently to water-soluble bilirubin diglucuronide, highlighting the fact that unconjugated bilirubin is poorly soluble in water. In case of hemolysis, biliary excretion of bilirubin is very much increased, with the risk of precipitation of calcium bilirubinate. This mechanism explains the high prevalence of these type of stones in chronic hemolytic disorders (22).

(b) Brown pigment stones: In contrast to the black, these are mostly developed in the lumen of the bile ducts. Their primary composition is calcium salts of unconjugated bilirubin and different amounts of cholesterol and proteins. They are associated with bile stasis and chronic bacterial infection of the bile ducts by *Escherichia coli*, *Bacteroides spp*, *Clostridium spp* and parasites like *Opisthorchis viverrini*, *Clonorchis sinensis*, *Ascaris lumbricoides* (Table 2.2, Addenda). Bacteria produce β glucuronidase, phospholipase A, and bile acid hydrolase which leads to an increase in the amounts of unconjugated bilirubin, palmitic and stearic acids, and unconjugated bile acids, which can join with calcium and thus form stones. Parasites may stimulate stone formation by the calcified overcoat of the parasite egg, which may serve as the nucleus of the future stone with the deposit of calcium bilirubinate (23).

Table 2.2 Factors for the formation of brown pigment stones

Genetic factors
Liver hypersecretion of bilirubin
Bile stasis
Bacterial infection

2.3 Pathophysiology of ACC

The primary cause of acute cholecystitis is obstruction. Of all individuals who have gallstones, only 1–3% will undergo an acute episode. Other obstructive causes include: primary tumors of the gallbladder or the biliary tract, polyps, parasites, metastatic tumors, or nodes in the vicinity of the gallbladder neck (24).

The extended gallbladder outlet obstruction by a stone is the initial and main factor leading to an ACC. The process corresponds to the physical obstruction of the gallbladder by a gallstone, which may be located at the neck or in the cystic duct. The following sequence of pathophysiologic steps is described in the production of an episode of ACC (Table 2.3, Addenda): the obstruction leads to distention and an increased gallbladder pressure, taking into account the fact that the progression to acute cholecystitis is determined by two main factors: (a) the degree of

Table 2.3 Steps in the development of calculous acute cholecystitis

Obstruction at the gallbladder's neck
↓
Increased endoluminal pressure
↓
Venous congestion, compromised blood irrigation, alterations in lymphatic drainage Ischemia of the mucosa
↓
Release of inflammatory mediators: prostaglandins I2 and E2
↓
Localized mucosal trauma
↓
Lysosome release of phospholipase
↓
Conversion of lecithin to lysolecithin
↓
Wall thickening + edema, vascular congestion and intramural hemorrhage
↓
Mucosal ulcers with focal areas of wall necrosis

obstruction and (b) the duration of the obstruction by the stone. Meanwhile the obstruction is partial and the duration short, the patient will most probably experience a biliary colic, but if the obstruction is complete and the duration long, an acute cholecystitis episode will develop. In this case, if the patient does not receive immediate treatment, the clinical picture will tend to progress and increase the severity of its evolution with a higher incidence of complications. The persistence of the obstruction leads to a sustained increase in the gallbladder endoluminal pressure, leading to venous congestion, a compromise in the blood irrigation, and the lymphatic drainage with mucosal ischemia. It is important to note that the inflammatory response and the release of its mediators (prostaglandins I2 and E2) generate the release of phospholipase from the lysosomes, which aids in the conversion of lecithin into lysolecithin, via enzymatic hydrolysis, within the supersaturated bile in the gallbladder lumen. Lysolecithin is a potent detergent and very harmful for the mucosa (25). The gallbladder wall may suffer from necrosis and gangrene, achieving a gangrenous or necrotizing cholecystitis.

Regarding the role of bacteria, this fact does not play neither an initial nor a major role in ACC, but it has been recognized that secondary infection may complicate up to 50% of the cases (26). Bacteria implicated in ACC are usually present in the bile before the onset of the disease, since bacterial growth is present in 20% to 70% of patients. They include:

(a) Gram negative bacilli (*Escherichia coli*, *Klebsiella spp*, *Enterobacter spp*).
(b) Gram positive cocci (*Enterococci*).
(c) Anaerobes (Bacteroides, *Clostridia spp*, *Fusobacterium spp*).

A major Achilles' heel is represented by the limitations of microbial cultures, situation that may be improved by the use of next-generation sequencing (27). The overgrowth of gas-producing bacteria within the gallbladder lumen may lead to emphysematous cholecystitis.

Histologically, infiltration of neutrophilic leukocytes, microabscesses, and secondary vasculitis will be the usual findings. Secondary bacterial infection, due to delay in diagnosis or inappropriate initial antibiotic treatment, may result in gallbladder empyema with accumulation of pus, perforation with localized or generalized peritonitis, and even sepsis (13). Other complications are liver abscess and intra-abdominal collections.

There are some specific forms of acute cholecystitis that need to be distinguished from ACC: (a) xanthogranulomatous, (b) emphysematous, (c) acalculous, and (d) torsion, due to inherent, acquired, and other physical causes.

2.4 Diagnosis of ACC

The diagnosis of ACC is based on the clinical presentation and imaging. Although ACC is a common disease for patients presenting in the Emergency Department, its diagnosis represents a major challenge for clinicians and surgeons, in order to decide the best treatment and management strategy. The cornerstone of a correct and precise diagnosis consists of the evidence of an acute inflamed gallbladder with stones in its lumen, preventing the passage of bile to the cystic duct and the main biliary duct due to impacted calculi.

The diagnosis of ACC is based on the clinical presentation and physical examination, laboratory, and imaging studies. Nonetheless, the gold standard for diagnosis is the confirmation of the presence of a stone obstructing the gallbladder infundibulum or the cystic duct together with the pathological examination of the specimen, performed through a cholecystectomy, usually in a minimal invasive approach.

Most patients who present with ACC have symptoms of right upper quadrant pain, but many times the pain may be referred in different locations as well as irradiation. When the inflammation worsens, the pain tends to be localized in the right upper quadrant. The patients may also refer a history of biliary colic or dyspepsia or even a previous diagnosis of cholelithiasis, but sometimes the acute presentation is the initial one. Nausea, vomiting, and anorexia are usually described in the acute episode.

The most typical physical sign is the presence of abdominal pain, usually in the upper abdomen and the right upper quadrant. The examination may evidence tenderness or Murphy's sign in the right upper quadrant; this sign was described in 1903 as a sign of cholelithiasis (28). A palpable mass is usually present in about 25% of patients after more than 24 h of symptoms. In occasions, ACC can derive in sepsis and organ failure, usually when a gangrenous or emphysematous cholecystitis is present. The additional presence of choledocholithiasis should be ruled out, since this situation may preclude a somewhat different approach.

According to the Tokyo Guidelines 2013 (29), the diagnostic criteria are based on the following three aspects:

(a) Local signs of inflammation: (1) Murphy sign, (2) right upper quadrant mass/pain or tenderness.
(b) Systemic signs of inflammation: (1) fever, (2) elevated protein C, (3) elevated white blood cell count.
(c) Imaging findings, characteristic of acute cholecystitis.

Ultrasonography should be considered as the first option as imaging modality (30). The typical and pathognomonic findings include: thickening of the gallbladder wall (5 mm or more), pericholecystic fluid, and ultrasonographic Murphy's sign (abdominal tenderness when the probe is pushed against the right upper quadrant or the palpable gallbladder). The simultaneous presence of these three signs is definitive for the diagnosis of acute cholecystitis. Other findings include an enlarged and distended gallbladder, an impacted stone, and debris echo (Figs. 2.1 and 2.2, Addenda_2). According to a meta-analysis published by Shea et al. (31), the diagnostic capability of ultrasonography for acute cholecystitis achieves a sensitivity of 88% and a specificity of 80%.

Ultrasonography is also useful when an emphysematous cholecystitis is suspected since an irregular thickening of the gallbladder wall and imaging of a ruptured gallbladder may be noted.

The suspected diagnosis of ACC includes one item in (a) and one item in (b), meanwhile

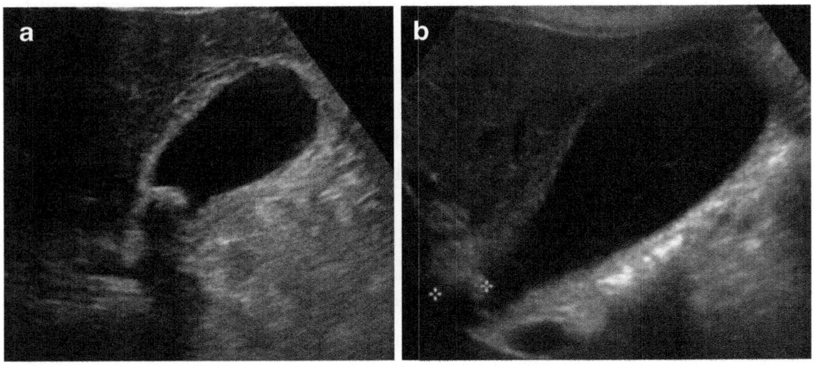

Fig. 2.2 (**a**): Distended gallbladder with impacted gallstone. (**b**): Distended gallbladder with impacted gallstone

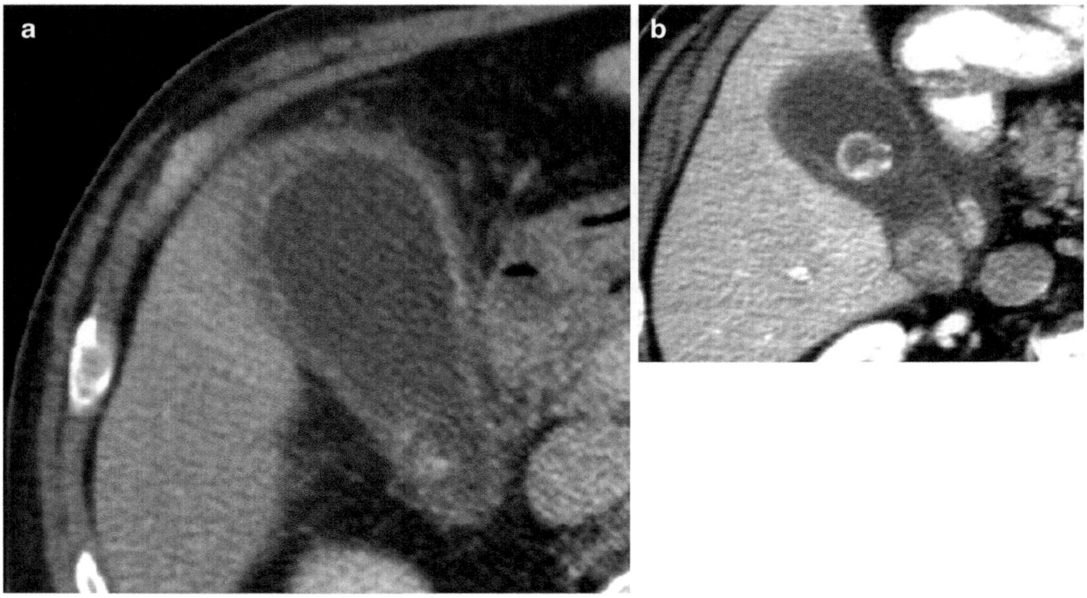

Fig. 2.3 (**a**): CT scan, showing a distended gallbladder with impacted gallstone. (**b**): CT Scan, with distended gallbladder with impacted stone and another one in its lumen

a definitive diagnosis of ACC includes one item in (a) and one in (b) plus (c). The level of serum bilirubin may be increased due to several factors: compression of the common bile duct by the inflamed infundibulum or the presence of contemporary common bile duct stones.

Some remarks should be added to these guidelines: some patients may present with few or minimal systemic symptoms and hence, underdiagnosed, and the use of protein C levels is seldom used for the diagnosis of ACC in many countries (32). From the point of view of laboratory tests, there are no specific ones for performing a diagnosis of ACC. The World Society of Emergency Surgery guidelines for ACC also recommend the use of clinical, laboratory, and imaging findings for the diagnosis (33).

Contrast-enhanced CT scans are usually not requested in the emergency setting, exception made in those conditions where a differential diagnosis needs to be ruled out. Some of the findings are: gallbladder distention, pericholecystic fat stranding, gallbladder wall thickening, subserosal edema, mucosal enhancement, transient focal enhancement of the liver adjacent to the gallbladder, pericholecystic fluid collections, pericholecystic abscess, gas collection within the gallbladder (Fig. 2.3, Addenda_2). It is recommended to rule out gangrenous cholecystitis (Fig. 2.4, Addenda_2) as well as emphysematous cholecystitis, where the main findings include gas in the wall or lumen, intraluminal membranes, irregular or absent wall, abscess/es, Fig. 2.5 Addenda_2 (30).

The use of magnetic resonance cholangiography maybe useful in the emergency setting to rule our common bile duct stones and hence, the chance of acute cholangitis. At a time, the use of HIDA scan (with 99 Tc-HIDA cholescintigraphy) was considered the most accurate test for the diagnosis of acute cholecystitis, with a sensitivity of 97% and specificity of 87% (34). The gallbladder was usually visualized within 30 min and the absence of the radiotracer uptake by 4 h was considered positive for cystic duct obstruction. Identification of the radiotracer in the pericholecystic space is suggestive of perforation. But since the availability of emergency ultrasound, HIDA scan is considered unnecessary.

The Tokyo Guidelines 2013 also collaborated in setting guidelines for establishing the severity of ACC in three grades (29):

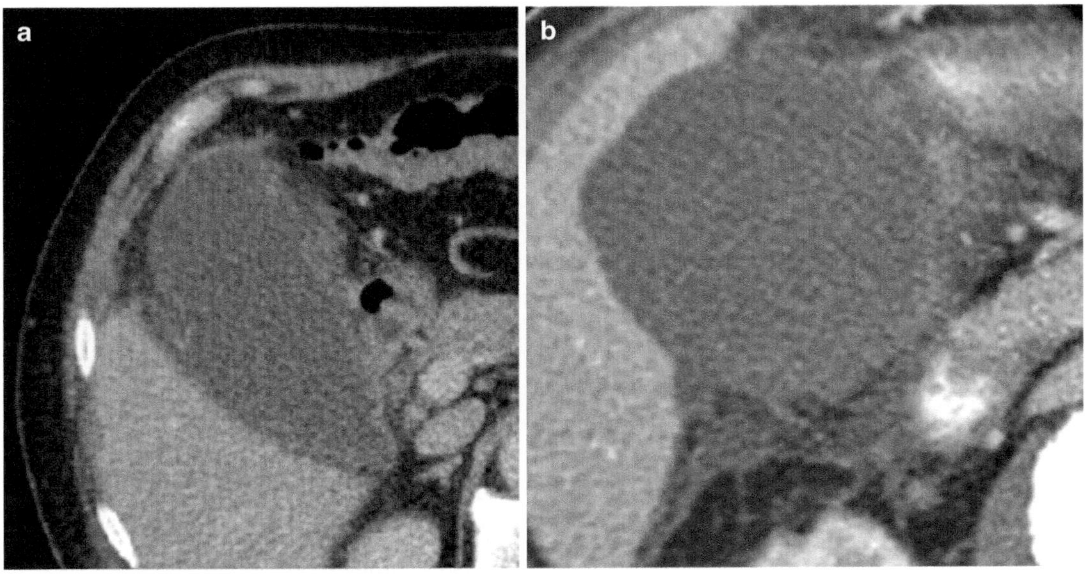

Fig. 2.4 (**a**, **b**): CT scan Gangrenous cholecystitis

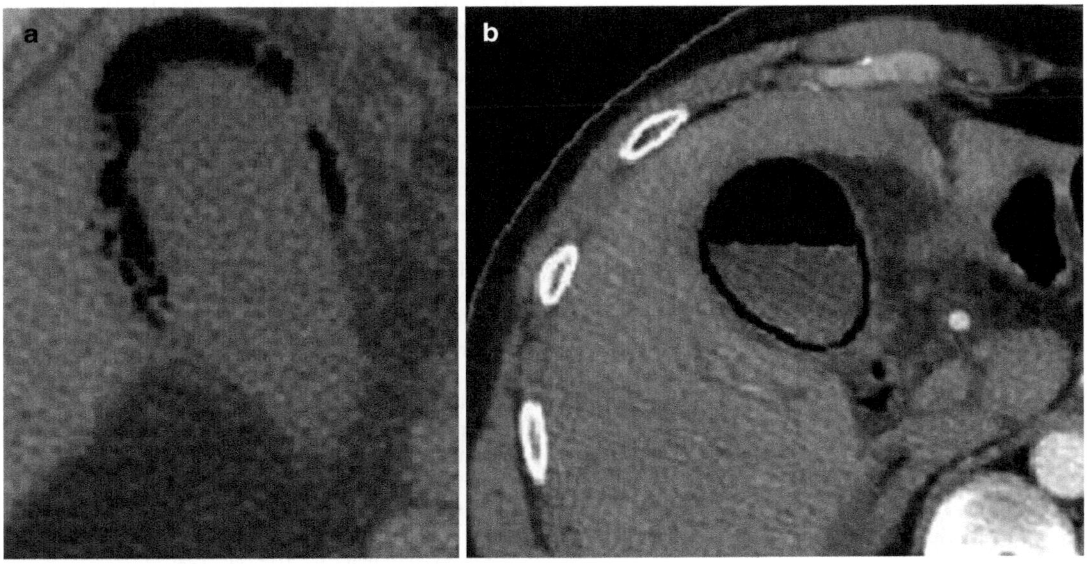

Fig. 2.5 (**a**, **b**): CT scan Emphysematous cholecystitis

- Mild (Grade I): Acute cholecystitis in a healthy individual with no organ dysfunction, mild inflammatory changes in the gallbladder, making cholecystectomy a safe and low-risk operative procedure.
- Moderate (Grade II): Acute cholecystitis in which the degree of acute inflammation is likely to be associated with increased operative difficulty in performing cholecystectomy (WBC > 18,000/mm^3, palpable tender mass, duration of complaints >72 h and/or suspicion of local complications gangrenous cholecystitis, pericholecystic abscess, hepatic abscess, biliary peritonitis, emphysematous cholecystitis).

– Severe (Grade III): Associated with organ dysfunction (cardiovascular, neurological, respiratory, renal, liver, and hematologic) and mandating intensive care with respiratory and circulatory support.

There are other grading scales for severity of acute cholecystitis, such as the one proposed by the American Association for the Surgery of Trauma, based on anatomic variables using clinical, imaging, operative, and pathologic criteria to assess the severity of acute cholecystitis in 5 Grades, excluding physiologic parameters. Grade 1 corresponds to acute cholecystitis; Grade 2, gangrenous or emphysematous cholecystitis; Grades 3 to 5 describe gallbladder perforation with local contamination, abscess or fistula and generalized peritonitis, respectively (35, 36). The Parkland score relies solely on the intraoperative macroscopic findings (37).

Keypoints
- ACC may eventually develop in about 20% of symptomatic patients when left untreated.
- The primary cause of ACC corresponds to the physical obstruction of the gallbladder by a gallstone, which may be located at the neck or in the cystic duct.
- Bacterial infection does not play neither an initial nor a major role in ACC, but secondary infection may complicate up to 50% of the cases.
- The diagnosis of ACC is based on the clinical presentation and imaging, being ultrasonography the most widely used in the emergency setting.
- Contrast-enhanced CT is useful in clinical conditions where a differential diagnosis needs to be ruled out.

References

1. Glenn F. Biliary tract disease since antiquity. Bull N Y Acad Med. 1971;47:329–50.
2. Glenn F, Graffe WR. Historical events in biliary tract surgery. Arch Surg. 1966;93:848–52.
3. Udekwu PO, Sullivan WG. Contemporary experience with cholecystectomy: establishing benchmarks two decades after the introduction of laparoscopic cholecystectomy. Am Surg. 2013;79:1253–7.
4. Friedman GD, Ravila CA, Fireman B. Prognosis of gallstones with mild or no symptoms: 25 years of follow- up in a health maintenance organization. J Clin Epidemiol. 1989;42:127–36.
5. McSherry CK, Ferstenberg H, Calhoun WF, Lahman E, Virshup M. The natural history of diagnosed gallstone disease in symptomatic and asymptomatic patients. Ann Surg. 1983;202:59–63.
6. Carter HR, Cox RL, Polk HC. Operative therapy for cholecystitis and cholelithiasis: trends over three decades. Am Surg. 1987;53:565–8.
7. Yeatman TJ. Emphysematous cholecystitis: an insidious variant of acute cholecystitis. Am J Emerg Med. 1986;4:163–6.
8. Lammert F, Gurusamy K, Ko CW, Miquel JF, Méndez Sánchez N, Portincasa P, van Epercum KJ, van Laarhoven CJ, Wang DQH. Gallstones. Nat Rev Dis Primers. 2016;2:1–17.
9. Shaffer EA. Epidemiology and risk factors for gallstone disease: has the paradigm changed in the 21st. century? Curr Gastroenterol Rep. 2005;7:132–40.
10. Volzke H, Baumeister SE, Alte D, Hoffman W, Schwahn C, Simon P, John U, Lerch MM. Independent risk factors for stone formation in a region with high cholelithiasis prevalence. Digestion. 2005;71:97–105.
11. Attili AF, Carulli N, Roda E, et al. Epidemiology of gallstone disease in Italy: prevalence data of the Multicenter Italian Study on Cholelithiasis (MICOL). Am J Epidemiol. 1995;141:158–65.
12. Stinton LM, Shaffer EA. Epidemiology of gallbladder disease: cholelithiasis and cancer. Gut Liver. 2012;6:172–87.
13. Elwood DR. Cholecystitis. Surg Clin N Am. 2008;88:1241–52.
14. Venneman NG, van Epercum KJ. Pathogenesis of gallstones. Gastroenterol Clin N Am 2010; 39: 171–183.
15. Wang HH, Portincasa P, Afdhal NZ, Wang DQH. Lith genes and genetic analysis of cholesterol gallstone formation. Gastroenterol Clin N Am. 2010;39:185–207.
16. Di Ciaula A, Wang DQH, Portincasa P. An update of the pathogenesis of cholesterol gallstone disease. Curr Opin Gastroenterol. 2018;34:71–80.
17. Katsika D, Grjibovski A, Einarsson C, et al. Genetic and environmental influences on symptomatic gallstone disease: a Swedish study of 43141 twin pairs. Hepatology. 2005;41:1138–43.
18. Wilkins T, Agabin E, Varghese J, Talukder A. Gallbladder dysfunction: cholecystitis, choledocholithiasis, cholangitis and biliary dyskinesia. Prim Care Clin. 2017;44:575–97.
19. Wang DQH, Adfahl NH. Gallstone disease. In: Feldman M, Friedman LS, Brandt LJ, editors. Sleisinger and Fordtran's gastrointestinal and liver disease. 9th ed. Philadelphia: Elsevier; 2010.

20. Somjen GJ, Gilat T. Contribution of vesicular and micellar carriers to cholesterol transport in human bile. J Lipid Res. 1985;26:699–704.
21. Wang DQH, Carey MC. Complete mapping of crystallization pathways during cholesterol precipitation from model bile: influence of physical-chemical variables from model bile: influence of a stable liquid-crystalline state in cold, dilute and hydrophilic bile salt-containing systems. J Lipid Res. 1996;37:606–30.
22. Haverfield EV, McKenzie CA, Forrester T, et al. UGT1A1 variation and gallstone formation in sickle cell disease. Blood. 2005;105:968–72.
23. Liu X, Hu J. Relationship between bilirubin free radical and formation of pigment gallstone. World J Gastroenterol. 2002;8:413–7.
24. Halpin V. Acute cholecystitis. BMJ Clin Evid. 2014;2014:0411.
25. Chung AYA, Duke MC. Acute biliary disease. Surg Clin N Am. 2018;98:877–94.
26. Knab LM, Boller AM, Mahvi DM. Cholecystitis. Surg Clin N Am. 2014;94:455–70.
27. Dyrhovden R, Ovebo KK, Nordahl MV, Nygaard RM, Ulvestad E, Kommedal O. Bacteria and fungi in acute cholecystitis. A prospective study comparing next generation sequencing to culture. J Infect. 80(1):16–23. https://doi.org/10.1016/j.jinf.2019.09.015. Accessed December 8, 2019
28. Murphy JB. The diagnosis of gallstones. Am Med News. 1903;82:825–33.
29. Yokoe M, Takada T, Strasberg SM, et al. TG13 diagnostic criteria and severity grading of acute cholecystitis. J HPB Sci. 2013;20:35–46.
30. Yokoe M, Hata K, Takada T, et al. Tokyo guidelines 2018: diagnostic criteria and severity grading of acute cholecystitis (with videos). J Hepatobiliary Pancreat Sci. 2018;25:41–54.
31. Shea JA, Berlin JA, Escarce JJ, et al. Revised estimates of diagnostic test sensitivity and specificity in suspected biliary tract disease. Arch Intern Med. 1994;154:2573–81.
32. Strasberg SM. Acute calculous cholecystitis. N Engl J Med. 2008;358:2804–11.
33. Ansaloni L, Pisano M, Coccolini F, et al. WSES guidelines on acute calculous cholecystitis. World J Emerg Surg. 2016;11(11):25–48.
34. Ralls PW, Coletti PM, Halls JM, et al. Prospective evaluation of 99m TC-IDA cholescintigraphy in the diagnosis of acute cholecystitis. Radiology. 1982;144(144):369–71.
35. Shafi S, Aboutanos M, Brown CVR, et al. American Association for Surgery of Trauma Committee on patient assessment and outcomes. Measuring anatomic severity of disease in emergency general surgery. J Trauma Acute Care Surg. 2014;76:884–7.
36. Tominaga GT, Saudenmayer KL, Shafi S, et al. The American Association for the Surgery of Trauma grading scale for 16 emergency general surgery conditions: disease-specific criteria characterizing anatomic severity grading. J Trauma Acute Care Surg. 2016;81:593–602.
37. Madni TD, Leshikar DE, Minshall CT, et al. The Parkland grading scale for cholecystitis. Am J Surg. 2018;215:625–30.

Pathophysiology and Diagnosis of Acute Acalculous Cholecystitis

3

Florin Botea, Alin Kraft, and Irinel Popescu

Abbreviat ions

AAC Acute acalculous cholecystitis
ACC Acute calculous cholecystitis

3.1 Introduction

Acute acalculous cholecystitis (AAC) is an acute necro-inflammatory infection of the gallbladder with a multifactorial pathogenesis, in the absence of cholelithiasis, sludge, or cystic duct obstruction on diagnostic imaging [1]. The condition was first described by Duncan in 1844. It accounts for approximately 2–15% of all cases of acute cholecystitis [1, 2] and is associated with high morbidity and mortality rates.

3.2 Epidemiology

AAC occurs in 0.2–0.4% of all critically ill patients [3] with predisposing multifactorial risk factors (Table 3.1). AAC has a predominance in elderly, as well as a male predominance ranging 40–80% and even more [4, 5], affecting patients much older and more predominantly of male sex than acute calculous cholecystitis (ACC) [6, 7]. However, AAC may also occur in young and middle-aged outpatient healthy individuals [2]. In children, AAC represents 50–70% of all cases of acute cholecystitis [8]. The incidence of AAC in outpatients is not well defined. Up to 77% of patients diagnosed with AAC during hospitalization may in fact have the onset at home without evidence of acute illness or trauma, but with significant vascular disease in up to 72% of these cases [9]. Although this would indicate that the actual incidence in outpatients may be in fact much higher than acknowledged, it may be also possible that some of these patients in this condition may have been misdiagnosed as AAC due to failure to reveal gallstones or microcrystals.

3.3 Etiology

AAC occurs more frequently as a complication of severe acute conditions (polytrauma, severe burns, shock, aortic dissection, or non-biliary operations—especially aortic surgery, acute myelogenous leukemia) [10–12]. AAC is also often associated with chronic conditions such as diabetes mellitus, cardiovascular disease, chronic kidney disease, vasculitis, acquired immunodeficiency syndrome, malignant tumors, bone marrow transplantation, and long-term total parenteral nutrition [13, 14]. Patients with cancer are at risk for AAC, including metastasis to the porta hepatis, therapy with interleukin-2, and

F. Botea · A. Kraft · I. Popescu (✉)
Fundeni Clinical Institute, Center of General Surgery and Liver Transplantation, Titu Maiorescu University, Bucharest, Romania

© Springer Nature Switzerland AG 2021

I. Di Carlo (ed.), *Difficult Acute Cholecystitis*, https://doi.org/10.1007/978-3-030-62102-5_3

Table 3.1 Risk factors and infections predisposing to acalculous cholecystitis

Risk factors for acalculous cholecystitis	Infections predisposing to acalculous cholecystitis	Risk factors that warrant broad empiric antimicrobial coverage
Systemic diseases: – Acute myelogenous leukemia – Diabetes mellitus – End-stage kidney disease – Immunosuppression – Infections/Sepsis	Bacteria: – *Coxiella burnetiid* – *Campylobacter jejuni* – *Salmonella species* (S. enterica, S typhi) – *Brucella species* – *Leptospira species* – *Mycobacterium tuberculosis* – *Vibrio cholerae*	Factors associated with mortality: – Age > 70 years – Comorbidities (e.g., liver disease, malignancy, chronic malnutrition) – Immunocompromising conditions (e.g., poorly controlled diabetes mellitus, chronic high-dose corticosteroid use, other immunosuppressive agents, neutropenia, advanced AIDS, B or T leukocyte deficiency) – Factors related to acalculous cholecystitis: high severity (i.e., sepsis); extensive peritoneal involvement or diffuse peritonitis; delay in initial intervention (source control) >24 h; inability to achieve adequate debridement or drainage control
Cardiovascular diseases: – Coronary heart disease – Heart failure – Aortic dissection – Hypotension – Cholesterol emboli – Vasculitis	Fungi: – *Candida species* – Isospora	
Iatrogenic factors: – Cardiopulmonary resuscitation – Mechanical ventilation – Nonbiliary surgery – Cystic duct obstruction by a percutaneous transhepatic catheter in the bile duct – Medications (e.g. opiates, sunitinib) – Multiple transfusions – Total parenteral nutrition – Bone marrow transplantation	Parasites: – *Ascaris lumbricoides* – *Echinococcus granulosus* – *Plasmodium species* – *Cryptosporidium*	
Surgical emergencies: – Burns – Major trauma	Viruses: – Cytomegalovirus – Epstein-Barr virus – Flavivirus – Hepatitis A and B – Dengue virus	Factors associated with antibiotic-resistant bacteria: – Nosocomial infections – Travel related: travel to areas with high rates of antibiotic-resistant organisms within the few weeks prior to infection onset; antibiotics received during travel – Known colonization with antibiotic-resistant organisms
HPB diseases: – Ampullary stenosis – Choledochal cyst – Hemobilia – Metastases involving portal vein	Miscellaneous: – Snake bites	
Miscellaneous: – Pregnancy – Childbirth		

lymphokine-activated killer cells for metastatic disease [15]. Local conditions that may often lead to AAC include dehydration, bile stasis, gallbladder dysmotility, or ischemia; systemic conditions that commonly lead to AAC include inflammation mediators [16], systemic bacterial (gram-negative or anaerobic) or viral (EBV, hepatotropic virus) infections, and sepsis [17, 18]. AAC usually develop as a secondary infection of the gallbladder during systemic sepsis, such as disseminated candidiasis, leptospirosis, chronic biliary tract carriers of typhoidal and nontyphoidal Salmonella, cholera, and tuberculosis [19–24], less often malaria, brucellosis, and dengue fever [25–27]. AAC due to extrahepatic biliary obstruction may have infectious, such as ascariasis and echinococcal cysts [28, 29], or noninfectious causes, such as haemobilia, choledochal cyst, ampullary stenosis, or percutaneous transhepatic catheter drainage [30–32]. Rare causes for AAC are photodynamic therapy for duodenal lesions or snakebite [33, 34].

AAC has been reported in 0.7–0.9% of patients following open abdominal aortic reconstruction, in 0.5% of patients following cardiac surgery, and in as many as 4% of patients who have undergone bone marrow transplantation [4, 35, 36].

3.4 Pathogenesis

3.4.1 Gallbladder Wall Ischemia

Although not completely understood, the pathogenesis of AAC is related to blood stasis and ischemia of the gallbladder wall, usually related to hypoperfusion, that lead to a local inflammatory response that induces necrosis of the gallbladder wall [14, 37]. Gallbladder ischemia is central to the pathogenesis of AAC. Hypoperfusion is due to hypotension (e.g., heart failure), dehydration (e.g., fever), and vasoactive drug administration [37].

Prolongation of ischemia has been associated with increased mucosal phospholipase A2, superoxide dismutase activities, and increased mucosal lipid peroxide content, associated with high rates of gallbladder necrosis and perforation [35, 38]. Gallbladder specimen arteriography reveals marked differences between ACC and AAC [39]: ACC is correlated with arterial dilatation and extensive venous filling, while AAC is correlated with multiple arterial occlusions and minimal-to-absent venous filling, underlining the key role of vascular occlusion and microcirculatory disruption in the pathogenesis of AAC. Additionally, reperfusion injury may worsen the ischemic injuries of the gallbladder wall [40].

An interrelationship between ischemia and stasis can result in hypoperfusion [41]. In this model, bacterial invasion of ischemic tissue becomes a secondary phenomenon [41].

3.4.2 Bile Stasis

Another cause of AAC is thought to be bile stasis and increased lithogenicity of bile, proven in both experimental and clinical studies [8]. Hospitalized patients often have bile stasis due to multiple factors including dehydration, absence of oral intake that leads to impaired enterohepatic circulation, long-term total parenteral nutrition, and impaired gut metabolism. Volume depletion leads to bile concentration, thus the bile becomes thick bile or sludge and, in correlation with the absence of a stimulus for gallbladder emptying, may obstruct the cystic duct. Moreover, the use of opioid analgesics induces the spasm of the sphincter of Oddi as adverse effect, increasing the intraluminal bile duct pressure, promoting bile stasis. Bile stasis may also be prompted by mechanical ventilation with positive end-expiratory pressure that also reduces portal perfusion by increasing hepatic venous pressure [42]. Ileus is also thought to induce in bile stasis, but experimental results are conflicting.

Critically ill patients are more predisposed because of increased bile viscosity due to fever and dehydration and because of prolonged absence of oral feeding resulting in a decrease or absence of cholecystokinin-induced gallbladder contraction.

Bile stasis may be aggravated by total parental nutrition [43]. Parenteral nutrition is associated with gallstone formation, as well as AAC, in both adults and children. During long-term total parental nutrition, the incidence of AAC may be as high as 30% [44], while gallbladder "sludge" occurs in 50% of these patients at 4 weeks and is omnipresent at 6 weeks [45]. Neither cholecystokinin administration, to stimulate gallbladder emptying, nor enteral alimentation can completely prevent AAC among critically ill patients [46].

Bile stasis may alter the chemical composition of bile, which may induce gallbladder mucosal injury. For example, lysophosphatidylcholine may induce acute cholecystitis in animal models with identical histopathological features to that of human AAC [47]; lysophosphatidylcholine has potent effects on gallbladder structure and functional water transport across mucosa [47]. Other bile compounds (e.g., beta-glucuronidase) have also been implicated in the pathogenesis of AAC [44].

3.4.3 Vasoactive Mediators

Vasoactive mediators also play a key role in the pathogenesis of AAC. Bacterial infection is most likely a secondary event, while the phenomena of primary importance seems to be the host response to splanchnic ischemia/reperfusion injury or gram-negative bacteremia. Intravenous injection of *Escherichia coli* lipopolysaccharide, a potent stimulus of inflammation and coagulation, produces AAC in several mammalian species [48, 49]. Human gallbladder mucosal cells stimulated in vitro with the same compound inducing the production of eicosanoids and platelet-activating factor [50]. AAC can also be induced by injecting plant polyphenols that activate factor XII directly and generate spasm of the cystic artery [51]. Platelet-activating factor induces splanchnic hypoperfusion in sepsis and other low-flow states [52]. The inflammation appears to be mediated by pro-inflammatory eicosanoids, as it is inhibited by nonspecific cyclooxygenase inhibitors [49].

In AAC, endothelial injury, gallbladder ischemia, and stasis lead to concentration of bile salts, gallbladder distension, and gallbladder wall necrosis. The majority of patients with AAC have multiple risk factors (Table 3.1) [36, 53–55].

3.4.4 Infection

In some cases, specific primary infections predispose to AAC (Table 3.1). More often, however, these infections cause a cholangiopathy without cholecystitis. Once AAC is established, secondary infection with enteric pathogens, including *Escherichia coli*, *Enterococcus faecalis*, *Klebsiella spp.*, *Pseudomonas spp.*, *Proteus spp.*, and *Bacteroides fragilis* and related strains is common [56]. Perforation occurs in severe cases [57]. AAC is associated with a higher incidence of gangrene and perforation compared to ACC.

Bacteremia is one of the major causes of morbidity and mortality in the ICU [58]. Early diagnosis of bacteremia and prompt initiation of antibiotic therapy improve the clinical outcomes in critically ill patients [14].

The incidence of bacteremia has increased over time despite the availability of suitable antibiotic therapy [59]. The most common bacterial species associated with AAC, identified by blood and/or bile cultures, are gram-negative *Enterobacteriaceae*, such as E. coli and *Klebsiella pneumoniae* [60], [61], followed by *Enterococcus species*, *Staphylococcus spp.*, *Streptococcus spp.*, and *Candida spp.* [14]. Particularly, AAC associated with acquired immunodeficiency syndrome (AIDS) or other immunosuppressive conditions may be due to opportunistic infections such as microsporidia, *Cryptosporidium,* or cytomegalovirus [62].

In pediatric patients, AAC occurs in young children and neonates, as well as older children [63]. Common precipitant factors are dehydration, acute bacterial infections, viral diseases, such as hepatitis, upper respiratory tract infections [64], and portal lymphadenitis with extrinsic cystic duct obstruction. Recent studies suggest that the pathogenesis may be similar to that in adults [63].

3.5 Clinical Manifestations

The clinical presentation of AAC varies based on the severity of illness and underlying predisposing conditions (Table 3.1). Early diagnosis is the key to improve prognosis because of the fast progression of AAC due to gangrene and perforation, with dismal prognosis [37]. AAC has to be suspected in a critically ill patient, often intubated and sedated, presenting sepsis or unexplained fever, jaundice, abdominal discomfort, or high transaminases (not justified for other reasons), especially in postoperative setting [6].

The presentation may be similar to ACC, with fever, severe right upper quadrant pain with tenderness at palpation, and positive Murphy's sign [6], sometimes presenting with a palpable right upper quadrant mass and/or crepitus (due to emphysematous cholecystitis) and rarely jaundice [9]. Murphy's sign is operator-dependent and involves an alert and cooperative patient; when present, is indicative of gallbladder inflammation. Presentation characterized by recurrent biliary symptoms for months or years usually has gallstone-related disease or functional gallbladder disorder. The presentation may be insidious; therefore, patients may have sepsis, shock, and peritonitis at presentation due to complications including gallbladder necrosis, gangrene, or perforation.

Jaundice typically results from sepsis-related cholestasis, partial biliary obstruction due to inflammation expanding to the common bile duct or due to extrinsic compression of the common bile duct by a phlegmon (Mirizzi-type syndrome).

Nowadays, the diagnosis rate of AAC is increasing due to several factors, such as increased number of severe forms, enhanced awareness on behalf of the medical staff, improved imaging techniques, and consideration of AAC in the differential diagnosis of complications in patients with major comorbidities [37].

As AAC occurs frequently in critically ill patients, it is important to recognize this condition:

- The potentially critically ill patient: is sweaty, anxious, pale, agitated, or confused; responds to moderate stimulation only (loud voice, physical prodding); uses the respiratory accessory muscles at a respiratory rate of 20–30 or under 8; has the heart rate over 100, the systolic blood pressure under 90, and the urinary out is under 0.5 ml/kg/h.
- The critically ill patient: has a severe general status; is dehydrated, unresponsive, or poorly responsive neurologically; has the respiratory rate under 8 or over 30, the heart rate under 50 or over 150, the systolic blood pressure under 60, oliguria or anuria. These patients might not withstand surgery when the Charlson Comorbidity Index (CCI) is at least 6 and the American Society of Anesthesiologists physical status classification (ASA-PS) is at least 3 (patients with severe systemic disease, with one or more moderate to severe diseases, that leads to significant functional limitations with one or more organ dysfunctions) [65–67].

3.6 Laboratory Tests

Laboratory tests in patients with AAC are nonspecific. Leukocytosis is present in 70–85% of patients [68]. Abnormal liver tests include conjugated hyperbilirubinemia and a mild increase in serum alkaline phosphatase and serum aminotransferases [9].

Blood cultures should be acquired in all patients with suspected AAC to guide narrowing of empiric antibiotics (Table 3.1). However, the culture findings may be negative or inconclusive in late-stage disease [13], and bile culture results are negative in nearly 50% of patients with AAC, probably due to concurrent antibiotic therapy.

3.7 Imaging

Imaging in AAC is not specific enough to make a stand-alone diagnosis. Imaging findings must be integrated in the context of clinical presentation.

3.7.1 Ultrasonography

Ultrasonography in patients with suspected AAC is mandatory [56, 69]. Features suggestive of AAC are similar as the ones for ACC, but without gallstones [70]:

- Thick wall (≥3.5–4 mm) (with distended gallbladder of ≥5 cm longitudinally and no ascites)–the most reliable feature seen in patients with AAC but is not specific [71].
- Ultrasonographic Murphy's sign.
- Pericholecystic fluid (halo)/subserosal edema.
- Other signs: intramural gas, mucosal membrane, sludge, hydrops (distension ≥8 cm longitudinally or 5 cm transversely, with clear fluid).

The reported sensitivity of ultrasound for AAC ranges from 30% to 92% [71], while the specificity is 89–100% [3]. False-positive results may be due to hypoalbuminemia, ascites, sludge, non-shadowing stones, or cholesterolosis, which can mimic a thickened gallbladder wall.

3.7.2 Computed Tomography

When diagnosis is uncertain at ultrasound, contrast-enhanced abdominal computed tomography (CT) scan is recommended to confirm AAC and/or to rule out other causes for acute abdominal pain.

CT scan findings in AAC include gallbladder wall thickening (>3 mm), intramural gas, lack of gallbladder wall enhancement, subserosal and/or pericholecystic edema, pericholecystic fluid, mucosal sloughing, hyperdense bile (sludge), and/or gallbladder distention (>5 cm) [71] (Figs. 3.1, 3.2, and 3.3). Of these findings, gas in the gallbladder wall or lumen and pericholecystic edema have the highest specificity for AAC (99, 95, and 92%, respectively), but with poor sensitivity (11, 38, and 22%, respectively). The accuracy of CT scan appears to be like that seen with ultrasonography [72].

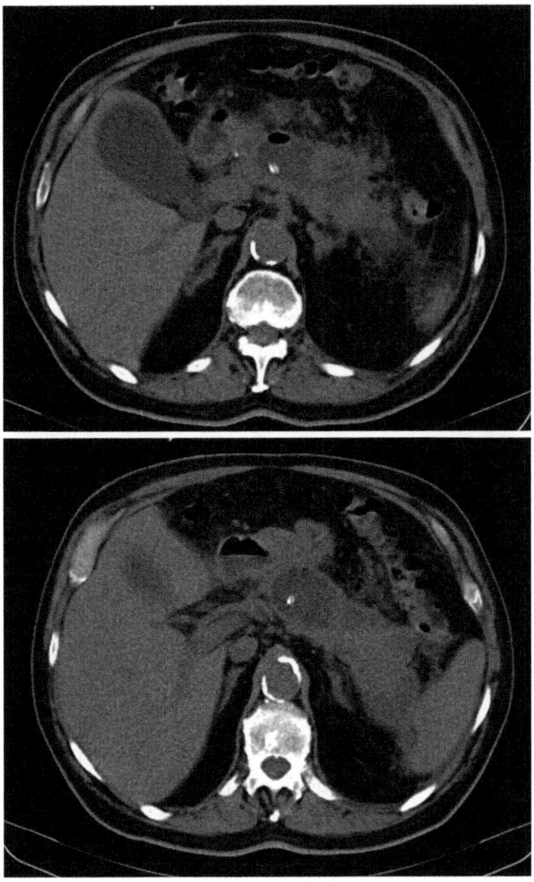

Fig. 3.1 Control CT after percutaneous drainage of an infected pancreatic pseudocyst due to recent episode of acute alcoholic pancreatitis, in a 69-year old patient, with multiple comorbidities (obesity, third degree hypertension, dyslipidemia, hepatic steatosis, acute on chronic kidney condition stage G3a)

3.7.3 Cholescintigraphy

In stable patients with unclear diagnosis at ultrasonography and abdominal CT scan, a hepatic technetium 99 m Tc iminodiacetic acid (HIDA) scan is recommended [73]. As cholescintigraphy (HIDA scan) takes hours to perform, it is not recommended in critically ill patients in whom a delay in therapy can be potentially fatal; other arguments for not recommending it in this setting are the frequent false-negative and false-positive results (due to fasting, liver disease, or total parenteral nutrition) [74].

Failure to opacify the gallbladder at 1 h is considered positive for AAC. Leakage into the pericholecystic space indicates gallbladder perforation. The sensitivity of cholescintigraphy for AAC is 67–100% [74, 75], while the specificity is 58–88% [75].

Cholescintigraphy associated with intravenous morphine administration (0.05 mg/kg) has led to a reappraisal of HIDA imaging for AAC [75, 76], especially when ultrasound is nondiagnostic, increasing the diagnostic accuracy to 95% [75, 77]. AAC is diagnosed if the gallbladder is not visualized in 30 min after morphine injection.

False-negative results are rare occurring in certain conditions, such as cystic duct patency despite a diseased gallbladder, bowel loop simulation of the gallbladder, bile leak from gallblad-

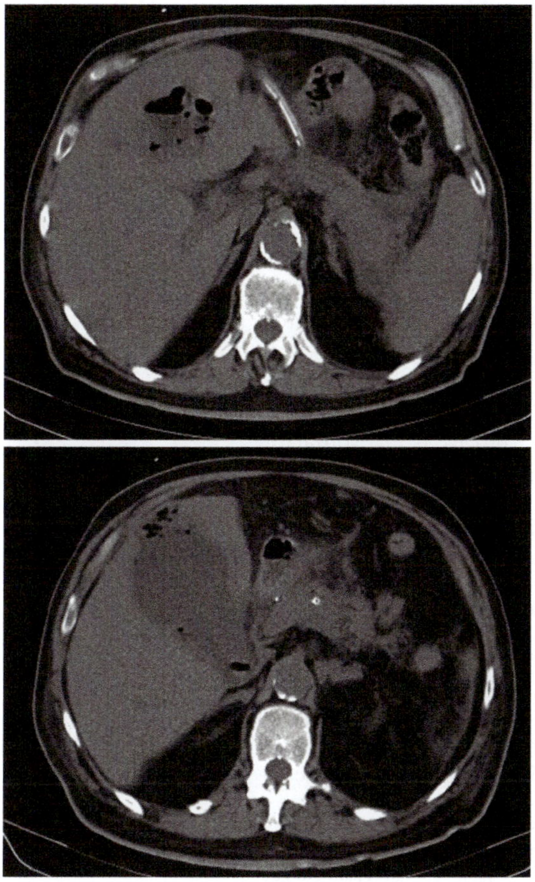

Fig. 3.2 Same patient as in Fig. 3.1: CT at 3 weeks showing gallbladder with significant distension (115/80 mm), with thickened, irregular walls, nonhomogenous mixed fluid, para-fluid and multiple air blob contents, associated with significant densification of the adjacent fat structures, with inflammatory infectious aspect; continuity solution present at the level of the gallbladder fundic area, with intrahepatic penetration in the fourth liver segment, with gaseous, fluid, and parafluid accumulation at this level, approximately 50/45 mm in size axially, without biliary lithiasis—acute acalculous cholecystitis with in-hospital onset, in a critically ill patient, with pericholecystic liver abscess

der perforation, and tracer activity in the kidneys simulating the gallbladder [78]. False-positive results may occur in several conditions, such as fasting, total parenteral nutrition, severe illness, severe hepatocellular disease, hyperbilirubinemia, rapid biliary to bowel transit, biliary sphincterotomy, and/or prior cholecystectomy. Other

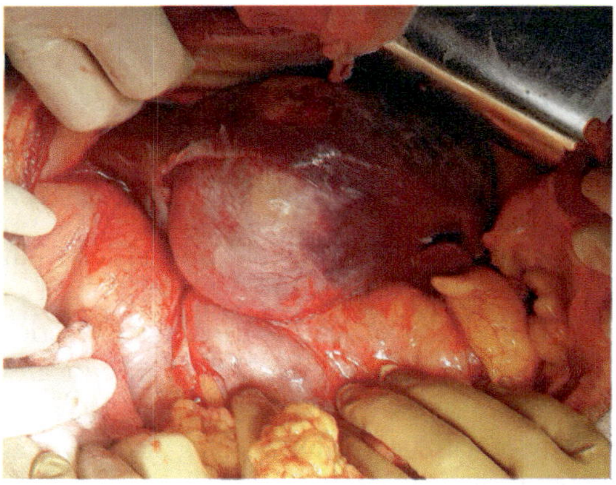

Fig. 3.3 Same patient as in Figs. 3.1 and 3.2: Intraoperative aspect of acalculous cholecystitis with pericholecystic liver abscess (superficialized on the diaphragmatic surface of segments 4–5), for which subtotal cholecystectomy, liver abscess evacuation, and multiple drainage was performed. The patient died in POD 10 due to recurrent acute pancreatitis and multiple peritoneal abscesses, despite ICU aggressive treatment and surgical reintervention

agents (diisopropyl and m-bromothymethyl iminodiacetic acid) used in cholescintigraphy have generally overcome the limitations of morphine cholescintigraphy.

3.7.4 Laparoscopy

Laparoscopy is recommended when the diagnosis of AAC is in question or if percutaneous cholecystostomy has failed to improve the patient's general status [79]. Bedside laparoscopy has been used with certain success for both diagnosis and therapy of AAC, but initial enthusiasm has diminished due to the bulky equipment that has to be brought to the ICU bedside. Nowadays, due to advances in intensive care, most patients will tolerate the transport to the operating room. For severe local forms of AAC, when complete laparoscopic cholecystectomy is not possible in a safe and expedient manner, a laparoscopic damage control procedure such as cholecystostomy or partial cholecystectomy may be performed to treat the patient's condition while minimizing the iatrogenic aggression.

3.8 Diagnosis

3.8.1 Positive Diagnosis

AAC remains difficult to diagnose mainly due to complicated clinical settings [14], the low prevalence, and the complexities to distinguish it from ACC [37].

The diagnosis of AAC is based upon a series of symptoms and clinical signs (e.g., critically ill patients with sepsis without a clear cause or jaundice) correlated with imaging findings that support such diagnosis, and the exclusion of other diagnoses. Imaging in AAC is not specific enough to make the diagnosis alone and must be interpreted in the clinical context. AAC is often diagnosed based on the following:

- Fever, abdominal pain, leukocytosis, and/or elevated liver tests.
- Risk factors for AAC (Table 3.1).
- Imaging features suggesting AAC.
- No evidence of other conditions that explain the clinical and imaging findings.

After diagnosis, imaging has a monitoring role of the development of AAC during medical and interventional treatment. Sometimes, gallstones are discovered by imaging late, during nonsurgical treatment, converting the diagnosis from AAC to ACC, case in which cholecystectomy becomes mandatory (Fig. 3.4).

3.8.2 Differential Diagnosis

The differential diagnosis of AAC includes other causes of sepsis (e.g., pneumonia, urinary tract infection), right upper quadrant pain, and/or jaundice. These include:

- Acute calculous cholecystitis.
- Noninfectious gallbladder hydrops (Fig. 3.5).
- Noninfectious thick gallbladder wall.

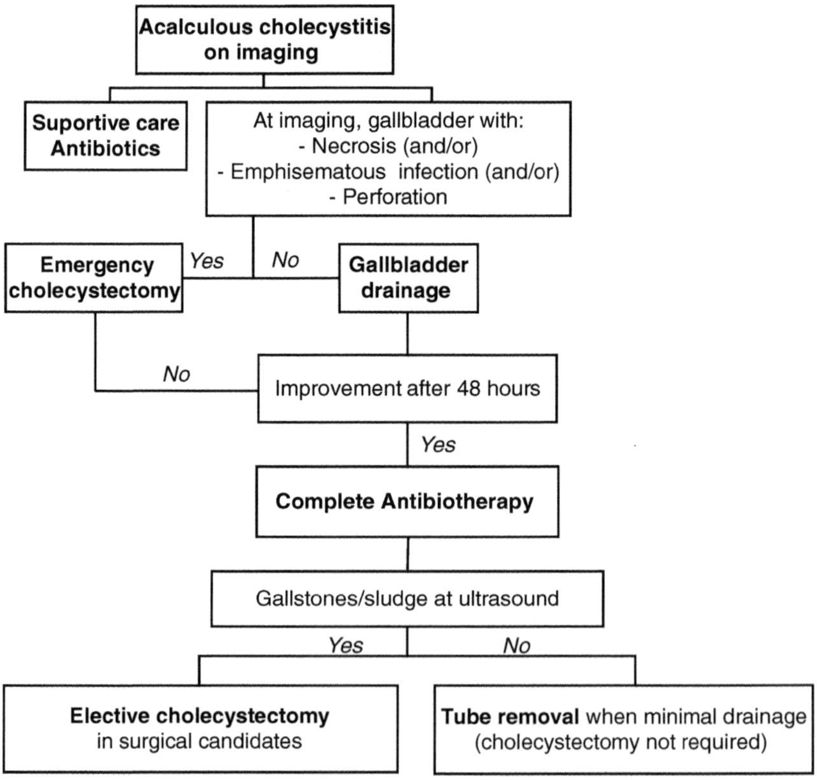

Fig. 3.4 Approach to the management of acalculous cholecystitis

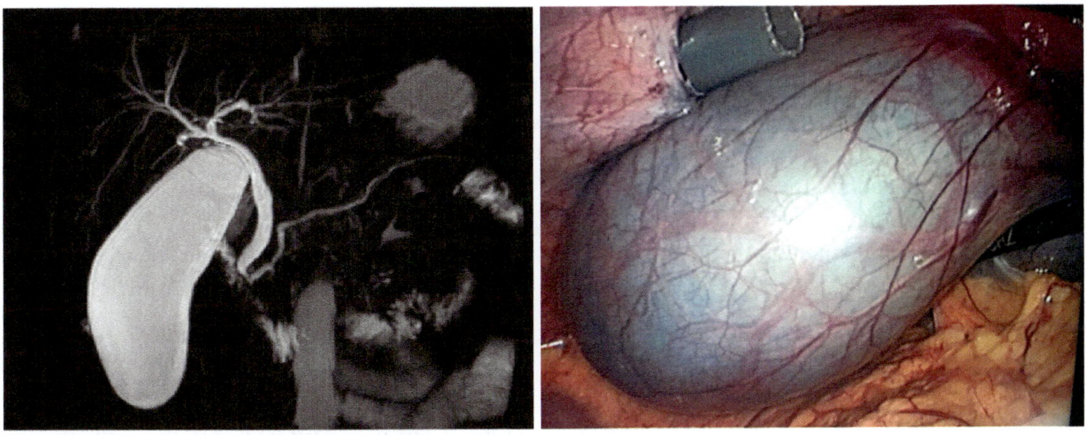

Fig. 3.5 Noninfectious gallbladder hydrops (13 cm) due to stenosis of the terminal common bile duct induced by autoimmune pancreatitis (MRI imaging and intraoperative aspect during laparoscopic cholecystectomy) in a 23-year-old female patient, with Crohn's disease, autoimmune pancreatitis, type 1 ANA autoimmune hepatitis, autoimmune thyroiditis. Surgery consisted in laparoscopic cholecystectomy, with favorable outcome

- Acute pancreatitis.
- Hepatic or subphrenic abscess.
- Right-sided pyelonephritis.
- Right-sided pneumonia.
- Other causes for right upper quadrant pain.
- Other causes for jaundice.
- Other causes for sepsis and abdominal pain.

These conditions can be ruled out by clinical examination, laboratory tests, and imaging also performed for AAC diagnosis. Laboratory evaluation should include a complete blood count, electrolytes, liver tests, and pancreatic enzymes. In addition, a urine analysis to exclude urosepsis, and a chest X-ray or CT scan to exclude pneumonia.

3.8.3 Complications

Because of the potential obscurity of the diagnosis, the underlying illnesses of the affected patients, and the potentially rapid progression of the disease to emphysematous and gangrenous cholecystitis, and gallbladder perforation, complications associated with this condition are frequent and usually severe [53, 69]. Gallbladder necrosis, gangrene, and perforation are frequently present at the time of diagnosis, especially in the critically ill patients, being associated with poor outcome [53, 69]. The incidence of gallbladder gangrene is higher in the AAC than in ACC (31% vs 5%, respectively) [80]. Gallbladder gangrene occurs in approximately 50% of patients with AAC, commonly leading to gallbladder perforation [71]. Particularly, emphysematous cholecystitis increases the risk for perforation. Perforation occurs in approximately 10% of patients with AAC [7, 35] that may result in abscess formation, free perforation with generalized peritonitis or cholecystoenteric fistula. When gallbladder gangrene occurs without perforation, the common complications are acute pancreatitis, obstruction of the main bile duct, and colonic perforation.

The incidence of cerebrovascular accidents is significantly higher in patients with acute AAC than in those with ACC (15% vs 6%) [80].

3.8.4 Mortality

AAC is associated with a high mortality rate, which depends on comorbidities and the swiftness of diagnosis. The cause of death in most patients with AAC is multiorgan failure due to sepsis [81]. The mortality rate is related to the initial clinical severity and a high prevalence of gangrene (approximately 50%) and perforation (approximately 10%) [37], but always greater than 1% reported in gallstone cholecystitis [70].

With treatment, the overall mortality rate is high (30%) [7, 71, 82], but it increases to up to 75% if diagnosis and treatment are delayed [83]. The mortality rate in critically ill patients is very high, up to 90%, while in outpatient cases may be as low as 10% [71, 84].

3.9 Conclusion

AAC is very difficult to diagnose and should be screened in all critically ill or injured patients with sepsis, especially in cases where the cause of sepsis is not clear, in case of hypoperfusion, onset of jaundice, and/or postoperative setting. Ultrasound is the main diagnostic tool, being repeatable, noninvasive, cost-effective, and bedside available. The diagnosis must be prompt, otherwise mortality increases significantly.

References

1. Treinen C, Lomelin D, Krause C, et al. Acute acalculous cholecystitis in the critically ill: risk factors and surgical strategies. Langenbeck's Arch Surg. 2015;400:421–7. https://doi.org/10.1007/s00423-014-1267-6.
2. Ganpathi IS, Diddapur RK, Eugene H, et al. Acute acalculous cholecystitis: challenging the myths. HPB (Oxford). 2007;9:131–4.
3. Huffman JL, Schenker S. Acute acalculous cholecystitis: a review. Clin Gastroenterol Hepatol. 2010;8:15–22.
4. Cadot H, Addis MD, Faries PL, et al. Abdominal aortic aneurysmorrhaphy and cholelithiasis in the era of endovascular surgery. Am Surg. 2002;68:839.
5. Ganpathi IS, Diddapur RK, Eugene H, Karim M. Acute acalculous cholecystitis: challenging the myths. HPB (Oxford). 2007;9:131.
6. Ryu JK, Ryu KH, Kim KH. Clinical features of acute acalculous cholecystitis. J Clin Gastroenterol. 2003;36:166–9.
7. Kim SB, Gu MG, Kim KH, Kim TN. Long-term outcomes of acute acalculous cholecystitis treated by nonsurgical management. Medicine. 2020;99(7):e19057.
8. Tsakayannis DE, Kozakewich HP, Lillehei CW. Acalculous cholecystitis in children. J Pediatr Surg. 1996;31:127–30.
9. Savoca PE, Longo WE, Zucker KA, et al. The increasing prevalence of AC in outpatients. Results of a 7-year study. Ann Surg. 1990;211:433.
10. Hamp T, Fridrich P, Mauritz W, et al. Cholecystitis after trauma. J Trauma. 2009;66:400.
11. Inagaki FF, Hara Y, Kamei M, Tanaka M, Yasuno M. Acute and chronic acalculous cholecystitis associated with aortic dissection. J Surg Case Rep. 2015;2015(8):rjv101.
12. Topeli A, Demiroglu H, Dundar S. Acalculous cholecystitis in patients with acute leukaemia. Br J Clin Pract. 1996;50:224–5.
13. Tana M, Tana C, Cocco G, Iannetti G, Romano M, Schiavone C. Acute acalculous cholecystitis and cardiovascular disease: a land of confusion. J Ultrasound. 2015;18(4):317–20.
14. Rincon JE, Rasane RK, Aldana JA, Zhang CX, Fonseca RA. Acute acalculous cholecystitis-associated bacteremia has worse outcome. Surg Infect (Larchmt). 2020. https://doi.org/10.1089/sur.2019.297
15. Chung-Park M, Kim B, Marmyola G, et al. Acalculous lymphoeosinophilic cholecystitis associated with interleukin-2 and lymphokine-activated killer cell therapy. Arch Pathol Lab Med. 1990;114:1073–5.
16. Afdhal NH. Acalculous cholecystitis. Up to date. 2016. https://www.uptodate.com/contents/acalculous cholecystitis?source=search_result&search=acalculo uscholecystitis&selectedTitle=1~28.
17. Souza LJ, Braga LC, Rocha Nde S, Tavares RR, et al. Acute acalculous cholecystitis in a teenager with hepatitis A viral infection: a case report. Braz J Infect Dis. 2009;13:74–6.
18. Basar O, Kisacik B, Bozdogan E, et al. An unusual cause of acalculous cholecystitis during pregnancy: hepatitis a virus. Dig Dis Sci. 2005;50(8):1532.
19. Mandak JS, Pollack B, Fishman NO, et al. Acalculous candidal cholecystitis: a previously unrecognized complication after cardiac transplantation. Am J Gastroenterol. 1995;90:1333–7.
20. Baelen E, Roustan J. Leptospirosis associated with acute acalculous cholecystitis. Surgical or medical treatment? J Clin Gastroenterol. 1997;25:704–6.
21. Khan FY, Elouzi EB, Asif M. Acute acalculous cholecystitis complicating typhoid fever in an adult patient: a case report and review of the literature. Travel Med Infect Dis. 2009;7:203–6.
22. McCarron B, Love WC. Acalculous nontyphoidal salmonellal cholecystitis requiring surgical intervention despite ciprofl oxacin therapy: report of three cases. Clin Infect Dis. 1997;24:707–9.
23. West BC, Silberman R, Otterson WN. Acalculous cholecystitis and septicemia caused by non-01 Vibrio cholerae: first reported case and review of biliary infections with Vibrio cholerae. Diagn Microbiol Infect Dis. 1998;30:187–91.
24. Vallejo EA. Acute tuberculous cholecystitis. Gastroenterology. 1950;16:501–4.

25. Abreu C, Santos L, Poínhos R, Sarmento A. Acute acalculous cholecystitis in malaria: a review of seven cases from an adult cohort. Infection. 2013;41(4):821–6.
26. Ashley D, Vade A, Challapali M. Brucellosis with acute acalculous cholecystitis. Pediatr Infect Dis J. 2000;19:1112–3.
27. Bhatty S, Shaikh N, Fatima M, Sumbhuani AK. Acute cholecystitis in dengue fever. J Pak Med Assoc. 2009;59:519–21.
28. Kuzu MA, Ozturk Y, Ozbek H, Soran A. Acalculous cholecystitis: ascariasis as an unusual cause. J Gastroenterol. 1996;31:747–9.
29. Mansour K. Acute cholecystitis with echinococcal cyst obstruction of the common bile duct. Postgrad Med J. 1963;39:542–3.
30. Sandblom P. Hemorrhage into the biliary tract following trauma: "Traumatic hemobilia". Surgery. 1948;24:571–86.
31. Lin SL, Shank M, Hung YB, et al. Choledochal cyst associated with acute acalculous cholecystitis. J Pediatr Gastroenterol Nutr. 2000;31:307–8.
32. Lillemoe KD, Pitt HA, Kaufman SL, et al. Acute cholecystitis occurring as a complication of percutaneous transhepatic drainage. Surg Gynecol Obstet. 1989;168:348–56.
33. Savoye G, Michel P, Hochain P, et al. Fatal acalculous cholecystitis after photodynamic therapy for high-grade dysplasia of the major duodenal papilla. Gastrointest Endosc. 2000;51:493–5.
34. Cello JP. AIDS cholangiopathy: spectrum of disease. Am J Med. 1989;86:539–46.
35. Hagino RT, Valentine RJ, Clagett GP. Acalculous cholecystitis after aortic reconstruction. J Am Coll Surg. 1997;184:245.
36. Wiboltt KS, Jeffrey RB Jr. Acalculous cholecystitis in patients undergoing bone marrow transplantation. Eur J Surg. 1997;163:519.
37. Soria-Aledo V, Galindo-Iñíguez L, Flores-Funes D, Carrasco-Prats M, Aguayo-Albasini JL. Is cholecystectomy the treatment of choice for acute acalculous cholecystitis? A systematic review of the literature. Rev Esp Enferm Dig. 2017;109(10):708–18.
38. Barie PS. Acalculous and postoperative cholecystitis. In: Barie PS, Shires GT, editors. Surgical intensive care. Boston: Little, Brown; 1993. p. 837–57.
39. Hakala T, Nuuiten PJ, Ruokonen ET, Alhava E. Microangiopathy in acute acalculous cholecystitis. Br J Surg. 1997;84:1249–52.
40. Taoka H. Experimental study on the pathogenesis of acute acalculous cholecystitis, with special reference to the roles of microcirculatory disturbances, free radicals and membrane-bound phospholipase A2. Gastroenterol Jpn. 1991;26:633–44.
41. Orlando R, Gleason E, Drezner AD. Acute acalculous cholecystitis in the critically ill patient. Am J Surg. 1983;145:472–6.
42. Parkman HP, James AN, Bogar LJ, et al. Effect of acalculous cholecystitis on gallbladder neuromuscular transmission and contractility. J Surg Res. 2000;88:186–92.
43. Lin KYK. Acute acalculous cholecystitis: a limited review of the literature. Mt Sinai J Med. 1986;53:305–9.
44. Kouromalis E, Hopwood D, Ross PE, et al. Gallbladder epithelial acid hydrolases in human cholecystitis. J Pathol. 1983;139:179–91.
45. Messing B, Bories C, Kuntslinger F, et al. Does total parenteral nutrition induce gallbladder sludge formation and lithiasis? Gastroenterology. 1983;84:1012–9.
46. Merrill RC, Miller-Crotchett P, Lowry P. Gallbladder response to enteral lipids in injured patients. Arch Surg. 1989;124:301–2.
47. Niderheiser DH. Acute acalculous cholecystitis induced by lysophosphatidyl choline. Am J Pathol. 1986;124:559–63.
48. Cullen JJ, Maes EB, Aggarwal S, et al. Effect of endotoxin on opossum gallbladder motility: a model of acalculous cholecystitis. Ann Surg. 2000;232:202–7.
49. Kaminski DL, Feinstein WK, Deshpande YG. The production of experimental cholecystitis by endotoxin. Prostaglandins. 1994;47:233–45.
50. Kaminski DL, Amir G, Deshpande YG, et al. Studies on the etiology of acute acalculous cholecystitis: the effect of lipopolysaccharide on human gallbladder mucosal cells. Prostaglandins. 1994;47:319–30.
51. Ratnoff OD, Crum JD. Activation of Hageman factor by solutions of ellagic acid. J Lab Clin Med. 1964;63:359–77.
52. Rehman T, Deboisblanc BP. Persistent fever in the ICU. Chest. 2014;145(1):158–65.
53. Shapiro MJ, Luchtefeld WB, Kurzweil S, et al. Acute acalculous cholecystitisin the critically ill. Am Surg. 1994;60:335.
54. Gofrit O, Eid A, Pikarsky A, et al. Cholesterol embolisation causing chronic AC. Eur J Surg. 1996;162:243.
55. Schwesinger WH, Diehl AK. Changing indications for laparoscopic cholecystectomy. Stones without symptoms and symptoms without stones. Surg Clin North Am. 1996;76:493.
56. Wang AJ, Wang TE, Lin CC, et al. Clinical predictors of severe gallbladder complications in acute acalculous cholecystitis. World J Gastroenterol. 2003;9(12):2821–3. https://doi.org/10.3748/wjg.v9.i12.2821.
57. Venkataramani A, Strong RM, Anderson DS, et al. Abnormal duodenal bile composition in patients with acalculous chronic cholecystitis. Am J Gastroenterol. 1998;93:434.
58. Nasa P, Juneja D, Singh O, et al. Incidence of bacteremia at the time of ICU admission and its impact on outcome. Indian J Anaesth. 2011;55:594–8.
59. Lachhab Z, Frikh M, Maleb A, et al. Bacteraemia in intensive care unit: clinical, bacteriological, and prognostic prospective study. Can J Infect Dis Med Microbiol. 2017;2017:4082938.
60. Ozyer U. Long-term results of percutaneous cholecystostomy for definitive treatment of acute acalcu-

lous cholecystitis: a 10-year single center experience. Acta Gastroenterol Belg. 2018;81:393–7.
61. Kuo CH, Changchien CS, Chen JJ, et al. Septic acute cholecystitis. Scand J Gastroenterol. 1995;30:272–5.
62. Wind P, Chevallier JM, Jones D, et al. Cholecystectomy for cholecystitis in patients with a cquired immune deficiency syndrome. Am J Surg. 1994;168:244.
63. Imamoglu M, Sarrhan H, Sari A, Ahmetoglu A. Acute acalculous cholecystitis in children: diagnosis and treatment. J Pediatr Surg. 2002;37:36–7.
64. Parithivel VS, Gerst PH, Banerjee S, et al. Acute acalculous cholecystitis in young patients without predisposing factors. Am Surg. 1999;65:366–8.
65. Charlson ME, Pompei P, Ales KL, MacKenzie CR. A new method of classifying prognostic comorbidity in longitudinal studies: development and validation. J Chronic Dis. 1987;40(5):373–83. https://doi.org/10.1016/0021-9681(87)90171-8.
66. Mayhew D, Mendonca V, Murthy BVS. A review of ASA physical status – historical perspectives and modern developments. Anaesthesia. 2019;74:373–9.
67. Okamoto K, Suzuki K, Takada T, et al. Tokyo Guidelines 2018: flowchart for the management of acute cholecystitis [published correction appears in J Hepatobiliary Pancreat Sci. 2019 Nov;26(11):534]. J Hepatobiliary Pancreat Sci. 2018;25(1):55–72.
68. Trowbridge RL, Rutkowski NK, Shojania KG. Does this patient have acute cholecystitis? JAMA. 2003;289:80.
69. Kalliafas S, Ziegler DW, Flancbaum L, Choban PS. Acute acalculous cholecystitis: incidence, risk factors, diagnosis, and outcome. Am Surg. 1998;64:471.
70. Javier BA, Eloísa SGC, Raquel GG, Carolina JA. Acute alithiasic cholecystitis: a not so rare disease. Rev Esp Enferm Dig. 2014;106(7):487–90.
71. Barie PS, Eachempati SR. Acute acalculous cholecystitis. Gastroenterol Clin N Am. 2010;39:343.
72. Mirvis SE, Whitley NO, Miller JW. CT diagnosis of acalculous cholecystitis. J Comput Assist Tomogr. 1987;11:83.
73. Westlake PJ, Hershfield NB, Kelly JK, et al. Chronic right upper quadrant pain without gallstones: does HIDA scan predict outcome after cholecystectomy? Am J Gastroenterol. 1990;85:986.
74. Shuman WP, Roger JV, Rudd TG, et al. Low sensitivity of sonography and cholescintigraphy in acalculous cholecystitis. AJR Am J Roentgenol. 1984;142:531–4.
75. Mariat G, Mahul P, Prévt N, et al. Contribution of ultrasonography and cholescintigraphy to the diagnosis of acute AC in intensive care unit patients. Intensive Care Med. 2000;26:1658.
76. Krishnamurthy S, Krishnamurthy GT. Cholecystokinin and morphine pharmacological intervention during 99mTc-HIDA cholescintigraphy: a rational approach. Semin Nucl Med. 1996;26:16–24.
77. Ziessman HA. Hepatobiliary scintigraphy in 2014. J Nucl Med Technol. 2014;42(4):249–59.
78. Dillehay G, Bar-Sever Z, Brown M, Brown R, Green R, Lee M, Lim K, et al. Appropriate use criteria for Hepatobiliary Scintigraphy in abdominal pain: summary and excerpts. J Nucl Med. 2017;58:9N.
79. Ceribelli C, Adami EA, Mattia S, Benini B. Bedside diagnostic laparoscopy for critically ill patients: a retrospective study of 62 patients. Surg Endosc. 2012;26(12):3612–5.
80. Gu MG, Kim TN, Song J, Nam YJ, Lee JY, Park JS. Risk factors and therapeutic outcomes of acute acalculous cholecystitis. Digestion. 2014;90(2):75–80.
81. Barie PS, Hydo LJ, Pieracci FM, et al. Multiple organ dysfunction syndrome in critical surgical illness. Surg Infect. 2009;10:369.
82. Eachempati SR, Barie PS. Acute acalculous cholecystitis. In: Eachempati SR, Reed II RL, editors. Acute Cholecystitis. Cham: Springer; 2015. https://doi.org/10.1007/978-3-319-14824-3_15.
83. Cornwell EE 3rd, Rodriguez A, Mirvis SE, Shorr RM. Acute acalculous cholecystitis in critically injured patients. Preoperative diagnostic imaging. Ann Surg. 1989;210:52.
84. Unal H, Korkmaz N, Kirbas I, Selcuk H, Yilmaz U. Acute acalculous cholecystitis associated with acute hepatitis B infection. Int J Infect Dis. 2009;13:e310–2.

4 Guidelines for the Management of Acute Cholecystitis

Antonio Tarasconi, Gianmaria Casoni Pattacini, Arianna Heyer, Vittoria Pattonieri, Gennaro Perrone, Carlo Mazzucchelli, Hariscine Keng Abongwa, and Fausto Catena

4.1 Introduction

Despite being a common disease, there are significant controversies regarding the diagnosis and management of acute calculous cholecystitis (ACC). The 2007 and 2013 Tokyo guidelines (TG) attempted to establish objective parameters for the diagnosis of ACC [1, 2]. While the TG have certainly improved the understanding of ACC, some criticisms have followed [3, 4]. There continue to be debates regarding the diagnostic value of single ultrasound (US) signs, as well as of laboratory tests. Historically, with regard to the treatment of ACC, the main controversy surrounded timing of surgery. The need for surgery versus conservative management has been less investigated, particularly in high-surgical-risk patients. A thorough discussion of the limitations of the Tokyo Guidelines goes beyond the aim of this chapter (see Chap. 5), but these limitations were the impetus for the World Society of Emergency Surgery (WSES) to convene a consensus conference. This consensus conference led to the creation of the 2016 WSES guidelines on ACC [5]. After the creation of these guidelines, the MICOL study [6] revealed the high incidence of gallstones and ACC in the elderly population and highlighted unique characteristics of this patient population. Because of these results, the WSES and SICG (Italian Society of Geriatric Surgery) joined forces to convene another consensus conference focusing on acute cholecystitis in the elderly population. Their efforts led to the creation of the 2017 WSES/SICG guidelines on ACC in the elderly population [7]. The aim of this chapter is to combine and briefly summarize the WSES guidelines on ACC and to provide a quick and easy-to-use tool for physicians treating this challenging disease.

4.2 Materials and Methods

The Scientific Board of the WSES organized the consensus conference on ACC in order to develop the WSES Guidelines on this topic. It is important to note that these guidelines should serve as an adjunct to clinical decision-making but do not replace clinical judgment in the context of an individual patient. The WSES President appointed four members to a Scientific Secretariat, eight members to an Organization Committee, and eight members to a Scientific Committee. Eight relevant key questions regarding diagnosis and treatment of ACC were developed to thoroughly analyze the topic. Before the

A. Tarasconi (✉) · V. Pattonieri · G. Perrone
C. Mazzucchelli · H. K. Abongwa · F. Catena
Emergency Surgery Department, Maggiore Hospital of Parma, University of Parma, Parma, Italy

G. C. Pattacini
Oncologic Surgery Department, San Martino Hospital, University of Genoa, Genova, Italy

A. Heyer
Sidney Kimmel Medical College, Thomas Jefferson University, Philadelphia, PA, USA

© Springer Nature Switzerland AG 2021
I. Di Carlo (ed.), *Difficult Acute Cholecystitis*, https://doi.org/10.1007/978-3-030-62102-5_4

consensus conference, a number of statements were developed for each of the main questions, along with the Level of Evidence (LoE) and the Grade of Recommendation (GoR) for each statement. The consensus conference on ACC was held in Jerusalem, Israel, on July 6th, 2015 during the 3rd World Congress of the WSES. Each statement was then voted upon by the audience, and comments on each statement were collected. Before the second part of the consensus conference, the president and representatives from the Organization Committee, Scientific Committee, and Scientific Secretariat modified the statements according to the findings of the first session. The revised statements were then presented again to the audience. During this process, a comprehensive algorithm for the treatment of ACC was developed based on the results of the first session of the consensus conference and voted upon for definitive approval.

The eight topics investigated during the first consensus conference were:

1. Diagnosis of ACC: Investigations.
2. Treatment of ACC: Best options.
3. Antibiotic therapy for ACC.
4. Patient selection for surgery: Risk stratification, i.e., definition of high-risk patients.
5. Timing for surgery for ACC.
6. Type of surgery for ACC.
7. Associated common bile duct stone: Suspicion and diagnosis at the presentation.
8. Alternative treatments for high-risk patients.

The methods used to inform the 2017 WSES/SICG guidelines mirror those used for the 2016 WSES guidelines. However, the consensus conference was held in 2017 during the 30th annual congress of SICG. The aim of the consensus conference was to investigate age-related factors that could influence diagnosis and management of ACC in people ages 65 and older.

Although the age cutoff of 65 was chosen arbitrarily, it is important to note that the definition of "old age" is a composite of various factors including chronological age, social factors, economic and cultural factors, and functional status. Six relevant key questions regarding diagnosis and treatment of ACC in elderly people were developed to thoroughly analyze the topic. The 2016 WSES Guidelines on ACC were used as the main point of reference.

The six topics investigated during the second consensus conference were:

1. Diagnosis: Which test is most useful in the elderly?
2. How to weigh pro and cons of surgery in elderly patients with ACC?
3. What is the most appropriate timing and the most appropriate surgical technique for elderly?
4. Alternative treatments in case of reduced benefit from surgery in elderly: Is there a role for percutaneous cholecystostomy?
5. Associated biliary tree stones: What test for suspicion, what treatment, when to treat it?
6. Antibiotic: What schedule for treatment?

4.3 Discussion

The results of the two consensus conferences and the associated guidelines are summarized in Tables 4.1 and 4.2.

4.3.1 Diagnosis

Although ACC is a common disease encountered in the Emergency Department, its diagnosis remains a major challenge. Evidence of an inflamed gallbladder containing stones is the diagnostic cornerstone. The diagnosis of ACC is based on clinical findings, laboratory data, and imaging studies. The diagnostic performance of an abdominal ultrasound (AUS) in the diagnosis of inflammation of the gallbladder is not as good as its performance in the diagnosis of gallstones, as indicated in a recent meta-analysis [8]. However, its widespread availability, lack of invasiveness, lack of exposure to ionizing radiation, and a short duration of examination make it the first-choice imaging investigation for the diagnosis of ACC. The same meta-analysis by Kieiwiet et al. [8] included studies on CT, MRI, and HIDA

Table 4.1 2016 WSES Guidelines, STATEMENTS

Diagnosis: Investigation	
1.1	There is no single clinical or laboratory finding with sufficient diagnostic accuracy to establish or exclude acute cholecystitis (LoE 2 GoR B). Combination of detailed history, complete clinical examination, and laboratory tests may strongly support the diagnosis of ACC (LoE 4 GoR C)
1.2	Abdominal ultrasound (AUS) is the preferred initial imaging technique for patients who are clinically suspected to have ACC because of its lower cost, better availability, lack of invasiveness, and high accuracy for gallbladder stones (LoE 2 GoR B)
1.3	AUS exploration is a fairly reliable investigation method but its sensitivity and specificity for diagnosing ACC are relatively low according to the adopted AUS criteria (LoE 3 GoRC)
1.4	Evidence on the diagnostic accuracy of computed tomography (CT) is scarce. While diagnostic accuracy of magnetic resonance imaging (MRI) might be comparable to that of AUS, insufficient data are available to support it. Hepatobiliary iminodiacetic acid scan (HIDA scan) has the highest sensitivity and specificity for acute cholecystitis, although its scarce availability, long time required to perform the test, and exposure to ionizing radiation limit its use (LoE 2 GoRB)
1.5	Combining clinical, laboratory, and imaging investigations is recommended, although the best combination is not yet known (LoE 4 GoRC)
Treatment: Best options	
2.1	There is no role for gallstones dissolution, drugs, or extracorporeal shock wave lithotripsy (ESWL) or a combination in the setting of ACC (LoE 2 GoR B)
2.2	Since there are no reports on surgical gallstone removal in the setting of ACC, surgery in the form of cholecystectomy remains the main option (LoE 4 GoR C)
2.3	Surgery is superior to observation of ACC in the clinical outcome and shows some cost-effectiveness advantages due to the gallstone-related complications and to the high rate of readmission and surgery in the observation group (LoE 3 GoR C)
2.4	Antibiotics should be suggested as supportive care; they are effective in treating the first episode of ACC but a high rate of relapse can be expected. Surgery is more effective than antibiotics alone in the treatment of ACC (LoE 2 GoR C)
2.5	Cholecystectomy is the gold standard for treatment of ACC (LoE 3 GoR C)
2.6	If surgery is not available, medications such as antibiotics and analgesic should be prescribed, and the patients should be referred to a surgical center (depending upon the general condition) due to the high rate of gallstone-related events (LoE 5 GoR D)
Antibiotic therapy	
3.1	Patients with uncomplicated cholecystitis can be treated without postoperative antibiotics when the focus of infection is controlled by cholecystectomy (LoE 1 GoR B)
3.2	In complicated acute cholecystitis, the antimicrobial regimens depend on presumed pathogens involved and risk factors for major resistance patterns (LoE 3 GoR B)
3.3	The results of microbiological analysis are helpful in designing targeted therapeutic strategies for individual patients to customize antibiotic treatment and ensure adequate antimicrobial coverage in patients with complicated cholecystitis and at high risk for antimicrobial resistance (LoE 3 GoR C)
Patient selection for surgery: Risk stratification	
4.1	Patient's age above 80 in ACC is a risk factor for worse clinical behavior, morbidity, and mortality (LoE 3 GoR B)
4.2	The coexistence of diabetes mellitus does not contraindicate urgent surgery but must be reconsidered as a part of the overall patient comorbidity (LoE 3 GoR C)
4.3	Currently, there is no evidence of any scores in identifying patient's risk in surgery for ACC. ASA, POSSUM, and APACHE II are correlated to surgical risk in patients with gallbladder perforation, higher accuracy being for APACHE II. However, APACHE II is built to predict morbidity and mortality in the patients admitted to ICU; its use as a preoperative score should be considered as an extension usage from the original concept. (LoE 4 GoR C)
Timing for surgery	
5.1	Early laparoscopic cholecystectomy is preferable to delayed laparoscopic cholecystectomy in patients with ACC as long as it is completed within 10 days of onset of symptoms (LoE 1 GoR A)

(continued)

Table 4.1 (continued)

5.2	Laparoscopic cholecystectomy should not be offered for patients beyond 10 days from the onset of symptoms unless symptoms suggestive of worsening peritonitis or sepsis warrant an emergency surgical intervention. In people with more than 10 days of symptoms, delaying cholecystectomy for 45 days is better than immediate surgery (LoE 2 GoR B)
5.3	Early laparoscopic cholecystectomy should be performed as soon as possible but can be performed up to 10 days of onset of symptoms. (level 1 evidence; grade A recommendation). However, it should be noted that earlier surgery is associated with shorter hospital stay and fewer complications (LoE 2 GoR B)
Type of surgery	
6.1	In ACC, a laparoscopic approach should initially be attempted except in case of absolute anaesthesiology contraindications or septic shock (LoE 2 GoR B)
6.2	Laparoscopic cholecystectomy for ACC is safe, feasible, with a low complication rate, and associated with shortened hospital stay (LoE 1 GoR A)
6.3	Among high-risk patients, in those with child A and B cirrhosis, advanced age > 80, or pregnant women, laparoscopic cholecystectomy for ACC is feasible and safe (LoE 3 GoR C)
6.4	Laparoscopic or open subtotal cholecystectomy is a valid option for advanced inflammation, gangrenous gallbladder, or any setting of the "difficult gallbladder" where anatomy is difficult to recognize and main bile duct injuries are more likely (LoE 2 GoR A)
6.5	In case of local severe inflammation, adhesions, bleeding in Calot's triangle, or suspected bile duct injury, conversion to open surgery should be strongly considered. (LoE 3 GoR B)
Associated common bile duct stones	
7.1	Elevation of liver biochemical enzymes and/or bilirubin levels is not sufficient to identify ACC patients with choledocholithiasis, and further diagnostic tests are needed (LoE 2 GoR B)
7.2	At AUS, the visualization of CBDS is a very strong predictor of choledocholithiasis. (LoE 5 GoR D). Indirect signs of stone presence such as increased diameter of common bile duct are not sufficient to identify ACC patients with choledocholithiasis, and further diagnostic tests are needed. (LoE 1 GoR A)
7.3	Liver biochemical tests, including ALT, AST bilirubin, ALP, gamma glutamyl transferase (GGT), AUS should be performed in all patients with ACC to assess the risk for CBS (LoE 2 GoR B)
7.4	Common bile duct stone risk should be stratified according to the proposed classification, modified from the American Society of Gastrointestinal Endoscopy and the Society of American Gastrointestinal Endoscopic Surgeon Guidelines (LoE 5 GoR D)
7.5	Patients with moderate risk for choledocholithiasis should undergo preoperative MRCP, EUS, intraoperative cholangiography, or laparoscopic ultrasound depending on the local expertise and availability. (LoE 1 GoR A)
7.6	Patients with high risk for choledocholithiasis should undergo preoperative ERCP, intraoperative cholangiography, laparoscopic ultrasound, depending on the local expertise and the availability of the technique. (LoE 1 GoR A)
7.7	CBDS could be removed preoperatively, intraoperatively, or postoperatively according to the local expertise and the availability of the technique (LoE 1 GoR A)
Alternative treatments for high-risk patients	
8.1	Gallbladder drainage, together with antibiotics, converts a septic cholecystitis into a nonseptic condition; however, the level of evidence is poor (LoE 4, GoR C)
8.2	Among standardized gallbladder drainage techniques percutaneous transhepatic gallbladder drainage (PTGBD) is generally recognized as the preferred technique due to the ease and the reduced costs (LoE 4, GoR C)
8.3	Percutaneous cholecystostomy could be considered as a possible alternative to surgery after the failure of conservative treatment in a small subset of patients unfit for emergency surgery due to their severe comorbidities (LoE 2 GoR B)
8.4	Delayed laparoscopic cholecystectomy could be offered to patients after reduction of operative and anesthesiology-related risks to reduce further hospitalization (LoE 5 GoR D)

Table 4.2 2017 WSES/SICG Elderly Guidelines, STATEMENTS

Diagnosis	
1.1	There is no single investigation with sufficient diagnostic power to establish or exclude acute cholecystitis without further testing even in elderly people (LoE 2 GoR B). Combination of symptoms, signs, and laboratory tests results may have better diagnostic accuracy in confirming the diagnosis of ACC (LoE 4 GoR D)
1.2	Abdominal ultrasound is the preferred initial imaging technique for elderly patients who are clinically suspected of having acute cholecystitis, in terms of lower costs, better availability, lack of invasiveness, and good accuracy for stones (LoE 3 GoR C)
1.3	Even in elderly patients, evidence on the diagnostic accuracy of CT are scarce and remain elusive while diagnostic accuracy of MRI might be comparable to that of abdominal ultrasound, but no sufficient data are provided to support this hypothesis. HIDA scan has the highest sensitivity and specificity for acute cholecystitis than other imaging modalities although its scarce availability, long time of execution, and exposure to ionizing radiations limit its use (LoE 3 GoR C)
1.4	Even in elderly patients, combining clinical, laboratory, and imaging investigations should be recommended, although the best combination is not yet known (LoE 5 GoR D)
1.5	No high-quality studies on specific diagnostic findings of acute cholecystitis in the elderly have been found; therefore, the stated recommendations of the WSES guidelines previously reported remain unchanged (LoE 4 GoR D)
Surgical risk assessment and treatment	
2.1	Old age (>65 years), by itself, does not represent a contraindication to cholecystectomy for ACC (LoE 3 GoR B)
2.2	Cholecystectomy is the preferred treatment for ACC even in elderly patients (LoE 3 GoR C)
2.3	The evaluation of the risk for elderly patient with ACC should include: 1. Mortality rate for conservative and surgical therapeutic options 2. Rate of gallstone-related disease relapse and the time to relapse 3. Age-related life expectancy 4. Consider patient frailty evaluation by the use of frailty scores 5. Consider estimation of specific risk (patient/type of surgery) by the use of surgical clinical scores (LoE 3 GoR C)
Timing and surgical technique	
3.1	In elderly patients with acute cholecystitis, laparoscopic approach should always be attempted at first except in the case of absolute anesthetic contraindications and septic shock (LoE 2 GoR B)
3.2	In elderly patients, laparoscopic cholecystectomy for acute cholecystitis is safe, feasible, with a low complication rate, and associated with shortened hospital stay (LoE 2 GoR B)
3.3	In elderly patients, laparoscopic or open subtotal cholecystectomy is a valid option for advanced inflammation, gangrenous gallbladder, and "difficult gallbladder" where anatomy is difficult to be recognized, and main bile duct injuries are highly probable (LoE 3 GoR C)
3.4	In elderly patients, conversion to open surgery may be predicted by fever, leucocytosis, elevated serum bilirubin, and extensive upper abdominal surgery. In case of local severe inflammation, adhesions, bleeding in the Calot's triangle, and suspect bile duct injury, conversion to open surgery should be considered (LoE 3 GoR C)
3.5	Even in elderly patients, early laparoscopic cholecystectomy should be performed as soon as possible but can be performed up to 10 days of onset of symptoms. However, it should be noted that earlier surgery is associated with shorter hospital stay and fewer complications (LoE 2 GoR B)
Alternative treatments	
4.1	Percutaneous cholecystostomy can be considered in the treatment of ACC patients (older than 65, with ASA III/IV, performance status 3 to 4, or septic shock) who are deemed unfit for surgery (LoE 2 GoR B)
4.2	If medical therapy failed, percutaneous cholecystostomy should be considered as a bridge to cholecystectomy in acutely ill (high-risk) elderly patients deemed unfit for surgery, in order to convert them in a moderate-risk patient, more suitable for surgery (LoE 3 GoR C)
4.3	As in the general population, even in elderly patients, percutaneous transhepatic cholecystostomy is the preferred method to perform percutaneous cholecystostomy (LoE 4 GoR D)

(continued)

Table 4.2 (continued)

4.4	As in the general population, even in elderly patients, percutaneous cholecystostomy catheter should be removed between 4 and 6 weeks after placement, if a cholangiogram performed 2–3 weeks after percutaneous cholecystostomy demonstrated biliary tree patency (LoE 3 GoR C)
Associated common bile duct stones	
5.1	Even in elderly patients, elevation of liver biochemical enzymes and/or bilirubin levels is not sufficient to identify ACC patients with choledocholithiasis, and further diagnostic tests are needed. (LoE 3 GoR C)
5.2	Even in elderly patients, the visualization of common bile duct stones on abdominal ultrasound is a very strong predictor of choledocholithiasis (LoE 5 GoR D). Even in elderly patients, indirect signs of stone presence such as increased diameter of common bile duct are not sufficient to identify ACC patients with choledocholithiasis, and further diagnostic tests are needed. (LoE 2 GoR B)
5.3	Liver biochemical tests, including ALT, AST, bilirubin, ALP, GGT, and abdominal ultrasound should be performed in all patients with ACC to assess the risk for common bile duct stones. (LoE 3 GoR C). Even in elderly patients, common bile duct stone risk should be stratified according to the proposed classification, modified from the American Society of Gastrointestinal Endoscopy and the Society of American Gastrointestinal Endoscopic Surgeon Guidelines (LoE 5 GoR D)
5.4	Even in elderly patients with moderate risk for choledocholithiasis preoperative magnetic resonance cholangiopancreatography (MRCP), endoscopic US, intraoperative cholangiography, or laparoscopic ultrasound should be performed depending on the local expertise and availability (LoE 2 GoR B)
5.5	Elderly patients with high risk for choledocholithiasis should undergo preoperative ERCP, intraoperative cholangiography, or laparoscopic ultrasound, depending on the local expertise and the availability of the technique (LoE 2 GoR B)
5.6	Even in elderly patients, common bile duct stones could be removed preoperatively, intraoperatively, or postoperatively according to the local expertise and the availability of the technique (LoE 2 GoR B)
Antibiotic therapy	
6.1	Elderly patients with uncomplicated cholecystitis can be treated without postoperative antibiotics when the focus of infection is controlled by cholecystectomy (LoE 2 GoR C)
6.2	In elderly patients with complicated acute cholecystitis, antibiotic regimens with broad spectrum are recommended as adequate empiric therapy significantly affects outcomes in critical elderly patients. The principles of empiric antibiotic therapy should be guided by most frequently isolated bacteria taking into consideration antibiotic resistance and the clinical condition of the patient (LoE 2 GoR B)
6.3	The results of microbiological analysis are helpful in designing targeted therapeutic strategies for individual patients with healthcare infections to customize antibiotic treatments and ensure adequate antimicrobial coverage (LoE 5 GoR D)

in addition to those on AUS. In a head-to-head comparison, the diagnostic accuracy of MRI was comparable with that of AUS. Data on the diagnostic accuracy of CT is limited, and CT exposes patients to ionizing radiation. CT is therefore usually indicated when sonography is nondiagnostic or patients have confusing signs and symptoms [9]. Although radiological investigation by HIDA may be required to reach diagnostic certainty, its utility is limited by its lack of availability, long examination duration, and inability to image the biliary tract. Furthermore, since symptomatic gallbladder stones are, in any case, an indication for laparoscopic cholecystectomy, the AUS diagnostic uncertainty may not be relevant in healthy patients and invasive radiological investigation, such as HIDA, should therefore be applied only in high-risk patients. To further complicate the diagnostic process, age-related changes involving pain perception [10, 11], biliary tract physiology [12], and stress response to tissue injury [13, 14] may modify the clinical picture of ACC occurring in an elderly patient. A full clinical examination should be performed and recorded and this should be combined with laboratory tests for inflammation and AUS. When there are uncertain findings on AUS imaging with clinical suspicion of ACC, there is no definitive evidence in favor of using a high cost although highly accurate investigation (HIDA or MRI) or of treating the patient empirically as if he or she had ACC. It is important to keep in mind that aging is a risk factor for gangrenous cholecystitis and that a higher rate of severe cholecystitis has been reported in the elderly patient group [15].

4.3.2 Surgical Therapy and Risk Stratification

ACC is a heterogeneous condition and the severity of inflammation and its life-threatening potential are strongly determined by the overall status of the patient. Regarding ACC treatment, different gallstone-removal techniques besides cholecystectomy have not been tested in the acute setting and there is a paucity of evidence about this technique. We found one prospective randomized study by Schmidt et al. (2016) comparing observation to surgery after ACC [16]. The sample size was 33 patients assigned to observation versus 31 assigned to surgery. After an average follow-up period of 14 years, 33% (11 patients) in the observation group experienced relapse of gallstone disease and all required surgery. On the basis of Schmidt et al.'s findings and a RCT on symptomatic but uncomplicated gallstone disease [17], Brazzelli et al. produced a clinical and cost-effectiveness analysis, comparing surgery to observation, using a UK-based economic model [18, 19]. They found that patients randomized to observation experienced a higher rate of gallstone-related complications (14% versus 2%) when compared to surgical group. These complications occurred more frequently in patients with ACC than in those with biliary colic only. Nowadays, laparoscopy is the gold standard for ACC surgery. Laparoscopic approach is safer than open approach for ACC: the morbidity and mortality, in the case of laparoscopic procedure are 10% and 1%, respectively, compared to 25% and 2% for open procedure [20]. Coccolini and colleagues in 2015 published a systematic review and meta-analysis with the focus of comparing open and laparoscopic cholecystectomy for ACC, and the morbidity and mortality analysis favors the use of the laparoscopic procedure [21]. Laparoscopic or open subtotal cholecystectomy is a valid option for advanced inflammation, gangrenous gallbladder, or any setting of a "difficult gallbladder" where the anatomy is difficult to recognize and main bile duct injuries are more likely. A recent systematic review with meta-analysis by Elshaer et al. [22] reported that subtotal cholecystectomy was performed using the laparoscopic (72.9%), open (19%), and laparoscopic converted to open (8%) techniques. They concluded that subtotal cholecystectomy is an important tool in the difficult cholecystectomy and achieves morbidity rates comparable to those reported for total cholecystectomy in simple cases. An alternative surgical strategy is the fundus-first approach, although the risk of lesions in this approach must be kept in mind [23, 24]. According to Giger et al., extensive inflammation, adhesions, and consequent increased exudate can make laparoscopic dissection of Calot's triangle and recognition of the biliary anatomy hazardous and difficult. Therefore, conversion to open surgery is strongly recommended to ensure patient safety in such difficult conditions [25]. In conclusion, gangrenous gallbladder, obscure anatomy, bleeding, bile duct injuries, adhesions, and previous upper abdominal surgery represent clinical conditions for which conversion to open cholecystectomy should be strongly considered. However, the recommendations regarding surgical treatment of ACC are limited to patients who may be good candidates for urgent surgery. Unfortunately, gray areas remain in cases of patients unfit for urgent surgery or for laparoscopic surgery due to general comorbid conditions. Furthermore, older patients require further considerations when suggesting surgery for ACC. However, a large retrospective cohort study including 29,918 patients with ACC demonstrated that the mortality rate of elderly patients (mean age 77.7 years) is significantly lower in those undergoing surgery during the same admission compared to those discharged home without receiving surgery during the initial admission [20]. The scientific evidence coming from the literature allows us to consider cholecystectomy during the initial admission as the preferred treatment for all patients with ACC, including the elderly. To achieve this, elderly patients require a more detailed and rapid evaluation compared to the general population to take into account the higher susceptibility of elderly patients. A systematic review of retrospective studies was performed in 2017 and focused its attention on the safety of early cholecystectomy in 592 elderly patients (mean age 81 years) with a high surgical risk (American Society of Anesthesiologist (ASA) status ≥3 in 44% of the included patients); the authors concluded that early cholecystectomy is feasible because the overall mortality was 3% and the morbidity was 23%, which was similar to that in the younger population (1% and 15%, respectively) [26]. In the setting of ACC and old age, a single "rule" for all patients cannot be applied, and research is necessary to stratify the surgical risk. ASA, P-POSSUM, and APACHE II showed the best correlation with surgical risk, but there is no validated way of stratifying risk in elderly patients, even though age is one of the factors considered for calculation of P-POSSUM and APACHE II scores. Frailty scoring systems may help in stratifying the risk.

4.3.3 Timing for Surgery

Several RCTs have investigated early laparoscopic cholecystectomy versus delayed laparoscopic cholecystectomy. Different trials have used varying definitions for early and delayed laparoscopic cholecystectomies. In general, early laparoscopic cholecystectomy has been defined either as being performed in patients with acute cholecystitis with symptoms for less than 72 h or as patients with acute cholecystitis with symptoms for less than 7 days but within 4–6 days of diagnosis, which roughly translates to 10 days from onset of symptoms. Although the historical rule of 72 h to perform cholecystectomy for ACC is no longer mandatory, surgery performed as soon as possible is associated with a better outcome [27–30]. Moreover, the expected reduction in reserve capacity in older patients should prompt rapid treatment if possible. One trial compared early laparoscopic cholecystectomy versus delayed laparoscopic cholecystectomy performed between 7 days and 45 days after initial diagnosis [28]. This trial demonstrated that the morbidity was higher, and the length of hospital stay was 5 days longer in the delayed laparoscopic cholecystectomy group compared to the early laparoscopic cholecystectomy group. Evidence from a large database review including approximately 95,000 patients with ACC demonstrated that patients who had surgery within 2 days of admission had fewer complications than those who underwent surgery between 2 and 5 days after admission, and those who had surgery between 6 days and 10 days of presentation. There was no significant difference in the groups between conversion to open surgery [30].

4.3.4 Antibiotic Therapy

Alongside surgical treatment, therapy with appropriate antibiotic agents is an important component in the management of patients with ACC [31, 32]. Antibiotics are always recommended in complicated cholecystitis and in delayed management of uncomplicated cholecystitis. In a recently published prospective RCT [33], a total of 414 patients treated at 17 French medical centers for grade I or II ACC and who received 2 g of amoxicillin plus clavulanic acid three times a day and once at the time of surgery were randomized after surgery. Patients were randomized to either no antibiotics after surgery or continuation with the preoperative antibiotic regimen three times daily for 5 days. Among patients with mild ACC who received preoperative and intraoperative antibiotics, lack of postoperative treatment with amoxicillin plus clavulanic acid did not result in a greater incidence of postoperative infections. The principles of empiric antibiotic treatment should be defined according to the most frequently isolated microbes, always taking into consideration the local trend of antibiotic resistance. Organisms most often isolated in biliary infections are gram-negative aerobes, *Escherichia coli*, and Klebsiella pneumonia and anaerobes, especially *Bacteroides fragilis* [34, 35]. Healthcare-related infections are commonly caused by more resistant strains. For these infections, broader spectrum regimens are recommended because adequate empiric therapy appears to be a crucial factor affecting postoperative complications and mortality rates, especially in critically ill patients [36]. The efficacy of antibiotics in the treatment of biliary infections depends on the concentration of the antibiotic in the biliary tract, which may be limited in patients with obstructed bile ducts [37]. The choice of antibiotic regimen may be problematic in the management of critically ill patients with ACC. In patients with severe sepsis or septic shock of abdominal origin, early, appropriate empirical antibiotic therapy has a significant impact on outcomes [38]. Recent international guidelines for the management of severe sepsis and septic shock (Surviving Sepsis Campaign) recommend intravenous antibiotics within the first hour after severe sepsis and septic shock are recognized, use of broad-spectrum agents with good penetration into the presumed site of infection, and reassessment of the antimicrobial regimen daily to optimize efficacy, prevent resistance, avoid toxicity, and minimize costs [39]. Identifying the causative organism(s) is an essential step in the management of ACC, especially in patients with infections at high risk for antibiotic resistance such as healthcare-associated infections. Management of antibiotics in the elderly patient is often a major challenge. Advancing age is accompanied by changes in the pharmacokinetics and pharmacodynamics of antibiotics that often can be exacerbated by renal effects of coexisting diseases. Moreover, elderly patients in institutions, such as nursing homes or geriatric hospitals, pose a particular challenge. Frailty combined with suboptimal hygiene (e.g., often the case in patients with dementia) can promote rapid dissemination of multidrug-resistant organisms (MDROs).

4.3.5 Associated Common Bile Duct Stones

Choledocholithiasis, i.e., the presence of common bile duct stones (CBDS), is reported to occur in 10–20% of cholelithiasis cases, with a lower incidence in ACC ranging from 5% to 15% [40–42]. Investigation for CBDS requires time and can delay surgical intervention. Due to the relatively low incidence of CBDS during ACC, the challenge is to identify patients with a high likelihood of CBDS who would benefit from further diagnostic tests and eventual stone removal. Historically, liver function tests have great utility in determining the presence of CBDS. However, the majority of published studies are not in patients with ACC and also include asymptomatic cholelithiasis. In fact, in ACC, liver function tests may be altered due to the acute inflammatory process of the gallbladder and the biliary tree and up to 15–50% of patients with ACC show elevation in liver enzymes without choledocholithiasis. Chang et al. showed that 51% and 41% of ACC patients without choledocholithiasis had elevated ALT and AST, respectively. However, increased bilirubin levels with leukocytosis may predict gangrenous cholecystitis [43]. The diagnostic accuracy increases for cholestasis tests such as serum bilirubin with the duration and the severity of obstruction. Specificity of serum bilirubin level for CBDS was 60% with a cutoff level of 1.7 mg/dL and 75% with a cutoff level of 4 mg/dL [44]. AUS, the preferred imaging technique to diagnose ACC, can simultaneously visualize the gallbladder and common bile duct. Although visualization of CBDS is a very strong predictor of choledocholithiasis, a retrospective analysis by Boys et al. concluded that AUS-identified common bile duct diameter is not sufficient to identify patients at significant risk for CBDS [45]. Several predictive scores of CBDS have been proposed and validated but none are specific for ACC. The implementation of these predictive scores in clinical practice is poor. The American Society of Gastrointestinal Endoscopy and the Society of American of Gastrointestinal Endoscopic Surgeons combined the various published validated clinical scores and proposed a risk stratification of CBDS into three different classes: low risk (<10%), moderate (10 to 50%), and high risk (>50%), based on the presence of predictive factors for having CBDS [46]. The ASGE guidelines seem to be the best available tool for the diagnosis and the management of

CBDS during ACC. However, according to this classification, high-risk patients have a >50% probability of having CBDS; this means that up to 49% of patients that undergo ERCP may have no CBDS. For this reason, we prefer a more cautious approach; only patients with evidence of CBDS on AUS should be considered at high risk of CBDS and should directly undergo diagnostic and therapeutic ERCP. Two preoperative imaging techniques are available for the detection of CBDS, MRCP, and EUS. Although these diagnostic tools could delay ACC treatment, they could also exclude the presence of CBDS with high diagnostic accuracy, thereby avoiding further invasive procedures such ERCP or intraoperative cholangiography and their complications. ERCP has both a diagnostic and therapeutic role in the management of choledocholithiasis but is an invasive procedure with severe potential complications. On the other hand, intraoperative cholangiography significantly increases the length of surgery [47] and requires dedicated staff in the operating room that may not be available, especially in the acute setting. Furthermore, intraoperative evidence of CBDS, either via cholangiography or laparoscopic ultrasound, leads to intraoperative management of common bile duct with additional operating time. A systematic review assessed the difference between the different techniques for CBDS removal (i.e., preoperative ERCP with sphincterotomy, intraoperative ERCP with sphincterotomy, laparoscopic or open common bile duct exploration, or postoperative ERCP with sphincterotomy) and found no differences in terms of morbidity, mortality, and success comparing these methods [48]. For these reasons, CBDS could be removed preoperatively, intraoperatively, or postoperatively according to the local expertise and technique availability.

4.3.6 Alternative Treatments for High-Risk Patients

Cholecystectomy for ACC in the elderly and in high-risk patients has always been considered a high-risk procedure with a reported mortality up to 19% [49]. Gallbladder drainage, also known as percutaneous cholecystostomy (PC), is a potential alternative to cholecystectomy in high-risk patients, but its role is difficult to determine because different definitions are used to identify "high-risk" patients. PC decompresses the infected bile or pus in the gallbladder, removing the infected collection without removing the gallbladder. The removal of the infected material, in addition to antibiotic therapy, can result in reduced inflammation and improvement of the clinical condition. A recently published Dutch trial, the CHOCOLATE trial, compared the results of PC and laparoscopic cholecystectomy in high-risk patients with ACC [50]. The trial was concluded early after a planned interim analysis due to a significantly higher percentage (65% vs. 12%) of major complications in the percutaneous catheter drainage group compared to the laparoscopic cholecystectomy (RR 0.19, 95% CI 0.10-0.37, $p < 0.001$). In the drainage group, 66% of patients required a reintervention compared with 12% in the cholecystectomy group ($p < 0.001$). Recurrent biliary disease occurred more often in the percutaneous drainage group (53% v 5%, $p < 0.001$), and the median length of hospital stay was longer (9 days v 5 days, $p < 0.001$). These results are in favor of early laparoscopic cholecystectomy even for high-risk patients. However, it is important to note that the definition of high-risk patients in this trial included patients with APACHE II score between 7 and 15, while patients with an APACHE II score > 15 were excluded. Furthermore, other exclusion criteria were: symptoms that lasted longer than 7 days at time of first presentation, pregnancy, decompensated liver cirrhosis, admission to the intensive care unit at the time of cholecystitis diagnosis, and mental illness prohibiting informed consent. In this setting, the patients that could really have benefitted from percutaneous drainage are actually excluded from the trial, and the results of the study should be interpreted with the caveat of significant exclusion criteria. A previous Cochrane systematic review by Gurusamy et al. investigated the role of cholecystostomy. Authors included only two randomized trials, both at high risk of bias, concluding that "we are unable to determine the role of percutaneous cholecystostomy in the clinical management of high-risk surgical patients with acute cholecystitis" [51]. Furthermore, De Mestral et al. published a large retrospective epidemiological analysis in 2012 showing that only 40% of patient underwent delayed laparoscopic cholecystectomy after percutaneous drainage, and the 1 year readmission rate for patients who did not undergo delayed laparoscopic cholecystectomy was 49% with an in-hospital mortality of 1% [52]. In light of the above findings, a patient-tailored approach is the best choice, and percutaneous drainage can be considered as a possible alternative to surgery or after the failure of conservative treatment in a small subset of patients unfit for emergency surgery due to severe comorbidities. However, it is important to remember the complications associated with percutaneous drainage.

4.4 Conclusions

Based on the evidence included in these guidelines, it is clear that early laparoscopic cholecystectomy is the best therapeutic approach for ACC and that postoperative antibiotics are not necessary for uncomplicated cholecystitis. The most important takeaway of these guidelines is the superiority of early laparoscopic cholecystectomy for all patients among treatment options for ACC. According to several high-quality studies, subtotal cholecystectomy, along with a low threshold for conversion from complete cholecystectomy to partial or open approach, should be recommended when severe, acute inflammation of the gallbladder is encountered at time of operation. Although the threshold for conversion strongly depends on the experience and skills of the surgeon, we support the development of an intraoperative score to help the surgeon decide whether to complete the operation by partial cholecystectomy and/or by open approach when "the critical view of safety" cannot be reached without adding risk. The recommendations on the surgical treatment of ACC are limited to patients who are good candidates for urgent surgery. Gray areas still remain in cases of patients not fit for urgent surgery or for laparoscopic surgery secondary to general conditions. However, age alone is not a contraindication for surgery. These WSES guidelines define the patient condition in lieu of the cholecystitis severity score as underlined in the TG13. This approach could favor a therapy tailored to the patient's individual condition. Data on criteria for defining a patient as high-risk, besides septic shock, are scarce and of low quality. This is certainly an area for research to improve the management of patients with ACC. The role of cholecystostomy, as a bridging therapy until cholecystectomy or as a definitive treatment in elderly patients, is uncertain. The high incidence of major complications post-percutaneous drainage, as shown by the CHOCOLATE trial, is important to consider when evaluating this intervention as a possible alternative to surgery or after the failure of conservative treatment in the small subset of patients unfit for emergency surgery due to their severe comorbidities.

Moreover, studies providing a high level of evidence on the management of associated common bile duct stones (CBDS) have also been published. AUS is an accurate technique to visualize CBDS, and patients with a high likelihood of CBDS as seen on AUS should have a preoperative ERCP, while patients with a moderate risk should have a noninvasive preoperative investigation. Because the majority of RCTs exclude elderly patients, evidence has to be extrapolated from that in the younger population. This indirectness causes significant uncertainty in developing guidelines for management of acute cholecystitis in the elderly population. Future research on management of acute cholecystitis should include elderly patients whenever ethical and possible. In addition, researchers should present a subgroup analysis of the results in elderly patients, to resolve areas of uncertainty across age groups. The development and validation of a reliable prognostic score in assessing frailty would greatly help in guiding the management on acute calculous cholecystitis.

References

1. Miura F, Takada T, Kawarada Y, Nimura Y, Wada K, Hirota M, Nagino M, Tsuyuguchi T, Mayumi T, Yoshida M, Strasberg SM, Pitt HA, Belghiti J, de Santibanes E, Gadacz TR, Gouma DJ, Fan ST, Chen MF, Padbury RT, Bornman PC, Kim SW, Liau KH, Belli G, Dervenis C. Flowcharts for the diagnosis and treatment of acute cholangitis and cholecystitis: Tokyo Guidelines. J Hepatobiliary Pancreat Surg. 2007;14:27–34.
2. Yokoe M, Takada T, Strasberg SM, Solomkin JS, Mayumi T, Gomi H, Pitt HA, Garden OJ, Kiriyama S, Hata J, Gabata T, Yoshida M, Miura F, Okamoto K, Tsuyuguchi T, Itoi T, Yamashita Y, Dervenis C, Chan AC, Lau WY, Supe AN, Belli G, Hilvano SC, Liau KH, Kim MH, Kim SW, Ker CG, Tokyo Guidelines Revision C. TG13 diagnostic criteria and severity grading of acute cholecystitis (with videos). J Hepatobiliary Pancreat Sci. 2013;20:35–46.
3. Lee SW, Yang SS, Chang CS, Yeh HJ. Impact of the Tokyo guidelines on the management of patients with acute calculous cholecystitis. J Gastroenterol Hepatol. 2009;24:1857–61.
4. Campanile FC, Catena F, Coccolini F, Lotti M, Piazzalunga D, Pisano M, Ansaloni L. The need for new "patient-related" guidelines for the treatment of acute cholecystitis. World J Emerg Surg. 2011;6:44.
5. Ansaloni L, Pisano M, Coccolini F, Peitzmann AB, Fingerhut A, Catena F, Agresta F, Allegri A, Bailey I, Balogh ZJ, Bendinelli C, Biffl W, Bonavina L, Borzellino G, Brunetti F, Burlew CC, Camapanelli G, Campanile FC, Ceresoli M, Chiara O, Civil I, Coimbra R, De Moya M, Di Saverio S, Fraga GP, Gupta S, Kashuk J, Kelly MD, Koka V, Jeekel H, Latifi R, Leppaniemi A, Maier RV, Marzi I, Moore F, Piazzalunga D, Sakakushev B, Sartelli M, Scalea T, Stahel PF, Taviloglu K, Tugnoli G, Uraneus S, Velmahos GC, Wani I, Weber DG, Viale P, Sugrue M, Ivatury R, Kluger Y, Gurusamy KS, Moore EE. 2016 WSES guidelines on acute calculous cholecystitis. World J Emerg Surg. 2016;11:25.
6. Festi D, Dormi A, Capodicasa S, Staniscia T, Attili AF, Loria P, Pazzi P, Mazzella G, Sama C, Roda E, Colecchia A. Incidence of gallstone disease in Italy: results from a multicenter, population-based Italian study (the MICOL project). World J Gastroenterol. 2008;14:5282–9.
7. Pisano M, Ceresoli M, Cimbanassi S, Gurusamy K, Coccolini F, Borzellino G, Costa G, Allievi N, Amato B, Boerma D, Calcagno P, Campanati L, Campanile FC, Casati A, Chiara O, Crucitti A, di Saverio S, Filauro M, Gabrielli F, Guttadauro A, Kluger Y, Magnone S, Merli C, Poiasina E, Puzziello A, Sartelli M, Catena F, Ansaloni L. 2017 WSES and SICG guidelines on acute calcolous cholecystitis in elderly population. World J Emerg Surg. 2019;14:10.
8. Kiewiet JJ, Leeuwenburgh MM, Bipat S, Bossuyt PM, Stoker J, Boermeester MA. A systematic review and meta-analysis of diagnostic performance of imaging in acute cholecystitis. Radiology. 2012;264:708–20.
9. Marincek B. Nontraumatic abdominal emergencies: acute abdominal pain: diagnostic strategies. Eur Radiol. 2002;12:2136–50.
10. Sanson TG, O'Keefe KP. Evaluation of abdominal pain in the elderly. Emerg Med Clin North Am. 1996;14:615–27.
11. Ragsdale L, Southerland L. Acute abdominal pain in the older adult. Emerg Med Clin North Am. 2011;29:429–48, x
12. Ross SO, Forsmark CE. Pancreatic and biliary disorders in the elderly. Gastroenterol Clin N Am. 2001;30:531–45.
13. Lavretsky H, Newhouse PA. Stress, inflammation, and aging. Am J Geriatr Psychiatry. 2012;20:729–33.
14. Diniz BS, Vieira EM. Stress, inflammation, and aging: an association beyond chance. Am J Geriatr Psychiatry. 2018;26:964–5.
15. Ambe PC, Weber SA, Christ H, Wassenberg D. Primary cholecystectomy is feasible in elderly patients with acute cholecystitis. Aging Clin Exp Res. 2015;27:921–6.
16. Schmidt M, Sondenaa K, Vetrhus M, Berhane T, Eide GE. Long-term follow-up of a randomized controlled trial of observation versus surgery for acute cholecystitis: non-operative management is an option in some patients. Scand J Gastroenterol. 2011;46:1257–62.
17. Schmidt M, Sondenaa K, Vetrhus M, Berhane T, Eide GE. A randomized controlled study of uncomplicated gallstone disease with a 14-year follow-up showed that operation was the preferred treatment. Dig Surg. 2011;28:270–6.
18. Brazzelli M, Cruickshank M, Kilonzo M, Ahmed I, Stewart F, McNamee P, Elders A, Fraser C, Avenell A, Ramsay C. Clinical effectiveness and cost-effectiveness of cholecystectomy compared with observation/conservative management for preventing recurrent symptoms and complications in adults presenting with uncomplicated symptomatic gallstones or cholecystitis: a systematic review and economic evaluation. Health Technol Assess. 2014;18:1–101, v-vi
19. Brazzelli M, Cruickshank M, Kilonzo M, Ahmed I, Stewart F, McNamee P, Elders A, Fraser C, Avenell A, Ramsay C. Systematic review of the clinical and cost effectiveness of cholecystectomy versus observation/conservative management for uncomplicated symptomatic gallstones or cholecystitis. Surg Endosc. 2015;29:637–47.
20. Riall TS, Zhang D, Townsend CM Jr, Kuo YF, Goodwin JS. Failure to perform cholecystectomy for acute cholecystitis in elderly patients is associated with increased morbidity, mortality, and cost. J Am Coll Surg. 2010;210:668–77, 77-9
21. Coccolini F, Catena F, Pisano M, Gheza F, Fagiuoli S, Di Saverio S, Leandro G, Montori G, Ceresoli M,

Corbella D, Sartelli M, Sugrue M, Ansaloni L. Open versus laparoscopic cholecystectomy in acute cholecystitis. Systematic review and meta-analysis. Int J Surg. 2015;18:196–204.
22. Elshaer M, Gravante G, Thomas K, Sorge R, Al-Hamali S, Ebdewi H. Subtotal cholecystectomy for "difficult gallbladders": systematic review and meta-analysis. JAMA Surg. 2015;150:159–68.
23. Tuveri M, Calo PG, Medas F, Tuveri A, Nicolosi A. Limits and advantages of fundus-first laparoscopic cholecystectomy: lessons learned. J Laparoendosc Adv Surg Tech A. 2008;18:69–75.
24. Kelly MD. Laparoscopic retrograde (fundus first) cholecystectomy. BMC Surg. 2009;9:19.
25. Giger U, Michel JM, Vonlanthen R, Becker K, Kocher T, Krähenbühl L. Laparoscopic cholecystectomy in acute cholecystitis: indication, technique, risk and outcome. Langenbeck's Arch Surg. 2004;390:373–80.
26. Loozen CS, van Ramshorst B, van Santvoort HC, Boerma D. Early cholecystectomy for acute cholecystitis in the elderly population: a systematic review and meta-analysis. Dig Surg. 2017;34:371–9.
27. Brooks KR, Scarborough JE, Vaslef SN, Shapiro ML. No need to wait: an analysis of the timing of cholecystectomy during admission for acute cholecystitis using the American College of Surgeons National Surgical Quality Improvement Program database. J Trauma Acute Care Surg. 2013;74:167–73; 73-4
28. Gutt CN, Encke J, Koninger J, Harnoss JC, Weigand K, Kipfmuller K, Schunter O, Gotze T, Golling MT, Menges M, Klar E, Feilhauer K, Zoller WG, Ridwelski K, Ackmann S, Baron A, Schon MR, Seitz HK, Daniel D, Stremmel W, Buchler MW. Acute cholecystitis: early versus delayed cholecystectomy, a multicenter randomized trial (ACDC study, NCT00447304). Ann Surg. 2013;258:385–93.
29. Johner A, Raymakers A, Wiseman SM. Cost utility of early versus delayed laparoscopic cholecystectomy for acute cholecystitis. Surg Endosc. 2013;27:256–62.
30. Zafar SN, Obirieze A, Adesibikan B, Cornwell EE 3rd, Fullum TM, Tran DD. Optimal time for early laparoscopic cholecystectomy for acute cholecystitis. JAMA Surg. 2015;150:129–36.
31. Fuks D, Cosse C, Regimbeau JM. Antibiotic therapy in acute calculous cholecystitis. J Visc Surg. 2013;150:3–8.
32. Gomi H, Solomkin JS, Takada T, Strasberg SM, Pitt HA, Yoshida M, Kusachi S, Mayumi T, Miura F, Kiriyama S, Yokoe M, Kimura Y, Higuchi R, Windsor JA, Dervenis C, Liau KH, Kim MH, Tokyo Guideline Revision C. TG13 antimicrobial therapy for acute cholangitis and cholecystitis. J Hepatobiliary Pancreat Sci. 2013;20:60–70.
33. Regimbeau JM, Fuks D, Pautrat K, Mauvais F, Haccart V, Msika S, Mathonnet M, Scotte M, Paquet JC, Vons C, Sielezneff I, Millat B, Chiche L, Dupont H, Duhaut P, Cosse C, Diouf M, Pocard M, FRENCH Study Group. Effect of postoperative antibiotic administration on postoperative infection following cholecystectomy for acute calculous cholecystitis: a randomized clinical trial. JAMA. 2014;312:145–54.
34. Sartelli M, Catena F, Ansaloni L, Leppäniemi A, Taviloglu K, van Goor H, Viale P, Lazzareschi DV, de Werra C, Marrelli D, Colizza S, Scibé R, Alis H, Torer N, Navarro S, Catani M, Kauhanen S, Augustin G, Sakakushev B, Massalou D, Pletinckx P, Kenig J, Di Saverio S, Guercioni G, Rausei S, Laine S, Major P, Skrovina M, Angst E, Pittet O, Gerych I, Tepp J, Weiss G, Vasquez G, Vladov N, Tranà C, Vettoretto N, Delibegovic S, Dziki A, Giraudo G, Pereira J, Poiasina E, Tzerbinis H, Hutan M, Vereczkei A, Krasniqi A, Seretis C, Diaz-Nieto R, Mesina C, Rems M, Campanile FC, Agresta F, Coletta P, Uotila-Nieminen M, Dente M, Bouliaris K, Lasithiotakis K, Khokha V, Zivanović D, Smirnov D, Marinis A, Negoi I, Ney L, Bini R, Leon M, Aloia S, Huchon C, Moldovanu R, de Melo RB, Giakoustidis D, Ioannidis O, Cucchi M, Pintar T, Jovine E. Complicated intra-abdominal infections in Europe: preliminary data from the first three months of the CIAO study. World J Emerg Surg. 2012;7:15.
35. Sartelli M, Catena F, Ansaloni L, Coccolini F, Corbella D, Moore EE, Malangoni M, Velmahos G, Coimbra R, Koike K, Leppaniemi A, Biffl W, Balogh Z, Bendinelli C, Gupta S, Kluger Y, Agresta F, Di Saverio S, Tugnoli G, Jovine E, Ordonez CA, Whelan JF, Fraga GP, Gomes CA, Pereira GA, Yuan KC, Bala M, Peev MP, Ben-Ishay O, Cui Y, Marwah S, Zachariah S, Wani I, Rangarajan M, Sakakushev B, Kong V, Ahmed A, Abbas A, Gonsaga RA, Guercioni G, Vettoretto N, Poiasina E, Diaz-Nieto R, Massalou D, Skrovina M, Gerych I, Augustin G, Kenig J, Khokha V, Trana C, Kok KY, Mefire AC, Lee JG, Hong SK, Lohse HA, Ghnnam W, Verni A, Lohsiriwat V, Siribumrungwong B, El Zalabany T, Tavares A, Baiocchi G, Das K, Jarry J, Zida M, Sato N, Murata K, Shoko T, Irahara T, Hamedelneel AO, Naidoo N, Adesunkanmi AR, Kobe Y, Ishii W, Oka K, Izawa Y, Hamid H, Khan I, Attri A, Sharma R, Sanjuan J, Badiel M, Barnabe R. Complicated intra-abdominal infections worldwide: the definitive data of the CIAOW study. World J Emerg Surg. 2014;9:37.
36. Solomkin JS, Mazuski JE, Bradley JS, Rodvold KA, Goldstein EJ, Baron EJ, O'Neill PJ, Chow AW, Dellinger EP, Eachempati SR, Gorbach S, Hilfiker M, May AK, Nathens AB, Sawyer RG, Bartlett JG. Diagnosis and management of complicated intra-abdominal infection in adults and children: guidelines by the surgical infection society and the Infectious Diseases Society of America. Clin Infect Dis. 2010;50:133–64.
37. Dhalluin-Venier V, Bazin C, Massias L, Farah RB, Boytchev I, Fritsch J, Choury AD, Prat F, Buffet C, Furlan V, Pelletier G. Effects of biliary obstruction on the penetration of ciprofloxacin and cefotaxime. Eur J Gastroenterol Hepatol. 2008;20:127–30.
38. Sartelli M, Catena F, Di Saverio S, Ansaloni L, Malangoni M, Moore EE, Moore FA, Ivatury R, Coimbra R, Leppaniemi A, Biffl W, Kluger Y, Fraga

GP, Ordonez CA, Marwah S, Gerych I, Lee JG, Trana C, Coccolini F, Corradetti F, Kirkby-Bott J. Current concept of abdominal sepsis: WSES position paper. World J Emerg Surg. 2014;9:22.
39. Dellinger RP, Levy MM, Rhodes A, Annane D, Gerlach H, Opal SM, Sevransky JE, Sprung CL, Douglas IS, Jaeschke R, Osborn TM, Nunnally ME, Townsend SR, Reinhart K, Kleinpell RM, Angus DC, Deutschman CS, Machado FR, Rubenfeld GD, Webb SA, Beale RJ, Vincent J-L, Moreno R. Surviving sepsis campaign: international Guidelines for Management of Severe Sepsis and Septic Shock: 2012. Crit Care Med. 2013;41:580–637.
40. Ko CW, Lee SP. Epidemiology and natural history of common bile duct stones and prediction of disease. Gastrointest Endosc. 2002;56:S165–9.
41. Peng WK, Sheikh Z, Paterson-Brown S, Nixon SJ. Role of liver function tests in predicting common bile duct stones in acute calculous cholecystitis. Br J Surg. 2005;92:1241–7.
42. Khalfallah M, Dougaz W, Bedoui R, Bouasker I, Chaker Y, Nouira R, Dziri C. Validation of the Lacaine-Huguier predictive score for choledocholithiasis: prospective study of 380 patients. J Visc Surg. 2012;149:e66–72.
43. Chang CW, Chang WH, Lin CC, Chu CH, Wang TE, Shih SC. Acute transient hepatocellular injury in cholelithiasis and cholecystitis without evidence of choledocholithiasis. World J Gastroenterol. 2009;15:3788–92.
44. Barkun AN, Barkun JS, Fried GM, Ghitulescu G, Steinmetz O, Pham C, Meakins JL, Goresky CA. Useful predictors of bile duct stones in patients undergoing laparoscopic cholecystectomy. Ann Surg. 1994;220:32–9.
45. Boys JA, Doorly MG, Zehetner J, Dhanireddy KK, Senagore AJ. Can ultrasound common bile duct diameter predict common bile duct stones in the setting of acute cholecystitis? Am J Surg. 2014;207:432–5; discussion 5
46. ASGE Standards of Practice Committee, Maple JT, Ben-Menachem T, Anderson MA, Appalaneni V, Banerjee S, Cash BD, Fisher L, Harrison ME, Fanelli RD, Fukami N, Ikenberry SO, Jain R, Khan K, Krinsky ML, Strohmeyer L, Dominitz JA. The role of endoscopy in the evaluation of suspected choledocholithiasis. Gastrointest Endosc. 2010;71:1–9.
47. Ford JA, Soop M, Du J, Loveday BP, Rodgers M. Systematic review of intraoperative cholangiography in cholecystectomy. Br J Surg. 2012;99:160–7.
48. Dasari BV, Tan CJ, Gurusamy KS, Martin DJ, Kirk G, McKie L, Diamond T, Taylor MA. Surgical versus endoscopic treatment of bile duct stones. Cochrane Database Syst Rev 2013;(9):CD003327.
49. Winbladh A, Gullstrand P, Svanvik J, Sandstrom P. Systematic review of cholecystostomy as a treatment option in acute cholecystitis. HPB (Oxford). 2009;11:183–93.
50. Loozen CS, van Santvoort HC, van Duijvendijk P, Besselink MG, Gouma DJ, Nieuwenhuijzen GA, Kelder JC, Donkervoort SC, van Geloven AA, Kruyt PM, Roos D, Kortram K, Kornmann VN, Pronk A, van der Peet DL, Crolla RM, van Ramshorst B, Bollen TL, Boerma D. Laparoscopic cholecystectomy versus percutaneous catheter drainage for acute cholecystitis in high risk patients (CHOCOLATE): multicentre randomised clinical trial. BMJ. 2018;363:k3965.
51. Gurusamy KS, Rossi M, Davidson BR. Percutaneous cholecystostomy for high-risk surgical patients with acute calculous cholecystitis. Cochrane Database Syst Rev 2013;(8):CD007088.
52. de Mestral C, Rotstein OD, Laupacis A, Hoch JS, Zagorski B, Nathens AB. A population-based analysis of the clinical course of 10,304 patients with acute cholecystitis, discharged without cholecystectomy. J Trauma Acute Care Surg. 2013;74:26–30; discussion -1

5 Tokyo Guidelines and Their Limits

Kohei Mishima and Go Wakabayashi

5.1 Diagnostic Criteria and Severity Grading of Acute Cholecystitis

The diagnostic criteria and severity grading of acute cholecystitis (AC) were discussed among global experts at the Tokyo Consensus Meeting held in 2006, and the first version of Tokyo Guidelines (TG07) was published in 2007 [1]. TG07 diagnostic criteria was revised in 2013 as Tokyo Guidelines 2013 (TG13) [2] in response to a validation study [3] of TG07. According to a validation survey [4] of TG13, the TG13 diagnostic criteria for acute cholecystitis (Table 5.1) had higher sensitivity and specificity than those of TG07, and continuous use of TG13 criteria was recommended in the updated version of Tokyo Guidelines (TG18) [5]. Regarding the severity grading system, while TG07 defined Grade III (severe) AC as AC with indication for emergent surgery, the revised TG13 described Grade III AC as AC associated with organ system dysfunction, which in some circumstances may require treatment in an intensive care unit [2]. According to a case series study of over 5000 patients, the prognosis for Grade III patients was significantly worse than that for Grades I and II [4]. The TG 13 severity grading of acute cholecystitis (Table 5.2) was recommended for continuous use in the TG18 severity grading of acute cholecystitis as a useful indicator from the perspective of predicting prognosis [5].

Table 5.1 TG18/TG13 diagnostic criteria for acute cholecystitis. From [5], with permission

A. Local signs of inflammation
(1) Murphy's sign, (2) RUQ mass/pain/tenderness
B. Systemic signs of inflammation
(1) Fever, (2) elevated CRP, (3) elevated WBC count
C. Imaging findings characteristic of acute cholecystitis
Suspected diagnosis: one item in A + one item in B
Definite diagnosis: one item in A + one item in B + C

5.2 Flowcharts for the Management of Acute Cholecystitis

5.2.1 Revisions of Flowcharts for the Management

Flowcharts for the management of acute cholecystitis (AC) were presented in TG07 [6] and revised in TG13 [7]. These flowcharts were useful to show recommended treatments according to the severity of AC. However, TG07 and TG13 did not cover issues like physical status, comorbidities, or other risk factors when choosing a treatment pathway according to severity. In

K. Mishima · G. Wakabayashi (✉)
Department of Surgery, Ageo Central General Hospital, Saitama, Japan
e-mail: gowaka@ach.or.jp

© Springer Nature Switzerland AG 2021

I. Di Carlo (ed.), *Difficult Acute Cholecystitis*, https://doi.org/10.1007/978-3-030-62102-5_5

addition, Grade III AC was considered not suitable for straightforward laparoscopic cholecystectomy (LC). In the TG18 guidelines [8], modified flowcharts (Figs. 5.1, 5.2, and 5.3) were proposed based on recent recommendations in the clinical setting and evidence reported after the publication of TG13 [9, 10]. The revision of flowcharts was aimed at improving the percentage of lives saved by allowing clinicians to determine how they can safely treat AC through the use of decision-making criteria even for severe cases.

Table 5.2 TG18/TG13 severity grading for acute cholecystitis. From [5], with permission

Grade III (severe) acute cholecystitis is associated with dysfunction of any one of the following organs/systems:
1. Cardiovascular dysfunction: hypotension requiring treatment with dopamine ≥5 μg/kg per min, or any dose of norepinephrine
2. Neurological dysfunction: decreased level of consciousness
3. Respiratory dysfunction: PaO2/FiO2 ratio < 300
4. Renal dysfunction: oliguria, creatinine >2.0 mg/dl
5. Hepatic dysfunction: PT-INR >1.5
6. Hematological dysfunction: platelet count <100,000/mm^3
Grade II (moderate) acute cholecystitis is associated with any one of the following conditions:
1. Elevated WBC count (>18,000/mm^3)
2. Palpable tender mass in the right upper abdominal quadrant
3. Duration of complaints >72 ha
4. Marked local inflammation (gangrenous cholecystitis, pericholecystic abscess, hepatic abscess, biliary peritonitis, emphysematous cholecystitis)
Grade I (mild) acute cholecystitis does not meet the criteria of Grade III or Grade II acute cholecystitis

5.2.2 The Updated Version of Tokyo Guidelines (TG18)

The selection of treatment strategy for patients at each severity grade was based on risk factors [8]. The risk factors adopted in TG18 were: Charlson comorbidity index (CCI) score [9] and the American Society of Anesthesiologists physical status classification (ASA-PS) score [10]. Early LC to treat AC of moderate and severe grades (Grade II and III) should be performed only at advanced centers where experienced surgeons practice. An advanced center should have both appropriate personnel and facilities to manage the level of patients being managed. Surgeons should have experience in advanced laparoscopic techniques, and intensive care unit should be available. LC can be performed to treat AC if the conditions described above for each Grade are satisfied.

5.2.3 Definition of Early Cholecystectomy

TG07 recommended that surgery for AC be performed soon after hospital admission, whereas TG13 recommended that surgery be performed soon after admission and within 72 h after onset. When managing AC, it is difficult to determine precisely how many hours have passed since disease onset. The meta-analysis of the case study reports [11] found that compared with delayed cholecystectomy, early cholecystectomy for cases within 72 h of patient presentation or symptom onset was associated with lower mortality rates, complication rates, incidence of bile duct injury, and switching to open surgery.

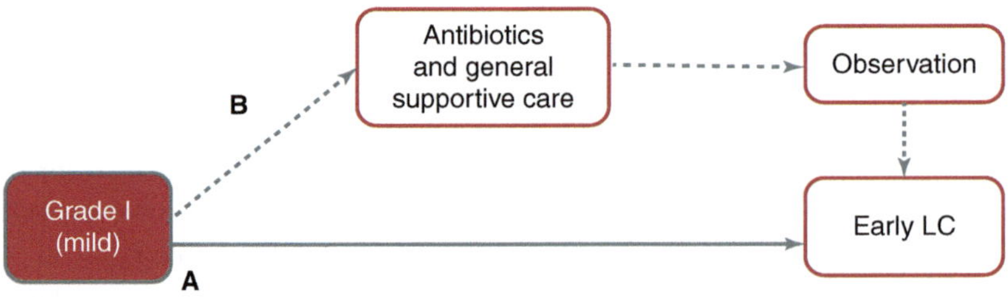

Fig. 5.1 TG18 flowchart for the management of Grade I AC [8]. A, CCI 5 or less and/or ASA class II or less (low risk); B, CCI 6 or greater and/or ASA class III or greater (not low risk)

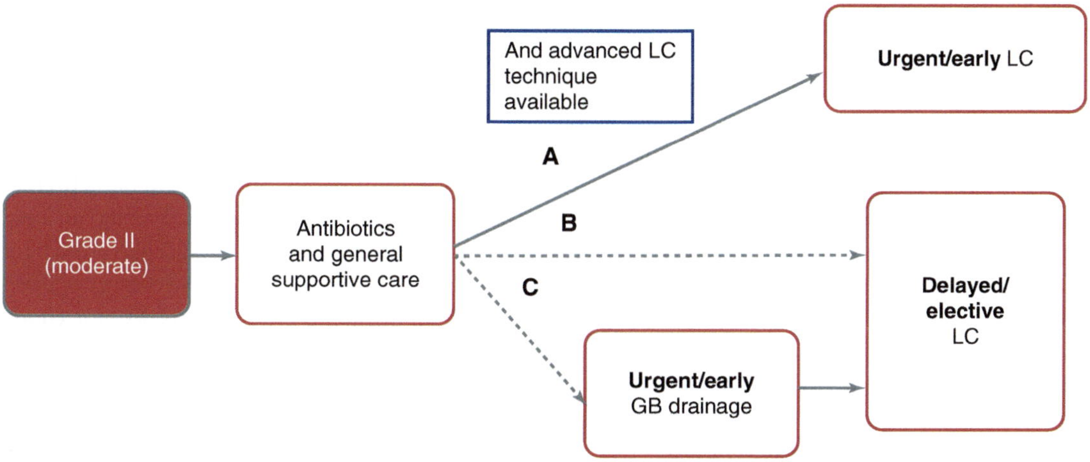

Fig. 5.2 TG18 flowchart for the management of Grade II AC [8]. A, CCI 5 or less and/or ASA-PS class II or less (low risk); B, CCI 6 or greater and/or ASA-PS class III or greater (not low risk); C, antibiotics and general supportive care fail to control inflammation

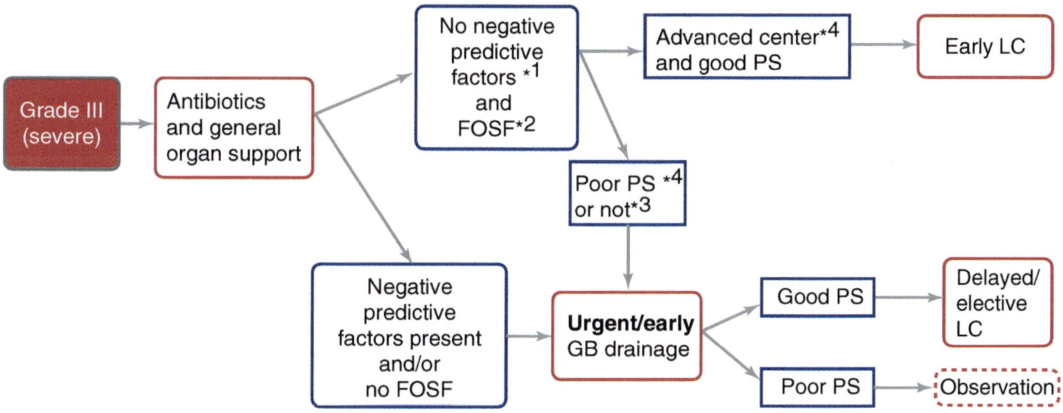

Fig. 5.3 TG18 flowchart for the management of Grade III AC [8]. *¹, negative predictive factors = jaundice (TBil ≥2), neurological dysfunction, respiratory dysfunction; *², FOSF: favorable organ system failure = cardiovascular or renal organ system failure which is rapidly reversible after admission and before early LC in AC; *³, advanced center = intensive care and advanced laparoscopic techniques are available; *⁴, poor PS = CCI (Charlson comorbidity index) 4 or greater, ASA-PS 3 or greater

Similar results were also obtained with early cholecystectomy for cases with time from onset 72 h to 1 week [12, 13]. Therefore, TG 18 recommended early surgery regardless of exactly how much time has passed since onset, if a patient is deemed capable of withstanding surgery for AC.

5.3 Surgical Management of Acute Cholecystitis

Compared to TG13, TG18 recommended that clinicians should consider early LC even for moderate or severe AC [8]. The backbone of this change was the improvement of the operative skill for early

LC and perioperative care. Regarding the improvement in operative skills, standardized procedures of safe LC were proposed [14]. The critical view of safety (CVS) is the most important concept in the safe LC [15]. Several landmarks are helpful for surgeons to safely proceed surgical procedures during the process for the establishment CVS. The baseline of the segment 4 of the liver and the Rouviere's sulcus are good landmarks for the start line of dissecting the serosa of gallbladder for avoiding the bile duct injury of the anterior and posterior branch of Glissonian pedicles [14]. A bailout procedure should be chosen when a CVS cannot be achieved because of the presence of severe fibrosis.

5.4 Management Strategies for Gallbladder Drainage

A standard drainage method for surgically high-risk patients with AC and the latest developed endoscopic gallbladder drainage techniques were described in the updated Tokyo Guidelines 2018 (TG18) [16]. Percutaneous transhepatic gallbladder drainage (PTGBD) should be considered the first alternative to surgical intervention in surgically high-risk patients with AC. Also, endoscopic transpapillary gallbladder drainage or endoscopic ultrasound-guided gallbladder drainage can be considered in high-volume institutes by skilled endoscopists.

5.5 The Limits of TG18

5.5.1 Introduction

Tokyo Guidelines flowcharts allow clinicians to understand treatment flow at a glance and have proven useful standardization of the management of AC [8]. There have been significant changes in clinical management, including advances in surgical techniques [14] and equipment and progress in multidisciplinary treatment [16]. However, there are still issues warranting resolution.

5.5.2 Is Early LC Feasible for Patients with Grade III AC?

The severity grading of TG18/13 [5] is regarded as a useful classification system to predict the mortality rate of AC [4]. TG18 flowcharts [8] recommended that early LC or GB drainage following initial systemic treatment be performed for patients with Grade III AC. However, it is difficult for clinicians to choose early LC for Grade III AC according to TG18 flowchart, since the flowchart did not include elements of surgical difficulty and accompanying cholangitis. Although bailout procedures can be performed in difficult cases [14], conversion from LC to open surgery and postoperative complications are significantly more likely for patients at higher severity grades [17, 18]. A set of severity grading criteria including surgical difficulty is needed to be produced in the future.

5.5.3 How to Manage Elderly Patients with AC?

The management of elderly patients with AC is still a complex challenge due to the balance of benefits from LC versus the increased risk of perioperative morbidity and mortality [13]. In TG18 flowcharts [8], ASA-PS and age-adjusted CCI were adopted to evaluate physical status of patients, and age-adjusted CCI $\geq$6 and ASA-PS $\geq$3 were proposed as surgical risk factors based on the result of a cohort study [9]. Most elderly patients are classified into high-risk patients in this criteria. On the other hand, one study reported no deaths after cholecystectomy for patients with ASA-PS $\geq$3 at advanced centers [19]. In the era of aging society, AC in elderly patients is becoming an increasingly frequent problem. More case series data is needed to be gathered for future analysis to compare the clinical outcomes of early LC in high-risk elderly patients and those of conservative therapy with or without PTGBD.

5.5.4 What Determines the Advanced LC Technique?

In the 1990s, AC is regarded as contraindicated for LC according to SAGES guidelines [20]. But as times have changed, advances in optical and surgical devices and improvements in surgical techniques have led to the expansion of indications for LC [14]. As LC for AC has been more widely performed, vasculo-biliary injury is known to occur in a certain population of cases [21]. Therefore, TG18 flowcharts [8] recommended that early LC for AC be performed by surgeons with advanced techniques at advanced centers. In addition, the chapter of surgical management of AC was added to describe safe steps in LC for AC [14]. However, clinical evidence is scarce on advanced techniques of LC at the moment and warrants further investigation.

5.5.5 Summary

Based on studies that have found the lifespan of guidelines to be around 5 years [22], the Tokyo Guidelines Revision Committee revised the guidelines in 2013 and 2018. TG18 should be validated from abovementioned viewpoints during the next several years and be revised according to newly published clinical evidence.

References

1. Hirota M, Takada T, Kawarada Y, Nimura Y, Miura F, Hirata K, et al. Diagnostic criteria and severity assessment of acute cholecystitis: Tokyo guidelines. J Hepatobiliary Pancreat Surg. 2007;14:78–82.
2. Yokoe M, Takada T, Strasberg SM, Solomkin JS, Mayumi T, Gomi H, et al. TG13 diagnostic criteria and severity grading of acute cholecystitis (with videos). J Hepatobiliary Pancreat Sci. 2013;20:35–46.
3. Yokoe M, Takada T, Mayumi T, Yoshida M, Hasegawa H, Norimizu S, et al. Accuracy of the Tokyo guidelines for the diagnosis of acute cholangitis and cholecystitis taking into consideration the clinical practice pattern in Japan. J Hepatobiliary Pancreat Sci. 2011;18:250–7.
4. Yokoe M, Takada T, Hwang TL, Endo I, Akazawa K, Miura F, et al. Validation of TG13 severity grading in acute cholecystitis: Japan-Taiwan collaborative study for acute cholecystitis. J Hepatobiliary Pancreat Sci. 2017;24:338–45.
5. Yokoe M, Takada T, Strasberg SM, Solomkin JS, Mayumi T, Gomi H, et al. Tokyo guidelines 2018: diagnostic criteria and severity grading of acute cholecystitis (with videos). J Hepatobiliary Pancreat Sci. 2018;25:41–54.
6. Miura F, Takada T, Kawarada Y, Nimura Y, Wada K, Hirota M, et al. Flowcharts for the diagnosis and treatment of acute cholangitis and cholecystitis: Tokyo guidelines. J Hepatobiliary Pancreat Surg. 2007;14:27–34.
7. Miura F, Takada T, Strasberg SM, Solomkin JS, Pitt HA, Gouma DJ, et al. TG13 flowchart for the management of acute cholangitis and cholecystitis. J Hepatobiliary Pancreat Sci. 2013;20:47–54.
8. Okamoto K, Takada T, Strasberg SM, Solomkin JS, Pitt HA, Gouma DJ, et al. Tokyo guidelines 2018: flowchart for the management of acute cholecystitis. J Hepatobiliary Pancreat Sci. 2018;25:55–72.
9. Endo I, Takada T, Hwang T-L, Akazawa K, Mori R, Miura F, et al. Optimal treatment strategy for acute cholecystitis based on predictive factors: Japan-Taiwan multicenter cohort study. J Hepatobiliary Pancreat Sci. 2017;24:346–61.
10. CholeS Study Group, West Midlands Research Collaborative. Population-based cohort study of variation in the use of emergency cholecystectomy for benign gallbladder diseases. Br J Surg. 2016;103:1716–26.
11. Cao AM, Eslick GD, Cox MR. Early laparoscopic cholecystectomy is superior to delayed acute cholecystitis: a meta-analysis of case–control studies. Surg Endosc. 2016;30:1172–82.
12. Ambe P, Weber SA, Christ H, Wassenberg D. Cholecystectomy for acute cholecystitis. How time-critical are the so called "golden 72 hours"? Or better "golden 24 hours" and "silver 25–72 hour"? A case control study. World J Emerg Surg. 2014;9:60.
13. Loozen CS, van Ramshorst B, van Santvoort HC, Boerma D. Early cholecystectomy for acute cholecystitis in the elderly population: a systematic review and meta-analysis. Dig Surg. 2017;34:371–9.
14. Wakabayashi G, Iwashita Y, Hibi T, Takada T, Strasberg SM, Asbun HJ, Endo I, et al. Tokyo guidelines 2018: surgical management of acute cholecystitis: safe steps in laparoscopic cholecystectomy for acute cholecystitis. J Hepatobiliary Pancreat Sci. 2018;25:73–86.
15. Strasberg SM, Hertl M, Soper NJ. An analysis of the problem of biliary injury during laparoscopic cholecystectomy. J Am Coll Surg. 1995;180:101–25.
16. Mori Y, Itoi T, Baron TH, Takada T, Strasberg SM, Pitt HA, Ukai T, et al. Tokyo guidelines 2018: management strategies for gallbladder drainage in patients with acute cholecystitis. J Hepatobiliary Pancreat Sci. 2018;25:87–95.
17. Asai K, Watanabe M, Kusachi S, Matsukiyo H, Saito T, Kodama H, et al. Risk factors for conversion of laparoscopic cholecystectomy to open surgery associ-

ated with the severity characteristics according to the Tokyo guidelines. Surg Today. 2014;44:2300–4.
18. Cheng WC, Chiu YC, Chuang CH, Chen CY. Assessing clinical outcomes of patients with acute calculous cholecystitis in addition to the Tokyo grading: a retrospective study. Kaohsiung J Med Sci. 2014;30:459–65.
19. Rodríguez-Sanjuán JC, Arruabarrena A, Sánchez-Moreno L, González-Sánchez F, Herrera LA, Gómez-Fleitas M. Acute cholecystitis in high surgical risk patients: percutaneous cholecystostomy or emergency cholecystectomy? Am J Surg. 2012;204:54–9.
20. The role of laparoscopic cholecystectomy (L.C.). Guidelines for clinical application. Society of American Gastrointestinal Endoscopic Surgeons (SAGES). Surg Endosc 1993;7:369–370
21. Tornqvist B, Waage A, Zheng Z, Ye W, Nilsson M. Severity of acute cholecystitis and risk of iatrogenic bile duct injury during cholecystectomy, a population-based case-control study. World J Surg. 2016;40:1060–7.
22. Shekelle PG, Ortiz E, Rhodes S, Morton SC, Eccles MP, Grimshaw JM, et al. Validity of the Agency for Healthcare Research and Quality clinical practice guidelines: how quickly do guidelines become outdated? JAMA. 2001;26:1461–7.

Preoperative Evaluation and Management of Acute Cholecystitis: Optimal Timing and Surgical Approach

6

Wesley Wendell B. Cruz and Ho-Seong Han

6.1 Introduction

Acute cholecystitis is defined as inflammation of the gallbladder, mainly due to bile obstruction with or without bacterial proliferation. Over 90% of cases are caused by an obstructing stone at the level of the cystic duct [1, 2]. Other causes include helminthic infections such as ascariasis, enlarged cystic node, or tumors [3]. Persistence of the inflammation and distention often leads to severe complications including hydrops, empyema, gangrene, and perforation, which if left untreated may lead to increased mortality and morbidity [4]. Ultrasound is the initial imaging of choice for patients with suspected acute cholecystitis. In equivocal cases, HIDA scan is preferred over MRI or CT scan due to its higher sensitivity and specificity. Guidelines have been established and validated in the diagnosis, treatment, and management of acute cholecystitis [5–7].

W. W. B. Cruz
Department of Surgery, Rizal Medical Center, Pasig, Philippines
e-mail: weecruzmd@ngcmed.com

H.-S. Han (✉)
Department of Surgery, Seoul National University Bundang Hospital, Seoul National University, College of Medicine, Seongnam-si, Gyeonggi-do, South Korea
e-mail: hanhs@snubh.org

6.2 Etiology and Pathogenesis

Gallstone formation has dated back as early as 3500 BC, as recorded from Egyptian and Chinese autopsies [8]. Bile, which is synthesized by the liver, is secreted and subsequently stored in the gallbladder. During storage, the gallbladder concentrates the bile, absorbing most of its water content. The bile is then secreted from the gallbladder, aiding in digestion. Alterations in absorption, such as oversaturation and concentration of bile, may precipitate its solid contents, thus forming biliary stones [9].

The most common cause of acute cholecystitis is an impacted stone at the level of the cystic duct or infundibulum. In developing countries in Asia, southern Africa and Latin America, helminthic infections (ascariasis) may also be commonly encountered [3]. Uncommon causes of cholecystitis may include strictures, kinking of the cystic duct, intussusception of a polyp, torsion of the gallbladder, or external compression from an overlying lymph node on the cystic duct [4].

In adults, approximately 10–20% will develop gallstones during their lifetime. Risk factors which may contribute to stone formation include family history, genetics, female sex, ethnicity, age, obesity, use of certain drugs, rapid weight loss and presence of other underlying diseases such as liver cirrhosis and Crohn's disease [8, 9].

Majority of cases are usually asymptomatic, with only ~20% presenting with symptoms such as abdominal pain, fever, nausea and/or vomiting.

© Springer Nature Switzerland AG 2021

I. Di Carlo (ed.), *Difficult Acute Cholecystitis*, https://doi.org/10.1007/978-3-030-62102-5_6

Abdominal pain may be characterized as persistent, localized in the right upper quadrant or epigastric area, with radiation to the right shoulder and back. Pain in cholecystitis is believed to be caused by increase in intraluminal pressure within the gallbladder due to an obstructing stone, leading to gallbladder distention. As a result of this distention, blood vessels within the gallbladder wall may be compressed, leading to ischemia and gangrene, with the most common site being the gallbladder fundus [10]. If left untreated, this may lead to gallbladder perforation and subsequent abscess formation or peritonitis, with complication rates as high as 22% and 16–25%, respectively [11].

Fever and leukocytosis (WBC >10,000/μL) are also usually seen in acute cholecystitis. Aside from causing obstruction, the gallstones itself may contribute to the inflammatory response by stimulating prostaglandins I_2 and E_2. Bacterial proliferation, found in 20% of cases of acute cholecystitis, is usually caused by Gram negative bacteria of gastrointestinal origin, such as *Klebsiella spp.* and Escherichia coli.

6.3 Imaging

Transabdominal ultrasound is the preferred initial imaging test for patients suspected to have acute cholecystitis, since it is readily available, inexpensive, and noninvasive [10, 11]. A diagnosis of acute cholecystitis may be reached based on ultrasonographic findings of: (1) impacted gallstones at the infundibulum or cystic duct; (2) gallbladder wall diameter of >4 mm; (3) fluid collection around the gallbladder; and (4) gallbladder diameter of >8 cm (long axis) × >4 cm (short axis) [12]. Sensitivity of ultrasound in the detection of acute cholecystitis is relatively high at 84%, with a positive sonographic Murphy's sign increasing the sensitivity to as much as 92%. Specificity is also high at 99% (97–100%) [9, 11, 12]. Aside from diagnosing cholecystitis, ultrasound also has high sensitivity in detecting gallbladder stones (92%) [13, 14].

Cholescintigraphy or hepatic 2,6-dimethyl-iminodiacetic acid (HIDA) scan (Fig. 6.1) is considered to be the "gold standard" in diagnosing acute cholecystitis. In HIDA scan, a radioactive tracer is injected intravenously, subsequently taken up by the liver and excreted into the bile ducts. The tracer is stored in the gallbladder for approximately 30 min after administration. A normal scan would demonstrate the liver, bile ducts, gallbladder, and duodenum after 1 h of administration; thus, non-visualization of the gallbladder and the cystic duct may indicate an impacted stone or obstruction at the cystic duct (Fig. 6.2). The sensitivity and specificity of HIDA scan in diagnosing acute cholecystitis is higher compared to ultrasound (97% vs 96% and 98% vs 90%, respectively) [15–18]. However, the main disadvantage of this imaging modality is the exposure to ionizing radiation, as well as its cost and availability.

A study conducted by Cho et al. last 2011 demonstrated HIDA scan as a predictive tool for assessing the severity of acute cholecystitis. In the study, acute cholecystitis was diagnosed when two or more clinical and operative findings were present. Clinical findings included: temperature >37.5 °C, leukocytosis >10,000/μL, right upper quadrant pain and tenderness, and symptom duration >48 h; whereas operative findings included: gallbladder wall >4 mm, presence of severe adhesions, distorted biliary anatomy, and gross inflammation of the gallbladder fossa. Results showed that non-visualization of the gallbladder during HIDA scan was seen in 86.4% of the patients diagnosed as acute cholecystitis. In cases of complicated acute cholecystitis (such as hydrops, empyema, pericholecystic abscess, and gangrenous gallbladder), the diagnostic accuracy of HIDA scan was higher at 92.7%, compared to 75.3% of uncomplicated acute cholecystitis. Gallbladder ejection fraction (GBEF) (Fig. 6.1d) was also included and shown to have a predictive value of 82.9%. A GBEF of <30% was significantly associated with increased difficulty during laparoscopic cholecystectomy, with associated increase in operative time, blood loss, and postoperative complication rates compared to those with GBEF 30% or higher (6.3% vs 2.6%; $p = 0.006$) [19].

In comparison, MRI with MRCP with or without contrast has been shown to have higher sensi-

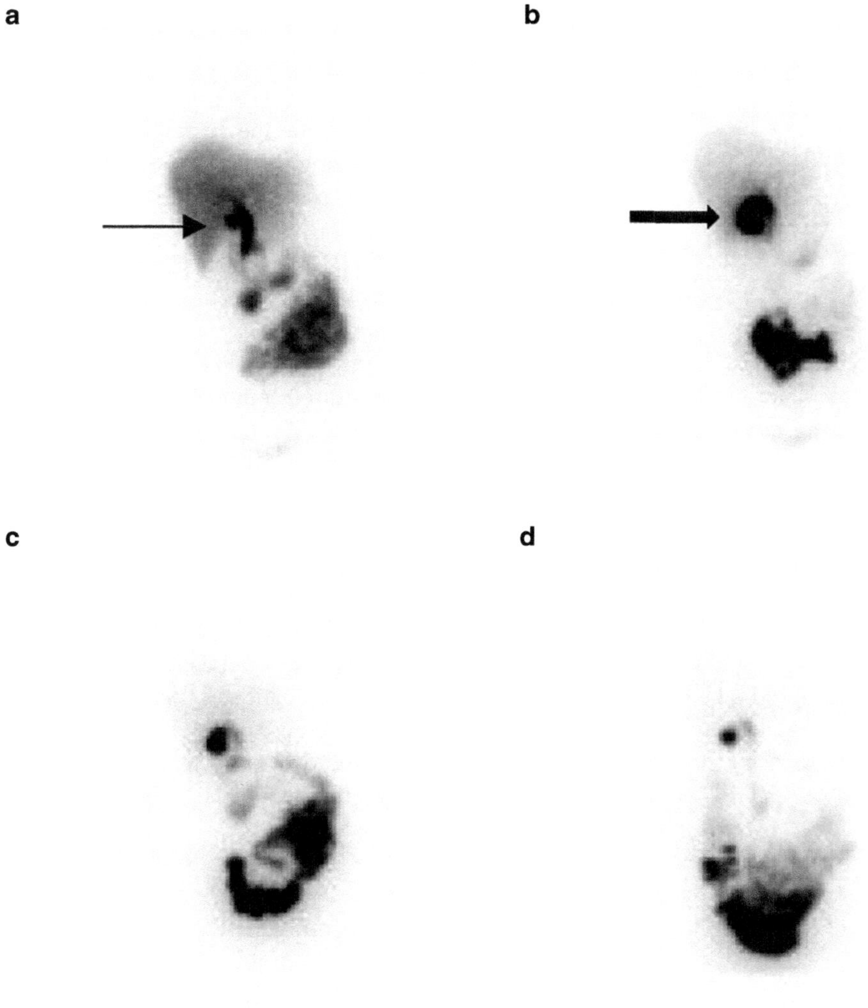

Fig. 6.1 HIDA scan of a 46-year-old female, (**a**) patent cystic duct at 30 min with normal liver uptake (narrow arrow), (**b**) visualized gallbladder at 60 min (thick arrow), (**c**) tracers are seen in the small bowel at 90 min, (**d**) retention of tracer in the gallbladder and common bile duct with ejection fraction (GBEF) of 73.25%

tivity than ultrasound at 85% but lower than that of HIDA scan [20]. MRI is able to detect inflammation, fluid retention, and fatty tissues around the gallbladder, while MRCP is able to provide images of the biliary tree even without contrast. Thus, MRI has been recommended as the diagnostic imaging of choice when ultrasound results are equivocal.

Use of CT scan in the diagnosis of acute cholecystitis is limited, since ultrasound and HIDA scan both have higher sensitivities in diagnosing suspected acute cholecystitis. As demonstrated in a study conducted by Fagenholz et al. (2015), ultrasound had a higher sensitivity in detecting gallbladder stones compared to CT scan (87% vs 60%, $p < 0.01$) [13, 21]. However, CT scan is still useful in diagnosing gangrenous cholecystitis, with relatively high diagnostic accuracy at 87.6%. It also has high specificity in the detection of presence of gas in the lumen or wall (100%), irregular or absent walls (97.6%), and abscess formation (96.6%) [22, 23].

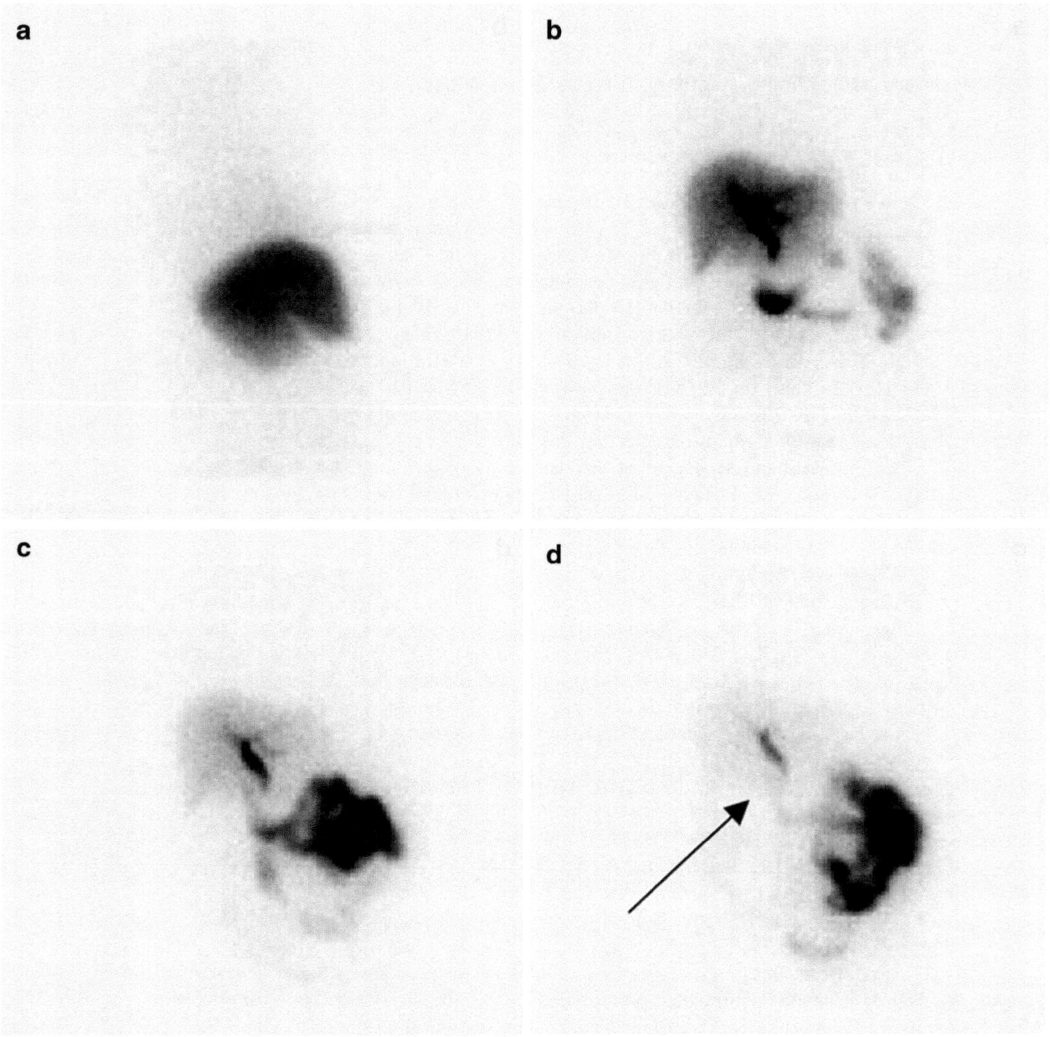

Fig. 6.2 HIDA scan of a 58-year-old male, (**a**) tracers with normal liver uptake, (**b**) tracers shown highlighting the main intrahepatic ducts and common bile duct at 30 min, (**c**) tracers are seen in the small bowel with some retention in the common bile duct, (**d**) most tracers are seen in the small bowel with decrease amount in the common bile duct. Non-visualization of the gallbladder and cystic duct up to 3 h (narrow arrow)

6.4 Diagnosis and Severity Grading

Prior to 2007, standard diagnostic criteria for acute cholecystitis were not available. Clinical history, physical examination, and routine laboratory tests were primarily used, resulting in a number of unnecessary cholecystectomies or missed diagnoses [10].

6.4.1 Diagnosis

In 2007, global experts at the Tokyo Consensus Meeting met and established the first version of the Tokyo Guidelines for the diagnosis, severity grading, and management of acute cholecystitis (TG7); in 2013, these guidelines were revisited and revised according to current literature and validity studies, and TG13 guidelines were

Table 6.1 TG18/13 Diagnostic Criteria for Acute Cholecystitis. From [5], with permission

A. Local signs of inflammation
(1) Murphy's sign
(2) Right upper quadrant mass/pain/tenderness
B. Systemic signs of inflammation
(3) Fever
(4) Elevated CRP
(5) Elevated WBC count
C. Imaging findings
(6) Imaging findings characteristic of acute cholecystitis
Definitive diagnosis: one item in A + one item in B + C
Suspected diagnosis: one item in A + one item in B

Acute hepatitis, other acute abdominal diseases, and chronic cholecystitis should be excluded
WBC white blood count, *CRP* C-reactive protein

Table 6.2 TG18/TG13 Severity Grading for Acute Cholecystitis. From [5], with permission

Grade III (severe) acute cholecystitis
"Grade III" acute cholecystitis is associated with dysfunction of any one of the following organs/systems:
1. Cardiovascular dysfunction: hypotension requiring treatment with dopamine ≥5 lg/kg per min, or any dose of norepinephrine
2. Neurological dysfunction: decreased level of consciousness
3. Respiratory dysfunction: PaO_2/FiO_2 ratio < 300
4. Renal dysfunction: oliguria, creatinine >2.0 mg/dl
5. Hepatic dysfunction: PT-INR >1.5
6. Hematological dysfunction: platelet count <100,000/mm^3
Grade II (moderate) acute cholecystitis
"Grade II" acute cholecystitis is associated with any one of the following conditions:
1. Elevated WBC count (>18,000/mm^3)
2. Palpable tender mass in the right upper abdominal quadrant
3. Duration of complaints >72 h
4. Marked local inflammation (gangrenous cholecystitis, pericholecystic abscess, hepatic abscess, biliary peritonitis, emphysematous cholecystitis)
Grade I (mild) acute cholecystitis
"Grade I" acute cholecystitis does not meet the criteria of "Grade III" or "Grade II" acute cholecystitis. It can also be defined as acute cholecystitis in a healthy patient with no organ dysfunction and mild inflammatory changes in the gallbladder, making cholecystectomy a safe and low-risk operative procedure

PaO_2 partial pressure of oxygen, *FiO_2* fraction of inspired oxygen, *PT-INR* prothrombin time-international normalized ratio, *WBC* white blood count

released. In 2017, Yokoe and Takada conducted a validation study on TG13 and demonstrated that the TG13 guidelines were useful in definitively diagnosing acute cholecystitis, with a sensitivity of 84.9%, but low specificity at 50.0%. These issues were then addressed in the revision of TG13, and subsequent numerous validation studies of TG13 in clinical practice have yielded higher sensitivity and specificity rates of 91.2% and 96.9%, respectively, with concomitant increase in accuracy rate from 92.7% to 94.0%; thus, these recommendations were adopted into the latest Tokyo Guidelines for 2018 (TG18) without any modification [5].

According to TG18, a definitive diagnosis of acute cholecystitis is made if all of the following criterion are met: Presence of local signs of gallbladder inflammation (A), presence of systemic signs of inflammation (B), and imaging findings characteristic of acute cholecystitis (C) (Table 6.1). Acute cholecystitis is suspected if local (A) and systemic (B) signs of inflammation are present but is not supported by any of the imaging modalities done (ultrasound, CT scan, or MRI).

6.4.2 Severity Assessment

Once the diagnosis of acute cholecystitis is made, the patients should then be categorized according to the severity of the disease (Table 6.2). Severe cholecystitis (Grade III) is defined as acute cholecystitis accompanied with end organ failure (cardiac, neurologic, pulmonary, renal, hepatic, or hematologic failure). Moderate cholecystitis (Grade II) should include any of the following conditions: signs of local inflammation, duration of signs and symptoms >72 h, a palpable tender mass at the right upper quadrant during physical examination, or leukocytosis of 18,000/mm^3. If the criterion for severe or moderate cholecystitis is not met, then the patient is categorized as mild cholecystitis [5].

6.4.2.1 Other Possible Factors to Be Considered in the Diagnosis and Severity Grading of Patients with Acute Cholecystitis

Preoperative assessment is a vital step in the approach of a patient with suspected acute cholecystitis, since several factors may contribute to increased risk and predisposition for acute cholecystitis. Cho et al. in 2010 identified risk factors which increased the risk for development of acute cholecystitis in patients with gallbladder stones ($p < 0.0001$) [24]. These factors included: (1) presence of comorbidities (cardiovascular disease, diabetes, and cerebrovascular accident (CVA); (2) age >60 years old; and (3) male gender [24, 25]. The study concluded that presence of these factors may be associated with early development of complications of acute cholecystitis.

Onoe et al. in a review of acute cholecystitis cases diagnosed according to TG18/TG13 proposed a predictive scoring system that would determine ease of achieving the critical view of safety based on preoperative factors. The following three factors were considered: (1) C-reactive protein >5.5 mg/dl (3 points); (2) symptom duration >72 h (2 points); and (3) impacted gallstones (1 point) on imaging. The higher the points, the less likely the critical view of safety (CVS) was identified during laparoscopic cholecystectomy ($p < 0.001$) [26]. Other risk factors proposed to be predictive of difficulties during cholecystectomy were ASA score > III ($p < 0.001$) and those with concomitant common bile duct (CBD) stones ($p < 0.001$) [27].

6.5 Treatment

The aim of treatment in patients diagnosed with acute cholecystitis is stabilization and optimization prior to definitive intervention. Resuscitation with intravenous fluids and correction of electrolytes is the initial step. The patient is placed on NPO (nothing-per-orem) as oral intake may aggravate contraction of the gallbladder, producing more pain. H2-blockers or Proton-pump inhibitors are started. Analgesics should be initiated, preferably nonsteroidal anti-inflammatory drugs (NSAIDS) to inhibit the cyclooxygenase pathway (Cox-1 and Cox-2) and decrease the mucous production in the gallbladder [7].

Initiation of anti-microbial empiric therapy for acute cholecystitis is dependent on severity grading. In mild (Grade I) acute cholecystitis, antibiotic therapy is recommended prior to surgery. In moderate (Grade II) and severe (Grade III) acute cholecystitis, antibiotics should be given once the diagnosis is made. In TG18/13, it is recommended that antibiotics be started immediately (within 1 h) for severe cases and urgently (within 6 h) for moderate cases [7]. Antibiotic treatment should be directed to the microorganisms of the gut, most commonly *Escherichia coli*, *Klebsiella spp*, *Enterococcus spp*., and the anaerobic organisms [28–32]. Bile samples should be taken for microbial culture and antibiotic sensitivity testing, and antibiotics promptly shifted once bile culture results become available [29]. Blood culture is not necessary unless warranted [28].

For mild and moderate cases, antibiotics should be stopped once source control (cholecystectomy) has been achieved. Several randomized control trial studies regarding continuation of antibiotics postoperatively showed no benefit in extending antibiotics in terms of decrease in postoperative infections [33, 34], and this has been supported by meta-analyses [35, 36]. It was also demonstrated from these meta-analyses that prolonged administration of antibiotics in fact lengthened hospital stay, increased overall costs, and increased microbial resistance [35, 36]. For severe cholecystitis cases, antibiotics are recommended to be continued for a duration of 4–7 days after cholecystectomy [7, 28].

6.5.1 Timing: Early vs Delayed Cholecystectomy

It has been a long-standing debate on whether surgery for acute cholecystitis be done during the same admission or after a prolonged interval, and up to the present time there is still some controversy in deciding between early and delayed cholecystectomy [37]. By definition, early cholecystectomy may range from time of admission up to 10 days from onset of the symptoms [38–40], while delayed cholecystectomy is defined as surgery scheduled 6–8 weeks after the initial symptoms with administration of antibiotics, with the rationale that at this time most of the inflammatory process has subsided.

In Tokyo Guidelines 2018/2013, early laparoscopic cholecystectomy (defined as 72 h to 1 week after onset of symptoms) was compared to delayed cholecystectomy in terms of operative time, bile duct injuries, length of hospital stay, and overall cost of treatment. It was determined that there was no statistical difference in outcomes between the early and delayed groups [7].

A meta-analysis done by Lyu et al., composed of 15 randomized trials with 1669 patients, compared early laparoscopic cholecystectomy and delayed laparoscopic cholecystectomy [39]. The primary outcomes considered were risk for bile duct injury and bile leak, and secondary outcomes included wound infection, complications, conversion to open cholecystectomy, and operative time. It was determined that there was no significant difference between the two treatment groups in terms of increased risk for bile leak and bile duct injuries, as well as the included secondary outcomes (wound infection, complications, and operative time). Postoperative length of stay also showed no difference between the two groups. A subgroup analysis was also performed, wherein early laparoscopic cholecystectomy was divided into three groups (3 days, 4 days, and 7 days from onset of symptoms) and then compared to delayed cholecystectomy. Even in subgroup analysis, the 3-day and 4-day groups showed no difference in terms of operative time; however, the 7-day group showed a longer operative time compared to the delayed group [39].

Early cholecystectomy for acute cholecystitis is therefore a safe and feasible option, regardless of severity grading, and this has been consistently supported by various trials and meta-analyses [37, 38, 40–46]. Aside from comparable outcomes between early and delayed intervention, early cholecystectomy also decreases the risk for recurrence of symptoms, total hospital cost, and total hospital stay.

6.5.1.1 Timing of Early Cholecystectomy: What Is "Early?"

As was previously stated, early surgery has been defined to range from the day of admission (onset of symptoms) to as long as the tenth hospital day. Blohm et al. (2017) analyzed data from 15,760 cholecystectomies performed for acute cholecystitis within an 8-year period. It was noted that adverse events increased as surgery was delayed, with complications the least in cholecystectomies done within 2–3 days from admission [47]. A 30-day and 90-day mortality risk was noted to be reduced for patients who were operated on within three days of admission. A similar study done by Polo et al. in 2015 assessed the optimal timing of early cholecystectomy for acute cholecystitis. It was discovered that on patients where cholecystectomy was performed on the day of admission and 3 days after admission, mortality and morbidity (postoperative sepsis, ICU admission, and reoperation) increased significantly. It was suggested that in the first 24 h of admission, patients often present with unstable hemodynamics, and therefore require initial resuscitation and stabilization prior to any surgical intervention [47, 48]. It has thus been recommended that early cholecystectomy be done within the first three days, after initial resuscitative measures have been instituted [47–49].

6.5.2 Laparoscopic Cholecystectomy for Acute Cholecystitis

Surgical removal of the gallbladder, or cholecystectomy, is the definitive treatment for acute cholecystitis. From the first recorded open cholecystectomy performed in July 1882 by Dr. Carl Langenbuch in Lazarus Hospital, Berlin, it has since become the gold standard treatment for benign gallbladder diseases [50, 51]. In September 12, 1985, Prof Dr. Med Erich Mühe of Böblingen, Germany, performed the first laparoscopic cholecystectomy [52]. With this novel approach, open cholecystectomy has then slowly shifted to laparoscopic cholecystectomy over the past decades, emerging as the current gold standard in the treatment of benign gallbladder diseases [53].

As stated in TG18/13, laparoscopic cholecystectomy is a safe approach for the treatment of mild (Grade 1) and moderate (Grade 2) acute cholecystitis. In a study conducted by Keus et al. which included 38 randomized control trials (2338 patients), there was no significant difference between open cholecystectomy and laparoscopic cholecystectomy in terms of complications and mortality [54]. The advantages of the laparoscopic group seen in the study were shorter operative time, shorter hospital stay, decreased requirement for postoperative analgesics, and decreased morbidity [55].

Safety within the confines of the operating room theater, of both the patient and the surgeon, has always been the primary concern and priority in any field of surgery [56, 57]. Strasberg's analysis and review was the first to describe the critical view of safety (CVS) as an intraoperative tool during laparoscopic cholecystectomy to decrease bile duct and vascular injury [58–61]. As was stated by Strasberg, the CVS is achieved by opening up the triangle of Calot (clearance of fibrous and fatty tissues and separation of the lower third of the gallbladder from the liver to expose the liver surface, with no structures being ligated or divided), until only two structures are seen going to the gallbladder, the cystic duct, and the cystic artery [58].

However, in cases of acute cholecystitis with concomitant intense inflammation around the gallbladder and hepatoduodenal ligament surrounding the biliary tree, difficult cholecystectomy during laparoscopy may be an unavoidable encounter, whether timing of surgery be early or delayed. Identification of the critical view of safety may therefore be quite a challenge in the face of an ongoing inflammatory process, wherein the distorted anatomy poses a significant risk for vasculo-biliary injuries (VBI) [58].

Several intraoperative imaging strategies are available which may be utilized in the identification of the vital structures and CVS. Intraoperative cholangiography (IOC) may be used to identify the cystic duct and its junction with the common bile duct. In cases where biliary injury may have already occurred, IOC may also help in identifying early injuries. Intraoperative indocyanine green (ICG) may also be used to identify the biliary anatomy. However, the main limitation of ICG is the presence of severe inflammation, which may preclude clear visualization of the ducts [62]. Intraoperative ultrasound may also be used for intraoperative assessment of the vascular and biliary anatomy [56].

In instances where a difficult laparoscopic cholecystectomy is encountered (and absence of available intraoperative imaging modalities or lack of expertise) and a critical view of safety cannot be achieved, bailout techniques were developed. Partial or subtotal cholecystectomy may be performed, wherein partial removal of the gallbladder fundus and body may be carried out, with closure of the gallbladder remnant done using a reconstituting (complete closure of the gallbladder remnant) or fenestrated (open gallbladder with closure of cystic duct) technique. Fundus first (dome-down) technique is also another option for the difficult gallbladder. If the extrahepatic biliary anatomy cannot be identified, the surgeon may proceed to partial or subtotal cholecystectomy after a fundus first approach. In terms of a difficult laparoscopic surgery, conversion to open is another bailout approach; however, studies demonstrate that conversion does not lower the risk of VBI but increases it by a hundredfold [63].

In cases of Grade II and Grade III acute cholecystitis, TG18/13 recommends that open cholecystectomy be the preferred approach, especially for the less experienced surgeons [7]. This approach is also reserved for patients who cannot tolerate laparoscopic surgeries.

In conclusion, it is still the prerogative of the attending surgeon to perform whatever approach, technique, or combinations of techniques applicable in the current situation, as long as patient safety is paramount [56, 57].

6.5.2.1 Other Treatment Alternatives Besides Cholecystectomy

Cholecystectomy may not always be an ideal option for a select group of patients. In patients with severe acute cholecystitis necessitating prolonged resuscitation with fluids and antibiotics, in patients with underlying medical conditions wherein general anesthesia is contraindicated, and in high-risk surgical patients, other techniques are recommended prior to definitive treatment [7]. Percutaneous biliary aspiration, with or without tube placement, to drain the infected bile contents can be done under local anesthesia either with or without sedation. Preferably, image-guided transhepatic gallbladder drainage is recommended due to less complications compared to percutaneous tube cholecystostomy. Another suggested method may be endoscopic transpapillary gallbladder drainage, but these are reserved for centers with an experienced endoscopist. Another safe and feasible approach is endoscopic ultrasound-guided gallbladder drainage through the antrum or bulb of the duodenum. A plastic stent or self-expanding metallic stent is then placed for internal drainage [64]. Once the patient recovers, elective cholecystectomy is then scheduled, either in the same admission or delayed setting (6–8 weeks).

References

1. Indar AA, Beckingham IJ. Acute cholecystitis. BMJ. 2002;325(7365):639–43.
2. Yokoe M, Takada T, Hwang T-L, Endo I, Akazawa K, Miura F, et al. Descriptive review of acute cholecystitis: Japan-Taiwan collaborative epidemiological study. J Hepatobiliary Pancreat Sci. 2017;24(6):319–28.
3. Bahú MGS, Baldisseroto M, Custodio CM, Gralha CZ, Mangili AR. Hepatobiliary and pancreatic complications of ascariasis in children: a study of seven cases. J Pediatr Gastroenterol Nutr. 2001;33(3):271–5.
4. Byrne JJ, Berger RL. The pathogenesis of acute cholecystitis. Arch Surg. 1960;81(5):812–6.
5. Yokoe M, Hata J, Takada T, Strasberg SM, Asbun HJ, Wakabayashi G, et al. Tokyo guidelines 2018: diagnostic criteria and severity grading of acute cholecystitis (with videos). J Hepatobiliary Pancreat Sci. 2018;25(1):41–54.
6. Yokoe M, Takada T, Hwang T-L, Endo I, Akazawa K, Miura F, et al. Validation of TG13 severity grading in acute cholecystitis: Japan-Taiwan collaborative study for acute cholecystitis. J Hepatobiliary Pancreat Sci. 2017;24(6):338–45.
7. Okamoto K, Suzuki K, Takada T, Strasberg SM, Asbun HJ, Endo I, et al. Tokyo guidelines 2018: flowchart for the management of acute cholecystitis. J Hepatobiliary Pancreat Sci. 2018;25(1):55–72.
8. Erlinger S. Gallstones in obesity and weight loss. Eur J Gastroenterol Hepatol. 2000;12(12):1347–52.
9. Stinton LM, Shaffer EA. Epidemiology of gallbladder disease: cholelithiasis and cancer. Gut Liver. 2012;6(2):172–87.
10. Mehrzad M, Jehle CC, Roussel LO, Mehrzad R. Gangrenous cholecystitis: a silent but potential fatal disease in patients with diabetic neuropathy. A case report. World J Clin Cases. 2018;6(15):1007–11.
11. Pinto A, Reginelli A, Cagini L, Coppolino F, Stabile Ianora AA, Bracale R, et al. Accuracy of ultrasonography in the diagnosis of acute calculous cholecystitis: review of the literature. Crit Ultrasound J. 2013;5 Suppl 1(Suppl 1):S11.
12. Ralls PW, Colletti PM, Lapin SA, Chandrasoma P, Boswell WD, Ngo C, et al. Real-time sonography in suspected acute cholecystitis. Prospective evaluation of primary and secondary signs. Radiology. 1985;155(3):767–71.
13. Tan E, Friesen J, Friesen B. Acute cholecystitis: computed tomography (CT) versus ultrasound (US). Open J Radiol. 2018;08:131–9.
14. Yarmenitis S. Ultrasound of the gallbladder and the biliary tree. Eur Radiol. 2002;12(2):270–82.
15. Shea JA, Berlin JA, Escarce JJ, Clarke JR, Kinosian BP, Cabana MD, et al. Revised estimates of diagnostic test sensitivity and specificity in suspected biliary tract disease. Arch Intern Med. 1994;154(22):2573–81.
16. Rodriguez LE, Santaliz-Ruiz LE, De La Torre-Bisot G, Gonzalez G, Serpa MA, Sanchez-Gaetan F, et al. Clinical implications of hepatobiliary scintigraphy and ultrasound in the diagnosis of acute cholecystitis. Int J Surg. 2016;35:196–200.
17. Kaoutzanis C, Davies E, Leichtle SW, Welch KB, Winter S, Lampman RM, et al. Abdominal ultrasound versus hepato-imino diacetic acid scan in diagnosing acute cholecystitis—what is the real benefit? J Surg Res. 2014;188(1):44–52.
18. Kaoutzanis C, Davies E, Leichtle SW, Welch KB, Winter S, Lampman RM, et al. Is hepato-imino diacetic acid scan a better imaging modality than abdominal ultrasound for diagnosing acute cholecystitis? Am J Surg. 2015;210(3):473–82.
19. Cho JY, Han H-S, Yoon Y-S, Ahn KS, Lee SH, Hwang J-H. Hepatobiliary scan for assessing disease severity in patients with cholelithiasis. Arch Surg. 2011;146(2):169–74.
20. Kiewiet JJS, Leeuwenburgh MMN, Bipat S, Bossuyt PMM, Stoker J, Boermeester MA. A systematic review and meta-analysis of diagnostic performance of imaging in acute cholecystitis. Radiology. 2012;264(3):708–20.
21. Fagenholz PJ, Fuentes E, Kaafarani H, Cropano C, King D, de Moya M, et al. Computed tomography is more sensitive than ultrasound for the diagnosis of acute cholecystitis. Surg Infect. 2015;16(5):509–12.

22. Bennett GL, Balthazar EJ. Ultrasound and CT evaluation of emergent gallbladder pathology. Radiol Clin N Am. 2003;41(6):1203–16.
23. Bennett GL, Rusinek H, Lisi V, Israel GM, Krinsky GA, Slywotzky CM, et al. CT findings in acute gangrenous cholecystitis. Am J Roentgenol. 2002;178(2):275–81.
24. Cho JY, Han H-S, Yoon Y-S, Ahn KS. Risk factors for acute cholecystitis and a complicated clinical course in patients with symptomatic cholelithiasis. Arch Surg. 2010;145(4):329–33.
25. Lee HK, Han H-S, Min SK, Lee J-H. Sex-based analysis of the outcome of laparoscopic cholecystectomy for acute cholecystitis. Br J Surg. 2005;92(4):463–6.
26. Onoe S, Maeda A, Takayama Y, Fukami Y, Kaneoka Y. A preoperative predictive scoring system to predict the ability to achieve the critical view of safety during laparoscopic cholecystectomy for acute cholecystitis. HPB. 2017;19(5):406–10.
27. Chun K-S, Han H-S, Yoon Y-S, Cho J, jh K, Ahn K. Overcoming the difficulties encountered when performing laparoscopic cholecystectomy: review of over one thousand laparoscopic cholecystectomies. Hepato-Gastroenterology. 2010;57:398–402.
28. Gomi H, Solomkin JS, Schlossberg D, Okamoto K, Takada T, Strasberg SM, et al. Tokyo guidelines 2018: antimicrobial therapy for acute cholangitis and cholecystitis. J Hepatobiliary Pancreat Sci. 2018;25(1):3–16.
29. Fuks D, Cossé C, Régimbeau JM. Antibiotic therapy in acute calculous cholecystitis. J Visc Surg. 2013;150(1):3–8.
30. Kaya M, Beştaş R, Bacalan F, Bacaksız F, Arslan EG, Kaplan MA. Microbial profile and antibiotic sensitivity pattern in bile cultures from endoscopic retrograde cholangiography patients. World J Gastroenterol. 2012;18(27):3585–9.
31. Capoor MR, Nair D, Rajni, Khanna G, Krishna SV, Chintamani MS, et al. Microflora of bile aspirates in patients with acute cholecystitis with or without cholelithiasis: a tropical experience. Braz J Infect Dis. 2008;12:222–5.
32. Tazuma S. Epidemiology, pathogenesis, and classification of biliary stones (common bile duct and intrahepatic). Best Pract Res Clin Gastroenterol. 2006;20(6):1075–83.
33. Regimbeau JM, Fuks D, Pautrat K, Mauvais F, Haccart V, Msika S, et al. Effect of postoperative antibiotic administration on postoperative infection following cholecystectomy for acute calculous cholecystitis: a randomized clinical trial. JAMA. 2014;312(2):145–54.
34. Loozen C, Kortram K, Kornmann V, Ramshorst B, Vlaminckx B, Knibbe C, et al. Randomized clinical trial of extended versus single-dose perioperative antibiotic prophylaxis for acute calculous cholecystitis: extended versus single-dose perioperative antibiotic prophylaxis for acute calculous cholecystitis. Br J Surg. 2017;104:e151–e7.
35. La Regina D, Di Giuseppe M, Cafarotti S, Saporito A, Ceppi M, Mongelli F, et al. Antibiotic administration after cholecystectomy for acute mild-moderate cholecystitis: a PRISMA-compliant meta-analysis. Surg Endosc. 2019;33(2):377–83.
36. Hajibandeh S, Popova P, Rehman S. Extended postoperative antibiotics versus no postoperative antibiotics in patients undergoing emergency cholecystectomy for acute calculous cholecystitis: a systematic review and meta-analysis. Surg Innov. 2019;26(4):485–96.
37. Lai PBS, Kwong KH, Leung KL, Kwok SPY, Chan ACW, Chung SCS, et al. Randomized trial of early versus delayed laparoscopic cholecystectomy for acute cholecystitis. Br J Surg. 1998;85(6):764–7.
38. Yamashita Y, Takada T, Hirata K. A survey of the timing and approach to the surgical management of patients with acute cholecystitis in Japanese hospitals. J Hepatobiliary Pancreat Surg. 2006;13(5):409–15.
39. Lyu Y, Cheng Y, Wang B, Zhao S, Chen L. Early versus delayed laparoscopic cholecystectomy for acute cholecystitis: an up-to-date meta-analysis of randomized controlled trials. Surg Endosc. 2018;32(12):4728–41.
40. Roulin D, Saadi A, Di Mare L, Demartines N, Halkic N. Early versus delayed cholecystectomy for acute cholecystitis, are the 72 hours still the rule?: a randomized trial. Ann Surg. 2016;264(5):717–22.
41. Cao AM, Eslick GD, Cox MR. Early cholecystectomy is superior to delayed cholecystectomy for acute cholecystitis: a meta-analysis. J Gastrointest Surg. 2015;19(5):848–57.
42. Gallagher TK, Kelly ME, Hoti E. Meta-analysis of the cost-effectiveness of early versus delayed cholecystectomy for acute cholecystitis. BJS Open. 2019;3(2):146–52.
43. Gurusamy K, Samraj K, Gluud C, Wilson E, Davidson BR. Meta-analysis of randomized controlled trials on the safety and effectiveness of early versus delayed laparoscopic cholecystectomy for acute cholecystitis. Br J Surg. 2010;97(2):141–50.
44. Gurusamy KS, Davidson C, Gluud C, Davidson BR. Early versus delayed laparoscopic cholecystectomy for people with acute cholecystitis. Cochrane Database Syst Rev 2013;(6):CD005440.
45. Imbisat M, Rizvi S, Ali I. An evaluation of early and delayed laparoscopic cholecystectomy for acute cholecystitis. Int Surg J. 2019;6(9):1–5.
46. Chang TC, Lin MT, Wu MH, Wang MY, Lee PH. Evaluation of early versus delayed laparoscopic cholecystectomy in the treatment of acute cholecystitis. Hepato-Gastroenterology. 2009;56(89):26–8.
47. Blohm M, Österberg J, Sandblom G, Lundell L, Hedberg M, Enochsson L. The sooner, the better? The importance of optimal timing of cholecystectomy in acute cholecystitis: data from the National Swedish Registry for Gallstone Surgery, GallRiks. J Gastrointest Surg. 2017;21(1):33–40.

48. Polo M, Duclos A, Polazzi S, Payet C, Lifante JC, Cotte E, et al. Acute cholecystitis—optimal timing for early cholecystectomy: a French Nationwide study. J Gastrointest Surg. 2015;19(11):2003–10.
49. Jensen KK, Roth NO, Krarup P-M, Bardram L. Surgical management of acute cholecystitis in a nationwide Danish cohort. Langenbeck's Arch Surg. 2019;404(5):589–97.
50. Hardy KJ. Carl Langenbuch and the Lazarus hospital: events and circumstances surrounding the first cholecystectomy. Aust N Z J Surg. 1993;63(1):56–64.
51. Acar T, Kamer E, Acar N, Atahan K, Bağ H, Hacıyanlı M, et al. Laparoscopic cholecystectomy in the treatment of acute cholecystitis: comparison of results between early and late cholecystectomy. Pan Afr Med J. 2017;26:49.
52. Reynolds W Jr. The first laparoscopic cholecystectomy. JSLS. 2001;5(1):89–94.
53. Soper NJ, Stockmann PT, Dunnegan DL, Ashley SW. Laparoscopic cholecystectomy the new 'Gold Standard'? Arch Surg. 1992;127(8):917–23.
54. Keus F, de Jong J, Gooszen HG, Laarhoven C. Laparoscopic versus open cholecystectomy for patients with symptomatic cholecystolithiasis. Cochrane Database Syst Rev 2006;(4):CD006231.
55. Poggio JL, Rowland CM, Gores GJ, Nagorney DM, Donohue JH. A comparison of laparoscopic and open cholecystectomy in patients with compensated cirrhosis and symptomatic gallstone disease. Surgery. 2000;127(4):405–11.
56. Gupta V, Jain G. Safe laparoscopic cholecystectomy: adoption of universal culture of safety in cholecystectomy. World J Gastrointest Surg. 2019;11(2):62–84.
57. Gupta V. ABCD of safe laparoscopic cholecystectomy: imbibing universal culture of safety in cholecystectomy. Indian J Surg. 2019;81(2):203–4.
58. Strasberg SM, Brunt LM. Rationale and use of the critical view of safety in laparoscopic cholecystectomy. J Am Coll Surg. 2010;211(1):132–8.
59. Strasberg SM, Hertl M, Soper NJ. An analysis of the problem of biliary injury during laparoscopic cholecystectomy. J Am Coll Surg. 1995;180(1):101–25.
60. Giménez ME, Houghton EJ, Zeledón ME, Palermo M, Acquafresca P, Finger C, et al. The critical view of safety prevents the appearance of biliary injuries? Analysis of a survey. Arq Bras Cir Dig. 2018;31(2):e1380.
61. Singh R, Brunt LM. Critical view of safety—its feasibility and efficacy in preventing bile duct injuries. Ann Laparosc Endosc Surg. 2018;3:1.
62. Ambe PC, Plambeck J, Fernandez-Jesberg V, Zarras K. The role of indocyanine green fluoroscopy for intraoperative bile duct visualization during laparoscopic cholecystectomy: an observational cohort study in 70 patients. Patient Saf Surg. 2019;13(1):2.
63. Mangieri CW, Hendren BP, Strode MA, Bandera BC, Faler BJ. Bile duct injuries (BDI) in the advanced laparoscopic cholecystectomy era. Surg Endosc. 2019;33(3):724–30.
64. Mori Y, Itoi T, Baron TH, Takada T, Strasberg SM, Pitt HA, et al. Tokyo guidelines 2018: management strategies for gallbladder drainage in patients with acute cholecystitis (with videos). J Hepatobiliary Pancreat Sci. 2018;25(1):87–95.

7 Perioperative Evaluation and Decision-Making, When to Operate and by Which Approach: Tube Cholecystostomy

Anthony Bacon, Travis Corgan, Tyler Pender, and Alexander Colonna

7.1 Introduction

Percutaneous cholecystostomy tubes (PCTs) have emerged as a safe and accepted therapeutic alternative to the treatment of acute cholecystitis in patients that present as prohibitive surgical candidates. Modern percutaneous techniques allow for minimally invasive and accurate placement of these tubes within the lumen of the diseased gallbladder. Following successful placement, the PCT is then used for gallbladder aspiration and drainage, trans-cystic biliary decompression, dilation of biliary strictures, and stenting of the bile ducts.

In the United States, it has been estimated that approximately 10–15% of the adult population have gallstones. Of this cohort, 1–4% will have gallstone-related symptoms manifest as biliary cholic. Among these, 20% will—approximately 400,000 patients—develop acute complications in the form of acute cholecystitis, choledocholithiasis, gallstone pancreatitis, or gallstone ileus [1–4]. Cholecystectomy remains the standard of care for resolution and prevention of recurrence of these complications. The reported incidence of cholecystectomy is broad, from 600,000 to 1.5 million operations per year in the United States. While there is large variability in the numbers quoted, the overwhelming consensus is that gallbladder pathology is pervasive and the need for intervention is common. That said, despite technical advancement in the surgical treatment of gallbladder disease, complications remain an issue. Overall, the reported complication rates range from 1% to 12%, with a 0.02–0.2% risk of common bile duct injury. While these are relatively low numbers, when applied to the large number of procedures per year, these complication rates become a significant factor in ongoing morbidity and increased cost of care.

PCTs have become a safe tool for the management of acute cholecystitis in patients deemed high risk for operative intervention at the time of their diagnosis. The primary factors influencing fitness for operative intervention include acute critical illness, severity of preexisting comorbid conditions, or a known higher risk of surgery specific complications including bile duct injury [5, 6]. With regard to this patient population, the literature governing the selection criteria of those who would most benefit from PCT placement is quite variable. While a general consensus may not exist, the recently updated 2018 Tokyo Guidelines are frequently used to help differentiate which cohort of patients would qualify and benefit from a PCT [7]. These guidelines established a grading system to classify the severity of acute cholecystitis, Table 7.1.

In general, patients presenting with Tokyo Grade I cholecystitis should be offered

A. Bacon · T. Corgan · T. Pender · A. Colonna (✉)
Department of Surgery, University of Utah, Salt Lake City, UT, USA
e-mail: tony.bacon@hsc.utah.edu; travis.corgan@hsc.utah.edu; tyler.pender@hsc.utah.edu; alexander.colonna@hsc.utah.edu

© Springer Nature Switzerland AG 2021
I. Di Carlo (ed.), *Difficult Acute Cholecystitis*, https://doi.org/10.1007/978-3-030-62102-5_7

Table 7.1 Tokyo grading for acute cholecystitis

Grade	Criteria
Mild (grade 1)	Acute cholecystitis that does not meet the criteria for a more severe grade mild gallbladder inflammation, no organ dysfunction
Moderate (grade 2)	The presence of one or more of the following: Elevated white-cell count (>18,000 cells per cubic millimeter) Palpable, tender mass in the right upper quadrant Duration >72 h Marked local inflammation including biliary peritonitis, pericholecystic abscess, hepatic abscess, gangrenous cholecystitis, emphysematous cholecystitis
Severe (grade 3)	The presence of one or more of the following: Cardiovascular dysfunction (hypotension requiring treatment with dopamine at ≥5 μg per kilogram of body weight per minute or any dose of dobutamine) Neurologic dysfunction (decreased level of consciousness) Respiratory dysfunction (ratio of partial pressure of arterial oxygen to the fraction of inspired oxygen <300) Renal dysfunction (oliguria; creatinine level, >2.0 mg/deciliter) Hepatic dysfunction (prothrombin time—international normalized ratio, >1.5) Hematologic dysfunction (platelet count, <100,000 per cubic millimeter)

cholecystectomy based on response to initial resuscitation. In patients presenting with Tokyo Grade II cholecystitis, every effort should be made to perform a cholecystectomy within 48 h of presentation. However, if the patient has symptoms for more than 3 days, comorbidities that would preclude the use of general anesthesia, advanced metastatic disease, or other history that would further complicate the cholecystectomy, then a PCT should be considered. This consideration can be based upon and standardized through use and application of empiric scoring systems which include, but are not limited to, the Charlson Comorbidity Index and American Society of Anesthesiologists (ASA) Classification. Use of these tools allow institutional development of treatment protocols based upon an individual patient population. In those patients with Tokyo Grade III cholecystitis, a PCT should be strongly considered unless the patient demonstrates a complete response to resuscitation and is otherwise healthy (Fig. 7.1).

7.2 Technique

A PCT is placed under radiologic guidance. Currently, ultrasonography is the most common method used due to its ease of use, portability, and low risk. However, computed tomography (CT) is also frequently used with modern multislice scanners providing a high level of spatial resolution. In contrast to ultrasound machines, CT scanners are more expensive and cumbersome. While this certainly is a factor in modality choice, CT is often more efficacious in those patients where the gallbladder is not easily visualized due to the extent of the acute inflammatory change, body habitus, overlying bowel loops, or other anatomic aberrations (Fig. 7.2).

During placement of a PCT, anesthesia in the form of conscious sedation is administered to the patient. This typically consists of a combination of rapid-onset, short-acting agents that include a narcotic (e.g., fentanyl) for analgesia as well as either a benzodiazepine (e.g., midazolam) or other sedative (e.g., propofol) for anxiolysis and amnesia. Local anesthetic is also frequently used to infiltrate the skin and subcutaneous tissues at the insertion site.

After appropriate level of sedation has been obtained, the Seldinger technique is used to place the PCT. First, an 18–22G needle is used to access the gallbladder. Aspiration of bile (or pus in the case of suppurative cholecystitis) and imaging confirms proper intralumenal placement. The gallbladder aspirate should be sent for microbiologic analysis to include Gram stain, culture, and antibiotic sensitivities. A guidewire is then inserted, and the access needle with-

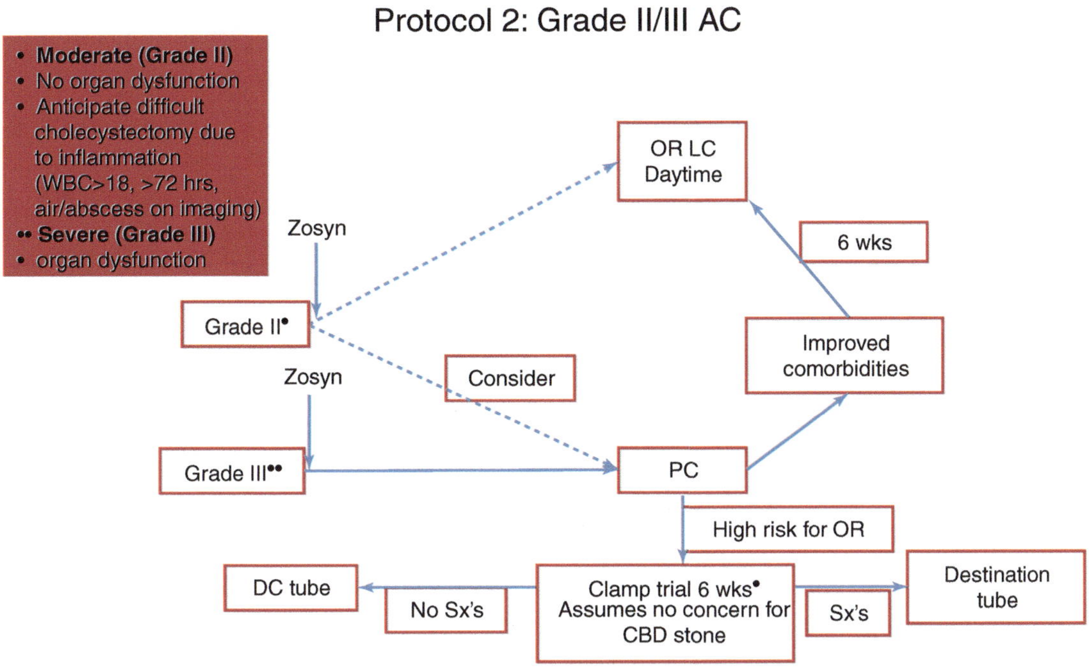

Fig. 7.1 Grade II/III Acute Cholecystitis Algorithm

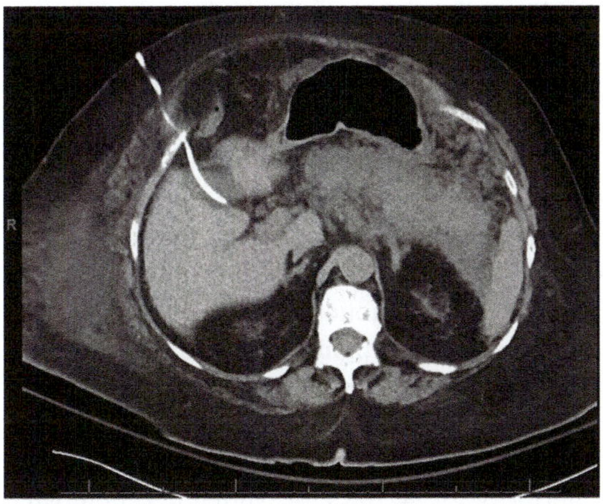

Fig. 7.2 Computed Tomography Guided Percutaneous Cholecystostomy Tube Placement. 74-year-old female with Tokyo Grade III acute cholecystitis, pancreatitis, septic shock, and hypercarbic respiratory failure

drawn. Then, depending on the type and size of the drain to be placed, the tract may need to be dilated. A drain—typically an 8F or 10F pigtail-type—is then advanced over the guidewire into the gallbladder lumen. Finally, a fluoroscopic cholecystogram is typically obtained to confirm placement, evaluate for cystic duct patency, and delineate the extra-cystic ductal anatomy in the porta hepatis [6] (Figs. 7.3 and 7.4).

7.3 Management After Placement

Once the percutaneous cholecystostomy tube (PCT) has been placed, the post-procedural care of the patient is typically managed by the general surgery service. Initial considerations include ensuring source control has been achieved, appropriate resuscitation from the systemic inflammatory response, and treatment of comorbidities. Later, the surgical team will need to determine appropriate discharge disposition and organize close follow-up that will necessarily include ongoing evaluation and management of the PCT, its discontinuation, or planning for interval cholecystectomy.

Intravenous antibiotics started upon diagnosis of acute cholecystitis should be continued.

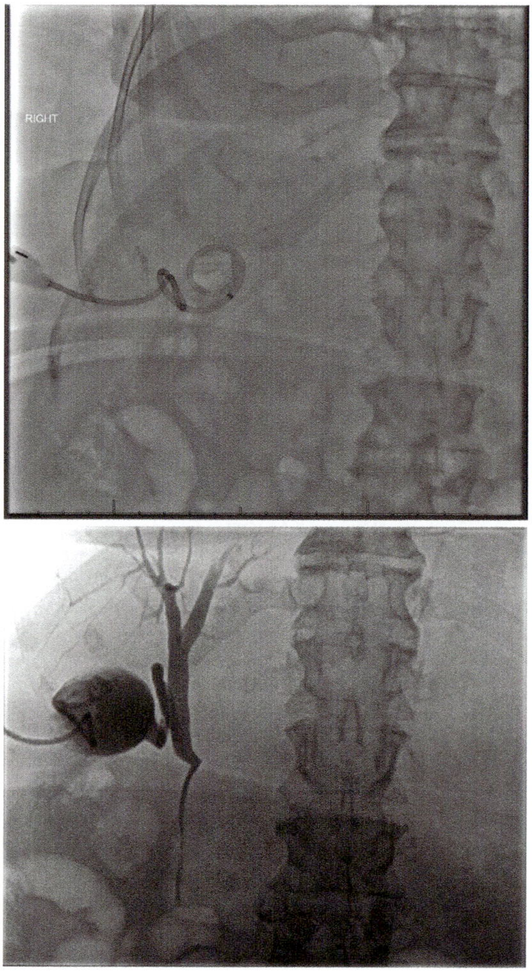

Figs. 7.3 and 7.4 Fluoroscopic Cholangiogram via Percutaneous Cholecystostomy. 74-year-old female with Tokyo Grade III acute cholecystitis, pancreatitis, septic shock, and hypercarbic respiratory failure

Immediately after successful placement, the patient may clinically worsen. Patients can demonstrate an escalation of the systemic inflammatory response that may be worse than on initial presentation; including fever, diaphoresis, tachycardia, and hypotension, and, in the worst case, evidence of end-organ hypoperfusion leading to organ dysfunction. This response is presumed to be secondary to transient bacteremia and systemic inflammation caused by the drain placement. Appropriate steps are necessarily taken to monitor the patient's hemodynamics based on the degree of their response. Should the patient

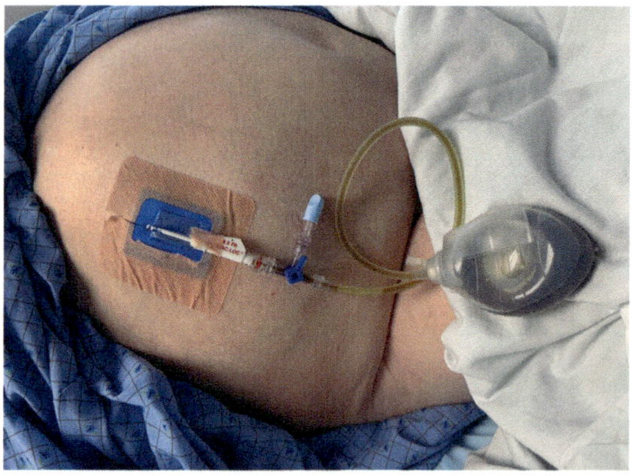

Fig. 7.5 Patient with Cholecystostomy Tube in Place

begin to decompensate, they will likely warrant a higher level of care with advanced therapies. Despite the potential for clinical decline, it is important to note most patients do not have these issues and experience symptomatic relief within 24 h of placement [8] (Fig. 7.5).

Once the patient has demonstrated clinical improvement, the decision must be made regarding the duration of antibiotic therapy. Traditionally, despite little high-quality data to guide decision-making, the duration of antibiotics following PCT has been 7–10 days or upon resolution of symptoms and/or various clinical parameters. However, given continually mounting concerns regarding antibiotic stewardship, the current overall trend in the management of intra-abdominal sepsis has been to decrease the duration of antibiotic therapy. This change in management paradigm was, in part, initiated as a result of the often-quoted Study to Optimize Peritoneal Infection Therapy (STOP-IT) trial. This randomized trial demonstrated the non-inferiority of 4 days of antibiotics compared to 8 days following abdominal surgical source control. It is crucial to note, however, that in this study only 10.8% of those patients had biliary infections. Further, the number treated with cholecystectomy was not reported [9]. That said, several smaller studies have shown the non-inferiority of antibiotic treatment regimens of less than a week in patients treated with PCT [10, 11]. With deference to this trend and the mounting data in support of shorter antibiotic duration, the 2018 Tokyo Guidelines suggest a duration of 4–7 days of antibiotics even for patients with systemic manifestations of cholecystitis (i.e., Grade III) following PCT placement [7].

The antibiotic regimen selected should be guided by the bile culture obtained during PCT placement as well as the local antibiogram. In general, coverage should initially consist of broad-spectrum agents that can be narrowed as dictated by the culture results. In patients with Grade III cholecystitis, an anti-pseudomonal agent is recommended [7]. Of note, there is debate about whether consideration should be given to a more prolonged course should cultures grow Gram positive organisms. In this case, there is conflicting evidence with respect to the optimal duration, with some advocating for 2-week duration. This represents an important exception to the 4- to 7-day paradigm. Finally, antibiotic selection and duration should be discussed with an interdisciplinary team prior to discharge [12]. In our practice, antibiotics are transitioned from IV to oral within 24 h provided the patient demonstrates clinical improvement. Patients are discharged on oral antibiotics for a total course of 4–7 days at the discretion of the attending surgeon.

With resolution of symptoms, a diet can be reintroduced and advanced as tolerated following PCT placement. The patient is appropriate for discharge with resolution of symptoms, normalization of physiology, and intake of adequate enteral nutrition. Clearly, the cohort of patients who receive a PCT will have factors making a routine discharge home not feasible. Each patient will necessarily need individualized case management and coordination, preferably by a multidisciplinary team.

An important consideration is ensuring the PCT is managed properly after discharge. Careful patient education prior to discharge is essential for both the patient and the healthcare system as most reinterventions are due to tube dislodgement [13, 14]. The patient or appropriate caregiver should be educated in how to care for the tube and its external apparatus in order to maintain proper positioning and patency. In addition, they should be instructed in how to record daily outputs as this will help the surgical team with future clinical decision-making.

In our practice, follow up is performed at 2 weeks from discharge from the hospital. An interim history is obtained, and physical exam performed. The drain output record is reviewed. In the event of output greater than 100 ml/day, the PCT is interrogated for distal obstruction via trans-PCT cholangiography. Provided output is less than 100 ml/day and the patient remains asymptomatic, the decision upon whether to perform an interval cholecystectomy or continue nonoperative management with the PCT as destination therapy can then be considered.

7.4 Interval Cholecystectomy

At the 2-week follow-up, if the patient has shown improvement and is deemed a potential candidate to proceed with interval cholecystectomy, steps are taken to optimize them for surgery. The primary areas to address include all comorbidities that initially prompted the placement of the PCT. A plan should be established with the patient to optimize their functional status with a specific exercise program. Diet plans and nutrition goals should be discussed. Any specialists or consultants necessary to achieve these goals should be involved.

In our practice, the patient will return for a second follow-up in 4 weeks (6 weeks after PCT placement) to be reevaluated. Should the patient remain a candidate for surgery, elective cholecystectomy can be scheduled at that time. We have shown that tube removal without interval cholecystectomy confers a 10.6% incidence of recurrent cholecystitis, so every effort is made to maintain patency of the tube until operation [13]. Otherwise, the patient will remain in the nonoperative management algorithm. The PCT should remain in place until the time of surgery because of the risk of recurrence [15]. Ultimately, the optimal timing of the surgery varies widely in the surgical literature. However, generally accepted criteria for interval cholecystectomy include complete resolution of symptoms and fitness to undergo general anesthesia. We do not offer the surgery until a minimum of 6 weeks after placement of the PCT but as soon as possible thereafter.

A recent study has shown that younger patients, those with fewer comorbidities, and those presenting with lower APACHE II scores were more likely to progress to interval cholecystectomy. During the postoperative period, 5% of these patients suffered a major postoperative complication with 12% of patients having complication manifest from prior comorbidity [14]. These data are similar to other studies reporting on the total perioperative morbidity for initial cholecystectomy in acute cholecystitis [16]. However, despite these promising statistics, the degree of acute and chronic inflammation may complicate the operation, making the critical view of safety harder to obtain. This subsequent technical difficulty is likely responsible for some studies suggesting a higher rate (10%) of biliary complications in cholecystectomy in patients who had undergone preoperative PCT [17]. While the literature is clear with respect to the benefit of proceeding with interval cholecystectomy in appropriate patients, the increased rate of complications shows the importance of ensuring these operations are under optimal operative conditions.

7.5 Nonoperative Management

If a patient presents at the 2-week follow-up and is deemed to have medical conditions precluding them from an interval cholecystectomy, they remain in the nonoperative management algorithm. The primary factor prompting ongoing nonoperative management is continuing medical comorbidities felt to elevate the risks of cholecystectomy beyond the morbidity of the PCT. Disseminated malignancy or a short life expectancy is an additional indication for definitive nonoperative management.

In the case that cholecystectomy is prohibitive, the PCT is then interrogated. If the output is low (less than 100 ml/day), the PCT is clamped. During the trial, patients are instructed to keep the PCT clamped unless they have recurrence of their original symptoms. In this case, they are instructed to unclamp the PCT in order to decompress the biliary system. Patients then return to clinic in 6 weeks with repeat imaging, dedicated right upper quadrant or CT.

While the data suggest decreased complications with PCT, its discontinuation, if appropriate, is seen as preferable with respect to patient comfort, risk of drain-related complication, and burden on the healthcare system [17]. While this is a generally agreed-upon principle, there is no consensus in the current literature on the ideal timing for PCT removal [18]. In our practice, the PCT is removed if the patient continues to have comorbidities or malignancy precluding operative intervention but remains asymptomatic during the subsequent clamp trial. However, patients with residual gallstones have a higher risk for recurrence even if asymptomatic during the 4 weeks of the clamp trial. In this setting, this risk in some studies is as high as 41% [19]. If available, percutaneous gallstone extraction can be offered. Conversely, despite having more comorbidities precluding safe interval cholecystectomy, patients with acalculous cholecystitis have a lower risk for recurrence [20].

If the patient develops recurrent symptoms during the clamp trial, the PCT is left in place and becomes destination therapy. The PCT is then used as needed to decompress the biliary system with the onset of recurrent symptoms. Close follow-up must be maintained to ensure the frequent decompression does not result in depletion of bile salts and subsequent nutritional deficiencies. In our practice, if the PCT is deemed to be destination therapy, care of the patient is transitioned from the general surgery to the interventional radiology service once out of the acute period. The intervention radiologists then maintain the drain with follow-up approximately every 12 weeks for PCT exchange [13].

Finally, an emerging alternative to committing patients to a destination PCT is endoscopic decompression of the gallbladder into the gastrointestinal lumen with self-expanding stent placement. Initial studies have shown a high success rate and comparable outcomes to PCT placement [21, 22]. While the goal of endoscopic decompression is to serve as a temporizing procedure prior to cholecystectomy, chronic inflammation and scar formation may make future operation difficult. Further investigation is needed to determine if endoscopic drainage and stent placement can serve as a stand-alone procedure.

7.6 Conclusion

PCT is an appropriate therapy for severe acute cholecystitis (Tokyo Grade III), or acute cholecystitis in patients who are at high risk for general anesthesia and cholecystectomy due to advanced malignancy or medical comorbidities (Tokyo Grade II). After the PCT is placed and the patient recovers from their acute illness, the treatment team will have to decide if the PCT will be a bridge to cholecystectomy or destination therapy. In select patients who are not operative candidates and meet criteria, the PCT may be eventually removed with acceptable rates of recurrence.

References

1. Simorov A, Ranade A, Parcells J, et al. Emergent cholecystostomy is superior to open cholecystectomy in extremely ill patients with acalculous cholecystitis: a large multicenter outcome study. Am J Surg. 2013;206(6):935e940; discussion 40-1
2. Viste A, Jensen D, Angelsen J, Hoem D. Percutaneous cholecystostomy in acute cholecystitis; a retrospective analysis of a large series of 104 patients. BMC Surg. 2015;15:17.
3. Welschbillig-Meunier K, Pessaux P, Lebigot J, et al. Percutaneous cholecystostomy for high-risk patients with acute cholecystitis. Surg Endosc. 2005;19(9):1256e1259.
4. Hassler KR, Jones MW. Laparoscopic cholecystectomy [Updated 2019 Mar 22]. In: StatPearls [Internet]. Treasure Island, FL: StatPearls Publishing; 2019. https://www.ncbi.nlm.nih.gov/books/NBK448145/.
5. Blythe J, Herrmann E, Faust D, Falk S, Edwards-Lehr T, Stockhausen F, Hanisch E, Buia A. Acute cholecystitis - a cohort study in a real-world clinical setting (REWO study, NCT02796443). Pragmat Obs Res. 2018;9:69–75.
6. Gulaya K, Desai SS, Sato K. Percutaneous cholecystostomy: evidence-based current clinical practice. Semin Intervent Radiol. 2016;33(4):291–6. https://doi.org/10.1055/s-0036-1592326.
7. Mayumi T, Okamoto K, Takada T, et al. Tokyo guidelines 2018: management bundles for acute cholangitis and cholecystitis. J Hepatobiliary Pancreat Sci. 2018;25(1):96–100.
8. Miura F, Takada T, Strasberg SM, et al. TG13 flowchart for the management of acute cholangitis and cholecystitis. J Hepatobiliary Pancreat Sci. 2013;20:47–54.
9. Sawyer RG, Claridge JA, Nathens AB, Rotstein OD, Duane TM, Evans HL, et al. Trial of short-course antimicrobial therapy for intraabdominal infection. N Engl J Med. 2015;372(21):1996–2005.
10. Walker C, Young K, Moosavi A, Molacek N, Dove J, Hunsinger M, et al. Cancel that PICC line order; cholecystostomy tube and short course of antibiotics. Am J Surg. 2019;217(3):485–9.
11. Loftus TJ, Brakenridge SC, Dessaigne CG, Sarosi GA Jr, Zingarelli WJ, Moore FA, et al. Antibiotics may be safely discontinued within one week of percutaneous cholecystostomy. World J Surg. 2017;41(5):1239–45.
12. Gomi H, Solomkin JS, Schlossberg D, Okamoto K, Takada T, Strasberg SM, et al. Tokyo guidelines 2018: antimicrobial therapy for acute cholangitis and cholecystitis. J Hepatobiliary Pancreat Sci. 2018;25(1):3–16.
13. Colonna AL, Griffiths TM, Robison DC, Enniss TM, Young JB, McCrum ML, et al. Cholecystostomy: are we using it correctly? Am J Surg. 2019;217(6):1010–5.
14. Yeo CS, Tay VW, Low JK, Woon WW, Punamiya SJ, Shelat VG. Outcomes of percutaneous cholecystostomy and predictors of eventual cholecystectomy. J Hepatobiliary Pancreat Sci. 2016;23(1):65–73.
15. Chou CK, Lee KC, Chan CC, Perng CL, Chen CK, Fang WL, et al. Early percutaneous cholecystostomy in severe acute cholecystitis reduces the complication rate and duration of hospital stay. Medicine (Baltimore). 2015;94(27):e1096.
16. Gutt CN, Encke J, Köninger J, Harnoss J-C, Weigand K, Kipfmüller K, et al. Acute cholecystitis. Ann Surg. 2013;258(3):385–93.
17. Mizrahi I, Mazeh H, Yuval JB, Almogy G, Bala M, Simanovski N, et al. Perioperative outcomes of delayed laparoscopic cholecystectomy for acute calculous cholecystitis with and without percutaneous cholecystostomy. Surgery. 2015;158(3):728–35.
18. Macchini DDL, Oldani M, Leni D, Padalino P, Romano F, Gianotti L. Timing of percutaneous cholecystostomy tube removal: systematic review. Minerva Chir. 2016;71:6.
19. McKay A, Abulfaraj M, Lipschitz J. Short- and long-term outcomes following percutaneous cholecystostomy for acute cholecystitis in high-risk patients. Surg Endosc. 2012;26(5):1343–51.
20. Abbas SH, Ghazanfar MA, Gordon-Weeks AN, Reddy SR, Soonawalla Z, Silva MA. Acalculous cholecystitis: is an elective interval cholecystectomy necessary. Dig Surg. 2018;35(2):171–6.

21. Penas-Herrero I, de la Serna-Higuera C, Perez-Miranda M. Endoscopic ultrasound-guided gallbladder drainage for the management of acute cholecystitis (with video). J Hepatobiliary Pancreat Sci. 2015;22(1):35–43.

22. Jang JW, Lee SS, Song TJ, Hyun YS, Park DY, Seo DW, et al. Endoscopic ultrasound-guided transmural and percutaneous transhepatic gallbladder drainage are comparable for acute cholecystitis. Gastroenterology. 2012;142(4):805–11.

Difficult Laparoscopic Cholecystectomy: Intraoperative Evaluation

8

Philip J. Townend, Rupaly Pande, Henry Bergmann, and Ewen A. Griffiths

8.1 Introduction

Since the 1990s, laparoscopic cholecystectomy has become the 'gold standard' treatment for gall stone disease [1]. Initially there was some controversy due to a higher reported rate of bile duct injury (BDI) and vasculobiliary injuries (VBI); however, this was principally a learning curve issue, and a large study of over half a million patients over a 30-year period has shown LC has become safer over time. It found that reported rates of BDI have reduced over time (1994–1999: 0.69% (range 0.52–0.84%) versus 2010–2015 0.22% (range 0.02–0.40%); $p = 0.011$) [2]. In addition, there has also been a decrease in conversion to open surgery rates. LC has subsequently been shown to be equally as safe with no increased risk of BDI, shorter hospital stay and decreased overall hospital costs even when some LC has increased operating times [3]. LC is now a very common operation which may vary in operative difficulty. For example, it can be a routine operation comfortably performed by a training grade surgeon (with appropriate supervision) but, at its most difficult, can tax even the most experienced specialist surgeon. The difficult LC is associated with higher operative duration, conversion to open surgery, 30-day complications and 30-day reintervention [4].

The difficult LC can often be predicted based on preoperative evaluation as discussed in previous chapters. The authors of this chapter recommend the use of the choles difficult laparoscopic cholecystectomy score which is preoperative score developed from two large, high-quality prospective series of cholecystectomy patients [5]. The score includes factors which were independently associated with difficulty and included increasing age, ASA score, male gender, diagnosis of CBD stone or cholecystitis, thick-walled gallbladders, CBD dilation, use of preoperative ERCP and non-elective operations. This can allow the surgical team (surgeon, anaesthetist, trainees, theatre staff, etc) to plan for extra theatre time and specialist equipment on standby, if necessary, or refer out to a specialist. There are times however when the operative conditions can come as a surprise, and the surgeon needs to know how to adapt to the hostile operating conditions. These cases can present in both emergency and elective settings.

This chapter will discuss the intraoperative evaluation the surgeon must undertake to tackle

P. J. Townend
Consultant Upper GI Surgeon, Department of Upper GI Surgery, Gold Coast University Hospital, Gold Coast Health, Gold Coast, QLD, Australia

R. Pande
Department of HPB Surgery, Queen Elizabeth Hospital, University Hospitals Birmingham NHS Foundation Trust, Birmingham, UK

H. Bergmann · E. A. Griffiths (✉)
Department of Upper GI Surgery, Queen Elizabeth Hospital, University Hospitals Birmingham NHS Foundation Trust, Birmingham, UK
e-mail: Ewen.griffiths@uhb.nhs.uk

© Springer Nature Switzerland AG 2021
I. Di Carlo (ed.), *Difficult Acute Cholecystitis*, https://doi.org/10.1007/978-3-030-62102-5_8

the difficult gallbladder (GB). We will also discuss some helpful grading systems for standardise assessment and evaluation of difficult cases, safe dissection approaches with respect to key anatomical features and specific operative scenarios which may challenge the surgeon. It must be remembered that the surgeon's primary objective is to avoid BDI and VBI. The secondary objective is to remove the gallbladder. Bail out options to avoid injury to the patient include performing a subtotal cholecystectomy (reconstituting or fenestrated) [6], cholecystostomy drainage tube insertion, open conversion or abandoning the operation entirely and referral to a specialist hepatobiliary surgeon.

8.2 Gallbladder Difficulty: Intraoperative Features

Whilst there are a variety of preoperative variables which are reliable predictors of the difficult LC, it is only when the gallbladder and liver are visualised laparoscopically (or not if the adhesions and inflammation are so extensive) that the true nature of how difficult the operation may be becomes apparent. Intraoperative features which are associated with a difficult cholecystectomy are shown in Table 8.1, categorised between those related to the gallbladder and those unrelated to the gallbladder. Very few of these factors are reversible, although it is recognised that there is still a place for delayed cholecystectomy in certain scenarios—that is, when a patient is admitted acutely with cholecystitis and treated conservatively and brought back in for a planned cholecystectomy after around 6–8 weeks of 'cooling' off to allow safe laparoscopic cholecystectomy [7, 8]. Scenarios where this might be appropriate include when the duration of cholecystitis is greater than 7 days (as cholecystectomy can be extremely challenging within this time frame) or when the patient is borderline fit for surgery and requires medical optimisation prior to surgery.

Obesity and non-alcoholic fatty liver disease are known to increase the difficulty of LC (due to access issues and difficultly in retracting the liver due to stiffness) and in the elective setting this should be addressed with appropriate lifestyle advice. A randomised trial of a 2-week very low calorie diet (VLCD) in obese patients has been shown to reduce operating times and make obtaining the critical view easier [9]. The authors of this chapter use this VLCD in patients with known fatty liver or whose BMI is over 35 to make laparoscopic surgery easier. Patients who comply with this VLCD have been shown to have easier operations due to the weight loss and easier retraction of the liver, so explaining the rationale for the diet and its importance is paramount [10]. There are a variety of VLCD plans which include either commercial shakes, calorie counting or a 'milk and yoghurt' diet plan.

Table 8.1 Intraoperative features that make laparoscopic cholecystectomy more difficult

Factors related to the gallbladder	Intra-abdominal factors unrelated to the gallbladder
Gallbladder adhesions (acute or chronic)	Adhesions (from previous operations)
Fibrosis and scarring of the gallbladder	Obesity and excessive visceral fat
Fibrosis and scarring of the hepato-cystic triangle	Non-alcoholic fatty liver disease
Atrophic or contracted gallbladder	Cirrhotic liver
Intrahepatic gallbladder	Biliary anomalies
Impacted stone in the neck of the gallbladder	Vascular anomalies
Cystic duct and CBD stones	Left-sided gallbladder
Gallbladder necrosis	Situs inversus
Mirizzi syndrome	Other liver pathology, for example large liver cysts
Abscess formation	
Perforated gallbladder	
Cholecystectomy tube in situ	
Cholecystoenteric fistula	

8.3 Intraoperative Gallbladder Difficulty Scores

Being able to stratify intraoperative difficulty with a simple scale of operative difficulty has the advantages of assisting in intraoperative strategy and planning; allowing comparison across different research studies; facilitating risk adjustment for surgical outcomes and providing an aid in training surgeons and monitoring of training progression. Several intraoperative scoring and other scoring systems have developed for the use in cholecystectomy. These include the Nassar scale [4, 11], Cuschieri scale [12], Parkland scale [13, 14], WSES score [15], the American Association for the Surgery of Trauma (AAST) [16] and Tokyo Guidelines Grading for cholecystitis [17] (Tables 8.2 and 8.3). Each of these have different systems of grading the operative difficulty, although broadly similar, and most have been correlated with post-operative outcomes. Only the Nassar score has been validated in two large prospective series of patients and is correlated with worsening outcomes (including operative duration, conversion to open surgery, 30-day mortality and 30-day complications) [4, 11]. In addition, a preoperative risk prediction score is available which correlates with the Nassar score intraoperatively [5]. Whilst the other scores do have utility, the authors would recommend the Nassar scale for these reasons. This simple operative difficulty scale can be used by multiple grades of surgeons (including trainees and consultants) and remain highly clinically relevant. It therefore provides a tool for reporting disease and intraoperative severity and can reliably be utilised in future research to adjust outcomes according to case mix and intraoperative difficulty. It is recommended that grading systems should be routinely used in all cholecystectomies and recorded in the operative report.

8.4 General Safe Dissection Approaches

Safe dissection approaches also include calm decision-making during the operation and the ability to adapt and change the operation and 'bail out if necessary' to avoid BDI or VBI (Fig. 8.1). It is important during difficult LC for the surgeon to orientate themselves multiple times during the procedure to important landmarks such as the duodenum, colon, hepatoduodenal ligament, bile duct, hepatic artery, Rouviere's sulcus, segment 4 of the liver and the more recently described R4U line [18]. This is especially true when attempting to dissect out the critical view of safety where risk of BDI is greatest. It has been shown that the most bile duct injuries during LC occur due to misperception of the anatomy as opposed to faults in technical skills or knowledge. An analysis of 252 laparoscopic bile duct injuries showed 97% of cases were due to a visual perception illusion and found only 3% due to faults in technique and skill [19]. We will discuss some useful anatomical landmarks to identify the 'safe' zones and 'danger' zones of dissection and the rationale for using them. We will also discuss the importance of the critical view of safety (CVS) in the difficult LC and the reason why it is preferable but not paramount to achieve in all cases, especially when there are other safer surgical alternatives.

8.5 Rouviere's Sulcus

Rouviere's sulcus was originally described by French anatomist Henre Rouviere in 1924, over 60 years before the first laparoscopic cholecystectomy [20]. It is found to the right of the hepatoduodenal ligament, is normally about 2–3 cm long, is anterior to the caudate lobe and usually contains the right portal structures (right portal vein, right hepatic artery and right hepatic duct) [21]. It is found in approximately 80% of patients. When the fundus of the gallbladder is retracted cephalad, the common bile duct will be found below the anterior leaf of the sulcus and the cystic duct and artery will lie above it. In 2002, Hugh developed a surgical checklist that was used for all operations including using Rouviere's sulcus as a reference point and to begin surgical dissection ventral to this [22]. Hugh published on a single surgeon series of 2000 consecutive LCs, which included a supervised environment with trainees performing the operations without a single major bile duct injury.

Table 8.2 Nassar, Cushieri, Parkland and WSES G10 scores for assessing and scoring intraoperative difficulty scores for cholecystectomy

Nassar scale [4, 11]	Cuschieri scale [12]	Parkland scale [13, 14]	*WSES G10 score* [15]
Grade 1: *Gallbladder*: Floppy, non-adherent *Cystic pedicle*: Thin and clear *Adhesions*: Simple up to the neck/Hartmann's pouch **Grade 2:** *Gallbladder*: Mucocele, packed with stones *Cystic pedicle*: Fat laden *Adhesions*: Simple up to the body **Grade 3:** *Gallbladder*: Deep fossa, acute cholecystitis, contracted, fibrosis, Hartmann's pouch adherent to CBD, impaction *Cystic pedicle*: Abnormal anatomy or cystic duct—Short, dilated or obscured *Adhesions*: Dense up to fundus; involving hepatic flexure or duodenum **Grade 4:** *Gallbladder*: Completely obscured, empyema, gangrene, mass *Cystic pedicle*: Impossible to clarify *Adhesions*: Dense, fibrosis, wrapping the gallbladder, duodenum or hepatic flexure difficult to separate	**Grade 1:** Easy/ uncomplicated cholecystectomy **Grade 2:** Medium difficulty, for example mild cholecystitis, cystic duct or artery obscured by adhesions or fatty tissue; mucocele may be present **Grade 3:** Difficult cholecystectomy due to either gangrenous cholecystitis; shrunken fibrotic gallbladder; severe cholecystitis; subhepatic abscess formation; Hartmann's pouch adherent to the CHD; cases in which the cystic duct or artery are difficult or impossible to dissect or liver cirrhosis with portal hypertension **Grade 4:** Conversion to open surgery is required	**Grade 1:** Normal gallbladder/no adhesions **Grade 2:** Minor adhesions at the neck **Grade 3:** Presence of ANY of the following: Hyperaemia, pericholecystic fluid, adhesions to the body, distended gallbladder **Grade 4:** Presence of ANY of the following: Adhesions obscuring majority of gallbladder or grade I–III with abnormal liver anatomy, intrahepatic gallbladder or impacted stone (Mirizzi) **Grade 5:** Presence of ANY of the following: Perforation, necrosis, inability to visualise the gallbladder due to adhesions	**Gallbladder appearance** Adhesions <50% of GB (1 point) Adhesions burying GB (3 points) **Distension/ contraction** Distended GB (or contracted shrivelled GB) (1 point) Unable to grasp with atraumatic laparoscopic forceps (1 point) Stone ≥1 cm impacted in Hartmann's pouch (1 point) **Access** BMI >30 (1 point) Adhesions from previous surgery limiting access (1 point) **Severe sepsis/ complications** Bile or pus outside GB (1 point) Time to identify cystic artery and duct >90 min (1 point) **Difficulty** (A) Mild <2 (B) Moderate = 2–4 (C) Severe = 5–7 (D) Extreme = 8–10
Correlation with outcome data available? Yes; outcome reports from a prospective single surgeon series of 4089 patients and validation in a large multicentre prospective cohort of 8820. Increasingly difficulty associated with worse clinical outcomes including 30-day complications, reintervention, length of stay and conversion to open surgery. Independent on multivariate analysis	**Correlation with outcome data available?** **No**	**Correlation with outcome data available?** Outcome data available for 50 patients showing increasing severity was associated with longer operating times, length of stay and post-operative bile leaks	**Correlation with outcome data available?** Conversion occurred in 33% of patients with G10 scores of ≥5 in a prospective multicentre study of 504 patients

Table 8.3 The American Association for the Surgery of Trauma (AAST) grading of Cholecystectomy Difficulty and the 2018 Tokyo Guidelines. Grading for cholecystitis

American Association for the Surgery of Trauma (AAST) grading of cholecystectomy difficulty [16, 31]	2018 Tokyo Guidelines Grading for cholecystitis [16, 17]
Grade 1 is acute cholecystitis **Grade 2** is gangrenous or emphysematous cholecystitis **Grade 3** is localised perforation **Grade 4** is GB perforation with pericholecystic abscess or gastrointestinal fistula **Grade 5** is GB perforation with generalised peritonitis	**Grade I**: Acute cholecystitis does not meet the criteria of "Grade III" or "Grade II" acute cholecystitis. It can also be defined as acute cholecystitis in a healthy patient with no organ dysfunction and mild inflammatory changes in the gallbladder, making cholecystectomy a safe and low-risk operative procedure **Grade II**: Acute cholecystitis is associated with any one of the following conditions: 1. Elevated WBC count (>18,000/mm^3) 2. Palpable tender mass in the right upper abdominal quadrant 3. Duration of complaints >72 h 4. Marked local inflammation (gangrenous cholecystitis, pericholecystic abscess, hepatic abscess, biliary peritonitis, emphysematous cholecystitis) **Grade III**: Acute cholecystitis is associated with dysfunction of any one of the following organs/systems: 1. Cardiovascular dysfunction: Hypotension requiring treatment with dopamine ≥5 μg/kg per min, or any dose of norepinephrine 2. Neurological dysfunction: Decreased level of consciousness 3. Respiratory dysfunction: PaO2/FiO2 ratio < 300 4. Renal dysfunction: Oliguria, creatinine >2.0 mg/dl 5. Hepatic dysfunction: PT-INR >1.5 6. Haematological dysfunction: Platelet count <100,000/mm^3
Correlation with outcome data available? Incidence of complications, LOS, ICU use and any adverse event increased with increasing anatomic grade when assessed in a retrospective cohort of 315 patients [16]	**Correlation with outcome data available?** Whilst the 2018 Tokyo guidelines for grading the severity of cholecystitis are based on a combination of laboratory and clinical features as well as intraoperative findings, multiple studies have associated increasing grades of cholecystitis to be associated with length of stay, conversion to open surgery, 30-day mortality and post-operative complications [17]

8.6 R4U Line

The 'R4U line' is a more recently described term that builds on the anatomical principals behind the dissection rules developed, starting dissection above Rouviere's sulcus (Fig. 8.2). It involves an imaginary line from Rouviere's sulcus to the base of segment 4 towards the umbilical fissure [18]. The base of segment 4 often forms a ledge over the left portal pedicle and extends to the left to end at the umbilical fissure. Above the R4U line is the safe zone of dissection containing the gallbladder, cystic duct and cystic artery. Below the R4U line is the 'danger zone' of dissection and contains the common bile duct, hepatic artery and portal vein. In the absence of Rouviere's sulcus, it can still be used as a reference point and give the surgeon an idea of where Rouviere's sulcus should be if it were present.

8.7 Critical View of Safety

When LC was introduced as an alternative to open cholecystectomy, there was an increase incidence of bile duct injuries [23]. The most common cause of bile duct injury or 'classic injury' being mistaking the CBD or aberrant right hepatic duct to be the cystic duct [24]. Strasberg et al. described the critical view of

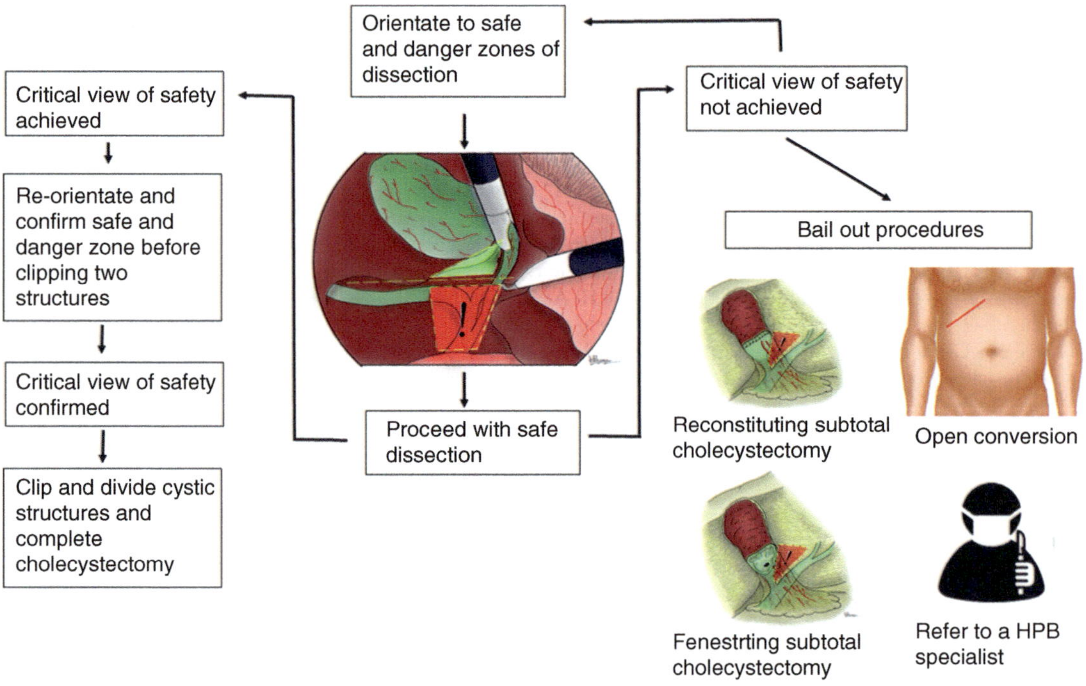

Fig. 8.1 Algorithm for safe dissection in the difficult laparoscopic cholecystectomy and appropriate bail out options should the critical view of safety not be achieved. The zone of safe dissection is shown with the danger zone. (Courtesy of H. Bergmann)

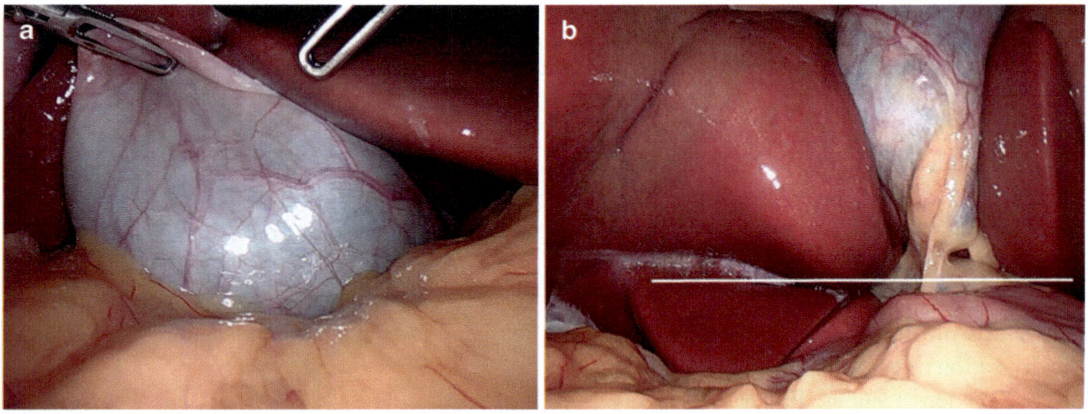

Fig. 8.2 (**a**)—Nassar Grade 1 cholecystectomy with a thin walled gallbladder and no inflammation or adhesions. (**b**)—Zone of safe dissection in laparoscopic cholecystectomy with the R4U line shown

safety (CVS) and how it should be achieved prior to clipping and dividing any ductal structure so to avoid BDI [25]. The CVS has three components:

1. The fibrous and fatty tissue is dissected off the hepatocystic (HC) triangle.
2. At least one-third of the gallbladder dissected from the gallbladder fossa/cystic plate.
3. Only two structures (cystic artery and cystic duct) are seen entering the gallbladder.

Using this method of dissection allows the surgeon to stay high and away from the cystic duct–

CBD junction and thus reducing the risk of BDI. Only once the CVS is achieved can the surgeon confidently identify the cystic duct and artery, prior to clipping and dividing them. The end result of CVS dissection is seeing the two structures entering the gallbladder and having a third of the gallbladder dissected free to avoid the risk of injuring a looping CBD. Most surgeons attempt to dissect out the HC triangle prior to taking the gallbladder off the cystic plate, particularly in the elective cases. However, in the setting of a difficult LC, sometimes the safer option will be to start dissecting the gallbladder off the liver half way up and creating a tunnel. This often allows better lateral retraction of the gallbladder and makes it safer and easier to dissect out the HC triangle and eventually achieve a critical view.

8.8 Specific Scenarios Which Make Cholecystectomy Difficult

8.8.1 Biliary and Vascular Anomalies

There are a wide variety of biliary and vascular anomalies which might make laparoscopic cholecystectomy more difficult.

The common biliary anomalies are illustrated in Fig. 8.3. Luckily, because current methods of teaching advocate high dissection and avoid precise identification of the common bile duct and biliary tree, lots of these anomalies go unnoticed by the surgeon. Those of particular note include where the cystic duct is either absent or fibrosed to the CBD as this makes operating hazardous. A wide cystic duct poses a challenge for safe ligation and in this case, when it is confirmed to be the cystic duct, either by the critical view or by intraoperative cholangiogram, ligation can be either with a large Hemolock clip or by suture ligation with an intra-corporeal knot or an endoloop (Fig. 8.4). It is worthy of note that a cystic duct which is larger than a standard clip should be suspected to be the CBD until proven otherwise. Accessory right hepatic ducts can be injured as they can be superficial and lie close to the gallbladder bed, and the management of these is out with the scope of this chapter. However, if any significant biliary abnormality is seen at cholecystectomy and the critical view is in doubt, an intraoperative cholangiogram is recommended.

The cystic artery is usually a single branch of the right hepatic artery in 80% of cases. Vascular anomalies of the cystic artery include the cystic artery passing anterior to the common hepatic/bile duct (17.9%); a short (<1 cm) cystic artery (9.5%); multiple cystic arteries (8.9%) or the cystic artery located inferior to the cystic duct (4.9%).

Anomalies of the right hepatic artery (RHA) are common and can make cholecystectomy difficult. A replaced RHA may be confused as the cystic artery and inadvertently ligated during cholecystectomy; if this is also associated with a CBD injury this has a poor prognosis as a simple biliary reconstruction may not be possible and a liver resection and more complex reconstruction may be required.

8.9 Acute Cholecystitis

When acute cholecystitis is present and an obstructing stone is found in the cystic duct or Hartmann's pouch, the gallbladder can be extremely distended (Fig. 8.5a). In this scenario, the gallbladder should be aspirated to allow grasping and retraction (Fig. 8.5b). Inflammatory adhesions are best dealt with a combination of blunt and sharp dissection (Fig. 8.5c). The surgeon should be cognisant of the risk of injury to the duodenum or transverse colon which can be stuck and fibrosed to the gallbladder in this area. This scenario is likely if the cholecystitis is advanced and has been going on for many days (>7 days) or if a fistula is present. Necrotising cholecystitis with gallbladder wall necrosis (Fig. 8.5d) is usually easy to separate from the liver if the correct plane is entered. However, as these operations are usually more bloody and have a risk of post-operative collections or bile leaks the surgeon should consider the need to place an abdominal drain at the conclusion of surgery.

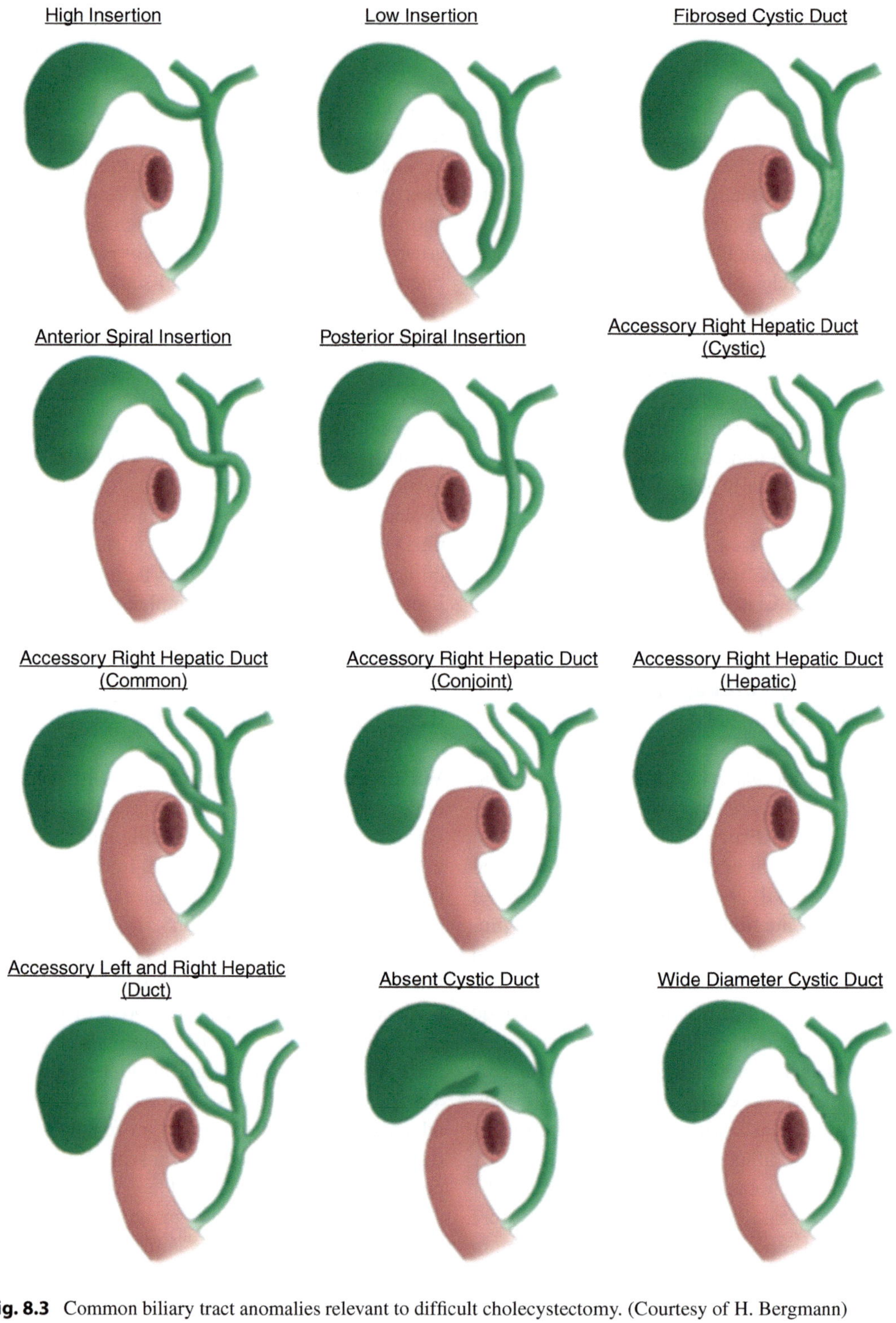

Fig. 8.3 Common biliary tract anomalies relevant to difficult cholecystectomy. (Courtesy of H. Bergmann)

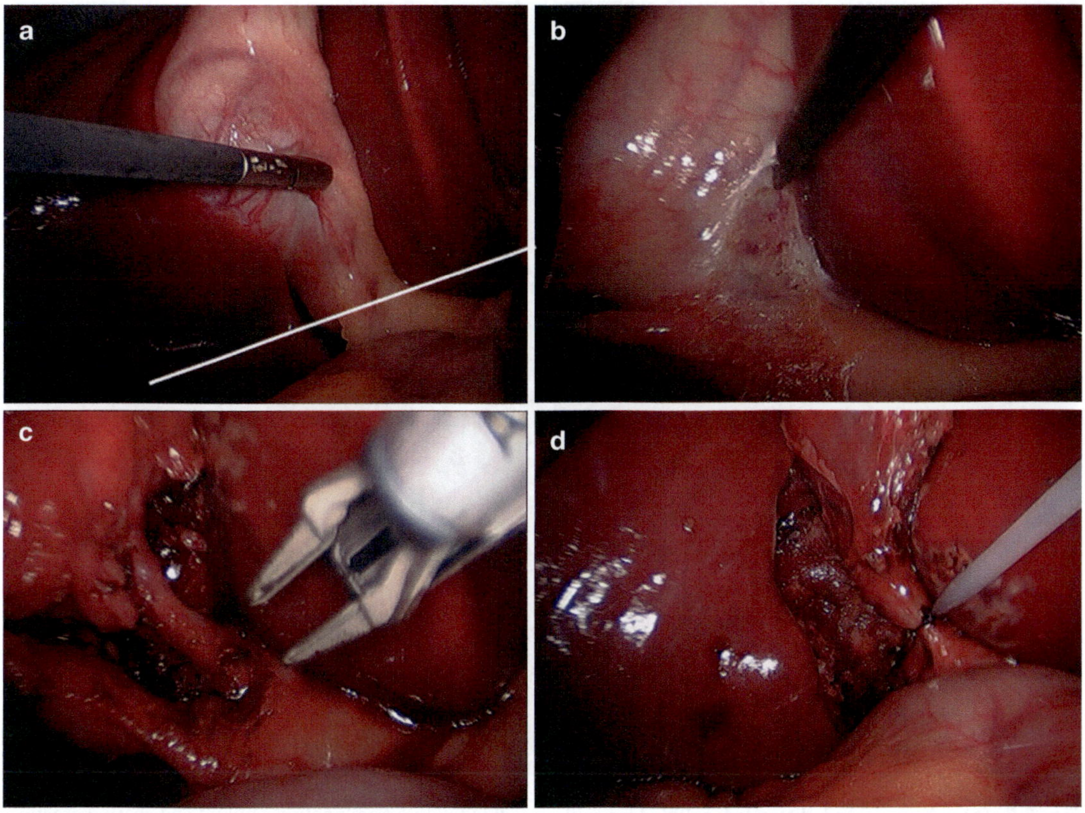

Fig. 8.4 (**a**)—R4U line drawn before dissection in a mildly inflamed gallbladder. (**b**)—Initial peritoneal dissection. (**c**)—Critical view of safety with the cystic artery about to be divided. (**d**)—The wide cystic duct was ligated by the use of an endoloop technique

8.10 Acute on Chronic Cholecystitis

Patients with a more chronic history can present with adhesions to the omentum and liver which are more fibrotic than inflammatory (Fig. 8.6a). This patient had a history of gallstones going back many years and the omentum had walled off the gallbladder almost completely. They presented with an acute attack of cholecystitis (acute on chronic cholecystitis). With careful laparoscopic dissection adhering to the rules set out above the critical view of safety was achieved (Fig. 8.6b).

8.11 Previous Cholecystostomy Drainage Tube

Radiological percutaneous cholecystostomy tubes have been increasingly used in the treatment of patients with severe acute cholecystitis, especially if the patient is unfit for surgery and not responding to non-operative treatment with intravenous antibiotics. These tubes are usually placed transhepatically by a radiologist to avoid the risk of bile leakage on drain removal. The drainage tube resolves the local and systemic sepsis and avoids the risks of emergency surgery. Some patients

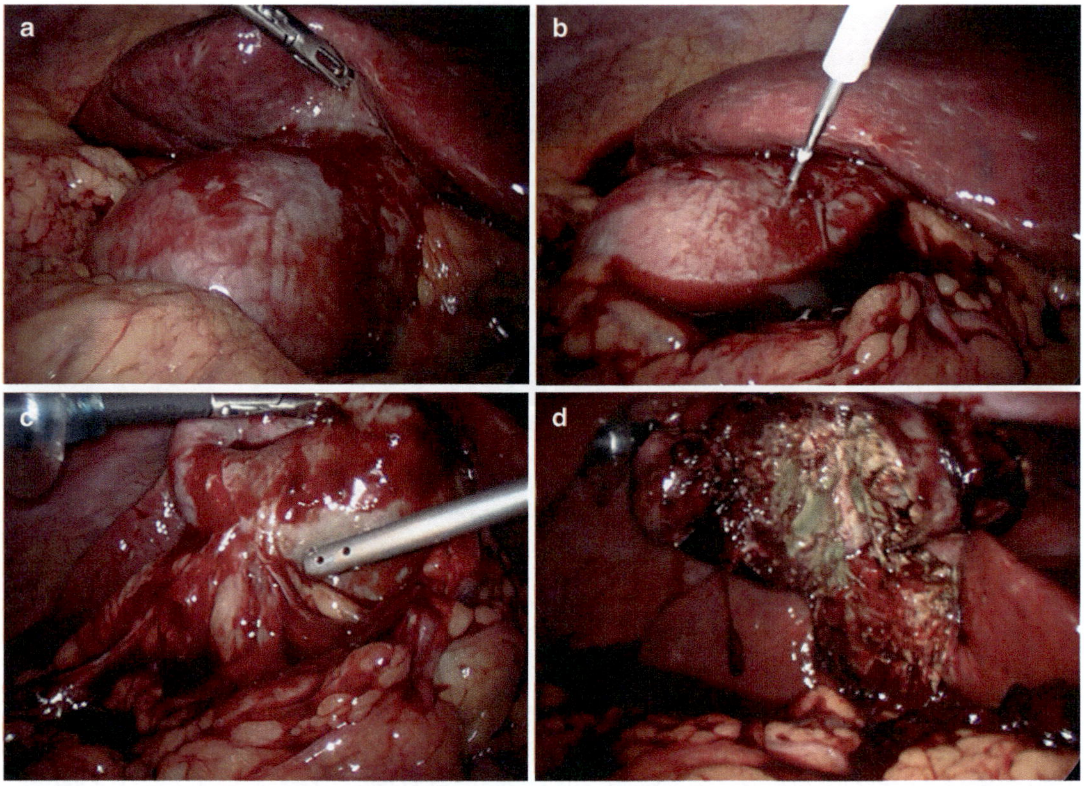

Fig. 8.5 (**a**)—A tense and distended gallbladder with severe acute cholecystitis present. (**b**)—The gallbladder is aspirated with a long aspiration needle to allow grasping and retraction. (**c**)—The inflammatory adhesions can be tackled with a combination of blunt and sharp dissection. (**d**)—Dissection of the liver reveals the necrotic gallbladder wall

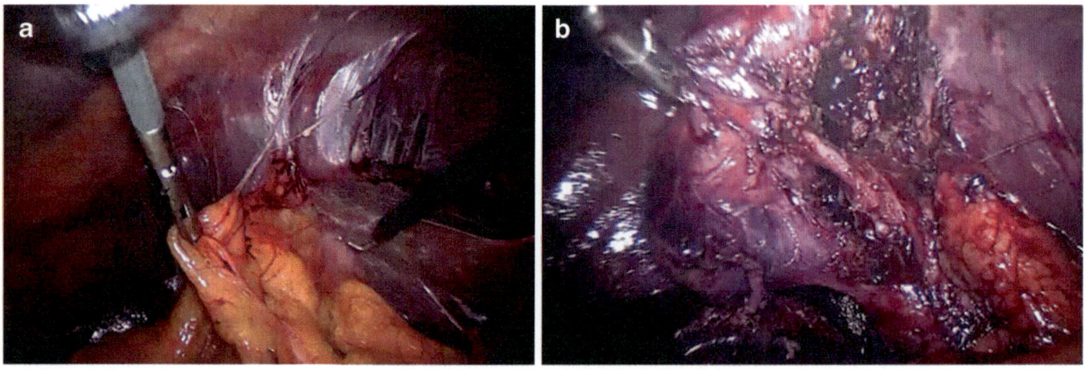

Fig. 8.6 (**a**)—Features of hepatic and omental adhesions in a patient presenting with acute on chronic cholecystitis. (**b**)—The critical view of safety has been achieved in this difficult cholecystectomy

with reversible pathology (for example myocardial infarction or pneumonia) will subsequently become fit for surgery. They will need careful assessment and pre-optimisation with an anaesthetist and other specialists. However, it is worth mentioning that in a randomised trial of 142 high-risk patients with acute cholecystitis randomised to either cholecystostomy (68 patients) or laparo-

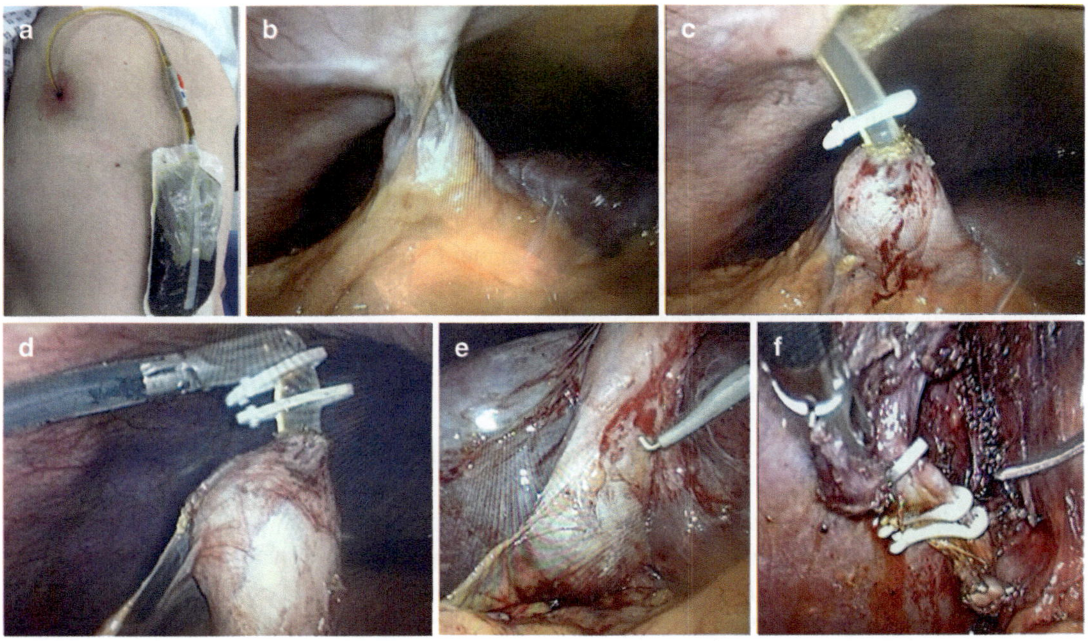

Fig. 8.7 (**a**)—External view of the draining cholecystostomy tube placed during a 'bail out procedure'. (**b**)—Fibrosis around the Foley catheter tube. (**c**)—The Foley catheter has been clipped to avoid bile leakage, so that the balloon did not deflate. (**d**)—The Foley catheter can be used to manipulate the gallbladder to aid in manipulation of the gallbladder and dissection. (**e**)—Features of chronic cholecystitis. (**f**)—Clipping of the wide cystic duct with Haemolock clips

scopic cholecystectomy (66 patients), surgery was clearly superior in that major complications, and need for reintervention, length of stay and hospital costs were reduced [26]. Therefore, it should be noted that cholecystostomy drainage is only a temporising measure and that surgeons should be involved in the assessment of these patients during the acute admission for consideration of definitive surgery.

In our unit, if the patient is fit for future surgery, we prefer to leave the cholecystostomy tube in situ and then discharge the patient for a delayed cholecystectomy. Extra time should be permitted for the surgery as it is often difficult with fibrosed tissue planes. Before performing surgery, it is wise to perform a cholangiogram via the cholecystostomy catheter to assess for CBD stones and unobstructed passage of contrast to the duodenum.

Figure 8.7a shows the external view of a patient who had a bail out cholecystostomy performed at another unit. In this patient, severe cholecystitis was observed at his initial operation and the surgeon decided to place a Foley catheter as a cholecystostomy drainage tube, rather than risk a very difficult cholecystectomy. After around 3 months of 'cooling' off, he underwent a laparoscopic cholecystectomy in our unit. Figure 8.7b shows fibrosis around the tube. The Foley catheter was clipped with a Hemolock clip to allow the balloon to remain inflated and avoid bile spillage (Fig. 8.7c). This allowed the cut Foley catheter to be grasped and manipulate the gallbladder to aid in the dissection (Fig. 8.7d). In this operation, difficult tissue planes are observed (Fig. 8.7e), but the operation is completed laparoscopically with the critical view of safety achieved and the cystic duct divided with Hemolock clips.

8.12 Suspected Gallbladder Cancer

The occurrence of incidental gallbladder cancer found at laparoscopic cholecystectomy in around 0.19% to 2.8% of cases depending on the published series [27]. The disease is rare in Europe and is more common in Chile, Japan and North India [27]. Only around 30% of gallbladder cancers are suspected preoperatively; patients at risk include patients with suspicious imaging features (focal GB wall thickening, intra-mural nodules, halo sign, intrahepatic duct dilation or loss of interface between the gallbladder and liver, enlarging 'polyps', a porcelain gallbladder, CT imaging showing liver invasion or incidental PET positive gallbladder lesions) or other features such as advanced age, weight loss or raised alkaline phosphatase. Some patients are only diagnosed on subsequent histopathological examination of the gallbladder specimen after the gallbladder is removed at laparoscopic cholecystectomy. Features of gallbladder cancer at laparoscopic cholecystectomy include the abnormal thickening of the gallbladder, peritoneal disease or liver metastases (Fig. 8.8). Some surgeons recommend intraoperative frozen section pathology to diagnose gallbladder cancer with a view to immediate open radical resection (wedge resection of the gallbladder bed and lymphadenectomy). However, we would recommend consulting with a specialist HPB surgeon, aborting the procedure (as the patient is usually not consented for radical liver resection) and performing appropriate staging investigations (spiral CT of the chest and abdomen with IV portovenous contrast) with subsequent HPB MDT/tumour board discussion.

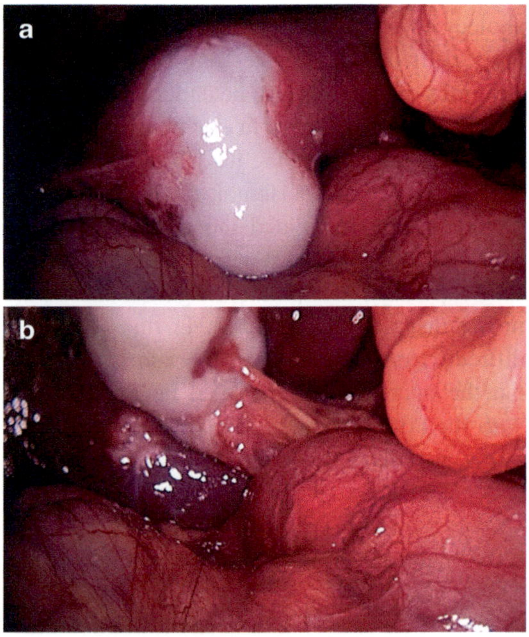

Fig. 8.8 (**a**) Incidental gallbladder cancer at laparoscopic cholecystectomy with abnormal thickening (**b**) Associated liver metastasis

8.13 Xanthogranulomatous Cholecystitis

Xanthogranulomatous cholecystitis (XGC) is often mistaken for, and may predispose to, gallbladder carcinoma [28]. It is usually a histological diagnosis and can be diagnosed on preoperative FNA sampling of the gallbladder via endoscopic ultrasound or on frozen section histology at surgery. Focal GB wall thickening favours gallbladder cancer whilst diffuse thickening favours XGC. The condition is associated with hostile operating conditions and a difficult cholecystectomy as the rates of inflammatory adhesions, fistulae to adjacent organs and postoperative infection rates are higher than a normal cholecystectomy as this reflects the chronic inflammatory nature of this condition. The disease has a high risk of conversions to open surgery for these reasons.

8.14 Mirizzi Syndrome

Mirizzi syndrome is a complication of longstanding cholelithiasis and makes cholecystectomy extremely challenging with a significant increase in the risk of intraoperative biliary injury [29]. It may only become apparent at operative surgery and poses particular risk to the surgeon and patients.

Mirizzi syndrome is subclassified in to five types [30]:

- Type 1: is obstruction of the extrahepatic bile duct by stone/s in the Hartmann's pouch or cystic duct.

- Type 2: is with a cholecystocholedochal fistula (diameter < 1/3 or the common hepatic duct wall).
- Type 3: is with a cholecystocholedochal fistula (diameter < 2/3 of the common hepatic duct wall).
- Type 4: is with a cholecystocholedochal fistula (involving the whole common hepatic duct wall).
- Type 5: any type associated with a cholecysto-enteral fistula (i.e. fistula to stomach, duodenum or hepatic flexure or transverse colon). This is sometimes sub-classified depending on whether gallstone ileus is present or not.

This modified Csendes classification is shown in Fig. 8.9.

The classic presentation of Type 1 Mirizzi is painless obstructive jaundice with evidence, at ultrasonography, of a gallstone impacted in the gallbladder infundibulum and obstruction of the CBD with consequent dilation of the intrahepatic biliary tree. ERCP and stent insertion may temporise the jaundice and also provide a landmark for protection of the CBD at surgery. Stent insertion will also reduce the risk of bile leakage after surgery.

Mirizzi syndrome can also cause a stricture which mimics biliary cancer. This occurs when the associated inflammatory process is predominant, and it involves the CBD and presents like a malignant stricture. CT, MRCP or ERCP may help differentiate the causes and guide appropriate referral and treatment.

Features of Mirizzi syndrome at surgery include an oedematous or atrophic gallbladder with distortion of Calot's triangle, an impacted gallstone in the infundibulum or the neck of the cystic duct or Hartmann's pouch, thick fibrosis around Calot's triangle, and adhesions under the liver space. Cholecystobiliary fistula should be suspected if the extraction of an impacted stone is followed by the leakage of bile from the common hepatic or common bile duct.

The surgical management of Mirizzi syndrome is outside the scope of this chapter, but can include removal of the gallbladder leaving in place the portion of the infundibulum adherent to the CBD or subtotal cholecystectomy (Type 1 Mirizzi) or cholecystectomy and T-tube insertion

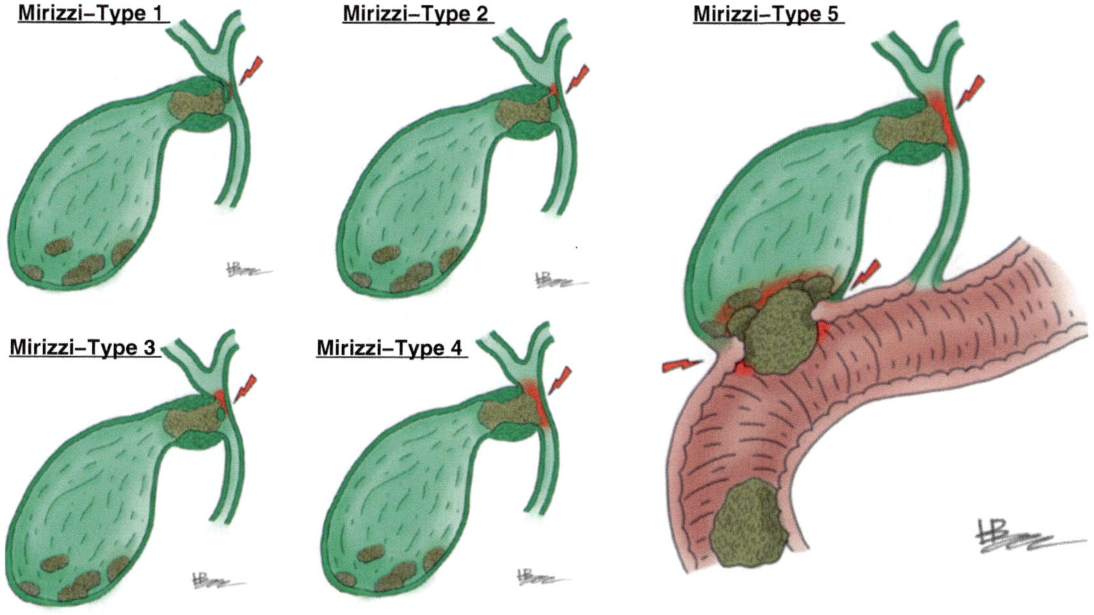

Fig. 8.9 Modified Csendes classification of Mirizzi syndrome. (Courtesy of H. Bergmann)

or bailing out of the cholecystectomy completely or techniques to resect gallbladder and reconstruct the biliary tree. The decision-making process will depend not only on the fitness of the patient, the condition of the gallbladder and type of Mirizzi but also on the level of skill and expertise of the surgeon. It is strongly recommended that involvement of a specialist HPB surgeon is obtained in these difficult cases.

8.15 Summary and Conclusion

Laparoscopic cholecystectomy can be an extremely challenging operation if operative conditions are hazardous. It is important that the surgeons try to predict the difficult case preoperatively (1) to allow extra operative time for the case, (2) consent the patient appropriately and (3) obtain specialist equipement or specialist help with the procedure. We would recommend routinely using one of the Operative Difficultly Scores, such as a the Nassar score for the documentation of operation difficulty. This will allow standardisation, and it will be helpful as a training tool and for surgical audit or morbidity discussions. We hope that this chapter has demonstrated various tips and tricks for dealing with some specific operative scenarios in the difficult case. The surgeon should have a vast array of techniques to use to safely deal with the difficult case, including using techniques to obtain the critical view, performing a subtotal cholecystectomy, placing a cholecystostomy drainage tube or converting to open surgery.

References

1. Haribhakti SP, Mistry JH. Techniques of laparoscopic cholecystectomy: nomenclature and selection. J Minim Access Surg. 2015;11(2):113–8.
2. Pucher PH, Brunt LM, Davies N, Linsk A, Munshi A, Rodriguez HA, Fingerhut A, Fanelli RD, Asbun H, Aggarwal R. Outcome trends and safety measures after 30 years of laparoscopic cholecystectomy: a systematic review and pooled data analysis. Surg Endosc. 2018;32(5):2175–83.
3. Lengyel BI, Panizales MT, Steinberg J, Ashley SW, Tavakkoli A. Laparoscopic cholecystectomy: what is the price of conversion? Surgery. 2012;152(2):173–8.
4. Griffiths EA, Hodson J, Vohra RS, Marriott P, Katbeh T, Zino S, Nassar AHM. Utilisation of an operative difficulty grading scale for laparoscopic cholecystectomy. Surg Endosc. 2019;33(1):110–21. https://doi.org/10.1007/s00464-018-6281-2.
5. Nassar AHM, Hodson J, Ng HJ, Vohra RS, Katbeh T, Zino S, Griffiths EA, et al. Predicting the difficult laparoscopic cholecystectomy: development and validation of a pre-operative risk score using an objective operative difficulty grading system. Surg Endosc. 2019;34(10):4549–61. https://doi.org/10.1007/s00464-019-07244-5.
6. Strasberg SM, Pucci MJ, Brunt LM, Deziel DJ. Subtotal cholecystectomy-“Fenestrating” vs “reconstituting” subtypes and the prevention of bile duct injury: definition of the optimal procedure in difficult operative conditions. J Am Coll Surg. 2016;222(1):89–96. https://doi.org/10.1016/j.jamcollsurg.2015.09.019.
7. Vohra RS, Pasquali S, Kirkham AJ, Marriott P, Johnstone M, Spreadborough P, Alderson D, Griffiths EA, et al. Population-based cohort study of variation in the use of emergency cholecystectomy for benign gallbladder diseases. Br J Surg. 2016;103(12):1716–26. https://doi.org/10.1002/bjs.10288.
8. Vohra RS, Pasquali S, Kirkham AJ, Marriott P, Johnstone M, Spreadborough P, Alderson D, Griffiths EA, et al. Population-based cohort study of outcomes following cholecystectomy for benign gallbladder diseases. Br J Surg. 2016;103(12):1704–15. https://doi.org/10.1002/bjs.10287.
9. Burnand KM, Lahiri RP, Burr N, Jansen Van Rensburg L, Lewis MPN. A randomised, single blinded trial, assessing the effect of a two week preoperative very low calorie diet on laparoscopic cholecystectomy in obese patients. HPB. 2016;18(5):456–61. https://doi.org/10.1016/j.hpb.2016.01.545.
10. Jones AD, Waterland PW, Powell-Brett S, Super P, Richardson M, Bowley D. Preoperative very low-calorie diet reduces technical difficulty during laparoscopic cholecystectomy in obese patients. Surg Laparosc Endosc Percutan Tech. 2016;26(3):226–9. https://doi.org/10.1097/SLE.0000000000000278.
11. Nassar AHM, Ashkar KA, Mohamed AY, Hafiz AA. Is laparoscopic cholecystectomy possible without video technology? Minim Invasive Ther Allied Technol. 1995;4:63–5. https://doi.org/10.3109/13645709509152757.
12. Hanna GB, Shimi SM, Cuschieri A. Randomised study of influence of two-dimensional versus three-dimensional imaging on performance of laparoscopic cholecystectomy. Lancet. 1998;351(9098):248–51. https://doi.org/10.1016/S0140-6736(97)08005-7.
13. Lee W, Jang JY, Cho JK, Hong SC, Jeong CY. Does surgical difficulty relate to severity of acute cho-

lecystitis? Validation of the parkland grading scale based on intraoperative findings. Am J Surg. 2019;219(4):637–41. https://doi.org/10.1016/j.amjsurg.2018.12.005.
14. Madni TD, Nakonezny PA, Barrios E, Imran JB, Clark AT, Taveras L, Cunningham HB, Christie A, Eastman AL, Minshall CT, Luk S, Minei JP, Phelan HA, Cripps MW. Prospective validation of the parkland grading scale for cholecystitis. Am J Surg. 2019;217(1):90–7. https://doi.org/10.1016/j.amjsurg.2018.08.005.
15. Sugrue M, Coccolini F, Bucholc M, Johnston A, Manatakis D, Ioannidis O, Bonilauri S, Gachabayov M, Isik A, Ghnnam W, Shelat V, Aremu M, Mohan R, Montori G, Walędziak M, Pisarska M, Kong V, Strzałka M, Fugazzola P, Nita GE, Nardi M, Major P, Negoi I, Allegri A, Konstantoudakis G, Di Carlo I, Massalou D, D'Amico G, Solaini L, Ceresoli M, Bini R, Zielinski M, Tomasoni M, Litvin A, De Simone B, Lostoridis E, Hernandez F, Panyor G, Machain GMV, Pentara I, Baiocchi L, Ng KC, Ansaloni L, Sartelli M, Arellano ML, Savala N, Couse N, McBride S. Intra-operative gallbladder scoring predicts conversion of laparoscopic to open cholecystectomy: a WSES prospective collaborative study. World J Emerg Surg. 2019;14:12. https://doi.org/10.1186/s13017-019-0230-9.
16. Hernandez M, Murphy B, Aho JM, Haddad NN, Saleem H, Zeb M, Morris DS, Jenkins DH, Zielinski M. Validation of the AAST EGS acute cholecystitis grade and comparison with the Tokyo guidelines. Surgery. 2018;163(4):739–46. https://doi.org/10.1016/j.surg.2017.10.041.
17. Yokoe M, Hata J, Takada T, Strasberg SM, Asbun HJ, Wakabayashi G, Kozaka K, Endo I, Deziel DJ, Miura F, Okamoto K, Hwang TL, Huang WSW, Ker CG, Chen MF, Han HS, Yoon YS, Choi IS, Yoon DS, Noguchi Y, Shikata S, Ukai T, Higuchi R, Gabata T, Mori Y, Iwashita Y, Hibi T, Jagannath P, Jonas E, Liau KH, Dervenis C, Gouma DJ, Cherqui D, Belli G, Garden OJ, Giménez ME, de Santibañes E, Suzuki K, Umezawa A, Supe AN, Pitt HA, Singh H, Chan ACW, Lau WY, Teoh AYB, Honda G, Sugioka A, Asai K, Gomi H, Itoi T, Kiriyama S, Yoshida M, Mayumi T, Matsumura N, Tokumura H, Kitano S, Hirata K, Inui K, Sumiyama Y, Yamamoto M. Tokyo guidelines 2018: diagnostic criteria and severity grading of acute cholecystitis (with videos). J Hepatobiliary Pancreat Sci. 2018;25(1):41–54. https://doi.org/10.1002/jhbp.515.
18. Gupta V, Jain G. Safe laparoscopic cholecystectomy: adoption of universal culture of safety in cholecystectomy. World J Gastrointest Surg. 2019;11(2):62–84. https://doi.org/10.4240/wjgs.v11.i2.62.
19. Way LW, Stewart L, Gantert W, Liu K, Lee CM, Whang K, Hunter JG. Causes and prevention of laparoscopic bile duct injuries: analysis of 252 cases from a human factors and cognitive psychology perspective. Ann Surg. 2003;237(4):–460, 9.
20. Peti N, Moser MAJ. Graphic reminder of Rouviere's sulcus: a useful landmark in cholecystectomy. ANZ J Surg. 2012;82(5):367–8.
21. Dahmane R, Morjane A, Starc A. Anatomy and surgical relevance of Rouviere's sulcus. Sci World J. 2013;2013:254287. https://doi.org/10.1155/2013/254287.
22. Hugh TB, Kelly MD, Mekisic A. Rouviere's sulcus: a useful landmark in laparoscopic cholecystectomy. Br J Surg. 1997;84(9):1253–4.
23. Strasberg SM, Brunt LM. Rationale and use of the critical view of safety in laparoscopic cholecystectomy. J Am Coll Surg. 2010;211(1):132–8. https://doi.org/10.1016/j.jamcollsurg.2010.02.053.
24. Davidoff AM, Pappas TN, Murray EA, Hilleren DJ, Johnson RD, Baker ME, Newman GE, Cotton PB, Meyers WC. Mechanisms of major biliary injury during laparoscopic cholecystectomy. Ann Surg. 1992;215(3):196–202. https://doi.org/10.1097/00000658-199203000-00002.
25. Strasberg SM, Hertl M, Soper NJ. An analysis of the problem of biliary injury during laparoscopic cholecystectomy. J Am Coll Surg. 1995;180(1):101–25.
26. Loozen CS, Van Santvoort HC, Van Duijvendijk P, Besselink MG, Gouma DJ, Nieuwenhuijzen GA, Kelder JC, Donkervoort SC, Van Geloven AA, Kruyt PM, Roos D, Kortram K, Kornmann VN, Pronk A, Van Der Peet DL, Crolla RM, Van Ramshorst B, Bollen TL, Boerma D. Laparoscopic cholecystectomy versus percutaneous catheter drainage for acute cholecystitis in high risk patients (CHOCOLATE): multicentre randomised clinical trial. BMJ. 2018;363:k3965. https://doi.org/10.1136/bmj.k3965.
27. Nitta T, Kataoka J, Ohta M, Fujii K, Takashima Y, Inoue Y, Ishibashi T. Surgical strategy for suspected early gallbladder carcinoma including incidental gallbladder carcinoma diagnosed during or after cholecystectomy. Ann Med Surg. 2018;33:56–9. https://doi.org/10.1016/j.amsu.2018.07.009.
28. Hale MD, Roberts KJ, Hodson J, Scott N, Sheridan M, Toogood GJ. Xanthogranulomatous cholecystitis: a European and global perspective. HPB. 2014;16(5):448–58. https://doi.org/10.1111/hpb.12152.
29. Clemente G, Tringali A, De Rose AM, Panettieri E, Murazio M, Nuzzo G, Giuliante F. Mirizzi syndrome: diagnosis and management of a challenging biliary disease. Can J Gastroenterol Hepatol. 2018;2018:6962090. https://doi.org/10.1155/2018/6962090.
30. Chen H, Siwo EA, Khu M, Tian Y. Current trends in the management of Mirizzi syndrome. Medicine (Baltimore). 2018;97(4):e9691. https://doi.org/10.1097/MD.0000000000009691.
31. Madni TD, Nakonezny PA, Imran JB, Taveras L, Cunningham HB, Vela R, Clark AT, Minshall CT, Eastman AL, Luk S, Phelan HA, Cripps MW. A comparison of cholecystitis grading scales. J Trauma Acute Care Surg. 2019;86(3):471–8. https://doi.org/10.1097/TA.0000000000002125.

9 Difficult Laparoscopic Cholecystectomy: Timing for Conversion

Samer AlMasri and Ali Hallal

9.1 Introduction

Cholelithiasis-related disease is a major cause of global morbidity with its prevalence varying based on several racial, ethnic, and geographical parameters. The disease is three to four times more prevalent in females, and its incidence increases with advancing age in both genders [1]. In the United States (US), 10–15% of the adult population have gallstone, yet more than 80% will remain asymptomatic [2, 3] However, gallstone-related disease constitutes approximately 2.2 million of all annual ambulatory care visits and represents an annual consumption of approximately $6.5 billion, creating a significant health burden in developed countries [3]. On the other hand, the incidence of gallstone-related disease is increasing worldwide in developing countries. This coincides with increase in calorie and fat consumption and sedentary lifestyles in these populations [4]

Laparoscopic cholecystectomy (LC) is the gold standard treatment for benign gallbladder disease and with the growing experience and advanced technical skills, the aforementioned procedure is one of the most commonly performed minimally invasive operation worldwide [5, 6]. Since its was first introduced in the mid-1980s, it has gained widespread popularity because of its advantages that clearly outweigh the open technique. LC is associated with less postoperative pain, shorter length of hospital stay, earlier return to work, and better cosmetic results [7–9]. This in turn leads to a dramatic shift in the surgical management of benign gallbladder disease. Consequently, an expanding number of reports demonstrated the safety and feasibility of this approach for the management of acute cholecystitis (AC) and other gallstone-related complications [5, 7–11].

When performed by well-trained surgeons, LC is an easily reproducible surgical approach that is safe and is associated with a minimal risk of major complications (<5%) [11]. However, there are several patient-related, disease-related, and even surgeon-related variables that can hinder the standard operative steps and increase operative morbidity. Insertion of a cholecystostomy tube, subtotal cholecystectomy, and conversion to the open approach (LOC) are all valid emergency alternatives. LOC, given that the operating surgeon is well familiar with the open approach, promises increased visibility and maneuverability that might aid in the safe removal of the gallbladder. Numerous prior studies have analyzed the incidence of LOC among various patient

S. AlMasri
Complex Surgical Oncology Research Fellow, Department of GI Surgical Oncology, University of Pittsburgh Medical Center, Pittsburgh, PA, USA
e-mail: almasaris@upmc.edu

A. Hallal (✉)
Associate Professor of Clinical Surgery, Department of Surgery, American University of Beirut Medical Centre, Beirut, Lebanon
e-mail: ah05@aub.edu.lb

© Springer Nature Switzerland AG 2021

I. Di Carlo (ed.), *Difficult Acute Cholecystitis*, https://doi.org/10.1007/978-3-030-62102-5_9

groups and the factors that would increase this risk. Underlying pathology, timing of cholecystectomy, distorted anatomy, adhesions, patients age, body mass index (BMI), gender, comorbidities, and surgeon experience in minimally invasive surgery (MIS) have all been shown to increase the risk of LOC [12–18].

In this chapter, we will be discussing the variables that have been shown to consistently increase the risk of LOC. Furthermore, we will analyze the previously published prediction models and risk scores that help in preoperative surgical planning and patient counseling. Our aim is to highlight the importance of when and why should this approach be considered as a valuable "bailout" technique based on an intraoperative decision rather than a failure on the surgeon's part. This mandate balancing the risk of continuing with the laparoscopic approach with the morbidity associated with LOC.

9.2 Risk Factors for Conversion

Preoperative recognition of the risk factors that can hinder a safe LC is crucial, as it increases surgeon awareness and therefore aids in proper patient counseling, guide operative planning, and ultimately optimize patient outcomes. Table 9.1 demonstrates the most commonly cited variables that have been shown to impact the risk of conversion. However, due to the prior significant clinical and methodological heterogeneity in published literature, several of these parameters have either been supported or refuted. Furthermore, there is a wide variation in the actual percentage of conversion reported across various institution that can be as low as 1% [16] or be as high as 32% [19]. This wide variation in the reported conversion rate is related to surgeon experience, patient selection, and procedure-related factors among various studies. Certainly, the conversion rate is decreasing compared to historical figures owing to better preoperative assessment, alternative treatment modalities availability, and enhanced overall surgeon experience. Nevertheless, we will be reviewing the variables that have been consistently proven to impact the risk of conversion across various settings.

Table 9.1 Risk factors for conversion (CBD: common bile duct)

Patient-related factors
Advanced age
Male gender
History of multiple upper abdominal operations
Obesity
Medical comorbidities
Disease-related factors
Acute cholecystitis
Gallbladder perforation
Gangrenous cholecystitis
Gallbladder empyema
Emphysematous cholecystitis
Imaging parameters (gallbladder wall thickness, pericholecystic fluid, CBD size)
Mirizzi syndrome
Gallstone pancreatitis and coledocholithiasis
Chronic cholecystitis
Minimally invasive surgical training (MIST)

9.2.1 Patient-Related Factors

9.2.1.1 Age and Gender

Male gender and advanced age (particularly <65) are two of the most commonly cited variables that have been shown to increase the risk of LOC across multiple prior systematic reviews, meta-analysis, prospective, and retrospective studies [12, 13, 15–21] It has been postulated that male gender is associated with increased severity of the underlying inflammatory process that would hinder safe dissection of the triangle of Calot and increase the risk of conversion [21, 22]. On the other hand, the increased risk of LOC seen in the elderly population can be explained by the fact that in this subcategory of patients, the underlying inflammatory process is more severe. In addition, an elderly patient may have had repeated prior attacks of biliary colic or untreated AC episodes. These variables may lead to the formation of dense adhesions and create anatomical hurdles that would hinder safe dissection during LC and ultimately drive the operating surgeon to abort the LC and convert to open [16, 23, 24].

9.2.1.2 Previous Abdominal Surgery

A history of prior abdominal operations is not a contraindication for LC. However, several studies have shown an increased risk of LOC in the setting of prior abdominal surgeries, particularly those that involve the upper abdomen [16, 25–27]. In a large single-center retrospective review of 4668 LC cases, AlMasri et al. (2018) [16] found that a history of prior abdominal surgeries, especially in the setting of a prior laparotomy for penetrating abdominal trauma, is a strong independent predictor of LOC (OR 4.66, $P = 0.002$). This translates to an increased formation of dense adhesions that obscure safe access and exposure to the hepatocystic triangle, increase the risk of bleeding, iatrogenic injury, and ultimately LOC.

Nevertheless, neither should the nature nor the number of prior abdominal operations preclude the laparoscopic approach. The laparoscopic approach should be the first therapeutic option in symptomatic gallbladder disease as long as the initial access to the abdominal cavity is performed safely and adhesiolysis carried out meticulously until the right upper quadrant is clearly delineated [27].

9.2.1.3 Obesity

Patients with an increased body mass index (BMI) have been reported to be prone to severe underlying inflammation of the gallbladder, making dissection in LC more difficult [24]. More importantly, obesity poses unique technical challenges for the operating surgeon secondary to trocar placement, obscured anatomy secondary to excess intraperitoneal fat, and even an inability to retract the liver sufficiently for adequate exposure [28]. However, while several prior studies have reported obesity (BMI ≥ 30 kg/m^2) to be associated with an increased risk of conversion [13, 19, 29], others found no such association [12, 14–16, 20, 28], and the authors concluded that the previously reported increased conversion rate observed in obese patients is attributable to surgeon experience and technical limitations eventually abolishing obesity as a risk factor for LOC. Currently, several reports propose techniques for safe initial trocar placement in the morbidly obese patient for a safe laparoscopic operation [30, 31].

9.2.1.4 Medical Comorbidities

Cardiopulmonary Disease

It is well established that the risk LOC is increased in patients with several medical comorbidities. Some of these are specific to LC and others can affect the risk of any laparoscopic procedure. It is believed that patients with cardiopulmonary disease are particularly susceptible to the hemodynamic changes that result from pneumoperitoneal insufflation pressures, as the increase in abdominal pressure is associated with an increase in peak airway pressures, a drop-in stroke volume, and therefore cardiac index [32]. This results in an increased risk of LOC due to the inherent risks that are associated with the laparoscopic approach.

In a large retrospective study involving 20,307 patients from the Danish cholecystectomy database, Harboe and Bardram (2011) [33] found that risk of conversion doubled for patients with American Society of Anesthesiology (ASA) score > 3 compared to patients with a lower ASA score. Furthermore, analysis of prospectively collected data from the National Surgical Quality Improvement Program (NSQIP) by Kaafarani et al. (2010) [34] identified 11,669 patient who underwent cholecystectomy at 117 VA hospitals. They found that patients with more cardiac, pulmonary, renal, and nutritional comorbidities, as reflected by a higher ASA class, had a higher incidence of conversion ($P < 0.05$). The aforementioned variables were also found to be more prevalent in patients who underwent OC from the start.

Finally, in a single institution retrospective study conducted by AlMasri et al. (2018) [16] that aimed to analyze the risk factors implicated in increasing the risk of LOC among 4668 LC cases. They found that chronic obstructive pulmonary disease is a significant independent predictor of LOC with an odds ratio (OR) of 6.03 ($P = 0.03$). Therefore, we can conclude from these studies that although a higher ASA class is not a contraindication for attempting LC, preoperative optimization of this subcategory of patients is crucial.

Liver Cirrhosis and Portal Hypertension

Patients with liver cirrhosis are twice more likely to develop gallstones compared to the general population. Furthermore, the morbidity and mortality associated with gallstone disease and its surgical treatment are increased in this subcategory of patients [35]. First, there is a significant increase in the risk of perioperative bleeding secondary to the extensive collateral circulation developed due to portal hypertension and the technical difficulties imposed by the fibrotic liver. Second, and due to the multi-organ dysfunction seen in liver cirrhosis, patients are prone to develop hepatic and renal decompensation under the stress of the surgery and anesthesia itself. Finally, patients with liver cirrhosis have impaired wound healing that increases the risk of postoperative surgical site infection [36] All these aforementioned complications lead the NIH to issue a consensus statement in 1992 that considered liver cirrhosis as an absolute contraindication for LC [37].

However, since then, there has been several publications that showed LC to be a safe surgical alternative in patients with gallstone disease and underlying liver cirrhosis. This is especially true for patients with Child A or B liver cirrhosis [37–40]. In 2003, Puggioni and Wong [38] performed a systematic analysis of articles published between 1993 and 2001 and included 400 cirrhotic patients. This meta-analysis found that LC was superior to OC; it was associated with decreased perioperative blood loss, operative time, and postoperative length of hospital stay with an overall conversion rate of 7%. Machado [40] demonstrated similar results after enrolling 1310 patients through a meta-analysis of articles published between 1994 and 2011. Among these patients, 17 had Child C liver cirrhosis, and these patients had a higher conversion rate (35%) compared to patients with Child A and B liver cirrhosis (4.5%) and increased overall morbidity.

Currently, the existing evidence is not sufficient for definitive conclusions in regard to the laparoscopic approach in cirrhotic patients. Although the conversion rate is higher, LC is neither contraindicated nor associated with a higher morbidity in patients with Child A and B liver cirrhosis. However, and particularly for patients with Child C cirrhosis, OC still has an important role. Nevertheless, the extent of liver disease should be established preoperatively for appropriate patient optimization and counseling. Laboratory workup should include liver function tests and coagulation studies to determine Child's classification and MELD score, as the latter has been shown to be an effective predictor of postoperative morbidity [41].

Diabetes Mellitus

Poorly controlled diabetes mellitus (DM) is theoretically associated with autonomic dysfunction and peripheral neuropathy; thus, patients with gallstone disease may not develop symptoms until late in the disease course leading to a delay in the diagnosis, an increased risk of conversion, and overall morbidity following LC [42, 43]. Although cholecystectomy should not be performed electively for asymptomatic gallstone disease [44], the question of whether DM increases the risk of conversion remains controversial as some studies support this postulate [27, 45] while others show no such association [13, 16, 20].

9.2.2 Disease-Related Factors

9.2.2.1 Acute Cholecystitis and Cholecystitis-Related Complications

AC is characterized by inflammation of the gallbladder secondary to obstruction of the biliary drainage, leading to an increased intraluminal pressure, distension, wall edema, increase in lymphatic and venous pressure, and eventually ischemia, necrosis, and perforation [46]. In 90% of the cases, cholelithiasis is identified, while in the remining 10%, no gallstones are seen and hence, the diagnosis is referred to as "acalculous cholecystitis" [46]. According to the most recent update of the Tokyo guidelines [47], the diagnosis of AC includes (1) local signs of inflammation (local tenderness, pain), (2) systemic signs of inflammation (leukocytosis, fever, elevated inflammatory markers), (3) radiological criteria for cholecystitis (pericholecystic fluid, thickened wall >3 mm, with/without presence of cholelithiasis), and (4) finally a positive murphy sign on physical exam or ultrasound evaluation.

The severity of the underlying inflammatory process in AC is a prime risk factor for LOC and overall morbidity following surgical intervention. This can be predicted preoperatively based on the status of admission (emergency or elective), systemic inflammatory markers, radiological criteria, and clinical presentation [13, 16, 18–20, 25–27, 34, 35]. All these aforementioned variables can predict a "difficult cholecystectomy" that would translate to technical limitations for safe dissection and thus increase the risk of LOC.

For instance, severe inflammatory cases, such as perforation of the gallbladder (seen in 6–18% of AC cases, Fig. 9.1), gangrenous cholecystitis (seen in 2–30% of AC cases) with secondary abscess or empyema formation, and emphysematous cholecystitis (seen in 1% of AC cases) [48–50], result in the formation of dense adhesions around the surgical field and possible encasement of the gallbladder by the omentum. On the other hand, the acutely inflamed gallbladder can become shrunken and contracted, shortening the cystic duct and distorting the anatomy of the hepatocystic triangle. Furthermore, the gallbladder might become adherent to adjacent visceral structures such as the common bile duct (CBD), duodenum, and colon. All of these variables combined pose significant technical challenges for the operating surgeon due to an increase in the risk of intraoperative bleeding, iatrogenic injury. That is the reason why, in the face of these challenges, the surgeon might choose to abort the laparoscopic approach and convert to open [48, 50–53]. The presence of any of the three aforementioned complications, based on reports from national registries [54, 55], increases the risk of conversion by threefold compared to uncomplicated AC.

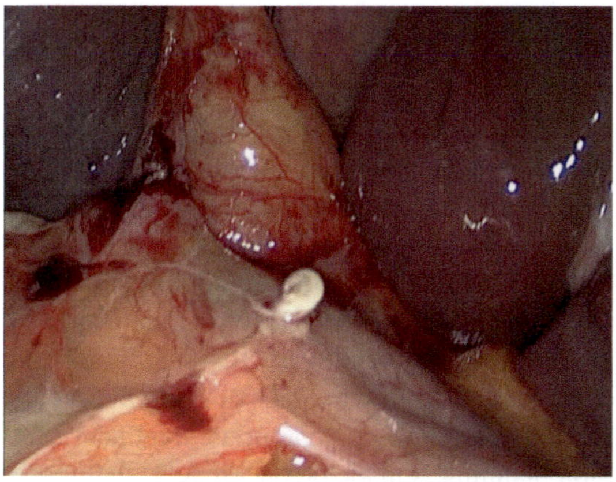

Fig. 9.1 Severe acute cholecystitis complicated by hydrops of the gallbladder. This patient had several gallstones impacted in the infundibulum and dense omental adhesions secondary to the severe underlying inflammatory process

9.2.2.2 Timing of Cholecystectomy

There has been considerable debate on whether the timing of cholecystectomy has any relation to the conversion risk. While some studies showed an increased risk of LOC if LC is delayed beyond 48–96 h of symptoms onset [12, 56], most other retrospective reviews and meta-analyses [26, 57–59] demonstrate that early LC (within 7 days of symptom onset) may be associated with shorter operation time, lower postoperative wound infection rates, and shorter length of hospital. However, delayed LC was not associated with an increase LOC risk. Roulin et al. (2016) [60] performed a prospective randomized controlled study that looked at the timing of cholecystectomy and its relation to clinical outcomes. They randomized 86 patients to either early (within 72 h of symptom onset) or late LC (6 weeks, initial antibiotic therapy). They found that patients with AC operated on within 72 h of symptom onset had lower overall morbidity, shorter median length of hospital stay, and shorter duration of antibiotic therapy. However, there was no difference in the conversion rate between early and delayed LC. Therefore, current evidence advocates early LC (within 72 h) of symptom onset rather than delayed or interval LC due to evidence supporting superior patient outcomes.

9.2.2.3 Mirizzi Syndrome

Mirizzi syndrome develops secondary to a large impacted stone in the infundibulum of the gallbladder that compresses the common hepatic duct leading to obstructive jaundice, cholangitis, and eventually chronic inflammation and fibrosis [61]. It is encountered in 0.3–3% of all LC cases and can be subdivided into two main subtypes [61, 62]. Type 1 is characterized by extrinsic compression of the CBD secondary to a large gallstone in the Hartmann's pouch, while in type 2, the stone erodes through the gallbladder wall into the CBD leading to the development of a cholecysto-coledochal fistula [63]. Preoperative recognition of this diagnosis is crucial, and a high index of suspicion is required to identify this disease entity preoperatively especially in the presence of an empyema, mucocele, or stone impaction. This can be suspected based on cholestatic elevation pattern of liver function tests (LFTs), or on magnetitic resonant cholangiopancreatography (MRCP), or on endoscopic retrograde cholangiopancreatography (ERCP) [64]. Furthermore, a differential diagnosis of gallbladder cancer involving the CBD should always be entertained, as a high association between gallbladder cancer and Mirizzi syndrome was previously demonstrated [65].

Initially, Mirizzi syndrome was considered a contraindication for LC [61], as it was associated with a significant risk of LOC (>50%) and increased morbidity [62]. However, with the advert of alternative laparoscopic approaches such as subtotal cholecystectomy and increased surgeon experience, the laparoscopic approach can be attempted in selected cases, with an acceptable elevated risk of conversion [66].

9.2.2.4 Imaging Parameters

Several findings on preoperative radiological evaluation have been shown to be associated with an increased risk of LOC across multiple prior publications [14, 18–20, 27, 42, 53, 67]. Thickened gallbladder wall, pericholecystic fluid, presence of CBD stone, and dilated CBD- or AC-related complications have all been shown to increase the risk of conversion following LC. In a prospective analytical study conducted by Yadav and Janugade (2019) [18] to determine the predictive factors for difficult LC, they found that a thickened gallbladder wall, impacted stone, and pericholecystic collection are all significant predictors of LOC. Fuks et al. (2012) [67] correlated preoperative CT findings with the risk of conversion prospectively. They demonstrated that the absence of gallbladder wall enhancement (suggestive of gangrenous cholecystitis) and the presence of gallstones in the infundibulum are significant predictors of LOC. Therefore, and based on the aforementioned studies, radiological findings that reflect a severe underlying inflammatory process should be considered as risk factors for an increased risk of LOC.

9.2.2.5 Coledocholithiasis and Gallstone Pancreatitis

CBD stones are detected in 11–25% of all patients with symptomatic cholelithiasis, with the reported incidence reaching 43% in individuals above 80 years of age [23, 68]. For patients with preoperative evidence of coledocholithiasis, clearance of the CBD using ERCP followed by LC is the gold standard treatment modality [69]. However, approximately 10% of patients who undergo LC are found to have CBD stones intraoperatively [68, 70] and with the availability of surgical expertise and the necessary resources, laparoscopic CBD exploration (LCBDE) can be safely performed without an increased risk of LOC [71] Two meta-analyses [72, 73] have demonstrated that patients who undergo LCBDE, as opposed to those who undergo postoperative ERCP as a two-staged approach, have comparable results in terms of overall morbidity and rate of CBD clearance. Therefore, and based on the above, the presence of CBD stone is neither a contraindication for LC, nor does it increase the risk of conversion, if appropriate treatment decision planning is made preoperatively.

Gallstone induced pancreatitis is the most common etiology for acute pancreatitis with varying disease severity [74, 75]. It has been shown that patients with mild–moderate gallstone pancreatitis should undergo early LC, owing to the increased (20–60%) risk of recurrence if the definitive operation is not performed at the initial admission [76, 77]. Furthermore, performing the cholecystectomy in these patients is neither associated with increased complication rate nor an increased risk of LOC [27, 76]. However, in the subcategory of patients with severe gallstone pancreatitis, there is consensus that LC be deferred (preferably 6 weeks after the index episode) until complete resolution of local and systemic inflammation is achieved [76, 77].

9.2.2.6 Chronic Cholecystitis

The chronicity of gallbladder inflammation, most commonly secondary to recurrent biliary colic's, has been shown to be associated with increased technical limitations during an otherwise straightforward LC, and thus may increase the risk of LOC (Fig. 9.2) [78–80]. It is believed that the fibrotic and desmoplastic reaction that results secondary to the chronic inflammatory process distorts normal tissue plane, rendering dissection around the hepatocystic triangle more difficult and surrounding visceral structures such as the CBD or duodenum more prone to iatrogenic injury [80, 81] This is thought to be the primary underlying factor for the increased risk of LOC witnessed in males and in the elderly population [16, 21–24]. Therefore, identifying patients with chronic cholecystitis preoperatively is crucial for surgeon preparation for intraoperative hurdles that will be encountered in chronic inflammatory cases.

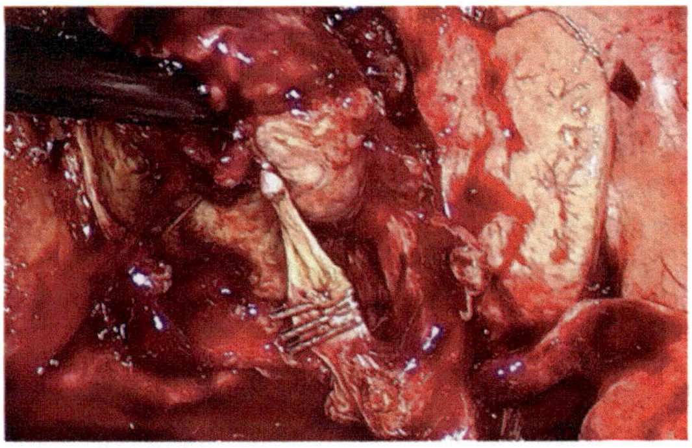

Fig. 9.2 Severe chronic cholecystitis causing dense adhesions and inflammatory fusion of the triangle of Calot

9.2.3 Surgeon-Related Factors

9.2.3.1 Minimally Invasive Surgical Training (MIST)

It has been well documented that the conversion rate from laparoscopic to open cholecystectomy is lower among well-experienced high-volume surgeons and minimally invasive surgical training propitiates this effect [15, 19, 81–84]. Nevertheless, the threshold of conversion varies between surgeons and is related to several subjective variables such as perceived intraoperative difficulty, expertise, and prior training in MIST [14].

In a single-center retrospective study that included 2810 LC cases, Coffin et al. (2017) [15] identified MIST as a significant predictor of conversion on univariate but not multivariate analysis. However, despite the presence of several known risk factors for conversion among the MIST surgeon group, the LOC rate remained significantly lower, indicating that expertise and MIST are independent predictors of conversion. Furthermore, it has been proposed that surgical experience standardizes the basic steps of LC, regardless of the underlying disease severity [83]. Therefore, a well-rounded, structured, educational MIST for surgical trainees can guarantee high patient safety profiles, decrease the conversion rate, and ultimately improve patient outcomes [84].

9.3 Risk Scores System and Prediction Models

Numerous studies have attempted to develop a validated risk score for predicting LOC based on several preoperative clinical, radiological, and laboratory parameters [14, 25, 29, 42, 85–87]. However, these risk scores have not been well implemented in clinical practice, owing to the retrospective nature of most of these studies, lack of prospective validation, and lastly heterogeneity in patient selection and surgeon experience [16, 88]. Moreover, with the current advert of variety of strategies and techniques for dealing with a "Difficult cholecystectomy," conversion to open surgery in the face of these challenges has become much less frequently encountered [88]. Beksac et al. (2016) [85] retrospectively reviewed 1335 LC cases to develop a predictive statistical model based on identified risk factors for conversion. Based on four parameters (age, gender, history of abdominal surgery, and alkaline phosphatase level), their model predicted conversion with a sensitivity of 70% and a specificity of 79%. However, given its retrospective nature and patient heterogeneity, implantation remains restricted.

Siddiqui et al. (2017) [87] attempted to develop a risk score based on seven ultrasound findings through a single-center retrospective review of 300 LC cases. They found that a score of >5 has a sensitivity of 80.7% and specificity of 91.7% in predicting a difficult LC and significantly increase the risk of LOC. However, they excluded patients who underwent emergent LC and patients who underwent conversion based in the presence of other comorbidities. As we have shown previously, both of these variables are known risk factors for LOC, thus disregarding them excludes a significant proportion of patients who underwent conversion, putting the generalizability of these results into question.

Lastly, Sutcliffe et al. (2016) [14] developed a validated risk score for LOC based on a prospectively maintained cholecystectomy database from the United Kingdom that included 8820 patients across 166 hospitals. The risk score (CLOC score) was derived from six significant predictors of conversion: ASA class, age, gender, indication for LC, thickness of gallbladder wall, and CBD diameter. They concluded that a score of more than six identified patients at a high risk of conversion (7.1%, with an area under the curve = 0.766 ($P < 0.001$), and therefore, should be operated on by experienced surgeons. However, this study failed to identify the precise indication for conversion. Moreover, they failed to account for several variables that have been shown to exacerbate the risk of LOC including patient comorbidities, prior surgical history, and even the utilization of the critical view of safety during LC. This again puts the generalizability of this risk score to the general population into question.

In summary, the studies that have aimed to develop a statistical model for prediction of conversion are limited by a small sample size, patient heterogeneity, retrospective nature, and failure to account for the "surgeon" variable. Therefore, the applicability of these models and their implementation into clinical practice is limited by the lack of validation and prospective evidence. Nevertheless, although these models can aid in operative planning, recognizing the aforementioned risk factors as significant predictors of conversion and making the necessary treatment decision are key factors in optimizing patient outcomes.

9.4 Conclusions

Conversion from laparoscopic to open cholecystectomy is multifactorial in origin and, as we have shown, is influenced by several patient-related, disease-related, and surgeon-related factors. In the setting of an intraoperative complications such as bleeding, or as a means to avoid iatrogenic injury and even if progress cannot be accomplished laparoscopically, the operating surgeon might consider abandoning the laparoscopic approach and converting to open [16, 29]. Several prior reports have shown that patients who do undergo conversion may have an increased length of hospital stay, surgical site infection rates, and possibly overall morbidity [12, 13, 16, 30]. However, conversion should still be considered as one of several alternative options to deal with the "difficult gallbladder." This modality, in the face of intraoperative challenges, should never be considered as a complication nor as a failure on part of the surgeon. Rather, it is a safe option to avoid complications and optimize patient outcomes. Preoperative identification of the cited risk factors for LOC is crucial for appropriate operative planning, surgeon preparation, and, most importantly, improved patient outcomes.

Acknowledgments We have no disclosures to make, financial or otherwise.

References

1. Ahmed A, Ranjan SK, Sinha DK, et al. Changing incidence of gall stone disease: a single centre study from Eastern India. IOSR J Dent Med Sci. 2015;14(12):50–3.
2. Shaffer EA. Epidemiology and risk factors for gallstone disease: has the paradigm changed in the 21st century? Curr Gastroenterol Rep. 2005;7:132–40.
3. Shaffer EA. Gallstone disease: epidemiology of gallbladder stone disease. Best Pract Res Clin Gastroenterol. 2006;20:981–96.
4. Chen CH, Huang MH, Yang JC. Prevalence and risk factors of gallstone disease in an adult population of Taiwan: an epidemiological survey. J Gastr Hepa. 2006;21(2):1737–43.
5. Coccolini F, Catena F, Pisano M, et al. Open versus laparoscopic cholecystectomy in acute cholecystitis. Systematic review and meta-analysis. Int J Surg. 2015;18:196–204.
6. Gaillard M, Tranchart H, Lainas P, et al. New minimally invasive approaches for cholecystectomy: review of literature. World J Gastrointest Surg. 2015;27:243–8.
7. Keus F, de Jong J, Gooszen HG, et al. Laparoscopic versus open cholecystectomy for patients with symptomatic cholecystolithiasis. Cochrane Database Syst Rev. 2006;18(4):CD006231.
8. Ros A, Gustafsson L, Krook H, et al. Laparoscopic cholecystectomy versus mini-laparotomy cholecystectomy. Ann Surg. 2001;234(6):741–9.
9. Comitalo JB. Laparoscopic cholecystectomy and newer techniques of gallbladder removal. JSLS. 2012;16:406–12.
10. Kiviluoto T, Siren J, Luukkonen P, et al. Randomized trial of laparoscopic versus open cholecystectomy for acute and gangrenous cholecystitis. Lancet. 1998;351:321–5.
11. Dalwani AG, Shaikh R, Das K, et al. Complications of laparoscopic cholecystectomy at Liaquat University, Jamshoro. World Appl Sci J. 2013;23:808–11.
12. Li W, Chu C, Cheung M. Factors for conversion in laparoscopic cholecystectomy for acute cholecystitis: is timing important? Surg Pract. 2009;13(2):42–7.
13. Sippey M, Grzybowski M, Manwaring ML, et al. Acute cholecystitis: risk factors for conversion to an open procedure. J Surg Res. 2015;199(2):357–61.
14. Sutcliffe RP, Hollyman M, Hodson J, et al. Preoperative risk factors for conversion from laparoscopic to open cholecystectomy: a validated risk score derived from a prospective UK database of 8820 patients. HPB (Oxford). 2016;18(11):922–8.
15. Coffin SJ, Wrenn SM, Callas PW, et al. Three decades later: investigating the rate of and risks for conversion from laparoscopic to open cholecystectomy. Surg Endosc. 2017;32(2):923–9.
16. Al Masri S, Shaib Y, Edelbi M, et al. Predicting conversion from laparoscopic to open cholecystectomy: a single institution retrospective study. World J Surg. 2018;42(8):2373–82.
17. Mannino M, Toro A, Teodoro M et al. Open conversion for laparoscopically difficult cholecystectomy is still a valid solution with unsolved aspects. World J Emerg Surg 2019;14(1).
18. Yadav P, Janugade HB. A clinical study to determine predictive factors for difficult laparoscopic cholecystectomy. J Med Sci Clin Res. 2019;7:1.
19. Fried GM, Barkun JS, Sigman HH, et al. Factors determining conversion to laparotomy in patients undergoing laparoscopic cholecystectomy. Am J Surg. 1994;167(1):35–9.
20. Philip Rothman J, Burcharth J, Pommergaard HC, et al. Preoperative risk factors for conversion of laparoscopic cholecystectomy to open surgery - a systematic review and meta-analysis of observational studies. Dig Surg. 2016;33:414–23.
21. Yol S, Kartal A, Vatansev C, et al. Sex as a factor in conversion from laparoscopic cholecystectomy to open surgery. JSLS. 2006;10:359–63.
22. Lein HH, Huang CS. Male gender: risk factor for severe symptomatic cholelithiasis. World J Surg. 2002;26:598–601.
23. Brunt LM, Quasebarth MA, Dunnegan DL, et al. Outcomes analysis of laparoscopic cholecystectomy in the extremely elderly. Surg Endosc. 2001;15:700–5.
24. Giger UF, Michel JM, Opitz I, et al. Risk factors for perioperative complications in patients undergoing laparoscopic cholecystectomy: analysis of 22,953 consecutive cases from the Swiss Association of Laparoscopic and Thoracoscopic Surgery database. J Am Coll Surg. 2006;203:723–8.
25. Ashfaq A, Ahmadieh K, Shah AA, et al. The difficult gallbladder: outcomes following laparoscopic cholecystectomy and the need for open conversion. Am J Surg. 2016;212:1261–4.
26. Goh JC, Tan JK, Lim JW, et al. Laparoscopic cholecystectomy for acute cholecystitis: an analysis of early versus delayed cholecystectomy and predictive factors for conversion. Minerva Chir. 2017;72:455–63.
27. Yang TF, Guo L, Wang Q. Evaluation of preoperative risk factor for converting laparoscopic to open cholecystectomy: a meta-analysis. Hepato-Gastroenterology. 2014;61:958–65.
28. Farkas D, Moradi D, Moaddel D, et al. The impact of body mass index on outcomes after laparoscopic cholecystectomy. Surg Endosc. 2012;26(4):964–9.
29. Goonawardena J, Gunnarsson R, de Costa A. Predicting conversion from laparoscopic to open cholecystectomy presented as a probability nomogram based on preoperative patient risk factors. Am J Surg. 2015;210:492–500.
30. Madan A, Menachery S. Safety and efficacy of initial trocar placement in morbidly obese patients. Arch Surg. 2006;141(3):300.
31. Clapp B. Optimal initial trocar placement for morbidly obese patients. JSLS. 2018;22(4):e2017.00101.

32. Alijani A, Hanna GB, Cuschieri A. Abdominal wall lift versus positive-pressure capnoperitoneum for laparoscopic cholecystectomy: randomized controlled trial. Ann Surg. 2004;239:388–94.
33. Harboe KM, Bardram L. The quality of cholecystectomy in Denmark: outcome and risk factors for 20,307 patients from the national database. Surg Endosc. 2011;25:1630–41.
34. Kaafarani HM, Smith TS, Neumayer L, et al. Trends, outcomes, and predictors of open and conversion to open cholecystectomy in Veterans Health Administration hospitals. Am J Surg. 2010;200:32–40.
35. de Goede B, Klitsie PJ, S Hagen M, et al. Meta-analysis of laparoscopic versus open cholecystectomy for patients with liver cirrhosis and symptomatic cholecystolithiasis. Br J Surg. 2013;100(2):209–16.
36. Strömberg J, Hammarqvist F, Sadr-Azodi O, et al. Cholecystectomy in patients with liver cirrhosis. Gastroenterol Res Pract. 2015;2015:1–6.
37. Gallstones and laparoscopic cholecystectomy. NIH Consens Statement. 1992;10(3):1–28.
38. Puggioni A, Wong LL. A meta-analysis of laparoscopic cholecystectomy in patients with cirrhosis. J Am Coll Surg. 2003;197:921–6.
39. Nguyen KT, Kitisin K, Steel J, et al. Cirrhosis is not a contraindication to laparoscopic cholecystectomy: results and practical recommendations. HPB (Oxford). 2011;13(3):192–7.
40. Machado NO. Laparoscopic cholecystectomy in cirrhotics. JSLS. 2012;16:392–400.
41. Delis S, Bakoyiannis A, Madariaga J, et al. Laparoscopic cholecystectomy in cirrhotic patients: the value of MELD score and child-Pugh classification in predicting outcome. Surg Endosc. 2010;24:407.
42. Lipman J, Claridge J, Haridas M, et al. Preoperative findings predict conversion from laparoscopic to open cholecystectomy. Surgery. 2007;142(4):556–65.
43. Karamanos E, Sivrikoz E, Beale E, et al. Effect of diabetes on outcomes in patients undergoing emergent cholecystectomy for acute cholecystitis. World J Surg. 2013;37:2257.
44. Aucott J, Cooper G, Bloom A, et al. Management of gallstones in diabetic patients. Arch Intern Med. 1993;153(9):1053.
45. Paajanen H, Suuronen S, Nordstrom P, et al. Laparoscopic versus open cholecystectomy in diabetic patients and postoperative outcome. Surg Endosc. 2011;25:764–70.
46. Yusoff IF, Barkun JS, Barkun AN. Diagnosis and management of cholecystitis and cholangitis. Gastroenterol Clin N Am. 2003;32:1145–68.
47. Yokoe M, Hata J, Strasberg SM, et al. Tokyo guidelines 2018: diagnostic criteria and severity of grading of acute cholecystitis. J Hepatobiliary Pancreat Surg. 2018;25:42–54.
48. Karim T, Patel G, Jain A, et al. Gallbladder perforation: a prospective study of its divergent appearance and management. Euroasian J Hepatogastroenterol. 2019;9(1):14–9.
49. Bouassida M, Mroua B, Zribi S, et al. Usefulness of laparoscopy in gangrenous cholecystitis. Surg Laparosc Endosc Percutan Tech. 2016;26(1):90–2.
50. Safwan M, Penny S. Emphysematous Cholecystitis. J Diagn Med Sonogr. 2016;32(3):131–7.
51. Bat O. The analysis of 146 patients with difficult laparoscopic cholecystectomy. Int J Clin Exp Med. 2015;8:16127–31.
52. Iwashita Y, Hibi T, Ohyama T, et al. An opportunity in difficulty: Japan–Korea–Taiwan expert Delphi consensus on surgical difficulty during laparoscopic cholecystectomy. J Hepatobiliary Pancreat Sci. 2017;24:191–8.
53. Kama NA, Doganay M, Dolapci M, et al. Risk factors resulting in conversion of laparoscopic cholecystectomy to open surgery. Surg Endosc. 2001;15:965–8.
54. Ambe PC, Jansen S, Macher-Heidrich S, et al. Surgical management of emphysematous cholecystitis: a register study of over 12,000 cases from a regional quality control database in Germany. Surg Endosc. 2016;30:5319–24.
55. Jansen S, Doemer J, Macher-Heidrich S, et al. Outcome of acute perforated cholecystitis: a register study of over 5,000 cases from a quality control database in Germany. Surg Endosc. 2017;31:1896–900.
56. Inoue K, Ueno T, Douchi D, et al. Risk factors for difficulty of laparoscopic cholecystectomy in grade II acute cholecystitis according to the Tokyo guidelines 2013. BMC Surg. 2017;17:11.
57. Thangavelu A, Rosenbaum S, Thangavelu D. Timing of cholecystectomy in acute cholecystitis. J Emerg Med. 2018;54(6):892–7.
58. Song G, Bian W, Zeng X, et al. Laparoscopic cholecystectomy for acute cholecystitis. Medicine. 2016;95(23):e3835.
59. Gurusamy KS, Davidson C, Gluud C, et al. Early versus delayed laparoscopic cholecystectomy for people with acute cholecystitis. Cochrane Database Syst Rev. 2013;6:CD005440.
60. Roulin D, Saadi A, Di Mare L, et al. Early versus delayed chole- cystectomy for acute cholecystitis, are the 72 hours still the rule? A randomized trial. Ann Surg. 2016;264:717.
61. Lai EC, Lau WV. Mirizzi syndrome: history, present and future development. ANZ J Surg. 2006;76:251–7.
62. Schäfer M, Schneiter R, Krahenbuhl L. Incidence and management of Mirizzi syndrome during laparoscopic cholecystectomy. Surg Endosc. 2003;17:1186–90.
63. Erben Y, Benavente-Chenhalls LA, Donohue JM, et al. Diagnosis and treatment of Mirizzi syndrome: 23-year Mayo Clinic experience. J Am Coll Surg. 2011;213:114.
64. Clemente G, Tringali A, De Rose A, et al. Mirizzi syndrome: diagnosis and management of a challenging biliary disease. Can J Gastroenterol Hepatol. 2018;2018:1–6.
65. Prasad T, Kumar A, Sikora S, et al. Mirizzi syndrome and gallbladder cancer. J Hepato-Biliary-Pancreat Surg. 2006;13(4):323–6.

66. Koike D, Suka V, Nagai M, et al. Laparoscopic management of Mirizzi syndrome without dissection of Calot's triangle. J Laparoendosc Adv Surg Tech A. 2017;27:141–5.
67. Fuks D, Mouly C, Robert B, et al. Acute cholecystitis: preoperative CT can help the surgeon consider conversion from laparoscopic to open cholecystectomy. Radiology. 2012;263:128–38.
68. Lee D, Ahn Y, Lee H. Prevalence and characteristics of clinically significant retained common bile duct stones after laparoscopic cholecystectomy for symptomatic cholelithiasis. Ann Surg Treat Res. 2016;91(5):239.
69. Williams E, Beckingham I, El Sayed G, et al. Updated guideline on the management of common bile duct stones (CBDS). Gut. 2017;66(5):765–82.
70. Collins C, Maguire D, Ireland A, et al. A prospective study of common bile duct calculi in patients undergoing laparoscopic cholecystectomy: natural history of choledocholithiasis revisited. Ann Surg. 2004;239:28–33.
71. Gurusamy KS, Koti R, Davidson BR. T-tube drainage versus primary closure after laparoscopic common bile duct exploration. Cochrane Database Syst Rev. 2013;6:CD005641.
72. Zhu HY, Xu M, Shen HJ, et al. A meta-analysis of single stage versus two-stage management for concomitant gallstones and common bile duct stones. Clin Res Hepatol Gastroenterol. 2015;39:584–93.
73. Nagaraja V, Eslick GD, Cox MR. Systematic review and meta-analysis of minimally invasive techniques for the management of cholecysto-choledocholithiasis. J Hepatobiliary Pancreat Sci. 2014;21:896–901.
74. Krishna S, Kamboj A, Hart P, et al. The changing epidemiology of acute pancreatitis hospitalizations. Pancreas. 2017;46(4):482–8.
75. Colvin S, Smith E, Morgan D. Acute pancreatitis: an update on the revised Atlanta classification. Abdom Radiol (NY). 2019;45(5):1222–31.
76. Giuffrida P, Biagiola D, Cristiano A, et al. Laparoscopic cholecystectomy in acute mild gallstone pancreatitis: how early is safe? Updates Surg. 2020;72(1):129–35.
77. Moody N, Adiamah A, Yanni F, et al. Meta-analysis of randomized clinical trials of early versus delayed cholecystectomy for mild gallstone pancreatitis. Br J Surg. 2019;106(11):1442–51.
78. Ekici U, Tatlı F, Kanlıöz M. Preoperative and postoperative risk factors in laparoscopic cholecystectomy converted to open surgery. Adv Clin Exp Med. 2019;28(7):857–60.
79. Chávez K, Márquez-González H, Aguirre I, et al. Prognostic risk factors for conversion in laparoscopic cholecystectomy. Updat Surg. 2017;70(1):67–72.
80. Panni R, Strasberg S. Preoperative predictors of conversion as indicators of local inflammation in acute cholecystitis: strategies for future studies to develop quantitative predictors. J Hepatobiliary Pancreat Sci. 2017;25(1):101–8.
81. Sakpal SV, Bindra SS, Chamberlain RS. Laparoscopic cholecystectomy conversion rates two decades later. JSLS. 2010;14:476–83.
82. Andrews S. Does concentration of surgical expertise improve outcomes for laparoscopic cholecystectomy? 9-year audit cycle. Surgeon. 2013;11:309–12.
83. Griniatsos J. Factors predisposing to conversion from laparoscopic to open cholecystectomy. Ann Laparosc Endosc Surg. 2018;3:12.
84. Bresadola V, Pravisani R, Pighin M, et al. Clinical strategies to aim an adequate safety profile for patients and effective training for surgical residents: the laparoscopic cholecystectomy model. Ann Med Surg (Lond). 2016;11:58–61.
85. Beksac K, Turhan N, Karaagaoglu E, et al. Risk factors for conversion of laparoscopic cholecystectomy to open surgery: a new predictive statistical model. J Laparoendosc Adv Surg Tech A. 2016;26(9):693–6.
86. Bourgouin S, Mancini J, Monchal T. How to predict difficult laparoscopic cholecystectomy? Proposal for a simple preoperative scoring system. Am J Surg. 2016;212(5):873–81.
87. Siddiqui M, Rizvi S, Sartaj S, et al. A standardized ultrasound scoring system for preoperative prediction of difficult laparoscopic cholecystectomy. J Med Ultrasound. 2017;25:227–31.
88. Nassar A, Hodson J, Ng H, et al. Predicting the difficult laparoscopic cholecystectomy: development and validation of a pre-operative risk score using an objective operative difficulty grading system. Surg Endosc. 2019;34(10):4549–61.

Difficult Laparoscopic Cholecystectomy: When to Convert to Open Technique

10

Fabrizio D'Acapito, Giuliano La Barba, Chiara Togni, and Giorgio Ercolani

10.1 Introduction

Laparoscopic cholecystectomy (LC) is the "gold standard" in the treatment of symptomatic gallbladder's lithiasis and is the most performed laparoscopic abdominal surgery in the world.

It is associated with a morbidity rate of around 10% with an increased risk of bile duct injury (0.1–1.5%) when compared to open surgery [1, 2].

In elective procedures, the laparoscopic conversion rate in the open cholecystectomy is low with a range in the literature between 2% and 15% [3–6], while it increases up to 25% when the patient is operated on for acute cholecystitis [7, 8].

There are conditions in which it is not possible to complete the cholecystectomy safely and in such cases deviations from the standard surgical procedure are mandatory.

In the literature, this condition is generically identified as "difficult gallbladder" and represents a challenge for the laparoscopic surgeon.

"Difficult gallbladder" (DGB) corresponds to a procedure with an increased surgical risk compared to standard cholecystectomies and has been reported with an incidence up to 26% in large series [9, 10].

The concept of "difficult gallbladder" is mainly based on intraoperative findings and strongly depends on the surgeon's skills. The pattern of "difficult gallbladder" is characterized by severe inflammation which makes dissection difficult, alters the anatomy, and increases the risk of bleeding [11, 12]. In 2016, among 2212 patients undergoing laparoscopic cholecystectomy in 10 years, Ashfaq A. et al. reported in 351 (15.8%) criteria of difficult gallbladder and among these the conversion rate was 19.9% [11].

In case of acute cholecystitis, chronic or scleroatrophic cholecystitis and cirrhotic liver are more frequently faced with a difficult gallbladder scenario (Fig. 10.1).

Acute cholecystitis is one of the main causes of acute abdominal hospitalization in the adult population and the most common indication for abdominal surgery in the elderly patient [13, 14]. Early laparoscopic cholecystectomy results in a shorter postoperative hospitalization period and lower healthcare costs [7, 15]. In a recent study by Kais H. et al., in 1658 laparoscopic cholecystectomies, the conversion rate increases more than tenfold depending on whether the surgery was

F. D'Acapito · G. La Barba
Department of Surgery, "Morgagni-Pierantoni" Hospital, Forlì, Italy
e-mail: fabrizio.dacapito@auslromagna.it; giuliano.labarba@auslromagna.it

C. Togni · G. Ercolani (✉)
Department of Surgery, "Morgagni-Pierantoni" Hospital, Forlì, Italy

Department of medical and surgical sciences, University of Bologna, Bologna, Italy
e-mail: chiara.togni2@studio.unibo.it; giorgio.ercolani2@unibo.it

© Springer Nature Switzerland AG 2021
I. Di Carlo (ed.), *Difficult Acute Cholecystitis*, https://doi.org/10.1007/978-3-030-62102-5_10

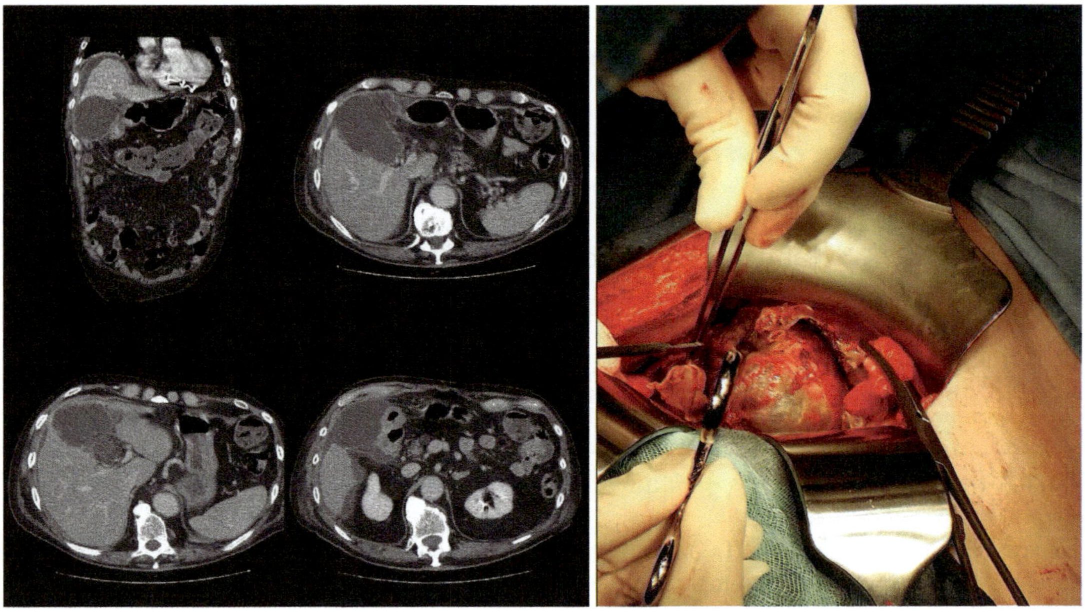

Fig. 10.1 Sample case: 89-year-old male. Admission to E.R. for abdominal pain for over 48 h. Abdominal U.S: acute acalculous cholecystitis with thickening of the walls and pericholecystic fluid. Medical therapy started. After 24 h worsening of clinical symptoms. CT scan: acute gangrenous cholecystitis, hydrops, peri-cholecystic abscess and perihepatic fluid , with irregularity of the gallbladder wall and the partial lack of contrast enhancement (perforation at the fundus level). Indication for emergency surgery. Laparoscopic approach but early conversion. Right subcostal laparotomy. Intraoperative evidence of: free corpuscular fluid in the abdomen; viscero-parietal and liver-diaphragmatic adhesion; abscess between cholecysts and «falciform ligament» and in the Morrison's pouch. The gallbladder is hydropic, with necrotic areas at the body and fundus level with at least two perforations. An anterograde cholecystectomy was performed leaving a small portion of gallbladder in the cholecystic bed

performed in election or for acute cholecystitis from 2.1% to 24.8%, respectively [16]. In order to univocally define the acute cholecystitis patterns, several scores have been proposed, the most widespread of which are the Tokyo Guidelines in their last revision dated 2018 (TG18). The TG 18 also suggest a treatment flowchart [17–20].

A recent Swedish study reported a doubled risk of bile duct injury (BDI) in acute cholecystitis and showed a statistically significant association between the severity of cholecystitis according to TG18 and BDI risk [21].

Chronic or scleroatrophic cholecystitis can lead to a difficult gallbladder pattern. The Swiss Society of Laparoscopic and Thoracoscopic Surgery analyzed a database of 22,953 patients and found a conversion rate for acute cholecystitis of 15.9% versus 6.4% for chronic cholecystitis. Both are significantly higher than for standard cholecystectomy [3].

Prevalence of gallstones in patients with cirrhosis is estimated at 29–46% and is three times higher than that in patients without cirrhosis [22]. Laparoscopic cholecystectomy in cirrhosis is associated with a morbidity rate between 5% and 23% and a mortality rate between 7% and 20%.

In a review on cholecystectomy in cirrhotic patients, Laurence J.M et al. reported that mortality rates in LC was 0.74% while in open cholecystectomy it was 2%, the conversion rate was 5.8% while the overall complication rate was 17.6% in LC and 47.7% in open [23]. In another review, Machado N.O. documented a conversion rate of 4.58%, 17% morbidity, and 0.45% mortality [24].

Cholecystectomy is more hazardous in cirrhosis because of hemorrhage related to portal hypertension, coagulopathy, and thrombocytopenia [23].

Surgeons around the world, after an initial period in which the majority of them were convinced that the cholecystectomy had to be completed in laparoscopy, soon realized that the procedure had to be converted to avoid complications [25].

A large-scale multinational survey involving more than 500 participants from Japan, Korea, and Taiwan achieved that the commonly used indicators of surgical difficulty during LC, such as the duration of surgery, estimated blood loss, and open conversion rate, are inappropriate as they are surgeon- and workplace-dependent. Safety measures and recognition of landmarks and gallbladder anatomy during LC are performed at the surgeons' discretion and are not yet standardized [26].

Laparoscopic surgeons have been found to have conversion rates to open surgery of one-fourth compared to others [27]. Laparoscopic surgeons tend to persist in laparoscopy even in case of significant lengthening of operating time caused by extensive viscerolysis, Calot fibrosis, or diffuse scarring of the gallbladder bed.

Another aspect to be considered is the training of young surgeons who have less experience in open cholecystectomy. Approximately 20% of surgeons find that conversion to open surgery does not make the procedure safer but sometimes more difficult [26].

In case of a difficult cholecystectomy, it is necessary to make sure to be as much as possible in the condition in which the conversion is an "elective" choice of the operator before being forced to do it as a result of major intraoperative complications.

10.2 Risk Factors to Open Conversion

Three types of factor have been identified in the literature that predispose to the conversion of the procedure and are classified as: patient-related, disease-related, and surgeon-related.

The "patient-related" factors are: age over 65 [28], male gender, BMI over 30, history of upper abdominal surgery, ASA score, cirrhosis [24, 29], diabetes mellitus (which can cause a delayed perception of symptoms) [30].

The "disease-related" factors are: gallbladder wall thicknesses (suggesting that a gallbladder wall thicker than 4–5 mm on preoperative ultrasound is a risk factor for conversion.); acute cholecystitis [29, 31], recurrent biliary colic, acute biliary pancreatitis; Mirizzi syndrome (found in 0.3–3%); GB cancer (which should be kept in mind in over 65-year-old patients, female gender, and high level of alkaline phosphatase); lithiasis of the main bile duct [6]; and the following laboratory data: CRP [32], WBC, albumin, and liver function tests [31].

"Surgeon-related" factors are the experience and skills of the surgeon [3, 33–35]. Using these factors, scores and models have been built to predict the conversion risk [6, 31, 36–38].

The pattern observed from these risk scores and models is that the risk of conversion increased when more risk factors were presented.

Defining risk factors for conversion and complications is important when planning the procedure and deciding who should perform the cholecystectomy [39].

In 2018, using the Delphi consensus methodology, Iwashita Y. identified 25 aspects of intraoperative difficulty associated to conversion; among these, diffuse scaring in the Calot's triangle area had the strongest impact on surgical difficulty. Surgeons agreed that the surgical difficulty increases as more fibrotic change and scarring develop [18].

A "universally recognized" codification of the steps of laparoscopic cholecystectomy is essential, in particular, in the difficult gallbladder to limit the risks of BDI and biliary-vascular injury (BVI) [17]. The training of young surgeons should aim at this result.

The primary target of laparoscopic cholecystectomy is "safety first, total cholecystectomy second," and the surgeon should always keep in mind this culture of safety and remain vigilant to stay ahead of dangerous situations. Safe management of the difficult gallbladder is possible with technical adjustment and careful use of bailout procedures.

10.3 Safe Steps in Laparoscopic Cholecystectomy in Difficult Gallbladder Pattern and When to Evaluate the Use of Bailout Procedures

We will develop the discussion by proposing a procedural algorithm built on the "Safe Step in Laparoscopic Cholecystectomy for Acute Cholecystitis" identified by Wakabayashi in the TG 2018, inserting moments of "time-out" in which the most common difficulties that can be found in the different steps will be identified, and codified solutions will be proposed (Fig. 10.2). In the next section of the chapter, we will examine in detail the bailout techniques.

The first assessment of the procedure should be made before carrying the patient to the operating room. It is necessary to assess with the anesthesiologist, depending on the anamnesis (COPD, cardiovascular diseases, previous surgery, especially of the upper abdomen, etc.) and the patient's condition at the time of surgery (grade of cholecystitis according to TG18), whether he is able to tolerate pneumoperitoneum for an adequate operative time, also evaluating in advance the possibility of a long and complex viscerolysis [12].

If the patient's condition is very damaged, consider the possibility of using percutaneous cholecystostomy as a definitive management or "bridge" to surgery [40].

10.4 In Operating Room

10.4.1 Step 1

A specific patient position is not considered as being better (French Vs American) [19].

In patients who have already been operated on, the site of the first port must be carefully chosen [41], also in variance with what is considered, the standard setting used in the surgical unit, in order to reduce the risk of being in an adhesion tangle that could lead to visceral iatrogenic lesions from the time of peritoneal access [12]. The method of placement of the first trocar should be tailored to the patient's characteristics. The open trocar insertion is a safe technique [42]. In cirrhotic patients, the first port was placed, with the open technique, in the midline sub-umbelically to avoid undetected enlarged collateral vessels [43].

Once the pneumoperitoneum has been established, it is necessary to evaluate the extent and characteristics of the adhesions to assess the complexity and risk of iatrogenic lesions from viscerolysis and the possibility of a significant increase in surgical time compared to an open procedure [44]. This is a good time to decide on an early conversion.

In a patient where the supramesocolic district is inaccessible due to adhesions, perhaps between the transverse colon and the parietal peritoneum, a right subcostal laparotomy could allow access to the cholecystic lodge avoiding prolonged and risky viscerolysis maneuvers. The same applies if there are adhesions that significantly hinder the setting of two or more trocar. Usually the lysis of adhesions caused by an acute cholecystitis is all the easier the earlier the intervention is performed compared to the onset, while the exacerbation on previous acute episodes usually leads to tenacious adhesions. During viscerolysis maneuvers, it is advisable to proceed as far as possible to dissect using cold scissors [41]. In case of the first episode of cholecystitis, especially if the intervention is performed early at the onset of symptoms, the adhesions are smoothed out. In case of relapse on chronic cholecystitis or in case of covered perforation, the adhesions can be tenacious. Viscerolysis should be performed particularly carefully to avoid injury to the duodenum, which may be attached to the gallbladder (Fig. 10.3).

10.4.2 Step 2

Once the gallbladder has been visualized, the possibility of its mobilization must be evaluated.

The mobilization of the gallbladder is a key point because it allows the correct exposure of the hepatocystic triangle. A correct mobilization involves a traction with fundus clamp towards

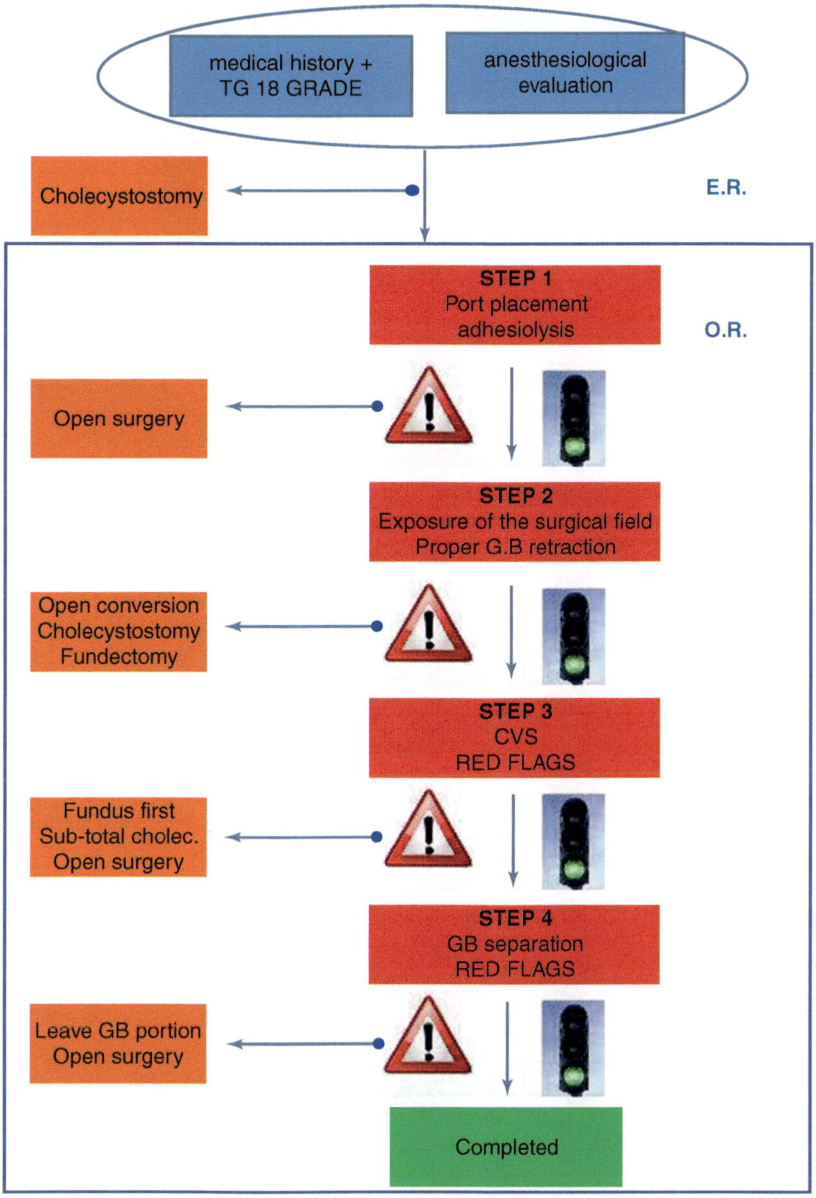

Fig. 10.2 Safe step in laparoscopic cholecistectomy: If the individual steps cannot be completed safely, Bail-out methods are suggested

the right shoulder of the patient associated with a traction with a second clamp positioned on the Hartmann pouch downwards and to the right [45]. Surgeons should keep in mind that decreasing the number of port and/or using smaller instruments may create technical challenges, due to more difficult retraction and triangulation [19]. In the case of an outstretched gallbladder (hydropic or emphysematous), prior needle aspiration results in decompression with minimal intraperitoneal contamination [46] (Fig. 10.4). Once aspirated, it is necessary to evaluate the thickness and consistency of the walls of the gallbladder. The use of an endograsper or the placement of one or more traction points on the bottom can mobilize the most demanding gallbladder. Usually the bleeding resulting from the trauma of the gallbladder wall is annoying but not significant.

The presence of large necrotic areas can preclude the possibility of performing a valid

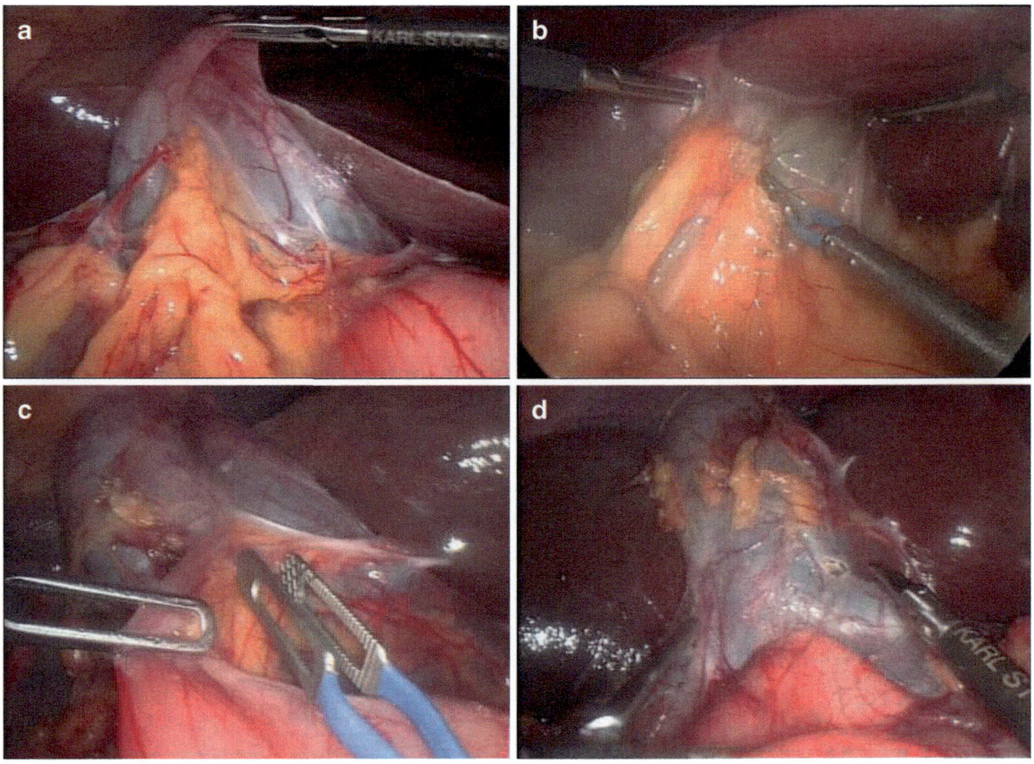

Fig. 10.3 Examples of different types of adhesions: (**a**) cholecysto-omental adhesions; (**b**) cholecysto-omental adhesions with acute cholecystitis edema; (**c**) bridge of adipose tissue binding the stomach to the gallbladder; (**d**) the first duodenal portion is fused to the gallbladder

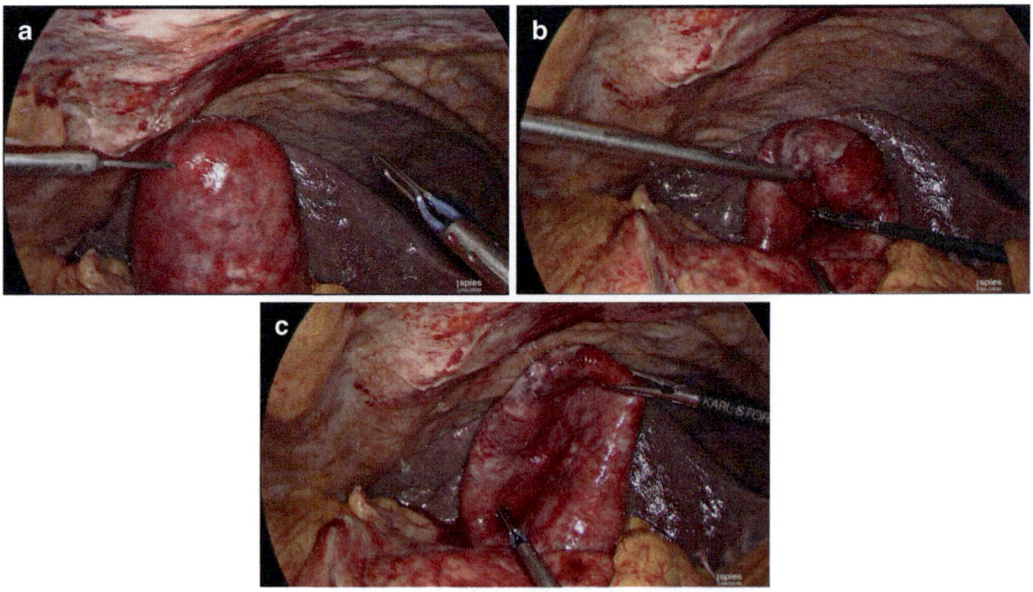

Fig. 10.4 Outstreatched gallbladder. (**a**) A suction needle is introduced from the port on the right side (always under direct vision). (**b**) The emptying of the gallbladder can be facilitated by cautious compression (milking) maneuvers performed with a clamp. (**c**) At the end of the procedure the prick area is grasped with the forceps in order to limit as much as possible the outflow of residual bile

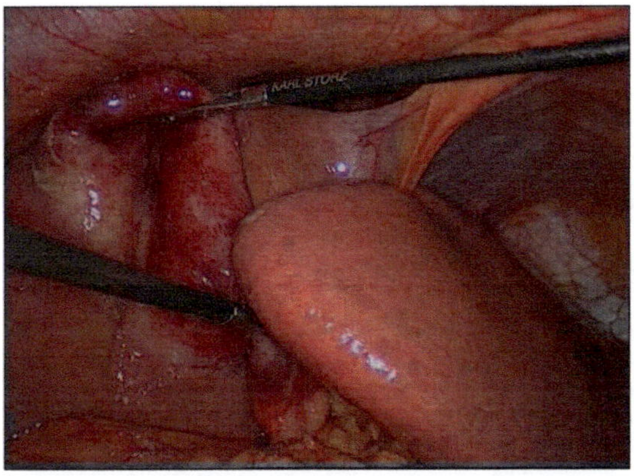

Fig. 10.5 Steatosic liver with segment 3 hypertrophy hiding the hepatocystic triangle

gallbladder traction, while the presence of perforations with constant outflow of pus, bile, and calculi can make the evaluation of the operating field very complex.

Even a bulky calculus impacted in the infundibulum can limit the possibility of mobilization of the gallbladder; often cautious maneuvers with the aspirator or with forceps allow the infundibular calculus to dislodge towards the gallbladder body [47].

Another element to take into account is the liver. The presence of segment 3 or 4 hypertrophy covering the hepatic pedicle may require the use of a retractor to visualize the cholecystic hilum or may force the use of incorrect traction to visualize the hepatocystic triangle (Fig. 10.5).

Liver texture is another important variable because tractions on a steatosic liver can lead to lacerations with subsequent bleeding while a cirrhotic liver can be very difficult to mobilize because it is hard and fibrotic [43]. The adhesions in the cirrhotic patient may be hypervascularized. Furthermore, the finding of signs of portal hypertension should lead to a careful reconsideration of the therapeutic strategy chosen for the high risk of bleeding [43].

10.4.3 Step 3

10.4.3.1 Critical View of Safety (CVS)

The CVS is not a dissection technique. It is the final view that is achieved after a thorough dissection of the hepatocystic triangle to delineate the cystic duct and the cystic artery before they are clipped and divided. The CVS should be seen clearly both from the front and the back to have a complete circumferential visualization of the cystic duct and the artery (doublet view). The anterior view is easily achievable by retracting the infundibulum inferolaterally towards the right (with segment 5 surface visible across window), while the posterior view requires the infundibulum to be retracted towards the umbilical fissure (with segment 4/quadrate lobe surface visible across window). Dissection has to lead to the creation of 2 windows, one between the cystic duct and the artery and one between the artery and the liver. The cystic plate must be clearly identified [48].

To obtain the CVS, the coded technique involves three steps [49]:

(a) Clearance of the hepatocystic (HC) triangle: The HC triangle should be cleared of all the fibrofatty and soft areolar tissue. Once adequately cleared of all fibrofatty tissue, the under surface of the liver is easily seen across this triangle.
(b) Exposure of the lower cystic plate: The gallbladder should be separated from its liver bed to expose at least the lower third of the cystic plate.
(c) Two and only two tubular structures should be seen entering the gallbladder: The cystic duct and the cystic artery [19] (Fig. 10.6).

Because of inflammation of the tissues of the hepatocystic triangle, the maneuvers often cause bleeding. For persistent bleeding, the surgeon must achieve hemostasis primarily by compression and by avoiding the excessive use of electrocautery or clipping [18]. The same gallbladder should be used as a compression instrument for parenchyma; the use of gauze and/or local hemostatic (e.g., oxidized cellulose) should also be considered [50]. There is a low level of evidence in favor of recommending a source of energy compared to another regarding safety. Bipolar, monopolar, and ultrasonic devices are appropriate source of energy for safe cholecystectomy [19]. If a monopolar energy device (most of the one with hook cautery) is used, it is important to keep it at a low setting; divide a small amount of

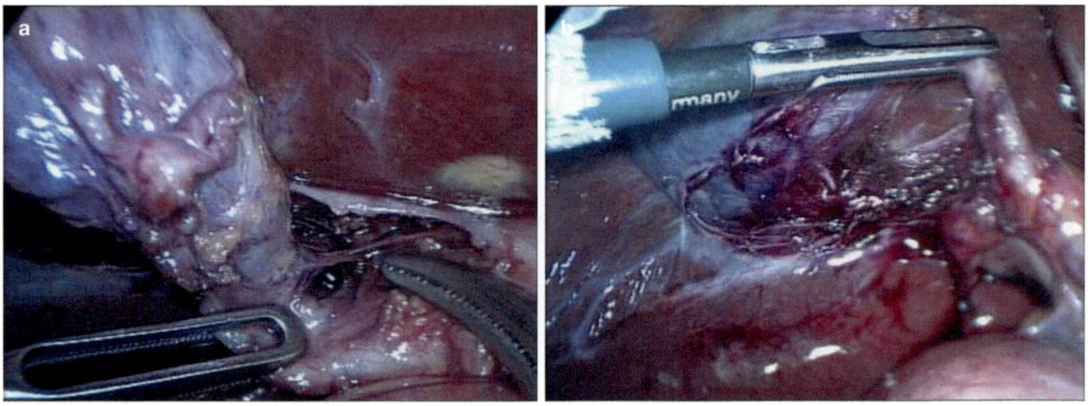

Fig. 10.6 The CVS should be seen clearly both from front (**a**) and the back (**b**) to have complete circumferential visualization of cystic duct and artery (doublet view). The HC triangle has been cleared of fibroadipose tissue, the gallbladder has been removed from the bottom third of the cystic plate, and 2 and only 2 structures are seen entering the gallbladder

tissue at a time after a gentle pull to avoid injury to deeper structures by the heel of the hook cautery; use intermittent short bursts of current at 2–3 s intervals in order to avoid thermal spread to the bile duct; and avoid blind use of cautery in the case of brisk bleeding [48, 51].

Bipolar cautery is useful to control bleeding in the HC triangle and in the liver bed.

Sometimes, the volumetric increase in Mascagni's lymph node (usually a landmark for cystic artery localization) makes it difficult to identify the cystic artery and gall bladder neck. In addition, in recurring inflammation, Rouviere's sulcus is often erased and not displayed correctly. In these cases, it is desirable to start the dissection very high in contact with the wall of the gallbladder, to which one must always remain attached, and then proceed on both sides to the gallbladder bed [52] (Fig. 10.7).

In chronic cholecystitis, inflammatory adhesions can melt the wall of the gallbladder to the wall of the common liver duct. If a biliary-cholecystic fistula is suspected at this stage, strongly consider a bailout technique [53].

In presence of severe acute and/or chronic inflammation, secure ductal identification by the critical view of safety (CVS) may be very challenging.

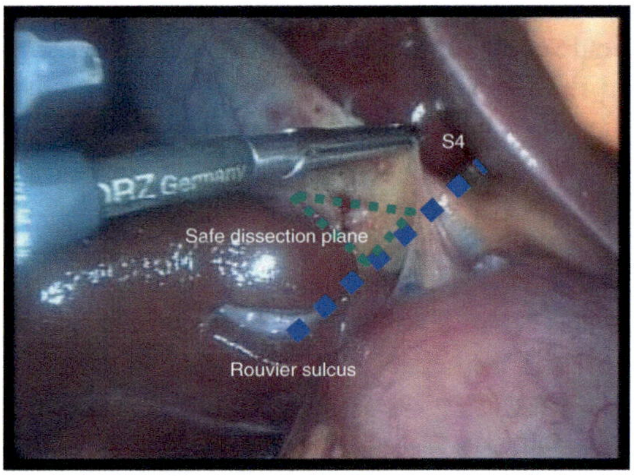

Fig. 10.7 Rouviere's sulcus. The sulcus indicates reliably the plane of the CBD; dissection may be started safely by division of the peritoneum immediately ventral to the sulcus and continued in a triangle bounded by the plane of the sulcus, the neck of the gallbladder and the liver surface

During "Step 3," it may also be useful to stop several times, widen the view of the surgical field, reevaluate our landmarks, and then resume the isolation maneuvers.

In accordance with the data in the literature, we have identified the warning signs, which we will call "red flags," to which particular attention should be paid during the acquisition of the CVS [47].

10.4.3.2 Red Flags

(a) More than two tubular structures entering GB [48].
(b) An unusually large presumed cystic artery (this may be the hepatic artery). The cystic artery is usually single, originates from RHA, and most commonly traverses the HC triangle. If the presence of a short cystic artery (<1 cm) is not noted during surgery, the right hepatic artery may be clipped and divided [54]. Keeping the dissection of the artery close to the gallbladder on the right side of the cystic lymph node may prevent injury to the right hepatic artery [47]. It may be useful to isolate a longer-than-usual tract of the artery to check whether it has penetrated the hepatic parenchyma or ended up in the gallbladder.
(c) Large artery pulsations behind the presumed cystic ducts (this duct may be common hepatic duct).
(d) A medium-large clip fails to occlude the ductal lumen (this duct may be the common hepatic duct) [55].
(e) Large ductal structure that can be traced behind the duodenum.
(f) Excessive fibrofatty/lymphatic tissue noted around the presumed cystic duct.
(g) Bile leak seen with intact GB: See dedicated paragraph.
(h) Bleeding requiring blood transfusion.

In persisting doubt, ask for a second opinion if available [56].

10.4.3.3 Warning

Alternative techniques to the standard exist and are implemented to obtain access to the cystic duct but they do not respect the principles of CVS.

The most widespread is the infundibular approach [57].

In the infundibular technique, cystic duct identification is based on the appearance of the infundibulum–cystic duct junction as a funnel. When this junction is circumferentially exposed, the surgeon confirms the identification of the cystic duct and then proceeds with its division. Complete dissection in the HC triangle is not performed at this stage. In certain situations, this technique can be misleading. When the cystic duct is fused with CBD due to acute or chronic inflammation, when the cystic duct is very short or effaced by a large stone impacted in the infundibulum, or when there is difficultly in exposing the HC triangle due to inadequate retraction, the CBD may be misidentified as the cystic duct. Circumferential dissection then goes around the CBD rather than around the cystic duct across the HC triangle. This leads to classic BDI where the bile duct is divided twice before the gallbladder can be completely separated from the liver. Therefore, this technique of cystic duct identification does not protect against biliary injury in difficult situations [48, 58–60].

The fundus first approach has been described as an alternative technique to complete LC in the presence of severe inflammation in the HC triangle. The gallbladder is dissected off its liver bed and then the cystic duct and the artery are identified and divided. However, the surgeons must be wary of this technique, they should have clear understanding of the cystic plate anatomy and pathological alteration affecting it, they should remain very close to the gallbladder throughout the dissection, and when such dissection does not seem possible, they should resort to bailout techniques like subtotal cholecystectomy (see dedicated paragraph).

Surgeons using this technique should be aware of this possible mishap [47].

Only after obtaining the CVS, surgeons should proceed to dissecting the artery and cystic duct [61].

10.4.4 Step 4

GB separation from its bed leaving behind the cystic plate attached to the liver.

Also, in this phase surgeons should pay attention especially in cirrhotic liver, scleroatrophic cholecystitis, and in partially intrahepatic and necrotic cholecystitis. It is better to leave a small portion of gallbladder in the cholecystic bed rather than enter the hepatic parenchyma in that site [43, 62].

Firstly, there might be troublesome bleeding from liver parenchyma, especially if the terminal tributaries of the middle hepatic vein (which lie in this location) are injured. This type of bleeding may sometimes require a conversion to open surgery for its control [62].

Secondly, sub-vesical bile ducts may be injured, causing a postoperative bile leak [63].

Such a breach is more likely to occur in chronic cholecystitis where the gallbladder may be densely adherent to the underlying liver without distinct dissection planes [64].

10.4.5 Special Issue: Bile Leak Seen with Intact GB

If bile appears in the operating field, you must identify the source of the leak. Do not proceed with blind dissections in search of the possible source [65], but try to obtain CVS. Once the cystic duct has been identified, perform an i.o. cholangiography to confirm and define the location and extent of the biliary injury [66, 67]. There is no evidence that IOC could prevent BDI [68–70], but IOC is recommended in order to define unclear anatomy [19]. In extreme cases, a cholangiography by direct puncture of the gallbladder can also be attempted. After the staging of the injury, you should make an evaluation of your experience in biliary surgery and decide how to proceed. In case of limited biliary surgery experience, it is preferable to drain the abdomen, even in laparoscopy, and refer the patient to a dedicated hospital. In case of partial lesion of the common bile duct, an attempt to suture on a tutor may be indicated, but always consider the technical experience of the surgeon and the stage of inflammation. In case of complete sections of CBD or complex lesions, it is advisable to stop the procedure, drain the abdomen, and send the patient to a reference center [67, 71].

If you convert the laparoscopic procedure into open surgery to define the extent of the lesion, you should not proceed with an extensive dissection of the hepatocystic triangle if you are not sure that the problem can be properly solved.

10.5 Bailout Procedures

In situation of a difficult gallbladder, when the target (cystic duct, cystic artery, and CBD) identification with the CVS cannot be properly achieved, it is not important to push ahead with the goal of a complete cholecystectomy while risking the patient's safety due to potential biliary/vascular injury. It is important to perform an alternative procedure that allows the surgeon to complete the procedure in a safe manner [47].

Bail-out techniques include: cholecystostomy, partial cholecystectomy and conversion to open surgery. In addition to these one should consider the fundus first approach, which is a hybrid way to try to complete the cholecystectomy laparoscopically, adopting the open surgery approach from the bottom of the gallbladder, with the possibility to conclude in a partial cholecystectomy.

The use of these methods should not be considered as a failure, but on the contrary as an integral and responsible part of the patient's path of care and as a way to safeguard his/her health.

The operating surgeon should not hesitate to seek a second opinion whenever needed, and this should be considered as a sign of good clinical practice rather than a sign of surgical incompetence.

10.5.1 Cholecystostomy

Tube cholecystostomy could be a simple bridge procedure to provide symptomatic relief until a definitive procedure can be performed. It can be done percutaneously, laparoscopically, or after conversion to open surgery [40, 72–74].

10.5.1.1 Percutaneous Cholecystostomy

A percutaneous cholecystostomy tube serves an important function for patients with cholecystitis who are unable to undergo immediate cholecystectomy safely. An increasing TG18 Grade and comorbidity status are the primary predictors of need for cholecystostomy [75]. If the patient is a poor candidate for general anesthesia, has had symptoms for more than 72 h, or has an advanced metastatic disease, PTC is considered [73, 74]. A trans hepatic approach is typically chosen to enter the gallbladder, with moderate sedation used for nearly all cases. Tube placement procedures were performed by the interventional radiologist with US or CT guidance.

10.5.1.2 Laparoscopically Cholecystostomy

During a laparoscopic approach, the decision to proceed with cholecystostomy is related to the finding of a gangrenous gallbladder and severe inflammation of the HC triangle in a patient in severe general condition. Laparoscopic cholecystostomy is performed when the intraoperative finding shows a condition in which a cholecystectomy cannot be performed safely [76]. The procedure can be facilitated by the use of the laparoscopic ultrasound guidance. An 18-gauge needle was inserted in subcostal position at the midclavicular line into the gallbladder. Once the bile has been aspirated, a guidewire is placed within the lumen of the gallbladder. Over the guidewire, a 14 F catheter is placed into the lumen of the gallbladder and secured to the skin. If there is a rupture on the gallbladder wall, it is easier to empty the gallbladder with the aspirator and then place a catheter with a balloon inside the gallbladder so that it can be safely fixed (without spillage) to the abdominal wall [77, 78].

10.5.1.3 Open Cholecystostomy

The same procedures performed in laparoscopy are also available in open surgery [47].

In most cases when a surgical cholecystostomy is performed, the preoperative assessment is probably not adequate.

10.5.2 Fundus First

In case of diffuse inflammation of Calot's triangle, continued dissection to obtain the CVS might result in BDI [79] and an anterograde approach may represent an alternative to immediate conversion to open cholecystectomy [80–82].

Requirements for a safe dome-down technique are: (a) clear understanding of the anatomy of the cystic and hilar plates [83]; (b) the dissection should be maintained along the subserosal-inner layer to avoid vascular and/or biliary injury [19].

The procedure involves the following steps:

1. The gallbladder is dissected away from the gallbladder bed from the fundus down towards the cystic duct [83].
2. Dissection then continues along the gallbladder [84]. The cystic artery is identified, isolated, ligated, and transected.
3. The cystic duct is positively identified and isolated, creating a 360-degree view of the gallbladder–cystic duct junction.
4. The cystic duct is ligated and divided.

This technique poses a technical challenge in handling the gallbladder, as it tends to twist once separated completely from the liver, and also in liver retracting.

In chronic cholecystitis with a small and contracted gallbladder, the longitudinal length of the cystic plate from the fundus to its attachment with right portal pedicle sheath becomes short. Without appreciating this pathologic shortening, the surgeon may enter into the right portal pedicle sheath soon after dissecting the fundus/body of the gallbladder. This may cause injury to the right portal pedicle structures causing serious VBI [64].

10.5.3 SubTotal Cholecystectomy

In 1954, McElmoyle first [85] described and illustrated the principles and technique of this operation when performed specifically for the prevention of bile duct or vascular injury during a difficult cholecystectomy. No attempt is made to dissect the cystic duct or artery when inflammation obscures the neck of the gallbladder. The gallbladder is opened and the redundant portions excised. The cystic duct and the portions of the body, neck, and infundibulum lying above and to the left side are left in situ as a shield to the vulnerable structures, then renamed "Shield of McElmoyle." The cystic duct is not closed; its mucosa is ablated and a drain is placed.

Thirty years later, Bornman and Terblanche [86] described their experience in managing difficult gallbladders in cases of severe cholecystitis. Bickel and Shtamler in 1993 describe their successful experience in the treatment of six patients with the use of laparoscopic subtotal cholecystectomy [87].

In literature, "partial," "subtotal," "insufficient," and "uncompleted" are different terms used to define the same concept. Strasberg in 2016 suggested that the term "subtotal" should be preferred since it expresses the nearly complete removal of the gallbladder.

It is important to remove all stones from the gallbladder, to ablate the mucosa of the gallbladder stump (with diathermy or argon plasma coagulator) and leave this stump as small as possible.

10.5.3.1 Technique [88]

The modern technique to perform these operations is clear and can be performed both laparoscopically and in open surgery. The gallbladder is opened along its long axis and emptied of stones, including those in the lumen of the gallbladder neck and cystic duct if possible. Surgeons are recommended to remove all stones from the peritoneal cavity, if necessary, by placing them in an endo-bag. The portion of the gallbladder adherent to the liver is usually left in situ and ablated. The latter may be done with electrocautery, a bipolar forceps, an argon beam, or saline-linked radiofrequency ablation. Alternatively, some or all of the gallbladder attached to the liver may be removed. When this is done, the gallbladder wall and cystic plate may be removed down to the bare liver or the cystic plate may be left in situ. In some cases, the gallbladder will be gangrenous. If so, the gangrenous portion should be excised without widening the extent of the subtotal resection. In a cirrhotic patient, the risk of bleeding from the liver bed may be theoretically avoided in subtotal cholecystectomy by not removing the posterior GB wall.

The area should be carefully drained. The gallbladder lip is usually somewhat larger and the lumen is closed by sutures [88, 89].

The patient must be informed that a gallbladder remnant may result in the formation of new stones with the risk of a new cholecystitis with a possibly challenging preoperative cholecystectomy [90].

10.5.3.2 Cross-Check the Different Techniques

Based on the meta-analysis of Elshaer and coworkers, on a sample of 1231 subtotal cholecystectomies, in 72.9% of cases the procedure was performed laparoscopically. They found low rate of postoperative BDI (0.08%) but higher rates of bile leak (18%), particularly in open procedures. These fistulas seem to resolve spontaneously in most cases within 2 weeks [89].

More patients whose surgery ended with a drainage left under the cholecystic bed because the stump of the neck of the gallbladder was not closed underwent postoperative ERCP compared to those in whom closure was successfully performed, but there was no change in the rate of complications [91].

Based on the meta-analysis of Elshaer and coworkers, it seems that a subtotal fenestrating cholecystectomy is more likely to be done when an open approach is used [89].

Paradoxically, in their data, bile leaks were more common after a laparoscopic procedure. Possibly, this is due to the improved ability to suture the cystic duct orifice when the procedure is done in open surgery [89].

Based on presently available information, it would seem that the fenestrating type of subtotal cholecystectomy would be preferable, but knowledge in this area is very incomplete.

There is no enough information regarding the incidence of symptomatic gallbladder remnants after subtotal cholecystectomies [91].

Laparoscopic subtotal cholecystectomies generally produced better outcomes compared with open subtotal cholecystectomies, but nonsignificant differences were found between the technique of closure or nonclosure of the cystic duct or gallbladder stump and removal compared to the nonremoval of the gallbladder posterior wall [89].

10.5.4 Open Conversion

In the past, difficult cholecystectomy was strongly associated with conversion to open surgery. More recently due to decreasing experience in open surgery, alternative tricks are considered before resorting to conversion [19, 92].

The need for conversion is often related to a problem of gallbladder mobilization or the need to control a massive bleeding.

It is important to realize that simply converting to an open procedure does not safeguard against bile duct/vascular injury [93]. A difficult procedure may remain difficult even after conversion to open surgery with no effect on postoperative complications [94].

When setting up the operating room for acute cholecystitis or when we suspect a difficult gallbladder, it is a good rule to prepare the operating bed for the placement of poles to anchor the retractor for the right hypochondrium.

When converting the procedure into open surgery, you need to have a few landmarks in mind.

(a) The abdomen should be deflated before incision, as the pneumoperitoneum distorts the abdominal wall anatomy. Subcostal laparotomy is made 2 to 3 fingerbreadths below the ribs (Fig. 10.8). The incision should allow ideal access to the hepatic pedicle; if necessary, it is preferable to extend it to the left [62].
(b) When the cause of conversion is the difficulty in identifying or releasing the gallbladder, the first point to find is the anterior margin of the liver. It is necessary to begin the release possibly starting from the right side of the gallbladder and then moving to the left. When the bottom of the gallbladder is discovered, if possible, it is grasped with a ring clamp and the release continues on the lower face of the gallbladder, descending towards the Winslow which the surgeon should explore using his index finger. The round ligament then is divided (except in cirrhotic patients), and a retractor is placed. In the most difficult cases, where adhesions due to inflammation or previous surgery have made the structures unrecognizable, more effort is required; the hepatic flexure of the colon and duodenum may be mobilized to the left.

    Placement of sponges behind the liver to lift it forward is often helpful with exposure.

    Use the Bismuth maneuver of straightening the hepatic peduncle for the correct identification of CBD: downward traction of the duodenum with a sponge and upward traction of the S4 base [52].
(c) When the rearrangement of the hepatic pedicle makes the management of the cystic pedicle dangerous, it is advisable to continue by anterograde approach [95].

    Depending on the adherent inflammation pattern, the detachment of the gallbladder from its bed can be started at the intermediate portion.

    In chronic cholecystitis with a small and contracted gallbladder, the longitudinal length of the cystic plate from the fundus to its attachment with the right portal pedicle sheath becomes short. This may cause injury to the right portal pedicle structures causing serious BDI/VBI when the surgeon enters into the right portal pedicle sheath.

    Despite the dome-down approach, if it is not possible to safely isolate and manage the cystic duct and cystic artery, consider performing a subtotal cholecystectomy.

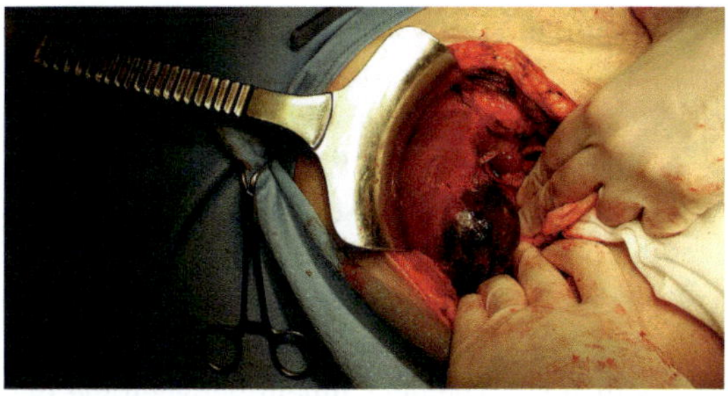

Fig. 10.8 Conversion to open surgery for acute gangrenous cholecystitis. Large right subcostal laparotomy allowing optimal control over the H-C triangle

(d) Recurrent episodes of cholecystitis can lead to the formation of biliodigestive fistulas (with the duodenum or colon). Cholecystic duodenal fistulas are the most common [96]. The finding is in most cases occasional, and the presence of a fistula must be suspected when you are locked on a very tight adhesion. We proceed by isolating the fistula on both sides. The detachment between the two organs will occur on the cholecystic side. Usually, the fistula is small, and once the healthy margins of the duodenum are prepared, a suture can be performed.

    Less often the situation can be more complex: the duodenum is fused between a scleroatrophic gallbladder and the CBD. It is advisable to empty the gallbladder and try a cholangiographic study before deciding what strategy to take.

    Cholecystocolic fistulae usually affect the bottom of the gallbladder. Their isolation is easier. They can be treated with either a mechanical suture or a direct suture on the colic side [97].

    Fistulas between gallbladder and bile duct deserve separate treatment and will not be the subject of this work.

(e) In case of bleeding from the HC triangle not controlled by compression, consider using the Pringle maneuver as an alternative to achieve temporary hemostasis and identify the source of bleeding. Sometimes it is enough to compress the pedicle between the fingers. Avoid placing stitches blindly or extensive blind coagulation.

In case of bleeding from the gallbladder bed, try compression with gauze and contact hemostatic. As far as possible try to identify whether the source of bleeding is from the roots of the suprahepatic vein [50].

10.6 Conclusions

Laparoscopic cholecystectomy is the gold standard for the treatment of gallbladder symptomatic lithiasis. To decrease the incidence of BDI during LC, an effective surgical education system is imperative [98]. While it is easy to underestimate LC as a basic general surgical procedure, the operation may actually be one of the most difficult challenges unexpectedly facing the general surgeon, who should adopt a mindset of "preparing for the worst." In nearly 20% of cases, there is a difficult gallbladder situation that makes the procedure a challenge for the surgeon.

We should always keep in mind that the procedure is performed for a benign pathology. Routine adoption of Culture of Safety in Cholecystectomy (COSIC) may help reduce the incidence of post cholecystectomy biliary/vascular injury [47].

While strict adherence to the CVS is important to decrease BDI, it is only one part of the COSIC, which mandates safety to be at the forefront. Besides achieving the CVS in cases of total cholecystectomy, COSIC also requires an appropriate selection and workup of the patient, the adjustment of the surgical technique in the setting of nonroutine cases, the use of bailout procedures, and the avoidance of complex cases when appropriate experience is not available [99].

A key concept when performing a difficult cholecystectomy is to promptly recognize that change in surgical strategy may result in minor risk of bile duct injury. The conversion of a laparoscopic cholecystectomy to an open procedure should not be experienced as a failure.

Despite overall low incidence of adverse events during LC, the high rate of LC leads to a significant absolute number of patients who suffer from long-term adverse events, one of the most significant being BDI. Otto Von Bismarck once said "Fools say they learn from experience; I prefer to learn from the experience of others."

References

1. Harboe KM, Bardram L. The quality of cholecystectomy in Denmark: outcome and risk factors for 20,307 patients from the national database. Surg Endosc. 2011;25:1630–41.
2. Navez B, Ungureanu F, Michiels M, et al. Surgical management of acute cholecystitis: results of a 2-year prospective multicenter survey in Belgium. Surg Endosc. 2012;26:2436–45.
3. Giger UF, Michel JM, Opitz I, et al. Risk factors for perioperative complications in patients undergoing

laparoscopic cholecystectomy: analysis of 22,953 consecutive cases from the Swiss Association of Laparoscopic and Thoracoscopic Surgery database. J Am Coll Surg. 2006;203:723–8.
4. Rosen M, Brody F, Ponsky J, et al. Predictive factors for conversion of laparoscopic cholecystectomy. Am J Surg. 2002;184:254–8.
5. Zhang W, Li J, Wu G, et al. Risk factors affecting conversion in patients undergoing laparoscopic cholecystectomy. ANZ J Surg. 2008;78(11):973–6.
6. Sutcliffe RP, Hollyman M, Hodson J, et al. Preoperative risk factors for conversion from laparoscopic to open cholecystectomy: a validated risk score derived from a prospective UK database of 8820 patients. J Hepatobiliary Pancreat Sci. 2016;18(11):922–8.
7. Gurusamy K, Samraj K, Gluud C, et al. Meta-analysis of randomized controlled trials on the safety and effectiveness of early versus delayed laparoscopic cholecystectomy for acute cholecystitis. Br J Surg. 2010;97:141–50.
8. Shingu Y, Komatsu S, Norimizu S, et al. Laparoscopic subtotal cholecystectomy for severe cholecystitis. Surg Endosc. 2016;30(2):526–31.
9. Simorov A, Ranade A, Parcells J, et al. Emergent cholecystostomy is superior to open cholecystectomy in extremely ill patients with acalculous cholecystitis: a large multicenter outcome study. Am J Surg. 2013;206(6):935–41.
10. Salky BA, Edye MB. The difficult cholecystectomy: problems related to concomitant diseases. Semin Laparosc Surg. 1998;5(2):107–14.
11. Ashfaq A, Ahmadieh K, Shah AA, et al. The difficult gall bladder: outcomes following laparoscopic cholecystectomy and the need for open conversion. Am J Surg. 2016;212:1261–4.
12. Santos BF, Brunt LM, Pucci MJ. The difficult gallbladder: a safe approach to a dangerous problem. J Laparoendosc Adv Surg Tech A. 2017;27:571–8.
13. Miettinen P, Pasanen P, Lahtinen J, et al. Acute abdominal pain in adults. Ann Chir Gynaecol. 1996;85:5–9.
14. Ukkonen M, Kivivuori A, Rantanen T, et al. Emergency abdominal operations in the elderly: a multivariate regression analysis of 430Consecutive patients with acute abdomen. World J Surg. 2015;39:2854–61.
15. Wilson E, Gurusamy K, Gluud C, et al. Cost-utility and value-of information analysis of early versus delayed laparoscopic cholecystectomy for acute cholecystitis. Br J Surg. 2010;97:210–9.
16. Kais H, Hershkovitz Y, Abu-Snina Y, et al. Different setups of laparoscopic cholecystectomy: conversion and complication rates: a retrospective cohort study. Int J Surg. 2014;12(12):1258–61.
17. Wakabayashi G, Iwashita Y, Hibi T, et al. Tokyo guidelines 2018: surgical management of acute cholecystitis: safe steps in laparoscopic cholecystectomy for acute cholecystitis (with videos). J Hepatobiliary Pancreat Sci. 2018;25:73–86.
18. Iwashita Y, Hibi T, Ohyama T, et al. Delphi consensus on bile duct injuries during laparoscopic cholecystectomy: an evolutionary cul-de-sac or the birth pangs of a new technical framework? J Hepatobiliary Pancreat Sci. 2017;24:591–602.
19. Conrad C, Wakabayashi G, Asbun HJ, et al. IRCAD recommendation on safe laparoscopic cholecystectomy. J Hepatobiliary Pancreat Sci. 2017;24:603–15.
20. Ansaloni L, Pisano M, Coccolini F, et al. 2016 WSES guidelines on acute calculous cholecystitis. World J Emerg Surg. 2016;11:25.
21. Tornqvist B, Waage A, Zheng Z, et al. Severity of acute cholecystitis and risk of iatrogenic bile duct injury during cholecystectomy, a population-based case-control study. World J Surg. 2016;40:1060–7.
22. Conte D, Fraquelli M, Fornari F, et al. Close relation between cirrhosis and gallstones: cross-sectional and longitudinal survey. Arch Intern Med. 1999;159:49–52.
23. Laurence JM, Tran PD, Richardson AJ, et al. Laparoscopic or open cholecystectomy in cirrhosis: a systematic review of outcomes and meta-analysis of randomized trials. HPB. 2012;14:153–61.
24. Machado NO. Laparoscopic cholecystectomy in cirrhotics. J Soc Laparoendosc Surg. 2012;16:392–400.
25. Pucher PH, Brunt LM, Davies N, et al. Outcome trends and safety measures after 30 years of laparoscopic cholecystectomy: a systematic review and pooled data analysis. Surg Endosc. 2018;32:2175–83.
26. Hibi T, Iwashita Y, Ohyama T, et al. The 'right' way is not always popular: comparison of surgeons' perceptions during laparoscopic cholecystectomy for acute cholecystitis among experts from Japan, Korea and Taiwan. J Hepatobiliary Pancreat Sci. 2017;24:24–32.
27. Kortram K, Reinders JS, van Ramshorst B, et al. Laparoscopic cholecystectomy for acute cholecystitis should be performed by a laparoscopic surgeon. Surg Endosc. 2010;24:2206–9.
28. Yang TF, Guo L, Wang Q. Evaluation of preoperative risk factor for converting laparoscopic to open cholecystectomy: a meta-analysis. Hepato-Gastroenterology. 2014;61(132):958–65.
29. Philip Rothman J, Burcharth J, Pommergaard HC, et al. Preoperative risk factors for conversion of laparoscopic cholecystectomy to open surgery—a systematic review and meta-analysis of observational studies. Dig Surg. 2016;33(5):414–23.
30. Paajanen H, Suuronen S, Nordstrom P, et al. Laparoscopic versus open cholecystectomy in diabetic patients and postoperative outcome. Surg Endosc. 2011;25(3):764–70.
31. Goonawardena J, Gunnarsson R, de Costa A. Predicting conversion from laparoscopicto open cholecystectomy presented as a probability nomogram based on preoperative patient risk factors. Am J Surg. 2015;210(3):492–500.
32. Terho PM, Leppäniemi AK, Mentula PJ. Laparoscopic cholecystectomy for acute calculous cholecystitis: a retrospective study assessing risk factors for conversion and complications. World J Emerg Surg. 2016;11:54.

33. Andrews S. Does concentration of surgical expertise improve outcomes for laparoscopic cholecystectomy? 9-year audit cycle. Surgeon. 2013;11(6):309–12.
34. Madani A, Watanabe Y, Feldman LS, et al. Expert intraoperative judgment and decision-making: defining the cognitive competencies for safe laparoscopic cholecystectomy. J Am Coll Surg. 2015;221(5):931–40 e8.
35. Beliaev AM, Booth M. An association between conversion of laparoscopic cholecystectomy to open surgery and intra-abdominal organ injury. ANZ J Surg. 2016;86(7–8):625.
36. Kologlu M, Tutuncu T, Yuksek YN, et al. Using a risk score for conversion from laparoscopic to open cholecystectomy in resident training. Surgery. 2004;135:282–7.
37. Lipman JM, Claridge JA, Haridas M, et al. Preoperative findings predict conversion from laparoscopic to open cholecystectomy. Surgery. 2007;142:556–63.
38. Sugrue M, Sahebally SM, Ansaloni L, et al. Grading operative findings at laparoscopic cholecystectomy- a new scoring system. World J Emerg Surg. 2015;10:14.
39. Hobbs MS, Mai Q, Knuiman MW, et al. Surgeon experience and trends in intraoperative complications in laparoscopic cholecystectomy. Br J Surg. 2006;93(7):844–53.
40. Stanek A, Dohan A, Barkun J, et al. Percutaneous cholecystostomy: a simple bridge to surgery or an alternative option for the management of acute cholecystitis? Am J Surg. 2018;216(3):595–603.
41. Balasuriya HD, Dunn DJ, Joseph MG. How to gain safe entry for laparoscopic cholecystectomy in the multi-scarred abdomen. ANZ J Surg. 2018;88(4):376–7.
42. Ahmad G, Gent D, Henderson D, et al. Laparoscopic entry techniques. Cochrane Database Syst Rev. 2015;8:CD006583.
43. Palanivelu C, Rajan PS, Jani K, et al. Laparoscopic cholecystectomy in cirrhotic patients: the role of subtotal cholecystectomy and its variants. J Am Coll Surg. 2006;203(2):145–51.
44. Ercan M, Bostanci EB, Ulas M, et al. Effects of previous abdominal surgery incision type on complications and conversion rate in laparoscopic cholecystectomy. Surg Laparosc Endosc Percutan Tech. 2009;19:373–8.
45. Eikermann M, Siegel R, Broeders I, et al. Prevention and treatment of bile duct injuries during laparoscopic cholecystectomy: the clinical practice guidelines of the European Association for Endoscopic Surgery (EAES). Surg Endosc. 2012;26(11):3003–39.
46. Giger U, Michel JM, Vonlanthen R, et al. Laparoscopic cholecystectomy in acute cholecystitis: indication, technique, risk and outcome. Langenbeck's Arch Surg. 2005;390:373–80.
47. Gupta V, Jain G. Safe laparoscopic cholecystectomy: adoption of universal culture of safety in cholecystectomy. World J Gastrointest Surg. 2019;11(2):62–84.
48. Strasberg SM, Brunt LM. Rationale and use of the critical view of safety in laparoscopic cholecystectomy. J Am Coll Surg. 2010;211:132–8.
49. Strasberg SM, Hertl M, Soper NJ. An analysis of the problem of biliary injury during laparoscopic cholecystectomy. J Am Coll Surg. 1995;180:101–25.
50. Masci E, Faillace G, Longoni M. Use of oxidized regenerated cellulose to achieve hemostasis during laparoscopic cholecystectomy: a retrospective cohort analysis. BMC Res Note. 2018;11(1):239.
51. Singh R, Brunt L. Critical view of safety-its feasibility and efficacy in preventing bile duct injuries. Ann Laparosc Endosc Surg. 2018;3:2.
52. Nuzzo G, Giuliante F, Giovannini I, et al. Le lesioni iatrogene della via biliare principale. Collana Monografica della Società Italiana di Chirurgia - N. 18, anno 2002.
53. Strasberg SM, Eagon CJ, Drebin JA. The "hidden cystic duct" syndrome and the infundibular technique of laparoscopic cholecystectomy--the danger of the false infundibulum. J Am Coll Surg. 2000;191:661–7.
54. Andall RG, Matusz P, du Plessis M, Ward R, Tubbs RS, Loukas M. The clinical anatomy of cystic artery variations: a review of over 9800 cases. Surg Radiol Anat. 2016;38:529–39.
55. Dixon E, Vollmer CM Jr, May GR. Management of benign biliary stenosis and injury. Switzerland: Springer; 2015. p. 165–86.
56. GuptaV. ABCD of safe laparoscopic cholecystectomy: imbibing universal culture of safety in cholecystectomy. Indian J Surg. 2018;81:203–4.
57. Vettoretto N, Saronni C, Harbi A, et al. Critical view of safety during laparoscopic cholecystectomy. JSLS. 2011;15:322–5.
58. Strasberg SM. Biliary injury in laparoscopic surgery: part 2. Changing the culture of cholecystectomy. J Am Coll Surg. 2005;201:604–11.
59. Strasberg SM. Error traps and vasculo-biliary injury in laparoscopic and open cholecystectomy. J Hepatobiliary Pancreat Surg. 2008;15:284–92.
60. Strasberg SM. Avoidance of biliary injury during laparoscopic cholecystectomy. J Hepato-Biliary-Pancreat Surg. 2002;9(5):543–7.
61. Nijssen MA, Schreinemakers JM, Meyer Z, et al. Complications after laparoscopic cholecystectomy: a video evaluation study of whether the critical view of safety was reached. World J Surg. 2015;39(7):1798–803.
62. Sanford DE. An update on technical aspects of cholecystectomy. Surg Clin North Am. 2019;99(2):245–58.
63. Schnelldorfer T, Sarr MG, Adams DB. What is the duct of Luschka?--a systematic review. J Gastrointest Surg. 2012;16(3):656–62.
64. Strasberg SM, Gouma DJ. 'Extreme' vasculobiliary injuries: association with fundus-down cholecystectomy in severely inflamed gallbladders. HPB (Oxford). 2012;14(1):1–8.
65. Parrilla P, Robles R, Varo E, et al. Liver transplantation for bile duct injury after open and laparoscopic cholecystectomy. Br J Surg. 2014;101(2):63–8.
66. Tornqvist B, Stromberg C, Persson G, et al. Effect of intended intraoperative cholangiography and early detection of bile duct injury on survival after cholecystectomy: population-based cohort study. BMJ. 2012;345:e6457.

67. Nuzzo G, Giuliante F, Giovannini I, et al. Bile duct injury during laparoscopic cholecystectomy. Results of an Italian national survey on 56591 cholecystectomies. Arch Surg. 2005;140:986–92.
68. Nuzzo G, Giuliante F, Giovannini I, et al. Re: role of intraoperative cholangiography in avoiding bile duct injury. J Am Coll Surg. 2007;205(4):e5–6; author reply e6.
69. Ford JA, Soop M, Du J, et al. Systematic review of intraoperative cholangiography in cholecystectomy. Br J Surg. 2012;99:160–7.
70. Sajid MS, Leaver C, Haider Z, et al. Routine on-table cholangiography during cholecystectomy: a systematic review. Ann R Coll Surg Engl. 2012;94:375–80.
71. Nuzzo G, Giuliante F, Giovannini I, et al. Advantages of multidisciplinary management of bile duct injuries occurring during cholecystectomy. Am J Surg. 2008;195(6):763–9.
72. Akhan O, Akinci D, Ozmen MN. Percutaneous cholecystostomy. Eur J Radiol. 2002;43(3):229e236.
73. Colonna AL, Griffiths TM, Robison DC, et al. Cholecystostomy: are we using it correctly? Am J Surg. 2019;217(6):1010–5.
74. Gurusamy KS, Rossi M, Davidson BR. Percutaneous cholecystostomy for high-risk surgical patients with acute calculous cholecystitis. Cochrane Database Syst Rev 2013;(8):CD007088.
75. Okamoto K, Suzuki K, Takada T, et al. Tokyo guidelines 2018: flowchart for the management of acute cholecystitis. J Hepatobiliary Pancreat Sci. 2018;25:55–72.
76. Haicken BN. Laparoscopic tube cholecystostomy. Surg Endosc. 1992;6(6):285–8.
77. Berber E, Engle KL, String A. Selective use of tube cholecystostomy with interval laparoscopic cholecystectomy in acute cholecystitis. Arch Surg. 2000;135(3):341–6.
78. Cherng N, Witkowski ET, Sneider EB, et al. Use of cholecystostomy tubes in the management of patients with primary diagnosis of acute cholecystitis. J Am Coll Surg. 2012;214(2):196–201.
79. Iwashita Y, Ohyama T, Honda G, et al. What are the appropriate indicators of surgical difficulty during laparoscopic cholecystectomy? Results from a Japan–Korea–Taiwan multinational survey. J Hepatobiliary Pancreat Sci. 2016;23:533–47.
80. Kelly MD. Laparoscopic retrograde (fundus first) cholecystectomy. BMC Surg. 2009;9:19.
81. Fullum TM, Kim S, Dan D, et al. Laparoscopic "dome-down" cholecystectomy with the LCS-5 harmonic scalpel. JSLS. 2005;9(1):51–7.
82. Huang SM, Hsiao KM, Pan H, et al. Overcoming the difficulties in laparoscopic management of contracted gallbladders with gallstones: possible role of fundus-down approach. Surg Endosc. 2011;25(1):284–91.
83. Honda G, Iwanaga T, Kurata M. Dissection of the gallbladder from the liver bed during laparoscopic cholecystectomy for acute or subacute cholecystitis. J Hepato-Biliary-Pancreat Surg. 2008;15(3):293–6.
84. Honda G, Iwanaga T, Kurata M, et al. The critical view of safety in laparoscopic cholecystectomy is optimized by exposing the inner layer of the subserosal layer. J Hepato-Biliary-Pancreat Surg. 2009;16(4):445–9.
85. McElmoyle WA. Cholecystectomy: a method for the difficult gall-bladder. Lancet. 1954;266(6826):1320–3.
86. Bornman PC, Terblanche J. Subtotal cholecystectomy: for the difficult gallbladder in portal hypertension and cholecystitis. Surgery. 1985;98:1):1–6.
87. Bickel A, Shtamler B. Laparoscopic subtotal cholecystectomy. J Laparoendosc Surg. 1993;3(4):365–7.
88. Strasberg SM, Pucci MJ, Brunt LM, et al. Subtotal cholecystectomy-"Fenestrating" vs "Reconstituting" subtypes and the prevention of bile duct injury: definition of the optimal procedure in difficult operative conditions. J Am Coll Surg. 2016;222(1):89–96.
89. Elshaer M, Gravante G, Thomas K, et al. Subtotal cholecystectomy for "difficult gallbladders": systematic review and meta-analysis. JAMA Surg. 2015;150(2):159–68.
90. Pernice LM, Andreoli F. Laparoscopic treatment of stone recurrence in a gallbladder remnant: report of an additional case and literature review. J Gastrointest Surg. 2009;13(11):2084–91.
91. Henneman D, da Costa DW, Vrouenraets BC, et al. Laparoscopic partial cholecystectomy for the difficult gallbladder: a systematic review. Surg Endosc. 2013;27(2):351–8.
92. Lengyel BI, Azagury D, Varban O, et al. Laparoscopic cholecystectomy after a quarter century: why do we still convert? Surg Endosc. 2012;26(2):508–13.
93. Mangieri CW, Hendren BP, Strode MA, et al. Bile duct injuries (BDI) in the advanced laparoscopic cholecystectomy era. Surg Endosc. 2019;33(3):724–30.
94. Borzellino G, Sauerland S, Minicozzi AM, et al. Laparoscopic cholecystectomy for severe acute cholecystitis. A meta-analysis of results. Surg Endosc. 2008;22(1):8–15.
95. Jenkins PJ, Paterson HM, Parks RW, et al. Open cholecystectomy in the laparoscopic era. Br J Surg. 2007;94(11):1382–5.
96. Tantia O, Bandyopadhyay SK, Sen B, et al. Pericholecystic fistula: a study of 64 cases. Int Surg. 2002;87(2):90–3.
97. Mourot J. Colecistectomia per via laparotomica per litiasi della colecisti. In: Tecniche Chirurgiche-Addominale. Paris: EMC (Elsevier Masson SAS); 2006. p. 40–920.
98. McKinley SK, Brunt LM, Schwaitzberg SD. Prevention of bile duct injury: the case for incorporating educational theories of expertise. Surg Endosc. 2014;28:3385–91.
99. Chen CB, Palazzo F, Doane SM, et al. Increasing resident utilization and recognition of the critical view of safety during laparoscopic cholecystectomy: a pilot study from an academic medical center. Surg Endosc. 2017;31:1627–35.

When Is It Safe to Continue Laparoscopically?

11

Cecilia Chambon, Pablo Valsangiacomo, and Luis Ruso Martinez

Abbreviations

BDI	Bile duct injury
CBD	Common bile duct
CVS	Critical view of safety
IOC	Intraoperative Cholangiography
HPB	Hepato-pancreatic-biliary

11.1 Introduction

Laparoscopic cholecystectomy is one of the most frequently performed surgical procedures in the world, with epidemiological differences and areas with different prevalence. This requires health systems to rationalize expenses, including excellence in quality of results and avoid legal medical litigation to surgeons.

The main purpose of biliary surgery safety is the removal of the gallbladder without bile duct injury (BDI) or the vascular structures of the liver pedicle, with a minimum invasion.

Laparoscopic surgery has solved this with an acceptable conversion rate, up to 15% [1].

The safety of a surgical procedure is determined by the ability to perform surgery without increasing the surgical risks and to resolve complications that may occur during the procedure.

Advances in the prevention of bile duct injuries can be summarized in: the development of the concept of "difficult cholecystectomy" and the derivations of it, the critical view of safety of Strasberg [2], conversion indicators, and technical alternatives to cholecystectomy. All these have been useful to the development of the concept of safe cholecystectomy and the idea of a culture of safety for this procedure.

The term "difficult cholecystectomy" is an extensive, complex, and difficult to define concept in the intraoperative time. It can be said that it is a set of pathological situations that technically prevent cholecystectomy in a regular manner. It refers to cholecystectomy under certain situations that do not allow safe dissection, leading to an extension of surgical time and the risk of complications. In a practical sense, we can say that "risk" is implicitly associated with "safety deficit" during a procedure that both factors have a proportional connection and that the resulting decision has an impact on the outcome of the surgery. There are well-established concepts, vast experience, and literature regarding preoperative risk factors for vascular and/or biliary surgical injury, as well as the intraoperative factors that determine the decision to convert or change tactic to more limited surgeries. Under these circumstances, it is considered that the incidence of complications of the main bile duct as well as vascular structures are 2 to 5 times

C. Chambon · P. Valsangiacomo · L. Ruso Martinez (✉)
Surgery Department 3, Hospital Maciel (ASSE), Medical School, University of Republic (UDELAR), Montevideo, Uruguay

© Springer Nature Switzerland AG 2021

I. Di Carlo (ed.), *Difficult Acute Cholecystitis*, https://doi.org/10.1007/978-3-030-62102-5_11

higher in laparoscopic cholecystectomy than in the open one [3].

The objective of this chapter is to analyze intraoperative indicators and the logistical context essential to safely continue with a laparoscopic cholecystectomy, mainly technical, linked to dissection and its difficulties. We will not analyze other factors such as the intolerance of pneumoperitoneum, the inability to achieve a correct working cavity, the failure of surgical instruments, or the expertise of the surgical team.

11.2 Technical Factors that Decrease Security

Cholecystectomy is a procedure that progresses with technical, systematized, and well-defined steps, involving prior theoretical knowledge and surgical skills. It is therefore important that the surgeon realizes when the dissection is becoming unsafe, the risk of injury, as well as the need to establish technical changes that will further lead the procedure to a correct outcome.

The impossibility of carrying on with surgery, anatomical disorientation, and decreased visualization, whatever the cause, are factors that take the procedure away from the safety path, increasing the risks.

There are factors that can affect the safety of a cholecystectomy; we can group them into anatomical, pathological, and technical factors.

The presence of inflammation, an impacted gallstone on the basin, or the impossibility of gallbladder traction affect the correct and safe identification and dissection of the hepatocystic triangle [4]. In order to maintain anatomical orientation as a safety element, several anatomical landmarks have been described, useful in cases where the hepatocystic triangle is not easily identified and that would allow anatomical-spatial reorientation in difficult cases, such as identifying the umbilical fissure or maintaining dissection above Rouviere's sulcus [5].

There are multiple anatomical variants of the bile duct and in relation to the upper biliary confluent, although between 53% and 63% of cases of their formation is modal [6]. Chaib [7] established five types of anatomical variants were characterized in the right liver duct (A1-5) and 6 types in the left liver duct (B1-6). Atypical branching patterns in both right and left liver ducts were found in 14% and 8%, respectively [7].

In our experience, the variation of the highest risk of bile injury is the abouchement of the right lateral duct (segments VI-VII) in the cystic duct (Fig. 11.1).

Regarding the ostium modalities of the cystic duct, they are also very variable; it can flow anywhere on the main bile duct, between CBS and Vater's ampulla [8].

Benson [9] described congenital anatomical variations of extrahepatic bile ducts and classified them in five main types, which are the most seen in surgical practice (Fig. 11.2).

In fact, only 33% of patients have the "classic" anatomical connection between cystic and extrahepatic bile ducts and related arteries, and in 75% of cases, the cystic has an angular input in the hepatic duct, which facilitates its identification and allows surgeons to describe the Calot's triangle [10].

In 20% of the cases, the cystic and hepatic duct come together in a long and parallel path, performing the actual abouchement further down the apparent junction, presenting a path attached in "shotgun pipe" [9, 11], which makes it difficult to identify the cystic duct and produces the bile injury.

In 5–8% of the cases, the cystic is tortuous and it can also be spiral shaped, describing variable entry angles in the common duct. The main bile duct can be surrounded from behind or front to flow to its left edge [11].

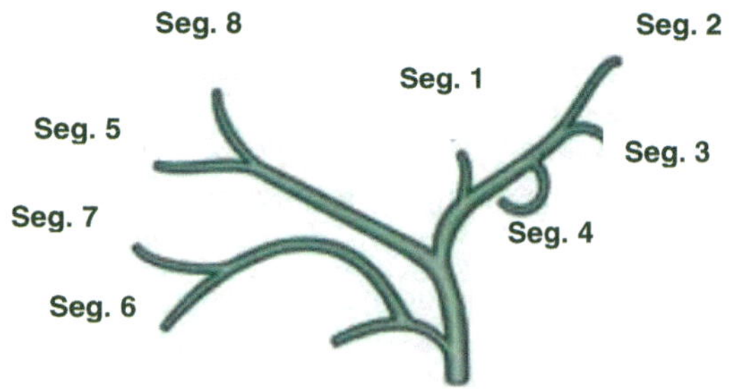

Fig. 11.1 Right lateral sectoral duct ending into the cystic duct. (Courtesy of L. Ruso Martinez)

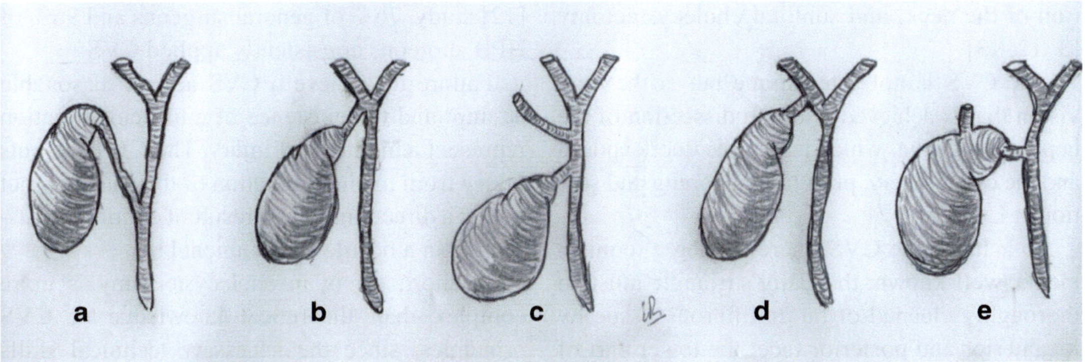

Fig. 11.2 Benson-Page [9] classification for anatomical variations of the cystic duct insertion. (**a**) Long cystic with low insertion in the choledoco; (**b**) cystic ending in the superior biliary confluent; (**c**) right sectorial duct (seg VI-VII) ending close to the cystic end; (**d**) cystic ending in the right hepatic duct; (**e**) "Modal"cystic, ending in common bile duct. (Courtesy of L. Ruso Martinez)

There are pathologies and intraoperative findings that allow us to predict difficulties as they determine by different ways of limitations in the basic principles of a safe cholecystectomy.

Acute cholecystitis generates inflammation of the hepatocystic triangle, which in determining a limitation to CVS is one of the most common causes of tactic change. The presence of acute inflammation causes edema of the adipose cell tissue of the hepatocystic triangle, which can sometimes be a facilitating factor for dissection and anatomical identification, although in others it can easily bleed to contact, limiting it. Gangrenous cholecystitis with gallbladder wall necrosis is a determinant finding in the tactic because it limits the alternative possibilities to total cholecystectomy.

On the other hand, chronic inflammation is a determinant factor of scarring fibrosis at the hepatocystic triangle level. The presence of a complete scleroatrophic gallbladder causes the retraction and difficulty in the grasp; an impacted gallstone on the basin makes it impossible to dissect and display the structures. Mirizzi's syndrome and cholecystoenteric fistula that determine particular and specific anatomical alterations become a technical and tactical challenge, independently of the approach.

All these findings have something in common, the difficulty of getting a CVS (Table 11.1).

Table 11.1 Intraoperative factors of technical difficulties

Thick wall gallbladder
Small gallbladder shrunken in the liver parenchyma
Chronicles/firm adhesions of the colon and duodenum in gallbladder bed
Cirrhotic liver
Misidentification of anatomical structures. Biliary and vascular variations
Permanent bleeding that decreases the vision of the operating field
Failure to progress dissection
Unreasonable dissection time

11.3 Safety Factors

The safety factors that allow to continue with the total cholecystectomy procedure come up from the analysis and knowledge of the technical limitations of it.

11.3.1 Critical View of Safety

Currently the CVS is the paradigm for performing a safe cholecystectomy. Recent recommendations (IRCAD Y SAGES) assume that CVS and training are the most relevant technical factors for decreasing bile duct injury (BDI) and also suggest as technical alternatives, dissection of the neck, and subtotal cholecystectomy [3, 12, 13].

The CVS is not a technique but is the final vision that is achieved after the dissection of the hepatocystic area, which leaves the duct exposed and the cystic artery, prior to its clipping and section [14, 15].

To achieve the CVS, there are three requirements, well-known: the Calot's triangle must be thoroughly cleaned of fat and fibrous tissue by its anterior and posterior face; the lower part of the gallbladder must be separated from the liver bed (dissection of the cystic plate) so that, finally, only two structures are visible entering the gallbladder. It is not necessary to expose the bile duct. Once the critical security vision is obtained, the cystic structures can be connected [14, 16, 17].

The creation of two holes in the hepatocystic area does not ensure the CVS, until the region is completely dissected, on both sides, with the total circumferential vision of the duct and the cystic artery (double view). This allows a safe identification of a possible third abnormal structure (arterial or biliary) that needs to be preserved.

However, it is difficult sometimes to dissect the structures of the Calot's triangle; to accomplish this can take an excessive time and beyond the conviction of the surgeon who is observing the correct structures, the presence of a Mirizzi's syndrome, gallstones in the Hartmann's pouch that hid the cystic, and the main bile duct; also scarring fibrosis and acute inflammatory edema, the existence of epiploic block, abscess, gallbladder necrosis, or perforation may decrease the safety of the procedure [18].

Likewise, it is a prerequisite to understand the concept of CVS and to be convinced of its usefulness. Nijssen [19] in a recent report shows a review of video and operative notes of laparoscopic cholecystectomy that CVS was achieved in only 10.8% of cases, although it was reported that it was accomplished in 80% of the cases. In a survey of experienced surgeons from 14 Latin American countries, only 21.8% answered correctly to the definition of CVS [20]. In the Ircad [12] study, 76% of general surgeons and 96% of HPB surgeons consistently applied CVS.

Failure to achieve a CVS after a reasonable attempt and the existence of a difficult situation represent a high risk of injury. The CVS prevents injury from misinterpretation of the anatomy, but not by a direct injury as a result of continuing dissection in a hostile environment [14].

In short, safety in cholecystectomy is more complex than theoretical knowledge of CVS principles, since the necessary technical skills and maneuvers may require a level of training which exceeds the safety of the procedure.

11.3.2 Primary Dissection of the Gallbladder–Cystic Junction

In situations of difficulty, such as anatomical identification or when CVS is not achieved, the technical alternative may be the location and primary circumferential dissection of the gallbladder–cystic junction. It starts with the peritoneal section on both sides of the gallbladder basin and continues with blunt dissection from right to left, until an orifice is made at the level of the gallbladder cystic angle. That being stablished and based on the fact that the safe dissection plane is the gallbladder wall, the dissection is maintained through the subsequent plane to avoid vascular or biliary injuries, continuing along the inner edge of the gallbladder, ligating it in an upward direction.

A limitation is that occasionally the cystic artery transgresses the cyst or it is parallel to it, or behind, to end at the gallbladder cystic angle. In these cases, the artery is bound, the presence of the cystic is confirmed, and the dissection is continued upwardly.

This reverse alternative of the infundibular technique avoids the "tunnel effect" well described by Strasberg [21]. It does not require the dissection of the Calot's triangle or the visualization of the main biliary tract, as the dissection is maintained in the area of the hepatocystic ligament at the Hartmann's pouch [22].

11.3.3 Imageology

Getting a bile duct mapping in a difficult surgical environment can be hard, but it is a tool that allows cholecystectomy to continue more safely.

11.3.4 Intraoperative Cholangiography (IOC)

IOC is the most widely used method for the assessment of the bile duct in the intraoperative. While there is no conclusive evidence that the IOC prevents BDI, it is a recommended tool for defining an unclear anatomy during a difficult cholecystectomy [12]. It is a technique that can be performed in 90–95% of cholecystectomies, but in cases of short or thin cystics it can be particularly difficult. Cholecysto cholangiography through infundibular gallbladder opening and puncture or placement of a Foley catheter is a good alternative to achieve biliary opacification.

The limitations of it are that it must be technically well done, visualizing the entire biliary tract, intra and extrahepatic, and the passage of contrast to the duodenum, which involves knowing the biliary anatomy and its variations for a correct interpretation, and being performed without extending the surgical time too long.

Less routine use: Laparoscopic ultrasound. It allows the assessment of biliary and vascular pieces, arterial and venous, with the advantage of being noninvasive and radiation free, although it requires adequate training.

Also, near-infrared fluorescence angiography. Recently implemented, it is effective and safe in several studies, but its use is not yet widespread.

11.3.5 Surgical Time

Surgical time is an indicator itself of difficult cholecystectomy. It depends on multiple factors, such as surgeon skills, surgical team experience, and expertise.

The decision whether to continue with laparoscopy or not does not depend on a time factor but on the balance between difficulties in dissection progress, risks of complications, and extended surgical time.

The time for a change of surgical tactical (cholecystostomy/conversion) varies from 30 to 90 min depending on the experience of the surgical team, bleeding, patient tolerance, and complications.

In a multicenter study, 41% of surgeons consider that the maximum time for laparoscopic cholecystectomy should be 180 min, while 26% do not consider time as a determinant factor for conversion [23]. Recent reports conclude that more than the duration of the cholecystectomy is the experience that determines whether to continue laparoscopically or not [24].

11.3.6 Abstention to Continue

It is an attitude of prudence in the course of an uncertain dissection and/or in the presence of sustained unidentified structures. Therefore, three possibilities come up from this: performing maneuvers to increase vision and facilitate dissection, consult another surgeon or if this is not feasible, and the adoption of alternative techniques.

11.3.7 Maneuvers to Increase Visualization

They are made to improve visualization of the surgical field and to improve dissection. Gallbladder puncture and evacuation, very common in cases of thick-walled gallbladders, of difficult grasp or gallstones impacted on the basin; in that case, if it is feasible, the gallbladder opening and removal of the calculi to continue the procedure safely. Placing a fifth trocar, is a maneuver to keep in mind, as well as the suspension of the round ligament or conversion to assisted hand, a less frequent procedure that requires experience and suitable equipment for its performance.

11.3.8 Second Opinion

A second opinion consult to a more experienced surgeon or HPB surgery specialist is present in all published recommendations on this topic. In addition, up to 18% prevention of biliary/vascular injuries has been reported when calling a second surgeon because of unexpected findings [25].

11.3.9 Alternatives to Cholecystectomy

While the ideal objective is total cholecystectomy, in cases where the safety of the procedure is at risk, there is the option of alternative procedures that allow the treatment of the pathology without exposing the patient to a high risk of bile or vascular injuries. The clinical judgment of the surgeon is essential to define when a dissection becomes difficult and therefore risky and determines the need for alternative procedures, taking into account their experience and expertise.

11.3.10 Conversion

It is clear that the conversion does not guarantee the security of the procedure and therefore many times is not the solution to the problem. In fact it is a controversial issue among those who find that the conversion is associated to three times more complications, mortality, surgical site infection, hospital stay, and readmission than total laparoscopic surgery, while other authors show that there are eight times more bile duct injuries in unconverted patients [26, 27].

11.3.11 Percutaneous Cholecystostomy

It is a timeserver procedure that causes symptomatic relief until final resolution.

11.3.12 Partial or Subtotal Cholecystectomy

In the face of a frozen pedicle with intense fibrosis, subtotal cholecystectomy is an option, avoiding dissection in a risky area.

Ideally, lithiasis should be removed and then the cauterization of the remaining gallbladder must be performed. These procedures can be performed laparoscopically or after conversion, with the surgeon's experience being a determinant factor. An increase in incidence of bile fistulas in subtotal cholecystectomies has been reported, compared to total cholecystectomy (6.3% vs 0.35%), probably related to the incomplete closure of the residual infundibulum. However, morbidity is relatively low requiring endoscopic resolution between 1.5% and 15% [28]. In a review of 1231 subtotal cholecystectomies, of which 73% were laparoscopic, 0.3% postoperative hemorrhage was found, 2.9% sub hepatic collection, and 0.08% BDI [29]. Therefore, laparoscopic subtotal cholecystectomy is a valid and safe option to avoid BDI during a difficult cholecystectomy. Although with a high biliary leakage rate of 18% [29].

11.3.13 Anterograde Cholecystectomy Technique or Fundus First Cholecystectomy

This technique performed during the conventional procedure is also applicable to laparoscopic approach, but it requires a clear knowledge of the anatomy and cystic plate area and hilum to avoid injury [30]. In our experience, despite the fact that it appears in recommendations of recent publications [12, 13], we consider it a risky technique because the possibility of confusing the dissection planes next to the liver hilum.

11.3.14 When Is It Safe to Continue Laparoscopically?

When difficulties are checked during cholecystectomy, the surgeon should think calmly if the procedure should be carried on laparoscopically.

It is possible to continue laparoscopic surgery in the presence of objective safety indicators when:

- There is the conviction of the surgical team that there is proper exposure of the hepatocystic area and that the visceral tractions are made in a technically correct way.
- An appropriate CVS is established.
- Circumferential dissection of the gallbladder cystic angle is achieved, and the cystic artery is visualized, with double vision of both structures.
- There is no doubt regarding the safety of the ongoing surgical procedure.

This determines that no "no return" maneuvers should be performed that require cholecystectomy of necessity before deciding whether to do the procedure or not. In this situation, intraoperative cholangiography, correctly interpreted, showing the entire bile tree can enable us to continue with the procedure.

Finally, to continue with laparoscopy to the extent that the correct identification of the anatomical structures is achieved, this is the synthesis of dissection plus image in a rational time span.

Failure to progress dissection, whatever its cause, may be the determinant factor in adopting an alternative laparoscopic technique, such as subtotal cholecystectomy or cholecystostomy.

Conversion will be an alternative if the team has experience in open gallbladder surgery. Our consideration will be limited when such experience is exclusively, or almost, laparoscopic. Prior to the decision, the infrastructure conditions must be verified to see if they are in place to continue via laparotomy.

Acknowledgments Professor Dr. Daniel Gonzalez MD. For reading the manuscript.

References

1. Hu ASY, Menon R, Gunnarsson R, de Costa A. Risk factors for conversion of laparoscopic cholecystectomy to open surgery—a systematic literature review of 30 studies. Am J Surg. 2017;214:920–30.
2. Strasberg SM, Hertl M, Soper NJ. An analysis of the problem of the biliary injury during laparoscopic cholecystectomy. J Am Coll Surg. 1995;180:101–25.
3. Wakabayashi G, Iwashita Y, Hibi T, Takada T, Strasberg SM, Asbun HJ, et al. Tokyo guidelines 2018: surgical management of acute cholecystitis: safe steps in laparoscopic cholecystectomy for acute cholecystitis (with videos). J Hepatobiliary Pancreat Sci. 2018;25:73–86. https://doi.org/10.1002/jhbp.517; Epub 2018 Jan 10.
4. Abdalla S, Pierre S, Ellis H. Calot's triangle. Clin Anat. 2013;26:493–501. https://doi.org/10.1002/ca.22170; Epub 2013 Mar 21.
5. Gupta V, Jain G. Safe laparoscopic cholecystectomy: adoption of universal culture of safety in cholecystectomy. World J Gastrointest Surg. 2019;11:62–84.
6. Huang TL, Cheng YF, Chen CL, Chen TY, Lee TY. Variants of the bile ducts: clinical application in the potential donor of living-related hepatic transplantation. Transpl Proc. 1996;128:1669–70.
7. Chaib E, Fligelman A, Ferreira F, Carneiro L. Bile duct confluence: anatomic variations and its classification. Surg Radiol Anat. 2014;36:105–9.
8. Couinaud C. Le pédicule hépatique. In: Couinaud C, editor. Le foie, études anatomiques et chirurgicales, vol. Cap. V: Edition Masson; 1957. p. 70–186.
9. Benson EA, Page RE. A practical reappraisal of the anatomy of the extrahepatic bile ducts and arteries. Br J Surg. 1976;63:853–60.
10. Adkins RB Jr, Chapman WC, Reddy VS. Embryology, anatomy, and surgical applications of the extrahepatic biliary system. Surg Clin North Am. 2000;80:363–79.
11. Smadja C, Blumgart LH. The biliary tract and the anatomy of biliary exposure. In: Blumgart LH, editor. Surgery of the liver and biliary tract, vol. 1. 2nd ed. London: Churchill Livingstone; 1994. p. 11–4.
12. Conrad C, Wakabayashi G, Asbun HJ, Dallemagne B, Demartines N, Diana M, et al. IRCAD recommendation on safe laparoscopic cholecystectomy. J Hepatobiliary Pancreat Sci. 2017;24:603–615. https://doi.org/10.1002/jhbp.491; Epub 2017 Oct 27.
13. Pucher PH, Brunt LM, Fanelli RD, Asbun HJ, Aggarwal R. SAGES expert Delphi consensus: critical factors for safe surgical practice in laparoscopic cholecystectomy. Surg Endosc. 2015;29(11):3074–85. https://doi.org/10.1007/s00464-015-4079-z; Epub 2015 Feb 11.

14. Strasberg SM, Brunt LM. Rationale and use of the critical view of safety in laparoscopic cholecystectomy. J Am Coll Surg. 2010;211:132–8. https://doi.org/10.1016/j.jamcollsurg.2010.02.053.
15. Singh R, Brunt L. Critical view of safety-its feasibility and efficacy in preventing bile duct injuries. Ann Laparosc Endosc Surg. 2018;3:2. https://doi.org/10.21037/ales.2017.12.04.
16. Strasberg SM. A teaching program for the "culture of safety in cholecystectomy" and avoidance of bile duct injury. J Am Coll Surg. 2013;217:751. https://doi.org/10.1016/j.jamcollsurg.2013.05.001; Epub 2013 May 23.
17. Álvarez L, Rivera D, Esmeral M, Garcia M, Toro D, Rojas O. Colecistectomía laparoscópica difícil, estrategias de manejo. Rev Colomb Cir. 2013;28:186–95.
18. Iwashita Y, Hibi T, Ohyama T, Honda G, Yoshida M, Miura F, et al. An opportunity in difficulty: Japan-Korea-Taiwan expert Delphi consensus on surgical difficulty during laparoscopic cholecystectomy. J Hepatobiliary Pancreat Sci. 2017;24:191–8. https://doi.org/10.1002/jhbp.440; Epub 2017 Mar 19.
19. Nijssen MA, Schreinemakers JM, Meyer Z, van der Schelling GP, Crolla RM, Rijken AM. Complications after laparoscopic cholecystectomy: a video evaluation study of whether the critical view of safety was reached. World J Surg. 2015;39:1798–803. https://doi.org/10.1007/s00268-015-2993-9.
20. Giménez ME, Houghton EJ, Zeledón ME, Palermo M, Acquafresca P, Finger C, Serra E. Visão crítica de segurança previne lesões biliares? Análise de um levantamento. ABCD Arq Bras Cir Dig. 2018;31:e1380. https://doi.org/10.1590/0102-672020180001e1380.
21. Strasberg SM. Error traps and vasculo-biliary injury in laparoscopic and open cholecystectomy. J Hepato-Biliary-Pancreat Surg. 2008;15:284–92. https://doi.org/10.1007/s00534-007-1267-9; Epub 2008 Jun 6.
22. Arbues G. Colecistectomia dificultosa. Rev Arg Cirugia 2016;(Suplemento1):S.7-S.45.pag.17.
23. Iwashita Y, Ohyama T, Honda G, Hibi T, Yoshida M, Miura F, et al. What are the appropriate indicators of surgical difficulty during laparoscopic cholecystectomy? Results from a Japan-Korea-Taiwan multinational survey. J Hepatobiliary Pancreat Sci. 2016;23:533–47.
24. Hibi T, Iwashita Y, Ohyama T, Honda G, Yoshida M, Takada T, et al. The "right" way is not always popular: comparison of surgeons' perceptions during laparoscopic cholecystectomy for acute cholecystitis among experts from Japan, Korea and Taiwan. J Hepatobiliary Pancreat Sci. 2017;24:24–32.
25. Iwashita Y, Hibi T, Ohyama T, Umezawa A, Takada T, Strasberg SM, et al. Delphi consensus on bile duct injuries during laparoscopic cholecystectomy: an evolutionary cul-de-sac or the birth pangs of a new technical framework? J Hepatobiliary Pancreat Sci. 2017;24:591–602.
26. Sippey M, Grzybowski M, Manwaring ML, Kasten KR, Chapman WH, Pofahl WE, et al. Acute cholecystitis: risk factors for conversion to an open procedure. J Surg Res. 2015;199:357–61. https://doi.org/10.1016/j.jss.2015.05.040; Epub 2015 Jun 12.
27. Malik AM. Difficult laparoscopic cholecystectomies. Is conversion a sensible option? J Pak Med Assoc. 2015;65:698–700.
28. Van De Graaf FW, Zaïmi I, Stassen LPS, Lange JF. Safe laparoscopic cholecystectomy: a systematic review of bile duct injury prevention. Int J Surg. 2018;60:164–72.
29. Elshaer M, Gravante G, Thomas K, Sorge R, Al-Hamali S, Ebdewi H. Subtotal cholecystectomy for "difficult gallbladders": systematic review and meta-analysis. JAMA Surg. 2015;150:159–68. https://doi.org/10.1001/jamasurg.2014.1219.
30. Honda G, Iwanaga T, Kurata M. Dissection of the gallbladder from the liver bed during laparoscopic cholecystectomy for acute or subacute cholecystitis. J Hepato-Biliary-Pancreat Surg. 2008;15:293–6. https://doi.org/10.1007/s00534-007-1260-3; Epub 2008 Jun 6.

Open Partial or Subtotal Cholecystectomy: Techniques and Indications

12

Maurizio Mannino, Elena Schembari, Adriana Toro, and Isidoro Di Carlo

12.1 Introduction

Laparoscopic cholecystectomy is the gold standard for gallstone disease [1]. Technical skills and learning curve are very important to reduce the risk of complications during the surgical procedure [2]. The complication most feared by surgeons is iatrogenic bile duct injury (BDI) which is associated with significant morbidity and mortality [3].

To reduce this complication, various measures have been proposed during laparoscopy: the use of a laparoscope at 30° and avoidance of tenting [4]; the use of a "critical vision" approach [5]; and the "dome-down" LC [6]. All these procedures have permitted to reduce BDI from 0.5% in 1990 to 0.3% in 2009 [7]. However, when the surgeon is not sure that he can manage the integrity of the biliary tract, the conversion to open surgery remains mandatory, especially in cases of difficult cholecystectomy as for acute cholecystitis [8].

Even today conversion to open surgery is part of the laparoscopic cholecystectomy which is required for patient safety. The conversion rate is between 5% and 7%. The causes of conversion are severe inflammation (55.3%), adhesion (26.0%), bleeding (5.3%), probable choledocholithiasis (4.3%), and inability to continue (5.3%) [9].

In all these cases in which the structures of the Calot's triangle (cystic duct, cystic artery, common bile duct) cannot be identified in a safe manner, open subtotal cholecystectomy has proved to be a safe, simple, and definitive procedure [10].

A recent systematic review has shown that male patients, aged between 60 and 65 years, sclerotic gallbladder or wall thickness (4–5 mm), and acute cholecystitis are at most risks of surgical conversion [11].

12.2 History

In 1882, the open cholecystectomy technique was described [12]. This technique was considered the standard technique until 1987 when laparoscopic technique was reported for the first time [12].

Many changes were proposed after the first technical description for the management of the difficulties that may arise during both open and laparoscopic surgery. Those difficult conditions can be classified into five categories: adhesions with greater neovascularization, difficulty in treating the liver, inadequate exposure of the

M. Mannino · I. Di Carlo (✉)
Department of Surgical Sciences and Advanced Technologies "GF Ingrassia", University of Catania, Cannizzaro Hospital, Catania, Italy
e-mail: idicarlo@unict.it

E. Schembari
Barts Health NHS Trust, London, UK

A. Toro
Department of General Surgery, E. Muscatello Hospital, Augusta (SR), Italy

© Springer Nature Switzerland AG 2021

I. Di Carlo (ed.), *Difficult Acute Cholecystitis*, https://doi.org/10.1007/978-3-030-62102-5_12

Calot's triangle, a high-risk gallbladder bed, and a high-risk hilum [13].

The first modified cholecystectomy was described by Hans Kehr in 1898 when he reported the case of a 27-year-old lady with acute cholecystitis who underwent surgery. He could not remove the hardened posterior wall of the gallbladder and its part close to the cystic duct because of the adhesions. So, he modified the traditional technique in order to avoid severe injuries. However, he also reported a severe postoperative bile fistula which required a further operation [14]. After the description of Kehr, several techniques have been described in order to manage difficult cases.

In 1938, Estes [15] advised performing a subtotal cholecystectomy when the level of inflammation was too high to make a clear identification of the cystic duct. A longitudinal incision was made along the gallbladder's wall up to 1–2 cm from the cystic duct, and the wall was swabbed with tincture of iodine. In this way, the removal of the impacted stones was possible. The redundant wall was trimmed, preserving the part attached to the liver bed. The cystic duct was not sutured, so there was no gallbladder remnant, and drains were placed [15].

In 1939, a technique was described which involved opening the gallbladder in the longitudinal direction, extraction of the stones, and the thermal ablation of both part of the wall of the gallbladder up to the sierosa which were sutured together to re-peritonealize the liver bed. This technique requires the suturing of the cystic duct and cystic artery as in total cholecystectomy [16].

In 1950, a variation of this technique was described. It contemplates the resection of the free wall of the gallbladder until the cystic duct. Since the cystic artery has to be sectioned at the inferior level of the gallbladder (within or on the wall of the gallbladder) near the cystic duct, it is recommended to suture the wall at the point to avoid vascular damages [17].

In 1954, McElmoyle [18] clearly illustrated his technique, underlying the difference with that one previously proposed by Pribram [19], Love [20], and Thorek [21]. In fact, these three authors advised to dissect and ligate artery and cystic duct and leaving a part of the gallbladder attached to the liver bed. Conversely, McElmoyle suggested that when it was safe, the dissection of the artery and cystic duct should be performed and associated with complete removal of the gallbladder wall. Otherwise, in difficult cases, the isolation of the artery and cystic duct should not be attempted, especially when there was not a visible surgical field. Consequently, the portion of gallbladder's wall closer to the important ducts and vessels was left in order to protect them from unsafe surgical maneuvers [18]. At the end of the McElmoyle's procedure, the edge of the remaining wall was sutured to control the bleedings, the mucosa was treated with phenol or electric cautery, and drains were placed [18]. Similarly to McElmoyle, other authors have supported the idea that it is safer to not close the cystic duct in order to avoid risky manipulations of the area [22].

Alternatively, a safe method is the closure of the cystic duct from inside by a purse-string as suggested by Bornman and Terblanche [23]. They also advised introducing a probe into a cystic duct for easier identification and ligation. However, the probe could be wrongly advanced in the common bile duct, especially if the cystic duct is short, leading to its erroneous ligation [24].

The Tokyo Guidelines 2018 [25] have summarized the technique of subtotal cholecystectomy, referring to the paper of Strasberg et al. [24]. According to this chapter, after emptying the gallbladder and cystic duct from stones and, eventually, a cholangiography or intraoperative ultrasound done, the posterior wall of the gallbladder is usually left in situ and ablated [25]. The ablation of the mucosa should minimize the recurrence of gallstones [26]. If there is a risk of bile duct injury (BDI), intraoperative cholangiography, intraoperative ultrasound, intraoperative indocyanine green fluorescence imaging may be useful, but there is no unified consensus on their usefulness. It is also possible a partial or total excision of the posterior wall but gangrenous gallbladder should be removed mandatorily. Oversewing the cut edges with a continuous suture is not mandatory but it could be helpful where the cystic artery branches reach the gallbladder, even if they are often thrombosed because of the inflammation. The suture from inside of the cystic duct is not compulsory but advisable. The number of drains depends on the degree of contamination. In the fenestrating subtotal cholecystectomy, the residual gallbladder lumen is open into the peritoneal cavity, while in the reconstituting one the lumen is closed with sutures or staplers [24].

12.3 Indication

Open conversion is required in 5–10% of cases with an increase in hospital days [38]. Between 0.2% and 1.1% of patients undergoing not converted laparoscopic difficult cholecystectomy reported bile duct lesions [27].

Open conversion is necessary in case of difficulty in identifying the bile duct, cystic duct, and cystic artery or in case of intraoperative complications (bile duct injury, hemorrhage, intestinal perforation, etc.).

In literature, several factors that can increase the possibility of converting into an open procedure are reported: age [28], male sex [29], obesity [30], cholecystitis [29], and ERCP [31].

The most common presentation of patients with acute cholecystitis is abdominal pain in the right hypochondrium, fever, and high white blood cells. The liver function tests can be normal.

During radiological examinations, it is possible to forecast the possibility to use the subtotal cholecystectomy technique. When the US or CT scan show a severe inflammation or complications as fluid collections or gas in the wall or the lumen of the gallbladder or free air in the peritoneum, an open technique with subtotal cholecystectomy can be necessary [10].

For this reason, many authors report scores to predict the possibility to convert to open surgery.

Sutcliffe et al. reporting CLOC score. This score is applicable before the laparoscopic surgery. Where a lower score ≤ 6 is a low risk, so patients can be treated by surgeons in the first phase of training. A higher score ≥ 6 is a high risk of conversion and the patient should be operated by experienced surgeons [32].

Sugrue et al. reported a 10-point intraoperative gallbladder scoring system (G10). The gallbladder surgery was considered easy if the G10 score < 2, moderate ($2 \leq 4$), difficult ($5 \leq 7$), and extreme ($8 \leq 10$). Conversion occurred in 33% of patients with G10 scores of ≥ 5. Completely buried GB, impacted stone, bile or pus outside GB, and fistula represent the four factors statistically predictive of conversion [33].

In literature, two techniques are reported for open cholecystectomy in difficult gallbladder: partial cholecystectomy and subtotal cholecystectomy. The difference between partial and subtotal cholecystectomy is not well explained in the literature because many authors have used the term partial and subtotal in a personal way. Partial should mean the removal of part of an organ while the subtotal should mean the removal of almost all of an organ.

Some authors suggest using the term subtotal to indicate the extent of the resection. If it is removed only upper part can be used the term fundectomy and eliminated the term partial [24].

12.4 Technique

The open techniques to remove gall bladder are summarized in three categories: the first reports to leave the cystic duct closed with clips or inside the Hartmann's suture bag and leaving the posterior mucosa adherent to the liver; the second technique reports to leave the cystic duct and the Hartmann's bag left open and drained; the third technique contemplates leaving the cystic duct open and the Hartmann's bag closed with stapler or suture [34].

The technique for subtotal cholecystectomy used by the authors is the following: a small right subcostal transverse incision (max 12 cm) is performed under general anesthesia (Fig. 12.1). After the gallbladder is incised by electrocautery at the fundus, the bile or pus is aspirated (Fig. 12.2a, b) and the stones evacuated. Then the fundus of the gallbladder are resected, and the anterior wall is transected until 1 cm before the cystic orifice in order to visualize it (Fig. 12.3). At this moment,

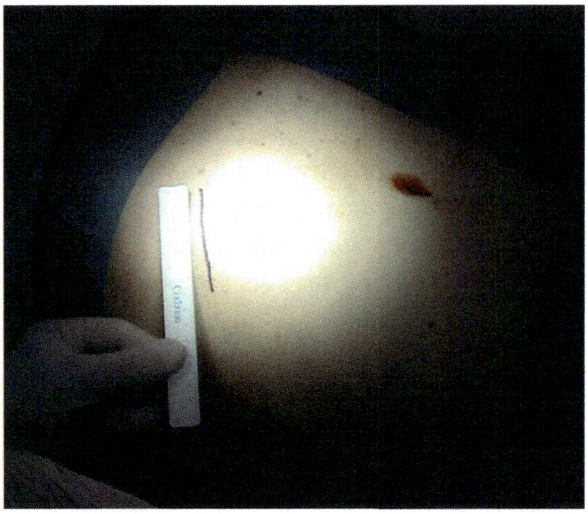

Fig. 12.1 Skin incision up to 12 cm. (median incision is 8 cm)

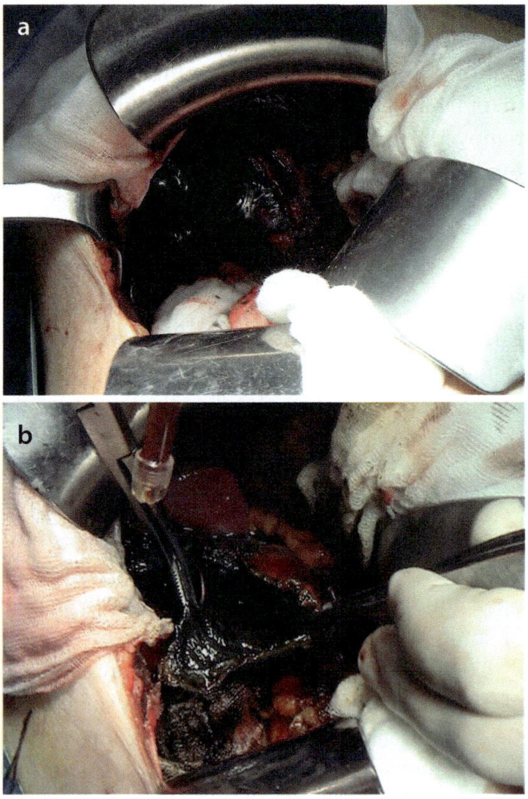

Fig. 12.2 (a) Intraoperative view of cholecystitis (b) The fundus is incised and resected, then the gallbladder is empty of all contest (bile, pus, stones)

the posterior wall is resected from the liver bed (also this, 1 cm before the cystic orifice). The remaining anterior and posterior infundibular tis-

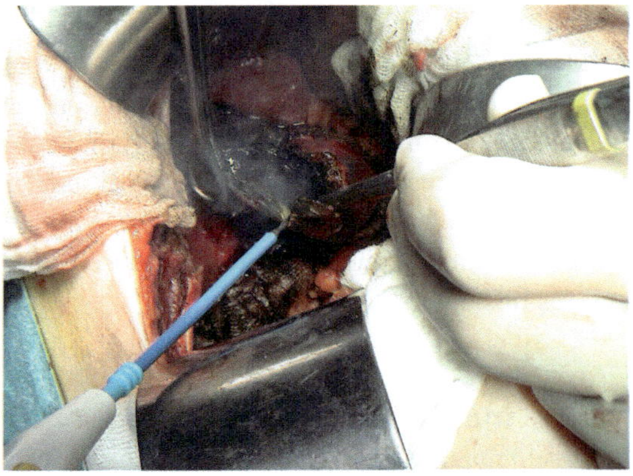

Fig. 12.3 Resection of anterior wall until the cystic orifice

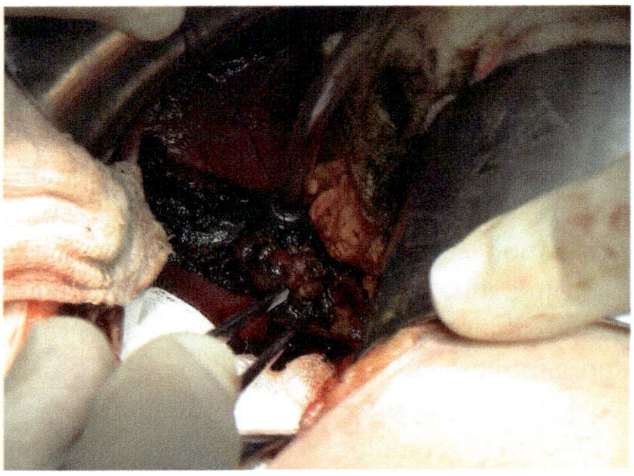

Fig. 12.4 Remaining infundibular anterior and posterior wall are sutured in order to safely avoid CBD lesion and to eliminate any residual cavity in the infundibulum

sue is closed hermetically by double running suture in order to avoid bile leakage or, more important, the formation of a new cavity [10] (Fig. 12.4). A small drainage can be left in place depending from the intraoperative situation.

It is described by many authors how the anterior wall of the inferior infundibulum should be sutured to the posterior wall left adherent to the liver bed, but this difficult technique could create a new cavity and be the origin for stones recurrence. Furthermore, performing this suture, it is possible to damage the hepatic parenchyma causing bleeding.

When a high grade of inflammation is present, the limits between seromuscularis tissue and mucosa are hard to be individuated. For this reason, in this case, it could be much cautious leaving in place the posterior wall of the gallbladder leaving open the cystic orifice.

Furthermore, the risk of a suture only with the mucosa can consequently create a subtle infundibulum wall that can be damaged by the traction practiced during the suture and causes necrotic degeneration or fistulas. This is why the technique of suturing the anterior wall to the posterior wall has to be practiced only when this last is separated from the liver bed, in order to create a stable structure with no risk of new biliary cavities [10].

12.5 Complications

During subtotal cholecystectomy, the dissection and ligation of the cystic duct is difficult, but needed, by some authors, to avoid a postoperative bile leakage [34].

Furthermore, patients undergoing subtotal cholecystectomy have a higher rate of biliary fistula, an overall increase in length of hospital stay with an additional cost due to ERCP, and biliary stenting. But debate is still open because the low incidence of biliary fistula and effective treatment with ERCP reduce morbidity and do not justify to exploration of the common bile duct or more difficult procedure to tie the cystic duct [35].

The use a 10 French endoprosthesis in the cystic duct stump to allow the complete closure of the persistent fistula in 6 weeks is reported in the literature, but is not commonly used [36].

Other authors show a technique in which a piece of omentum is plugged into the gallbladder stump to avoid bile leakage. This technique is used when it is not possible to close the cystic duct due to a difficult gallbladder [37]. Also, this technique is not commonly used.

The closure of the residual gallbladder (Hartmann's pocket) can be considered the safest method, but if not well performed it can cause the formation of the gallbladder residue which reduces the incidence of biliary fistula but in which the formation of the bile stones is possible [38]. In literature, there are no indications on the incidence of symptomatic residual gallbladder after subtotal or partial cholecystectomy because there is no long follow-up, and the residual gallbladder can give clinical signs after many years of surgical treatment [38]. In the cases of the patients with residual gallbladder can be necessary a new surgical procedure to remove the residual gallbladder [24].

The advantages of subtotal cholecystectomy are the reduction of recurrent gallstone formation because all the gallbladder mucosa is eliminated and the necrotic parts of the gallbladder are removed, avoiding the formation of empyema [35].

The disadvantages of subtotal cholecystectomy reported in the literature are the increased incidence of infection and intra-abdominal injury [35], cystic stump syndrome (continuous discharge of mucus from the retained gallbladder mucosa), subphrenic collections, or persistent drainage from the drainage site [39].

References

1. Abdelrahim WE, Elsiddig KE, Wahab AA, et al. Subtotal laparoscopic cholecystectomy influences the rate of conversion in patients with difficult laparoscopic cholecystectomy: case series. Med Surg (Lond). 2017;19:19–22.
2. Halbert C, Pagkratis S, Yang J, et al. Beyond the learning curve: incidence of bile duct injuries following laparoscopic cholecystectomy normalize to open in the modern era. Surg Endosc. 2016;30:2239–43.
3. Fullum TM, Downing SR, Ortega G, et al. Is laparoscopy a risk factor for bile duct injury during cholecystectomy? JSLS. 2013;17:365–70.
4. Hunter JG. Avoidance of bile duct injury during laparoscopic cholecystectomy. Am J Surg. 1991;162:71–6.
5. Strasberg SM. Avoidance of biliary injury during laparoscopic cholecystectomy. J Hepato-Biliary-Pancreat Surg. 2002;9:543–7.
6. Kato K, Matsuda M, Onodera K, et al. Laparoscopic cholecystectomy from fundus downward. Surg Laparosc Endosc. 1994;4:373-4.
7. Hogan AM, Hoti E, Winter DC, et al. Quality of life after iatrogenic bile duct injury: a case control study. Ann Surg. 2009;249:292–5.
8. Buddingh KT, Hofker HS, ten Cate Hoedemaker HO, et al. Safety measures during cholecystectomy: results of a nationwide survey. World J Surg. 2011;35:1235–41.
9. Knight JS, Mercer SJ, Somers SS, et al. Timing of urgent laparoscopic cholecystectomy does not influence conversion rate. Br J Surg. 2004;91:601–4.
10. Di Carlo I, Pulvirenti E, Toro A, Corsale G. Modified subtotal cholecystectomy: results of a laparotomy

procedure during the laparoscopic era. World J Surg. 2009;33:520–5.
11. Philip Rothman J, Burcharth J, Pommergaard HC, et al. Preoperative risk factors for conversion of laparoscopic cholecystectomy to open surgery - a systematic review and meta-analysis of observational studies. Dig Surg. 2016;33:414–23.
12. Jenkins PJ, Paterson HM, Parks RW, et al. Open cholecystectomy in the laparoscopic era. Br J Surg. 2007;94:1382–5.
13. Palanivelu C, Rajan PS, Jani K, et al. Laparoscopic cholecystectomy in cirrhotic patients: the role of subtotal cholecystectomy and its variants. J Am Coll Surg. 2006;203:145–51.
14. Kehr H. Introduction to the differential diagnosis of the separate forms of gallstone diseases: based upon his own experience gained from 433 laparotomies for gallstones. Philadelphia: P Blakiston's Son and Co.; 1901.
15. Estes WL. Acute gangrenous cholecystitis and the use of partial cholecystectomy in its treatment. Am J Surg. 1938;40:197–204.
16. Pribram BO. Mukoklase und drainagelose Gallenchirurgie. Zentralbl Chir. 1928;55:773–9.
17. Lerner AI. Partial cholecystectomy. Can Med Assoc J. 1950;63:54–6.
18. McElmoyle WA. Cholecystectomy: a method for the difficult gall-bladder. Lancet. 1954;266:1320–3.
19. Pribram BO. The electrosurgical operation in gallbladder diseases: results of 13 years' experience. Lancet. 1939;234:927e929.
20. Baily H, Love RJM. Electrosurgical obliteration of gallbladder without drainage: Thorek's operation. Br Med J. 1939;30:682e683.
21. Thorek M. Electrosurgical obliteration of gallbladder without drainage: a means of reducing mortality. Am J Surg. 1936;32:417e434.
22. Philips JA, Lawes DA, Cook AJ, et al. The use of laparoscopic subtotal cholecystectomy for complicated cholelithiasis. Surg Endosc. 2008;22:1697–700.
23. Bornman PC, Terblanche J. Subtotal cholecystectomy: for the difficult gallbladder in portal hypertension and cholecystitis. Surgery. 1985;98:1–6.
24. Strasberg SM, Pucci MJ, Brunt LM, Deziel DJ. Subtotal cholecystectomy-"Fenestrating" vs "Reconstituting" subtypes and the prevention of bile duct injury: definition of the optimal procedure in difficult operative conditions. J Am Coll Surg. 2016;222:89–96.
25. Wakabayashi G, Iwashita Y, Hibi T, et al. Tokyo Guidelines 2018: surgical management of acute cholecystitis: safe steps in laparoscopic cholecystectomy for acute cholecystitis (with videos). J Hepatobiliary Pancreat Sci. 2018;25:73–86.
26. Kuwabara J, Watanabe Y, Kameoka K, et al. Usefulness of laparoscopic subtotal cholecystectomy with operative cholangiography for severe cholecystitis. Surg Today. 2014;44:462–5.
27. Navez B, Ungureanu F, Michiels M, et al. Surgical management of acute cholecystitis: results of a 2-year prospective multicenter survey in Belgium. Surg Endosc. 2012;26:2436–45.
28. Ballal M, David G, Willmott S, et al. Conversion after laparoscopic cholecystectomy in England. Surg Endosc. 2009;23:2338–44.
29. Lipman JM, Claridge JA, Haridas M, et al. Preoperative findings predict conversion from laparoscopic to open cholecystectomy. Surgery. 2007;142:556–63.
30. Goonawardena J, Gunnarsson R, de Costa A, et al. Predicting conversion from laparoscopic to open cholecystectomy presented as a probability nomogram based on preoperative patient risk factors. Am J Surg. 2015;210:492–500.
31. Reinders JS, Gouma DJ, Heisterkamp J, et al. Laparoscopic cholecystectomy is more difficult after a previous endoscopic retrograde cholangiography. HPB (Oxford). 2013;15:230–4.
32. Sutcliffe RP, Hollyman M, Hodson J, et al. Preoperative risk factors for conversion from laparoscopic to open cholecystectomy: a validated risk score derived from a prospective U.K. database of 8820 patients. HPB (Oxford). 2016;18:922–8.
33. Sugrue M, Sahebally SM, Ansaloni L, Zielinski MD. Grading operative findings at laparoscopic cholecystectomy- a new scoring system. World J Emerg Surg. 2015;10:14.
34. Hirajima S, Koh T, Sakai T, et al. Utility of laparoscopic subtotal cholecystectomy with or without cystic duct ligation for severe cholecystitis. Am Surg. 2017;83:1209–13.
35. Davis B, Castaneda G, Lopez J. Subtotal cholecystectomy versus total cholecystectomy in complicated cholecystitis. Am Surg. 2012;78:814–7.
36. Gholson CF, Dungan C, Neff G, et al. Suspected biliary complications after laparoscopic and open cholecystectomy leading to endoscopic cholangiography: a retrospective comparison. Dig Dis Sci. 1998;43:534–9.
37. Matsui Y, Hirooka S, Kotsuka M, et al. Use of a piece of free omentum to prevent bile leakage after subtotal cholecystectomy. Surgery. 2018;164:419–23.
38. Elshaer M, Gravante G, Thomas K, et al. (2015) subtotal cholecystectomy for "difficult gallbladders": systematic review and meta-analysis. JAMA Surg. 2015;150(2):159–68. https://doi.org/10.1001/jamasurg.2014.1219.
39. Sharp CF, Garza RZ, Mangram AJ, Dunn EL. Partial cholecystectomy in the setting of severe inflammation is an acceptable consideration with few long-term sequelae. Am Surg. 2009;75:249–52.

13 Laparoscopic Subtotal Cholecystectomy and Other Laparoscopic Techniques

Elena Schembari, Maurizio Mannino, Adriana Toro, Piero Marco Fisichella, and Isidoro Di Carlo

13.1 Introduction

When laparoscopic cholecystectomy (LC) is difficult due to a severe inflammation degree that makes the Calot's triangle dissection challenging, conversion to open surgery was suggested in the past. Nowadays, thanks to the increasing surgeons' laparoscopic experience, several tricks have been described to have a better visualization of the operative field in order to finalize the total cholecystectomy by laparoscopy. Moreover, when a "critical view of safety" (CVS) is not possible, other laparoscopic techniques have been advised to manage the difficult cases that can be treated by subtotal cholecystectomy or other techniques that do not resect the gallbladder in its entirety but leave a part of the gallbladder wall in place. This chapter will explore all these possible solutions and suggest that a change in surgical laparoscopic strategy can give better results than the open conversion.

13.2 Tricks

Many tricks have been reported in literature to make a cholecystectomy easier. Santos et al. [1] described the trocars' position in obese patients. The camera trocar should not be inserted at the umbilicus but 15 cm below the xiphoid process. The reason is that in these patients the umbilicus is located lower in the abdomen, and consequently the placement of the camera trocar in this site would make more distant and difficult the visualization of the gallbladder. Even previous median laparotomies are contraindications for umbilical access; in these cases, the first trocar should be placed in the upper left or right quadrant in order to remove adhesions in the umbilical region and allowing a safe insertion of the camera trocar.

Moreover, in obese patients with a substantial amount of intra-abdominal fat and the omentum covering the gallbladder, the traditional reverse Trendelenburg position slightly turned on the left side could not be enough to achieve a good visualization of the gallbladder and an instrument should be used to take them away from the surgical field.

In addition, the use of a further 5 mm trocar should be considered as a valid option for facilitating the surgeon's performance as for bulky left lobe of the liver that can be found not only in obese patients but also in normal weight subjects.

E. Schembari
Barts Health NHS Trust, London, UK

M. Mannino · I. Di Carlo (✉)
Department of Surgical Sciences and Advanced Technologies "GF Ingrassia", University of Catania, Cannizzaro Hospital, Catania, Italy
e-mail: idicarlo@unict.it

A. Toro
Department of General Surgery, E. Muscatello Hospital, Augusta (SR), Italy

P. M. Fisichella
Feinberg School of Medicine, Northwestern University, Evanston, IL, USA

© Springer Nature Switzerland AG 2021
I. Di Carlo (ed.), *Difficult Acute Cholecystitis*, https://doi.org/10.1007/978-3-030-62102-5_13

A 30° or 45° laparoscope should be preferred to a 0° one because this facilitates the vision during the lateral and medial dissections.

Decompression of gallbladder by needle aspiration is advised when its distension is too exaggerated and interferes with the field of view [2].

During the dissection, the intensity of diathermy should be regulated according to the size of the patient and the surgeon's skills. High levels of energy can not only damage closer organs such as duodenum and stomach during adhesiolysis but also burn the liver with possible postoperative bile leakages. Undoubtedly, modern energy devices (Harmonic, Thunderbeat) facilitate the hemostasis in patients with acute cholecystitis or cirrhosis, even if there are some risks of serious injuries due to the thermal spread [1]. Persistent mild bleedings should be managed by compression, while uncontrolled clipping and electrocautery should be avoided [2].

Another fundamental step during the dissection is the correct exposure of the Calot's triangle. An adequate retraction of the infundibulum towards the lateral and caudal parts of the patient allows the opening of the triangle. Without this maneuver, the cystic duct would lay parallel to the common bile duct and distinguishing these two structures could be challenging, with an obvious increased risk of damaging the common bile duct. The assistant could make this phase easier, facilitating the visualization of the infundibulum by pulling up and to the right patient's shoulder the fundus of the gallbladder. Moreover, thanks to this maneuver, the incision of the medial peritoneal attachment of the gallbladder can be safely performed. This in conjunction with the lateral attachment incision will result in a further opening of the Calot's triangle and give access to gallbladder's wall through the inflammatory capsule [1].

When the cystic artery is short or enters high into the gallbladder, it hinders a reliable achievement of CVS. In such occasions, it has been advised to cut it. The aim of this procedure is to allow clear visualization of the cystic duct which will be the only tubular structure in the Calot's triangle. However, before performing this division, the surgeon must be sure that the identified structure is the cystic artery. This represents a crucial step because, basing this assessment just on the presence of pulsation or its size, the cystic artery could be confused with the right hepatic artery or with the cystic duct. In order to avoid this unpleasant and dangerous misidentification, removing all the tissue (such as fat) which surrounds the cystic artery is fundamental, and this vascular structure should be followed from its origin to its entrance into the gallbladder [3].

However, surgical decision-making remains the most fundamental element in the management of difficult cholecystectomy [4]. Unclear anatomy, bleedings, bile leakage, and the use of several clips are all factors that should encourage the young surgeon to ask for some help. Converting to open cholecystectomy can be useful to get out of Dodge, but it is not always the best solution to make a cholecystectomy easier. In fact, having the opinion of a colleague with good expertise in laparoscopic surgery can be more effective rather than converting to open surgery. Moreover, there are other strategies that can be used to overcome these difficult situations because the safety of patients has to ever guide the surgeon's behavior.

13.3 Alternative Strategies

The surgeon should always bear in mind that cholecystectomy is usually performed for benign disease [4]. Dangerous maneuvers, which can lead to serious injuries and sometimes life-threating situations, should not be carried out especially because there are other solutions that are safe and effective. So, the decision of changing the surgical strategy should be made before doing vascular or biliary injuries.

The CVS is not the only technique to isolate the cystic duct, but the infundibular technique could be also adopted (Fig. 13.1). According to this method, the dissection of the cystic duct is made on the front and back of the Calot's triangle once the cystic duct is found, and it is traced on to the union with the gallbladder. A typical flare or funnel shape is evident when the cystic duct joins the gallbladder. However, this technique seems to

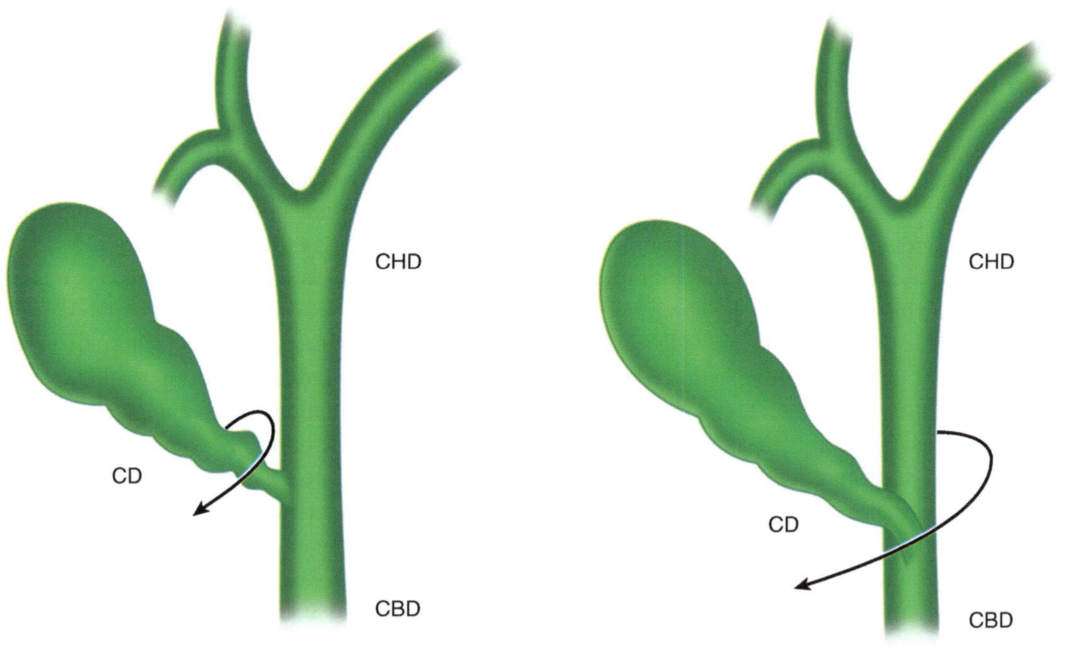

Fig. 13.1 The infundibular technique of laparoscopic cholecystectomy. Left: typical anatomy, where the dissection is made around the cystic duct (CD), which can be easily distinguished and is far away from the common hepatic duct (CHD) and the common bile duct (CBD). Right: due to the inflammatory process, the CHD could be adherent to the CD and misidentified as this. So, the circular dissection is more likely to be wrongly made around the block CBD–CD rather than just around the CD, causing biliary injuries

create a flaw in the visualization of the cystic duct. In fact, it has been demonstrated that, in case of severe inflammation, it is hidden, and the risk of misidentifying the common bile duct as the cystic duct and biliary injury is high. In these situations, the dissection around the left and the right sides of the common bile duct instead of anteriorly and posteriorly to the Calot's triangle can be done but very cautiously and only in expert hands. As a result, this technique is unreliable, even if it is performed by expert surgeons, and should be avoided [5].

In 1994, LC from "fundus downward" or "fundus first" was proposed by Kato et al. [6]. When the exposure of the cystic duct was difficult, the gallbladder dissection should start from the fundus and the cystic duct should be clipped and cut at the end of the procedure. This technique was slightly modified by Uyama et al. [7], who lifted the liver bed up to the diaphragm by a suture, obtaining a good view of the operative field. However, because of the contraction of the Calot's triangle occurring during an inflammatory process, the lower end of the gallbladder becomes closer to the common hepatic duct, the right hepatic artery, and the right or main portal veins. So, gallbladder and common hepatic duct can be perceived by the surgeon as one structure, the route of the dissection will be wrong, and, at the end of the procedure, the common hepatic duct will be divided [8].

The impossibility of obtaining a CVS is a clear signal that a bailout procedure should be considered [2]. Thanks to a subtotal cholecystectomy (SC), it is possible to treat the disease at once, avoiding a second operation. Indeed, subtotal cholecystectomy in the case of portal hypertension or cholecystitis is a well-known technique [9]. Generally speaking, "subtotal" means almost complete removal of an organ, while "partial" refers to the removal of a portion of an organ. These two terms have been used in literature to describe the same extension of an incomplete gallbladder resection. However, Strasberg [10] suggested that the term "subtotal" was more accurate to describe this type of surgical procedure and avoid confusion. The term "fundectomy" should be adopted referring to the removal of the top part of the gallbladder. As a result, the word "partial" should not be used anymore. Furthermore, the terms "reconstituting" and "fenestrating" refer to the presence or absence of a gallbladder remnant that in the majority of cases concerns the posterior wall. The remaining portion of the gallbladder wall can be left open or closed, when it is sutured this has to be done as close as possible to the cystic duct. Otherwise the residual sutured stump, called "remnant," will result in a new and smaller gallbladder.

Overall, some differences come to light when the articles about subtotal cholecystectomy are examined. In fact, the authors of the published articles have controversial opinions about how to perform some steps of this procedure.

One of the most critical steps of the subtotal cholecystectomy is the handling of the cystic duct. Some authors prefer to isolate and close the cystic duct with surgical clips, suture ligation, Endoloop (Ethicon), purse-string suture, or intracorporeal sutures for closure [11, 12].

Palanivelu et al. [13] introduced the concept of tailored subtotal cholecystectomy by laparoscopy. In fact, they classified laparoscopic subtotal cholecystectomy (LSC) in three types which were performed according to the risk of damaging liver bed or hilum. So, in type I, they suggested to not remove the posterior wall of the gallbladder when its dissection from the liver bed was difficult for an increased risk of bleeding. The remnant mucosa could be removed (mucosectomy) or electrofulgurated. Type II should be performed when recognizing the hilar structures was complicate, the entire gallbladder was removed, and the infundibulum was cut close to the cystic duct and sutured with a continuous suture of polyglactin 3–0. Finally, when high-risk hilum and gallbladder bed coexisted, a combination of LSC I and II should be performed and this was called LSC III.

When LSC is performed, there are two possible options to manage the remnant gallbladder stump. The first option is to close it, reconstituting the gallbladder as in open surgery described by Strasberg. Several methods can be used to do it like an absorbable suture [14], a purse-string suture [11], endoloop [15], or an EndoGIA stapler [12]. All these techniques have to be used carefully, and they can be applied only when a safe distance between the cystic duct and the common bile ducts exists. Otherwise, the risk is to have the traction and consequently involvement of the CBD and all related immediate or late complications. This closure can be performed also when the posterior wall of the gallbladder is not excised [10]; in this case, it is completely cauterized with the only exception of the part that will be sutured. The second option is to leave it open (fenestrating LSC), closing the cystic duct [16, 17] or leaving it open. Drains are usually placed [18, 19].

Recently, the association of "fundus first" LC and subtotal cholecystectomy has been proposed [20, 21]. According to Harilingam et al. [20], the procedure starts with the opening of the fundus to drain its content (pus, bile, stones). After dividing the gallbladder into two halves, the posterior wall is used to make traction and pulling up the liver and the anterior wall is transected at the level of Hartmann's pouch. Then, the posterior wall is divided from the liver bed, but, when this dissection is difficult, it is cauterized. The cystic duct or the small gallbladder remnant is closed with an intracorporeal stitch or endoloop. The rationale of this technique is that viewing the gallbladder from the inside could make the dissection safe, reducing the risk of biliary and vascular injuries. Moreover, an intraoperative cholangiography could be performed. Nasr et al. [21] proposed the traditional fundus first technique, but they ended the dissection at the so-called "Critical Point of Surgical Control" (CPSC) of the gallbladder. The CPSC is the junction between the gallbladder neck and the cystic duct where the cystic artery comes into the gallbladder. When they arrived at CPSC, an endoloop was applied to control the hilum of the gallbladder. However, due to the small number of patients involved in these studies [20, 21], it is not possible to conclude if these techniques have better outcomes than the others [2].

13.4 Outcomes

Overall, postoperative bile leakage was more frequent after laparoscopic subtotal cholecystectomy compared with open conversion, while rates of retained stones, subhepatic collections, wound infections, reoperations and mortality were all lower [22]. Moreover, the incidence of postoperative complications after subtotal cholecystectomy (SC) is similar to that after a total cholecystectomy (TC) and, taking into account that SC is usually performed in difficult cases, this means that SC is a safe and simple method to manage complex situations. It is important to highlight the lower rate of common bile duct injury after SC rather than TC, which is one of the most important reasons why the SC is performed because it avoids hazardous maneuvers in the Calot's triangle [22]. In fact, vascular injuries can cause acute liver failure, while biliary obstruction dues to the wrong closure of the CBD could lead to secondary biliary cirrhosis and chronic liver failure. In both cases, liver transplantation is the only treatment [23, 24].

The most common complication of LSC is bile leak, which varies from 10.6% [25] to 18% [22]. This incidence is higher after laparoscopy maybe because the cystic duct (CD) can be closed with a tighter knot during an open procedure. The increased rate of bilomas and bile leaks after SC can be consequent to the inflammation because, when the inflammatory process is resolved, the edema disappears and the sutures used to close CD or Hartmann's pouch can become looser [22]. Bile leaks are more common when CD or Hartmann's pouch is left open rather than when they are closed [22, 25]. Leaving drainages in place is useful to monitor the evolution of the leakage also because the majority of bile fistulas can resolve spontaneously [22]. Otherwise, percutaneous drainage or ERCP can be used to address the problem [25].

The fundus-down technique is associated with a high incidence of vasculo-biliary injury, especially in difficult cases like severe inflammation with the fusion of the structures because it is easier to misidentify the correct plane [26]. For this reason, performing the dissection close to the gallbladder has been advised [2].

The incidence of recurrent or residual gallstones after intentional incomplete cholecystectomy has been estimated between 0.0% and 16% [18, 27]. During SC, stones placed in the gallbladder stump or cystic duct could not be identified, this could explain the increased incidence of retained stones after SC than TC. The difference in the rate of this complication is not statistically significant between cystic duct/gallbladder stump open and close, even if this appears to be slightly higher when cystic duct/gallbladder stump is left open [22]. In long-term follow-up, recurrent symptomatic stones can form in the gallbladder remnant in only 5% of patients, giving symptoms of cholecystolithiasis [2, 10, 25]. There is no evidence that increasing the number of LSC and reducing laparotomic conversions causes a rise in the rate of residual or recurrent gallstones. The size of the remnant could influence the probability of stone formation. Gallstones relapse is more possible if a "fundectomy" is done instead of a true subtotal cholecystectomy [28]. According to the intraoperative findings that some symptomatic gallbladder remnants had an internal diameter of only about 1 cm, the section during an SLC should be performed very close to the cystic duct [10, 29]. Gallstones recurrence is a complication that a surgeon should consider in patients with symptoms related to biliary colic after an SC. Diagnosis of stone recurrence in a gallbladder remnant is quite complex, and it arises mainly from ultrasonography (US), computed tomography (CT), magnetic resonance cholangiopancreatography (MRCP), endoscopic retrograde cholangiopancreatography (ERCP) (which is also useful to treat residual gallstones of the common bile duct), and endoscopic ultrasonography (EUS). The surgical treatment represents the best option. The laparoscopic approach should be performed by expert surgeons because of the scar around the Calot's triangle following the previous operation [27, 28].

One of the disadvantages of LSC is that in the case of cancer that has not diagnosed preoperatively, there is the risk of tumor dissemination in the abdominal cavity and remnant tumors. A tumor should be excluded before surgery [30], even if the unexpected rate of gallbladder cancer has been reported to be very low, around 0.2–0.8% [31].

13.5 Conclusions

Severe inflammation could make LC difficult with an increased risk of vasculo-biliary injuries. A bailout procedure should be adopted when a CVS cannot be achieved because of severe fibrosis which hides the structures of the Calot's triangle. To avoid these damages, several rescue procedures have been proposed over time but only a few have been recommended. The first one is the laparoscopic subtotal cholecystectomy. This is superior to open conversion and TC in terms of postoperative complications and biliary injuries. So, SLC is a procedure that should be definitively considered in difficult situations. Conversely, there is no clear evidence about the safety of the fundus first technique even when it is combined with SLC. The open conversion is a controversial issue because the decision to convert into open depends on the surgeon's experience [2]. Most surgeons trained in the past 20 years have little experience in open cholecystectomy [8], so open conversion does not make surgery easier. Otherwise, open conversion does not exclude the opportunity to perform an SC when the intraoperative findings discourage a TC [2].

References

1. Santos BF, Brunt LM, Pucci MJ. The difficult gallbladder: a safe approach to a dangerous problem. J Laparoendosc Adv Surg Tech. 2017;27:571–8.
2. Wakabayashi G, Iwashita Y, Hibi T, et al. Tokyo Guidelines 2018: surgical management of acute cholecystitis: safe steps in laparoscopic cholecystectomy for acute cholecystitis (with videos). J Hepatobiliary Pancreat Sci. 2018;25:73–86.
3. Mascagni P, Spota A, Felli E, et al. Conclusive identification and division of the cystic artery: a forgotten trick to optimize exposure of the critical view of safety in laparoscopic cholecystectomy. J Am Coll Surg. 2019;229:e5–7.
4. Pucci MJ, Brunt LM, Deziel DJ. Safety first, total cholecystectomy second. J Am Coll Surg. 2016;223:543–4.
5. Strasberg SM, Eagon CJ, Drebin JA. The "hidden cystic duct" syndrome and the infundibular technique of laparoscopic cholecystectomy - the danger of the false infundibulum. J Am Coll Surg. 2000;191:661–7.
6. Kato K, Matsuda M, Onodera K, et al. Laparoscopic cholecystectomy from fundus downward. Surg Laparosc Endosc. 1994;4:373–4.
7. Uyama I, Iida S, Ogiwara H, et al. Laparoscopic retrograde cholecystectomy (from fundus downward) facilitated by lifting the liver bed up to the diaphragm for inflammatory gallbladder. Surg Laparosc Endosc. 1995;5:431–6.
8. Strasberg SM. Error traps and vasculo-biliary injury in laparoscopic and open cholecystectomy. J Hepatobiliary Pancreat Surg. 2008;15:284–92.
9. Bornman PC, Terblanche J. Sub-total cholecystectomy: for the difficult gall bladder in portal hypertension and cholecystitis. Surgery. 1985;98:1–6.
10. Strasberg SM, Pucci MJ, Brunt LM, Deziel DJ. Subtotal cholecystectomy–"Fenestrating" vs "Reconstituting" subtypes and the prevention of bile duct injury: definition of the optimal procedure in difficult operative conditions. J Am Coll Surg. 2016;222:89–96.
11. Michalowski K, Bornman PC, Krige JEJ. Laparoscopic subtotal cholecystectomy in patients with complicated acute cholecystitis or fibrosis. Br J Surg. 1998;85:904–6.
12. Chowbey PK, Sharma A, Khullar R, et al. Laparoscopic subtotal cholecystectomy: a review of 56 procedures. J Laparoendosc Adv Surg Tech A. 2000;10:31–4.
13. Palanivelu C, Rajan PS, Jani K, et al. Laparoscopic cholecystectomy in cirrhotic patients: the role of subtotal cholecystectomy and its variants. J Am Coll Surg. 2006;203:145–51.
14. Nakajima J, Sasaki A, Obuchi T, et al. Laparoscopic subtotal cholecystectomy for severe cholecystitis. Surg Today. 2009;39:870–5.
15. Singhal T, Balakrishnan S, Hussain A, et al. Laparoscopic subtotal cholecystectomy: initial experience with laparoscopic management of difficult cholecystitis. Surgeon. 2009;7:263–8.
16. Bickel A, Shtamler B. Laparoscopic subtotal cholecystectomy. J Laparoendosc Surg. 1993;3:365–7.
17. Hubert C, Annet L, van Beers BE, Gigot JF. The "inside approach of the gallbladder" is an alternative to the classic Calot's triangle dissection for a safe operation in severe cholecystitis. Surg Endosc. 2010;24:2626–32.
18. Beldi G, Glättli A. Laparoscopic subtotal cholecystectomy for severe cholecystitis. Surg Endosc. 2003;17:1437–9.

19. Sinha I, Smith ML, Safranek P. Laparoscopic subtotal cholecystectomy without cystic duct ligation. Br J Surg. 2007;94:1527–9.
20. Harilingam MR, Shrestha AK, Basu S. Laparoscopic modified subtotal cholecystectomy for difficult gall bladders: a single-centre experience. J Minim Access Surg. 2016;12:325–9.
21. Nasr MM. An innovative emergency laparoscopic cholecystectomy technique; early results towards complication free surgery. J Gastrointest Surg. 2017;21:302–11.
22. Elshaer M, Gravante G, Thomas K, et al. Subtotal cholecystectomy for "difficult gallbladders": systematic review and metaanalysis. JAMA Surg. 2015;150:159e168.
23. Parrilla P, Robles R, Varo E, et al. Liver transplantation for bile duct injury after open and laparoscopic cholecystectomy. Br J Surg. 2014;101:63–8.
24. Silva Filho JFRE, Coelho GR, Leite Filho JAD, et al. Liver transplantation for bile duct inijury after cholecystectomy. Arq Gastroenterol. 2019;56:300–3.
25. Henneman D, Da Costa DW, Vrouenraets BC, et al. Laparoscopic partial cholecystectomy for the difficult gallbladder: a systematic review. Surg Endosc. 2013;27:351–8.
26. Strasberg SM, Gouma DJ. "Extreme" vasculobiliary injuries: association with fundus-down cholecystectomy in severely inflamed gallbladders. HPB. 2012;14:1–8.
27. Chowbey PK, Bandyopadhyay SK, Sharma A, et al. Laparoscopic reintervention for residual gallstone disease. Surg Laparosc Endosc Percutan Tech. 2003;13:31–5.
28. Pernice LM, Andreoli F. Laparoscopic treatment of stone recurrence in a gallbladder remnant: report of an additional case and literature review. J Gastrointest Surg. 2009;13:2084–91.
29. Di Carlo I, Pulvirenti E, Toro A, Corsale G. Modified subtotal cholecystectomy: results of a laparotomy procedure during thelaparoscopic era. World J Surg. 2009;33:520e525.
30. Kuwabara J, Watanabe Y, Kameoka K, et al. Usefulness of laparoscopic subtotal cholecystectomy with operative cholangiography for severe cholecystitis. Surg Today. 2014;44:462–5.
31. Ouchi K, Mikuni J, Kakugawa Y, et al. Laparoscopic cholecystectomy for gallbladder carcinoma: results of a Japanese survey of 498 patients. J Hepatobiliary Pancreat Surg. 2002;9:256–60.

The Indocyanine Green Role in Acute Cholecystitis

14

Rene Aleman, Fernando Dip, Emanuele Lo Menzo, and Raul J. Rosenthal

Objectives

This chapter aims to:

- Define difficult acute cholecystitis.
- Review the appropriate management of difficult acute cholecystitis.
- Review the outcomes following the adequate approach to difficult acute cholecystitis.

14.1 Introduction

Cholecystectomy continues to be among the most commonly performed surgeries in the United States (US) and developed countries. Currently, more than 90% of the cholecystectomies performed in the US are performed laparoscopically, and an open approach is no longer considered standard of care. LC is recognized as the therapeutic gold standard of benign gallbladder (GB) disease, and it has been associated with short hospital stay and fewer postoperative complications when compared to the open approach [1]. Current and ongoing advances in optical and surgical devices, improvement in surgical techniques, and the introduction of novel technologies have skewed this recommendation.

Acute cholecystitis is a common complication of gallstone disease, imposing a latent risk of developing surgical complications such as bleeding and bile duct injuries (BDI), if managed improperly [2]. The incidence of BDIs during LC ranges from 0.2% to 1.1% [3–5]. The implications of BDI following LC extend beyond the significant medical complications and encompass increased medical costs, litigation, and decrease in quality of life [6–8]. The first treatment guidelines for AC based on severity criteria were published in 2007 and provided a thorough understanding on how to adequately manage AC in accordance to clinical appearance.

Up until now, LC has been widely implemented as surgical therapy for AC. However, it is well known that patients undergoing LC for AC have twice the risk of sustaining a BDI when compared to patients without AC. Several techniques have been described to limit BDIs in this particular setting. Among these, the use of intraoperative cholangiography (IOC) has been shown to decrease severity of the BDI, but not necessarily their occurrence [9].

This chapter focuses on the surgical aspects of adequate management of AC through LC.

R. Aleman · F. Dip · E. Lo Menzo · R. J. Rosenthal (✉)
Cleveland Clinic Florida, Weston, FL, USA
e-mail: alemanr@ccf.org; lomenze@ccf.org; Rosentr@ccf.org

© Springer Nature Switzerland AG 2021

I. Di Carlo (ed.), *Difficult Acute Cholecystitis*, https://doi.org/10.1007/978-3-030-62102-5_14

14.2 Acute Cholecystitis

14.2.1 Severity of Acute Cholecystitis

The first treatment guidelines for AC of different levels of severity were published in 2007. Since then, there have been several updates and modifications. The 2018 Tokyo Guidelines (TG18) have indicated three levels of severity for AC. These levels are summarized in Table 14.1.

The recognition of the severity level of AC remains paramount for safe operative planning. Based on this severity stratification, the surgeon can objectively analyze the potential pitfalls and technical shortcomings of surgical intervention. All of these will undoubtedly have an impact on the ease of the surgery and patient outcomes. Prior to the introduction of the critical view of safety for the dissection of Calot's triangle and the evolution of visual optics in laparoscopic equipment, LC for AC was not considered the gold standard [10, 11].

The performing surgeon should be aware that an intra-abdominal image translated into even a high-resolution two-dimensional screen presents shortfalls based on the different haptic feedback and visual misperceptions. The improvement of optoelectronic instrumentation and increased surgical experience has decreased the learning curve for this and many other surgical procedures. Nonetheless, it is imperative to identify the risk factors associated with the levels of severity for AC. Similar to other laparoscopic procedures, the surgical difficulty of AC is proportional to the severity of the inflammation and fibrosis, and the risk of developing a BDI has been shown to increase in accordance with the severity of AC [9].

Table 14.1 Levels of severity for AC—according to TG18

Level I	Mild
Level II	Moderate—Conditional to the availability of advanced laparoscopic techniques
Level III	LC to be performed after GB drainage—If both the patient and facilities meet strict conditions, LC can be performed as a straightforward procedure

AC Acute cholecystitis, *TG18* Tokyo Guidelines 2018, *LC* Laparoscopic cholecystectomy, *GB* Gallbladder

The TG13 was the initial attempt to establish a complexity scale of AC based on intraoperative findings during LC. As a result, an initial expert consensus was reached by more than 400 surgeons from Japan, Korea, and Taiwan [12]. Following this initial publication, a Delphi survey was then performed. The survey consists of the opinion of 614 international surgeons when confronted with 29 scenarios that might involve the risk of BDI along with possible preventive measures [13].

14.2.2 Risk of Iatrogenic Bile Duct Injury

The incidence of BDI is considered to be 2 to 5 times higher for LC when compared to the open approach [14, 15]. Thus, it is important for the operating surgeon to identify the preoperative risk. Considering the high number of LCs performed in a single institution due to AC, it is important to promptly and adequately identify these risk factors leading up to a potentially difficult LC. Mainly, inflammatory tissue surrounding the GB affects both the correct identification of structures and their safe isolation. The stage of inflammation also plays a key role, with advance and severe inflammation affecting the visualization more than early and mild inflammation. All these factors also affect the operation time. The GB's pathological process that directly affects the complexity of the procedure includes GB wall thickening, impacted stones at the GB's neck with potential mass effect on common bile duct, duration of elevated C-reactive protein (CRP), nonvisualized GB on preoperative studies, body temperature, abscess formation, and body mass index (BMI) [16]. In contrast, the risks associated with conversion to an open approach include mostly observational and numerical variables: A GB wall thickening >4–5 mm on preoperative ultrasonography (USG), age >60 or 65 years old, male gender, AC TG18 level II/III, a contracted GB on USG, previous abdominal surgery, BMI, and American

Society of Anesthesiologists (ASA) score [16]. Furthermore, elevated white blood cells (WBCs), low albumin, high bilirubin, pericholecystic fluid, and diabetes mellitus (DM) are predictive factors associated with conversion to an open procedure [17–20]. As a final note on the timing of surgical intervention for AC, the available evidence shows that the rate of complications and the probability of conversion to open procedure increase significantly if the LC is performed more than 72 h after the onset of symptoms [21, 22]. This is especially important in diabetic and immunocompromised patients, in which the onset of intensity of symptoms is typically delayed, increasing the overall risks in these patient populations.

In summary, the level of surgical difficulty can be estimated by the aforementioned factors, principally the preoperative imaging studies, blood tests, and AC TG18 level. Nevertheless, both prolongation of the operative time and the rates for open conversion are greatly dependent on both the surgeon's skill and experience.

14.3 Surgical Management

14.3.1 Intraoperative Difficulty Indicators

In spite of the previously mentioned preoperative identifiers, the intraoperative objective findings are the main factors determining the complexity of the LC, are imperative, and are considered appropriate indicators of surgical difficulty during LC [12].

The intraoperative difficulty indicators became part of the AC TG18 practice guidelines. These indicators were the result of a multinational survey conducted in Japan, Korea, and Taiwan [12]. A total of 26 Japanese expert hepatobiliary surgeons generated a list of intraoperative findings that contribute to surgical difficulty using the nominal group technique. Subsequently, 61 experts were surveyed addressing LC experience, surgical strategy, and perceptions of 30 objective intraoperative findings. Of relevance, the objective intraoperative findings were categorized into factors related to inflammation and additional findings of the GB, and other intra-abdominal factors. The former factors were further subdivided into appearance around the GB, appearance of the Calot's triangle area, appearance of the GB, and additional findings of the GB and its surroundings. These factors were measured using a difficulty scale that ranged from 0 to 6; 0 being the easiest and 6 being the most difficult. A score ≥4 is highly suggestive of a difficult LC. Regarding the appearance around the GB, the presence of diffuse scarring tissue scored an average of 4. In regard to the appearance of the Calot's triangle area, both partial and diffuse scarring in the Calot's triangle area scored 4 and 5, respectively. Similarly, when considering the appearance of the GB, diffuse scarring in the GB bed (including atrophy of the GB with no lumen due to severe contraction) was the most prevalent finding with a score of 4. In terms of additional findings of the GB and its surroundings, five findings were identified as high indicators of a difficult LC. These included necrotic changes around the GB/Calot's triangle/GB bed, abscess formation toward the liver parenchyma, cholecystoenteric fistula, cholecystocholedochal fistula, and impacted gallstone in the confluence of the cystic duct (CD), common hepatic duct (CHD), and common bile duct (CBD); they were all graded as high-risk difficulty indicators with scores of 4, 4, 5, 6, and 5, respectively. As to the intra-abdominal factors unrelated to inflammation, anomalous bile duct, collateral vein formations due to liver cirrhosis, and inversion of the GB in its bed due to liver cirrhosis, were all given a score of 4. Figure 14.1 summarizes the most relevant difficulty risk identifiers in accordance with scoring from high to low.

14.3.2 Safe Steps

The preoperative risk stratification and planning should never be rescinded by any surgeon, regardless of their expertise and years of practice. Thus, in accordance with the Delphi consensus on how to perform a safe LC in the presence of AC, the authors propose a rather modified

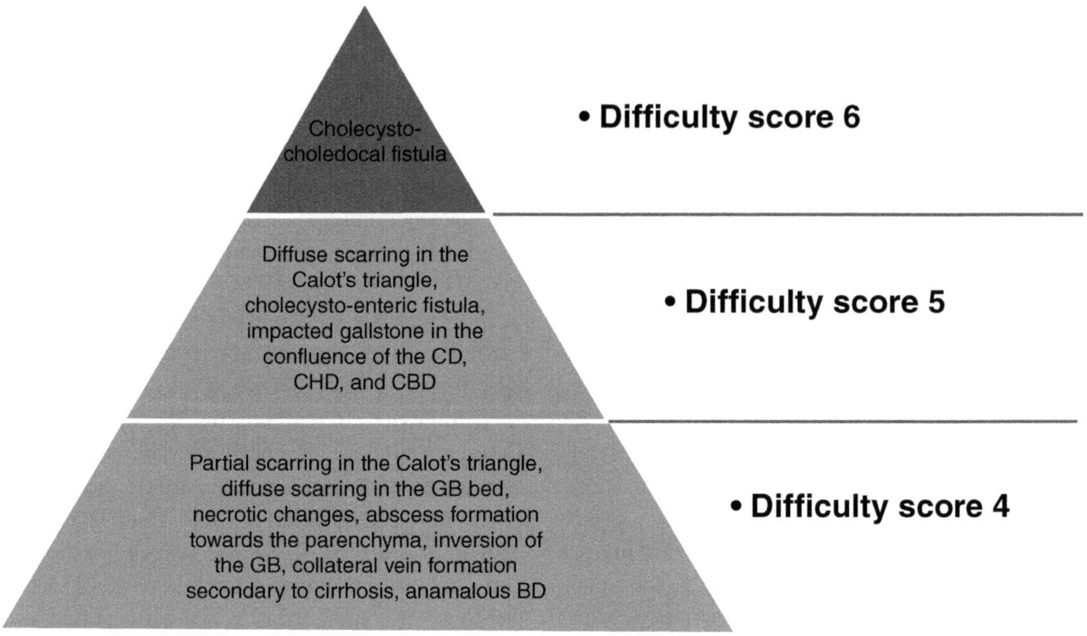

Fig. 14.1 Most commonly encountered difficulty indicators during LC

approach in views of recent and novel technologies that aid in the navigation of said procedure. Table 14.2 compares and contrasts the standard of care steps, to the new recommendations.

Evidently, the steps are seemingly different from one another. However, the proposed steps are based on both the Delphi consensus on BDI during LC and in the implementation of technologies such as fluorescence guided surgery, with the application of intraoperative incisionless fluorescent cholangiography (IOIFC) [13, 23]. The addition of IOIFC would aid in the identification of the main extrahepatic bile structures prior and during dissection with a contrast visual feedback. The advantages of this technology are obvious as often the implementation of other imaging modalities like IOC would have determined an unwanted injury already. Similarly, the CVS can be not sufficient by itself to avoid BDIs.

Initially proposed by Strasberg and colleagues, the CVS was popularized as the most commonly implemented surgical technique used to prevent BDIs [10, 24]. Although widely praised by surgeons, the CVS requires a long-time curve for residents in training and reflects in prolonged operative time [25]. Equally, the role of intraoperative cholangiography during LC continues to raise questions in regard to applicability and true benefit in the prevention of BDIs. The heterogeneous results on intraoperative cholangiography have deemed this imaging technique to be optional [24, 26]. It is important, however, to recognize that imagery feedback from surgical tools can, in fact, reduce the extent of a BDI. Perioperative cholangiography, magnetic resonance cholangiopancreatography (MRCP), laparoscopic ultrasound, and IOIFC have proven to prevent BDI, yet may require further supporting evidence [27].

14.3.3 Avoiding BDIs

Although not the focus of this chapter, operating surgeons should be knowledgeable on how to proceed in the face of a potential or an actual occurrence of a BDI. Firstly, the surgeon must be capable of identifying the type of BDI, based on Bismuth/Strasberg's classification of BDIs. The importance of appropriately classifying the type of BDI relies on the implications of the management of iatrogenic BDIs. Overall, surgical mor-

Table 14.2 Safe steps for an LC in the presence of AC

Delphi consensus steps [14]	New recommendations
Step 1 If a distended GB interferes with the field of view, decompress by needle aspiration	*Step 1* Administration of peripheral ICG
Step 2 Effective retraction of the GB to develop a plane in the Calot's triangle area and identify its boundaries	*Step 2* Exposure of the hepatoduodenal ligament
Step 3 Start dissection from the posterior leaf of the peritoneum covering the neck of the GB and exposing the GB surface above Rouvière's sulcus	*Step 3* Initial anatomical evaluation: Identification of the biliary tree structures following lysis of adhesions
Step 4 Maintaining the plane of dissection on the GB surface throughout the procedure	*Step 4* Identification of the CD and CBD junction
Step 5 Dissecting the lower part of the GB (at least one-third) to obtain the critical view of safety (CVS)	*Step 5* Identification of the CD and its junction to the GB
Step 6 Creating the CVS	*Step 6* Identification of the CHD
	Step 7 Identification of the CBD
	Step 8 Identification of the cystic artery and optional performance of an arteriography
	Step 9 Time-out before transection and reidentification of Calot's triangle structures
	Step 10 Evaluation of the liver bed and identification of accessory ducts

LC Laparoscopic cholecystectomy, *AC* Acute cholangitis, *GB* Gallbladder, *ICG* Indocyanine green, *CD* Cystic duct, *CBD* Common bile duct, *CHD* Common hepatic duct, *CVS* Critical view of safety

tality rates have been reported up to 5%, while re-stenosis rates range from 5% to 28% [28]. This should be considered prior to any type of surgical re-intervention. Additionally, these suggestions should be followed by a set of perioperative points that have been determined crucial for the avoidance of BDIs [16].

These points can be considered as a summarized confluence of the steps to follow while performing an LC, the difficulty indicators during LC, and the levels of severity for AC. The points to follow are based on tissue appearance, surgical technique, imaging tools, and bailout procedures. Figure 14.2 briefly demonstrates the highlights of said points.

Evidently, there is more to these points than just prioritizing them during the performance of the surgery. Firstly, there is an unequivocal time frame—as previously mentioned in this chapter—on the performance of surgery. LC in the setting of AC should be performed no longer than 72 h following the presenting symptoms. Failure to do so will result in extensive inflammation and fibrosis surrounding relevant structures, causing difficulties in the identification of the biliary tree anatomy and achieving CVS [29]. Secondly, meticulous surgical technique will undoubtedly provide the grounds for the prevention of BDI. The CVS must be achieved regardless of the imaging tools available in the surgical setting. Although it is a technique with limitations, it has most definitely proven its effectiveness in reducing BDI occurrences [24]. In contrast, imaging tools are dependent on the availability of them

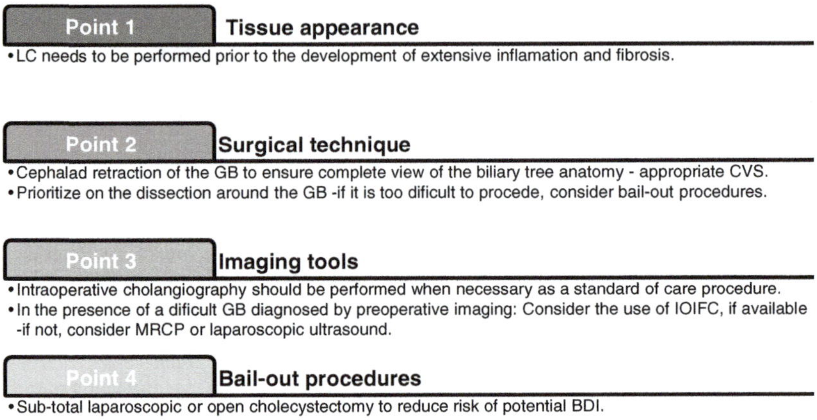

Fig. 14.2 Critical points to prevent BDIs

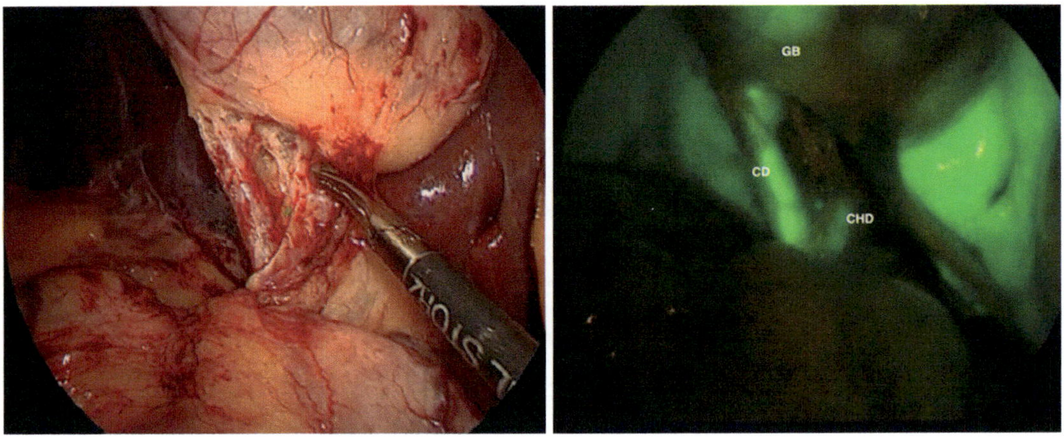

Critical view of safety during an LC. Comparison between white light imaging (WLI—left) and near-infrared (NIR—right) light filter. Lysis of adhesions can be performed with NIR filter. IOIFC aids in the identification of the gallbladder and biliary structures guiding the surgeon (GB: Gallbladder; CD: Cystic duct; CHD: Common hepatic duct). Cystic artery arteriography can be performed intraoperatively by an additional administration of 3 mL of intravenous ICG

where the procedure is being performed. Further detail of aiding imaging tools is discussed later in this chapter. Lastly, bailout procedures must be considered to ensure BDI when a difficult LC has been identified. In the presence of severe fibrosis surrounding Calot's triangle, subtotal LC or open conversion must be considered [30]. Recall that objective intraoperative findings can be identified as indicators of surgical difficulty. There are still no criteria available for the conversion or performance of a subtotal LC, yet the pioneering imaging tools might rescind the need for said criterion.

14.4 Groundbreaking Alternative

Ever since LC was first described, the incidence of BDI has held a steady range between 0.3% and 0.52% [31, 32]. Mainly, the reason behind said steady incidence is the misidentification of biliary tree anatomy. Even in the presence of the CVS, both training and experienced surgeons practice LCs with the risk of developing BDIs. Imaging tools, including but not limited to, intraoperative cholangiography, MRCP, and laparoscopic ultrasound have all been developed to ease surgical performance and achieve a risk-free procedure. The literature regarding these tools is inconsistent, and although applicable in the clinical setting, these have shown to be impractical, costly, or impose an unnecessary exposure to patients. Comparatively, near-infrared (NIR) fluorescence cholangiography performed with ICG and NIR light has been described as a feasible, simple, and cost-effective technique to perform a safe LC [33].

Intraoperative incisionless fluorescent cholangiography (IOIFC) has recently emerged as a safe, simple, cost-effective technique. Furthermore, IOIFC has been proven to be statistically superior to white light in visualizing extrahepatic biliary structures during LC [23]. In the only multicenter randomized control trial available on the subject, pre-dissection and post-dissection rates favored IOIFC in the correct identification of relevant structures during LC. More so, this study revalidated the premise of IOIFC being a useful teaching tool to teach LC and hence decreasing the learning curve of this procedure [34]. In terms of performing LC in the presence of a difficult AC, the authors consider that the application of IOIFC among the already validated practice consensus will indubitably provide a greater benefit and further the risk of BDI incidence. Unfortunately, IOIFC has yet to establish itself as standard of care. Nevertheless, it is a promising tool that should be considered by the performing surgeon in the presence of either straightforward or challenging cases.

14.5 Technique

In accordance to what is steadily becoming standard of care while performing an LC, the authors have a present practice that promotes an injury-free procedure. The Delphi consensus thoroughly describes six key steps in the performance of a safe LC [13]. However, in hopes to reduce iatrogenic events associated to BDI, the use of IOIFC has been implemented into a new set of ten key steps that aim to prevent said occurrences (Table 14.2).

The technique should proceed as follows. Following induction of general anesthesia, a 2 cm supraumbilical incision is made. A Hasson cannula is placed, and a 15-mmHg pneumoperitoneum is established. Upon exploration of the abdominal cavity, three 5 mm trocars are inserted under direct vision in this order: Subxiphoid, right upper quadrant, and right mid quadrant. The gallbladder is then grasped and lifted over the liver. Fluorescent cholangiography is performed at this moment in surgery to correctly identify all relevant structures to the procedure (Table 14.2). The dissection initiates laterally, and the peritoneum surrounding the gallbladder is taken down. This is continued toward the infundibulum of the gallbladder and extended toward the liver on its medial side to allow visualization of the CD and cystic artery. The dissection is continued upon the separation of both structures. In continuance with the dissection, the cystic artery is medially approached toward the liver bed. At this point, the critical view of safety should be achieved. This view should portray overall visibility of the gallbladder and liver, in between the cystic artery and CD, just medial to the artery and under the lower border of the liver. The cystic artery is then clipped twice proximally and once distally. The CD is clipped in a similar fashion and both structures are posteriorly divided. The gallbladder is taken off the liver bed and placed in a retrieval bag for extraction, under direct vision, from the umbilicus. Irrigation continues and adequate cauterization of the liver bed.

This is a short description of the technique; however, further literature should be consulted elsewhere for detailed approach on the safe and adequate performance of an LC.

14.6 Conclusions

In the setting of AC, LC should be performed in a step-by-step manner. It is paramount for the performing surgeon to recognize all perioperative implications prior to surgery. An adequate and thorough understanding of the level of severity of the AC, the difficulty level of performing said LC, the risk indicators, safe steps, and the cardinal points for preventing BDI should provide the ideal guide for a safe LC. The authors recognize that novel imaging tools might not be present in every operative room. Thus, this chapter emphasizes the effort of the operating surgeons to prioritize the prompt recognition and following of these recommendations.

References

1. Yamashita Y, Takada T, Strasberg SM, et al. TG13 surgical management of acute cholecystitis. J Hepatobiliary Pancreat Sci. 2013;20:89–96.
2. Halldestam I, Enell E-L, Kullman E, Borch K. Development of symptoms and complications in individuals with asymptomatic gallstones. Br J Surg. 2004;91:734–8.
3. Giger UF, Michel J-M, Opitz I, Inderbitzin DT, Kocher T, Krähenbühl L. Risk factors for perioperative complications in patients undergoing laparoscopic cholecystectomy: analysis of 22,953 consecutive cases from the Swiss Association of Laparoscopic and Thoracoscopic Surgery Database. J Am Coll Surg. 2006;203:723–8.
4. Harboe KM, Bardram L. The quality of cholecystectomy in Denmark: outcome and risk factors for 20,307 patients from the national database. Surg Endosc. 2011;25:1630–41.
5. Navez B, Ungureanu F, Michiels M, et al. Surgical management of acute cholecystitis: results of a 2-year prospective multicenter survey in Belgium. Surg Endosc. 2012;26:2436–45.
6. Truant S, Boleslawski E, Lebuffe G, Sergent G, Pruvot F-R. Hepatic resection for post-cholecystectomy bile duct injuries: a literature review. HPB. 2010;12:334–41.
7. Andersson R, Eriksson K, Blind P-J, Tingstedt B. Iatrogenic b – a cost analysis. HPB. 2008;10:416–9.
8. Way LW, Stewart L, Gantert W, Liu K, Lee CM, Whang K, Hunter JG. Causes and prevention of laparoscopic bile duct injuries: analysis of 252 cases from a human factors and cognitive psychology perspective. Ann Surg. 2003;237:460–9.
9. Törnqvist B, Waage A, Zheng Z, Ye W, Nilsson M. Severity of acute cholecystitis and risk of iatrogenic bile duct injury during cholecystectomy, a population-based case-control study. World J Surg. 2016;40:1060–7.
10. Strasberg SM, Hertl M, Soper NJ. An analysis of the problem of biliary injury during laparoscopic cholecystectomy. J Am Coll Surg. 1995;180:101–25.
11. The role of laparoscopic cholecystectomy (L.C.). Guidelines for clinical application. Society of American Gastrointestinal Endoscopic Surgeons (SAGES). Surg Endosc. 1993;7:369–70.
12. Iwashita Y, Ohyama T, Honda G, et al. What are the appropriate indicators of surgical difficulty during laparoscopic cholecystectomy? Results from a Japan-Korea-Taiwan multinational survey. J Hepatobiliary Pancreat Sci. 2016;23:533–47.
13. Iwashita Y, Hibi T, Ohyama T, et al. Delphi consensus on bile duct injuries during laparoscopic cholecystectomy: an evolutionary cul-de-sac or the birth pangs of a new technical framework? J Hepatobiliary Pancreat Sci. 2017;24:591–602.
14. Morgenstern L. Twelve hundred open cholecystectomies before the laparoscopic era. Arch Surg. 1992;127:400.
15. Flum DR, Dellinger EP, Cheadle A, Chan L, Koepsell T. Intraoperative cholangiography and risk of common bile duct injury during cholecystectomy. JAMA. 2003;289:1639–44.
16. Wakabayashi G, Iwashita Y, Hibi T, et al. Tokyo guidelines 2018: surgical management of acute cholecystitis: safe steps in laparoscopic cholecystectomy for acute cholecystitis (with videos). J Hepatobiliary Pancreat Sci. 2018;25:73–86.
17. Cho KS, Baek SY, Kang BC, Choi H-Y, Han H-S. Evaluation of preoperative sonography in acute cholecystitis to predict technical difficulties during laparoscopic cholecystectomy. J Clin Ultrasound. 2004;32:115–22.
18. Shamiyeh A, Danis J, Wayand W, Zehetner J. A 14-year analysis of laparoscopic cholecystectomy: conversion—when and why? Surg Laparosc Endosc Percutan Tech. 2007;17:271–6.
19. Cho JY, Han H-S, Yoon Y-S, Ahn KS, Lee SH, Hwang J-H. Hepatobiliary scan for assessing disease severity in patients with cholelithiasis. Arch Surg. 2011;146:169–74.
20. Cwik G, Skoczylas T, Wyroślak-Najs J, Wallner G. The value of percutaneous ultrasound in predicting conversion from laparoscopic to open cholecystectomy due to acute cholecystitis. Surg Endosc. 2013;27:2561–8.
21. Low JK, Barrow P, Owera A, Ammori BJ. Timing of laparoscopic cholecystectomy for acute cholecystitis: evidence to support a proposal for an early interval surgery. Am Surg. 2007;73:1188–92.
22. Zhu B, Zhang Z, Wang Y, Gong K, Lu Y, Zhang N. Comparison of laparoscopic cholecystectomy for acute cholecystitis within and beyond 72 h of symptom onset during emergency admissions. World J Surg. 2012;36:2654–8.
23. Dip F, LoMenzo E, Sarotto L, et al. Randomized trial of near-infrared incisionless fluorescent cholangiography. Ann Surg. 2019;270:992–9.
24. Sanjay P, Kulli C, Polignano FM, Tait IS. Optimal surgical technique, use of intra-operative cholangiography (IOC), and management of acute gallbladder

disease: the results of a nation-wide survey in the UK and Ireland. Ann R Coll Surg Engl. 2010;92:302–6.
25. Vettoretto N, Saronni C, Harbi A, Balestra L, Taglietti L, Giovanetti M. Critical view of safety during laparoscopic cholecystectomy. JSLS. 2011;15:322–5.
26. Törnqvist B, Strömberg C, Akre O, Enochsson L, Nilsson M. Selective intraoperative cholangiography and risk of bile duct injury during cholecystectomy. Br J Surg. 2015;102:952–8.
27. Pesce A, Piccolo G, La Greca G, Puleo S. Utility of fluorescent cholangiography during laparoscopic cholecystectomy: a systematic review. World J Gastroenterol. 2015;21:7877–83.
28. Strasberg SM, Callery MP, Soper NJ. Laparoscopic hepatobiliary surgery. Prog Liver Dis. 1995;13:349–80.
29. Honda G, Hasegawa H, Umezawa A. Universal safe procedure of laparoscopic cholecystectomy standardized by exposing the inner layer of the subserosal layer (with video). J Hepatobiliary Pancreat Sci. 2016;23:E14–9.
30. Hussain A. Difficult laparoscopic cholecystectomy: current evidence and strategies of management. Surg Laparosc Endosc Percutan Tech. 2011;21:211–7.
31. Pucher PH, SAGES Safe Cholecystectomy Task Force, Michael Brunt L, et al. Outcome trends and safety measures after 30 years of laparoscopic cholecystectomy: a systematic review and pooled data analysis. Surg Endosc. 2018;32:2175–83.
32. Rystedt J, Lindell G, Montgomery A. Bile duct injuries associated with 55,134 cholecystectomies: treatment and outcome from a national perspective. World J Surg. 2016;40:73–80.
33. Dip F, Roy M, Lo Menzo E, Simpfendorfer C, Szomstein S, Rosenthal RJ. Routine use of fluorescent incisionless cholangiography as a new imaging modality during laparoscopic cholecystectomy. Surg Endosc. 2015;29:1621–6.
34. Roy M, Dip F, Nguyen D, Simpfendorfer CH, Menzo EL, Szomstein S, Rosenthal RJ. Fluorescent incisionless cholangiography as a teaching tool for identification of Calot's triangle. Surg Endosc. 2017;31:2483–90.

How to Avoid Common Bile Duct Injuries and Their Classification

15

Ioannis Triantafyllidis and David Fuks

Abbreviations

BDI	Bile duct injuries
CBD	Common bile duct
CHD	Common hepatic duct
CVS	Critical view of safety
ERCP	Endoscopic retrograde cholangiopancreatography
ICG	Indocyanine green;
IOC	Intraoperative cholangiography
IOUS	Intraoperative ultrasonography
LC	Laparoscopic cholecystectomy
PTC	Percutaneous transhepatic cholangiography
RHD	Right hepatic duct

15.1 Introduction

Laparoscopic cholecystectomy has become the gold standard for the management of symptomatic cholelithiasis and other gallbladder diseases. However, several reports demonstrated that the incidence of bile duct injuries (BDI) has risen from 0.2–0.3% in the era of conventional open cholecystectomy to 0.5–0.8% in the era of laparoscopic cholecystectomy [1–4]. Wrong or incomplete dissection of Calot's triangle, especially in cases of significant inflammation at the surgical site, or aberrant anatomy of the bile duct may result in bile duct injuries (BDI) [5, 6]. Iatrogenic BDI are associated with significant postoperative morbidity and mortality, decreased long-term survival, and quality of life and their management constitute a surgical challenge. The goal in these cases is the restoration of the biliary tree and the prevention of complications such as strictures, recurrent cholangitis and secondary biliary cirrhosis, abscess, and fistulae. Management depends on the timing of recognition of injury, the extent of bile duct injury, the patient's condition, and the availability of experienced hepatobiliary surgeons. Technical difficulty of repair, operative risk, and long-term outcome of bile duct injuries vary considerably and are mainly associated with the location and the extent of the injury. Consequently, several classifications with therapeutic and prognostic implications have been established [1–4]. However, as the precise causes of injury are becoming better understood, technical refinements for prevention are emerging. Prevention should be the goal and this requires adherence to strict principles of meticulous and safe dissection of the identified structures.

I. Triantafyllidis (✉)
Department of General Surgery, Konstantopoulio-Patision General Hospital of Nea Ionia, Athens, Greece

D. Fuks
Department of Digestive Oncologic and Metabolic Surgery, Institut Mutualiste Montsouris, Université Paris Descartes, Paris, France

© Springer Nature Switzerland AG 2021

I. Di Carlo (ed.), *Difficult Acute Cholecystitis*, https://doi.org/10.1007/978-3-030-62102-5_15

15.2 Risk Factors for Biliary Injury

There are many factors that increase the incidence of BDI during laparoscopic cholecystectomy. First of all, the camera provides a monocular view from a direction quite different from that of open surgery, thus the CBD is not usually seen from this angle. The high rate of biliary injury in early reports was due in part to inexperience in the procedure. This was called the “learning curve” effect [7]. Indeed, experience contributes to BDI, but several other factors are responsible, as well.

Biliary injuries are more likely to occur during difficult laparoscopic cholecystectomies [8, 9]. The incidence of BDI when laparoscopic cholecystectomy is performed for acute cholecystitis (0.51%) was reported to be three times higher than that for elective laparoscopic cholecystectomy and twice as high as that for open cholecystectomy for acute cholecystitis [9, 10]. Severity of coexisting inflammation in the operating field with dense scarring contribute as well to intraoperative bleeding that obscures the field. Furthermore, the presence of abundant adipose tissue around the hepatoduodenal ligament, especially in obese patients, increases the difficulty of surgery and promotes BDI. Adverse factors include higher age (>65 years), male gender, morbid obesity and long duration of symptoms prior to surgery, upper abdominal surgery, history of attacks of acute cholecystitis, or previously established cholecystostomy [10].

Aberrant anatomy or anatomic variants and anomalies undoubtedly contribute to biliary injuries. The aberrant right hepatic duct anomaly is the most common problem because the duct may be mistakenly regarded as the cystic duct and ligated or cut. Excessive, more than is necessary, dissection around the hepatoduodenal ligament during cholecystectomy may lead to damage to the axial arteries running along the CBD. Vascular damage is the cause of postoperative biliary strictures due to ischemia.

Last but not least, maintenance of laparoscopic equipment is of paramount importance. Focal loss of insulation on electrocautery instruments may lead to thermal injuries [6].

15.3 Prevention of Bile Duct Injuries

Laparoscopic cholecystectomy is performed in an area adjacent to many vital structures such as the portal vein, hepatic artery, and extrahepatic biliary tract, and thus, thorough knowledge of the relevant anatomy as is of paramount importance for a safe procedure. The surgeon should be aware of anatomical variations and the anatomical distortion due to acute or chronic inflammation.

A number of factors predictive of difficult cholecystectomy have been universally recognized and should be identified in both acute cholecystitis and elective cases. The presence of these risk factors should alert surgeons with limited experience, for careful patient selection. On the other hand, the experienced surgeon should be prepared for the possibility of conversion to an open cholecystectomy, or need for various bailout procedures, such as the establishment of a tube cholecystectomy, subtotal or fundus first cholecystectomy, either laparoscopic or open [10–12]. The exposure and cautious dissection of Calot’s triangle with judicious use of energy and meticulous attention to technique in order to achieve “the critical view of safety (CVS)” is an essential step of laparoscopic cholecystectomy.

It is important for the operating surgeon to be able to recognize when the dissection is becoming unsafe with a high potential for BDI. More than two tubular structures entering the gallbladder, unusually large presumed cystic artery or artery pulsations behind the presumed cystic duct which cannot be occluded with medium–large clips and is surrounded by excessive fibrofatty tissue, bile leakage with intact gallbladder, and/or bleeding requiring blood transfusion, are important indicators of unsafe dissection [10–14]. In such cases, the dissection should be stopped temporarily and reconsider alternative technical plans for a safe dissection, seek for a second opinion from another surgeon, preferably an experienced one. Various intraoperative imaging techniques, such as intraoperative cholangiography (IOC), laparoscopic ultrasound, and near-infrared fluorescent cholangiography, may be used to assess the biliary anatomy, as well [10, 13, 14]. Intraoperative team communication is obviously significant but the surgeon should know when to call for help and recognize the need for conversion or an alternative procedure, such as subtotal cholecystectomy [15]. However, converting to an open procedure does not safeguard against BDI (Table 15.1).

Table 15.1 Essential steps to reduce BDI during laparoscopic cholecystectomy

Preoperative evaluation of predictors of a difficult cholecystectomy [male gender, obesity, age >65 years, previous attacks of biliary colic, increased interval between onset and presentation (>72–96 h), upper abdominal surgery, prior attempted cholecystectomy, fever, high ASA score, raised CRP and white blood cell count, thickened gallbladder wall (>5 mm), small contracted or distended gallbladder with impacted stone, cirrhosis etc]
Use an angled (30^0 or 45^0) laparoscope
Use high-quality imaging equipment
Cooperation with a dedicated and experiences assistant
Application of appropriate lateral traction of the fundus
Use Rouviere's sulcus and the base of segment IV as landmarks to aid orientation
Dissection and correct exposure of the Calot's triangle end establishment of CVS: (a) hepatocystic triangle is cleared of fat and fibrous tissues; (b) the lower one-third of the gallbladder is separated from the liver to expose the cystic plate; (c) two and only two structures should be seen entering in the gallbladder
Judicious use of energy devices at Calot's triangle
Dissection of the liver bed along the cystic plate
Avoid dissection on the left side of the hepatoduodenal ligament
Knowledge of anatomical variations, both biliary and vascular Early recognition if dissection becomes unsafe Seek a second opinion from another surgeon I difficult or unexpected situations
Use of intraoperative imaging when the anatomy is not clarified; obtain intraoperative cholangiograms, liberally
Implement bail-out procedures, such as subtotal cholecystectomy, or fundus-first cholecystectomy in cases of severe inflammation and/or inability to perform CVS
Do not hesitate to convert to open cholecystectomy in cases where CVS cannot be achieved and bail-out strategies could not be implemented

Adaptation of well-proven principles of open surgery is the best prevention of biliary lesions in laparoscopic cholecystectomy as well as the readiness to convert early to the open procedure.

15.3.1 Critical View of Safety and Technical Points

A surgeon is always required to apply reliable surgical techniques to achieve division of the cystic duct and artery in either open or laparoscopic cholecystectomy. Misidentification of the extrahepatic bile duct anatomy during LC is the main cause of bile duct injury [5]. Meticulous dissection of the Calot's triangle and preparation of all relevant structures are the cornerstone of a safe laparoscopic cholecystectomy.

The CVS technique, which was first described by Strasberg et al. in 1995 [5], was introduced to reduce the risk of bile duct injury. A recent Society of American Gastrointestinal and Endoscopic Surgeons (SAGES) expert Delphi consensus deemed the CVS as being the most important factor for overall safety [15]. Nowadays, the CVS technique is the gold standard to perform a safe cholecystectomy with identification of the vital structures such as the cystic duct.

The reviewed literature suggests that judicious establishment of CVS could decrease bile duct injury rate, from an average 0.4% to nearly 0% [16].

To establish CVS, two windows need to be created during dissection of Calot's triangle: one window between the cystic artery, cystic duct, and gallbladder, and another one between the cystic artery, gallbladder, and liver. The CVS technique is aimed especially at mobilizing the gallbladder neck from the liver in the appropriate cystic plate to obtain a circumferential identification of the cystic duct and its transition into the gallbladder [5]. The guiding structure for dissection should be the wall of the gallbladder. Proper retraction of the fundus cephalad and of the infundibulum posteriorly and laterally is necessary, and tenting by excessive lateral pulling on the gallbladder should be avoided. Cephalad traction on the fundus compresses Calot's triangle, while lateral traction on Hartmann's pouch tents up the CBD, which may then be mistaken for the cystic duct, especially when that duct is very short. The cystic duct should be dissected in a retrograde fashion, starting at gallbladder proceeding with the identification of the cystic duct–gallbladder junction on both sides and the visualization of the cystic duct–common bile duct junction prior to clipping. Calot's triangle should be dissected from all fibrous and fatty tissues. At the end of the dissection, only the cystic duct and artery cystica should enter the gallbladder and the bottom of the liver bed should be visible. The CBD is not necessary to be exposed. Failure to achieve the CVS is an absolute indication for conversion or additional bile duct imaging [6]. The CVS should be described in the operative report.

Connor et al. and Wakabayashi et al. elegantly describe five key initial steps in performing safe laparoscopic cholecystectomy: (1) retract the gallbladder laterally to a 10 o'clock position relative to the principle plane of the liver (Cantlie's line); (2) confirm Hartmann's pouch is retracted up and towards segment IV; (3) identify Rouviere's sulcus which marks the level of the right posterior portal pedicle and is identifiable in >80% of the patients. An imaginary line drawn along the sulcus and carried across to the base of segment IV shows the level ventral to which dissection is "safe" and dorsal to which it is not; (4) dissect the posterior peritoneum of the hepatobiliary or hepatocystic triangle; and (5) confirm the critical view is obtained [12, 17].

Energy devices should be used cautiously in the of Calot's triangle with low cautery settings (<30 W), coagulation of small pieces of tissue at one time, and being sure that the coagulating surface is free of any adjacent tissue [6]. There are few data on the comparison between different energy devices in LC with respect to safety. Nevertheless, there was no significant difference between the use of ultrasonic and electrocautery energy with respect to postoperative bile leakage [15]. Sharp dissection increases the risk of bleeding, which presents added problems in controlling the bleeding when clips must be used blindly, or thermocoagulation is applied near the porta hepatis. Instruments should be kept in the field of vision at all times during dissection and instrument changes. Before ligation and division of any structure, its anatomical position should be defined clearly. Clips should be applied so that their tips are seen projecting beyond the duct, free of any extraneous material. In cases of thickened cystic duct, use of ligature loops or intracorporeal ligation is recommended instead of clips. Two loops should be applied on the side of the cystic duct to be retained. Applying extra clips is not the answer and may, in fact, lead to tenting injury [6].

15.3.2 Role of Intraoperative Cholangiography, Ultrasonography, and Fluorescence Imaging

Intraoperative cholangiography (IOC) is the most frequently applied technique for intraoperative assessment of the biliary anatomy. Although, for years, it has been speculated that IOC may decrease both the incidence and the severity of BDI, reports on the protective effect of routine IOC against BDI are conflicting, ranging from no benefit to a 40% risk reduction [18]. Van de Graaf et al. [19] in their systematic review compared routine versus selective use of IOC, and no clear conclusions could be drawn. IOC has been demonstrated to be a helpful tool in both prevention and intraoperative recognition of BDI. However, routinely application of this modality is not definitively recommended due to limited available supporting evidence. Accordingly, Ford et al. in their review made a similar conclusion: no robust evidence currently exists to either support or abandon the use of IOC in the prevention of BDI [20]. Additionally, IOC is prone to failure with a median reported success rate at 89%, involves radiation exposure, and requires additional equipment and manpower. An IOC has to be correctly performed and interpreted to assist the surgeon in identifying the CBD, and injuries may occur even if an IOC has been performed. A normal cholangiogram reveals flow of the contrast media into the duodenum, visualization of the proximal hepatic duct along with the right anterior and posterior sectoral ducts and left main duct, no filling defects within CBD, and presence of spiral valves within cystic duct. Advocates for omission of IOC also state that this technique might even be harmful to the patients due to the additional operative time and the risk of iatrogenic major BDI [19]. Moreover, the interpretation of an intraoperative cholangiography with potentially distorted anatomy clearly depends on the expertise of the surgeon. Thus, it may be argued that the absolute risk reduction associated with IOC does not warrant the added time and cost. Perhaps even more relevant than whether IOC in itself is useful is the question of whether it should be performed routinely or selectively.

Intraoperative ultrasonography (IOUS) is another imaging modality to identify and clarify the anatomy at Calot's triangle and hepatoduodenal ligament, less invasive than IOC. It has the potential to achieve high accuracy, with reports of completely visualizing the biliary tract in 92–100% of cases, with a failure rate that is lower than IOC [19, 21]. Although, the learning curve in the performance and interpretation of the ultrasonogram constitutes a major disadvantage [22, 23]. All evidence shows excellent results with laparoscopic IOUS in delineating the biliary anatomy. The advantages of laparoscopic IOUS over IOC are the shorter procedure time, its noninvasive nature, and lack of use of radiation. Furthermore, it may be performed prior to dissection in Calot's triangle and repeated in uncertain cases [24].

Indocyanine green (ICG) enhanced fluorescence near-infrared imaging is an emerging minimally invasive and easy modality for the visualization of the easier intraoperative recognition of the biliary anatomy. ICG can be injected into the human blood stream and becomes fluorescent once excited with specific light in the near-infrared spectrum, as it is exclusively by the liver after intravenous administration and has a very well-known pharmacokinetic and safety profile. ICG imaging allows repeatable and real-time exploration of the biliary system, something that is not possible with radiological IOC and provides relevant high detection rates of biliary tree structure, with specifically high detection rates of the cystic duct. Real-time simultaneous imaging of the bile ducts and the arterial anatomy (i.e., hepatic and cystic arteries) also can be obtained. Neither radiological support nor additional intervention such as opening the cystic or CBD is required, making it an easy, real-time, and flexible technique to use during surgery. However, the routine use of ICG fluorescence laparoscopy has not gained wide clinical acceptance yet due to a lack of high-quality clinical data. Furthermore, increased costs are involved in terms of the light source, camera, and fluorescent dye [25].

15.4 Classification of Bile Duct Injuries (BDI)

Several classification systems, such as Bismuth's classification, Hanover classification, Neuhaus classification, Siewert classification, Stewart-Way classification, and Strasberg classification, have been used to stratify bile duct injuries [5, 26–30]. Although the abovementioned systems are useful for standardization of outcome reporting and management decision-making, most of them fail to take into consideration significant prognostic factors, such as the mode of presentation, associated vascular injuries—particularly injuries to the right hepatic artery—, any longitudinal strictures of the common bile duct due to failed repair attempts, the presence of concomitant sepsis or secondary biliary cirrhosis, or segmental liver atrophy [31].

Classification of bile duct injuries is of paramount importance before planning any intervention because the type of treatment and optimal timing of treatment vary significant among the various types of BDI [32]. Relaparotomy should never be undertaken before adequate classification. Many injuries can be treated endoscopically with or without percutaneous drainage of any collections (i.e., bilomas). It is extremely important to identify the exact location of a BDI in order to select the optimal strategy for their management [32, 33].

Despite the presence of so many classification systems, the Bismuth and Strasberg systems remain the most popular and are used widely with the former being the first established in 1982 [27].

15.4.1 Bismuth Classification

Bismuth proposed a classification system of post-cholecystectomy benign biliary strictures (Fig. 15.1, Table 15.2) which was based on the lowest level at which healthy biliary mucosa is available for anastomosis, measured from the confluence of the right and left hepatic ducts [27]. It reveals a good correlation with the final outcome after attempted repair. Bismuth classification intended to help the surgeon to choose the appropriate technique for the repair and, although, it was established for biliary strictures, it is commonly implemented to acute BDI. This classification included five types (I to V) of bile duct injuries according to the level of the injury, the distance from the biliary bifurcation, the involvement of the bifurcation, or an anomalous right sectoral duct [34].

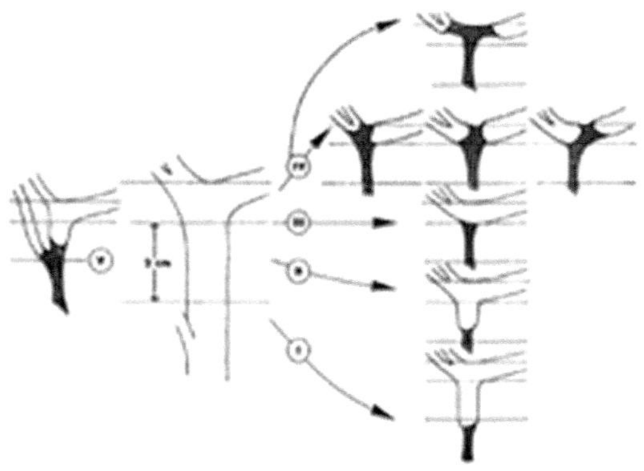

Fig. 15.1 Bismuth classification. (From [34], with permission)

Table 15.2 Bismuth classification

Type	Injury type
I	Low CHD stricture, with a length of the CBD stump of >2 cm
II	Proximal CHD stricture with a length of the CBD stump <2 cm
III	Hilar stricture, no residual CBD, but the hepatic ducts' confluence is preserved
IV	Hilar stricture, with involvement of the confluence and loss of communication between right and left hepatic ducts
V	Involvement of an aberrant right sectorial hepatic duct alone or with concomitant stricture of the CHD or CBD

Type I is associated with low common hepatic duct strictures, with a common hepatic bile duct stump longer than 2 cm, and can be repaired without opening the left hepatic duct and without lowering the hilar plate. Type II refers to proximal strictures, with a stump shorter than 2 cm, and requires opening of the left hepatic duct for a satisfactory anastomosis. Lowering the hilar plate is not always necessary, although it may improve the exposure. Type III lesions in the hilum, in which only the ceiling of the biliary confluence is intact, require lowering the hilar plate and anastomosis on the left ductal system. There is no need to open the right duct if the communication between the ducts is wide. With type IV lesions, the biliary confluence is interrupted and requires either reconstruction or two or more anastomoses, after lowering the hilar plate. Type V lesions are strictures of the hepatic duct (type I, II, or III) associated with a stricture on a separate aberrant right sectorial hepatic duct alone and that branch must be included in the repair [27, 34].

Although, this classification is applicable while evaluating long-term complications following bile duct injuries, it does not include the wide spectrum of all possible biliary injuries.

Sikora et al. [35] proposed that progression of fibrosis results in an intermediate stage between type III and type IV—according to Bismuth—strictures, where the floor of the confluence of the right and left hepatic ducts is scarred, although complete hilar isolation has not occurred. Consequently, hilar benign biliary strictures need to be subclassified, based on whether the floor of the confluence is healthy or scarred, as assessed by cholangiography or intraoperatively, because it influences the degree of operative difficulty and morbidity. Thus, patients with type III—according to Bismuth classification—strictures are subclassified into type IIIA hilar strictures, where the floor of the confluence was healthy and type IIIB hilar strictures, where the scarring involved the floor of the confluence. It is proposed that type IIIB strictures should be subclassified along with type IV strictures.

15.4.2 Strasberg Classification

Strasberg et al. [5, 36] reviewed the patterns of biliary injury and proposed a simplified, holistic classification based on the location of the injury in the biliary tract, combining not only the injuries proposed by Bismuth but also the early injuries. Although, this classification is very useful in determining the prognosis of an attempted repair, it does not take into consideration any additional vascular injuries. According to this system, there are five types (Fig. 15.2, Table 15.3) of common BDI (A–E).

Type A injuries occur due to leakage from the cystic duct stump or minor accessory radicals

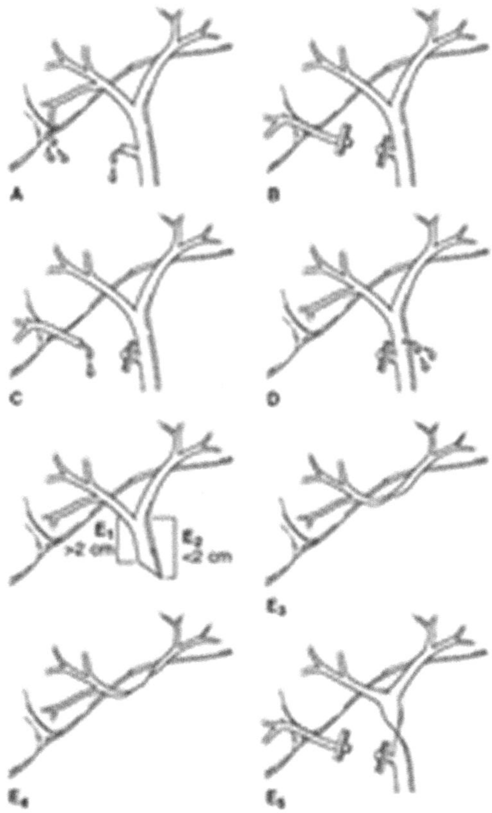

Fig. 15.2 Strasberg classification [5, 36]

Table 15.3 Strasberg classification

Type	Injury type
A	Injury of small bile ducts in communication with the main biliary system, with leakage from cystic duct or from small ducts in the liver bed
B	Occlusion of an aberrant hepatic duct (almost invariably the right posterior sectoral duct)
C	Sectioning without ligation of an aberrant right hepatic duct
D	Lateral injury of the CBD
E1	CBD injury at a distance>2 cm from the hepatic duct confluence
E2	CBD injury at a distance<2 cm from the hepatic duct confluence
E3	Hilar injury with preservation of the confluence of the hepatic ducts
E4	Hilar injury with involvement of the confluence and loss of communication between the right and left hepatic ducts
E5	Injury to an aberrant right sector hepatic duct or associated with a concomitant injury to the CBD

draining directly into the gallbladder (ducts of Luschka) and present as a biliary leakage and/or subhepatic biloma. Type B injuries are defined as ligation and division of an anomalous segmental duct—typically the duct draining segment VI—or right posterior sectoral duct (draining both segments VI and VII). This injury is often facilitated by the associated anomaly where the cystic duct drains into the right posterior duct. Type B injuries are usually subclinical or may have a delayed onset with abdominal pain or cholangitis involving the occluded liver segment. The occluded liver parenchyma will atrophy over time. Type C injuries occur in the same anatomic setting as type B injuries, though the proximal ductal segment is just divided and not occluded. Consequently, it leaks freely into the peritoneal cavity. This type of injury is often misdiagnosed, as ERCP typically misses the leaking segment because it is not opacified via the main biliary tree. Cholangiography should be carefully inspected to make sure all liver segments are visualized. In cases where the right posterior segments are not depicted, PTC may be not only diagnostic but will also allow leakage control. In type D injuries, a lateral injury—without major tissue loss—to the main bile duct occurs. This type of injury results either in an early leakage or in a delayed stricture and may be diagnosed accurately by ERCP, which can also provide a definitive treatment. Type E injuries are defined by complete disruption of the main bile duct due to transection, excision, and/or ligation of the extrahepatic biliary tree. Injuries that include a free biliary leakage will prevent early bile peritonitis and sepsis. Injuries with occlusion of the proximal hepatic drainage may present in a delayed fashion with jaundice and/or cholangitis. Type E injuries are further stratified to five subtypes (E1 to E5), according to Bismuth's classification system. E1 and E2 injuries result from a transected CBD or a stricture more or less than 2 cm from the biliary bifurcation, respectively. E3 injuries refer to a stricture of the biliary bifurcation with right and left hepatic ducts in communication. In type E4, the stricture of the biliary bifurcation results in separation of right and left hepatic ducts, whereas in type E5 a stricture of the main bile duct is associated with a transected right posterior sectoral duct. The majority of type E injuries will require PTC to definitively reveal the anatomic details of the injury and to establish stable biliary drainage.

Neither the Strasberg nor the Bismuth classification clearly describes one of the most serious injuries, namely that which presents as a biliary leak with separation of the right and left ducts resulting from excision of the extrahepatic biliary tree. For that, Connor et al. [31] proposed a sixth subdivision in type E injuries (E6), which is associated with complete excision of the extrahepatic ducts involving the confluence of the left and right hepatic ducts.

15.4.3 Siewert Classification

Siewert et al. [37] proposed four different types of BDI (Table 15.4). The most severe case is the lesion with a structural defect of the CBD or CHD with (IVa) or without (IVb) concomitant vascular injury. Tangential lesions without structural loss of the duct should be denominated as type III (stratified as IIIa and IIIB, according to the presence or not of additional vascular injury, respectively). Type II comprehends late strictures without obvious intraoperative trauma to the duct. Type I includes immediate biliary fistulae of usually good prognosis.

Table 15.4 Siewert classification

Type	Injury type
I	Immediate biliary fistulae
II	Late strictures without obvious intraoperative trauma to the duct
III IIIa IIIb	Tangential lesions without structural loss of the duct With additional vascular injury Without additional vascular injury
IV Iva IVb	Lesion with a structural defect of the CBD or CHD With additional vascular injury Without additional vascular injury

Table 15.5 Mattox classification

Type	Injury type
I	Contusion of the gallbladder or portal triad
II	Partial gallbladder avulsion from liver bed; cystic duct intact Laceration or perforation of the gallbladder
III	Complete gallbladder avulsion from liver bed Cystic duct laceration/transection
IV	Partial or complete right hepatic duct laceration Partial or complete left hepatic duct laceration Partial common hepatic duct laceration (≤ 50%) Partial common bile duct laceration (≤ 50%)
V	> 50% transection of common hepatic duct > 50% transection of common bile duct Combined right and left hepatic duct injuries Intraduodenal or intrapancreatic bile duct injuries

15.4.4 Mattox Classification

The Mattox classification (Table 15.5) of BDI takes into consideration a variety of injure patterns such as contusion, laceration, perforation, and transection of the biliary tree [38, 39].

15.4.5 McMahon Classification

McMahon et al. suggested that the type of injury may be subdivided into bile duct laceration, bile duct transection or excision, and bile duct stricture [40]. The level of stricture may be further graded according to the Bismuth's classification. Based on this classification, lacerations under 25% of the bile duct diameter or cystic–common bile duct junction ("buttonhole tear") were classified as minor ductal injury, whereas transection of CBD or CHD, or lacerations over 25% of bile duct diameter and postoperative bile duct stricture were classified as major injury [40]. Minor injury can usually be managed by simple suture repair and/or insertion of a T-tube, and major injury usually requires hepaticojejunostomy.

15.4.6 Amsterdam Academic Medical Center's Classification

Bergman et al. [41] from the "Amsterdam Academic Medical Center" identified four types of BDI (A–D). Type A is a leakage from the cystic duct or an aberrant or from peripheral hepatic radicles. Type B represents major bile duct leakage with or without concomitant biliary strictures, whereas type C corresponds to bile duct strictures without bile leakage. Type D refers to complete transection of the bile duct with or without excision of some portion of the biliary tree. The site of the ductal lesion was determined by its most proximal border (Table 15.6). Majority of type A and most type B lesions are amenable to stenting during ERCP, whereas majority of type C and all type D lesions require surgical intervention.

15.4.7 Neuhaus Classification

Neuhaus classification (Fig. 15.3) encompasses minor leaks from the gallbladder fossa or the cystic duct (type A) and major BDI including: occlusion of the CBD, CHD, right or left hepatic ducts by clips, either incomplete or complete (types B1 and B2, respectively), lateral lesions of the CBD, either small (<5 mm) or extended (>5 mm) (types C1 and C2, respectively), complete transections of the CBD or CHD, either without or with structural defect (types D1 and D2, respectively), and late strictures with stenosis of the extrahepatic bile ducts (type E). The latter group of BDI (E) is further stratified into four types: E1 and E2 with short (<5 mm) or long (>5 mm) stenosis of the CBD, respectively, E3 when the stenosis affects the confluence of the hepatic ducts, and E4 when there is stenosis of the right hepatic or a segmental duct (Table 15.7) [26, 42].

Table 15.6 Amsterdam Academic Medical Center's classification

Type	Injury type
A	Cystic duct leaks or leakage from aberrant or peripheral hepatic radicles
B	Major bile duct leaks with or without concomitant biliary strictures
C	Bile duct strictures without bile leakage
D	Complete transection of the duct with or without excision of some portion of the biliary tree

The advantage of the Neuhaus' classification may be the ability to discriminate different injury patterns and recurrent cholangitis in the long term. Treatment strategies may be tailored according to the anatomical type of injury. However, this classification does not account for any concomitant vascular injuries [42].

15.4.8 Csendes Classification

Csendes et al. [43] proposed another classification, consisted of four types (I–IV) which has the advantage of classifying the severity of the lesions and proposing the appropriate management (Table 15.8). This system describes the mechanism of injury in detail and hence is useful while applying preventive strategies. However, it does not account for vascular injuries.

Type I corresponds to a small tear of the hepatic duct or right hepatic branch caused by dissection with the hook or scissors during the dissection of Calot's triangle. Type II, which is a new type of injury which was seldom seen during open surgery, corresponds to lesions of the cysticocholedochal junction due to excessive traction, the use of a Dormia catheter, section of the cystic duct very close or at the junction with the CBD, or to a burning of the cysticocholedochal junction by electrocautery. Type III corresponds to a partial or complete section of the CBD whereas type

Type A	**Peripheral bile leak** (in communication with the CBD) A1: Cystic duct leak A2: Bile leak from the liver bed	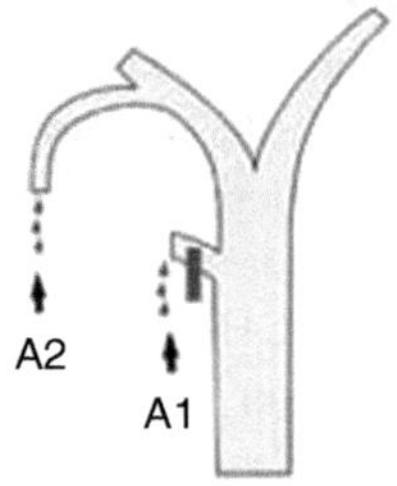
Type B	**Occlusion of the CBD** (or right resp. left hepatic duct, i.e. Clip, ligation) B1: Incomplete B2: Complete	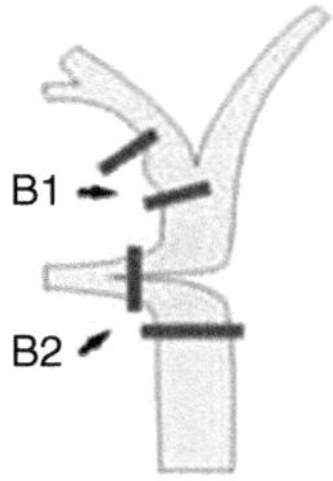
Type C	**Lateral injury of the CBD** C1: Small lesion (< 5 mm) C2: Extended lesion (> 5 mm)	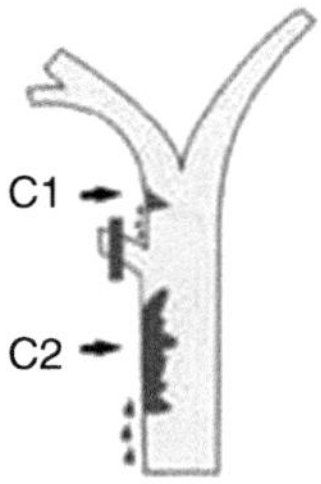
Type D	**Transsection of the CBD** (or right hepatic duct not in communication with the CBD) D1: Without structural defect D2: With structural defect	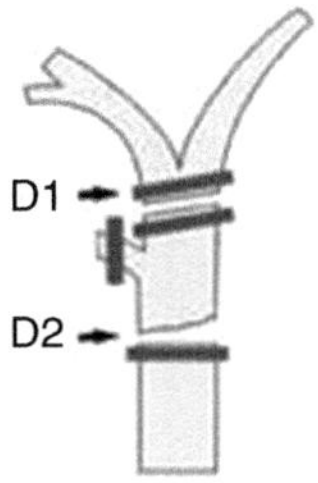
Type E	**Stenosis of the CBD** E1: CBD with short stenosis (< 5 mm) E2: CBD with long stenosis (> 5 mm) E3: Confluence E4: RIght hepatic duct/Segmental duct	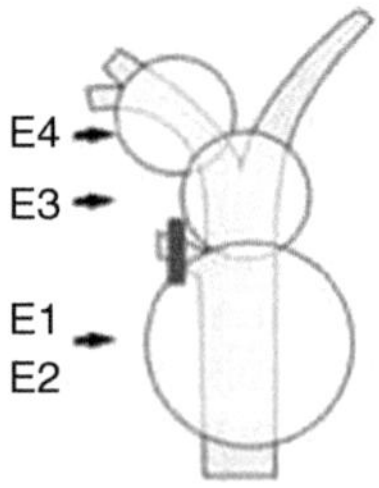

Fig. 15.3 Neuhaus classification. (From [26], with permission)

Table 15.7 Neuhaus classification

Type	Injury type
A	Peripheral bile leak from the cystic duct (A1) or an accessory hepatic duct within gallbladder fossa (A2)
B	Occlusion of the CBD, or right/left hepatic duct (i.e clip, ligation): incomplete (B1) or complete (B2)
C	Lateral injury of CBD over a distance of up to 5 mm (small lesion, C1) or more than 5 mm (extended lesion, C2)
D	Transection of the CBD, or right hepatic duct not in communication with the CBD) without (D1) or with structural defect (D2)
E	Stenosis of the CBD
E1	CBD with short stenosis (<5 mm)
E2	CBD with long stenosis (>5 mm)
E3	Confluence
E4	Right hepatic duct or segmental duct

Table 15.8 Csendes classification

Type	Injury type
I	A small tear of the hepatic duct or right hepatic branch caused by dissection with the hook or scissors during the dissection of Calot's triangle
II	Lesions of the cysticocholedochal junction due to excessive traction, the use of a Dormia catheter, section of the cystic duct very close or at the junction with the CBD, or to a burning of the cysticocholedochal junction by electrocautery
III	A partial or complete section of the CBD
IV	Resection of more than 10 mm of the CBD

IV corresponds to resection of more than 10 mm of the CBD [43].

15.4.9 Stewart-Way Classification

Stewart-Way classification (Fig. 15.4) details the mechanisms and possible reasons for various classes of injuries and makes provision for combined biliovascular injuries, as well. This classification arose from the analysis of operative reports, providing the human mistakes and cognitive processes involved in the mechanisms of BDI. Stewart-Way classification groups BDI according to anatomic pattern and causation (Table 15.9) and encompasses four classes [44].

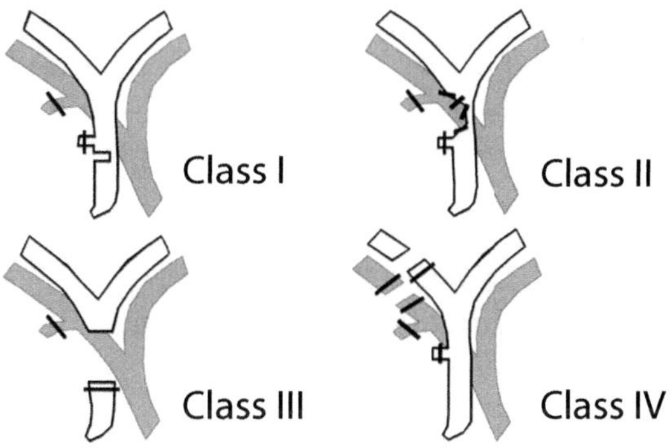

Fig. 15.4 Stewart-Way classification. (From [44], with permission)

Table 15.9 Stewart-Way classification

Type	Injury type
I	Small incisions or incomplete intersections of the CBD Cholangiogram incision in cystic duct extended into CBD
II	Lateral damage or stricture of the CBD caused by thermal injury or clips
III	Total transection or excision of the or CBD, CHD or the right or left hepatic ducts
IV	RHD mistaken for cystic duct, RHA mistaken for cystic artery RHD and RHA transected Lateral damage to the RHD from cautery or clips placed on duct

Class I injury occurs when CBD is mistaken for the cystic duct, but the error is recognized, usually by intraoperative cholangiography, before CBD is divided, or when the incision made in the cystic duct for the cholangiography is extended on to CBD. Class II injuries involve lateral damage to CHD from clips or cautery used too close to the duct. This often occurs in cases where visibility is limited due to inflammation or bleeding and results in stricture and/or fistula formation. Class III injury, the most common type, occurs when CBD is not recognized and mistaken for the cystic duct. The CBD, CHD, right or left hepatic ducts are transected, and a variable portion including the junction of the cystic and CBD is excised. Class IV injuries involve damage to the RHD or a right segmental hepatic duct, either because this structure is mistaken for the cystic duct or because it is injured during dissection or from cautery and/or clips placed on duct, often with injury of the right hepatic artery because it is mistaken for cystic artery (Fig. 15.4) [44].

15.4.10 Lau–CUHK (Chinese University of Hong Kong) Classification

This system stratifies the biliary injuries in an ascending order of severity from type 1 to 5 and emphasizes attention to operative detail to prevent these injuries. Type 1 injuries describe leaks from cystic duct stump or small ducts in liver bed. Type 2 refers to partial common hepatic or bile duct wall injuries without (2A) or with (2B) tissue loss, whereas type 3 to common bile or hepatic duct transection without (3A) or with (3B) tissue loss. Right or left hepatic duct or sectorial duct injuries without (4A) or with (4B) tissue loss constitute type 4 injuries. All bile duct injuries associated with vascular injuries encompass type 5 injuries (Table 15.10) [45].

15.4.11 Kapoor Classification

Kapoor [46] in a letter to the editor published a classification similar to ATOM [47] established by EAES, in that letters pertaining to the type of injury were used (nominal), rather than a categorical sequence. The proposed classification consisted of three types of injury (B,C,D) describing bile leakage, circumference involvement, and duct injury, respectively (Table 15.11). Every type has two subdivisions: By for open duct and Bn for ligated or clipped ducts, Cf when full circumference was involved due to either transection or excision and Cp when partial circumference was involved (clip, cautery, hole, excision), and Ds for significant duct (CBD,CHD, RHD, right sectoral, or segmental duct) injury and Di for insignificant duct (cystic duct, subsegmental duct, subvesical duct) injury. Vascular injury was included (the letter V is added when there is associated vascular injury), but there was no clear description of the level of the injury. However, the proposed classification is simple and easy to remember, reproduce, and interpret.

Table 15.10 Lau - CUHK classification

Type	Injury type
1	Leaks from cystic duct stump or small ducts in liver bed
2	Partial CBD/CHD wall injuries without (2A) or with (2B) tissue loss
3	CBD/CHD transection without (3A) or with (3B) tissue loss
4	Right or left hepatic duct or sectorial duct injuries without (4A) or with (4B) tissue loss
5	Bile duct injuries associated with vascular injuries

Table 15.11 Kapoor classification

Type	Injury type
B	Bile leak By-yes (open duct) Bn-no(ligated/clipped duct)
C	Circumference involved Cf-full circumference (transection or excision) Cp-partial circumference (clip, cautery, hole, excision)
D	Duct injured Ds-significant duct (CBD, CHD, RHD, right sectoral or segmental duct) Di-insignificant duct (cystic duct, subsegmental duct, subvesical duct)

15.4.12 Hannover Classification

Hannover classification delineated the injury patterns, including information regarding distal bile duct injuries and concomitant vascular injuries within the liver hilum. This classification provides discriminators for the localization of tangentially or completely transected bile ducts above or below the bifurcation of the hepatic duct, which is a major drawback of other classification systems. Furthermore, it is reproducible and ensures uniformity of reporting. In this classification, BDI were divided into five types from A to E [48].

According to Hannover classification, a type A injury describes a peripheral biliary leakage, either originating from the cystic duct (A1) or from the gallbladder bed (A2) with reconnection to the main bile duct system. This type of injury corresponds to type A and 1 injury according to Strasberg and Siewert classification, respectively, but Hannover classification further distinguishes a type A1 injury that leads to biliary leakage from the cystic duct and type A2 that is leakage from the liver bed of the gallbladder. Both Siewert and Strasberg classification systems do not clarify whether the leakage is from the cystic duct or the liver bed. Additionally, Bismuth and Stewart-Way systems do not delineate these types of lesions.

A type B injury describes either an incomplete (B1) or complete (B2) occlusion of the common or main bile duct or the right hepatic duct by clips or ligation without injury. Type C corresponds to a tangential injury of the CBD or CHD with further subdivisions: C1 for small punctiform lesions (<5 mm), C2 for extensive lesions (>5 mm) below the confluence, C3 for extensive lesions at the level of the hepatic bifurcation, and C4 for extensive lesions above the level of the confluence. Type D refers to a completely transected bile duct with further stratification as follows: D1 without defect below the hepatic bifurcation, D2 with defect below the hepatic bifurcation, D3 at hepatic duct confluence level (with or without defect), and D4 above the hepatic bifurcation level (with or without defect). Vascular injuries are included in type C and type D (Fig. 15.5). Type E injury is associated with strictures of the main bile duct at a late postoperative state at varying distances from the confluence and is classified into four subtypes: E1 when the stricture is short circular (<5 mm) at the main bile duct, E2 when the stricture is longitudinal

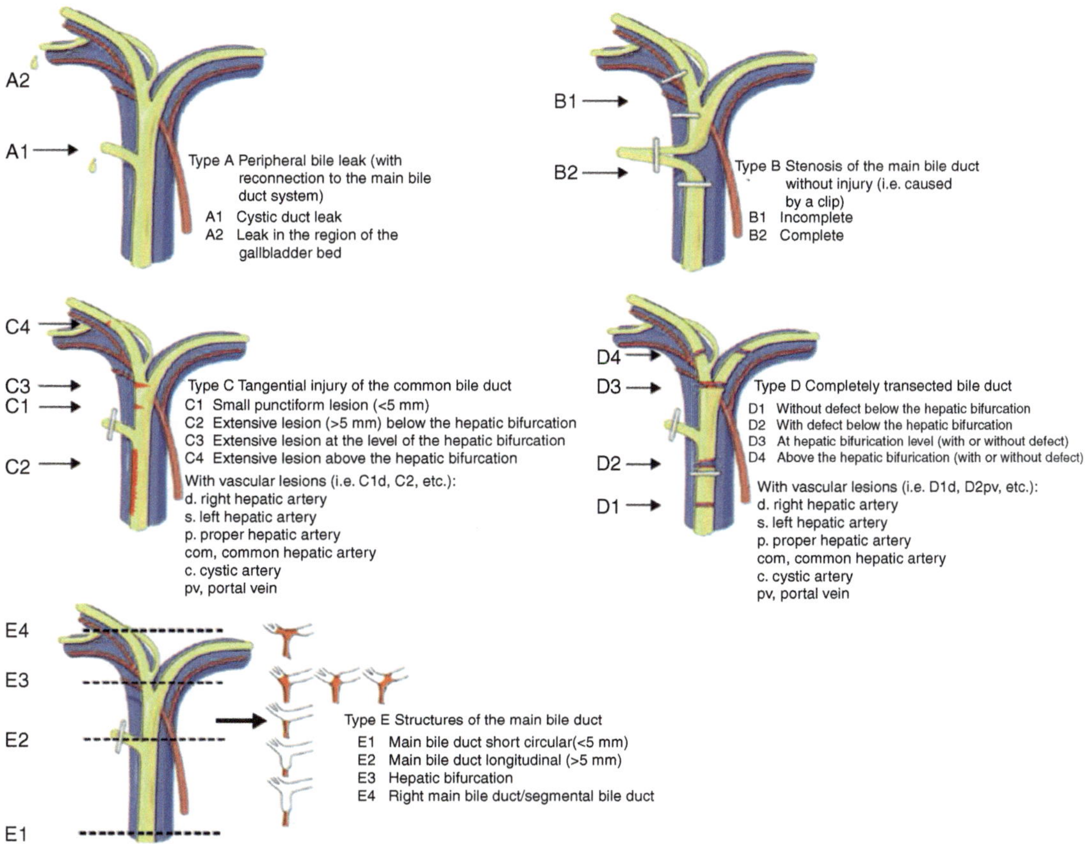

Fig. 15.5 Hanover classification. (From [28], with permission)

Table 15.12 Hannover classification

Type	Injury type
A	Peripheal bile leakage (in communication with main biliary system)
A1	Bile leakage from the cystic duct
A2	Bile leakage from the gallbalder fossa
B	CHD or CBD stricture without damage (eg caused by a clip)
B1	Incomplete
B2	Complete
C	Lateral CHD or CBD injury
C1	Small spot injury (<5 mm)
C2	Large injury (>5 mm) below the hepatic ducts confluence
C3	Large injury at the level of the hepatic ducts confluence
C4	Large injury above the hepatic ducts confluence
D	Total transsection of CHD or CBD
D1	Without ductal loss below the hepatic ducts confluence
D2	With ductal loss below the hepatic ducts confluence
D3	At the level of the hepatic ducts confluence
D4	Above the hepatic ducts confluence (with or without ductal loss)
E	CHD or CBD stricture/stenosis
E1	Short, circular (<5 mm) CBD stricture
E2	Longitudinal CBD stricture (>5 mm)
E3	Stricture at the level of the hepatic bifurcation
E4	Stricture of the right hepatic duct or segmental duct

(>5 mm) at the main bile duct, E3 when affects the hepatic confluence, and E4 when affects the right main bile duct or a segmental bile duct (Table 15.12) [48].

15.4.13 Cannon Classification

Cannon et al. [49] devised a simple, three-tier classification scheme with the primary goal of stratifying injuries based on the financial cost of definitive management. Grade I injuries consisted of leaks from the cystic duct stump, duct of Luschka, or accessory right hepatic ducts. Grade II injuries consisted of all other levels of biliary injury, including those to the common bile duct or intrahepatic bile ducts. Grade III includes all combined vascular and biliary injuries. However, this system does not provide the precise anatomic information afforded by current classification schemes, though its simplicity makes it applicable to routine clinical practice.

15.4.14 ATOM Classification

Several classifications have been proposed to stratify the type of injury and to standardize the treatment strategy [47]. For each classification, however, one or more relevant features of BDI necessary to thoroughly describe its complexity are lacking [50–52]. For this reason, the European Association for Endoscopic Surgery (EAES) proposed an all-inclusive BDI nominal classification system (ATOM), which includes the anatomy of damage and occurrence of vascular injury (A), the timing of detection (To), and the mechanism of damage (M) [47, 50–52] (Table 15.13).

The parameter "anatomic characteristics of the injury" includes the anatomic level on the biliary tree of the initial injury and concomitant vasculobiliary injury [47]. The biliary tree is divided into the main and nonmain biliary ducts. The main biliary duct (MBD in the EAES classification) (including the CBD, the CHD, and the right and left hepatic ducts) derived from the Bismuth, Strasberg, Neuhaus, Connor, McMahon, and Lau classifications [5, 6, 26, 31, 34, 40, 45]. The anatomic localization is as follows: type 1, low main BDI ≥2 cm distal to inferior border of superior hepatic confluence; type 2, middle main BDI <2 cm distal to inferior border of superior hepatic confluence; type 3, high main BDI involving the superior hepatic confluence but the left–right communication is preserved, usually on the roof; type 4, high main BDI involving the superior hepatic confluence but left–right communication is interrupted, including the E6 injury of Connor and Garden [31]; type 5, left or right hepatic duct injuries without injury to the superior confluence; and type 6, isolated segmental hepatic duct injury [53].

The nonmain biliary duct (NMBD in the EAES classification) includes the cystic aberrant and accessory (hepatic bed, subhepatic, or Luschka) ducts, corresponding to Strasberg types A and C, Neuhaus A, Lau 1, and Amsterdam type

Table 15.13 EAES classification matrix for bile duct injuries

Anatomical characteristics							Time of detection			Mechanism	
Anatomic level	Type and extent of injury					Vasculobiliary injury (yes = VBI+) and name of injured vessel (RHA, LHA, CHA, PV, MV); (no = VBI-)	Ei (de visu, bile leak, IOC)	Ep	L	Me	ED
	Occlusion		Division								
	C	P[a]	C	P[b]	LS[b]						
MBD											
1											
2											
3											
4											
5											
6											
NMBD											

For each injury, the surgeon fills in the following matrix: (1) single injury (yes/no); (2) multiple injuries (yes/no). Then one matrix is filled in for each injury, as appropriate. For example, an injury made by an energy-driven (ultrasonic) dissector involving the superior biliary confluence with interruption of the right and left hepatic ducts, detected (intraoperatively) during the operation by the presence of bile would be classed as MBD4 CVBI Ei, ED. The Connor Garden E6 injury is in fact a type 4 with LS: MBD 4 LS

EAES European Association for Endoscopic Surgery, *MBD* main biliary duct, *NMBD* nonmain biliary duct (Luschka duct, aberrant duct, accessory duct), *level 1* ≥ 2 cm from lower border of superior biliary confluent, *level 2* < 2 cm from lower border of superior biliary confluent, *level 3* involves the superior biliary confluent but communication right left is preserved, *level 4* involves superior biliary confluent but communication right left is interrupted, *level 5a* right or left hepatic duct, *level 5b* right sectorial duct but bile duct still in continuity, *C* complete, *P* partial, *LS* loss of substance, *Me* mechanical, *ED* energy driven, *VBI* vasculobiliary involvement, *RHA* right hepatic artery, *LHA* left hepatic artery, *CHA* common hepatic artery, *PV* portal vein, *MV* marginal vessels, *Ei* early intraoperative, *Ep* early postoperative, *L* late, *OC* intra-operative cholangiogram

[a]Indicate percentage of circumference, if known

[b]Indicate length, if known

A [5, 26, 33, 34, 42, 45]. The type as well as the circumferential and longitudinal extent of injury depends on whether the injured bile duct was initially occluded (O) (ligation, clip, sealed) or divided (D) and leaked. In both of these, the lowercase letter "c" is added to stand for complete interruption (ligation, clip, sealing, or division), while a partial interruption (ligation, clip, sealing, or division) is labeled "p," followed by the percentage of the circumference involved whenever this detail is known, whether there was a loss of substance between two divisions, irrespective of whether one or both of the extremities was occluded or divided (LS; the length in centimeters, whenever known, is indicated in parentheses). Concomitant vasculobiliary injury (VBI) is defined as an injury to both a bile duct and a nearby vessel [5]. Our definition also includes vascular injury that occurs alone in the index operation but results in injury, such as septic complications, stricture, or liver atrophy.

The parameter "time of detection" is classified as early (E), either intraoperative or late (L). The early detection group is further stratified according to the intraoperative (Ei) or immediate postoperative detection, whereas the former is usually discovered by the presence of bile in the operative field or at intraoperative cholangiography [27, 31, 45].

The parameter "mechanism of injury" may be classified as mechanical (Me) (e.g., scissors) or energy driven (ED) (e.g., cautery or ultrasonic) injury. The EAES classification label for BDI thus includes a series of acronyms: MBD for main bile duct (followed by a number 1–6, corresponding to the anatomic level on the main bile duct), NMBD for nonmain bile duct, followed by the relevant acronyms (Table 15.13): O or D, each with the suffix c or p (%), LS (cm), VBI (RHA, LHA, CHA, PV, marginal vessel [MV]), Ei, Ep, or L, and Me or ED. If for some reason a parameter is unknown, the suffix "?" is added [47].

Although, the classification may appear complex, ATOM is the only classification that allows true comparisons with the others because it is all-inclusive, and there are no missing details (as in the case with others) [50–52]. It includes objective data and not subjective terms, such as major, minor, peripheral, central, significant, and insignificant. It allows comparisons of mechanisms and timing of BDI between the other classifications. Last but not least, it emphasizes the underlying mechanism that led to the injury, the most relevant aspect for didactic purposes aiming at prevention [50–53].

15.5 Conclusions

Preventive strategies and safe surgery are of utmost importance to minimize BDI during laparoscopic cholecystectomy. Although many methods used in the prevention of BDI have demonstrated promising results, there is no consensus regarding a systematic reporting system of BDI. Currently, CVS seems to be the cornerstone for a safe laparoscopic cholecystectomy. In difficult cases, a sufficient attention to alternative techniques should be apprehended. In such cases, intraoperative imaging may delineate the biliary anatomy.

In order to define the type of BDI, several classifications have been proposed, but none is universally accepted. The heterogeneity of these classifications reduces their clinical utility and each of them has limitations. Although, they are useful for standardization of outcome and predictive quality, important short-term prognostic factors, including recognition of injury, mode of presentation, previously attempted repairs, presence of concomitant sepsis, and stability of the patient, are not accounted in most of the classification systems, and the documentation of an associated vascular injury has been described only recently. Furthermore, their complexity makes their routine incorporation into clinical use difficult. Among them, Bismuth's and Strasberg's classifications are most commonly used by clinicians. Recently, EAES devised an all-inclusive, semantics-based, nominal classification "ATOM" (Anatomic, Time Of detection, Mechanism) combining all existing classification items, which enables combination of all information on BDI, irrespective of the original classification used.

Acknowledgments *Ethical approval*: N/A.
Sources of funding: None.
Conflicts of interest: None.

References

1. National institutes of health consensus development conference statement on gallstones and laparoscopic cholecystectomy. Am J Surg. 1993;165:390–8.
2. Ludwig K, Bernhardt J, Steffen H, et al. Contribution of intraoperative cholangiography to incidence and outcome of common bile duct injuries during laparoscopic cholecystectomy. Surg Endosc. 2002;16:1098–104.
3. Tracey JY, Moossa AR. Surgical treatment of benign lesions and strictures of the bile ducts. Chirurg. 2006;77:315–24.
4. Tantia O, Jain M, Khanna S, et al. Iatrogenic biliary injury: 13,305 cholecystectomies experienced by a single surgical team over more than 13 years. Surg Endosc. 2008;22:1077–86.
5. Strasberg SM, Hertl M, Soper NJ. An analysis of the problem of biliary injury during laparoscopic cholecystectomy. J Am Coll Surg. 1995;180:101–25.
6. Strasberg SM. Avoidance of biliary injury during laparoscopic cholecystectomy. J Hepatobiliary Pancreat Surg. 2002;9:543–7.
7. Davidoff AM, Pappas TN, Murray EA, et al. Mechanisms of major biliary injury during laparoscopic cholecystectomy. Ann Surg. 1992;215:196–202.
8. Schol FP, Go PM, Gouma DJ. Risk factors for bile duct injury in laparoscopic cholecystectomy: analysis of 49 cases. Br J Surg. 1994;81:1786–8.
9. Russell JC, Walsh SJ, Mattie AS, et al. Bile duct injuries, 1989–1993. A statewide experience. Connecticut laparoscopic cholecystectomy registry. Arch Surg. 1996;131:382–8.

10. Gupta V, Jain G. Safe laparoscopic cholecystectomy: adoption of universal culture of safety in cholecystectomy. World J Gastrointest Surg. 2019;11(2):62–84.
11. Buddingh KT, Hofker HS, ten Cate Hoedemaker HO, et al. Safety measures during cholecystectomy: results of a nationwide survey. World J Surg. 2011;35:1235–41; discussion 42-3
12. Wakabayashi G, Iwashita Y, Hibi T, et al. Tokyo guidelines 2018: surgical management of acute cholecystitis: safe steps in laparoscopic cholecystectomy for acute cholecystitis (with videos). J Hepatobiliary Pancreat Sci. 2018;25:73–86.
13. Panni RZ, Strasberg SM. Preoperative predictors of conversion as indicators of local inflammation in acute cholecystitis: strategies for to future studies to develop quantitative predictors. J Hepatobiliary Pancreat Sci. 2018;25:101–8.
14. Philip Rothman J, Burcharth J, Pommergaard HC, et al. Preoperative risk factors for conversion of laparoscopic cholecystectomy to open surgery - a systematic review and meta-analysis of observational studies. Dig Surg. 2016;33:414–23.
15. Pucher PH, Brunt LM, Fanelli RD, et al. SAGES expert Delphi consensus: critical factors for safe surgical practice in laparoscopic cholecystectomy. Surg Endosc. 2015;29:3074–85.
16. Conrad C, Wakabayashi G, Asbun HJ, et al. IRCAD recommendation on safe laparoscopic cholecystectomy. J Hepatobiliary Pancreat Sci. 2017;24:603–15.
17. Connor SJ, Perry W, Nathanson L, et al. Using a standardized method for laparoscopic cholecystectomy to create a concept operation-specific checklist. HPB. 2014;16:422–9.
18. XChuang K, Corley D, Postlethwaite DA, et al. Does increased experience with laparoscopic cholecystectomy yield more complex bile duct injuries? Am J Surg. 2012;203(4):480–7.
19. van de Graaf FW, Zaïmi I, Stassen LPS, et al. Safe laparoscopic cholecystectomy: a systematic review of bile duct injury prevention. Int J Surg. 2018;60:164–72.
20. Ford JA, Soop M, Du J, et al. Systematic review of intraoperative cholangiography in cholecystectomy. Br J Surg. 2012;99(2):160–7.
21. Dili A, Bertrand C. Laparoscopic ultrasonography as an alternative to intraoperative cholangiography during laparoscopic cholecystectomy. World J Gastroenterol. 2017;23(29):5438–50.
22. Falcone RA Jr, Fegelman EJ, Nussbaum MS, et al. A prospective comparison of laparoscopic ultrasound vs intraoperative cholangiogram during laparoscopic cholecystectomy. Surg Endosc. 1999;13(8):784–8.
23. Soper NJ. Intraoperative detection: intraoperative cholangiography vs. intraoperative ultrasonography. J Gastrointest Surg. 2000;4(4):334–5.
24. Buddingh KT, Nieuwenhuijs VB, van Buuren L, et al. Intraoperative assessment of biliary anatomy for prevention of bile duct injury: a review of current and future patient safety interventions. Surg Endosc. 2011;25:2449–61.
25. Liu YY, Liao CH, Diana M, et al. Near-infrared cholecystocholangiography with direct intragallbladder indocyanine green injection: preliminary clinical results. Surg Endosc. 2018;32(3):1506–14.
26. Neuhaus P, Schmidt SC, Hintze RE, et al. Classification and treatment of bile duct injuries after laparoscopic cholecystectomy. Chirurg. 2000;71:166–73.
27. Bismuth H. Postoperative strictures of the bile ducts. In: Blumgart LH, editor. The biliary tract. Edinburgh: Churchill Livingstone; 1982. p. 209–18.
28. Bektas H, Kleine M, Tamac A, et al. Clinical application of the hanover classification for iatrogenic bile duct lesions. HPB Surg 2011;2011:612384.
29. Weber A, Feussner H, Winkelmann F, et al. Long-term outcome of endoscopic therapy in patients with bile duct injury after cholecystectomy. J Gastroenterol Hepatol. 2009;24:762–9.
30. Misawa T, Saito R, Shiba H, et al. Analysis of bile duct injuries (Stewart-way classification) during laparoscopic cholecystectomy. J Hepato-Biliary-Pancreat Surg. 2006;13:427–34.
31. Connor S, Garden OJ. Bile duct injury in the era of laparoscopic cholecystectomy. Br J Surg. 2006;93:158–68.
32. Trerotola SO, Savader SJ, Lund GB, et al. Biliary tract complications following laparoscopic cholecystectomy: imaging and intervention. Radiology. 1992;184:195–200.
33. Keulemans YC, Bergman JJ, de Wit LT, et al. Improvement in the management of bile duct injuries? J Am Coll Surg. 1998;187:246–54.
34. Bismuth H, Majno PE. Biliary strictures: classification based on the principles of surgical treatment. World J Surg. 2001;25:1241–4.
35. Sikora SS, Srikanth G, Sarkari A, et al. Hilar benign biliary strictures: need for subclassification. ANZ J Surg. 2003;73:484–8.
36. Sahajpal AK, Chow SC, Dixon E, et al. Bile duct injuries associated with laparoscopic cholecystectomy: timing of repair and long-term outcomes. Arch Surg. 2010;145:757–63.
37. Siewert JR, Ungeheuer A, Feussner H. Bile duct lesions in laparoscopic cholecystectomy. Chirurg. 1994;65:748–57.
38. Moore EE, et al. Organ injury scaling. VI: extrahepatic biliary, esophagus, stomach, vulva, vagina, uterus (nonpregnant), uterus (pregnant), fallopian tube, and ovary. J Trauma. 1995;39(6):1069–70.
39. Mattox KL, Feliciano DV, Moore EE. Trauma. 3rd ed. Stamford, CT: Applenton & Lange; 1996. p. 515–9.
40. McMahon AJ, Fullarton G, Baxter JN, et al. Bile duct injury and bile leakage in laparoscopic cholecystectomy. Br J Surg. 1995;82:307–13.
41. Bergman JJ, van den Brink GR, Rauws EA, et al. Treatment of bile duct lesions after laparoscopic cholecystectomy. Gut. 1996;38:141–7.
42. Schmidt SC, Settmacher U, Langrehr JM, et al. Management and outcome of patients with combined bile duct and hepatic arterial injuries after laparoscopic cholecystectomy. Surgery. 2004;135:613–8.

43. Csendes A, Navarrete C, Burdiles P, et al. Treatment of common bile duct injuries during laparoscopic cholecystectomy: endoscopic and surgical management. World J Surg. 2001;25:1346–51.
44. Stewart L, Robinson TN, Lee CM, et al. Right hepatic artery injury associated with laparoscopic bile duct injury: incidence, mechanism, and consequences. J Gastrointest Surg. 2004;8:523–31.
45. Lau WY, Lai EC. Classification of iatrogenic bile duct injury. Hepatobiliary Pancreat Dis Int. 2007;6(5):459–63.
46. Kapoor VK. New classification of acute bile duct injuries. Hepatobiliary Pancreat Dis Int. 2008;7:555–6.
47. Fingerhut A, Dziri C, Garden OJ, et al. ATOM, the all-inclusive nominal EAES classification of bile duct injuries during cholecystectomy. Surg Endosc. 2013;27(12):4608–19.
48. Bektas H, Schrem H, Winny M, et al. Surgical treatment and outcome of iatrogenic bile duct lesions after cholecystectomy and the impact of different clinical classification systems. Br J Surg. 2007;94:1119–27.
49. Cannon RM, Brock G, Buell JF. A novel classification system to address financial impact and referral decisions for bile duct injury in laparoscopic cholecystectomy. HPB Surg. 2011;2011:371245.
50. Balla A, Quaresima S, Corona M, et al. ATOM classification of bile duct injuries during laparoscopic cholecystectomy: analysis of a single institution experience. J Laparoendosc Adv Surg Tech A. 2019;29(2):206–12.
51. Gouma DJ. Commentary: the classification and injury patterns of iatrogenic bile duct injury during laparoscopic cholecystectomy. In: Dixon E, Vollmer Jr CM, May GR, editors. Management of benign biliary stenosis and injury: a comprehensive guide. Cham: Springer International Publishing; 2015. p. 223–7.
52. Velidedeoglu M, Arikan AE, Uludag SS, et al. Clinical application of six current classification systems for iatrogenic bile duct injuries after cholecystectomy. Hepato-Gastroenterology. 2015;62:577–84.
53. Li J, Frilling A, Nadalin S, et al. Surgical management of segmental and sectoral bile duct injury after laparoscopic cholecystectomy: a challenging situation. J Gastrointest Surg. 2010;14:344–51.

Iatrogenic Lesions of the Biliary Tree: The Role of a Multidisciplinary Approach

16

Sergio Calamia, Duilio Pagano, and Salvatore Gruttadauria

16.1 Background

The gold standard for symptomatic cholelithiasis is laparoscopic cholecystectomy (LC), one of the most widely performed abdominal surgical procedures worldwide. Unfortunately, when compared to open cholecystectomy, it is correlated to a relevant incidence of surgical bile duct injury (SBDI), representing 0.1% to 0.2% in the era of open cholecystectomy and 0.4% to 0.7% in the era of minimally invasive cholecystectomy [1, 2].

The indicators and factors in question and that can contribute to the increase of SBDIs are: [3, 4].

- Incorrect recognition of the common biliary duct anatomy;
- Presence of a right or aberrant bile duct such as a cystic duct followed by its excision, division or occlusion;
- Excessive gallbladder traction and consequent retraction of common biliary duct;
- Devascularization or thermal damage to the main biliary tree;
- The operating surgeon's experience and learning curve effects;
- Local operating factors, including inflammation, the presence of a pathological accumulation of adipose tissue, the onset of hemorrhage during the surgical dissection, and too deep a dissection of the gallbladder bed; and
- Equipment problems such as laser use or clip failure.

These elements can lead to complex clinical conditions in which SBDI following cholecystectomy can easily represent an iatrogenic catastrophe, associated with worsening clinical outcomes, and quality of life.

16.2 Surgical Decision-Making

To define the optimal treatment, it is crucial when the extent of the main SBDI lesion, the patient's clinical status, and a rapid availability of a tertiary hepatobiliary referral center are recognized.

The localized inflammatory state is one of the main determinants of the prognosis of definitive repair surgery. Ideally, the inflammatory changes

S. Calamia · D. Pagano
Department for the Treatment and Study of Abdominal Diseases and Abdominal Transplantation, IRCCS–ISMETT (Istituto Mediterraneo per i Trapianti e Terapie ad alta specializzazione)/ University of Pittsburgh Medical Center Italy, Palermo, Italy
e-mail: scalamia@ismett.edu; dpagano@ismett.edu

S. Gruttadauria (✉)
Department for the Treatment and Study of Abdominal Diseases and Abdominal Transplantation, IRCCS–ISMETT (Istituto Mediterraneo per i Trapianti e Terapie ad alta specializzazione)/ University of Pittsburgh Medical Center Italy, Palermo, Italy

Department of Surgery and Surgical and Medical Specialties, University of Catania, Catania, Italy
e-mail: sgruttadauria@ismett.edu

© Springer Nature Switzerland AG 2021

I. Di Carlo (ed.), *Difficult Acute Cholecystitis*, https://doi.org/10.1007/978-3-030-62102-5_16

can alter the complexity of surgical repair and/or reconstruction procedures. Consequently, an immediately intraoperative repair by an experienced hepatobiliary surgeon is recommended.

When an SBDI is suspected, the surgeon must evaluate the cholangiographic biliary anatomy in order to avoid further dissections. This is essential, otherwise further biliary duct devascularization or lesion may occur [5, 6]. In several cases, an open procedure is necessary to obtain a proper identification of the biliary anatomy.

In cases of technically complex biliary lesions to be treated, it is useful to place several laparoscopic drainages to avoid the formation of abdominal collections and to place a percutaneous trans-hepatic drainage of the biliary tree, so as to transform the SBDI into a monitored biliary leakage. At that point, it is appropriate to refer the patient to a hepatobiliary surgical referral center [7, 8]. A literature review shows that in cases in which the lesions are repaired by an expert surgeon, complications are significantly reduced (94% success for an experienced hepatobiliary surgeon versus 17% for an inexperienced surgeon), hospital stay (222 days vs. 78 days), and mortality decreased (0% vs 1.6%) [9].

The aim of the intervention is to restore the integrity of the damaged biliary tract in order to prevent the onset of short- or long-term complications, such as biliary leakage or stenosis, chronic cholangitis, abdominal abscesses, or secondary cirrhosis. The best time to repair the damaged biliary tract is during the first surgery but, unfortunately, in only 25%–32.4% of cases is the lesion recognized on that occasion. Much more often, an SBDI will occur in the first postoperative days after LC.

The clinical symptoms are fever, mild hyperbilirubinemia, and pain related to biloma or biliary peritonitis. Usually, bile is seen exiting externally from a drain or surgical incision. When lesions involving common bile or hepatic duct occlusion without intraperitoneal bile loss, jaundice with or without abdominal pain is the principal symptom. Sometimes, patients can experience recurrent cholangitis or end-stage liver disease (cirrhosis) from a remote SBDI later, typically months after surgery.

Some patients can experience sepsis from intra-abdominal fluid collections or recurrent cholangitis. It is first mandatory to check for sepsis, eventually drain the abdominal collections, and define the type and description of SBDI and other associated damages. An urgent laparotomy is justified only in cases of severe biliary peritonitis not responsive to percutaneous drainage or other conservative maneuvers. In a clinical picture of peritonitis, biliary tree repair is statistically disadvantageous. It is therefore appropriate, if possible, to postpone the surgery 4–6 weeks, when the inflammation and local infection are better controlled.

16.3 Surgical Bile Duct Injury Classification

SBDIs are classified according to anatomic picture and clinical entity of biliary transection. Here we present the classification proposed by Dr. Stewart et al. [10].

16.3.1 Stewart-Way Class I Injuries

The lesion is localized to the duct that joins the gallbladder to the common hepatic duct (cystic duct) and/or to a peripheral duct on the hepatic parenchymal bed. A leakage of the cystic stump occurs because of a defective clip application, clip slipping, tissue necrosis close to the clip application for the diathermic injury, or an obstructive common bile duct (CBD) stone. Generally, the damage is recognized during surgery and can therefore be quickly repaired using an absorbable fine monofilament suture if necessary. There is no indication for placing a catheter with a T-tube, as insertion of the tube itself would result in an extension of the lesion and would increase the risk of stenosis [11]. If the lesion is detected after surgery, the gold standard is an endoscopic treatment through sphincterotomy, possibly by inserting a nasal tube or an internal biliary stent to reduce the gradient of the intraductal pressure maintained by the Oddi sphincter and remove the biliary flow from the damaged spot. The success rates of endoscopic sphincterotomy are very high (near 100%) [12].

To promote faster healing, most authors recommend the insertion of biliary stents, as opposed to sphincterotomy, for reducing the intraductal biliary tree pressure and for a prompt leakage covering. Not performing sphincterotomy also means avoiding related complications. Placing a nasal tube in a timely way obviates the need for several endoscopic retrograde cholangiopancreatographies (ERCPs). Otherwise, it might lead to several disadvantages: accidental movement of the tube, worsening of patient comfort, and increase in hospital length of stay.

ERCP has limits in cases of aberrant or sectioned bile ducts, or in cases in which the ducts do not communicate with the CHD (for example, aberrant right hepatic duct), or in cases of complete transection of the bile duct. In these cases, percutaneous trans-hepatic cholangiography (PTHC or PTC) is necessary in order to visualize the damaged duct and to define the lesion and the necessary biliary drainage.

16.3.2 Stewart-Way Class II Injuries

The lesion is a lateral damage of the CHD, resulting in stenosis and/or leakage. The treatment of biliary loss requires a multidisciplinary approach with endoscopy and drainage with radiological guidance as the first therapeutic approach. Stewart-Way Class II lesions with stenosis can be treated with multiple plastic stents and self-expanding covered metal or biodegradable stents, related to the SBDI severity [13]. Surgery is clearly reserved for cases in which conservative treatment fails.

16.3.3 Stewart-Way Class III Injuries

This lesion type includes a complete CBD/CHD transection. The treatment is mostly operational, though in some specific cases a minimally invasive extra-anatomic reconstruction (radiological or/and endoscopic therapies) can provide a safe and definitive option.

Some studies have proposed a combined endoscopic and radiological technique for the treatment of complete transection of the main bile duct, thus avoiding having to perform a highly risky intervention [14].

In the event that surgery is required, an end-to-end ductal repair can be performed without tension. End-to-end biliary duct repair of laparoscopic SBDI is burdened by a high rate of biliary stenosis. On the other hand, hepaticojejunostomy with a Roux-en-Y limb is certainly easier and allows you to perform an anastomosis without tension. For biliary lesion of diathermy, anastomosis has to be performed proximally to the biliary tree confluence to reduce the rate of sclerotic changes related to diathermic jeopardizing of the collateral vascular supply of CBD/CHD.

16.3.4 Stewart-Way Class IV Lesions

This fourth type of biliary lesion is localized in the right/left hepatic duct or in the sectoral duct and are often nonoperatively managed with a drainage and/or a stenting via ERCP or PTC.

A bile duct transection might require a reconstruction of the RHD with a hepaticojejunostomy and Roux-en-Y limb.

16.4 Surgical Treatment and ISMETT Clinical Experience

To define a correct reparative surgery, there are some basic rules to follow. First, the identification of size of the damaged biliary duct and the related extension of the local acute inflammatory and sclerotic changes. The detection timing should not lead the surgical team to delay the operative procedures and is a crucial factor: a specific assessment by a multidisciplinary team of surgeons, anesthesiologists, skilled nurses, interventional radiologists, endoscopic gastroenterologists, and physical and respiratory therapists, specifically trained for the care of patients with hepatobiliary disease. The aim of these meetings is to review individual clinical cases and must estimate the life expectancy and, above all, the social and family living conditions. An aggressive treatment plan must be weighed against the patients' needs and family organization. Only in the case of a partial or a complete CBD transection, a rapid direct end-to-end suture can be performed if the distal bile duct is free and without intensive inflammation. To avoid tension, a Kehr T-tube can protect the suture [15, 16]. Alternatively, an internal Y biliary drainage is useful to split the anastomosis by inserting the two branches into the RHD and LHD and leading its main branch in the duodenum. These tubes should be removed with an endoscopic procedure after healing of the biliary anastomosis. When a direct suture is not suitable, or only in cases of severe biliary sclerotic inflammatory changes, a hepaticojejunostomy with a Roux-en-Y limb is recommended [17–19].

If dense adhesions with infected and friable tissues can alter the anatomy of the hepatic hilum, and a hepaticojejunostomy with a Roux-en-Y limb cannot be safely performed, it has been suggested to combine endoscopic biliary stenting as a bridge treatment, followed by a biliary repair with hedged patches to reduce bile loss and sepsis. Recently, treatment of an SBDI with a hepaticojejunostomy with a Roux-en-Y limb reconstruction even with minimally invasive surgical approaches has been proposed. The robotic approach has demonstrated good results and a similar safety and feasibility to the laparoscopic technique in achieving the primary hepatic patency of the hepaticojejunostomy for bile duct repair [20–22].

SBDIs are often associated with vascular lesions [21]. The incidence of post-cholecystectomy vascular lesions is 16.7%–47%, typically with the interruption of the right hepatic artery due to the close CHD anatomical relationships. Unlike biliary lesions, it usually does not lead to significant early complications. Therefore, without a proper computed tomographic evaluation, it can likely remain unnoticed in most patients.

Generally, due to portal flow and arterial blood supply from collateral arteries, hepatic artery ligation can be tolerated without major clinical consequences [23]. During surgical SBDI repair, an associated lesion of arterial supply can lead to a more complex reconstruction, an increase in intraoperative bleeding, and biliary stenosis. Liver ischemia or end-stage liver disease due to biliary stenosis can cause partial liver atrophy/necrosis and may require a major hepatic resection or liver transplant. A rapid recognition of concomitant vascular lesions is necessary in order to propose surgical repair and major clinical sequelae [24].

Our case series of SBDIs and types of treatment performed are presented in Table 16.1. We have adopted a study protocol for SBDI patients. It involves the radiological study with triphasic computed tomography and magnetic resonance cholangiography to confirm the diagnosis of SBDI, classify it, and exclude any associated vascular lesions. In our experience, percutaneous catheter dilatation of trans-hepatic biliary drainage (PTBD) or ERCP is recommended first as a treatment for post-LC biliary stenosis and/or leaks for diagnostics and children. The surgical procedure is reserved for cases in which radiological or endoscopic procedures have proved ineffective or in cases of serious vascular damage. At ISMETT, 54 patients with SBDI have been transferred from other centers over the past 20 years. The majority of patients were surgically treated (26, 48%), while in 20 cases (37%) patients were treated with ERCP. In 8 of 54 cases (15%), percutaneous treatment was performed. Our experience further suggests that, in this light, a rapid tertiary referral hepatobiliary surgical treatment can reduce the role of surgery on the

Table 16.1 Total number of patients admitted with a post-cholecystectomy iatrogenic lesion

N	54
Period	No. (%)
1999–2005	6 (11)
2006–2010	7 (13)
2011–2015	21 (39)
2015–2020	20 (37)
Type of treatment	No. (%)
Surgical procedures	26 (48)
Endoscopic procedures	20 (37)
Percutaneuous procedures	8 (15)

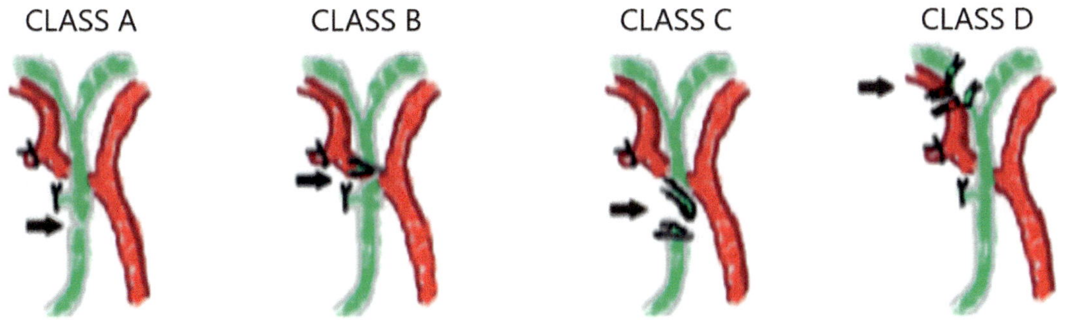

Fig. 16.1 Stewart-Way classification of bile duct injuries

patient and allows extension of the minimally invasive indications for patients with a complex SBDI (Fig. 16.1).

References

1. Pesce A, Portale TR, Minutolo V, Scilletta R, Li Destri G, Puleo S. Bile duct injury during laparoscopic cholecystectomy without intraoperative cholangiography: a retrospective study on 1,100 selected patients. Dig Surg. 2012;29(4):310–4.
2. Adamsen S, Hansen OH, Funch-Jensen P, Schulze S, Stage JG, Wara P. Bile duct injury during laparoscopic cholecystectomy: a prospective nationwide series. J Am Coll Surg. 1997;184:571–8.
3. Davidoff AM, Pappas TN, Murray EA, et al. Mechanisms of major biliary injury during laparoscopic cholecystectomy. Ann Surg. 1992;215(3):196–202.
4. Way LW. Bile duct injury during laparoscopic cholecystectomy. Ann Surg. 1992;195(Editorial):215.
5. Lillemoe KD. Benign post-operative bile duct strictures. Baillieres Clin Gastroenterol. 1997;11:749–79. https://doi.org/10.1016/S0950-3528(97)90020-8.
6. Lillemoe KD, Martin SA, Cameron JL, et al. Major bile duct injuries during laparoscopic cholecystectomy. Follow-up after combined surgical and radiologic management. Ann Surg. 1997;225:459–68; discussion 468-71. https://doi.org/10.1097/00000658-199705000-00003.
7. Sicklick JK, Camp MS, Lillemoe KD, et al. Surgical management of bile duct injuries sustained during laparoscopic cholecystectomy: perioperative results in 200 patients. Ann Surg. 2005;241:786–92.
8. Reuver PR, Rauws EA, Bruno MJ, et al. Survival in bile duct injury patients after laparoscopic cholecystectomy: a multidisciplinary approach of gastroenterologists, radiologists, and surgeons. Surgery. 2007;142(1):1–9.
9. Stewart L, Way LW. Bile duct injuries during laparoscopic cholecystectomy. Factors that influence the results of treatment. Arch Surg. 1995;130:1123–8.
10. Rainio M, Lindström O, Udd M, Haapamäki C, Nordin A, Kylänpää L. Endoscopic therapy of biliary injury after cholecystectomy. Dig Dis Sci. 2018;63(2):474–80.
11. Siiki A, Vaalavuo Y, Antila A, et al. Biodegradable biliary stents preferable to plastic stent therapy in post-cholecystectomy bile leak and avoid second endoscopy. Scand J Gastroenterol. 2018;5:1–5.
12. Podda M, Polignano FM, Luhmann A, Wilson MS, Kulli C, Tait IS. Systematic review with meta-analysis of studies comparing primary duct closure and T-tube drainage after laparoscopic common bile duct exploration for choledocholithiasis. Surg Endosc. 2016;30(3):845–61.
13. Donatelli G, Vergeau BM, Derhy S, et al. Combined endoscopic and radiologic approach for complex bile duct injuries (with video). Gastrointest Endosc. 2014;79(5):855–64.
14. Fiocca F, Salvatori FM, Fanelli F, et al. Complete transection of the main bile duct: minimally invasive treatment with an endoscopic-radiologic rendezvous. Gastrointest Endosc. 2011;74(6):1393–8.
15. Schizas D, Papaconstantinou D, Moris D, et al. Management of segmental bile duct injuries after cholecystectomy: a systematic review. J Gastrointest Surg. 2019;23(2):408–16.
16. Flores-Rangel GA, Chapa-Azuela O, Rosales AJ, Roca-Vasquez C, Böhm-González ST. Quality of life in patients with background of iatrogenic bile duct injury. World J Surg. 2018;42(9):2987–91.
17. Jabłonska B. End-to-end ductal anastomosis in biliary reconstruction: indications and limitations. Can J Surg. 2014;57(4):271–7.
18. Kapoor BS, Mauri G, Lorenz JM. Management of biliary strictures: state-of-the-art review. Radiology. 2018;289(3):590–603.
19. Renz BW, Bösch F, Angele MK. Bile duct injury after cholecystectomy: surgical therapy. Visc Med. 2017;33(3):184–90.

20. Cuendis-Velázquez A, Morales-Chávez C, Aguirre-Olmedo I, et al. Laparoscopic hepaticojejunostomy after bile duct injury. Surg Endosc. 2016;30(3):876–82.
21. Cuendis-Velázquez A, Trejo-Ávila M, Bada-Yllán O, et al. A new era of bile duct repair: robotic-assisted versus laparoscopic hepaticojejunostomy. J Gastrointest Surg. 2019;23(3):451–9.
22. Giulianotti PC, Quadri P, Durgam S, Bianco FM. Reconstruction/repair of iatrogenic biliary injuries: is the robot offering a new option? Short clinical report. Ann Surg. 2018;267(1):e7–9.
23. Tropea A, Pagano D, Biondi A, Spada M, Gruttadauria S. Treatment of the iatrogenic lesion of the biliary tree secondary to laparoscopic cholecystectomy: a single center experience. Updat Surg. 2016;68: 143–8.
24. Fong ZV, Pitt HA, Strasberg SM, Loehrer AP, Sicklick JK, Talamini MA, Lillemoe KD, Chang DC. California cholecystectomy group diminished survival in patients with bile leak and ductal injury: management strategy and outcomes. J Am Coll Surg. 2018;226(4):568.

This series includes monographs dealing with important topics in surgical pathology, cytopathology hematology, and diagnostic laboratory medicine. It is aimed at practicing hospital based pathologists and their residents providing them with concise up-to- date reviews and state of the art summaries of current problems that these physicians may encounter in their daily practice of clinical pathology.

Current Clinical Pathology

Series Editor
Antonio Giordano, Philadelphia, USA

Stefano Sioletic • Luigi Coppola
Editors

Next-Generation Sequencing in Solid Tumor Histopathology

Practical Insights and Applications

Springer

Editors
Stefano Sioletic
Department of Pathology
San Camillo-Forlanini Hospital
Rome, Italy

Luigi Coppola
Department of Pathology
Sandro Pertini Hospital
Rome, Italy

ISSN 2197-781X ISSN 2197-7828 (electronic)
Current Clinical Pathology
ISBN 978-3-032-18789-5 ISBN 978-3-032-18790-1 (eBook)
https://doi.org/10.1007/978-3-032-18790-1

© The Editor(s) (if applicable) and The Author(s), under exclusive license to Springer Nature Switzerland AG 2026

This work is subject to copyright. All rights are solely and exclusively licensed by the Publisher, whether the whole or part of the material is concerned, specifically the rights of translation, reprinting, reuse of illustrations, recitation, broadcasting, reproduction on microfilms or in any other physical way, and transmission or information storage and retrieval, electronic adaptation, computer software, or by similar or dissimilar methodology now known or hereafter developed.
The use of general descriptive names, registered names, trademarks, service marks, etc. in this publication does not imply, even in the absence of a specific statement, that such names are exempt from the relevant protective laws and regulations and therefore free for general use.
The publisher, the authors and the editors are safe to assume that the advice and information in this book are believed to be true and accurate at the date of publication. Neither the publisher nor the authors or the editors give a warranty, expressed or implied, with respect to the material contained herein or for any errors or omissions that may have been made. The publisher remains neutral with regard to jurisdictional claims in published maps and institutional affiliations.

This Springer imprint is published by the registered company Springer Nature Switzerland AG
The registered company address is: Gewerbestrasse 11, 6330 Cham, Switzerland

If disposing of this product, please recycle the paper.

To our families, for their patience and support

increasing rapidity, reshaping the practice of pathology as we enter the third decade of the twenty first century.

Today, histopathology has entered an era in which morphology, immunophenotype, and genomic profiling must be considered together as complementary and inseparable dimensions of diagnosis. This integration is further enhanced by emerging computational tools and artificial intelligence algorithms that assist in both morphological pattern recognition and molecular data interpretation.

This evolution is not only technological but also deeply clinical. For years, molecular diagnostics relied on single-gene assays, which were useful for identifying alterations such as EGFR mutations or BCR-ABL fusions. Yet these methods covered only a limited number of genes, missed structural variants and non-coding regions, and could not capture the genomic complexity of tumors. Next-generation sequencing (NGS) addressed these limitations by allowing the simultaneous analysis of thousands of genes, or even whole exomes and genomes, thereby providing a comprehensive view of the alterations driving cancer biology. International guidelines from organizations such as European Society for Medical Oncology (ESMO) and National Comprehensive Cancer Network (NCCN) now recommend NGS panels as standard practice in several tumor types, including lung and colorectal carcinomas as well as rarer cancers such as sarcomas and cholangiocarcinomas, confirming the transition of NGS from research tool to clinical requirement.

The clinical utility of NGS now extends beyond the identification of actionable alterations. It enables the recognition of hereditary cancer syndromes, guiding surveillance and preventive strategies for individuals and families at increased genetic risk. It has also become a valuable tool for monitoring minimal residual disease (MRD), offering greater sensitivity than conventional methods and allowing earlier detection of relapse. In oncology practice, it further informs immunotherapy by revealing biomarkers such as tumor mutational burden (TMB), microsatellite instability (MSI), and neoantigens that can predict response. These applications confirm that NGS has been integrated across multiple stages of patient management, from diagnosis and classification to treatment selection and disease monitoring.

Pathologists, through their combined training in histology and molecular diagnostics, are uniquely positioned to provide this synthesis. Their role is particularly critical when dealing with intratumoral heterogeneity, where a single biopsy may not capture the full spectrum of molecular alterations. At every step of the process, from tissue block selection to cellularity assessment and final interpretation, morphological evaluation directs molecular analysis. This expertise is indispensable when molecular findings appear discordant with morphological features, as clinical context is essential for accurate interpretation. Pathologists also safeguard testing quality by recognizing pre-analytical factors that influence molecular results, including fixation time and decalcification procedures.

The incorporation of sequencing into daily diagnostic practice is accompanied by significant challenges. The composition of panels and the platforms employed vary widely among laboratories, leading to inconsistency in the spectrum of alterations that can be identified. Subspecialties often require

AF809960

Current Clinical Pathology

Series Editor

Antonio Giordano, Philadelphia, USA

This series includes monographs dealing with important topics in surgical pathology, cytopathology hematology, and diagnostic laboratory medicine. It is aimed at practicing hospital based pathologists and their residents providing them with concise up-to- date reviews and state of the art summaries of current problems that these physicians may encounter in their daily practice of clinical pathology.

Stefano Sioletic • Luigi Coppola
Editors

Next-Generation Sequencing in Solid Tumor Histopathology

Practical Insights and Applications

Springer

Editors
Stefano Sioletic
Department of Pathology
San Camillo-Forlanini Hospital
Rome, Italy

Luigi Coppola
Department of Pathology
Sandro Pertini Hospital
Rome, Italy

ISSN 2197-781X ISSN 2197-7828 (electronic)
Current Clinical Pathology
ISBN 978-3-032-18789-5 ISBN 978-3-032-18790-1 (eBook)
https://doi.org/10.1007/978-3-032-18790-1

© The Editor(s) (if applicable) and The Author(s), under exclusive license to Springer Nature Switzerland AG 2026

This work is subject to copyright. All rights are solely and exclusively licensed by the Publisher, whether the whole or part of the material is concerned, specifically the rights of translation, reprinting, reuse of illustrations, recitation, broadcasting, reproduction on microfilms or in any other physical way, and transmission or information storage and retrieval, electronic adaptation, computer software, or by similar or dissimilar methodology now known or hereafter developed.
The use of general descriptive names, registered names, trademarks, service marks, etc. in this publication does not imply, even in the absence of a specific statement, that such names are exempt from the relevant protective laws and regulations and therefore free for general use.
The publisher, the authors and the editors are safe to assume that the advice and information in this book are believed to be true and accurate at the date of publication. Neither the publisher nor the authors or the editors give a warranty, expressed or implied, with respect to the material contained herein or for any errors or omissions that may have been made. The publisher remains neutral with regard to jurisdictional claims in published maps and institutional affiliations.

This Springer imprint is published by the registered company Springer Nature Switzerland AG
The registered company address is: Gewerbestrasse 11, 6330 Cham, Switzerland

If disposing of this product, please recycle the paper.

To our families, for their patience and support

Preface

In the era of precision medicine, the histopathologist has assumed a central role as the physician responsible for integrating morphology with molecular analysis. Building on a long tradition of tissue interpretation, pathology now incorporates genomic profiling as an essential component of diagnosis. The integration of morphology and genomic data is not merely a technical refinement but a fundamental transformation in how diseases are defined, classified, and treated. This synthesis is now essential, as precision medicine relies on both morphological expertise and molecular interpretation to achieve accurate diagnosis and guide patient care.

This dual expertise has deep historical roots that long predate the molecular era. In the seventeenth century, Marcello Malpighi pioneered the use of the microscope for the study of tissues, uncovering structures invisible to the naked eye. In the eighteenth century, Giovanni Battista Morgagni established the clinicopathologic method by correlating postmortem findings with clinical symptoms, thereby laying the foundations of modern pathology. At the beginning of the nineteenth century, Xavier Bichat introduced the concept of tissues as distinct anatomical and functional units, even before microscopy had reached full refinement. These early milestones progressively shifted the understanding of disease from notions of humoral imbalance to the recognition of structural alterations. Later, the introduction of tissue fixation techniques, particularly formalin fixation in the late nineteenth century, proved essential for the preservation of morphology and, ultimately, for the development of molecular analysis.

The decisive transformation occurred in the mid-nineteenth century with Rudolf Virchow's cellular pathology, which established the cell as the fundamental unit of disease and provided a scientific foundation for histopathology. From then on, the pathologist was defined as the physician who interpreted cellular and tissue architecture under the microscope. During the twentieth century, this role broadened as special stains, electron microscopy with its ultrastructural insights, and later immunohistochemistry transformed the ability to classify tumors and determine lineage. For many decades, microscopic evaluation combined with immunophenotyping was sufficient for most oncologic diagnoses. By the late twentieth century, polymerase chain reaction (PCR) and fluorescence in situ hybridization (FISH) had entered routine use, laying the foundation for the sequencing technologies that would follow. Since then, molecular tools have been adopted with increasing rapidity, reshaping the practice of pathology as we enter the third decade of the twenty-first century.

Today, histopathology has entered an era in which morphology, immunophenotype, and genomic profiling must be considered together as complementary and inseparable dimensions of diagnosis. This integration is further enhanced by emerging computational tools and artificial intelligence algorithms that assist in both morphological pattern recognition and molecular data interpretation.

This evolution is not only technological but also deeply clinical. For years, molecular diagnostics relied on single-gene assays, which were useful for identifying alterations such as EGFR mutations or BCR-ABL fusions. Yet these methods covered only a limited number of genes, missed structural variants and non-coding regions, and could not capture the genomic complexity of tumors. Next-generation sequencing (NGS) addressed these limitations by allowing the simultaneous analysis of thousands of genes, or even whole exomes and genomes, thereby providing a comprehensive view of the alterations driving cancer biology. International guidelines from organizations such as European Society for Medical Oncology (ESMO) and National Comprehensive Cancer Network (NCCN) now recommend NGS panels as standard practice in several tumor types, including lung and colorectal carcinomas as well as rarer cancers such as sarcomas and cholangiocarcinomas, confirming the transition of NGS from research tool to clinical requirement.

The clinical utility of NGS now extends beyond the identification of actionable alterations. It enables the recognition of hereditary cancer syndromes, guiding surveillance and preventive strategies for individuals and families at increased genetic risk. It has also become a valuable tool for monitoring minimal residual disease (MRD), offering greater sensitivity than conventional methods and allowing earlier detection of relapse. In oncology practice, it further informs immunotherapy by revealing biomarkers such as tumor mutational burden (TMB), microsatellite instability (MSI), and neoantigens that can predict response. These applications confirm that NGS has been integrated across multiple stages of patient management, from diagnosis and classification to treatment selection and disease monitoring.

Pathologists, through their combined training in histology and molecular diagnostics, are uniquely positioned to provide this synthesis. Their role is particularly critical when dealing with intratumoral heterogeneity, where a single biopsy may not capture the full spectrum of molecular alterations. At every step of the process, from tissue block selection to cellularity assessment and final interpretation, morphological evaluation directs molecular analysis. This expertise is indispensable when molecular findings appear discordant with morphological features, as clinical context is essential for accurate interpretation. Pathologists also safeguard testing quality by recognizing pre-analytical factors that influence molecular results, including fixation time and decalcification procedures.

The incorporation of sequencing into daily diagnostic practice is accompanied by significant challenges. The composition of panels and the platforms employed vary widely among laboratories, leading to inconsistency in the spectrum of alterations that can be identified. Subspecialties often require distinct molecular targets and diagnostic priorities, while access to testing remains uneven, with marked disparities between academic centers and community hospitals as well as between high-income and low-income countries. Training in molecular pathology is heterogeneous, and many pathologists continue to find it difficult to incorporate molecular alterations and signaling pathways into the traditional framework of histopathology. This difficulty reflects not a lack of relevance but differences in educational background, the rapid pace of technological development, and disparities in economic and cultural resources. Moreover, the technical and interpretive demands of NGS require robust bioinformatics support, and the management of incidental findings introduces new ethical questions concerning consent, disclosure, and data privacy. Reimbursement policies and regulatory standards also differ widely between countries, creating further obstacles to implementation.

The purpose of this book is to address these realities. It is not intended as a general or subspecialty textbook of anatomic pathology, for which comprehensive references already exist. Instead, it focuses on the molecular alterations and signaling pathways identifiable through NGS and on the practical challenges encountered in daily diagnostic work. These include the management of scant or degraded material, the need to correlate molecular findings with morphology and ancillary techniques, and the limited availability of advanced sequencing platforms in many routine settings. Particular attention is given to tumor types in which NGS is still evolving or not yet fully standardized, allowing readers to appreciate both the opportunities and the limitations of the method.

Each chapter is structured either around the molecular alterations characteristic of specific tumors or around broader theoretical concepts, with emphasis on decision-making algorithms and the resolution of common diagnostic problems. The text is designed not only for molecular pathology specialists but also for general surgical pathologists, who are increasingly required to interpret NGS reports and integrate them into daily diagnostic responsibilities, even in institutions without dedicated molecular facilities.

Finally, the concluding sections address rapidly emerging technologies such as liquid biopsy, single-cell and spatial transcriptomics, and epigenomic and proteogenomic profiling, which are expected to enter routine practice in the near future and with which pathologists must become conversant.

Rome, Italy — Stefano Sioletic
Rome, Italy — Luigi Coppola
Pennsylvania, PA, USA — Antonio Giordano

Contents

Part I

Principles of High-Throughput Sequencing in Histopathology

(DIN) above 8 is considered as optimal for library preparation for DNA extracted from blood and FFPE tissues. For RNA, the majority of the library prep kits needs a RIN (RNA Integrity Number). A RIN score of 8 or above indicates high quality. Some kits are available on the market that allow library preparation with a RIN below 8 (low RNA input designed kits). Any contaminants or low-quality DNA/RNA will impact the accuracy of your sequencing data.

Library Preparation [5–8]

There are some library preparation kits that can work with remarkably small input quantities of nucleic acids (particularly DNA) while maintaining high sensitivity. Although these offer a wide variety of choices for molecular lab professionals, the choice should be tailored on the specific diseases and case mix treated within the hospitals or depending on the level of skills and infrastructure (particularly the NGS machines available) of the genomic laboratory. In fact, some NGS sequencers have specific requirements for library insert sizes and adapters: therefore, the reagents for library preparation must be compatible with the instrumentation in use. The following steps are very crucial for library preparation: fragmentation, end repair, and adapter ligation.

The details of the abovementioned three steps are summarized in the following table (Table 1.1).

It is important to underline that some commercial DNA library preparation kits are available. These kits are applicable to genome types or applications and can start with different input quantities.

The available kits can be used for short-read vs. long-read platforms, depending on the laboratory infrastructure and activities (research or clinical-translational setting, respectively).

Many kits are compatible with low DNA input amounts (less than 1 ng) to help with the processing of low abundance samples. Nevertheless, the small input amount can affect the quality of downstream sequencing coverage. Samples with damaged or fragmented DNA (such as FFPE samples or cell-free DNA) are also challenging to process for NGS. There are several commercial kits able to solve issues like damaged, fragmented, or low-quality DNA samples.

Regarding the risk to generate biases by using PCR-based methods for library preparation, some companions have released PCR-free kits that reduced assay times and increased genome coverage across regions difficult to sequence.

Regarding the RNA library preparation, there are few main differences compared to the DNA workflow. Generally, most RNA-sequencing protocols require that extracted RNA is converted to cDNA via reverse transcription. This process is necessary because some NGS instruments require PCR-amplified libraries. The RNA can then be fragmented into smaller parts for adapter ligation and amplification (if required) during library preparation.

Since many different species of RNA are present within the extracted total RNA, the RNA type of interest should be enriched through different strategies. Noteworthy, up to 90% of all RNA within cells is ribosomal RNA (rRNA): therefore, many RNA-sequencing (RNA-seq) pipelines require rRNA removal or depletion to increase the relative abundance of the RNA species of interest. In this regard, rRNA can be removed from the sample by hybridization capture using rRNA-specific probes and magnetic bead separation. This method is particularly helpful for long noncoding RNA sequencing as they lack additional structural features suitable for enrichment.

To isolate mRNA transcripts, rRNA depletion can be achieved by poly(A) enrichment that works also on other species with poly(A) tails): in this case, a specific rRNA depletion step is not necessary. For smaller RNAs with poly(A) tails (snoRNAs), size selection enrichment can be performed with some commercial tools.

There are several library preparation commercially available for short- and long-read RNA sequencers: the protocols should be adapted to the instrumentation used.

Table 1.1 Main steps of library preparation setting

Stage	Procedure	Modality	Limits
Fragmentation This step is dependent on	Genomic DNA is broken into smaller fragments Falling within an optimal size range	*Enzymatic (DNA)* Restriction endonucleases *Physical (DNA)* Acoustic shearing Sonication *Chemical (RNA)* Heating with a divalent metal cation	Equipment availability DNA insert size Sample input
End repair	5′ and 3′ overhangs on the NA fragments are repaired using enzymes which create blunt ends Phosphorylation of the 5′ ends makes them suitable for adapter ligation Certain sequencing platforms, such as Illumina, require adding a single adenine to generate a 3′ overhang before adapter ligation	Polymerases	–
Adapter ligation	Synthetic oligonucleotides (adapters) are linked to both ends of the DNA fragments: They interact with oligos on the sequencer flow cells ensuring the library is recognized and sequenced Adapters are also used as a barcode (as a short index sequence) allowing multiplexing. As an example, unique molecular identifiers (UMIs) are often included prior to amplification to identify PCR biases and correct every sequencing errors	Adapters + ligase enzyme	–
Amplification	This step is optional It is generally used when lower sample inputs for library preparation are necessary	The sequencing library is amplified by polymerase chain reaction (PCR)	PCR amplification can introduce GC bias, duplicates, or artifacts that can impact downstream analysis PCR-free protocols are preferred to allow high library Complexity, particularly for whole-genome sequencing (WGS) and SNP variant detection
Purification	This step is crucial to ensure sequencing efficiency The unwanted products (excess adapter oligos, Primers, and dimers) are removed Only the nucleic acid fragments generated with the library preparation maintained for the sequencing step Size selection is necessary to separate fragments of the precise Size and generate a uniform library Type of sequencer chemistries determines the optimal library size	Agarose gel Magnetic bead	
Quality control	Quality control pipeline allows to verify the library quantity and its size distribution This guarantees that the library fragments are within the optimal size range and avoids possible coverage biases The purity of the library is assessed to exclude any contamination from adapter	Capillary electrophoresis based methods Real time	

Sequencing Tools [8–16]

First Generation Sequencing (Sanger Method)

Since the introduction of Sanger sequencing (SS-capillary sequencing) in 1977, sequencing methods and technologies have significantly advanced. Sanger's chain termination technique disrupts the DNA synthesis process using dideoxynucleotides labeled with radioactive isotopes. Following this, gel electrophoresis is employed to determine the DNA sequence based on the position of the electrophoretic bands. Overall, this method allows for the reading of DNA fragments ranging from 300 to 1,000 base pairs.

Capillary sequencing remains in use today with some updates in instrumentation settings and is the most cost-effective option for obtaining one or two reads to confirm a sequence (few dollars per template). This method is valued for its high accuracy and quality output: While it is accurate and quick, its throughput is relatively low. However, its high costs and laboriousness make it impractical for whole-genome sequencing and large-scale projects.

Second-Generation Sequencing (Next-Generation Sequencing (NGS))

NGS was initiated with the launch of the Roche GS20 by 454 Life Sciences in 2005. This platform utilized pyrosequencing technology, significantly enhancing the volume of DNA that could be sequenced simultaneously. The pyrosequencing method is based on the release of pyrophosphate during DNA synthesis, which is then converted to ATP, generating a light signal. The intensity of this light signal corresponds to the amount of pyrophosphate produced, which is specific to each DNA base.

Year by year various new NGS methodologies emerged. For instance, the Ion Torrent method, introduced in 2011, detects the release of hydrogen ions, while the sequencing by synthesis (SBS) approach was first implemented by Illumina in 2007. Since 2010, the newest NGS instruments had lowered the cost of sequencing to less than 200$ per genome nowadays. Many companies like Illumina, Element Biosciences, Ultima Genomics, and MGI claim the ability to produce a $100–$200 genome.

NGS instruments produce millions of sequencing reactions simultaneously—billions in some cases—yielding outputs ranging from megabases to terabases of sequence in a single run. As a result, whole human genomes can now be sequenced in about 1 day.

Third-Generation Sequencing

In 2011, Pacific Biosciences (PacBio) launched the third-generation single-molecule real-time (SMRT) sequencing. Unlike second-generation, SMRT sequencing does not require DNA amplification and can sequence extremely long single DNA molecules with a high degree of accuracy. In 2014, Oxford Nanopore Technologies released the biological nanopore based methodology to sequence long reads: in 2022, this technology sequenced the first fully complete human genome, with the capability to cover about 10% of the sequence that short-read technologies cannot effectively sequence.

The following table summarizes the main characteristics of both the commercially available instrumentations and sequencing methods. For companions, like Illumina, with multiple instrumentations models, only those used for IVD are reported (Table 1.2).

Third-Generation Sequencing: Long-Read Sequencers (LRS)

In 2023, long-read sequencing was recognized as the Nature Method of the Year. Recent advancements in long-read technologies have allowed researchers to investigate genomes with unprecedented resolution. Notable improvements in genome assemblies include the publication of a new, complete human genome in 2022 and a draft human pangenome in 2023, both driven by long-read sequencing.

Table 1.2 Main characteristics of instrumentations available on the market for second-generation massive parallel sequencing

Instrumentation	Company	Method of sequencing	Output per run	Max run duration	Max read length	Intended use
MiSeqDx	Illumina	Sequencing by synthesis	≥5 Gb	24 h	2 × 150 bp	In vitro diagnostic use IVD assay development Targeted enrichment cancer companion Diagnostics Metagenomics
NextSeq™ 550Dx*	Illumina	Sequencing by synthesis	16.25–120 Gb	≤35 h	2 × 150 bp	In vitro diagnostic use IVD assay development Targeted Enrichment Noninvasive prenatal testing comprehensive Genomic profiling Metagenomics
NovaSeq™ 6000Dx	Illumina	Sequencing by synthesis	1–6 Tb	≤45 h	2 × 150 bp	In vitro diagnostic use Targeted enrichment IVD assay development
Ion torrent GeneXus™	Thermo fisher scientific	Ion semiconductor sequencing	15–60 Gb	24 h	400 bp	Whole-genome sequencing (WGS) Whole exome sequencing (WES) Targeted genome sequencing
Ion GeneStudio™ S5 prime	Thermo fisher scientific	Ion semiconductor sequencing	20–25 Gb	8.5 h	600 bp	Exome sequencing Targeted transcriptomesequencing Whole transcriptome sequencing
DNBSEQ-E25	MGI	DNA nanoball	7.5 Gb	20 h	2 × 150 bp	Remote site sequencing, pathogen and microbiome study, small whole-genome sequencing, targeted sequencing, forensics, and education
DNBSEQ-G50	MGI	DNA nanoball	150 Gb	28–40 h	2 × 150 bp	Small genome sequencing Low-pass WGS Target sequencing RNA-Seq
DNBSEQ-G400RS FluoXpert	MGI	DNA nanoball	1440 Gb	31–109 h	2 × 300 bp	WGS WES Transcriptome seq, single-cell seq, methylation seq, 16 s sequencing, STOmics seq, small RNA seq, metagenomics, large/small panel seq
DNBSEQ-T7	MGI	DNA nanoball	7 Tb	24 h	2 × 150 bp	Deep WGS Deep WES Transcriptome seq Targeted panel projects Single-cell seq, stereo-seq

(continued)

Table 1.2 (continued)

Instrumentation	Company	Method of sequencing	Output per run	Max run duration	Max read length	Intended use
G4	Singular genomics	Rapid sequencing by synthesis	Up to 480 Gb	24 h	2 × 150 bp	RNA gene expression Single cell RNA-seq, total RNA-seq, exome sequencing target enrichment WGS
ONSO	PacBio	Sequencing by binding	120–150 Gb	48 h	2 × 150 bp	Cancer research Gene editing WES Single-cell analysis
AVITI system	Element biosciences	Avidity based chemistry (ABC)	300 Gb (600 Gb dual flow cell run)	38 h	2 × 150 bp 2 × 300 bp	Single-cell RNA seq WES WGS Targeted seq SARS-CoV-2
UG100™	Ultima genomics	Mostly natural sequencing by synthesis	3 Tb	<20 h	2 × 300 bp	Single-cell RNA seq WES WGS Multi-omics Clinical assays

Long-read sequencing enables the analysis of DNA sequences significantly longer than the typical 25–300 bp standard of short-read sequencing (SRS). Long-read technology can produce reads ranging from 5 kb (5000 bp) to 4 Mb (4,000,000 bp).

By sequencing a single long molecule, long-read technology mitigates the amplification bias happening in short-read methods and creates better overlaps for accurate sequence assembly, also providing information on an additional 5–10% of the genome that cannot be clearly addressed by short-read sequencing alone, although these benefits diminish for reads longer than approximately 20 kb. This capability enhances the resolution of highly repetitive genomic sequences and aids in assembling large and complex genomes: in this way, also the deciphering of large genomic rearrangements can be achieved.

Nevertheless, LRS still shows some limits, including higher costs and a greater likelihood of errors per read. Long-read sequencing may always be relatively more expensive than SRS.

There are two sequencing companies that dominate the long-read market.

1. **PacBio** are the proprietors of single-molecule real-time (SMRT) technology. A single DNA polymerase is attached to a zero-mode waveguide chip (a nanostructure for fluorescence detection). Within each zero-mode waveguide chip, two adapters are attached to both ends of the DNA molecule to form a circular single-stranded structure. DNA polymerase is used to sequence a complementary strand and fluorescence measured to identify the corresponding nucleotides. SMRT technology can produce data from 10 kb up to 25 kb in length. The latest platform, Revio, can produce 360 GbS of HiFi in about 24 h corresponding to 1300 human genomes per year. PacBio has introduced the Revio system, which offers 15 times the output of the Sequel II/IIe and can operate four independent SMRT cells, each containing 25 million zero-mode waveguides (ZMWs). Each SMRT cell is capable of generating sufficient HiFi data to sequence a human genome with high accuracy, at a cost of approximately $995.

In addition to the Revio, PacBio has launched a lower-throughput benchtop instrument named Vega. The Vega system is cheaper and produces 60 Gb of data per run.

On a single read, error rates can be relatively high, around 10%, due to the rapid addition of some bases being missed and incorrect bases occasionally interacting with the active site before being discarded. There is no fixed read length: the system can read well over 200,000 bases. However, the success of long reads relies on high-quality DNA: the strategy is evolved to sequencing the same circular DNA multiple times to generate a high-accuracy consensus. With approximately ten passes, it is now possible to achieve an accuracy of 99.9%. This method is referred to as HiFi sequencing.

2. **Oxford Nanopore Technologies (ONT)** are the principal nanopore long-read sequencing company. Sequencing is based on measuring changes in ionic current: as molecules pass through the pore, larger structures block the flow more strongly, producing distinct base-specific signals. Since each nucleotide produces a unique signal, bases can be identified in real time directly from these disturbance.

Nanopore sequencing is a rapid and versatile method that ONT has adapted for a wide range of applications, including portable sequencers designed for fieldwork and on-site pathogen detection. While this approach enables real-time sequencing of DNA, RNA, and modified bases, it is associated with a relatively high error rate due to challenges in controlling the speed at which DNA molecules pass through the nanopore. Unlike SMRT sequencing, where errors are random and often linked to polymerase degradation, nanopore errors tend to be systematic and more frequent. ONT instruments sequence single DNA or RNA molecules directly as they move through a nanopore embedded in a membrane. Typical read lengths range from 5 to 50 kb, but much longer reads have been reported, with the current record exceeding 4 Mb.

ONT flow cells contain arrays of independent chambers, each with its own nanopore and membrane. The system integrates several optimized components—including the biological pore, ionic conditions, the membrane, and a motor protein that unwinds and guides DNA at a controlled rate—allowing accurate current measurements for base calling.

Although nanopore sequencing does not require a primer, library preparation is still necessary. This process attaches a leader strand, a motor protein, and a cholesterol tether to direct DNA into the pore.

Libraries can be prepared via ligation with DNA ligase or a rapid transposon-based workflow.

Signal detection is powered by application-specific integrated circuits (ASICs), with each ASIC monitoring multiple nearby pores but recording one at a time. Because a single pore accommodates more than 20 nucleotides simultaneously, each signal reflects a composite of bases, making base calling computationally complex. ONT continuously refines its algorithms and machine-learning models to improve this process. Users can choose between different accuracy levels: fast mode for near real-time results or super-high-accuracy mode (up to Q26) for post-run base calling, delivering single nucleotide variant (SNV) performance comparable to other platforms.

Indel detection remains less accurate, but ONT excels in identifying structural variants and diverse DNA/RNA modifications.

ONT has also trained its models to recognize current shifts caused by base modifications, enabling the direct detection of epigenetic changes during standard sequencing runs.

ONT company offers a portfolio of sequencers with varying throughput: from the portable version (viz., MinION) which produces about 10 Gb per run (up to 48 Gb in optimal conditions) to the higher-throughput platforms, the GridION one, using multiple flow cells simultaneously, providing scalable sequencing power.

The following table summarizes them main difference among LRS instrumentations (Table 1.3).

Based on the above summarized information, the choice of any of these instrumentations should be based on the following:

(a) Laboratory settings: basic research, clinical-translational research, diagnostic genomic laboratory.
(b) Laboratory technological infrastructure.
(c) Laboratory professionals: number of laboratory specialists skilled in NGS-based methods.

Table 1.3 Main characteristics of instrumentations available on the market for third-fourth-generation massive parallel sequencing

Instrumentation	Company	Method of sequencing	Output per run	Max run duration	Max read length	Intended use
Vega	PacBio	Single-molecule real-time (SMRT)	~60 Gb HiFi	24 h	15–20 kb	Amplicon Microbial genome, whole genome Methylation seq targeted seq RNA-seq Small genome seq
Sequel II/IIe	PacBio	Single-molecule real-time (SMRT)	~30 Gb HiFi	Up to 30 h	15–20 kb	WGS RNA-seq Targeted seq complex populations Epigenetics, metagenome seq
MinION MK1D	Oxford Nanopore technologies	Nanopore	Up to 50 Gb	Up to 72 h	20 bp to 4 Mb	Low-pass WES/WGS Metagenomics Targeted sequencing, whole transcriptome Smaller transcriptomes multiplexing for smaller samples
PromethION 24–48	Oxford Nanopore technologies	Nanopore	Up to 7–14 Tb	Up to 72 h	20 bp to 4 Mb	Human, plant, and animal WGS Large genome assembly Targeted sequencing Transcriptomics Single cell highly multiplexed seq High depth metagenomics, epigenetics
AXELIOS1	ROCHE	Sequencing by expansion (SBX)	Not available	up to 5–6 genomes in 1 hour at >30x; in 1 hour of sequencing	DNA: 200–300 BP (SHORT READS); 500–1500 (LONG READS); RNA 500–1500 bp+	WGS; WES; Transcriptome seq; MRD; Methylation; Fragment-omics

(d) Volume of samples managed per month: this is crucial to guarantee an acceptable cost-effective rate.

(e) Type of assays necessary for clinical purposes: WES, WGS, clinical exome sequencing, or targeted panel.

(f) **Turnaround time (TAT)**: Cancer panels are different, for example, from prenatal assays and therefore the TAT are not equal for the different settings. If for a NIPT testing 3–4 days of analysis from the sample collection are desirable, for cancer profiling (FFPE or blood), the sample reporting should be available within three working weeks, from the sample check-in, in order to allow clinicians to administer targeted therapies when necessary. These requirements are generally established based on national-regional recommendations. Therefore, the laboratory equipment should be set up depending on the hospital and patients' need in order to offer the best diagnostic service. The most recently released NGS platform of Roche is designed to sequence up to 15 genomes in approximately four hours.: hovewer, this technology is still RUO and, therefore, the implementa-

Table 1.4 Comparison between short and long read-based sequencing characteristics

Type of sequencing	Reference	Read length	Accuracy	Costs	Lim Limitations
Short-read NGS sequencing	Illumina	50–300 bp	Error rate < 1%	Generally lower, high throughput (millions of reads per run)	Struggles with repetitive or structurally complex regions Fragmented de novo assemblies
Long-read NGS sequencing	PacBio, Oxford Nanopore	From several kb up to >100 kb	PacBio HiFi ~99% Lower for ONT	Higher per sample, lower throughput compared to short reads	Higher error rate in some technologies (e.g., standard nanopore) Requires larger amounts of high-quality DNA

tion in routine clinical diagnostics requires rigorous validation steps.

(g) **In vitro diagnostic rules**: About this specific regulatory rules for clinical diagnostics, also the genomic will comply with IVDR from year 2028. Meanwhile, laboratory providing genomic testing should be certified at least under ISO:9001 rules, possibly under ISO:15189 for some NGS-based methods, particularly when laboratory developed tests are set up. In the near future, most of NGS reagents, bioinformatic software, and instruments will be mandatorily released under IVD compliance.

Both SRS (sequence genomic reads up to 600 bp in length) and LRS (sequence genomic reads up to 4 mb in length) could be appropriately used for the specific pipeline of sequencing. However, it is important to consider how the advantages of each method suit your research question. To finally summarize the major pros and cons in using SRS versus LRS, the following information are necessary (Table 1.4):

In definitive, any laboratory should adapt technological solutions to the experimental needs. For genetic or molecular diagnostic laboratories, at least one IVD-Dx instrumentation should be used as reference. All in house developed assays or commercial research use methods, using materials adapted for diagnostic settings should be rigorously verified and certified at least under ISO175189 in order to offer to the patients the best qualified laboratory developed test.

References

1. Farooq S, Khan R, Farooq R, Shafqat R, Razaq A. Advances in DNA extraction techniques: a comprehensive review of methods and applications. Plant Cell Biotechnol Mol Biol. 2024;25(27–28):58–75.
2. Ralf A, Moghaddam N, Ribeiro A, Morling N. Forensic DNA extraction methods for human hard tissue: a systematic literature review and meta-analysis. Forensic Sci Int Genet. 2022;59:102705. https://doi.org/10.1016/j.fsigen.2022.102705.
3. O'Rourke SM, Hawkey J, Edwards DJ, et al. Comparison of six DNA extraction methods for isolation of high molecular weight DNA suitable for shotgun metagenomics and Nanopore sequencing. BMC Genomics. 2023;24:507. https://doi.org/10.1186/s12864-023-09537-5.
4. Behnaz R, Sholeh J, Ghasemi A, et al. Evaluation and comparison of genomic DNA extraction methods and PCR optimization on archival formalin-fixed and paraffin-embedded tissues. Diagnostics (Basel). 2022;12(5):1219. https://doi.org/10.3390/diagnostics12051219.
5. van Dijk EL, Jaszczyszyn Y, Thermes C. Library preparation methods for next-generation sequencing: tone down the bias. Exp Cell Res. 2014;322(1):12–20. https://doi.org/10.1016/j.yexcr.2014.01.008.
6. Jones MB, Highlander SK, Anderson EL, et al. Library preparation methodology can influence genomic and functional predictions in human microbiome research. Proc Natl Acad Sci USA. 2015;112(45):14024–9. https://doi.org/10.1073/pnas.1519288112.
7. Sanna G, Blois S, Pala A, et al. Comparative analysis of library preparation approaches for SARS-CoV-2 genome sequencing on the Illumina MiSeq platform. Int J Mol Sci. 2023;24(3):2374. https://doi.org/10.3390/ijms24032374.
8. The Sequencing Buyer's Guide. 7th Ed. https://frontlinegenomics.com/the-sequencing-buyers-guide-2025
9. Goodwin S, McPherson JD, McCombie WR. Coming of age: ten years of next-generation sequencing tech-

nologies. Nat Rev Genet. 2016;17(6):333–51. https://doi.org/10.1038/nrg.2016.49.
10. Wang B, Tseng E, Regulski M, et al. Comparative analysis of PacBio and Oxford Nanopore sequencing technologies for genome assembly. Gigascience. 2021;10(3):giab014. https://doi.org/10.1093/gigascience/giab014.
11. Tedersoo L, Anslan S. Perspectives and benefits of high-throughput long-read sequencing in microbial ecology. Appl Environ Microbiol. 2021;87(17):e00626–1. https://doi.org/10.1128/AEM.00626-21.
12. Maggiolini FAM, Pagliaroli G, Esposito S, et al. Long-read sequencing and structural variant detection: unlocking the hidden genome in rare genetic disorders. Diagnostics (Basel). 2025;15(14):1803. https://doi.org/10.3390/diagnostics15141803.
13. Cobbaert C, Schweiger C, Buchta C, Streichert T, Vanstapel F, Mullier F, Biaggini L, Capoluongo E, Bossuyt P, Bhattoa HP, Melvin T, Neumaier M. EFLM Committee on European Regulatory Affairs (EFLM C-ERA) and endorsed by the DGKL Board. Urgent call to the European Commission to simplify and contextualize IVDR article 5.5 for tailored and precision diagnostics. Clin Chem Lab Med. 2025; https://doi.org/10.1515/cclm-2025-1033.
14. van Dijk EL, Jaszczyszyn Y, Naquin D, Thermes C. The third revolution in sequencing technology. Trends Genet. 2018;34(9):666–81. https://doi.org/10.1016/j.tig.2018.05.008.
15. Amarasinghe SL, Su S, Dong X, Zappia L, Ritchie ME, Gouil Q. Opportunities and challenges in long-read sequencing data analysis. Genome Biol. 2020;21:30. https://doi.org/10.1186/s13059-020-1935-5.
16. Amarasinghe SL, Ritchie ME, Gouil Q. Long-read sequencing: current technologies and applications in cancer research. Nat Rev Cancer. 2023;23(2):115–31. https://doi.org/10.1038/s41568-022-00514-5.

Basics of Solid Tumor Pathology and Oncology

2

Carlo Della Rocca

Definition and Classification of Solid Tumors

The term *solid tumors* refers to a broad group of neoplasms characterized by the formation of masses of atypical tissue in organs or body structures, excluding those arising from the hemolymphopoietic system [3–5]. The term "tumor" in itself does not necessarily imply malignancy: it simply denotes an abnormal cellular proliferation, which may have very different clinical implications [3]. The fundamental distinction is between benign and malignant tumors, a central concept for understanding both the biology and clinical management of neoplastic diseases [3, 5].

Benign tumors are generally characterized by slow and localized growth. The cells that compose them usually maintain a high degree of differentiation, closely resembling the cells of the tissue from which they originate, and they tend to respect surrounding anatomical structures [3]. Although they may reach considerable size, often with significant clinical consequences due to compressive or space-occupying effects, they generally do not infiltrate adjacent tissues and do not give rise to metastases. Surgical removal is often curative. Classic examples include uterine leiomyoma and subcutaneous lipoma [3].

Malignant tumors, by contrast, typically show more rapid growth, marked cellular atypia, and the ability to invade and damage or destroy surrounding tissues [3, 4]. The defining characteristic of malignant tumors is their capacity to metastasize, that is, to disseminate to distant sites via hematogenous, lymphatic, and/or canalicular routes [3–5]. Today, the concept of malignancy can no longer be defined solely on morphological and clinical grounds, because tumor biology—the primary determinant of the aggressiveness of a neoplasm—is the result of genetic and epigenetic alterations that confer upon neoplastic cells the ability to proliferate autonomously, evade growth control mechanisms, resist apoptosis, induce angiogenesis, and adapt to the microenvironment [3, 10].

The distinction between benign and malignant tumors, although conceptually clear, may in practice show intermediate zones. Some neoplasms with apparently benign behavior may acquire aggressive features over time or be "clinically" malignant from the outset because of their anatomical location, while certain malignant tumors may remain clinically indolent for prolonged periods [3, 4]. Over time, this has made it clear that a purely morphological classification, although indispensable, is not sufficient to define the true nature and evolution of a tumor [3–5].

C. D. Rocca (✉)
Department of Medical and Surgical Sciences and Biotechnology, Faculty of Pharmacy and Medicine, Sapienza University of Rome, Umberto I University Hospital, Rome, Italy
e-mail: carlo.dellarocca@uniroma1.it

© The Author(s), under exclusive license to Springer Nature Switzerland AG 2026

S. Sioletic, L. Coppola (eds.), *Next-Generation Sequencing in Solid Tumor Histopathology*, Current Clinical Pathology, https://doi.org/10.1007/978-3-032-18790-1_2

ogy report is a fully fledged clinical document that contains essential information not only on the nature and type of tumor but also on its biological characteristics, which directly guide therapeutic choices [3, 4, 15].

Traditionally, the histopathologist provided a descriptive report identifying the histological type and degree of differentiation—diagnostic elements that were certainly useful for prognosis and surgical planning [3, 4]. With the advent of molecular medicine, however, the role of the pathologist has evolved and transformed: they are now the physician-custodian and interpreter of the tumor tissue, responsible for assessing its quality, selecting it for ancillary investigations, and translating morphological and genetic features into clinically actionable information [6–8, 16].

The first level of histopathological contribution concerns determination of the tumor type and grade. The degree of differentiation, presence of necrosis, mitotic rate, and depth of invasion are parameters that help estimate the biological aggressiveness of the neoplasm and, consequently, the need for adjuvant or neoadjuvant treatment. Similarly, assessment of surgical margins makes it possible to determine whether excision is complete or whether postoperative radiotherapy or further surgery is indicated [3, 4, 15].

The second, more advanced level concerns immunophenotypic and molecular characterization. Immunohistochemical analysis allows the identification of hormone receptors and growth factor receptors—such as estrogen receptor (ER), progesterone receptor (PR), and HER2 in breast carcinoma—which directly influence the choice of endocrine or biological therapies and also carry prognostic and predictive value [3, 5, 15]. Likewise, evaluation of PD-L1 expression and other immune markers is indispensable for selecting patients eligible for immunotherapy [8, 13, 15].

The third level of contribution is molecular, currently realized mainly through NGS and other molecular biology techniques. These investigations enable the detection of driver genetic alterations (such as mutations in EGFR, KRAS, BRAF, and rearrangements involving ALK, ROS1, or NTRK) that represent genuine therapeutic targets [9, 10, 14, 15]. In this setting, the pathologist does not simply "report" a test result but evaluates its clinical relevance and its consistency with the morphological picture, contributing to the validation and overall interpretation of the genomic data [6, 7, 16]. Without this indispensable interpretive role of the pathologist, molecular data have limited clinical value [6, 8].

The pathologist's contribution also extends to the management of pre-analytical quality, an often underestimated yet crucial aspect. Fixation time, decalcification procedures for calcified tissues, and choice of fixative and paraffin-embedding techniques all have a decisive impact on nucleic acid preservation and therefore on the success and reliability of molecular analyses [7, 8, 14]. Only strict control of these steps can guarantee the reproducibility and trustworthiness of the results [8].

Within the multidisciplinary oncology setting, the histopathologist participates actively in tumor boards, working together with all the other clinicians involved in defining the treatment plan. In these meetings, the pathologist's expertise is essential for correlating the tumor's biological features with the expected response to different therapeutic modalities and for interpreting any critical issues that may emerge during the therapeutic course, including in light of revisions or further in-depth analysis of tissue findings [6, 14, 15].

In light of these considerations, it is evident that histopathology has moved beyond the confines of diagnosis to assume a strategic role throughout the entire continuum of care for the cancer patient. The pathologist now represents the point of convergence between morphological and molecular data, between tumor biology and clinical practice, embodying the principle of precision medicine: not treating disease in the abstract, but treating the individual patient in the biological specificity of their neoplasm [5, 6, 10, 14].

Personalized Medicine and Targeted Therapies

The advent of precision medicine represents one of the most profound transformations in the history of modern oncology [9–14]. For decades, cancer treatment relied mainly on empirical approaches—surgery, radiotherapy, and cytotoxic chemotherapy. Today, the growing understanding of tumor molecular biology has enabled much more refined patient stratification and the adoption of targeted therapies capable of acting selectively on the mechanisms driving tumor growth and progression [9–11]. Precision medicine is rooted in the recognition that tumors with similar morphology may differ profoundly at the molecular level and therefore show heterogeneous responses to traditional therapies [10, 14, 16].

The contribution of pathology to this paradigm shift has been fundamental. Appropriate tissue selection, evaluation of tumor cellularity, and integrated interpretation of morphological, immunophenotypic, and molecular features form the essential basis of precision oncology [6–8, 14, 16]. A pivotal evolution in this field has been the introduction of genomic profiling, particularly next-generation sequencing (NGS). NGS has enabled the transition from single-gene assays to the simultaneous analysis of hundreds to thousands of genes and, when required, even whole-exome or whole-genome sequencing [7, 9–11].

NGS permits the identification of driver alterations—point mutations, gene fusions, copy-number variations, deletions, and characteristic mutational signatures—that refine tumor classification and directly inform therapeutic decision-making [9–11, 14]. Well-established examples include EGFR inhibitors for EGFR-mutated lung carcinoma, ALK and ROS1 inhibitors for tumors harboring the corresponding rearrangements, HER2-targeted therapy for HER2-amplified or overexpressing neoplasms, BRAF inhibitors for melanomas with the V600E mutation, and TRK inhibitors for neoplasms with NTRK gene fusions [9–11, 15]. The use of these highly specific agents depends entirely on accurate identification of the relevant biomarkers—a responsibility that lies at the core of modern pathology practice [6, 10, 14, 16].

Precision medicine, however, extends beyond targeted therapies. Immunotherapy, particularly immune checkpoint inhibitors, has emerged as a major therapeutic pillar. Its efficacy is partly predictable through biomarkers such as PD-L1 expression, microsatellite instability (MSI), and tumor mutational burden (TMB) [8, 10, 11, 13]. The evaluation of these biomarkers requires rigorous pathological assessment, involving morphology, immunohistochemistry, and molecular methods, underscoring once again the centrality of pathology to therapeutic decision-making [7, 8, 15].

A further dimension of precision oncology is the identification of hereditary cancer syndromes through germline genomic analysis. The detection of pathogenic variants in genes such as BRCA1, BRCA2, MLH1, and APC allows implementation of targeted prevention, risk-reduction, and surveillance strategies in affected families, extending the benefits of molecular diagnostics beyond the individual patient [3, 11, 15]. At the same time, NGS is transforming the monitoring of minimal residual disease (MRD), enabling earlier and more sensitive detection of tumor recurrence—particularly via circulating tumor DNA (ctDNA) assays [9, 11, 13].

Precision medicine is therefore not a collection of isolated technological advances but a comprehensive clinical framework in which therapeutic decisions derive from an integrated understanding of tumor biology [10, 13, 14, 16]. Within this framework, the pathologist plays a pivotal role: he is the professional who connects morphology and molecular data, tissue samples with therapeutic options, and biological complexity with clinical actionability [6–8, 14, 16]. The figure of the pathologist, originally defined as the interpreter of tissue under the microscope, is evolving into that of a mediator between biology, technology, and clinical medicine—an indispensable role for realizing the full potential of precision oncology [6, 10, 13].

Acknowledgements The content of the manuscript is solely the work of the author. Final proofreading, including English language and style review, was assisted by a generative AI tool (ChatGPT-5.1 Thinking), used exclusively to improve clarity and readability.

The author is grateful to **Dr. Caterina Chiappetta** for critically reviewing the manuscript.

References

Books and Classification Systems

1. Alaggio R, et al. The 5th edition of the World Health Organization classification of Haematolymphoid Tumours. Leukemia. 2022;36:1703–19.
2. Berney DM. An introduction to the WHO 5th edition 2022 classification of testicular Tumours. Histopathology. 2022;80:984–91.
3. Kumar V, Abbas AK, Aster JC. Robbins and Cotran – pathologic basis of disease. 10th ed. Philadelphia: Elsevier; 2021.
4. Rosai J. Rosai and Ackerman's surgical pathology. 11th ed. Philadelphia: Elsevier; 2017.
5. WHO Classification of Tumours Editorial Board. In: 5th edn, editor. WHO classification of Tumours. Lyon: IARC; 2025.

Pathologist's Role, Tissue Management, Diagnostic Integration

6. Angerilli V, Galuppini F, Pagni F, et al. The role of the pathologist in the next-generation era of tumour molecular characterisation. Diagnostics (Basel). 2021;11:339.
7. Schmid S, et al. How to read a next-generation sequencing report – what the oncologist needs to know. ESMO Open. 2022;7:100563.
8. Souza da Silva R, et al. Tissue management in precision medicine: what the pathologist needs to know. Front Mol Biosci. 2022;9:983102.

NGS, Genomic Profiling, Precision Medicine

9. Ghoreyshi N, et al. Next-generation sequencing in cancer diagnosis and management. J Cancer Res Clin Oncol. 2025;151:1123–42.
10. Horak P, Fröhling S, Glimm H. Integrating next-generation sequencing into clinical oncology: strategies, promises and pitfalls. EClinicalMedicine. 2016;3–4:13–20.
11. Isaic A, et al. Next-generation sequencing: a review of its transformative impact on cancer diagnosis, treatment and monitoring. Diagnostics. 2025;15:2425.
12. Sahoo OS, et al. Role of next-generation sequencing in revolutionizing oncology practice. Mol Exp Findings. 2024;

Guidelines and Recommendations (ESMO, NCCN)

13. ESMO Precision Medicine Working Group. ESMO recommendations in precision medicine and on the ESMO Scale for Clinical Action ability of molecular Targets (ESCAT). ESMO Guidelines (2023–2025)
14. Mosele MF, et al. Recommendations for the use of next-generation sequencing (NGS) for patients with advanced cancer: a report from the ESMO precision medicine working group. Ann Oncol. 2020;31:1491–505.
15. NCCN – National Comprehensive Cancer Network. NCCN Clinical Practice Guidelines in Oncology. Plymouth Meeting, PA: NCCN (updated annually). https://www.nccn.org/ (2024)
16. Van de Haar J, et al. ESMO recommendations on clinical reporting of genomic test results for solid cancers. Ann Oncol. 2024;35:245–60.

Genetic Profiling in Solid Tumors: Identification of Driver Mutations, Oncogenic Fusions, and Molecular Biomarkers

3

Priya D. Velu and James P. Solomon

Introduction

Over the past few decades, the landscape of cancer treatment has profoundly changed. In the not-so-distant past, oncologists selected therapeutic regiments based primarily on clinical and pathologic features. Histologic subtype, stage, and grade of the tumor determined whether patients were candidates for surgery, radiation, or cytotoxic chemotherapy. However, today's oncology practice is markedly different. Personalized and targeted approaches have rapidly become standard of care, with therapies designed to target specific oncogenic alterations, recruit the patient's own immune system to identify and eliminate cancer cells, and even account for the patient's underlying genetic profile. Effective utilization of personalized medicine relies upon the clinical laboratory's ability to detect specific molecular alterations and biomarkers present in the tumor or patient. Thus, it is critical for today's pathologists, oncologists, and other healthcare providers to understand how the application of modern sequencing technology affects clinical practice.

The clinical impact of tumor profiling is perhaps most dramatically illustrated in non-small cell lung cancer (NSCLC). In the past, NSCLC was subdivided based on histological subtypes: adenocarcinoma, squamous cell carcinoma, and other less common subtypes, with treatment regimens depending on histological diagnosis. Today, however, the identification of targetable alterations in oncogenes such as *EGFR*, *ERBB2*, and *BRAF*, or oncogenic fusions involving *ALK*, *RET*, and *ROS1*, has transformed the treatment landscape of NSCLC to one where molecular targeted therapies can significantly extend survival and improve quality of life for patients harboring these alterations [1–5]. Similar advances are occurring across the spectrum of solid tumor oncology [6].

While single-gene assays remain useful in some clinical situations requiring rapid therapeutic decision-making, comprehensive genomic profiling using next-generation sequencing (NGS) has largely supplanted these approaches. Many clinical laboratories today use targeted gene panels that sequence a predefined set of cancer-related genes with established clinical relevance. These panels typically cover 20–500 genes and can use amplicon-based or hybrid-capture approaches. A well-designed targeted panel can identify clinically relevant alterations in most tumors, but some academic and commercial laboratories are also increasingly implement-

P. D. Velu (✉) · J. P. Solomon
Department of Pathology and Laboratory Medicine, Weill Cornell Medicine, New York, NY, USA
e-mail: prv9013@med.cornell.edu; jas9373@med.cornell.edu

© The Author(s), under exclusive license to Springer Nature Switzerland AG 2026

S. Sioletic, L. Coppola (eds.), *Next-Generation Sequencing in Solid Tumor Histopathology*, Current Clinical Pathology, https://doi.org/10.1007/978-3-032-18790-1_3

ing exome sequencing, genome sequencing, and/or transcriptomic sequencing in select clinical situations. Comprehensive genomic profiling assesses single-nucleotide variants (SNVs) and small insertions and deletions (indels) in oncogenes and tumor suppressor genes. It is also capable of evaluating copy number alterations, may include RNA sequencing for the identification of oncogenic fusions and splice variant transcripts, and also may assess molecular biomarkers such as tumor mutational burden (TMB), microsatellite instability (MSI), or homologous recombination repair deficiency (HRD) [6].

With the previous chapters describing the technical aspects of NGS technology, and following chapters highlighting specific disease entities, this chapter focuses on the application of modern sequencing technologies in the clinical laboratory for comprehensive genomic profiling of solid tumors, and specific clinical applications for all of the clinically relevant alterations mentioned above will be explored.

Molecular Drivers of Oncogenesis: Oncogenes and Tumor Suppressor Genes

Understanding genomic profiling begins with recognizing the fundamental alterations that drive tumor formation and progression. Oncogenic drivers broadly fall into two categories: gain-of-function alterations in oncogenes and loss-of-function alterations in tumor suppressor genes. Many genes play a distinct role in carcinogenesis, with each exhibiting different mutation patterns and clinical considerations.

Oncogenes

Oncogenes are mutated genes that become aberrantly activated, leading to uncontrolled cell growth and proliferation through activation of cellular signaling pathways. Proto-oncogenes, the normal counterparts of oncogenes, typically are part of precise regulation mechanisms and cell signaling pathways important for normal cellular function [7]. Normally, a growth factor receptor binds to its ligand, a growth factor, resulting in receptor dimerization, transphosphorylation, and activation of kinase domains. These activated kinases in turn activate downstream signaling pathways such as the mitogen activated kinase (MAPK) pathway [8]. While an exhaustive description of all cellular signaling pathways that play a role in cancer exceeds the scope of this chapter, it is important to recognize that mutations can occur in many genes along the numerous pathways, resulting in constitutive activation and oncogenesis. Several types of alterations in proto-oncogenes can lead to constitutive activation, including SNVs, indels, amplifications, or structural variants (oncogenic fusions), and thus comprehensive molecular profiling should be able to account for these types of variants.

Since oncogene activation results in constitutive activation of cell signaling pathways, these alterations are often amenable to pharmacologic inhibition. Therefore, the identification of the oncogenic driver in a tumor is critically important, as it determines a patient's eligibility for either an approved targeted therapy or a clinical trial.

Probably the best example of a targetable alteration is *EGFR* activation in lung cancer. In the 1990s and early 2000s, researchers recognized the biological importance of *EGFR* activation of the MAPK pathway as an oncogenic driver in NSCLC [9]. Thus, targeting this pathway with the *EGFR* tyrosine kinase inhibitor, gefitinib, was developed as a treatment strategy. It received FDA approval for treatment of NSCLC after 2 other systemic therapies had failed. Clinical outcomes, however, were inconsistent: some patients responded, while others showed no benefit [10]. Retrospective analyses revealed that only tumors harboring *EGFR* mutations responded to the drug [5]. In retrospect, the explanation is obvious that tumors with downstream alterations in the MAPK pathway would not benefit from *EGFR* inhibition, as the constitutive pathway activation occurs beyond the point of EGFR blockade. Clinical findings and causation were confirmed in the prospective IPASS trial, where patients with known *EGFR* status were randomized to receive either gefitinib or conventional chemotherapy. Patients with *EGFR* mutations who received gefitinib demonstrated significantly improved survival compared to those receiving chemotherapy, whereas patients without *EGFR* mutations had better outcomes with conventional chemotherapy [11]. Based on this landmark study, *EGFR* mutational status in NSCLC became one of the first biomarkers where testing for specific genetic mutations at the DNA level guided targeted therapy decisions.

Tumor Suppressor Genes

Tumor suppressor genes encode proteins that restrain cell growth, promote apoptosis, or maintain genomic integrity. Unlike oncogenes, which generally require one allele to be mutated at a specific location for constitutive activation of downstream signaling pathways, tumor suppressor genes typically require loss of both alleles to eliminate their function. Several common mechanisms can knock out tumor suppressor activity. Nonsense or frameshift alterations can result in premature protein truncation. Missense mutations in key residues can abolish protein-protein, DNA-binding or other activities required for tumor suppressor function. Copy number deletions can eliminate an entire allele. While mutations and copy number alterations can be detected by many clinical assays, other processes affecting tumor suppressor gene function can be elusive. Epigenetic silencing through promoter hypermethylation can lead to transcriptional repression, or posttranslational mechanisms such as protein degradation or sequestration can also occur. These latter processes may be more difficult to detect with the current armamentarium of tumor profiling assays [12].

Direct therapeutic targeting of tumor suppressor genes has proven challenging. It is considerably easier to inhibit a constitutively active pathway than it is to repair defective tumor suppressor activity. However, synthetic lethal approaches have emerged as a promising strategy. In synthetic lethality, a second defect is added, and the combination of the two proves lethal to the cell, whereas either defect alone is tolerated. For example, in tumors with *BRCA1/2* alterations or other mutations affecting the homologous recombination repair pathway, poly ADP-ribose polymerase (PARP) inhibitors have emerged as an effective therapeutic strategy. PARP enzymes are important for the detection and repair of single-strand DNA breaks, and they also play a role in other DNA repair processes [13]. PARP inhibitors in conjunction with the *BRCA1/2* loss leads to accumulation of unrepaired DNA that ultimately leads to cell death. Clinically, PARP inhibitors are currently used in the treatment of *BRCA*-mutated ovarian, breast, pancreatic, and prostate cancers, exemplifying the therapeutic potential of synthetic lethality in solid tumors.

Copy Number Alterations

Although missense mutations in key residues of oncogenes are one mechanism of constitutive activation of oncogenic pathways, gene amplification provides an alternative means of activation. Amplification of oncogenes results in multiple gene copies that activate downstream pathways through overexpression. Multiple methods exist for detecting copy number alterations, each with distinct advantages and limitations.

Immunohistochemistry

Overexpression of oncogenes can be detected by immunohistochemistry, with the best example of this being HER2 overexpression in breast cancer caused by amplification of the *ERBB2* gene. There are well-established guidelines defining the interpretation of HER2 immunohistochemistry in multiple tumor types [14]. Levels of 3+ positive allow for patients to be treated with trastuzumab, while lower levels allow patients to be treated with antibody-drug conjugates such as fam-trastuzumab-deruxtecan-nxki [15]. Immunohistochemistry has the benefit of being

Oncogenic Fusion Detection

Gene fusions have beenrecognized as oncogenic drivers for decades. The classic example is the t (9;22) translocation seen in chronic myelogenous leukemia that leads to the Philadelphia chromosome and the *BCR::ABL1* chimeric protein. This fusion results in constitutive activation of the ABL1 tyrosine kinase, which subsequently leads to downstream activation of the JAK/STAT, MAPK, and other cell signaling pathways, driving cell proliferation and survival [22].

Oncogenic fusions are also increasingly recognized in solid tumors, where most result in translated chimeric proteins that lead to constitutive activation of signaling pathways. Oncogenic fusions in solid tumors are clinically important for several reasons. First, some fusions are characteristic or diagnostic of certain pathologic entities. Many sarcomas, for example, are defined by certain oncogenic fusions [23]. However, probably more important is the fact that many oncogenic fusions are amenable to targeted therapies. While numerous fusions are targetable in specific tumor types, an increasing number of basket trials are being performed, where therapies are not directed toward a particular histologic subtype of tumor, but instead on any tumor type harboring specific molecular alterations. Probably the most notable example would be the *NTRK1/2/3* fusions, where extremely successful basket trials led to FDA-approved therapy for all solid tumors.

There are three neurotrophic tyrosine receptor kinase genes, *NTRK1*, *NTRK2*, and *NTRK3*, that, like other receptor tyrosine kinases, normally respond to their respective growth factor ligands by dimerizing, cross-phosphorylating, and activating downstream cell signaling pathways. Each of these genes can participate in fusions where the C-terminal tyrosine kinase domain fuses to the N-terminal portion of another protein, resulting in a constitutively active chimeric protein that drives tumorigenesis. *NTRK* fusions can have an extremely diverse array of N-terminal fusion partners, with some being relatively common, while others are exceedingly rare with only isolated case reports in the literature. Novel N-terminal fusion partners continue to be reported with regularity.

NTRK fusions are classically associated with a few rare tumor subtypes: secretory carcinoma of the breast and secretory carcinoma of the salivary gland in adults and infantile fibrosarcoma and congenital mesoblastic nephroma in the pediatric population. In these rare entities, *NTRK* fusions are present in the vast majority of cases, and identification of the fusion often confirms the diagnosis. However, what makes these fusions particularly compelling is that they are also rarely seen in common tumor types. For example, they are identified in approximately 0.2% of lung cancers, 0.3% of colorectal cancers, 0.3% of pancreatic cancers, and 2% of thyroid cancers, among many other tumor histological subtypes [24, 25].

In a landmark basket trial, Drilon et al. examined the Trk-inhibitor larotrectinib for the treatment of tumors harboring NTRK fusions. Fifty-five consecutive patients with locally advanced or metastatic *NTRK* fusion positive cancer were included, including pediatric and adult patients with diverse solid tumor types. The results demonstrated remarkable efficacy irrespective of patient age and tumor type. The vast majority of patients responded to therapy, with many experiencing marked reduction in tumor size. Notably, some patients with unresectable tumors who had exhausted multiple lines of therapy experienced such dramatic responses that tumors became resectable, leading to a potential cure [26]. Given the findings of this clinical trial, the FDA approved larotrectinib for systemic treatment of any solid tumor harboring an *NTRK* fusion. Additional *NTRK* inhibitors, including entrectinib and repotrectinib, are also now available [27, 28].

The availability of directed therapy makes the identification of *NTRK* fusions in solid tumors essential. However, several challenges complicate their detection. *NTRK* fusions occur across many tumor types, necessitating screening of virtually every case with a diagnosis of cancer. Additionally, three *NTRK* genes exist with numerous potential fusion partners, so assays would need to account for this genetic diversity. Finally, given the rarity of *NTRK* fusions, hundreds of tumors may need to be screened for every positive case, and thus an ideal assay should be highly sensitive to avoid missing true positives and highly specific to minimize the false positives given the low prevalence. There are multiple methods available in the clinical laboratory for detecting oncogenic fusions, each with distinct advantages and limitations.

Immunohistochemistry

Immunohistochemistry (IHC) can identify the protein overexpression that often accompanies oncogenic fusions. Although this method does not directly detect the chimeric fusion transcript, overexpression has proven to be a sensitive and specific marker for oncogenic fusions in many contexts. IHC is rapid, often completed within 1 day, cost-effective, and readily implemented in surgical pathology laboratories. A significant limitation is the limited throughput. A different antibody tested on a separate tissue section is required for each fusion to be assessed. Additionally, the sensitivity and specificity for fusion detection can vary considerably [29]. While the ALK D5F3 antibody can be used as a standalone test for ALK fusions [30, 31], other antibodies may not have comparable performance. The ROS1 antibody, for example, may show positivity in some tissues with high background levels of ROS1 protein, as ROS1 may be overexpressed in some lung tissues [32]. The pan-Trk antibody (clone EPR17341) reacts with a conserved proprietary peptide in the C-terminal portion of all three Trk proteins, TrkA, TrkB, and TrkC. However, the sensitivity and specificity have been suboptimal. Some studies report 88% sensitivity and 81% specificity for *NTRK* fusions compared to RNA-based sequencing, with false negatives observed for some *NTRK3* fusions and false positives observed in sarcomas and neural-derived tumors [25].

Fluorescence In Situ Hybridization

FISH, previously described for copy number detection, can also detect structural variants in fresh tissue or FFPE specimens. FISH probes for fusion detection can be either fusion probes or break-apart probes. Fusion probes have one probe for each fusion partner. In normal cells, signals appear separately, but when a fusion occurs involving both partners, the signals merge to create a fused signal. In contrast, break-apart probes consist of two signals that flank the region or gene partner of interest in close proximity. In normal cells, the signal is fused, but once a structural variant occurs involving that region, the two signals "break apart," and separate signals are seen in the tumor cells. FISH offers high sensitivity and performs well even in samples with low tumor content, as visual inspection allows identification of signals specifically within the tumor cells. Additionally, turnaround time is only a few days, and the tissue requirements are low. However, like IHC, the throughput is limited, as separate FISH probes are required for each fusion interrogated [33].

Optical Genomic Mapping

Optical genomic mapping is a newer methodology that directly visualizes structural variants in DNA molecules. In this approach, ultrahigh molecular weight DNA is isolated from blood, bone marrow, or fresh tissue, and specific sequence motifs are fluorescently labeled. DNA molecules then pass through a microfluidic device to linearize the molecules, which then flow through the device by electrophoresis. As they flow through, the DNA molecules are imaged, and based on the pattern of fluorescent labeling, they can be aligned to the reference genome to identify structural variants. The main limitation of this technology is the requirement for ultrahigh molecular weight DNA. While this approach is emerging as a valuable technique for characterizing fusions and structural variants in hematologic malignancies, where high quality DNA is extracted from fresh blood and bone marrow samples, its utility in solid tumors, where poor quality DNA extracted from FFPE specimens, is limited [34].

Next-Generation Sequencing Approaches

DNA-based sequencing can identify structural variants such as translocations, but since short read sequencing analyzes many small DNA fragments, these structural variants can only be detected if the fusion breakpoints are explicitly covered. Many DNA-based cancer gene panels only cover exonic regions, as they are mainly designed for detecting protein-coding alterations affecting the function of oncogenes and tumor suppressor genes. However, the breakpoints of structural variants can occur anywhere in the genome, including in intronic regions between exons. These intronic regions can span hundreds of kilobases and often contain repetitive regions that can be difficult to align bioinformatically.

In messenger RNA, these intronic regions are spliced out by the cellular splicing machinery. If sequencing mRNA rather than DNA, the breadth of coverage of the assay can be much lower, reducing costs of sequencing and bioinformatic requirements. In addition, RNA sequencing provides direct evidence that RNA is being transcribed and processed, increasing the confidence that a detected fusion is functional. However, RNA sequencing does have limitations. RNA is more labile than DNA, making it more susceptible to degradation in FFPE specimens. Tissue blocks that are a few years old often have completely degraded RNA.

The clinical significance of DNA versus RNA sequencing is illustrated by a study from Benayed et al. In this study, the authors examined 2522 cases of lung adenocarcinoma using the hybridization capture-based DNA sequencing panel MSK-IMPACT. Of the sequenced cases, 589 were negative for oncogenic drivers by DNA sequencing. For these driver-negative cases, 232 were subsequently analyzed using anchored multiplex RNA sequencing for oncogenic fusion detection. Of the 232 cases tested, 36 harbored targetable oncogenic fusions that had not been detected by DNA sequencing and demonstrated the increased utility of RNA-based approaches [35].

One thing that is important to note, though, is that not all RNA sequencing is equivalent, and understanding the technical differences among them can be clinically important.

The chemistry for three of the most commonly used clinical assays are shown in Fig. 3.1. In RNA-based sequencing assays, RNA is first converted to cDNA, which then undergoes library preparation for sequencing. Amplicon-based sequencing uses primer pairs designed for each fusion covered by the assay, with one primer binding to each of the fusion partners. If an amplicon is produced, it is sequenced and compared to the reference sequence for the expected fusion. Amplicon-based assays can cover hundreds of known fusions, but because they require a primer for each of the fusion partners, they can only detect the fusion if both partners are included in the assay. The benefit of amplicon-based chemistry is rapid turnaround time and lower nucleic acid input requirements.

In contrast, anchored multiplex PCR employs chemistry capable of detecting fusions in a partner-agnostic manner. Adapters containing universal primer sites are ligated to the cDNA fragments. A PCR reaction using one gene-specific primer and one universal primer complementary to the site on the adapter then amplifies the cDNA fragment. A second, nested PCR reaction using a second gene-specific primer is then performed for specificity. The resulting amplicons can then be sequenced [36].

Hybridization capture-based RNA sequencing uses hybrid-capture probes that are complementary to the coding regions of the gene partner of interest. These probes are able to isolate all RNA transcripts containing a portion of that gene, including any chimeric fusion transcripts. All transcripts are then sequenced to identify any transcripts that support an oncogenic fusion. Like anchored multiplex PCR, hybridization capture-based sequencing is fusion partner agnostic, and only one fusion partner needs to be covered by the assay.

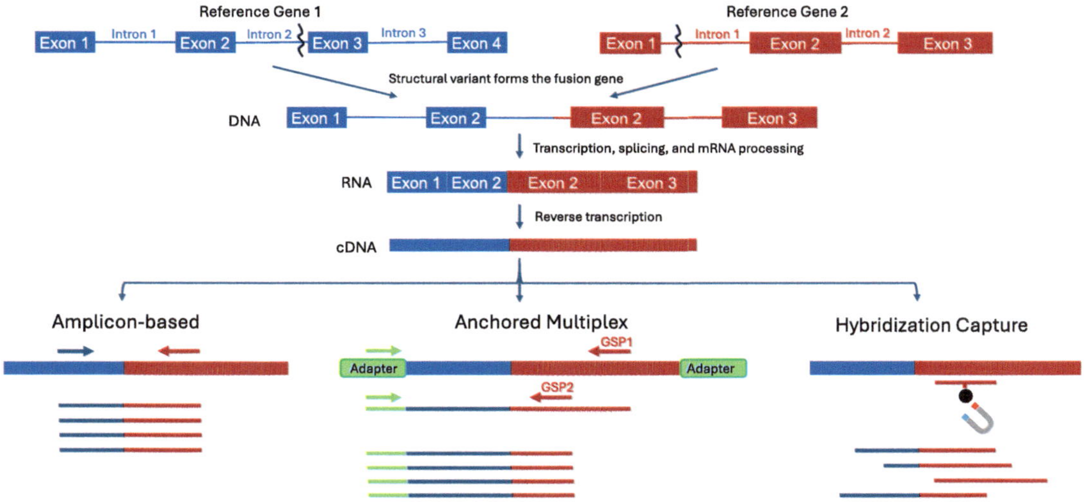

Fig. 3.1 Three commonly used RNA sequencing platforms for oncogenic fusion detection. An illustrative example of a fusion is shown. A structural variant affecting two genes occurs, which could be a large deletion, inversion, or translocation, with breakpoints within introns 1 and 2, respectively. The fusion gene that is formed at the DNA level is then transcribed into RNA, and the introns are removed by cellular splicing machinery to form the messenger RNA that is evaluated by sequencing. In all three platforms, the extracted RNA is first converted to cDNA in the laboratory by reverse transcription. In amplicon-based library preparation, a pair of primers, with one primer for each fusion partner, amplifies the fused gene across the breakpoint, and these amplicons are subsequently sequenced. In anchored multiplex sequencing, adapters, shown in green, are ligated to each end of the cDNA fragments. A series of two nested PCR reactions is then performed, each reaction using one universal primer that hybridizes to a region of the adapter and one gene-specific primer (GSP). Lastly, hybridization capture-based sequencing uses probes complementary to the fusion partner of interest to isolate any transcripts of that gene, including any fusion transcripts. While amplicon-based sequencing requires primers for both fusion partners, both anchored multiplex PCR and hybridization capture-based platforms can identify fusions in a partner-agnostic manner

The technical differences among these assays carry significant clinical implications. Studies have shown that common fusions with well-established breakpoints are able to be detected by all three platforms. However, fusions with novel partners or unusual breakpoints may be missed by amplicon-based sequencing if those partners are not covered by the assay [37, 38].

One single-institutional study described a testing algorithm for NSCLC using amplicon-based DNA and RNA sequencing followed by reflex hybridization capture-based RNA sequencing when initial testing was negative for oncogenic drivers. A total of 1211 NSCLC cases were included in the study, and of these, 321 were negative for oncogenic driver alterations in the initial amplicon-based testing. Reflex testing with hybridization capture-based RNA sequencing was performed on 120 of these, with nine cases harboring clinically significant oncogenic fusions in *ALK*, *BRAF*, *NRG1*, *NTRK3*, *ROS1*, and *RET*. None of these fusions were detected by the amplicon-based assay because they all had rare or novel fusion partners or unusual breakpoints. Overall, this demonstrates that hybridization capture-based RNA sequencing has higher clinical sensitivity for detection of oncogenic fusions with rare or novel fusion partners, maximizing patient eligibility for appropriate targeted therapies or clinical trials [39].

Molecular Biomarkers

In addition to alterations affecting specific genes, there are several molecular biomarkers that have emerged that provide important clinical information and guide treatment decisions. Microsatellite instability and tumor mutational burden status have important implications for patient response to immunotherapy, while homologous recombination deficiency status is associated with response to platinum-based chemotherapy and PARP inhibitors. These molecular biomarkers are assessed by examining global phenotypic changes across the sequencing assay.

Tumor Mutational Burden

Immune checkpoint blockade targeting PD-1 and PD-L1 has revolutionized cancer therapy.

The underlying principle is that tumors with more mutations generate more neoantigens for immune system recognition. When the immune system identifies tumor cells, it can cause tumor cell death, which means that it will be creating more "neoantigens" for the immune system to recognize. Once tumor cells are recognized by the immune system, CD8+ T-cells can be recruited to attack the tumor. Cancer cells are therefore under evolutionary pressure to evade immune surveillance, and cells that are able to effectively downregulate immune recognition through PD-1/PD-L1 signaling or CTLA4 signaling gain survival advantage [40].

Immunotherapies can block these inhibitory interactions and thereby enhance immune system activity. Tumors with higher numbers of neoantigens, as measured by tumor mutational burden, have demonstrated better responses to immunotherapy.

Tumor mutational burden (TMB) is defined as the number of mutations per megabase. The gold standard for tumor mutational burden has traditionally been matched tumor-normal whole exome sequencing. This approach definitively determines which alterations are somatic versus germline, and thereby the entire complement of somatic protein-coding alterations can be determined [41].

While this methodology may provide the most accurate TMB determination, performing whole exome sequencing solely for TMB is not practical. Instead, TMB is often extrapolated from targeted panel sequencing. Foundation Medicine's panel has been FDA-approved as a companion diagnostic for pembrolizumab using a TMB threshold of ten mutations per megabase. However, many other panels can also calculate TMB, and studies have demonstrated variability in TMB calculation [42]. While some have criticized the differences among various panels for determining TMB and used this evidence to push for more regulatory oversight and centralization, it may be that these issues in reality are inherent problems with the biomarker itself and how it is being used. Tumor mutational burden is a continuous number, and reducing it to a single threshold may not account for the complex biology behind it. The range and distribution of tumor mutational burden values vary among different tumor types, and thus a single threshold may be suboptimal [43, 44]. Moreover, tumor biology, microenvironment, and CD8 T-cell infiltration likely play a significant role in how strong of an effect TMB has on efficacy of immunotherapy [45]. Lastly, studies have demonstrated that patient ancestry can affect tumor mutational burden calculation, potentially affecting its accuracy in underrepresented patient populations [46]. In conclusion, while TMB is certainly correlated with response to immunotherapy, there are several inherent issues with the biomarker. Thus, some argue that development of new assays, algorithms, and improvements to this biomarker assessment should be encouraged, not hampered by stifling regulation and oversight.

Microsatellite Instability

Microsatellites, or short tandem repeats (STRs), are highly polymorphic repeated sequences of one to six base pairs of DNA that are scattered throughout both coding and noncoding regions of the genome. There are about one million known STRs in the human genome that comprise about 3% of its sequence, and variations in STR length contributes to normal genetic diversity and are associated with complex traits. However, pathologic expansion of the number of repeats can occur in some diseases such as Huntington's disease or fragile X syndrome. Such repeats are prone to mutations due to slippage of polymerases during DNA synthesis but normally maintain stable lengths through the mismatch repair (MMR) system. When MMR proteins are deficient or absent, replication errors can accumulate that leads to shorter or longer than expected STRs. This phenotype of aberrant STR lengths is referred to as microsatellite instability (MSI).

The MMR system is a highly conserved DNA repair mechanism in prokaryotes and eukaryotes and consists of four key proteins, MLH1, MSH2, MSH6, and PMS2, that interact as heterodimers to repair mismatched nucleotides. These errors can occur from innate processes such as genetic recombination or from external insults such as physical or chemical damage. MSH2/MSH6 binds to mismatched nucleotides and MLH1/PMS2 coordinate excision and synthesis of corrected bases at the mismatch site. Deficient MMR can result from epigenetic mechanisms, like *MLH1* gene promoter hypermethylation, or by genetic inactivation [47].

Immunohistochemistry (IHC) to detect nuclear expression of these four proteins is the most accessible and widely used method for determining MSI due to its low cost and speed. Dysfunction of MLH1 or MSH2 renders their respective heterodimers inactive so that loss of expression of MLH1 or MSH2 also results in loss of expression of PMS2 or MSH6, respectively. Loss of expression of one or more proteins is considered deficient MMR (dMMR) by IHC. However, non-truncating inactivating mutations in MMR genes that preserve antigenicity will appear as falsely proficient MMR (pMMR).

The gold standard method for detecting MSI is PCR amplification of five mononucleotide microsatellite markers, BAT25, BAT26, D2S123, D5S346, and D17S250, along with two pentanucleotide markers to identify sample mix-up and/or contamination. Fluorescently labeled primers that flank these markers are used to generate PCR fragments that can be analyzed through capillary electrophoresis to detect size variations between paired normal tissue and tumor tissue. Tumors with instability in one marker are defined as MSI-Low (MSI-L), and tumors with instability in two or more markers are MSI-High (MSI-H). Those with stability in all markers are designated as stable, or MSS. Similarly, the real-time PCR MSI test on the Idylla automated cartridge system uses fluorescently labeled molecular beacons with melting curve analysis to determine mutations in seven microsatellite markers (ACVR2A, BTBD7, DIDO1, MRE11, RYR3, SEC31A, and SULF2). Here, MSS is defined as less than two mutant markers and MSI as two or more mutant markers [48, 49].

NGS-based MSI detection is increasingly being offered on large targeted cancer gene panels that also report biomarkers like tumor mutation burden. The advantage of NGS is its ability to assess length variations in hundreds to thousands of microsatellites across the genome simultaneously. Most algorithms compare the number of differently sized repeats at each microsatellite locus in a tumor sample against matched normal tissue or a reference population of normal controls. Specifically, within a sample, the number of repeats is determined in every NGS read that fully spans a specific STR locus to determine the distribution of allelic lengths at the locus. Samples that are MSI-H would be expected to generate much more variable allelic lengths with decreased mean allele length since polymerase slippage more frequently results in deletions than insertions. However, NGS can mischaracterize cases with subtle MSI phenotypes, such as in endometrial carcinoma, and PCR capillary electrophoresis methods are preferred instead. STRs located in regions of low sequence complexity or in GC-rich areas can also present challenges for NGS approaches [50–53].

Homologous Recombination Repair Deficiency

DNA can be damaged in many ways, but the most critical events to repair are unintended simultaneous breaks affecting both strands of DNA, or double-strand breaks (DSBs). These can be repaired with high fidelity through the homologous recombination repair (HRR) pathway or suboptimally through more error-prone mechanisms like nonhomologous end joining (NHEJ). HRR utilizes the homologous chromosome as the template for repair, and deficient HRR can result in significant genomic instability with characteristic features. The most well-known genes involved in HRR are *BRCA1* and *BRCA2*, and the most common way homologous recombination deficiency (HRD) occurs is through biallelic inactivation of such genes. This can be leveraged for cancer treatment using the concept of synthetic lethality: drugs inactivating the poly (ADP-ribose) polymerase (PARP) family of proteins involved in base excision repair cause accumulations of single-strand breaks (SSBs) and collapse of replication forks that result in DSBs. These DSBs undergo inefficient NHEJ if there is HRD, resulting in broad genomic instability and subsequent cell death. PARP inhibitors are first-line treatments for breast, ovarian, pancreatic, and prostate cancers with HRD in specific contexts [54, 55].

The HRD score, the most common biomarker to assess HR deficient from HR proficient tumors, is derived from three independent features that reflect structural instability in the genome. It sums the number of observations of each feature in the sample genome: (1) loss of heterozygosity (LOH) limited to subchromosomal regions >15 mB; (2) large scale state transitions (LST) or chromosomal breaks and rearrangements between flanking regions >10 Mb; and (3) telomeric allelic imbalance (TAI) or subchromosomal regions with allelic imbalance that extends to telomeres. This has historically been determined using DNA copy number estimations from single-nucleotide polymorphism (SNP) arrays but has increasingly moved toward whole genome and whole exome sequencing. Targeted NGS platforms have also attempted to derive an HRD score based on much smaller genome coverage [56–59].

Conclusion

Comprehensive genomic profiling is rapidly becoming standard of care for diagnosis, prognosis, and therapeutic decision-making in solid tumors. Assays today are able to identify many attributes of tumor molecular pathology with significant clinical impact, and oncologists and other treating clinicians are increasingly relying on these clinical tests. As the field continues to advance, these tests will continue to be refined, bringing new technologies and new biomarkers into the clinical laboratory.

References

1. Skoulidis F, Heymach JV. Co-occurring genomic alterations in non-small-cell lung cancer biology and therapy. Nat Rev Cancer. 2019;19(9):495–509. https://doi.org/10.1038/s41568-019-0179-8.
2. Soda M, Choi YL, Enomoto M, Takada S, Yamashita Y, Ishikawa S, et al. Identification of the transforming EML4-ALK fusion gene in non-small-cell lung cancer. Nature. 2007;448(7153):561–6. https://doi.org/10.1038/nature05945.
3. Davies KD, Le AT, Theodoro MF, Skokan MC, Aisner DL, Berge EM, et al. Identifying and targeting ROS1 gene fusions in non-small cell lung cancer. Clin Cancer Res. 2012;18(17):4570–9. https://doi.org/10.1158/1078-0432.Ccr-12-0550.
4. Wang R, Hu H, Pan Y, Li Y, Ye T, Li C, et al. RET fusions define a unique molecular and clinicopathologic subtype of non-small-cell lung cancer. J Clin Oncol. 2012;30(35):4352–9. https://doi.org/10.1200/jco.2012.44.1477.
5. Paez JG, Jänne PA, Lee JC, Tracy S, Greulich H, Gabriel S, et al. EGFR mutations in lung cancer: correlation with clinical response to gefitinib therapy. Science. 2004;304(5676):1497–500. https://doi.org/10.1126/science.1099314.
6. Mosele MF, Westphalen CB, Stenzinger A, Barlesi F, Bayle A, Bièche I, et al. Recommendations for the use of next-generation sequencing (NGS) for patients with advanced cancer in 2024: a report from the ESMO Precision Medicine Working Group. Ann Oncol. 2024;35(7):588–606. https://doi.org/10.1016/j.annonc.2024.04.005.
7. Kontomanolis EN, Koutras A, Syllaios A, Schizas D, Mastoraki A, Garmpis N, et al. Role of oncogenes and tumor-suppressor genes in carcinogenesis: a review. Anticancer Res. 2020;40(11):6009–15. https://doi.org/10.21873/anticanres.14622.
8. Alharbi KS, Javed Shaikh MA, Afzal O, Alfawaz Altamimi AS, Almalki WH, Alzarea SI, et al. An overview of epithelial growth factor receptor (EGFR) inhibitors in cancer therapy. Chem Biol Interact. 2022;366:110108. https://doi.org/10.1016/j.cbi.2022.110108.
9. Scaltriti M, Baselga J. The epidermal growth factor receptor pathway: a model for targeted therapy. Clin Cancer Res. 2006;12(18):5268–72. https://doi.org/10.1158/1078-0432.Ccr-05-1554.
10. Kris MG, Natale RB, Herbst RS, Lynch TJ Jr, Prager D, Belani CP, et al. Efficacy of gefitinib, an inhibitor of the epidermal growth factor receptor

tyrosine kinase, in symptomatic patients with non-small cell lung cancer: a randomized trial. JAMA. 2003;290(16):2149–58. https://doi.org/10.1001/jama.290.16.2149.
11. Mok TS, Wu YL, Thongprasert S, Yang CH, Chu DT, Saijo N, et al. Gefitinib or carboplatin-paclitaxel in pulmonary adenocarcinoma. N Engl J Med. 2009;361(10):947–57. https://doi.org/10.1056/NEJMoa0810699.
12. Lee EY, Muller WJ. Oncogenes and tumor suppressor genes. Cold Spring Harb Perspect Biol. 2010;2(10):a003236. https://doi.org/10.1101/cshperspect.a003236.
13. Rose M, Burgess JT, O'Byrne K, Richard DJ, Bolderson E. PARP inhibitors: clinical relevance, mechanisms of action and tumor resistance. Front Cell Dev Biol. 2020;8:564601. https://doi.org/10.3389/fcell.2020.564601.
14. Wolff AC, Hammond MEH, Allison KH, Harvey BE, Mangu PB, Bartlett JMS, et al. Human epidermal growth factor receptor 2 testing in breast cancer: American society of clinical oncology/college of American pathologists clinical practice guideline focused update. J Clin Oncol. 2018;36(20):2105–22. https://doi.org/10.1200/jco.2018.77.8738.
15. Wolff AC, Somerfield MR, Dowsett M, Hammond MEH, Hayes DF, McShane LM, et al. Human epidermal growth factor receptor 2 testing in breast cancer: ASCO-College of American Pathologists Guideline Update. J Clin Oncol. 2023;41(22):3867–72. https://doi.org/10.1200/jco.22.02864.
16. Wolf J, Seto T, Han JY, Reguart N, Garon EB, HJM G, et al. Capmatinib in MET exon 14-mutated or MET-amplified non-small-cell lung cancer. N Engl J Med. 2020;383(10):944–57. https://doi.org/10.1056/NEJMoa2002787.
17. Cappuzzo F, Marchetti A, Skokan M, Rossi E, Gajapathy S, Felicioni L, et al. Increased MET gene copy number negatively affects survival of surgically resected non-small-cell lung cancer patients. J Clin Oncol. 2009;27(10):1667–74. https://doi.org/10.1200/jco.2008.19.1635.
18. Solomon JP, Yang SR, Choudhury NJ, Ptashkin RN, Eslamdoost N, Falcon CJ, et al. Bioinformatically expanded next-generation sequencing analysis optimizes identification of therapeutically relevant MET copy number alterations in >50,000 tumors. Clin Cancer Res. 2022;28(21):4649–59. https://doi.org/10.1158/1078-0432.Ccr-22-1321.
19. Ross DS, Zehir A, Cheng DT, Benayed R, Nafa K, Hechtman JF, et al. Next-generation assessment of human epidermal growth factor receptor 2 (ERBB2) amplification status: clinical validation in the context of a hybrid capture-based, comprehensive solid tumor genomic profiling assay. J Mol Diagn. 2017;19(2):244–54. https://doi.org/10.1016/j.jmoldx.2016.09.010.
20. Shen R, Seshan VE. FACETS: allele-specific copy number and clonal heterogeneity analysis tool for high-throughput DNA sequencing. Nucleic Acids Res. 2016;44(16):e131. https://doi.org/10.1093/nar/gkw520.
21. Ma L, Chung WK. Quantitative analysis of copy number variants based on real-time LightCycler PCR. Curr Protoc Hum Genet. 2014;80:7.21.1–7..8. https://doi.org/10.1002/0471142905.hg0721s80.
22. Ren R. Mechanisms of BCR-ABL in the pathogenesis of chronic myelogenous leukaemia. Nat Rev Cancer. 2005;5(3):172–83. https://doi.org/10.1038/nrc1567.
23. Zhu G, Benayed R, Ho C, Mullaney K, Sukhadia P, Rios K, et al. Diagnosis of known sarcoma fusions and novel fusion partners by targeted RNA sequencing with identification of a recurrent ACTB-FOSB fusion in pseudomyogenic hemangioendothelioma. Mod Pathol. 2019;32(5):609–20. https://doi.org/10.1038/s41379-018-0175-7.
24. Rosen EY, Goldman DA, Hechtman JF, Benayed R, Schram AM, Cocco E, et al. TRK fusions are enriched in cancers with uncommon histologies and the absence of canonical driver mutations. Clin Cancer Res. 2020;26(7):1624–32. https://doi.org/10.1158/1078-0432.Ccr-19-3165.
25. Solomon JP, Linkov I, Rosado A, Mullaney K, Rosen EY, Frosina D, et al. NTRK fusion detection across multiple assays and 33,997 cases: diagnostic implications and pitfalls. Mod Pathol. 2020;33(1):38–46. https://doi.org/10.1038/s41379-019-0324-7.
26. Drilon A, Laetsch TW, Kummar S, DuBois SG, Lassen UN, Demetri GD, et al. Efficacy of larotrectinib in TRK fusion-positive cancers in adults and children. N Engl J Med. 2018;378(8):731–9. https://doi.org/10.1056/NEJMoa1714448.
27. Doebele RC, Drilon A, Paz-Ares L, Siena S, Shaw AT, Farago AF, et al. Entrectinib in patients with advanced or metastatic NTRK fusion-positive solid tumours: integrated analysis of three phase 1-2 trials. Lancet Oncol. 2020;21(2):271–82. https://doi.org/10.1016/s1470-2045(19)30691-6.
28. Rais T, Shakeel A, Naseem L, Nasser N, Aamir M. Repotrectinib: a promising new therapy for advanced nonsmall cell lung cancer. Ann Med Surg (Lond). 2024;86(12):7265–9. https://doi.org/10.1097/ms9.0000000000002717.
29. Solomon JP, Hechtman JF. Detection of NTRK fusions: merits and limitations of current diagnostic platforms. Cancer Res. 2019;79(13):3163–8. https://doi.org/10.1158/0008-5472.Can-19-0372.
30. Wynes MW, Sholl LM, Dietel M, Schuuring E, Tsao MS, Yatabe Y, et al. An international interpretation study using the ALK IHC antibody D5F3 and a sensitive detection kit demonstrates high concordance between ALK IHC and ALK FISH and between evaluators. J Thorac Oncol. 2014;9(5):631–8. https://doi.org/10.1097/jto.0000000000000115.
31. Uruga H, Mino-Kenudson M. ALK (D5F3) CDx: an immunohistochemistry assay to identify ALK-positive NSCLC patients. Pharmgenomics Pers Med.

2018;11:147–55. https://doi.org/10.2147/pgpm.S156672.
32. Dülger O, Öz B. Comparison of different ROS1 immunohistochemistry clones and consistency with fluorescence in situ hybridization results in non-small cell lung carcinoma. Balkan Med J. 2023;40(5):344–50. https://doi.org/10.4274/balkanmedj.galenos.2023.2022-12-88.
33. Cheng L, Zhang S, Wang L, MacLennan GT, Davidson DD. Fluorescence in situ hybridization in surgical pathology: principles and applications. J Pathol Clin Res. 2017;3(2):73–99. https://doi.org/10.1002/cjp2.64.
34. Levy B, Baughn LB, Akkari Y, Chartrand S, LaBarge B, Claxton D, et al. Optical genome mapping in acute myeloid leukemia: a multicenter evaluation. Blood Adv. 2023;7(7):1297–307. https://doi.org/10.1182/bloodadvances.2022007583.
35. Benayed R, Offin M, Mullaney K, Sukhadia P, Rios K, Desmeules P, et al. High yield of RNA sequencing for targetable kinase fusions in lung adenocarcinomas with no mitogenic driver alteration detected by DNA sequencing and low tumor mutation burden. Clin Cancer Res. 2019;25(15):4712–22. https://doi.org/10.1158/1078-0432.Ccr-19-0225.
36. Zheng Z, Liebers M, Zhelyazkova B, Cao Y, Panditi D, Lynch KD, et al. Anchored multiplex PCR for targeted next-generation sequencing. Nat Med. 2014;20(12):1479–84. https://doi.org/10.1038/nm.3729.
37. Park HJ, Baek I, Cheang G, Solomon JP, Song W. Comparison of RNA-based next-generation sequencing assays for the detection of NTRK gene fusions. J Mol Diagn. 2021;23(11):1443–51. https://doi.org/10.1016/j.jmoldx.2021.07.027.
38. Qu X, Yeung C, Coleman I, Nelson PS, Fang M. Comparison of four next generation sequencing platforms for fusion detection: Oncomine by ThermoFisher, AmpliSeq by illumina, FusionPlex by ArcherDX, and QIAseq by QIAGEN. Cancer Genet. 2020;243:11–8. https://doi.org/10.1016/j.cancergen.2020.02.007.
39. Dillard A, Xu K, Sun Y, Lin HH, Shen C, Song E, et al. Comparison of targeted RNA-sequencing platforms for oncogenic fusion detection in non-small-cell lung cancer. J Mol Diagn. 2025;27(6):438–45. https://doi.org/10.1016/j.jmoldx.2025.02.007.
40. Yi M, Zheng X, Niu M, Zhu S, Ge H, Wu K. Combination strategies with PD-1/PD-L1 blockade: current advances and future directions. Mol Cancer. 2022;21(1):28. https://doi.org/10.1186/s12943-021-01489-2.
41. Sha D, Jin Z, Budczies J, Kluck K, Stenzinger A, Sinicrope FA. Tumor mutational burden as a predictive biomarker in solid tumors. Cancer Discov. 2020;10(12):1808–25. https://doi.org/10.1158/2159-8290.Cd-20-0522.
42. Vega DM, Yee LM, McShane LM, Williams PM, Chen L, Vilimas T, et al. Aligning tumor mutational burden (TMB) quantification across diagnostic platforms: phase II of the friends of cancer research TMB harmonization project. Ann Oncol. 2021;32(12):1626–36. https://doi.org/10.1016/j.annonc.2021.09.016.
43. Aggarwal C, Ben-Shachar R, Gao Y, Hyun SW, Rivers Z, Epstein C, et al. Assessment of tumor mutational burden and outcomes in patients with diverse advanced cancers treated with immunotherapy. JAMA Netw Open. 2023;6(5):e2311181. https://doi.org/10.1001/jamanetworkopen.2023.11181.
44. Fernandez EM, Eng K, Beg S, Beltran H, Faltas BM, Mosquera JM, et al. Cancer-specific thresholds adjust for whole exome sequencing-based tumor mutational burden distribution. JCO Precis Oncol. 2019;3:1–12. https://doi.org/10.1200/po.18.00400.
45. McGrail DJ, Pilié PG, Rashid NU, Voorwerk L, Slagter M, Kok M, et al. High tumor mutation burden fails to predict immune checkpoint blockade response across all cancer types. Ann Oncol. 2021;32(5):661–72. https://doi.org/10.1016/j.annonc.2021.02.006.
46. Nassar AH, Adib E, Abou Alaiwi S, El Zarif T, Groha S, Akl EW, et al. Ancestry-driven recalibration of tumor mutational burden and disparate clinical outcomes in response to immune checkpoint inhibitors. Cancer Cell. 2022;40(10):1161–72.e5. https://doi.org/10.1016/j.ccell.2022.08.022.
47. Vilar E, Gruber SB. Microsatellite instability in colorectal cancer-the stable evidence. Nat Rev Clin Oncol. 2010;7(3):153–62. https://doi.org/10.1038/nrclinonc.2009.237.
48. Bacher JW, Flanagan LA, Smalley RL, Nassif NA, Burgart LJ, Halberg RB, et al. Development of a fluorescent multiplex assay for detection of MSI-high tumors. Dis Markers. 2004;20(4–5):237–50. https://doi.org/10.1155/2004/136734.
49. Ukkola I, Nummela P, Kero M, Ristimäki A. Diagnostic performance of Idylla MSI test in colorectal cancer biopsies. Diagn Pathol. 2023;18(1):39. https://doi.org/10.1186/s13000-023-01328-6.
50. Zhao P, Li L, Jiang X, Li Q. Mismatch repair deficiency/microsatellite instability-high as a predictor for anti-PD-1/PD-L1 immunotherapy efficacy. J Hematol Oncol. 2019;12(1):54. https://doi.org/10.1186/s13045-019-0738-1.
51. Bartels S, Grote I, Wagner M, Boog J, Schipper E, Reineke-Plaass T, et al. Concordance in detection of microsatellite instability by PCR and NGS in routinely processed tumor specimens of several cancer types. Cancer Med. 2023;12(16):16707–15. https://doi.org/10.1002/cam4.6293.
52. Tanudisastro HA, Deveson IW, Dashnow H, MacArthur DG. Sequencing and characterizing short tandem repeats in the human genome. Nat Rev Genet. 2024;25(7):460–75. https://doi.org/10.1038/s41576-024-00692-3.
53. Trabucco SE, Gowen K, Maund SL, Sanford E, Fabrizio DA, Hall MJ, et al. A novel next-generation sequencing approach to detecting microsatellite instability and pan-tumor characterization of 1000 microsatellite instability-high cases in 67,000 patient samples. J Mol Diagn. 2019;21(6):1053–66. https://doi.org/10.1016/j.jmoldx.2019.06.011.

54. Stewart MD, Merino Vega D, Arend RC, Baden JF, Barbash O, Beaubier N, et al. Homologous recombination deficiency: concepts, definitions, and assays. Oncologist. 2022;27(3):167–74. https://doi.org/10.1093/oncolo/oyab053.
55. Doig KD, Fellowes AP, Fox SB. Homologous recombination repair deficiency: an overview for pathologists. Mod Pathol. 2023;36(3):100049. https://doi.org/10.1016/j.modpat.2022.100049.
56. Wagener-Ryczek S, Merkelbach-Bruse S, Siemanowski J. Biomarkers for homologous recombination deficiency in cancer. J Pers Med. 2021;11(7):612. https://doi.org/10.3390/jpm11070612.
57. de Luca XM, Newell F, Kazakoff SH, Hartel G, McCart Reed AE, Holmes O, et al. Using whole-genome sequencing data to derive the homologous recombination deficiency scores. NPJ Breast Cancer. 2020;6:33. https://doi.org/10.1038/s41523-020-0172-0.
58. Kim YN, Gulhan DC, Jin H, Glodzik D, Park PJ. Recent advances in genomic approaches for the detection of homologous recombination deficiency. Cancer Res Treat. 2024;56(4):975–90. https://doi.org/10.4143/crt.2024.154.
59. Hsiao SJ, Black D, Devereaux KA, Hagemann IS, Jennings LJ, Mandelker D, et al. Recommendations for clinical molecular Laboratories for Detection of homologous recombination deficiency in cancer: a joint consensus recommendation of the Association for Molecular Pathology, Association of Cancer Care Centers, and College of American Pathologists. J Mol Diagn. 2025;27(8):685–704. https://doi.org/10.1016/j.jmoldx.2025.05.003.

4 Gastrointestinal and Pancreatic Pathology

Jessica Gasparello, Claudio Luchini, and Matteo Fassan

Abbreviations

ARID1A	AT-Rich Interaction Domain 1A
ASCL2	Achaete-Scute Family BHLH Transcription Factor 2
ACRG	Asian Cancer Research Group
ADCs	antibody-drug conjugates
AJCC	American Joint Committee on Cancer
ASCO	American Society of Clinical Oncology
APC	adenomatous polyposis coli
BRAF	V-Raf Murine Sarcoma Viral Oncogene Homolog B
CIN	chromosome instability
CPS	combined positive score
CMS	consensus molecular subtypes
CRC	colorectal cancer
CNVs	copy number variants
CIN	chromosomal instable
CDKN2A	Cyclin Dependent Kinase Inhibitor 2A
ChIP	chromatin immunoprecipitation
CTNNA1	Catenin Alpha 1
CDH1	Cadherin 1
CGP	comprehensive genomic profiling
DSBR	double-strand break repair
EMT	epithelial to mesenchymal transition
ERBB2	v-erb-b2 avian erythroblastic leukemia viral oncogene homolog 2
ESMO	European Society of Medical Oncology
ESCAT	ESMO Scale for Clinical Actionability of molecular Targets
EORTC	European Organization of Research and Treatment of Cancer
EGFR	epidermal growth factor receptor
EBV	Epstein-Barr virus
FAP	familial adenomatous polyposis
FGFR2	fibroblast growth factor receptor 2

J. Gasparello
Department of Medicine (DIMED), University of Padua, Padua, Italy
e-mail: jessica.gasparello@unipd.it

C. Luchini
Surgical Pathology Unit, Verona University Hospital Trust, Verona, Italy

Department of Diagnostics and Public Health, Section of Pathology, University of Verona, Verona, Italy

Arc-Net Research Center, University of Verona, Verona, Italy
e-mail: claudio.luchini@univr.it

M. Fassan (✉)
Department of Medicine (DIMED), University of Padua, Padua, Italy

Surgical Pathology Unit, Azienda ULSS2, Marca Trevigiana, Treviso, Italy

Veneto Institute of Oncology (IOV-IRCCS), Padua, Italy
e-mail: matteo.fassan@unipd.it

© The Author(s), under exclusive license to Springer Nature Switzerland AG 2026

S. Sioletic, L. Coppola (eds.), *Next-Generation Sequencing in Solid Tumor Histopathology*, Current Clinical Pathology, https://doi.org/10.1007/978-3-032-18790-1_4

FFPE	formalin-fixed, paraffin-embedded
FISH	fluorescence in situ hybridization
FAMMM	familial atypical multiple mole melanoma syndrome
GEPs	gene expression profiles
GC	gastric
GS	genomically stable
GEJ	gastroesophageal junction cancers
GAPPS	gastric adenocarcinoma and proximal polyposis of the stomach
HRD	homologous repair deficiency
HER2	human epidermal growth factor receptor 2
HRR	homologous recombination repair
HNPCC	hereditary nonpolyposis colorectal cancer
HBOC	hereditary breast and ovarian cancer syndrome
HDGC	hereditary diffuse gastric cancer
HR	homologous recombination
indels	insertions or deletions
IHC	immunohistochemistry
ICIs	immune checkpoint inhibitors
IGCLC	International Gastric Cancer Linkage Consortium
KRAS	Kirsten Rat Sarcoma Viral Proto-Oncogene
JAK2	Janus Kinase 2
NGS	next-generation sequencing
lncRNAs	long noncoding RNAs
MRD	minimal residual disease
MSI	microsatellite instability
MTAP	methylthioadenosine phosphorylase
MYC	V-Myc Avian Myelocytomatosis Viral Oncogene Homolog
MAPK	Mitogen-activated protein kinases
MMR	DNA mismatch repair mechanism
mGC	metastatic gastric cancer
mAbs	monoclonal antibodies
MLH1	MutL Homolog 1
MSH2	MutS Homolog 2
MSH6	MutS Homolog 6
mRNAs	messenger RNAs
MAP	MUTYH-associated polyposis
NRAS	neuroblastoma RAS viral v-ras oncogene homolog
NTRK	neurotrophic receptor tyrosine kinase
NGS	next-generation sequencing
NRG1	Neuregulin 1
OS	overall survival
PC	pancreatic cancers
POLE	polymerase epsilon
QM	quasi-mesenchymal
RFS	recurrence-free survival
RHOA	Ras Homolog Family Member A
PD-1	programmed cell death protein 1
PanIN	pancreatic intraepithelial neoplasia
PD-L1	programmed death-ligand 1
PCR	polymerase chain reaction
PARPi	poly ADP-ribose polymerase inhibitors
SNVs	single-nucleotide variants
scRNA-seq	single-cell RNA sequencing
TMB	tumor mutational burden
TF	transcription factor
TGF-β	transforming growth factor-beta
TME	tumor microenvironment
TCGA	The Cancer Genome Atlas
TRKi	tyrosine kinase inhibitors
TMB-H	high tumor mutational burden
UICC	Union for International Cancer Control
WNT	wingless-type MMTV integration site family
WGS	whole-genome sequencing
WES	whole-exome sequencing

Introduction

The landscape of tumor treatment has undergone a dramatic transformation in the last decade. Conventional therapeutic approaches, such as chemotherapy and radiation therapy, are now complemented or replaced by advanced treatment modalities, including antibody-drug conjugates (ADCs), cell-based therapies, and gene therapies, which enable personalized targeting of tumors [1]. This revolution has also had an impact on gastrointestinal malignancies, encompassing colorectal cancer (CRC), esophageal and gastric cancer (GC), gastroesophageal junction cancers (GEJ), and pancreatic cancers (PC), albeit with notable distinctions. The fundamental prerequisite for personalized cancer treatment is acquiring a comprehensive biological understanding of cancer pathophysiology and identifying the molecular alterations driving cancer onset and progression. Consequently, the primary driving force for the emergence of precision oncology was the development of next-generation sequencing (NGS), a technology that facilitates rapid and cost-effective molecular characterization of tumors [2].

Next-Generation Sequencing in Gastrointestinal Tumors: Clinical Practice

The advent of NGS has caused a paradigm shift in the landscape of molecular testing techniques in oncology. Over the past decade, NGS has transitioned gradually from the research field to routine clinical practice [3]. We are currently in the middle of the clinical genomics era, wherein NGS has become an indispensable diagnostic tool. NGS is routinely employed in clinical practice to identify somatic driver mutations and germline mutations for the detection of hereditary cancer syndromes [4]. Moreover, it is used for the early detection of resistance mechanisms, to monitor the minimal residual disease (MRD), and for the quantification of mutational burden to predict the response to immunotherapy [5, 6]. As a result, NGS is an indispensable tool for treatment guidance and follow-up. Several commercial and in-house NGS panels are now available with different coverage and turnaround times. NGS-based diagnostics encompass two distinct approaches: (i) hotspot or targeted panels capable of sequencing parts (frequently mutated exons) of genes (typically less than 50) commonly altered in cancer and (ii) comprehensive genomic profiling (CGP) which involves the sequencing of the entire coding regions (all exons and in some cases "hot" introns or promoters) of multiple (from 50 to approximately 500) cancer-relevant genes [7]. CGP panels are designed for the identification of the most common genomic aberrations, including single-nucleotide variants (SNVs), copy number variants (CNVs), small insertions or deletions (indels), and gene rearrangements. These panels also detect genetic signatures, including microsatellite instability (MSI), tumor mutational burden (TMB), and homologous repair deficiency (HRD). Despite the European Society of Medical Oncology's (ESMO) 2020 recommendation for the implementation of CGP for select tumor types, at least in academic centers, the integration of CGP into the clinical workflow remains challenging due to infrastructure requirements, turnaround times, expertise, and reimbursement policies [8–10]. In light of the aforementioned issues, the cost-benefit balance remains ambiguous [9]. Several independent studies conducted in different solid tumors have demonstrated the low actionability of CGP results. For instance, Hilal et al. in a study of 2017 observed that the CGP assay identified actionable genomic variants in 92% of patients. However, only 12% of patients received targeted therapy, and only 2% obtained clinical benefits [11]. In a more recent work, in 2025, when the number of druggable alterations progressively increased, Schettini and colleagues, within the "MOZART" study, considered 304 adult patients with heavily pretreated metastatic cancers who were treated between January 2019 and March 2021 [12]. The 78% of them harbored potentially actionable genomic alterations, but only 34.5% were actionable ESCAT (ESMO Scale for Clinical Actionability of molecular Targets) Tier I or II alterations, and the prevalence, as expected, varied according to cancer type [13]. Of the 304 patients, only 20.4% were treated according to CGP panel results [12].

Comprehensive Genomic Profiling in Gastrointestinal and Pancreatic Tumors in Clinical Practice

In the gastrointestinal setting, the employment of CGP is being extensively studied [14–17]. A survey of the European Organization of Research and Treatment of Cancer (EORTC)

Gastrointestinal Tract Cancer Working Group, involving 45 oncologists from 41 European institutions, reveals that in upper gastrointestinal cancers (including esophageal, stomach, pancreatic, duodenal, gallbladder and bile duct, as well as liver and small bowel cancers), comprehensive tissue gene panels for advanced unresectable or metastatic tumors are a routine practice in 84% of the interviewed centers. In the 70% of the centers, CGP analyses are performed as a standard of care and reimbursed, while in the remaining cases, tests are funded through clinical trials. The most prevalent approach involves the employment of custom panels, which encompass a range of 50–500 genes, along with the Illumina TruSight Oncology 500 HT (comprising 523 genes). This approach accounts for 22% of all cases, followed by the FoundationOne CDx (324 genes), employed in 20% of the centers. Unfortunately, the percentage of patients treated with targeted agents, based on CGP data, is still limited—indeed, the majority of centers report that less than 25% of molecularly tested patients are treated based on the comprehensive genetic testing [14]. Thus, also in gastrointestinal oncology, the real "Achilles heel" still remains the actionability. Despite the evident advantage of CGP in identifying a considerably higher number of genetic alterations, including actionable mutations, the extent to which patients benefit from comprehensive profiling receiving targeted drugs based on NGS data remains uncertain. The clinical utility of the CGP approach in gastrointestinal and pancreatic malignancies appears to be multifaceted and closely dependent on tumor features, such as the site of neoplasm and its stage. It is also related to access to therapies and insurance coverage. For instance, despite the advent of novel targetable therapies, these treatments may not be utilized as frontline options. At the 2025 ASCO (American Society of Clinical Oncology) Gastrointestinal Cancers Symposium, a study was presented that retrospectively evaluated the impact of CGP testing on treatment outcome for patients with advanced gastrointestinal cancer. The study cohort is heavily influenced by advanced-stage colon cancers, which represent about half (48%) of all investigated cases. Druggable mutations were identified in 59.74% of patients, leading to FDA-approved targeted therapies for 44.16%, while 79.22% of patients were eligible for clinical trials. It is noteworthy that the impact of CGP was considerably less when first-line treatments were considered. Indeed, a modest 6.49% of patients received a first-line treatment based on the CGP outcome [18]. However, the practical application of molecular testing to guide patient treatment is currently limited in the case of pancreatic cancers. Lowery et al. reported that of the 336 patients who were tested with a panel of 410 cancer-associated genes, only 1% received a matched therapy based upon the sequencing results [19].

Genomic Landscape and Druggable Targets of Gastrointestinal and Pancreatic Malignancies

Despite the conventional classification of cancers based on anatomic site, histological features, morphologic grade, and the AJCC/UICC TNM stage, the advent of NGS and the subsequent The Cancer Genome Atlas (TCGA) program, launched in 2006, have enabled the identification of previously inconceivable cancer heterogeneity [20]. TGCA has facilitated the multiomic characterization of 33 cancer types, encompassing genomic, epigenomic, transcriptomic, and proteomic profiles. This comprehensive characterization has unveiled molecular subtypes within different cancer types, providing crucial insights into disease progression and prognosis. Moreover, these findings have significantly enhanced the development of targeted therapeutic approaches, offering patients more precise and effective treatment options.

Colorectal Cancer

Colorectal Cancer: TGCA Classification

According to the CRC molecular classification, four different consensus molecular subtypes (CMS) were identified [21]. CMS1, also defined as "MSI immune," encompasses 14% of all CRCs. CMS1 is characterized by microsatellite instability, marked immune activation, an increase in the expression of genes associated with a diffuse immune infiltrate, *V-Raf Murine Sarcoma Viral Oncogene Homolog B (BRAF)* mutations, and a widespread hypermethylation status. CMS1 tumors were frequently diagnosed in females with right-sided lesions and presented with higher histopathological grade [22]. In cases of nonmetastatic disease, the CMS1 subtype has a relatively favorable prognosis. Conversely, in the metastatic setting, CMS1 is characterized by worse survival than CMS2–4. CMS2 (canonical subtype) accounts for 37% of all CRC cases and is characterized by epithelial differentiation and strong upregulation of WNT (wingless-type MMTV integration site family) and MYC (V-Myc Avian Myelocytomatosis Viral Oncogene Homolog) downstream targets, which are involved in CRC cancerogenesis. It presents a high number of copy number alterations, including gains of oncogenes and losses of tumor suppressor genes. The majority of cases were documented on the left side, and the prognosis was relatively favorable in both local disease and metastatic settings. CMS2 demonstrated the most favorable overall survival (OS) compared with CMS1 and CMS3–4 [23]. CMS3 (metabolic subtype) constitutes 13% of CRC cases and is defined by *KRAS (Kirsten Rat Sarcoma Viral Proto-Oncogene)* mutations, resulting in RAS and MAPK (Mitogen-activated protein kinases) signaling hyperactivation. CMS3 is characterized by the enrichment of mRNAs involved in metabolic processes, including glutamine, fatty acid, and lysophospholipid metabolism. Compared with CMS1 and CMS2, CMS3 is characterized by less hypermethylation and chromosome instability (CIN). The majority of CMS3 cancers do not have identifiable therapeutic gene targets, despite the potential benefit of adjuvant chemotherapy [24]. CMS4 (mesenchymal subtype) is characterized by the upregulation of genes involved in epithelial to mesenchymal transition (EMT) and in molecular signatures associated with the activation of transforming growth factor-beta (TGF-β) signaling and angiogenesis. This could provide the rationale for the observed increased aggressiveness of CMS4. CMS4 cancers have been shown to exhibit a poorer OS and are often diagnosed at advanced stages (III and IV) [23].

Colorectal Cancer: Genomic Alterations According to ESCAT

Molecular testing is a standard procedure in the management of CRC patients, particularly in cases of advanced or metastatic disease. In the 2020 Recommendations for the use of NGS for patients with metastatic cancers, the ESMO Precision Medicine Working Group identified the search for *KRAS*, *NRAS* (*neuroblastoma RAS viral v-ras oncogene homolog*) and *BRAF* mutations, analysis of *ERBB2* (*v-erb-b2 avian erythroblastic leukemia viral oncogene homolog 2*) amplification, the study of the expression of DNA mismatch repair mechanism (MMR) proteins, and the search for *NTRK* (*neurotrophic receptor tyrosine kinase*) fusions as essential molecular biomarkers to be tested (Fig. 4.1) [25]. Hotspot *RAS* mutations encompassing *KRAS* (exon 2: codons 12 and 13; exon 3 and 4) and *NRAS* (exons 2, 3, 4) have been shown to predict resistance to EGFR (epidermal growth factor receptor) monoclonal antibodies (mAbs) in metastatic CRC. In the majority of cases, *BRAF* mutations (ESCAT IA) are almost exclusive and do not overlap with *RAS* mutations [13]. *BRAF* mutations have been identified as a significant negative prognostic marker for patients diagnosed with mCRC. Furthermore, the results of the BREAKWATER phase III trial demonstrated that the combination of encorafenib (a BRAF inhibitor) and cetuximab resulted in a substantial survival benefit in patients harboring *BRAF* V600E

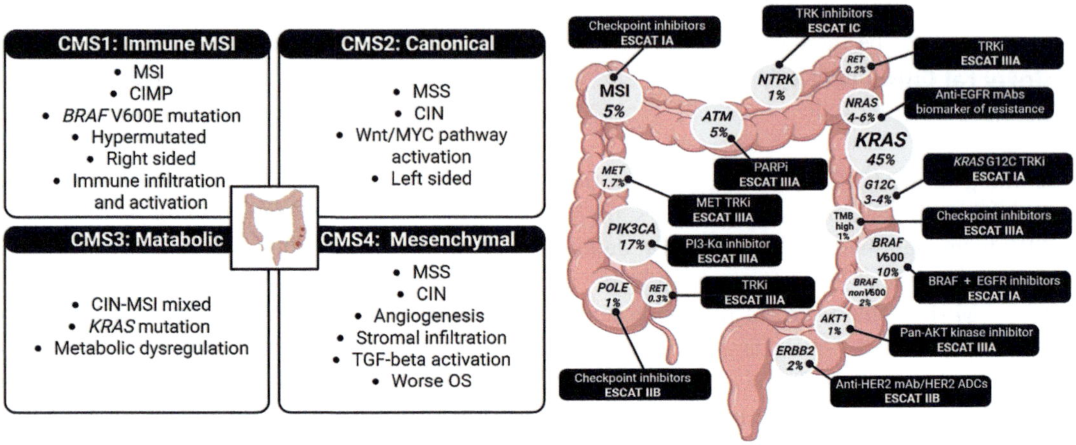

Fig. 4.1 The molecular landscape of colorectal cancer. In the left part of the figure, the four molecular CRC subtypes (consensus molecular subtypes (CMS)) are summarized, reporting principal molecular features. Principal actionable alterations in advanced CRC, according to the 2020 and 2024 guidelines of the ESMO Precision Medicine Working Group. *CIN* chromosomal instability, *CIMP* CpG island methylator phenotype, *MSS* microsatellite stable, *MSI* microsatellite instability, *OS* overall survival, *ADCs* antibody-drug conjugates, *PARPi* poly(ADP-ribose) polymerase1 inhibitor, *TRKi* receptor kinase (TRK) inhibitors

mutation [26]. In the context of CRC patients, the amplification of the *ERBB2* oncogene (ESCAT IIB) is present in less than 5% of cases, representing a druggable target using an antibody-drug conjugate: trastuzumab deruxtecan. Trastuzumab deruxtecan (DESTINY-CRC01 [27]) may be administered in combination with tyrosine kinase inhibitors (TRKi), such as lapatinib (HERACLES trial [28]) or tucatinib (MOUNTAINEER trial [29]) or pertuzumab (MyPathway trial [30]). The amplification of *ERBB2* and the subsequent hyper-expression of HER2 (human epidermal growth factor receptor 2) have been firmly established as negative predictive biomarkers in mCRC, thereby impeding the effectiveness of anti-EGFR targeted therapy. Rearrangements of the neurotrophic receptor tyrosine kinase (*NTRK*)—*NTRK1*, *NTRK2,* and *NTRK3* genes (ESCAT IC)—are of relevance in CRC, although their prevalence is very low (1.5%). *NTRK* rearrangements are predictive biomarkers for the response to TRK inhibitors as larotrectinib, which has been shown to be effective in a broad range of cancers [31]. MSI is a change (deletion or insertion) in repeated units in the microsatellite sequences in a tumor compared with normal tissue. Approximately 15% of the CRCs are MSI due to the hereditary mutations related to Lynch syndrome (3%) or somatic inactivation of the mismatch repair proteins. Despite the fact that the activity of the mismatch repair machinery is typically confirmed through immunohistochemistry (IHC), an NGS panel capable of detecting alterations in microsatellite loci can be useful for identifying patients with MSI (ESCAT 1A) who are eligible for immune checkpoint inhibitors (ICIs), as pembrolizumab [32] or the doublet nivolumab plus ipilimumab [33]. The recent revised version (2024) of the Recommendations for the use of NGS in metastatic cancers [25] also introduced two novel biomarkers to be tested in mCRC: *KRAS* G12C and *polymerase epsilon* (*POLE*) gene (ESCAT IIB). *KRAS* G12C is considered to be an ESCAT IA alteration, as demonstrated by the randomized phase III CodeBreak 300 trial, which showed that the combination of sotorasib (a *KRAS* G12C inhibitor) and an anti-EGFR monoclonal antibody (mAb) resulted in improved progression-free survival (PFS) in patients treated with this combination. The presence of hotspot inactivating missense mutations in the exonuclease domain of the *POLE* gene (ESCAT IIB) in MMR-proficient tumors has been identified as a marker of high tumor mutational burden (TMB-H). These mutations have been shown to be associated with a better response to programmed cell death protein 1 (PD-1) inhibitors. *POLE* mutations have been documented in less than 1% of CRCs. To date, there are several other genetic alterations affecting CRC for which there is an unmet medical need. Some of the most frequent mutations, including *transformation-related protein 53 (TP53)* and *Adenomatous Polyposis Coli (APC)* mutations, which occur in more than 70% of CRC patients, remain undruggable [34].

Germline Alterations in Colorectal Cancer

It is estimated that approximately 90% of CRC cases are classified as sporadic or familial. Familial cases are characterized by the absence of a clear Mendelian inheritance pattern, but rather by familial clustering due to the sharing of genetic and environmental factors. The remaining 10% of cases arose in a variegated context of hereditary CRC syndromes, which can be classified on the basis of their penetrance. The most prevalent inherited CRC syndrome, and perhaps the best characterized, is hereditary nonpolyposis colorectal cancer (HNPCC) [35]. HNPCC, otherwise referred to as Lynch syndrome (prevalence 3% of all CRC), is due to mutations in genes that encode for proteins involved in DNA mismatch repair. The most frequent of these are *MutL Homolog 1* (*MLH1*) and *MutS Homolog 2* (*MSH2*), and the less frequent are *MutS Homolog 6* (*MSH6*) and *PMS1 Homolog 2* (*PMS2*). Alterations in MMR proteins by IHC or the definition of microsatellite status by PCR are tested in all CRC patients as predictive and prognostic biomarkers. Nonmetastatic MSI/dMMR CRC, whether sporadic or Lynch syndrome-related, has been shown to exhibit a less aggressive clinical behavior and a more favorable prognosis in comparison with MSS cases. Concurrently, MSI/dMRR are hypermutated, resulting in the expression of abundant neoantigens with the ability to elicit the immune response. These tumors were found to be enriched in tumor-infiltrating lymphocytes and to be more responsive to PD-L1/PD-1 blockade-based immunotherapy. Consequently, MSI/dMMR is considered an ESCAT IA alteration. Although Lynch syndrome is the most prevalent, several other hereditary syndromes are associated with CRC, including familial adenomatous polyposis (FAP), due to mutations in the *APC* gene, *MUTYH*-associated polyposis (MAP), presenting mutations in the *MUTYH* gene, juvenile polyposis syndrome (*BMPR1A*, *SMAD4*), Cowden syndrome (*PTEN*), Peutz-Jeghers syndrome (*STK11*), and Li-Fraumeni syndrome (*TP53* gene) [36]. The genetic alterations responsible for hereditary pathologies encompass a range of alterations, including frameshift, nonsense, and splice site mutations, as well as substantial deletions and rearrangements. Evidence indicates that the genetic basis of CRC predisposition is distributed over a large number of genes, despite the fact that only a small number of these are subject to recurrent mutation. Current testing strategies are based on the evaluation of only a small number of focused genes. The MMR genes, *APC,* and *MUTYH* are routinely evaluated, whereas others are only tested in selected cases due to the lack of information about the actual risks for pathogenic variant carriers and the unavailability of surveillance programs. The advent of NGS multigene panels has also revolutionized the testing of hereditary alterations, improving turnaround times and reducing costs [37]. Concurrently, NGS gives rise to challenges in the context of genetic counseling and familial management, as it leads to the identification of novel variants that require the elucidation of their implications for the patients and their family members. As with somatic mutations, achieving an optimal balance between the benefits and costs for patients remains the primary challenge.

Gastric and Gastroesophageal Junction Cancers

Gastric Cancer: TGCA Classification

The 2014 classification of gastric cancer conducted by TCGA Research Network is considered to be a landmark achievement in the field of molecular classification of GC [38]. Notwithstanding the plethora of studies that have been reproduced in recent years, including the 2015 Asian Cancer Research Group (ACRG) study, the TGCA classification remains the most comprehensive molecular characterization of gastric adenocarcinoma [39]. The TCGA database provides a classification of GC into four subtypes: Epstein-Barr virus-associated GC (EBV; 8.8%), microsatellite instable GC (MSI; 21.7%), genomically stable GC (GS; 19.7%), and chromosomal instable GC (CIN; 49.8%). EBV-positive GCs are more prevalent in males (81%) and predominantly manifest in the stomach body-fundus (62%). The distinctive molecular fingerprint of EBV-related GC is characterized by the presence of *PIK3CA* (80%), *ARID1A* (55%), and *BCOR* (23%) point mutations. Additionally, recurrent *Janus Kinase 2 (JAK2)* and *ERBB2*, *CD274* (PD-L1) and *PDCD1LG2* (PD-L2), and extreme DNA hypermethylation involving the *CDKN2A* (*Cyclin Dependent Kinase Inhibitor 2A*) promoter are also observed. From a clinical perspective, the EBV subtype has been shown to be associated with a more favorable prognosis in terms of both recurrence-free survival (RFS) and OS [40]. MSI tumors, characterized by mismatch repair deficiency, exhibited a higher prevalence among elderly patients (>65 years) and female patients (56%). The MSI subgroup is characterized by high hypermethylation at the *MLH1* promoter and also shows high PD-L1 expression, rendering MSI-GCs highly responsive to ICIs. The TGCA study also reported frequent alterations in the *RNF43* and *NF1* genes. CIN GCs are distinguished by a high prevalence of *TP53* mutations (71%), pronounced aneuploidy, and recurrent copy number changes in key receptor tyrosine kinase oncogenes such as *HER2*, *EGFR*, fibroblast growth factor receptor 2 (*FGFR2*), and *MET* [41]. This particular subgroup of GCs manifests more frequently in the gastroesophageal junction/cardia (65%). Patients presenting with CIN GCs have a moderate prognosis, which is worse than that of patients with the EBV subtype, although it is better than that of patients with the GS subtype. They generally present the greatest benefit from adjuvant chemotherapy. Genomically stable GCs are diagnosed at an earlier age (i.e., <60 years) and are characterized by *CDH1 (Cadherin 1)*, *ARID1A* (*AT-Rich Interaction Domain 1A*), and *RHOA (Ras Homolog Family Member A)* point mutations. Furthermore, the presence of *RHOA* mutations was found to be mutually exclusive with the *CLDN18-ARHGAP* fusion. The presence of the GS subtype has been demonstrated to be associated with a more unfavorable prognosis, and there is a lack of evidence to suggest that adjuvant chemotherapy is beneficial.

Gastric and Gastroesophageal Cancer: Genomic Alterations According to ESCAT

Amplification of the *ERBB2* gene has been observed in approximately 15% of GC cases and is categorized as an ESCAT score 1A alteration. Indeed, patients presenting HER2 overexpression benefit from treatment with the anti-HER2 antibody trastuzumab combined with standard platinum-fluoropyrimidine chemotherapy, according to the ToGA study (Fig. 4.2) [42]. The guidelines for GC management state that the HER2 assessment is to be conducted by IHC [1, 43]. Patients presenting with a 3+ score or a 2+ score accompanied by fluorescence in situ hybridization (FISH) analysis of *ERBB2* amplification are eligible for treatment with trastuzumab. In light of the high intratumoral heterogeneity of HER2 expression, which in several cases hampers the response to the treatment, bulk analyses, as NGS, are not the most appropriate. Additionally, programmed death-ligand 1 (PD-L1) is recognized as an ESCAT 1B marker. In such cases, the assessment is determined by the IHC evaluation, which allows the definition

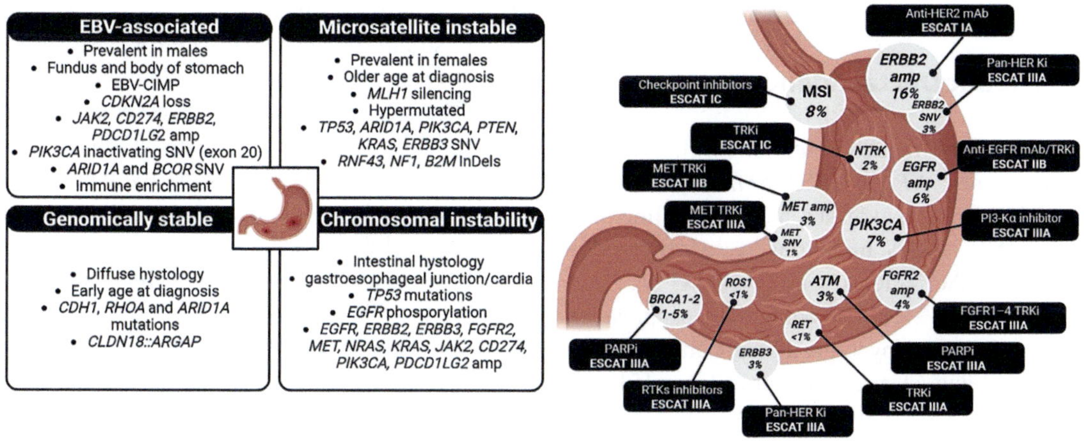

Fig. 4.2 The molecular landscape of gastric cancer. In the left part of the figure, the four molecular GC subtypes (defined by TCGA Research Network) are summarized, reporting principal molecular features. Principal actionable alterations in advanced GC, according to the 2020 and 2024 guidelines of the ESMO Precision Medicine Working Group. *EBV* Epstein-Barr virus, *SNV* single-nucleotide variant, *CIMP* CpG island methylator phenotype, *amp* amplification, *PARPi* poly(ADP-ribose) polymerase1 inhibitor, *TRKi* receptor kinase (TRK) inhibitors

of the combined positive score (CPS). The CheckMate 649 trial demonstrated that a CPS cutoff of ≥5 represents a validated threshold for OS benefit of nivolumab (an ICI) when administered in addition to standard platinum-fluoropyrimidine first-line chemotherapy [44]. Furthermore, MSI/MMR status is a prognostic indicator that should be utilized to predict the response to immune checkpoint inhibitors (ICIs). Its assessment in patients with locally advanced/metastatic GCs is crucial for the tailoring of treatment accordingly. As has already been reported for CRC, the preferred option for defining MSI is the analysis of MMR proteins through IHC, with the molecular analysis of microsatellite loci only being required for cases where there is a doubtful MMR protein expression or pre-analytical issues. With regard to the presence of agnostic markers, the incidence of *NTRK* fusion in GC is extremely low (0.05%) [45]. Moreover, the response to cetuximab and crizotinib was found to be limited in cases of, respectively, *EGFR*- and *MET*-amplified, metastatic gastric cancer (mGC) [46, 47]. In such a landscape, there are no recommendations for NGS multigene profiling in advanced GC, with no change between the 2020 recommendations and the most recent 2024 ones.

Germline Alterations in Gastric Cancer

The majority of GC cases are sporadic, with only 10% of patients displaying a familial history of GC. However, inherited genetic alterations predisposing to GC were identified in up to 3% of cases [41]. A higher hereditary GC cancer risk is predominantly driven by germline loss-of-function mutations involving *CDH1* and *CTNNA1* (*Catenin Alpha 1*) genes, which predispose to hereditary diffuse gastric cancer (HDGC) [48]. In addition to HDGC, the presence of gastric adenocarcinoma and proximal polyposis of the stomach (GAPPS) has been demonstrated to elevate the risk of GC development [49]. This condition has been found to be associated with pathogenic alterations within region 1B of the *APC* gene promoter. At present, the recommendation for genetic testing for GC is restricted to families that fulfil at least one of the criteria defined by the International Gastric Cancer Linkage Consortium (IGCLC) guidelines. Nevertheless, the use of NGS panels testing multiple genes has the potential to detect unknown pathogenic variants associated with hereditary diseases, even in cases where genetic findings are not suspected.

Pancreatic Ductal Adenocarcinoma

Pancreatic Ductal Adenocarcinoma

PDAC carries frequent mutations within four key driver genes: *KRAS*, *TP53*, *SMAD4*, *CDKN2A*, and alterations in at least ten core signaling pathways [50]. *KRAS* mutations were observed in 93% of PDAC patients, with G12D (41%), G12V (27%), and G12R (19%) being the most prevalent SNVs, followed by other hotspot mutations on codon 12 and 61 at a lower prevalence [51, 52]. Furthermore, these mutations are among the earliest alterations, arising in precursor lesions such as pancreatic intraepithelial neoplasia (PanIN) [53, 54]. In the low percentage of PDAC that are *KRAS* wild-type, alterations in other RAS pathway genes (e.g., *HRAS*, *NRAS*, *MAP2K*, and *MAPK*) have been reported [55, 56]. Indeed, the activation of the RAS pathway is recognized as the predominant molecular driver of PDAC, even in cases where *KRAS* itself is not mutated. Other recurrent mutations include alterations on the tumor suppressor *TP53*, *CDKN2A*, and *SMAD4*. A number of other genetic variants have been identified, with frequencies below 20%. These include *RNF43*, *TGFβR2*, *GNAS*, *RREB1*, and *PBRM1* [57]. In addition, alterations in genes involved in chromatin modification (*KDM6A* and *ARID1A*) have been observed. These alterations are associated with a poor prognosis [58]. Copy number alterations, including amplifications of *MYC*, *AKT2*, and *GATA6* at >2% prevalence, in addition to frequent homozygous deletions of *CDKN2A* and *SMAD4* at ≥30% prevalence, have been reported in PDAC patients. Even though molecular PDAC is well characterized, a clear and definitive molecular classification, such as that which is available for CRCs and GCs, has yet to be established. Recently, the PDAC molecular classification has evolved considerably. This evolution is evidenced by a number of seminal studies that have identified distinct molecular subtypes based on genetic alterations or gene expression. In relation to the classification system based on genomic aberrations, one of the most recent developments is the classifier proposed by Connor et al. (2017), which subdivided PDAC into four subtypes: (i) age-related, (ii) double-strand break repair (DSBR), (ii) mismatch repair (MMR), and (iv) unknown etiology [59]. The age-related subtype is associated with the gradual accumulation of damage during cell division, while DSBR is primarily caused by alterations in homologous recombination repair (HRR) of double-strand breaks. Furthermore, DSBR is associated with the enhancement of CD8+ T cell infiltration accompanied by increased expression of co-regulatory molecules, as CTLA-4, PD-L1, PD-L2, and IDO-1. Defective MMR/MSI is very rare in PDAC (1–2%) and is more often encountered in *KRAS*/*TP53* wild-type tumors [60]. It presents an immunological landscape that is similar to that presented by DSBR. With regard to the unknown etiology subtype, the etiology remains obscure. Advancements in molecular analysis technologies have facilitated the identification of additional molecular markers, such as the transcriptomic profile, thereby enabling more comprehensive characterization. The history of PDAC classifiers based on gene expression is extensive and begins with the work of Collisson et al. (2011), who proposed a classifier based on three subtypes: classical (high expression of adhesion-related genes, epithelial genes, and high GATA6), quasi-mesenchymal (QM-PDAC, high expression of stromal-related genes), and exocrine-like (high expression of tumor cell-derived digestive enzymes) [61]. This initial classification has subsequently been followed by several others, yet none of these have achieved universal acceptance [61]. The achievement of a definitive classification is hindered by intratumoral heterogeneity, the different processing methods, and the overlap among the different subtypes.

Pancreatic Ductal Adenocarcinoma: Genomic Alterations According to ESCAT

Notwithstanding the majority of PDACs exhibiting mutations in *KRAS*, only a limited number of them are suitable for pharmaceutical intervention. The CodeBreaK 100 trial has demon-

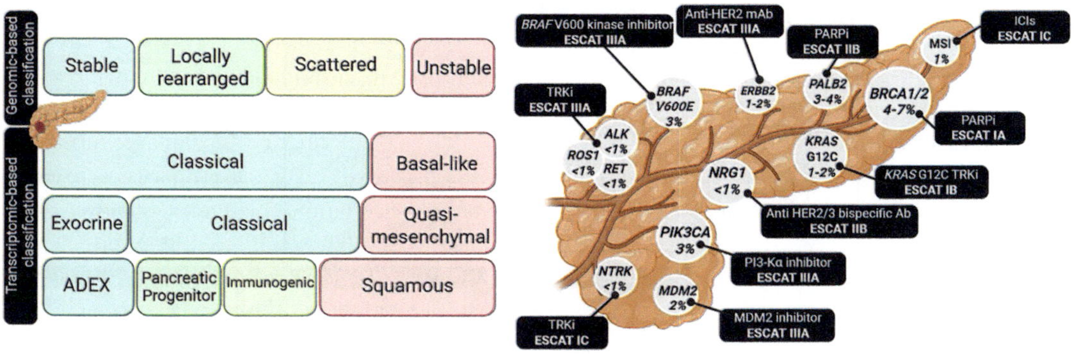

Fig. 4.3 The molecular landscape of pancreatic ductal adenocarcinoma. In the left part of the figure, some of the most relevant genomic or transcriptomic PDAC subclassifications are summarized. Principal actionable alterations in advanced PDAC, according to the 2020 and 2024 guidelines of the ESMO Precision Medicine Working Group. *ADEX* aberrantly differentiated endocrine exocrine, *PARPi* poly(ADP-ribose) polymerase1 inhibitor, *TRKi* receptor kinase (TRK) inhibitors

strated that the G12C (approximately 1–2% of PDAC) mutation can currently be treated with sotorasib [62]. It is for this reason that *KRAS* G12C is the only *KRAS* mutation considered to be an ESCAT IB alteration. In such a context, polymerase chain reaction (PCR) techniques, including allele-specific PCR and PCR followed by Sanger or pyrosequencing, are employed (Fig. 4.3). Conversely, NGS is more useful in the 5–10% of cases resulting in *KRAS* wild-type for the search of tumor-agnostic targets, such as fusion genes [63], including *Neuregulin 1* (*NRG1*) fusions (ESCAT IIB; zenocutuzumab, eNRGy trial [64]) and *BRAF* V600E mutation (ESCAT IC, dabrafenib plus trametinib) [65]. Furthermore, given the high number and length of exons constituting the *BRCA1* and *BRCA2* genes (ESCAT IA), NGS is also recommended in this setting to identify patients who could benefit from treatment with platinum-based chemotherapy and poly ADP-ribose polymerase inhibitors (PARPi) (POLO trial) [66].

Germline Mutations Linked to Pancreatic Ductal Adenocarcinoma

Although the majority of PDAC cases are sporadic, approximately 10–12% of them have a hereditary or familial basis. The term "familial pancreatic cancer" is employed to denote cases in which two or more relatives are diagnosed with PDAC. The most prevalent germline pathogenic variants were identified in the *ATM*, *BRCA1*, *BRCA2*, *PALB2*, and *CDKN2A* genes. It is known that alterations in *ATM*, *BRCA1*, *BRCA2*, and *PALB2* genes occur in families affected by hereditary breast and ovarian cancer syndrome (HBOC) [67]. Germline pathogenic variants in the tumor suppressor *CDKN2A* (prevalence of 1% of patients with PDAC), leading to its inactivation, have been reported in families affected by familial atypical multiple mole melanoma syndrome (FAMMM) [68]. The identification of germline pathogenic variants can have important implications for targeted therapies. The *BRCA1* and *BRCA2* genes are involved in the homologous recombination (HR) complex. The presence of pathogenic variants in these two genes constitutes the majority of germline findings in patients with PDAC. This has immediate implications for oncological treatment. In addition, *PALB2*, another gene implicated in HR, was identified as being altered in 3—4% of familial PDAC cases. As demonstrated in the NCT03140670 clinical trial, patients diagnosed with platinum-sensitive advanced disease who have alterations in either *BRCA1*, *BRCA2*, or *PALB2* can be considered candidates for treatment with the PARPi rucaparib. According to the ESCAT scale of actionabil-

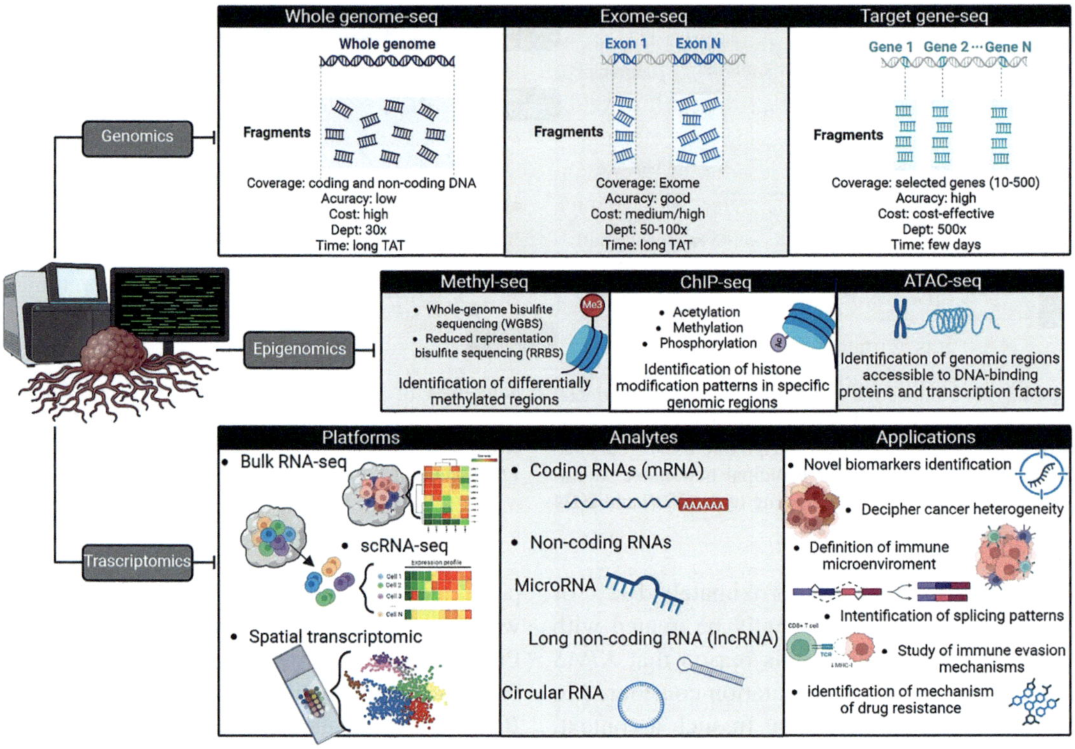

Fig. 4.4 Principal NGS-based platform for the study of gastrointestinal and pancreatic neoplasms. *TAT* turnaround time, *Chip* chromatin immunoprecipitation, *ATAC* Assay for Transposase-Accessible Chromatin using sequencing, *scRNA-seq* single-cell RNA seq, *mRNA* messenger RNA

ity, germline pathogenic/likely pathogenic variants of the genes *BRCA1/2* and *PALB2* are designated as ESCAT IA and ESCAT II B markers, respectively [8]. In such contexts, it is evident that the implementation of expanded tumor mutation profiling panels facilitates not only the identification of therapeutic targets but also the opportunity for germline testing [69].

Next-Generation Sequencing in Gastrointestinal and Pancreatic Cancer Research

Since its advent, NGS has revolutionized the approach to cancer pathogenesis studies. The high-throughput sequencing capacity and the ability to perform whole-genome sequencing (WGS) and whole-exome sequencing (WES) now allow the identification of almost all somatic alterations in cancer tissues and facilitate the identification of carcinogenic mechanisms (Fig. 4.4) [70]. In fact, in premalignant lesions, where genetic alterations are often present at low allele frequencies and thus difficult to detect by the classical Sanger sequencing method, NGS can produce deep data sets, facilitating the identification of gene alterations that exhibit low allele frequencies.

The ability to study other molecular templates through NGS, such as RNA or noncoding RNAs, introduces the possibility of studying epigenetic mechanisms that regulate gene expression, which are now well known as carcinogenic factors. Global gene expression encompassing the entire transcriptome including coding messenger RNAs (mRNAs) and noncoding microRNAs (e.g., lncRNAs and miRNAs) provides valuable information about regulatory regions, overall transcript expression levels, splicing patterns, and posttranscriptional regulation. In some cases, protein-coding mRNA (mRNA-seq) is preferred as a substrate for transcriptomic profiling of tumors because it provides direct information on up- or downregulated cellular processes, is more cost-effective, and reduces the amount of data to be analyzed. mRNA-seq employs an enrichment technique based on polyadenylated [poly(A)] RNAs, representing only a small fraction of total RNA [71]. Therefore, transcriptomic profiling using noncoding RNAs such as microRNAs (miRNA-seq) or long noncoding RNAs (lncRNAs) has gained interest, considering that both miRNAs and lncRNAs play regulatory roles in gene expression, either by binding directly to DNA promoter regions or indirectly through posttranscriptional gene regulation.

Transcriptomic subtyping captures not only gene mutations but also epigenetics, cancer cell intrinsic properties, and the composition of the tumor microenvironment (TME). In recent years, RNA-seq has become a robust technique for the characterization of the TME. Furthermore, the development of computational methods has enabled the resolution of the composition of the tumor immune infiltrate, thus facilitating precision immunotherapy. Algorithms such as CIBERSORT and ESTIMATE are tools that employ gene expression data to predict tumor purity and the presence of infiltrating stromal/immune cells in tumor tissues [72, 73]. The CIBERSORT algorithm was used to estimate the TME infiltration patterns of 1524 GCs and to correlate the TME phenotypes with genomic characteristics and clinicopathologic features. Three TME phenotypes were defined and correlated with the response to the checkpoint blockade [74].

Considering the importance of the TME in cancer treatment, transcriptomic profiling of bulk RNA appears to be clinically meaningful; however, gene expression profiles (GEPs) of tumor cells may be diluted, especially in samples rich in RNA from the TME. To address this issue, novel NGS-based platforms capable of separately characterizing tumor cell and stroma GEPs have been introduced. Single-cell RNA sequencing (scRNA-seq) has provided new insights into the cellular heterogeneity of such tissues [75]. ScRNA-seq has enabled the identification of rare cell populations, often masked in bulk profiling, and the expression of genes of interest in specific cell types. However, scRNA-seq requires tissue dissociation, which is not always feasible, especially in formalin-fixed, paraffin-embedded (FFPE) samples. Spatial transcriptomics quantifies hundreds to thousands of genes simultaneously in the native context of the tissue, preserving the naive tissue architecture, and can provide useful information about intercellular communication [76].

Several factors have been identified as contributors to the modification of gene expression in cancer cells. At the pre-transcriptional level, DNA methylation has been identified as a pivotal biochemical process that plays a regulatory role in gene expression. Methylation is a process that involves the addition of a methyl group (CH3) to DNA, predominantly affecting cytosine bases, part of CpG dinucleotides. Methylation processes have been demonstrated to exert a substantial influence on both temporal and spatial regulation of gene expression [77]. An aberrant methylation pattern has been identified as a hallmark of cancer. The methylation of the gene promoters has been demonstrated to play a pivotal role in the initiation and progression of cancer. Furthermore, it has been observed to influence drug response and the development of resistance to therapy. NGS has emerged as a valuable tool for the analysis of epigenetic alterations across the cancer genome. In most cases, the preferred approach is based on targeted methylation, which allows for the search of methylation aberrations in specific DNA regions of interest that are more prone to epigenetic regulation [78]. However, at the date NGS-based approaches providing a genome-wide methylation profiling are also available. In both cases, the chemical conversion of the unmethylated cytosine residues to uracil through bisulfite treatment is required to differentiate methylated cytosines, which remain unmodified, from unmethylated ones, which are read as thymine after high-throughput sequencing. Genome-wide approaches provide an extraordinary opportunity to obtain an extensive overview of the methylation landscape of the entire genome. This approach facilitates the discovery of novel methylation sites and regions and, consequently, novel epigenomic markers. However, the high amount of required DNA, the associated technical complexity, and the high analytical costs act as deterrents for many researchers, especially those lacking a robust bioinformatics system capable of handling the huge volume of sequencing data generated. Recently, methylation profiling has also demonstrated a diagnostic importance for non-ductal pancreatic malignancies, potentially applicable in the future also on small biopsies for improving diagnostic algorithms [79].

Methylation is not the unique epigenetic regulator; DNA interacts with several proteins, such as transcription factors. In addition, chemical modifications of histone proteins, which wrap DNA to form chromatin, contribute to regulate gene expression. Chromatin immunoprecipitation (ChIP) has historically been employed to identify protein-DNA interactions. Nonetheless, the advent of NGS has enabled the development of ChIP-seq, a technique that can provide a comprehensive genome-wide view of protein-DNA interactions [80]. A genome-wide ChIP-Seq analysis was conducted to identify DNA-protein interactions in colorectal cancer paired tissues (tumor and adjacent tissues from the same patient). The analysis reported KLF3 as an oncogenic transcription factor (TF) in CRC, along with the increase in histone H3 acetylation (H3K27ac) on the *ASCL2* (*Achaete-Scute Family BHLH Transcription Factor 2*) oncogene, resulting in its high expression [81].

Conclusion

The advent of NGS has dramatically transformed the approach to gastrointestinal and pancreatic tumors, both in terms of diagnosis and biomedical research. With the advent of NGS, the potential for multiplex gene testing has emerged, leading to significant cost reductions and reduced processing times. The advent of multigene panels has given rise to a new era in which the assessment of genetic mutations has evolved from a focus on a limited number of genes to a comprehensive evaluation of over 500 genes, along with the analysis of specific molecular mechanisms such as mismatch repair and homologous recombination. To date, the utilization of broad panels has been predominantly recommended within academic centers. Nonetheless, the true impact of these panels on the definition of therapeutic interventions remains to be fully elucidated, exhibiting a substantial degree of variability according to the specific neoplasm type. Concomitantly, NGS has enabled the exploration of multiple genes, thereby facilitating the identification of hereditary mutations that predispose individuals to cancer. The primary issue in this context arises from the extensive amount of data provided by NGS. Indeed, as a consequence of the capacity to test for the presence of mutations in the entire gene, a number of previously unidentified variants have been identified. However, given the paucity of literature, the implications for patients and their families remain largely unknown. In the context of research, NGS has initiated a period of significant advancement, providing researchers with a wide array of platforms. In the contemporary era, a range of NGS platforms are available, analyzing different templates and taking into account the tumor complexity. These platforms offer the possibility to define neoplasms from a variety of molecular perspectives. In addition to the less recent technologies of WES and WGS, a number of NGS platforms have emerged that facilitate the study of transcriptomics, thereby accounting for the heterogeneity of neoplasms (scRNA-seq) and the relationships that neoplastic cells have with the adjacent microenvironment (spatial transcriptomics). Furthermore, NGS facilitates the analysis of epigenetic alterations (methylation, acetylation, chromatin remodeling, and promoter-transcription factor interactions) that contribute to differential gene expression and are implicated in carcinogenic mechanisms. This will facilitate the advancement of research beyond the established mutational model of neoplasms. In this context, a new fundamental issue is raised: which is the more appropriate approach to apply, in order to obtain as much molecular information as possible, in a context in which the major limiting factor continues to remain the low quantity of tissue and the low quality of the nucleic acids obtained from FFPE samples

Competing Interests MF received funds or held consulting from Amgen, Astellas, AstraZeneca, BMS, Diapath, Eli Lilly, GSK, Incyte, IQVIA, Janssen Pharma, MSD, Novartis, Pierre Fabre, Pfizer, Sanofi, and Roche. CL reports honoraria from Astellas (consulting and advisory board), and from Bayer, Gilead Sciences, MSD and Medica s.r.l. (consulting and speaker bureau).

References

1. Falzone L, Salomone S, Libra M. Evolution of cancer pharmacological treatments at the turn of the third millennium. Front Pharmacol. 2018;9:1300. https://doi.org/10.3389/fphar.2018.01300.
2. Sadee W, Wang D, Hartmann K, Toland AE. Pharmacogenomics: driving personalized medicine. Pharmacol Rev. 2023;75(4):789–814. https://doi.org/10.1124/pharmrev.122.000810.
3. Kim JW, et al. Clinical implementation of next-generation sequencing testing and genomically-matched therapy: a real-world data in a tertiary hospital. Sci Rep. 2025;15(1):2171. https://doi.org/10.1038/s41598-024-84909-9.
4. Gu J, Ricker C, Barzi A. Value of germline multi-gene panel next generation sequencing (NGS) in identification of hereditary cancer syndromes (HCS) in colorectal cancer population (CRC). J Clin Oncol. 2018;36(15_suppl):1587. https://doi.org/10.1200/JCO.2018.36.15_suppl.1587.
5. Zhu L, et al. Minimal residual disease (MRD) detection in solid tumors using circulating tumor DNA: a systematic review. Front Genet. 2023;14:1172108. https://doi.org/10.3389/fgene.2023.1172108.
6. Dupain C, et al. Tumor mutational burden assessment and standardized bioinformatics approach using custom NGS panels in clinical routine. BMC Biol. 2024;22(1):43. https://doi.org/10.1186/s12915-024-01839-8.
7. Singh RR. Target enrichment approaches for next-generation sequencing applications in oncology. Diagnostics. 2022;12(7):1539. https://doi.org/10.3390/diagnostics12071539.
8. Mosele MF, et al. Recommendations for the use of next-generation sequencing (NGS) for patients with advanced cancer in 2024: a report from the ESMO precision medicine working group. Ann Oncol. 2024;35(7):588–606. https://doi.org/10.1016/j.annonc.2024.04.005.
9. De Micheli V, et al. Impact of comprehensive genomic profiling and molecular tumour board on costs and access to tailored therapies: real-world observational study. BMJ Open. 2025;15(5):e099134. https://doi.org/10.1136/bmjopen-2025-099134.
10. Paraskevas T, Papapanou M, Sergentanis TN, Kyriopoulos I, Athanasakis K. Comprehensive genomic profiling: a public health system perspective. Expert Rev Mol Diagn. 2025;25(4):101–9. https://doi.org/10.1080/14737159.2025.2471794.
11. Hilal T, et al. Comprehensive genomic profiling in routine clinical practice leads to a low rate of benefit from genotype-directed therapy. BMC Cancer. 2017;17(1):602. https://doi.org/10.1186/s12885-017-3587-8.
12. Schettini F, et al. Next-generation sequencing-based evaluation of the actionable landscape of genomic alterations in solid tumors: the "MOZART" prospective observational study. Oncologist. 2025;30(1):oyae206. https://doi.org/10.1093/oncolo/oyae206.
13. Mateo J, et al. A framework to rank genomic alterations as targets for cancer precision medicine: the ESMO scale for clinical actionability of molecular targets (ESCAT). Ann Oncol. 2018;29(9):1895–902. https://doi.org/10.1093/annonc/mdy263.
14. Alsina M, et al. Current practices and challenges in implementing precision medicine for upper gastrointestinal cancers in European academic centers: an EORTC survey. ESMO Gastrointestinal Oncology. 2024;5:100074. https://doi.org/10.1016/j.esmogo.2024.100074.
15. Sato Y, et al. Clinical outcomes of comprehensive genomic profiling tests for gastrointestinal cancers: experience from Tokushima University Hospital. J Med Invest. 2023;70(1.2):154–9. https://doi.org/10.2152/jmi.70.154.
16. Ricagno G, et al. Real-world performance and clinical outcome of comprehensive genomic profiling of gastrointestinal tumors: high-volume, single-center experience. J Clin Oncol. 2024;42(3_suppl):727. https://doi.org/10.1200/JCO.2024.42.3_suppl.727.
17. Alyaqoub FS, et al. Genomic profiling of gastrointestinal cancers by comprehensive tumor-normal sequencing. J Clin Oncol. 2021;39(3_suppl):109. https://doi.org/10.1200/JCO.2021.39.3_suppl.109.
18. Grover A, Makani NS. Impact of next-generation sequencing in advanced gastrointestinal cancer. J Clin Oncol. 2025;43(4_suppl):814. https://doi.org/10.1200/JCO.2025.43.4_suppl.814.
19. Lowery MA, et al. Real-time genomic profiling of pancreatic ductal adenocarcinoma: potential actionability and correlation with clinical phenotype. Clin Cancer Res. 2017;23(20):6094–100. https://doi.org/10.1158/1078-0432.CCR-17-0899.
20. Wang Z, Jensen MA, Zenklusen JC. A practical guide to the cancer genome atlas (TCGA). In: Mathé E, Davis S, editors. *Statistical Genomics* Methods in Molecular Biology, vol. 1418. New York, NY: Springer New York; 2016. p. 111–41. https://doi.org/10.1007/978-1-4939-3578-9_6.
21. Guinney J, et al. The consensus molecular subtypes of colorectal cancer. Nat Med. 2015;21(11):1350–6. https://doi.org/10.1038/nm.3967.

22. Rejali L, et al. Principles of molecular utility for CMS classification in colorectal cancer management. Cancer. 2023;15(10):2746. https://doi.org/10.3390/cancers15102746.
23. Ten Hoorn S, De Back TR, Sommeijer DW, Vermeulen L. Clinical value of consensus molecular subtypes in colorectal cancer: a systematic review and meta-analysis. JNCI J Natl Cancer Inst. 2022;114(4):503–16. https://doi.org/10.1093/jnci/djab106.
24. Thanki K, et al. Consensus molecular subtypes of colorectal cancer and their clinical implications. Int Biol Biomed J. 2017;3(3):105–11.
25. Mosele F, et al. Recommendations for the use of next-generation sequencing (NGS) for patients with metastatic cancers: a report from the ESMO precision medicine working group. Ann Oncol. 2020;31(11):1491–505. https://doi.org/10.1016/j.annonc.2020.07.014.
26. Kopetz S, et al. Encorafenib, cetuximab and chemotherapy in BRAF-mutant colorectal cancer: a randomized phase 3 trial. Nat Med. 2025;31(3):901–8. https://doi.org/10.1038/s41591-024-03443-3.
27. Siena S, et al. Trastuzumab deruxtecan (DS-8201) in patients with HER2-expressing metastatic colorectal cancer (DESTINY-CRC01): a multicentre, open-label, phase 2 trial. Lancet Oncol. 2021;22(6):779–89. https://doi.org/10.1016/S1470-2045(21)00086-3.
28. Tosi F, et al. Long-term clinical outcome of trastuzumab and lapatinib for HER2-positive metastatic colorectal cancer. Clin Colorectal Cancer. 2020;19(4):256–262.e2. https://doi.org/10.1016/j.clcc.2020.06.009.
29. Strickler JH, et al. Tucatinib plus trastuzumab for chemotherapy-refractory, HER2-positive, RAS wild-type unresectable or metastatic colorectal cancer (MOUNTAINEER): a multicentre, open-label, phase 2 study. Lancet Oncol. 2023;24(5):496–508. https://doi.org/10.1016/S1470-2045(23)00150-X.
30. Meric-Bernstam F, et al. Pertuzumab plus trastuzumab for HER2-amplified metastatic colorectal cancer (MyPathway): an updated report from a multicentre, open-label, phase 2a, multiple basket study. Lancet Oncol. 2019;20(4):518–30. https://doi.org/10.1016/S1470-2045(18)30904-5.
31. Demetri GD, et al. Updated integrated analysis of the efficacy and safety of Entrectinib in patients with *NTRK* fusion-positive solid tumors. Clin Cancer Res. 2022;28(7):1302–12. https://doi.org/10.1158/1078-0432.CCR-21-3597.
32. André T, et al. Pembrolizumab in microsatellite-instability–high advanced colorectal cancer. N Engl J Med. 2020;383(23):2207–18. https://doi.org/10.1056/NEJMoa2017699.
33. Overman MJ, et al. Durable clinical benefit with nivolumab plus ipilimumab in DNA mismatch repair–deficient/microsatellite instability–high metastatic colorectal cancer. J Clin Oncol. 2018;36(8):773–9. https://doi.org/10.1200/JCO.2017.76.9901.
34. Longo F, et al. P-175 next-generation sequencing in colorectal cancer patients: characterization and prognostic implications. Ann Oncol. 2023;34:S78. https://doi.org/10.1016/j.annonc.2023.04.231.
35. Stjepanovic N, et al. Hereditary gastrointestinal cancers: ESMO clinical practice guidelines for diagnosis, treatment and follow-up†. Ann Oncol. 2019;30(10):1558–71. https://doi.org/10.1093/annonc/mdz233.
36. Rebuzzi F, Ulivi P, Tedaldi G. Genetic predisposition to colorectal cancer: how many and which genes to test? Int J Mol Sci. 2023;24(3):2137. https://doi.org/10.3390/ijms24032137.
37. Simbolo M, et al. Next-generation sequencing for genetic testing of familial colorectal cancer syndromes. Hered Cancer Clin Pract. 2015;13(1):18. https://doi.org/10.1186/s13053-015-0039-9.
38. The Cancer Genome Atlas Research Network. Comprehensive molecular characterization of gastric adenocarcinoma. Nature. 2014;513(7517):202–9. https://doi.org/10.1038/nature13480.
39. Cristescu R, et al. Molecular analysis of gastric cancer identifies subtypes associated with distinct clinical outcomes. Nat Med. 2015;21(5):449–56. https://doi.org/10.1038/nm.3850.
40. Sohn BH, et al. Clinical significance of four molecular subtypes of gastric cancer identified by the cancer genome atlas project. Clin Cancer Res. 2017;23(15):4441–9. https://doi.org/10.1158/1078-0432.CCR-16-2211.
41. Lordick F, et al. Gastric cancer: ESMO clinical practice guideline for diagnosis, treatment and follow-up. Ann Oncol. 2022;33(10):1005–20. https://doi.org/10.1016/j.annonc.2022.07.004.
42. Bang Y-J, et al. Trastuzumab in combination with chemotherapy versus chemotherapy alone for treatment of HER2-positive advanced gastric or gastro-oesophageal junction cancer (ToGA): a phase 3, open-label, randomised controlled trial. Lancet. 2010;376(9742):687–97. https://doi.org/10.1016/S0140-6736(10)61121-X.
43. Rüschoff J, et al. HER2 testing in gastric cancer: a practical approach. Mod Pathol. 2012;25(5):637–50. https://doi.org/10.1038/modpathol.2011.198.
44. Janjigian YY, et al. First-line nivolumab plus chemotherapy versus chemotherapy alone for advanced gastric, gastro-oesophageal junction, and oesophageal adenocarcinoma (CheckMate 649): a randomised, open-label, phase 3 trial. Lancet. 2021;398(10294):27–40. https://doi.org/10.1016/S0140-6736(21)00797-2.
45. Dong K, et al. Prevalence and detection methodology for preliminary exploration of NTRK fusion in gastric cancer from a single-center retrospective cohort. Hum Pathol. 2024:S0046817724000637. https://doi.org/10.1016/j.humpath.2024.04.011.
46. Maron SB, et al. Targeted therapies for targeted populations: anti-EGFR treatment for *EGFR* -amplified gastroesophageal adenocarcinoma. Cancer Discov.

2018;8(6):696–713. https://doi.org/10.1158/2159-8290.CD-17-1260.
47. Lennerz JK, et al. *MET* amplification identifies a small and aggressive subgroup of Esophagogastric adenocarcinoma with evidence of responsiveness to Crizotinib. J Clin Oncol. 2011;29(36):4803–10. https://doi.org/10.1200/JCO.2011.35.4928.
48. Blair VR, et al. Hereditary diffuse gastric cancer: updated clinical practice guidelines. Lancet Oncol. 2020;21(8):e386–97. https://doi.org/10.1016/S1470-2045(20)30219-9.
49. Iwatsuki M, Matsumoto C, Mimori K, Baba H. The comprehensive review of gastric adenocarcinoma and proximal polyposis of the stomach (GAPPS) from diagnosis and treatment. Ann Gastroenterol Surg. 2023;7(5):725–32. https://doi.org/10.1002/ags3.12708.
50. Jones S, et al. Core signaling pathways in human pancreatic cancers revealed by global genomic analyses. Science. 2008;321(5897):1801–6. https://doi.org/10.1126/science.1164368.
51. Hu H, et al. Mutations in key driver genes of pancreatic cancer: molecularly targeted therapies and other clinical implications. Acta Pharmacol Sin. 2021;42(11):1725–41. https://doi.org/10.1038/s41401-020-00584-2.
52. Ciulla C, Luchini C. Genomic determinants of biological aggressiveness and poor prognosis of pancreatic cancers: KRAS and beyond. Expert Rev Mol Diagn. 2024;24(5):355–62. https://doi.org/10.1080/14737159.2024.2348676.
53. Liffers S-T, et al. Molecular heterogeneity and commonalities in pancreatic cancer precursors with gastric and intestinal phenotype. Gut. 2023;72(3):522–34. https://doi.org/10.1136/gutjnl-2021-326550.
54. Braxton AM, et al. 3D genomic mapping reveals multifocality of human pancreatic precancers. Nature. 2024;629(8012):679–87. https://doi.org/10.1038/s41586-024-07359-3.
55. Luchini C, et al. KRAS wild-type pancreatic ductal adenocarcinoma: molecular pathology and therapeutic opportunities. J Exp Clin Cancer Res. 2020;39(1):227. https://doi.org/10.1186/s13046-020-01732-6.
56. Philip PA, et al. Molecular characterization of KRAS wild-type tumors in patients with pancreatic adenocarcinoma. Clin. Cancer Res. Off J Am Assoc Cancer Res. 2022;28(12):2704–14. https://doi.org/10.1158/1078-0432.CCR-21-3581.
57. Electronic address: andrew_aguirre@dfci.harvard.edu and Cancer Genome Atlas Research Network. Integrated genomic characterization of pancreatic ductal adenocarcinoma. Cancer Cell. 2017;32(2):185–203.e13. https://doi.org/10.1016/j.ccell.2017.07.007.
58. Fan Z, Xiao Y, Du Y, Zhang Y, Zhou W. Pancreatic cancer subtyping – the keystone of precision treatment. Front Immunol. 2025;16:1563725. https://doi.org/10.3389/fimmu.2025.1563725.
59. Connor AA, et al. Association of Distinct Mutational Signatures with Correlates of increased immune activity in pancreatic ductal adenocarcinoma. JAMA Oncol. 2017;3(6):774. https://doi.org/10.1001/jamaoncol.2016.3916.
60. Luchini C, et al. Comprehensive characterisation of pancreatic ductal adenocarcinoma with microsatellite instability: histology, molecular pathology and clinical implications. Gut. 2021;70(1):148–56. https://doi.org/10.1136/gutjnl-2020-320726.
61. Collisson EA, et al. Subtypes of pancreatic ductal adenocarcinoma and their differing responses to therapy. Nat Med. 2011;17(4):500–3. https://doi.org/10.1038/nm.2344.
62. Skoulidis F, et al. Sotorasib for lung cancers with *KRAS* p.G12C mutation. N Engl J Med. 2021;384(25):2371–81. https://doi.org/10.1056/NEJMoa2103695.
63. Gkountakos A, Singhi AD, Westphalen CB, Scarpa A, Luchini C. Fusion genes in pancreatic tumors. Trends Cancer. 2024;10(5):430–43. https://doi.org/10.1016/j.trecan.2024.01.009.
64. Kim D-W, et al. The phase I/II eNRGy trial: Zenocutuzumab in patients with cancers harboring *NRG1* gene fusions. Future Oncol. 2024;20(16):1057–67. https://doi.org/10.2217/fon-2023-0824.
65. Shin JE, An HJ, Park HS, Kim H, Shim BY. Efficacy of dabrafenib/trametinib in pancreatic ductal adenocarcinoma with BRAF NVTAP deletion: a case report. Front Oncol. 2022;12:976450. https://doi.org/10.3389/fonc.2022.976450.
66. Golan T, et al. Maintenance Olaparib for germline *BRCA* -mutated metastatic pancreatic cancer. N Engl J Med. 2019;381(4):317–27. https://doi.org/10.1056/NEJMoa1903387.
67. Marmolejo DH, et al. Overview of hereditary breast and ovarian cancer (HBOC) guidelines across Europe. Eur J Med Genet. 2021;64(12):104350. https://doi.org/10.1016/j.ejmg.2021.104350.
68. Jacobs MF, Stoffel EM. Genetic and other risk factors for pancreatic ductal adenocarcinoma (PDAC). Fam Cancer. 2024;23(3):221–32. https://doi.org/10.1007/s10689-024-00372-5.
69. Russo A, et al. Implementation of preventive and predictive BRCA testing in patients with breast, ovarian, pancreatic, and prostate cancer: a position paper of Italian scientific societies. ESMO Open. 2022;7(3):100459. https://doi.org/10.1016/j.esmoop.2022.100459.
70. Kerle IA, et al. Translational and clinical comparison of whole genome and transcriptome to panel sequencing in precision oncology. NPJ Precis Oncol. 2025;9(1):9. https://doi.org/10.1038/s41698-024-00788-3.
71. Zhao W, He X, Hoadley KA, Parker JS, Hayes DN, Perou CM. Comparison of RNA-Seq by poly (a) capture, ribosomal RNA depletion, and DNA microarray for expression profiling.

BMC Genomics. 2014;15(1):419. https://doi.org/10.1186/1471-2164-15-419.
72. Newman AM, et al. Robust enumeration of cell subsets from tissue expression profiles. Nat Methods. 2015;12(5):453–7. https://doi.org/10.1038/nmeth.3337.
73. Yoshihara K, et al. Inferring tumour purity and stromal and immune cell admixture from expression data. Nat Commun. 2013;4(1):2612. https://doi.org/10.1038/ncomms3612.
74. Zeng D, et al. Tumor microenvironment characterization in gastric cancer identifies prognostic and immunotherapeutically relevant gene signatures. Cancer Immunol Res. 2019;7(5):737–50. https://doi.org/10.1158/2326-6066.CIR-18-0436.
75. Heumos L, et al. Best practices for single-cell analysis across modalities. Nat Rev Genet. 2023;24(8):550–72. https://doi.org/10.1038/s41576-023-00586-w.
76. Chelebian E, Avenel C, Wählby C. Combining spatial transcriptomics with tissue morphology. Nat Commun. 2025;16(1):4452. https://doi.org/10.1038/s41467-025-58989-8.
77. Nishiyama A, Nakanishi M. Navigating the DNA methylation landscape of cancer. Trends Genet. 2021;37(11):1012–27. https://doi.org/10.1016/j.tig.2021.05.002.
78. Liu C, Tang H, Hu N, Li T. Methylomics and cancer: the current state of methylation profiling and marker development for clinical care. Cancer Cell Int. 2023;23(1):242. https://doi.org/10.1186/s12935-023-03074-7.
79. Verschuur AVD, et al. DNA methylation profiling enables accurate classification of nonductal primary pancreatic neoplasms. Clin Gastroenterol Hepatol Off Clin Pract J Am Gastroenterol Assoc. 2024;22(6):1245–1254.e10. https://doi.org/10.1016/j.cgh.2024.02.007.
80. Nakato R, Sakata T. Methods for ChIP-seq analysis: a practical workflow and advanced applications. Methods. 2021;187:44–53. https://doi.org/10.1016/j.ymeth.2020.03.005.
81. Li Q-L, et al. Genome-wide profiling in colorectal cancer identifies PHF19 and TBC1D16 as oncogenic super enhancers. Nat Commun. 2021;12(1):6407. https://doi.org/10.1038/s41467-021-26600-5.

5 Next-Generation Sequencing in Hepatobiliary Carcinomas

Stefano Sioletic and Andrea Baiocchini

Introduction

Next-generation sequencing (NGS) has redefined diagnostic practice in hepatobiliary malignancies, moving from morphology-based evaluation to molecular classification. Hepatocellular carcinoma (HCC) and cholangiocarcinoma, once classified only by anatomical site and histological appearance, are now recognized as heterogeneous diseases composed of distinct molecular subgroups with specific therapeutic implications.

In hepatobiliary pathology, NGS serves three key objectives: detecting actionable genomic alterations that directly influence therapeutic decisions, improving risk stratification by identifying molecularly aggressive subsets, and enabling serial monitoring through circulating tumor DNA.

The pathologist's role now extends beyond morphologic evaluation and includes molecular consultation within multidisciplinary tumor boards, where sequencing data informs therapeutic decisions alongside histopathology, radiology, and clinical findings. Pathologists must therefore assume a central role in ensuring that limited material is used optimally to capture the most clinically relevant alterations. Decisions on whether to prioritize DNA-based panels for hotspot mutations, RNA sequencing for fusion detection, or combined strategies require an understanding of both tumor biology and practical laboratory constraints (Table 5.1).

S. Sioletic (✉) · A. Baiocchini
Department of Pathology, San-Camillo Forlanini Hospital, Rome, Italy
e-mail: abaiocchini@scamilloforlanini.rm.it

© The Author(s), under exclusive license to Springer Nature Switzerland AG 2026

S. Sioletic, L. Coppola (eds.), *Next-Generation Sequencing in Solid Tumor Histopathology*, Current Clinical Pathology, https://doi.org/10.1007/978-3-032-18790-1_5

Table 5.1 NGS technical requirements in hepatobiliary cancers. Key aspects include minimum tumor cellularity, proper tissue selection and handling, and tumor-specific sampling challenges. DNA panels are used for common mutations, while RNA sequencing is essential for fusion detection. Adequate fixation, limited cold ischemia, and recent FFPE blocks improve test success. Quality metrics such as coverage, turnaround time, and success rates help ensure reliable clinical reporting [11, 45]

NGS technical requirements for hepatobiliary malignancies
Specimen adequacy
Minimum 20% tumor cellularity for reliable variant detection at standard sequencing depths
Macrodissection or laser capture microdissection when stromal contamination exceeds 80%
Core biopsies: One to two fragments (18-gauge) typically adequate for targeted panels
Strategic tissue allocation: Diagnosis confirmation molecular profiling research applications
Pre-analytical challenges by tumor type
Hepatocellular carcinoma: Cirrhotic fibrosis, steatosis, coagulopathy limiting biopsy size
Cholangiocarcinoma: Extensive desmoplastic stroma, superficial endoscopic sampling
Combined tumors: Heterogeneous architecture requiring representative sampling of both components
Platform selection strategy
DNA-based panels (300–600 genes): Point mutations, copy number variants, >500× coverage depth
Suitable for TERT promoter, TP53, CTNNB1, KRAS hotspot detection
Input requirement: 10–50 ng DNA
RNA sequencing: Mandatory for fusion detection regardless of breakpoint location
Essential for FGFR2, NTRK, RET, ALK rearrangements
Input requirement: 50–200 ng RNA
Hybrid DNA/RNA approach: Comprehensive profiling when tissue permits (recommended for small duct ICC)
Sample quality requirements
Fixation: 6–24 h in 10% neutral buffered formalin (optimal nucleic acid preservation)
Cold ischemia: <30 min for RNA integrity (critical for fusion detection)
Block age: <3 years preferred for reliable RNA-based assays
Special considerations: Modified extraction protocols for steatotic tissue, EDTA decalcification when bone involvement suspected
Quality metrics
Target achievement: >90% of genomic targets reaching minimum coverage depth
Turnaround time: 10–14 working days for comprehensive panels, 5–7 days for targeted assays
Success rates: 80–90% for adequate FFPE blocks, 60–75% for challenging specimens
Amendment rate: <2% for validated clinical pipelines

Hepatocellular Carcinoma

Hepatocellular carcinoma (HCC) accounts for over 90% of primary hepatic tumors and presents unique molecular diagnostic challenges due to the cirrhotic microenvironment present in most cases, which affects both tissue quality and molecular interpretation.

Large-scale genomic studies have characterized the molecular architecture of hepatocellular carcinoma, revealing a landscape dominated by recurrent alterations [48]. TERT promoter mutations represent the most frequent molecular event, occurring in 50–60% of cases through characteristic C228T and C250T substitutions that generate de novo ETS binding sites at positions −124 and −146 from the transcription start site [33]. TERT promoter mutations provide critical prognostic information, as these alterations correlate with the progression from high-grade dysplastic nodules to early HCC. This marks a molecular transition that often precedes morphological evidence of invasion. TERT promoter regions are not covered by standard exome sequencing panels, requiring targeted amplicon-based assays or specialized panels that include noncoding regulatory regions. In the clinical setting of a well-differentiated hepatocellular proliferation arising in cirrhosis, where the distinction between a high-grade dysplastic nodule and early HCC remains uncertain, the presence of TERT promoter mutations strongly supports malignancy [33].

TP53 alterations, present in 40–50% of HCCs, demonstrate geographic and etiologic associations [47, 50]. In regions with endemic aflatoxin

B1 exposure, the characteristic R249S mutation predominates, representing a molecular signature of this carcinogenic exposure that can be traced through the distinctive G to T transversion at codon 249 [17]. This mutation eliminates normal p53 tumor suppressor function and confers gain-of-function properties that enhance cellular survival under oxidative stress, promote metabolic reprogramming favoring glycolysis, and drive chromosomal instability [12].

TP53-mutant HCCs typically present morphologically as poorly differentiated tumors. The transcriptomic profile of these tumors places them within the proliferation class, characterized by upregulation of cell cycle genes, expression of progenitor markers including EpCAM and keratin 19 detectable by immunohistochemistry, and elevated serum alpha-fetoprotein levels that often exceed 400 ng/mL [6, 19].

CTNNB1 mutations, identified in 20–35% of HCCs, define a molecularly and morphologically distinct subgroup with implications for treatment selection. These mutations cluster within exon 3, affecting the degradation domain through deletions of critical serine/threonine phosphorylation sites at codons 33, 37, 41, and 45 or missense mutations at adjacent residues that prevent phosphorylation-dependent ubiquitination [34]. β-catenin stabilization drives constitutive Wnt pathway activation, producing a morphological phenotype that the pathologist can recognize through the combination of well-differentiated trabecular or pseudoglandular architecture and nuclear β-catenin accumulation accompanied by diffuse glutamine synthetase expression detectable by immunohistochemistry [16, 39]. Identifying CTNNB1 mutations extends beyond classification, as these tumors exhibit an immunologically cold microenvironment characterized by T-cell exclusion mediated through defective CCL5 and CXCL10 production, rendering them resistant to immune checkpoint inhibitors [37].

Chromatin remodeling complex alterations represent a class of molecular drivers in HCC with therapeutic implications. ARID1A loss, detected in 10–15% of cases with enrichment in alcohol-associated tumors, represents a key chromatin remodeling alteration in HCC. Complete nuclear loss can be assessed through immunohistochemistry, with retention in stromal and endothelial cells serving as internal positive controls [15]. The functional consequences include disrupted SWI/SNF complex assembly, impaired DNA damage repair creating synthetic lethality with PARP inhibitors, and metabolic vulnerabilities targetable with EZH2 inhibitors [52]. Additional chromatin remodeling alterations include ARID2 mutations, present in 5–8% of HCCs particularly those arising in hepatitis C cirrhosis, which alter interferon signaling and immune infiltration patterns that may influence immunotherapy response [15]. BAP1 loss, observed in approximately 5% of cases, defines an aggressive molecular subtype characterized morphologically by poor differentiation, high nuclear grade with prominent nucleoli, and early recurrence [22].

Molecular findings with histopathological variants reveal genotype-phenotype correlations that guide diagnosis and management. Steatohepatitic HCC, characterized by more than 50% steatotic tumor cells, shows a distinct molecular profile with reduced frequency of canonical drivers including CTNNB1, TERT, and TP53 mutations, instead demonstrating IL-6/JAK/STAT pathway activation that may confer sensitivity to JAK inhibitors [8]. Macrotrabecular-massive HCC harbors TP53 mutations in 70–80% of cases along with FGF19 amplification in 15% and VEGFA overexpression, suggesting potential benefit from anti-angiogenic therapy and FGFR4 inhibitors [55]. The lymphocyte-rich variant, showing dense lymphocytic infiltration exceeding 50% of tumor volume, displays high PD-1/PD-L1 expression without specific driver mutations [9]. Fibrolamellar carcinoma, arising in young patients without cirrhosis and showing characteristic lamellar fibrosis surrounding tumor cells, harbors the pathognomonic DNAJB1-PRKACA fusion detectable through RNA sequencing or FISH [18].

Transcriptomic profiling has developed molecular classification systems that provide a framework for understanding HCC biology [6, 19]. The proliferation class, representing approximately 50% of HCCs, shows TP53 mutations in the majority of cases, chromosomal instability with frequent copy number alterations, elevated alpha-fetoprotein often exceeding 400 ng/mL, and poor prognosis with median survival under 2 years in advanced disease [6]. Within this group, the S2 subclass distinguished by progenitor features including EpCAM and keratin 19 expression may benefit from more aggressive therapeutic approaches [19]. The nonproliferation class demonstrates preserved hepatocytic differentiation with albumin production and cytochrome P450 expression, CTNNB1 mutations in a substantial subset, better prognosis with potential for long-term survival even in advanced stages, and resistance to conventional chemotherapy but possible sensitivity to metabolic targeting [6, 19]. The immune class, comprising 25–30% of HCCs, can be subdivided into active immune tumors with preserved cytotoxic function likely to respond to single-agent checkpoint blockade and exhausted immune tumors with T-cell dysfunction requiring combination immunotherapy approaches [41].

Identifying rare but actionable alterations justifies comprehensive profiling in HCC, where the overall frequency of targetable fusions remains below 1%. NTRK fusions, while occurring in fewer than 0.5% of cases, confer sensitivity to TRK inhibitors with response rates exceeding 75%, making their detection potentially transformative for individual patients [43]. Similarly, RET fusions, ALK rearrangements, and ROS1 fusions, though each present in less than 1% of HCCs, remain actionable with FDA-approved targeted therapies [36]. Fusion detection uses RNA sequencing or comprehensive DNA panels with adequate intronic coverage, as standard DNA-based hotspot panels will miss these alterations. For young patients with HCC, particularly those without cirrhosis or typical risk factors, comprehensive fusion testing becomes important given the higher likelihood of identifying actionable rearrangements.

When tissue sampling is limited by tumor accessibility, bleeding risk, or insufficient cellularity, liquid biopsy offers an alternative approach for molecular profiling. Liquid biopsy in HCC management addresses the challenge of inadequate tissue, particularly in patients with bleeding diathesis from liver dysfunction who cannot safely undergo biopsy [26, 51]. Circulating tumor DNA detection rates in HCC vary with disease burden: sensitivity reaches 70–80% in advanced disease but drops to 40–50% in early-stage tumors, necessitating careful patient selection for this approach [51]. Serial ctDNA monitoring during systemic therapy can detect resistance mutations before radiographic progression, particularly important for patients receiving targeted therapies where specific resistance mechanisms may guide next-line treatment selection [26] (Table 5.2).

Table 5.2 Molecular classification systems in HCC. Comprehensive overview of transcriptomic, immune, and driver-based classifications showing frequency, key molecular features, morphologic correlates, and therapeutic implications for precision medicine approaches [6, 15, 19, 48]

Classification	Subtype	Frequency	Key molecular alterations	Morphologic features
Major molecular drivers				
Key driver mutations	TERT promoter	50–60%	C228T and C250T substitutions	Transition from dysplastic nodules
			Positions −124 and−146 from TSS	Well to moderate differentiation
			De novo ETS binding sites	Precedes morphological invasion
			Early event in carcinogenesis	
	TP53	40–50%	R249S (aflatoxin-related)	Poorly differentiated
			G to T transversion at codon 249	High nuclear grade
			Gain-of-function properties	Proliferation class
			Whole-genome doubling events	AFP often >400 ng/mL
	CTNNB1	20–35%	Exon 3 mutations	Well-differentiated
			Deletions at S33, S37, T41, S45	Trabecular/ pseudoglandular
			β-Catenin stabilization	Nuclear β-catenin (IHC)
			Wnt pathway activation	Diffuse glutamine synthetase
	ARID1A loss	10–15%	Complete nuclear loss (IHC)	Variable differentiation
			Disrupted SWI/SNF complex	Nuclear loss in tumor cells
			Impaired DNA damage repair	Retained in stroma (control)
			Alcohol-associated enrichment	
	BAP1 loss	~5%	Complete loss detectable by IHC	Poor differentiation
			Homologous recombination deficiency	High nuclear grade
				Prominent nucleoli
Transcriptomic classification				
Gene expression classes	Proliferation class	~50%	TP53 mutations (majority)	Poor differentiation
			Chromosomal instability	S2 subclass: EpCAM+, CK19+
			Copy number alterations	Progenitor features
			AFP >400 ng/mL	
	Nonproliferation class	~50%	CTNNB1 mutations (substantial subset)	Well-differentiated
			Preserved differentiation	Hepatocytic features preserved
			Albumin production	
			Cytochrome P450 expression	
Immune classes	Active immune	25–30%	Preserved cytotoxic function	Lymphocytic infiltration
			High immune infiltration	Interface activity
			PD-1/PD-L1 expression	
	Exhausted immune	Subset	T-cell dysfunction	Variable infiltration
			Multiple checkpoint expression	

(continued)

Table 5.2 (continued)

Classification	Subtype	Frequency	Key molecular alterations	Morphologic features
Histological variants with molecular features				
WHO (2019) subtypes	Steatohepatitic HCC	5–10%	Reduced CTNNB1, TERT, TP53	>50% steatotic tumor cells
			IL-6/JAK/STAT activation	Ballooning degeneration
				Mallory-Denk bodies
	Macrotrabecular-massive	5–10%	TP53 mutations: 70–80%	Trabeculae >6 cells thick
			FGF19 amplification: 15%	>50% of tumor volume
			VEGFA overexpression	High nuclear grade
	Lymphocyte-rich	<5%	High PD-1/PD-L1 expression	>50% lymphocytic infiltration
			No specific driver mutations	Dense inflammatory infiltrate
	Fibrolamellar	<1%	DNAJB1-PRKACA fusion	Young patients, no cirrhosis
			Pathognomonic alteration	Lamellar fibrosis
				Oncocytic cells
Rare actionable alterations				
Fusion genes	NTRK/RET/ALK/ROS1	<1% each	Gene rearrangements	Variable presentation
			Higher frequency in young patients	No specific morphology
			Non-cirrhotic HCC enriched	

Cholangiocarcinoma

Cholangiocarcinoma presents a distinctive diagnostic setting in which anatomical location, morphological features, and molecular profile converge to define classification and guide therapeutic strategy. The distinction between intrahepatic small duct type, intrahepatic large duct type, and extrahepatic cholangiocarcinoma goes beyond anatomy, reflecting distinct molecular architectures that influence therapeutic choices and clinical outcomes [49].

The molecular dichotomy between small duct and large duct cholangiocarcinomas reflects their distinct cells of origin and pathogenic mechanisms. Small duct intrahepatic cholangiocarcinomas (iCCA), arising from peripheral bile ductules and canals of Hering, frequently present as mass-forming lesions in non-cirrhotic liver and harbor targetable alterations in approximately 40–50% of cases [4]. These tumors show a molecular profile dominated by IDH1/IDH2 mutations and FGFR2 fusions that are almost always mutually exclusive, suggesting they define distinct biological subgroups [4, 25]. In contrast, large duct intrahepatic and extrahepatic cholangiocarcinomas, originating from segmental or hilar bile ducts, present with periductal infiltration or intraductal growth patterns and display molecular features resembling pancreatic ductal adenocarcinoma, with KRAS mutations, TP53 alterations, and CDKN2A loss predominating [25, 30]. This molecular dichotomy guides testing strategies: small duct iCCAs are best evaluated with RNA-based sequencing for comprehensive fusion detection, whereas large duct tumors can often be adequately characterized using DNA-based panels focused on recurrent point mutations.

IDH1 mutations, present in 15–25% of small duct iCCAs, represent a paradigm for precision oncology in biliary malignancies [1, 2, 54]. These mutations, most often at codon R132 (particularly R132C), create an abnormal enzyme that produces the oncometabolite 2-hydroxyglutarate. This compound builds up to high levels and blocks α-ketoglutarate-dependent enzymes [54]. Global DNA hypermethylation and histone modifications create a CpG island methylator phenotype that blocks hepatocyte differentiation while promoting biliary lineage commitment.

Morphologically, IDH-mutant cholangiocarcinomas often display a characteristic appearance with clear cell change due to glycogen accumulation and a distinctive pattern of infiltration with preservation of portal tracts within the tumor mass [5]. Detection of IDH1 mutations has direct therapeutic relevance, as ivosidenib improves progression-free survival, leading to FDA approval as a targeted therapy option [54].

FGFR2 fusions constitute the second major class of targetable alterations in small duct iCCA, occurring in approximately 10–15% of cases [1, 2, 13]. The diversity of FGFR2 fusion partners now exceeds 150 different genes [3]. These fusions preserve the intact FGFR2 kinase domain while acquiring novel 5′ partners that provide constitutive dimerization domains, with BICC1-FGFR2 representing the most common fusion at approximately 30% of cases [13]. The morphological features associated with FGFR2-rearranged tumors include a distinctive anastomosing growth pattern creating a "honeycomb" appearance at low power, minimal desmoplastic stroma compared to typical cholangiocarcinomas, and frequent intraductal growth components that may be mistaken for intraductal papillary neoplasm [14]. Detection of FGFR2 fusions requires RNA sequencing or break-apart FISH, as DNA-based panels often miss these alterations due to the large intronic regions where breakpoints occur [31]. Multiple trials of FGFR inhibitors, including pemigatinib, infigratinib, and futibatinib, have reported objective response rates of 35–40%, with median progression-free survival approaching 9 months [1, 2, 13, 20, 21].

BRAF V600E mutations, while occurring in only 3–5% of iCCAs, represent another actionable alteration [46]. These mutations are enriched in tumors with papillary or micropapillary architecture and may show immunohistochemical positivity with the VE1 antibody, though molecular confirmation remains necessary for treatment selection.

Alterations in chromatin remodeling complexes have recently gained attention as potential therapeutic targets in cholangiocarcinoma. Loss of ARID1A, demonstrable by immunohistochemistry as complete nuclear absence in tumor cells with preserved expression in surrounding stromal elements, is observed in 10–15% of iCCAs [15]. In a similar manner, BAP1 inactivation occurs in 5–10% of cases, can also be detected immunohistochemically, and identifies tumors with homologous recombination deficiency [22].

Large duct intrahepatic and extrahepatic cholangiocarcinomas exhibit a molecular landscape dominated by alterations characteristic of pancreaticobiliary malignancies. KRAS mutations, present in 30–40% of these tumors, predominantly affect codons G12 and G13, with G12D and G12V representing the most common variants [24]. The pathologist evaluating a periductal-infiltrating cholangiocarcinoma with extensive desmoplasia should anticipate finding KRAS mutations along with cooperating alterations in TP53, CDKN2A, and SMAD4 that collectively drive aggressive biological behavior [24, 42]. KRAS-mutant cholangiocarcinomas typically show abundant desmoplastic stroma, frequent perineural invasion, and single-file infiltration of hepatic parenchyma.

Etiological factors influence the molecular profile of cholangiocarcinoma and create geographic variations. Liver fluke-associated cholangiocarcinomas, endemic in Southeast Asia due to *Opisthorchis viverrini* infection, frequently harbor TP53 mutations in 70–80% of cases [10]. These tumors also exhibit ARID1A loss in 20–25% and ERBB2 amplification in 15–20%, the latter providing a rationale for HER2-targeted therapy with trastuzumab-based regimens [20, 21]. By contrast, FGFR2 fusions and IDH1/IDH2 mutations are virtually absent.

Cholangiocarcinomas arising in primary sclerosing cholangitis follow a progression model resembling sporadic colorectal cancer, with early KRAS mutations in precursor biliary intraepithelial neoplasia, followed by sequential acquisition of TP53 mutations, CDKN2A deletion, and SMAD4 loss during progression to invasive carcinoma [32].

Transcriptomic profiling has revealed two principal cholangiocarcinoma classes with distinct therapeutic implications [40]. The inflam-

Conclusion

Molecular profiling has profoundly altered the diagnostic approach to hepatobiliary malignancies. Clinically actionable alterations occur in nearly half of cholangiocarcinomas, with growing numbers identified in hepatocellular carcinoma subsets. Yet integrating these discoveries into clinical practice requires diagnostic pathways that take into account the frequent limitations of tissue sampling and the biological heterogeneity of these tumors.

Testing strategies must reflect the biology of each tumor subtype. Small duct intrahepatic cholangiocarcinomas harbor FGFR2 fusions in 10–15% of cases, detectable only through RNA sequencing due to breakpoint dispersion across large intronic regions [31]. Large duct cholangiocarcinomas, which are typically characterized by KRAS and TP53 mutations, can often be adequately assessed through DNA-based panels alone.

In hepatocellular carcinoma, gene fusions are overall rare, occurring in less than 1% of cases; however, comprehensive profiling remains advisable in younger patients without underlying cirrhosis, in whom the prevalence of targetable fusions is markedly higher.

Liquid biopsy has emerged as a critical complementary approach, particularly valuable given that 30–40% of patients present with unresectable disease [26, 51]. Circulating tumor DNA (ctDNA) detection varies with tumor type and disease burden. In advanced HCC, ctDNA is detectable in most of the cases, allowing comprehensive profiling when biopsy is unsafe due to coagulopathy or varices [51]. Perihilar cholangiocarcinomas have lower detection rates of 30–40%, likely due to preferential drainage into bile rather than systemic circulation [27].

Serial ctDNA analysis during FGFR inhibitor therapy detects emerging resistance mutations, particularly V564F gatekeeper and N549H/K molecular brake variants, with sufficient lead time for therapeutic adjustment [13]. This lead time allows preemptive therapeutic adjustment, including a switch to futibatinib, which retains activity against selected resistance variants through covalent binding. However, polyclonal resistance emerges in approximately one-third of cases, underscoring the complexity of maintaining disease control even with real-time molecular monitoring [13].

Molecular findings in cholangiocarcinoma are interpreted within a tiered framework of clinical actionability. Level I alterations, such as IDH1 mutations responsive to ivosidenib and FGFR2 fusions targetable with multiple approved inhibitors, show proven benefit in randomized trials and mandate immediate therapeutic action [1, 13]. Level II alterations, including ERBB2 amplification and BRAF V600E mutations, demonstrate activity in prospective studies and can justify treatment, though reimbursement may require additional documentation [20, 21, 46]. Level III alterations, such as microsatellite instability and homologous recombination deficiency, show benefit in other tumor types and may support off-label therapy or clinical trial enrollment.

Future directions in hepatobiliary molecular diagnostics focus on technologies that improve sensitivity. Single-cell sequencing uncovers intratumoral heterogeneity and resistant subclones missed by bulk analysis. Spatial transcriptomics links genetic alterations to their microenvironmental context. Long-read sequencing resolves complex structural variants difficult for short-read platforms, while methylation profiling highlights epigenetic alterations, particularly relevant in IDH-mutant tumors. Machine learning tools are emerging for variant interpretation and outcome prediction, though they remain under validation in hepatobiliary cohorts. The challenge is no longer limited to detecting molecular alterations, but to interpreting their functional significance. Only by aligning molecular profiling with clinical application can genomic complexity be translated into strategies that improve patient outcomes.

References

1. Abou-Alfa GK, Macarulla T, Javle MM, Kelley RK, Lubner SJ, Adeva J, Cleary JM, Catenacci DV, Borad MJ, Bridgewater J, Harris WP, Murphy AG, Oh D-Y, Whisenant J, Lowery MA, Goyal L, Shroff RT, El-Khoueiry AB, Fan B, Wu B, Chamberlain CX, Jiang L, Gliser C, Pandya SS, Valle JW, Zhu AX. Ivosidenib in IDH1-mutant, chemotherapy-refractory cholangiocarcinoma (ClarIDHy): a multicentre, randomised, double-blind, placebo-controlled, phase 3 study. Lancet Oncol. 2020a;21(6):796–807.
2. Abou-Alfa GK, Sahai V, Hollebecque A, Vaccaro G, Melisi D, Al-Rajabi R, Paulson AS, Borad MJ, Gallinson D, Murphy AG, Oh D-Y, Dotan E, Catenacci DV, Van Cutsem E, Ji T, Lihou CF, Zhen H, Féliz L, Vogel A. Pemigatinib for previously treated, locally advanced or metastatic cholangiocarcinoma: a multicentre, open-label, phase 2 study. Lancet Oncol. 2020b;21(5):671–84.
3. Arai Y, Totoki Y, Hosoda F, Shirota T, Hama N, Nakamura H, Ojima H, Furuta K, Shimada K, Okusaka T, Kosuge T, Shibata T. Fibroblast growth factor receptor 2 tyrosine kinase fusions define a unique molecular subtype of cholangiocarcinoma. Hepatology. 2014;59(4):1427–34.
4. Banales JM, Marin JJG, Lamarca A, Rodrigues PM, Khan SA, Roberts LR, Cardinale V, Carpino G, Andersen JB, Braconi C, Calvisi DF, Perugorria MJ, Fabris L, Boulter L, Macias RIR, Gaudio E, Alvaro D, Gradilone SA, Strazzabosco M, Marzioni M, Coulouarn C, Fouassier L, Raggi C, Invernizzi P, Mertens JC, Moncsek A, Ilyas SI, Heimbach J, Koerkamp BG, Bruix J, Forner A, Bridgewater J, Valle JW, Gores GJ. Cholangiocarcinoma 2020: the next horizon in mechanisms and management. Nat Rev Gastroenterol Hepatol. 2020;17(9):557–88.
5. Borger DR, Tanabe KK, Fan KC, Lopez HU, Fantin VR, Straley KS, Schenkein DP, Hezel AF, Ancukiewicz M, Liebman HM, Kwak EL, Clark JW, Ryan DP, Deshpande V, Dias-Santagata D, Ellisen LW, Zhu AX, Iafrate AJ. Frequent mutation of isocitrate dehydrogenase(IDH)1andIDH2in cholangiocarcinoma identified through broad-based tumor genotyping. Oncologist. 2011;17(1):72–9.
6. Boyault S, Rickman DS, de Reyniès A, Balabaud C, Rebouissou S, Jeannot E, Hérault A, Saric J, Belghiti J, Franco D, Bioulac-Sage P, Laurent-Puig P, Zucman-Rossi J. Transcriptome classification of HCC is related to gene alterations and to new therapeutic targets. Hepatology. 2007;45(1):42–52.
7. Brunt E, Aishima S, Clavien PA, Fowler K, Goodman Z, Gores G, Gouw A, Kagen A, Klimstra D, Komuta M, Kondo F, Miksad R, Nakano M, Nakanuma Y, Ng I, Paradis V, Nyun Park Y, Quaglia A, Roncalli M, Roskams T, Sakamoto M, Saxena R, Sempoux C, Sirlin C, Stueck A, Thung S, Tsui WMS, Wang XW, Wee A, Yano H, Yeh M, Zen Y, Zucman-Rossi J, Theise N. cHCC-CCA: consensus terminology for primary liver carcinomas with both hepatocytic and cholangiocytic differentiation. Hepatology. 2018;68(1):113–26.
8. Calderaro J, Couchy G, Imbeaud S, Amaddeo G, Letouzé E, Blanc J-F, Laurent C, Hajji Y, Azoulay D, Bioulac-Sage P, Nault J-C, Zucman-Rossi J. Histological subtypes of hepatocellular carcinoma are related to gene mutations and molecular tumour classification. J Hepatol. 2017;67(4):727–38.
9. Calderaro J, Rousseau B, Amaddeo G, Mercey M, Charpy C, Costentin C, Luciani A, Zafrani ES, Laurent A, Azoulay D, Lafdil F, Pawlotsky JM. Programmed death ligand 1 expression in hepatocellular carcinoma: relationship with clinical and pathological features. Hepatology. 2016;64(6):2038–46.
10. Chan-On W, Nairismägi ML, Ong CK, Lim WK, Dima S, Pairojkul C, Lim KH, McPherson JR, Cutcutache I, Heng HL, Ooi L, Chung A, Chow P, Cheow PC, Lee SY, Choo SP, Tan IB, Duda D, Nastase A, Myint SS, Wong BH, Gan A, Rajasegaran V, Ng CC, Nagarajan S, Jusakul A, Zhang S, Vohra P, Yu W, Huang D, Sithithaworn P, Yongvanit P, Wongkham S, Khuntikeo N, Bhudhisawasdi V, Popescu I, Rozen SG, Tan P, Teh BT. Exome sequencing identifies distinct mutational patterns in liver fluke-related and non-infection-related bile duct cancers. Nat Genet. 2013;45(12):1474–8.
11. Cho M, Ahn S, Hong M, Bang H, Van Vrancken M, Kim S, Lee J, Park SH, Park JO, Park YS, Lim HY, Kang WK, Sun JM, Lee SH, Ahn MJ, Park K, Kim DH, Lee S, Park W, Kim KM. Tissue recommendations for precision cancer therapy using next generation sequencing: a comprehensive single cancer center's experiences. Oncotarget. 2017;8(26):42478–86.
12. Gouas D, Shi H, Hainaut P. The aflatoxin-induced TP53 mutation at codon 249 (R249S): biomarker of exposure, early detection and target for therapy. Cancer Lett. 2009;286(1):29–37.
13. Goyal L, Meric-Bernstam F, Hollebecque A, Valle JW, Morizane C, Karasic TB, Abrams TA, Furuse J, Kelley RK, Cassier PA, Klümpen HJ, Chang HM, Chen LT, Tabernero J, Oh DY, Mahipal A, Moehler M, Mitchell EP, Komatsu Y, Masuda K, Ahn D, Epstein RS, Halim AB, Fu Y, Salimi T, Wacheck V, He Y, Liu M, Benhadji KA, Bridgewater JA. Futibatinib for FGFR2-rearranged intrahepatic cholangiocarcinoma. N Engl J Med. 2023;388(3):228–39.
14. Graham RP, Barr Fritcher EG, Pestova E, Schulz J, Sitailo LA, Vasmatzis G, Murphy SJ, McWilliams RR, Hart SN, Halling KC, Roberts LR, Gores GJ, Couch FJ, Zhang L, Borad MJ, Kipp BR. Fibroblast growth factor receptor 2 translocations in intrahepatic cholangiocarcinoma. Hum Pathol. 2014;45(8):1630–8.
15. Guichard C, Amaddeo G, Imbeaud S, Ladeiro Y, Pelletier L, Maad IB, Calderaro J, Bioulac-Sage P, Letexier M, Degos F, Clément B, Balabaud C, Chevet E, Laurent A, Couchy G, Letouzé E, Calvo F, Zucman-Rossi J. Integrated analysis of somatic mutations and focal copy-number changes identifies key

49. Valle JW, Lamarca A, Goyal L, Barriuso J, Zhu AX. New horizons for precision medicine in biliary tract cancers. Cancer Discov. 2017;7(9):943–62.
50. Villar S, Ortiz-Cuaran S, Abedi-Ardekani B, Gouas D, Nogueira da Costa A, Plymoth A, Khuhaprema T, Kalalak A, Sangrajrang S, Friesen MD, Groopman JD, Hainaut P. Aflatoxin-induced TP53 R249S mutation in hepatocellular carcinoma in Thailand: association with tumors developing in the absence of liver cirrhosis. PLoS One. 2012;7(6):e37707.
51. von Felden J, Garcia-Lezana T, Schulze K, Losic B, Villanueva A. Liquid biopsy in the clinical management of hepatocellular carcinoma. Gut. 2020;69(11):2025–34.
52. Wu JN, Roberts CWM. ARID1A mutations in cancer: another epigenetic tumor suppressor? Cancer Discov. 2013;3(1):35–43.
53. Xue R, Chen L, Zhang C, Fujita M, Li R, Yan S-M, Ong CK, Liao X, Gao Q, Sasagawa S, Li Y, Wang J, Guo H, Huang Q-T, Zhong Q, Tan J, Qi L, Gong W, Hong Z, Li M, Zhao J, Peng T, Lu Y, Lim KHT, Boot A, Ono A, Chayama K, Zhang Z, Rozen SG, Teh BT, Wang XW, Nakagawa H, Zeng M-S, Bai F, Zhang N. Genomic and transcriptomic profiling of combined hepatocellular and intrahepatic cholangiocarcinoma reveals distinct molecular subtypes. Cancer Cell. 2019;35(6):932–947.e938.
54. Zhu AX, Macarulla T, Javle MM, Kelley RK, Lubner SJ, Adeva J, Cleary JM, Catenacci DVT, Borad MJ, Bridgewater JA, Harris WP, Murphy AG, Oh D-Y, Whisenant JR, Lowery MA, Goyal L, Shroff RT, El-Khoueiry AB, Chamberlain CX, Aguado-Fraile E, Choe S, Wu B, Liu H, Gliser C, Pandya SS, Valle JW, Abou-Alfa GK. Final overall survival efficacy results of ivosidenib for patients with advanced cholangiocarcinoma with IDH1 mutation. JAMA Oncol. 2021;7(11):1669.
55. Ziol M, Poté N, Amaddeo G, Laurent A, Nault J-C, Oberti F, Costentin C, Michalak S, Bouattour M, Francoz C, Pageaux GP, Ramos J, Decaens T, Luciani A, Guiu B, Vilgrain V, Aubé C, Derman J, Charpy C, Zucman-Rossi J, Barget N, Seror O, Ganne-Carrié N, Paradis V, Calderaro J. Macrotrabecular-massive hepatocellular carcinoma: a distinctive histological subtype with clinical relevance. Hepatology. 2018;68(1):103–12.

Applications and Innovations in High-Throughput Sequencing: Thoracic Pathology

6

Giuseppe Perrone and Lorenzo Nibid

Introduction

With the advent of the genomic era, an expanding repertoire of biomarkers has been approved or is currently under evaluation in advanced clinical trials to optimize the therapeutic management of patients with lung cancer (LC). As a consequence of this rapidly evolving scenario, conventional RT-PCR-based approaches are inadequate to simultaneously cover all druggable alterations starting from scant diagnostic specimens (25–30% of cases). This underscores the critical need to maximize the information obtained from limited diagnostic material (tissue and/or liquid biopsy) in order to inform evidence-based clinical decision-making.

By enabling comprehensive genomic profiling from limited tissue samples, NGS facilitates the identification of actionable mutations, which are critical for guiding targeted therapy decisions in current clinical practice, and supports the detection of emerging markers for immunotherapy response and resistance, thereby playing a central role in the implementation of precision medicine. Moreover, considering the new molecular-based entities in thoracic pathology, NGS technique could be also useful as a diagnostic support.

G. Perrone
Research Unit of Anatomical Pathology, Department of Medicine and Surgery, Campus Bio-Medico University of Rome, Rome, Italy
e-mail: g.perrone@policlinicocampus.it

L. Nibid (✉)
Anatomical Pathology Operative Research Unit, Fondazione Policlinico Universitario Campus Bio-Medico, Rome, Italy
e-mail: lorenzo.nibid@policlinicocampus.it

NGS in NSCLC Predictive Molecular Pathology

In recent years, there has been an expansion in the treatment options of non-small cell lung cancer (NSCLC) with the advent of targeted therapies and immuno-oncology therapies in both early and advanced stage. Lung tumors are heterogeneous, with distinct oncogenic drivers and tumor microenvironments. Recent advancements in cost-effective parallel high-throughput molecular diagnostics might drive personalized therapy beyond adenocarcinoma subtypes associated with the most targetable genetic alterations. Prior to precision medicine, patients were treated uniformly without considering the differences in clinicopathological characteristics and genetic backgrounds of different patients. Today, the right choice of molecular diagnostics is increasingly important, following the careful classification of pathological diagnostics.

While stand-alone single-gene assays remain valid, increasing requirements for synchronous testing for multiple targets make massive parallel

© The Author(s), under exclusive license to Springer Nature Switzerland AG 2026

S. Sioletic, L. Coppola (eds.), *Next-Generation Sequencing in Solid Tumor Histopathology*, Current Clinical Pathology, https://doi.org/10.1007/978-3-032-18790-1_6

sequencing technology the preferred option. According to recommendations of the European Society of Medical Oncology (ESMO) published in 2020 and revised in 2024, the adoption of NGS panels in thoracic pathology is mainly reserved to non-squamous NSCLC. Recommendations were based on the ESMO Scale for Clinical Actionability of molecular Targets (ESCAT) where level I means that the match of an alteration and a drug has been validated in clinical trials and should drive treatment decision in daily practice. Level II means that a drug that matches the alteration has been associated with responses in phase I/II or in retrospective analyses of randomized trials. Level III includes alterations that are validated in another cancer, but not in the disease-to-treat. Level IV includes hypothetically targetable alterations based on preclinical data (Table 6.1). In general, ESMO recommended NGS analysis in order to detect level I alterations.

Table 6.1 ESCAT levels in main mutations and fusions described in NSCLC

Non-squamous NSCLC		
Gene alteration	**Prevalence**	**ESCAT level**
EGFR mutations	38%[a]	I
ALK fusions	5%	I
MET mutations (exon 14 skipping)	3%	I
MET amplifications	3%	II
BRAF V600E mutations	2%	I
ROS1 fusions	1–2%	I
NTRK fusions	0.23–3%	I
RET fusions	1–2%	I
KRAS G12C mutations	12%	I
ERBB2 mutations/ amplifications	2–5%	II
NRG1 fusions	1.7%	II
BRCA1 and BRCA2 mutations	1.2%	III
PIK3CA mutations	1.2–7%	III
Squamous cell carcinoma of the lung		
Gene alteration	**Prevalence**	**ESCAT level**
NTRK fusions	0.23–3%	I
PIK3CA mutations	16%	III
BRCA1 and BRCA2 mutations	1.2%	III

[a]High variability depending on ethnic groups

While ALK and ROS1 mutations do not show ethnic prevalence, one can observe a four times elevated EGFR prevalence in the Asian population compared to the Western population. KRAS and MET mutations occur in older age populations with smoker status and adenocarcinoma. Moreover, a distinct excess of KRAS mutations in the Caucasian population is observable in the absence of clear gender preference. It is widely accepted that KRAS mutation in lung cancer is smoking-associated, but it is only proven for G12C. BRAF mutations occur in smokers without age or ethical tendencies. The BRAF V600 mutations are detected with a higher incidence for females; other BRAF mutations have a higher incidence for the opposite sex. HER2 mutations have a higher likelihood for female and never-smoker patients [1, 2].

Currently, commercially available NSG panels are heterogeneous in terms of reference range: narrow NGS panel, which focuses on hot spot druggable mutations (up to 10–15 genes) with direct therapeutic implications; broad NGS panel, including molecular analysis up to 50 cancer-related genes electing NSCLC patients to clinically approved treatments and/or experimental strategies under investigation in clinical trials; extended NGS cancer panel expanding the spectrum of referenced molecular biomarkers to tumor-related biology and resistance mechanism (up to 200 genes); and comprehensive genomic profiling (CGP) investigating more than 400 cancer-related genes, thanks to the integration of complex genomic signatures [microsatellite instability (MSI) status, tumor mutational burden (TMB), and homologous recombination deficiency (HRD) measurement]. CGP could be potentially the best choice, offering valuable predictive and prognostic insights in advanced-stage NSCLC; despite that, the high costs, the strict tissue sample requirements, and the low success rate in case of suboptimal specimens make this CGP difficult to apply in real-life clinical practice. Therefore, CGP should be performed as a complementary analysis in specific subsets of patients that are ineligible for available approved treatments and patients with an unexpected resistance to therapy [31]. Therefore, broad NGS panel (about 50 genes) including TP53, STK11, KEAP1, and PTEN genes could represent the best compromise between CGP and single-gene approaches, offering data on prediction to treatment response, prognosis, and risk of progression in target therapy and immunotherapy. In general, there is no universally perfect NGS platform; rather, the appropriate platform must be selected for each patient's specific sample. Therefore, a multidisciplinary team (including clinicians, pathologists, molecular biologists, technicians) may represent a key weapon to unveil genomic assessment of tumor patients.

Advanced Stage

At the time of diagnosis, all advanced non-squamous NSCLC should be screened at least for EGFR (exon 18: G719x; exon 19: ex19del; exon 20: T790M, S768I, ex20ins; exon 21: L858R, L861Q), KRAS (G12C), BRAF (V600E), and ERBB2 mutations, for MET exon 14 skipping, and for ALK, ROS1, RET, NTRK1, NTRK2, and NTRK3 rearrangements [2].

EGFR mutations represent the first driver alterations identified in advanced non-squamous NSCLC [3]. Most of them are in-frame activating deletions in exon 19 and point hot spot activating mutations in exon 21 (L858R), followed by acquired resistant mutations in exon 20 (T790M). Several randomized phase III trials have shown that EGFR tyrosine kinase inhibitors (TKIs) improve outcome in patients with EGFR-mutated NSCLC [4–7]. The efficacies of afatinib and osimertinib were assessed in prospective, non-randomized trials, reporting a high overall response rate (ORR) and improving progression-free survival (PFS) [8]. In addition, in patients with exon 20 insertions of EGFR, the PAPILLON trial demonstrated a longer PFS in patients treated with amivantamab (a bispecific monoclonal antibody targeting both EGFR and MET receptor) plus chemotherapy than in the chemotherapy alone arm [9]. In pretreated KRAS (G12C) NSCLC patients, sotorasib demonstrated a PFS improvement with no benefits in terms of overall survival (OS) [10]. In randomized trials, anaplastic lymphoma kinase (ALK) inhibitors (i.e. crizotinib, ceritinib, alectinib, brigantinib) confirmed an improvement of clinical outcomes across patients with ALK-rearranged NSCLC [11–14]. Moreover, findings from the phase III randomized LIBRETTO-431 trial showed that selpercatinib, a selective RET TKI, led to significantly longer PFS than platinum-based chemotherapy with or without pembrolizumab in the first line among patients with advanced RET fusion-positive NSCLC [15]. A significant ORR and clinical meaningful benefit have been shown in phase I/II studies in patients with NSCLC with METex14 mutations treated with MET TKIs such as crizotinib, capmatinib, or tepotinib, with BRAF (V600E) mutations that received dabrafenib-vemurafenib and with ROS1 fusions treated with crizotinib, ceritinib, or entrectinib [16–20]. No randomized trials were developed for these aberrations. Based on these results, crizotinib obtained the breakthrough designation from the FDA for METex14-mutated NSCLC and entrectinib for ROS1-positive NSCLC by the FDA, and dabrafenib-vemurafenib was approved for NSCLC with BRAF (V600E) mutation by both the FDA and the European Medicines Agency (EMA). Fusions involving neurotrophic tyrosine receptor kinase genes (NTRK1–3) occur with a low prevalence across different cancer types. Tropomyosin receptor kinase (TRK) inhibitors (larotrectinib, entrectinib) have demonstrated durable responses in NTRK fusion-positive tumors including NSCLC, leading to agnostic drug approvals by the EMA and FDA [21, 22]. Zenocutuzumab, an antihuman epidermal growth factor receptor 2 (HER2)/HER3 bispecific antibody, demonstrated benefits in terms of ORR in patients with advanced NRG1-positive NSCLC; therefore, zenocutuzumab received the breakthrough therapy designation by the FDA for NRG1 fusion-positive advanced NSCLC [23]. Several other drivers with therapeutic potential have been identified including MET amplifications and ERBB2 mutations and amplifications [24–26].

Although NTRK fusions and PIK3CA or BRCA 1–2 mutations are reported in squamous cell carcinoma, given the prevalence and ESCAT

patients with resectable early-stage NSCLC. This approach led to a significantly higher rate of pathological complete response (pCR) compared to chemotherapy alone. Similarly, the AEGEAN trial, which investigated durvalumab combined with neoadjuvant chemotherapy, included molecular screening to rule out the presence of driver oncogenes. The addition of durvalumab resulted in a notably greater rate of pCR to placebo [38, 39].

In the adjuvant setting, targeted therapies such as osimertinib and alectinib are now approved for patients with resected stage IB to IIIA NSCLC, based on findings from the ADAURA and ALINA trials, respectively. In both studies, complete surgical resection was a prerequisite for enrollment. The ADAURA trial focused on patients with classical EGFR mutations. Participants were permitted to receive adjuvant chemotherapy prior to starting osimertinib or to begin osimertinib therapy directly after surgery. The study demonstrated a strong improvement in disease-free survival (DFS) both with and without prior chemotherapy. Differently, the ALINA trial enrolled patients with ALK-rearranged tumors. Alectinib treatment led to substantially better DFS outcomes than chemotherapy alone, with durable benefits observed over time [40, 41].

Liquid Biopsy

Given the rapidly evolving landscape of testing biomarkers, tissue specimens may not be enough due to low neoplastic cell abundance and high fragmented nucleic acids, impacting successful rate of genomic analysis on diagnostic routine samples. In this scenario, liquid biopsy became an alternative, dynamic, and easy to recover source of nucleic acid for genomic profiling of NSCLC. Multiple tumor-derived analytes can be isolated and analyzed from liquid biopsy, such as ctDNA, circulating tumor cells (CTCs), extracellular vesicles (EVs), tumor-educated platelets (TEPs), circulating tumor RNA (ctRNA), and micrRNAs.

The 2021 IASLC NSCLC Liquid Biopsy Consensus states that plasma ctDNA can be considered a useful tool for genotyping newly diagnosed patients with advanced NSCLC and that the results are often complementary to those from tissue analysis. Also, ctDNA mutations have been found to be of some significance in lung cancer, but their mutations are not associated with early screening of tumors but rather tend to guide the selection of treatment regimens. Since it has been found that drug-resistant recurrence in many patients is associated with mutations in ctDNA, ctDNA testing may be used as an adjunctive means of detecting therapeutic efficacy and providing more rational clinical drug use [43]. In detail, among the analytes detectable in blod using Torrent-based assays, ctDNA is currently the only clinically approved target to identify actionable alterations in NSCLC patients. Spanning from early-stage detection to minimal residual diseases evaluation, liquid biopsy samples allow for dynamically capturing of the clonal evolution predicting treatment response or detecting novel resistance mechanisms. Unfortunately, biological issues (heterogeneous shedding of ctDNA in peripheral blood) and challenging handling procedures (pre-analytical and analytical) afflict molecular testing on liquid biopsy samples in diagnostic stage supporting the integration between liquid biopsy-based genotyping and standard tissue based molecular profiling. Due to the fluctuating and low ctDNA abundance in peripheral blood, highly sensitive methodologies play a key role detecting druggable alterations with low mutant allele frequency (MAF) in blood samples. Nevertheless, NGS technologies have been proven to simultaneously detect several molecular alterations (SNVs, INDELs, CNVs, aberrant rearrangements) across multiple targets starting from low input of nucleic acids. Moreover, the expression of ctDNA is highly correlated with the volume and size of the tumors, and thus ctDNA detection may be synergistic with imaging and more helpful in understanding the course of the patient's disease.

Although CTCs do not play a significant role in early cancer screening, the number of CTCs detected correlates strongly with tumor efficacy and prognosis. In fact, patients with high CTC counts before or after treatment had a significantly worse prognosis than those with low CTCs. The CSCO Small Cell Lung Cancer Diagnostic and Treatment Guidelines state that tracking CTCs can assist in accurately determining the disease's clinical stage, which will help in selecting the best course of action, directing each patient's unique course of care, keeping an eye on the tumor's metastasis and recurrence, assessing the effectiveness of the treatment, and forecasting the prognosis for survival.

miRNAs, as a prognostic biomarker for lung cancer, have also become an important component of liquid biopsies for lung cancer. In addition, miRNAs have been found to be involved in a variety of pathogenetic processes in cancer, such as proliferation, migration, and drug resistance. Therefore, miRNAs have the potential to become an effective biomarker for understanding tumor progression as well as treatment efficacy. In addition to this, the amount of ctDNA also reflects the different stages of lung cancer, and the detection rate of ctDNA rises with tumor stage, with ctDNA detected in 100% of plasma specimens from patients with stage II–IV NSCLC [42].

Immunohistochemistry

Of multiple predictive biomarker testing methods, immunohistochemistry (IHC) is widely available, cost-efficient, and technically less challenging, providing clinically meaningful results with a rapid turnaround time. In fact, several IHC assays for predictive biomarkers have already been implemented in routine pathology practice.

- Programmed death ligand 1 (PD-L1) is expressed on tumor cells and acts as a suppressor of the antitumor immune response through interaction with PD-1, which is expressed on immune cells. These would normally recognize and attack neo-antigen presenting tumor cells. This can be therapeutically exploited by inhibiting PD-L1 through PD-L1-binding antibodies, thus giving the patient's immune system the chance to recognize and destroy the malignant cells. The effectiveness of pharmaceutical PD-L1 inhibition depends on the amount of PD-L1 on the surface of tumor cells, with PD-L1-positive tumors showing a better response to (chemo) immunotherapy compared to PD-L1-negative tumors. PD-L1 expression in tumor cells is routinely assessed by PD-L1 immunohistochemistry (IHC), for which different antibody clones and protocols are used by pathologists. Different commercially available assays and PD-L1 clones (Ventana, SP263; Dako, 22C3) are available, and large comparability studies have shown that these assays provide both comparable and reliable results, given that measures of quality assurance (e.g., ring trials) are adequately employed and rigorously followed. Moreover, an external positive control should be included in all tested tissue slides. The PD-L1 tumor proportion score (TPS) is adopted in NSCLC and represents the ratio between PD-L1-positive tumor cells and all tumor cells in the respective sample (at least 100 viable tumor cells needed); high TP scores are associated with better response to immune checkpoint inhibitors targeting PD-1 or PD-L1 and higher overall survival in NSCLC patients (Fig. 6.1). However, the evaluation of PD-L1 staining is challenging due to biological heterogeneity, slightly different performance of antibody clones, and relevant interobserver variation. It has been highlighted that distinguishing "true positive" from "false-positive" artifacts can be difficult, especially in specimens with lower percentages of positive cells and faint staining. This is of utmost clinical relevance since under- or overscoring might result in under- or overtreatment of NSCLC patients.
- Several different IHC assays were used for detecting ALK protein expression secondary to ALK rearrangements in the lung. ALK protein is not expressed in normal lung parenchyma but is usually expressed secondary to gene rearrangements, and the promoter of the fusion partner likely drives the expression. Of the four most commonly used antibody clones, the clone ALK1 is not sensitive enough to

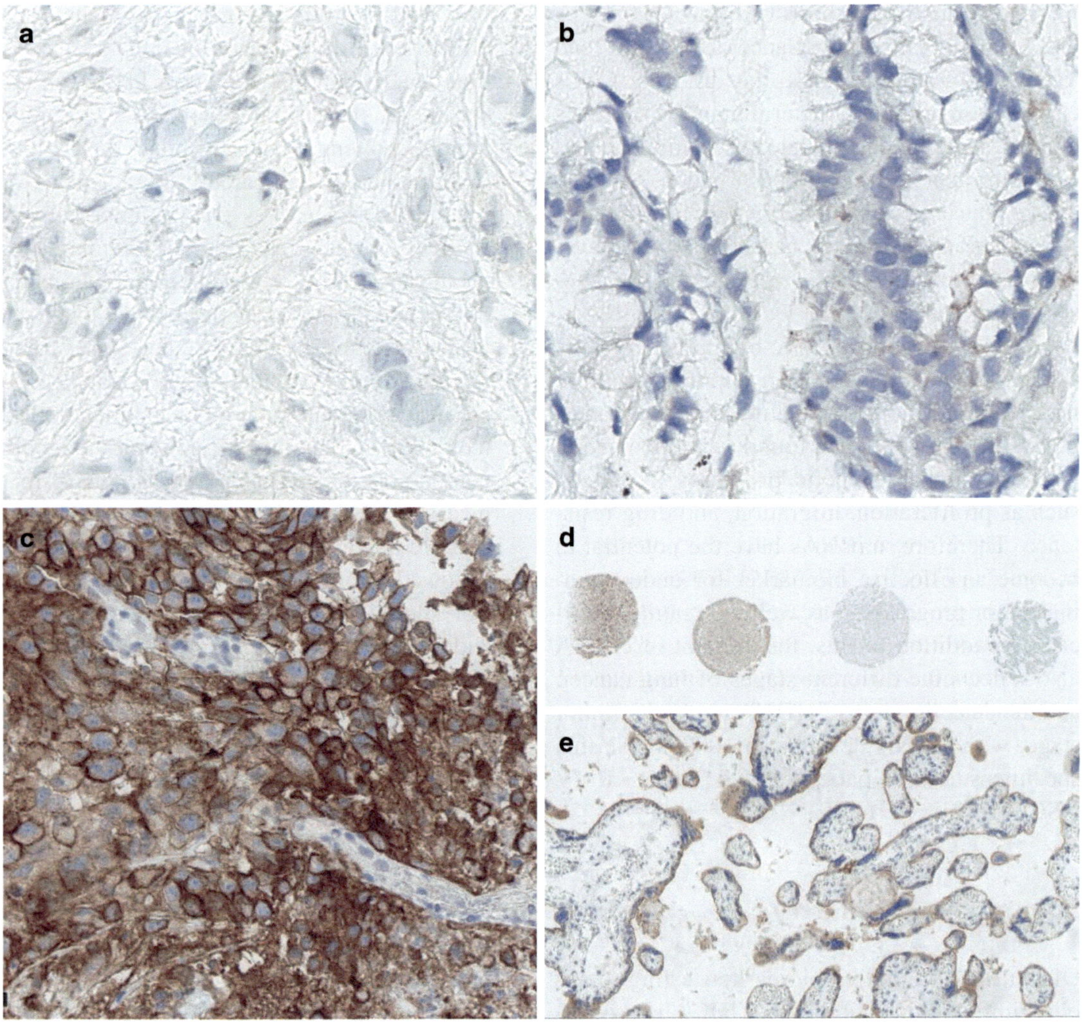

Fig. 6.1 (**a**) PD-L1 TPS 0%, lung adenocarcinoma, 40x. (**b**) PD-L1 TPS 2%, mucinous adenocarcinoma of the lung, 40x. (**c**) PD-L1 TPS 90%, lung adenocarcinoma, 20x. (**d**) Cell line control for PD-L1—note the high positive, medium positive, low positive, and negative cell lines. (**e**) Placenta as external PD-L1 control

detect the low-level expression of ALK protein secondary to gene rearrangements. Furthermore, increasing sensitivity with an enhanced detection system will likely result in the greatest amount of background staining with ALK1; thus, the clone is not preferred as a screening tool. The monoclonal anti-ALK antibody 1A4 (Origene, Rockville, MD, USA) was considered as a promising candidate for ALK rearrangement screening in lung cancer; however, it has been shown that the clone 1A4 antibody suffers from lower specificity (70%). Thus, tumors that are positive for ALK with 1A4 IHC require confirmation by another technology such as FISH or NGS. The performance of the other two clones, 5A4 and D5F3, in detecting ALK rearrangements appears to be equally good. As laboratory developed tests, the clone 5A4, in particular that produced by Novocastra (currently Leica Biosystems), carries very high sensitivity and specificity (92.9–100% and 98.1–100%, respectively) equivalent to, if not better than, those of the clone D5F3 (Cell Signalling Technology, Billerica, MA, USA) (75.9–100% and 95.0–100%, respectively). An immunoassay [Ventana ALK (D5F3) CDx Assay, Ventana Medical Systems, Tucson, AZ, USA] with the clone D5F3 coupled to the automated immunostaining platform BenchMark XT has been developed and approved by the US Food and Drug Administration and European Medicine Agency for the identification of patients with non-small cell lung cancer who are eligible for anti-ALK target therapy (at least 50 viable tumor cells). Positive ALK IHC typically shows strong granular cytoplasmic staining, while weaker cytoplasmic staining may be seen in alveolar macrophages, neural elements, glandular epithelium, extracellular mucin, and areas of necrotic tumor as well as ALK-negative NSCLC. Binary IHC scoring has been proposed, with 3+ as the cut-off for positivity: the ALK IHC-positive and IHC-negative categories corresponded to ALK FISH-positive and FISH-negative cases, respectively. When tumors exhibit 1+ or 2+ intensity, the results need to be confirmed with ALK FISH or NGS.

- Most studies on ROS1 IHC have used the D4D6 rabbit monoclonal antibody (Cell Signaling Technology, Danvers, MA, USA) applied at dilutions ranging from 1:50 to 1:250 with various antigen retrieval methods and amplification and detection systems in automated instruments or with manual testing. ROS1 overexpression in ROS1-rearranged lung cancers is typically cytoplasmic, but staining patterns vary and may be dependent upon the fusion partner. A granular cytoplasmic staining with focal or diffuse globular aggregates of protein has been associated with the CD74-ROS1 fusion, while membranous staining has been observed in tumors with the EZR-ROS1 fusion. ROS1 expression may be seen in tumors without ROS1 rearrangements, most often in a focal or patchy, weak pattern, but in some cases, it can be diffuse and/or strong. Moreover, ROS1 expression is occasionally present in nonneoplastic hyperplastic type II pneumocytes and in alveolar macrophages. To note, the performance of ROS1 IHC detecting ROS1rearrangements is not as good as that of ALK (D5F3) IHC. Therefore, all IHC-positive results need to be confirmed by FISH or another testing method before consideration of treatment with a ROS1 inhibitor [44].
- The occurrence of an NTRK1, NTRK2, or NTRK3 fusion acts as a biomarker for efficient treatment with NTRK inhibitors, irrespectively, of the tumor type. However, the occurrence of the NTRK1–3 fusions in lung carcinomas is extremely rare. Pan-TRK clone EPR17341, as a Class I IVD assay, is intended for use in diagnosis of disease. Nonetheless, the pan-TRK assay can be utilized as a screening method for NTRK fusions. Despite more recent studies reporting lower sensitivity (75–88%) for pan-TRK IHC, particularly for NTRK3 (55–79%), clinical practice evidence on the role of IHC in the screening of patients with NTRK1, NTRK2, and NTRK3 gene fusion is currently limited; therefore, a confirmatory molecular technique is always still needed in case of NSCLC [45].
- IHC may be used to detect other predictive biomarkers in NSCLC. Of those, EGFR mutation specific antibodies recognize the protein conformation change due to the mutation, but do not bind to the wild-type EGFR protein. Other available IHC assays detect RET rearrangement, MET amplification and exon 14 skipping mutation, and FGFR rearrangements. Despite that, these are not recommended for predictive testing in NSCLC [44].

Pre-analytics

The successful outcome of a histopathological and molecular diagnostic examination does not depend solely on the analytical methods employed but also on the quality of the sample under investigation: a suboptimal sample will therefore lead to an unusable or suboptimal result according to the "garbage-in garbage-out" principle.

Given the crucial role of molecular profiling in oncology, it is necessary to enhance the control of factors that determine the success of the diagnos-

contexts. Therefore, NGS becomes increasingly advantageous as the number of biomarkers required for testing grows, indicating that the expanding range of clinically actionable molecular alterations is likely to enhance the economic viability of this technology.

Despite the seemingly higher upfront investment, the cost of the NGS panel constitutes only about 1% of the overall expenditures associated with the therapeutic pathway of a patient affected by NSCLC. Thus, the diagnostic phase is not the primary limiting factor in terms of economic sustainability. Rather, investing in the development of NGS infrastructure—particularly through the creation of pathology networks—can ensure access to appropriate technical expertise, streamline diagnostic workflows, and support broader implementation of precision medicine approaches. Optimizing institutional workflows and implementing NGS facility networks could further increase the use of this method, reducing costs and TAT and improving patient care [47].

Role of Molecular Pathology in Diagnostics of Thoracic Tumors

Molecular pathology and NGS analysis represent useful supports in case of lung cancers with multiple pulmonary sites assessment and in rare thoracic neoplasms diagnosis.

Lung Cancers with Multiple Pulmonary Sites

Surveys of experts reveal that there was marked variability in how different people would classify lung cancers with multiple pulmonary sites, thus undermining the primary goal of TNM classification, which is to provide a nomenclature for tumor extent that creates homogeneous cohorts of tumors.

Four patterns of presentation are associated with multiple pulmonary sites of lung cancer. First (i), patients can present with second primary lung cancers. The demographic characteristics, outcomes, and recurrence patterns for each tumor are similar to those of single "typical" lung cancers according to the stage and histologic type. Second (ii), some patients with a solid primary lung cancer have one or more separate solid tumor nodules of the same histologic type (referred to as intrapulmonary metastasis in the pathology community). The behavior of these tumors is similar to that of a similar solitary tumor; outcomes are slightly inferior and affected by how they are treated. A third (iii) pattern of disease involves patients presenting with multiple lung cancer nodules with prominent ground glass or lepidic (GG/L) features. This group has different demographic characteristics, excellent outcomes, and infrequent recurrences outside the lung parenchyma. The ground glass and solid components seen by CT generally correspond to lepidic and invasive histologic patterns, respectively. The nature of these lesions and their relationship to one another are not yet fully understood; they are viewed as separate tumors with an in situ or invasive component that has arisen from a predominant noninvasive component. The results of clonality studies comparing multiple such tumors in the same patient are conflicting. The patients with such lung adenocarcinomas that present as multiple nodules with ground glass features have a decreased propensity for nodal or systemic spread and an increased propensity to the development of additional subsolid cancers. Furthermore, they often exhibit a more indolent behavior. In this case, the patients are often women and nonsmokers. These lesions are easy to recognize clinically (by CT imaging) and pathologically (by a prominent lepidic component). Thus, this pattern of disease has many distinct features. A fourth (iv) pattern of disease involves a form of lung cancer that is radiologically similar to a pneumonia (so-called pneumonic-type lung cancer). There are typically areas of ground glass as well as solid consolidation. This pattern of clinical presentation typically correlates with invasive mucinous adenocarcinoma, which characteristically shows a goblet and/or columnar cell morphologic pattern with abundant intracytoplasmic mucin. A detailed study of a patient with diffuse pneumonic adenocarcinoma suggested different clonality in each of the five lobes examined; how to interpret this case is controversial. Most of these patients have an invasive mucinous adenocarcinoma, while the rest have mixed or nonmucinous adenocarcinomas. Extrathoracic and nodal involvement is infrequent, but the prognosis is distinctly worse than that for patients with multiple GG/L nodules.

A different histologic type is generally sufficient to establish two malignant pulmonary lesions as **separate primary lung cancers (SPLCs)**, provided that adequate tissue is available. Similarly, different appearance by a detailed histologic assessment (proportion of subtypes, grade, cytologic and stromal features, etc.) of resected specimens can establish tumors as second primary cancers. However, the same (or predominant) histologic type does not by itself clearly establish that the lesions are manifestations of the same tumor. In case of invasive mucinous adenocarcinoma (IMA), a variant of adenocarcinoma, comprising 3–10% of lung adenocarcinomas, most cases are peripheral and present as multifocal nodules, typically with features of consolidation or nodularity on imaging. Multifocality is often present, with nodules in different lobes and sometimes in the contralateral lung, but, unlike nonmucinous adenocarcinomas, in which multiple tumor nodules not infrequently represent synchronous primary tumors, most multifocal IMAs are thought to represent intrapulmonary metastatic disease. This viewpoint has been supported by recent molecular studies showing identical genetic abnormalities within the separate pulmonary nodules of IMAs, the most frequently seen being shared KRAS mutations and NRG1 fusions, in line with the distinct prevalence of genomic alterations in IMAs which includes the dominance of KRAS mutations, presence of NRG1 fusions, and lack of EGFR mutation. Nevertheless, rare multifocal cases of IMA featuring different mutation types have been reported, particularly in the context of background usual interstitial pneumonia.

In case of **intrapulmonary metastases (IPMs)**, among clinically staged patients, overall survival (OS) decreased progressively by location of the separate tumor nodule relative to the primary tumor (same lobe > same lung [different lobe] > other lung). However, OS seems to have been primarily affected by the treatment given, and there was no difference in OS by separate tumor nodule location among only surgically managed patients or among nonsurgically managed patients. Other confounding factors include varying proportions of incidentally discovered nodules (not identified preoperatively) and selection factors leading some patients to be managed surgically and others nonsurgically. Therefore, distinction of these two scenario is pivotal for accurate staging and treatment of the disease. Historical studies, clonality studies, and outcomes studies indicate that the large majority of second cancers of the same histologic type are likely to be second primary lung cancers. Similarly, the same morphologic appearance by a more detailed histologic assessment as already noted should not be taken by itself as clear evidence that two lesions are manifestations of the same tumor; it is only suggestive that two lesions may be related. Assessment of biomarkers (driver gene mutations) is only suggestive, as there is a substantial rate of discordance among different samples of the same tumor and concordance among clearly separate tumors. Thus, mutational profiling should not be considered definitive and must be considered together with other information. More detailed genetic assessments (comparative genomic hybridization, next-gen sequencing) are promising. In fact, the NGS analysis revolutionized the discrimination of lung cancers with multiple pulmonary sites, but lacking explicit protocol accessible for medical practitioners. The first mutation analysis studies (on TP53 and KRAS) in the 1990s observed different distribution patterns in two distinct lung tumors: (1) mutation in only one of the tumors, (2) different mutations in the tumors, (3) same mutation in both tumors, and (4) no mutations detected (not informative). Distribution patterns 1 and 2 denote acquired genetic differences between the compared tumors and are therefore regarded as double primary lung cancers. Distribution pattern 3 shows the same mutation and was used as definitive evidence for lung cancer with IPM. Since 2007, EGFR mutations were frequently evaluated. With technical advances of NGS, panels with a larger number of genes were also applied. Mutation profiling in most studies revealed carcinomas with either strong arguments for an undisputable non-clonal relation or the same mutation suggesting clonal progression. Several studies comparing tumors with the same morphology (indistinguishable histology) revealed mutational profiles supporting independent primary tumors. A comparison of primary lung carcinoma and metastases has been recently reviewed. Generally, substantial concordance was observed between primary and metastatic tumors for EGFR, KRAS, BRAF, CDKN2A, and TP53 mutations. Moreover, careful analysis revealed that intra tumoral spatially heterogeneous distribution of EGFR mutation is extremely rare. This notion supports the hypothesis that when comparing tumors with unknown relation to each other, the test result of the same mutation is suggestive of a clonal relation (i.e., a primary tumor-metastases relation), especially when the mutation in question is a likely truncal driver. From a clonality testing point of view, the prevalence of a mutation in the population needs also to be taken into account. For example, the EGFR and KRAS genes have a high prevalence of hot spot mutations. In Western countries, the fraction of KRAS mutations is approximately 26%. The distribution of the hot spot mutations varies with G12C (40%), G12D (21%), and G12V (17%), resulting in a prevalence of around 10%, 5%, and 4.5%, respectively. In Asian countries, the prevalence of KRAS mutation is around 12%; the distribution of its hot spot mutations is slightly different, with G12C (30%), G12D (18%), and G12V (15%). For EGFR mutations, the estimated Asian and European prevalence rates are around 49% and 13%, respectively. In Asia and Europe, exon 19 deletions account for 49% and 48% of cases of EGFR mutations, respectively, whereas exon 21 L858R substitutions account for 41% and 30% of such cases, respectively. In contrast, the TP53 tumor suppressor gene has a high prevalence (60%) of somatic mutations in NSCLC. Importantly, there is a wide distribution of point mutations over the TP53 gene; this reduces the prevalence of each individual mutation. Nevertheless, in smoking-related lung cancer, the prevalence of certain hot spot mutations is higher: the frequency is 6%, 6%, 4%, and 4% for codons 248, 273, 245, and 249, respectively. The concept of field cancerization is another important consideration. Before multiple tumors in the lung arise in a patient, the whole lung is exposed to toxins (pro-carcinogens), metabolized to carcinogens by that patient's unique, genetically determined xenobiotic enzymes. Assuming particulate enzyme isoforms have a propensity to generate particulate mutations, the different foci of cancer arising in the same "field" may harbor the same mutation. The prevalence for that specific (driver) mutation (obtained at the population level) may, consequently, be an underestimate of the change in an individual. Therefore, in a comparison of two pulmonary adenocarcinomas within a patient, the finding of the same hot spot mutation may be on the basis of the combination of prevalence and the way toxic exposure is handled and, therefore, not a definite proof for a clonal relation. To further inspect this phenomenon, **at least two different genes or orthogonal approaches need to be considered**. According to the literature, roughly one in every ten patients with the same driver mutation in more than one tumor probably had independent primaries when additional genetic data points were evaluated. This frequency is not negligible and signifies the possible flaw in relying on single, common driver gene alterations for the IPM versus SPLC comparison. Strong evidence exists, with various molecular approaches, that the finding of discordant driver mutations in two tumors within a patient consistently points toward independent primary tumors. Meanwhile, even though the presence of the same driver mutations suggests a higher probability of IPMs, there is still a noteworthy chance (10%), particularly in cases involving hot spot mutations with a high prevalence, that the condition could indeed represent independent primary tumors. A more informative approach would be to investigate an expanded panel of genes by targeted NGS. Several recent studies have demonstrated the added value of that approach in clarifying clonal relationships nodules.

On the basis of current literature, a combined four-step histologic and molecular classification algorithm for differentiating between separate primary cancers and IPMs is proposed. Briefly, histologic classification alone is sufficient to establish SPLCs or IPMs in a few specific conditions, such as adenocarcinoma in situ, minimally invasive adenocarcinoma, lepidic predominant adenocarcinoma, or mucinous adenocarcinomas; in multiple pulmonary mucinous adenocarcinomas, noteworthily, the presence of notable distinct histologic features may warrant molecular studies to search for unique driver mutations to indicate SPLCs (Step 1). For tumors that cannot be categorized into SPLCs or IPMs solely by histologic classification, a comprehensive histologic evaluation with peer review is recommended (Step 2). In cases with discordant results from histology review, further molecular analysis including major driver mutations (such as KRAS, EGFR, and ALK mutations) is suggested (Step 3). Other than cases with different driver mutations assigned to be SPLCs, cases with either the same or no driver mutation detected by simple molecular analysis are recommended to be further examined by advanced molecular methods, such as large-scale NGS panels, whole-exome sequencing, or whole-genome sequencing; tumors with one or more than one shared somatic mutations other than driver mutations would then be regarded as IPMs, whereas tumors with different TP53 mutation status are probable SPLCs (Step 4) [50].

Molecular Pathology in Diagnostics [51]

Molecular evaluation of certain genes is sometimes included in essential and desirable diagnostic criteria of the World Health Organization Classification of Thoracic Tumours. That implies the need for adoption of wide NGS panel and/or specific molecular or immunohistochemical probes in selected cases (Table 6.3).

Most common of these entities are reported as follows:

Bronchiolar Adenoma/Ciliated Muconodular Papillary Tumor A benign peripheral lung tumor composed of bilayered bronchiolar-type epithelium containing a continuous basal cell layer. BRAF driver mutation is the most common, with other mutually exclusive driver alterations, including in EGFR, KRAS, HRAS, and ALK. Positive BRAF immunohistochemistry or BRAF mutation is included within desirable diagnostic criteria.

Pulmonary Chondromas A benign neoplasm of hyaline cartilage. Gain of chromosome 6 and loss of 1q have been reported, and functional deficiency of succinate dehydrogenase is the underlying mechanism of Carney triad (gastrointestinal stromal tumors, pulmonary chondromas, paragangliomas), driven by hypermethylation of SDHC. Carney-associated chondromas show frequent loss of SDHB by immunohistochemistry, in contrast to hamartomas, and this can be a useful diagnostic adjunct when the distinction is difficult.

Thoracic SMARCA4-Deficient Undifferentiated Tumor A high-grade malignant neoplasm that significantly involves the thorax of adults and shows undifferentiated or rhabdoid phenotype and deficiency of SMARCA4, a key member of the BAF chromatin-remodeling complex. Tumorigenesis is driven by biallelic inactivation of SMARCA4, including mainly nonsense and frameshift mutations, with missense mutations, splice-site mutations, or deletions being less common. TP53 inactivation is common, and some cases show additional mutations in KRAS, STK11, and/or KEAP1. NF1 mutation is present in a subset. Sequencing can confirm the presence of SMARCA4 mutation, but it is not necessary for the diagnosis, because immunohistochemistry shows complete loss in most cases and is sufficient to document SMARCA4 deficiency. However, sequencing can be helpful to clarify the significance of reduced expression of SMARCA4. The mutation may not be detectable, depending on the methods used, despite SMARCA4 (BRG1) immunohistochemical loss. Because the second hit is

Table 6.3 Molecular-based data useful for histopathological diagnosis in thoracic tumors of the lung, pleura, and thymus according WHO Classification of Thoracic Tumours (fifth Ed.)

Diagnosis	Molecular alteration	Desirable	Essential
Thoracic SMARCA4-deficient undifferentiated tumor	SMARCA4-BRG1 deficiency (IHC)	X	V
	SMARCA2-BRM deficiency (IHC)	V	X
Hyalinizing clear cell carcinoma of the lung	EWSR1-ATF1 fusion	V	X
Myoepithelioma and myoepithelial carcinoma of the lung	WSR1 fusions	V	X
Adenoid cystic carcinoma of the lung	MYB-NFIB fusion	V	X
Mucoepidermoid carcinoma of the lung and thymus	CRTC1-MAML2 fusion	V	X
Lymphoepithelial carcinoma of the lung and thymus	EBER (ISH)	V	X
NUT carcinoma of the lung and thymus	NUTM1 rearrangement (IHC/FISH/RT-PCR/NGS)	X	V
Mesothelioma in situ	BAP1 loss (IHC) And/or CDKN2A homozygous deletion (FISH/NGS) or MTAP loss (IHC)	X	V
Diffuse pleural mesothelioma	BAP1 loss (IHC) And/or CDKN2A homozygous deletion (FISH/NGS) or MTAP loss (IHC)	V	X
Congenital peribronchial myofibroblastic tumor	ETV6-NTRK3 rearrangement	X	X
Primary pulmonary myxoid sarcoma with EWSR1-CREB1 fusion	EWSR1-CREB1 fusions	V	X
Pulmonary blastoma	β-Catenin (IHC) and CTNNB1 mutation	V	X
Pleuropulmonary blastoma	Germline DICER1 mutation	V	X
Pulmonary artery intimal sarcoma	MDM2 amplification	V	X
Perivascular epithelioid cell tumors of the lung	TSC2 mutations	V	X
Bronchiolar adenoma/ciliated muconodular papillary tumor	BRAF (IHC/mutation)	X	X
Pulmonary chondroma	Loss of SDHB (IHC)	X	X

often copy-neutral loss of heterozygosity, SMARCA4 FISH assay is of limited utility. Detection of SMARCA4 (BRG1) deficiency by immunohistochemistry is mentioned within the essential diagnostic criteria, while detection of SMARCA2 (BRM) deficiency by immunohistochemistry is a desirable diagnostic criteria.

Adenoid Cystic Carcinoma of the Lung A malignant biphasic salivary gland-type tumor consisting of epithelial and myoepithelial cells. There are three main architectural growth patterns: tubular, cribriform, and solid. The main genomic alterations, including a fusion of the MYB oncogene and NFIB transcription factor t(6;9)(q22-q23;p23-p24) and less commonly t(8;9)/MYBL1-NFIB gene fusion, can occur in 30–100% of adenoid cystic carcinomas of the head and neck and tracheobronchial tree (desirable diagnostic criteria). Loss of heterozygosity of chromosomes 3p14 and 9p has been reported rarely in bronchial adenoid cystic carcinoma. High-resolution comparative genomic hybridization analysis showed losses at 3p, 4p, and 15q and gains at 12q15 (the MDM2 site). Despite immunoreactivity for KIT, KIT mutations are absent.

Hyalinizing Clear Cell Carcinoma of the Lung A low-grade malignant epithelial tumor with cords, trabeculae, and nests of clear and eosinophilic cells infiltrating within a background of myxohyaline and cellular fibrous stroma. The EWSR1-ATF1 fusion is present in all reported cases, and it is included within the desirable diagnostic criteria. One case reports an EWSR1-CREM fusion by FISH, which is also found in head and neck primaries.

Myoepithelioma and Myoepithelial Carcinoma of the Lung Very rare tumors that share morphological, immunophenotypic, and genetic features with their counterparts in the soft tissue, salivary gland, bone, and skin. The term "myoepithelioma" is applied to benign myoepithelial tumors, whereas malignant myoepithelial tumors are designated "myoepithelial carcinoma." WSR1 gene rearrangements are common in myoepithelial tumors (desirable diagnostic criteria), identified in about 50% of cases, with diverse fusion partners, including POU5F1, PBX1, ZNF444, KLF17, PBX3, and ATF1; occasional cases show alternative FUS gene rearrangements. A subset of myoepithelial carcinomas harbor homozygous deletions of SMARCB1.

Mucoepidermoid Carcinoma (MEC) of the Lung and Thymus A malignant salivary gland-type tumor that is composed of mucin-secreting cells, squamoid cells, and intermediate-type cells. Testing for CRTC1-MAML2 gene fusion by FISH can help to establish the diagnosis of MEC (desirable diagnostic criteria). The t(11;19)(q21;p13) involves the CRTC1 and MAML2 genes, located on chromosomes 19p13 and 11q21, respectively. CRTC1-MAML2 fuses exon 1 of CRTC1 with exons 2–5 of MAML2.

Lymphoepithelial Carcinoma of the Lung and Thymus A poorly differentiated squamous cell carcinoma admixed with variable amounts of lymphoplasmacytic infiltrate, frequently associated with EBV. TP53, KRAS, and EGFR mutations as well as ALK and ROS1 translocations are typically absent, suggesting a molecular tumorigenesis distinct from that of conventional non-small cell lung carcinomas. This diagnosis should be considered when a pulmonary nonkeratinizing SCC is encountered in a young never-smoker, particularly if the patient is from Asia. EBER in situ hybridization is positive in EBV-associated tumors (desirable criteria), but negative in EBV-independent tumors; the result does not affect diagnosis of cases with typical lymphoepithelial carcinoma morphology (especially in the thymus), but EBER positivity supports the diagnosis in lymphocyte-poor cases.

NUT Carcinoma of the Lung and Thymus A poorly differentiated carcinoma genetically defined by the presence of nuclear protein in testis (NUTM1) gene rearrangement. NUT carcinoma is characterized by chromosomal translocation t(15;19)(q14;p13.1) and resulting fusion of NUTM1 to BRD4 (> 75% of cases) or by fusion of NUTM1 to genes coding for BRD4-interacting proteins, such as BRD3 (9q34.2; ~15% of cases), NSD3 (8p11.23; ~5%), and others (ZNF532, ZNF592, and other unidentified gene[s]; ~5%). Demonstration of NUTM1 rearrangement is required (essential diagnostic criteria), such as by positive immunostaining (e.g., with clone C52B1) for nuclear NUT expression in >50% of nuclei, which achieves 100% specificity and 87% sensitivity. In the remaining cases, cytogenetic analysis, in situ hybridization (FISH), RT-PCR, or next-generation sequencing may be necessary (Fig. 6.2).

Mesothelioma In Situ A preinvasive single-layer surface proliferation of neoplastic mesothelial cells. BAP1 inactivation and CDKN2A homozygous deletion are considered to be early events in mesothelioma development. The diagnosis of mesothelioma in situ cannot be made on H&E stains. Loss of BAP1 nuclear expression by immunohistochemistry and/or CDKN2A homozygous deletion identified either by FISH or by MTAP immunohistochemistry (cytoplasmic staining) must be demonstrated using a validated assay with appropriate internal controls and external quality assurance (essential diagnostic criteria). Loss of these markers in isolation of other data does not exclude malignancy. This workup should be limited to patients with non-resolving pleural effusions or for whom there is clinical suspicion of mesothelioma.

Diffuse Pleural Mesothelioma A tumor of malignant mesothelial cells showing diffuse

28. Vansteenkiste JF, et al. Safety and efficacy of Buparlisib (BKM120) in patients with PI3K pathway-activated non-small cell lung cancer: results from the phase II BASALT-1 study. J Thorac Oncol. 2015;10:1319–27.
29. Cheung AHK, et al. EGFR mutation exists in squamous cell lung carcinoma. Pathology. 2020;52:323–8.
30. Lim TKH, et al. KRAS G12C in advanced NSCLC: prevalence, co-mutations, and testing. Lung Cancer. 2023;184:107293.
31. Nibid L, et al. Feasibility of comprehensive genomic profiling (CGP) in real-life clinical practice. Diagnostics (Basel). 2023;13:782.
32. Huang C, et al. Management of non-small Cell Lung Cancer Patients with MET exon 14 skipping mutations. Curr Treat Options Oncol. 2020;21:1–15.
33. Yang M, et al. Non-small cell lung cancer with MET amplification: review of epidemiology, associated disease characteristics, testing procedures, burden, and treatments. Front Oncol. 2023;13:1241402.
34. Rosen EY, et al. Overcoming MET-dependent resistance to selective RET inhibition in patients with RET fusion⇓positive lung cancer by combining selpercatinib with crizotinib. Clin Cancer Res. 2021;27:34–42.
35. Qin K, Hong L, Zhang J, Le X. MET amplification as a resistance driver to TKI therapies in lung cancer: clinical challenges and opportunities. Cancers (Basel). 2023;15:612.
36. Pezzuto F, et al. The significance of co-mutations in EGFR -mutated non-small cell lung cancer: optimizing the efficacy of targeted therapies? Lung Cancer. 2023;181:107249.
37. Ashrafi A, et al. Current landscape of therapeutic resistance in lung cancer and promising strategies to overcome resistance. Cancers (Basel). 2022;14:4562.
38. Forde PM, et al. Neoadjuvant Nivolumab plus chemotherapy in Resectable lung cancer. N Engl J Med. 2022;386:1973–85.
39. Heymach JV, et al. Perioperative Durvalumab for Resectable non–small-cell lung cancer. N Engl J Med. 2023;389:1672–84.
40. Wu Y-L, et al. Alectinib in resected ALK-positive non–small-cell lung cancer. N Engl J Med. 2024;390:1265–76.
41. Wu Y-L, et al. Osimertinib in resected EGFR-mutated non–small-cell lung cancer. N Engl J Med. 2020;383:1711–23.
42. Ma L, et al. Liquid biopsy in cancer: current status, challenges and future prospects. Sign Transduct Targeted Therapy. 2024;9:1–36.
43. Rolfo C, et al. Liquid biopsy for advanced NSCLC: a consensus statement from the International Association for the Study of Lung Cancer. J Thorac Oncol. 2021;16:1647–62.
44. Mino-Kenudson M. Immunohistochemistry for predictive biomarkers in non-small cell lung cancer. Transl Lung Cancer Res. 2017;6:570–87.
45. Strohmeier S, et al. Applicability of pan-TRK immunohistochemistry for identification of NTRK fusions in lung carcinoma. Sci Rep. 2021;11
46. Agrawal L, Engel KB, Greytak SR, Moore HM. Understanding Preanalytical variables and their effects on clinical biomarkers of oncology and immunotherapy. Semin Cancer Biol. 2017;52:26.
47. Eccher A, et al. Pathology laboratory archives: conservation quality of nucleic acids and proteins for NSCLC molecular testing. J Pers Med. 2024;14
48. Nibid L, et al. RNA-Seq analysis in non-small cell lung cancer: what is the best sample from clinical practice? J Pers Med. 2024;14:851.
49. Marchiò C, et al. Part I—pre-analytical phase. Pathologica J Italian Soc Anatom Pathol Diagn Cytopathol. 2025;117:5–17.
50. Chou TY, et al. Differentiating separate primary lung adenocarcinomas from intrapulmonary metastases with emphasis on pathological and molecular considerations: recommendations from the International Association for the Study of Lung Cancer pathology committee. J Thorac Oncol. 2025;20:311–30.
51. BlueBooksOnline. https://tumourclassification.iarc.who.int/chapters/35.

Next-Generation Sequencing in Malignant Mesenchymal Tumors

7

Stefano Sioletic, Elena Bellan, and Paola Dal Cin

Malignant Soft Tissue Tumors

Stefano Sioletic and Paola Dal Cin

Introduction

Soft tissue tumors constitute a rare group of malignancies, representing approximately 1% of adult cancers and 7–15% of pediatric malignancies [38, 192]. These neoplasms have traditionally been classified according to their presumed line of differentiation, such as adipocytic characteristics in liposarcoma. However, the cellular origin remains uncertain for many entities limiting the diagnostic utility of morphology alone. The current [207] classification systematically categorizes soft tissue tumors based on integrated morphological, immunohistochemical, and molecular features, with additional consideration of tumor size, anatomical location, and depth of invasion, delineating over 100 distinct mesenchymal tumor subtypes. Benign soft tissue masses vastly outnumber malignant tumors in clinical practice [49, 190, 207]. For the purposes of this review, both intermediate categories are discussed alongside classic malignant soft tissue tumors, collectively designated as sarcomas.

Clinically, many sarcomas demonstrate aggressive and unpredictable behavior. Even when localized disease undergoes complete surgical resection, 40–50% of patients with high-grade lesions develops metastatic disease within 5 years [35, 86]. Prognostic assessment has traditionally relied on tumor grade, size, and stage; however, these parameters often fail to capture the underlying biological complexity [75]. This limitation has driven increasing clinical interest in molecular classification, alongside hematologic malignancies, which can reveal subtype-defining genomic alterations while correlating with clinical outcomes and therapeutic responsiveness [84, 204].

Due to their distinctive biology and frequent association with recurrent chromosomal aberrations, sarcomas were among the earliest tumor groups to incorporate cytogenetic analysis as a diagnostic tool [121]. Long before the clinical implementation of sequencing technologies, conventional karyotyping and FISH provided insights into the genomic architecture of several sarcoma subtypes [179].

Conventional karyotyping proved essential for identifying pathognomonic rearrangements, including t(11;22) in Ewing sarcoma and its variant translocations, t(12;16) in myxoid liposarcoma, and t(X;18) in synovial sarcoma, directly from metaphase spreads. Nevertheless, cytogenetics has important limitations, including the requirement for fresh, viable, dividing tumor cells, the risk of normal stromal cell overgrowth, and lack of resolution for detecting cryptic or small-scale chromo-

S. Sioletic (✉)
Department of Pathology, San Camillo-Forlanini Hospital, Rome, Italy

E. Bellan
Department of Integrated Diagnostics, Azienda Ospedale–Università Padova, Padua, Italy

P. D. Cin
Pathology, Harvard Medical School, Boston, MA, USA
e-mail: pdalcin@bwh.harvard.edu

© The Author(s), under exclusive license to Springer Nature Switzerland AG 2026

S. Sioletic, L. Coppola (eds.), *Next-Generation Sequencing in Solid Tumor Histopathology*, Current Clinical Pathology, https://doi.org/10.1007/978-3-032-18790-1_7

somal alterations [140]. FISH analysis remains a key tool for confirming known rearrangements in nondividing cells from both fresh samples or histologic sections, particularly for core biopsy specimens [36]. However, its utility is limited by the ability to use only three fluorochromes simultaneously and by its inability to detect novel alterations or additional aberrations beyond those specifically targeted by employed probes.

These limitations have led to the implementation of both RNA- and DNA-based next-generation sequencing (NGS) assays, which enable sensitive and comprehensive detection of fusion genes, point mutations, and copy number alterations simultaneously [45, 132, 173].

The initial morphologic evaluation remains essential for guiding differential diagnosis, selecting appropriate immunohistochemical markers, and identifying candidates for molecular testing. Molecular profiling provides critical information on lineage commitment, oncogenic drivers, and therapeutic vulnerabilities and has redefined sarcoma classification by distinguishing distinct categories of pathogenesis beyond traditional morphology-based criteria [58, 143].

Based on these principles, sarcomas can be broadly categorized into those with simple genomic profiles, driven by specific genetic alterations, and those with complex genomic architecture characterized by extensive chromosomal instability.

Sarcomas with simple genomic profiles harbor specific genetic drivers, whether chromosomal translocations producing fusion oncoproteins, activating mutations in kinases, or focal oncogene amplifications, while maintaining relatively stable, near-diploid karyotypes [148, 197]. At the opposite extreme, complex genomic sarcomas display widespread chromosomal instability and aneuploidy and lack dominant drivers, frequently resulting from catastrophic events including chromothripsis [89, 143]. A separate category comprises epigenetically deregulated sarcomas, defined by their dependence on chromatin dysregulation or metabolic reprogramming for malignant transformation [182].

This molecular heterogeneity reflects the multistep nature of sarcoma development. While oncogenesis typically initiates with a primary driver event, secondary alterations in tumor suppressors, chromatin modifiers, or metabolic regulators significantly influence biological behavior and clinical outcomes [87, 194]. These additional changes, though not always subtype-defining, determine therapeutic sensitivity, metastatic potential, and overall prognosis [48]. The genetic heterogeneity observed in high-grade sarcomas reflects this progressive accumulation of alterations and requires comprehensive molecular characterization beyond simple driver identification. Characterizing both driver events and coexisting molecular alterations enables accurate diagnosis, prognostic assessment, and identification of therapeutic targets.

Current molecular platforms enable simultaneous identification of fusion transcripts, point mutations, copy number alterations, and methylation patterns from single tissue samples. Such integrated analysis detects both primary drivers and secondary modifiers that influence tumor progression and therapeutic response [41].

This chapter organizes molecular testing strategies according to genomic and epigenomic alterations rather than conventional histopathologic categories. The structure reflects diagnostic priorities: sarcomas with simple genomic profiles requiring fusion detection and targeted mutation analysis, epigenetically deregulated sarcomas benefiting from chromatin modifier profiling and methylation assessment, and complex genomic sarcomas requiring broad mutational profiling to identify actionable events within chaotic genomes. Each category demands specific molecular approaches, from RNA sequencing for fusion detection to methylation arrays for epigenetic characterization, guiding optimal test selection for accurate diagnosis and therapeutic planning (Fig. 7.1).

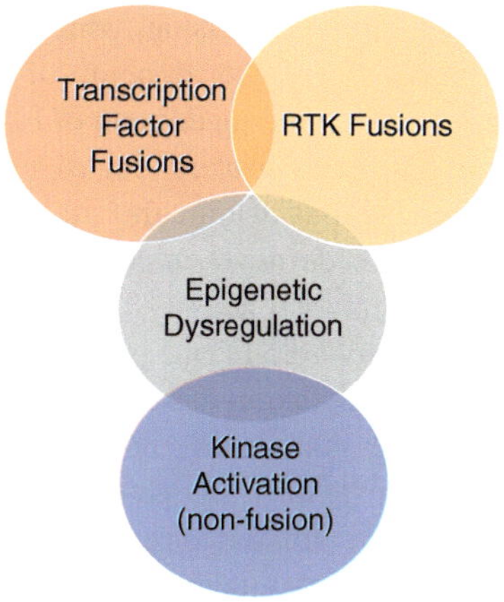

Fig. 7.1 Overlapping molecular mechanisms in soft tissue sarcomas. While tumors are classified by their primary driver mechanism, many exhibit features from multiple categories. The central intersection represents the epigenetic dysregulation that occurs as a consequence of various primary alterations, emphasizing that these categories represent a continuum rather than discrete entities. *RTK* receptor tyrosine kinase

Sarcomas with Simple Genomic Profiles

Sarcomas with simple genomic profiles represent a biologically distinct group of mesenchymal malignancies. They are often diagnosed in children and adolescents but may also occur across all age groups [207]. These tumors typically harbor a single, recurrent genetic alteration, most commonly a gene fusion, an activating mutation, or, more rarely, a focal amplification. Their karyotypes are typically near-diploid, with limited background chromosomal complexity and a relatively low mutational burden [41, 143]. Their characteristic molecular alterations frequently serve as specific diagnostic biomarkers, supporting morphological interpretation and defining the tumor entity.

Their genomic simplicity contrasts with considerable clinical heterogeneity. Some display indolent behavior with excellent outcomes following appropriate treatment, while others demonstrate aggressive biological characteristics and poor clinical outcomes despite intensive multimodal therapy [197]. Such clinical diversity indicates that single oncogenic drivers, though necessary for tumorigenesis, cannot predict prognosis alone. Additional factors modulate tumor behavior, including epigenetic regulation, interactions with the tumor microenvironment, cellular context, and secondary molecular events that accumulate during tumor evolution.

In selected cases, these alterations also represent actionable therapeutic targets, enabling the development of molecularly targeted therapies with significantly improved outcomes for specific sarcoma subtypes, particularly those harboring kinase fusions or activating mutations [65].

Based on the structural and functional nature of their driver alterations, they can be subdivided into three major categories:

Fusion-driven sarcomas with chimeric transcription factors: These tumors harbor gene rearrangements that generate aberrant transcriptional regulators, disrupting normal gene expression programs through constitutive activation, transcriptional repression, or chromatin remodeling [205].

RTK fusion-driven sarcomas: Characterized by rearrangements involving receptor tyrosine kinases that result in ligand-independent kinase activation and sustained proliferative signaling [12].

Non-fusion kinase-activated sarcomas: Defined by activating point mutations, oncogene amplifications, or tumor suppressor loss that dysregulate kinase signaling pathways without structural gene rearrangements [93].

This mechanistic division has limitations as many sarcomas show overlapping features. Fusion-positive tumors commonly display epigenetic remodeling, while kinase-activated neoplasms often demonstrate significant transcriptional dysregulation. These overlaps indicate that sarcomagenesis typically involves converging molecular events and interconnected pathways rather than isolated, linear oncogenic processes.

Fusion-Driven Sarcomas (Chimeric Transcription Factors)

Approximately 30% of adult sarcomas and a substantial proportion of pediatric sarcomas harbor recurrent gene rearrangements [207]. These chimeric proteins combine domains from two different genes: a transactivation domain from one partner and a DNA-binding domain from another. The resulting proteins disrupt normal development through three main mechanisms. First, they constitutively activate proliferative genes. Second, they suppress normal differentiation. Third, they remodel chromatin to create stable epigenetic changes. The fusion profiles serve as precise diagnostic markers and increasingly inform prognosis and treatment selection.

Fusion-driven transcription factors alter cellular programs through multiple mechanisms beyond simple activation or repression [199]. The specific combination of fusion partners, cellular context, and epigenetic landscape determines the phenotypic outcome. A single fusion may produce different tumors depending on the cell of origin and microenvironment, just as morphologically similar neoplasms may harbor distinct fusions with varying clinical behaviors [37].

While FISH and reverse transcriptase PCR (RT-PCR) remain useful in specific contexts, they cannot detect cryptic rearrangements, intronic breakpoints, or alternatively spliced fusion transcripts that RNA sequencing readily identifies. RNA-based NGS, particularly anchored multiplex PCR and hybrid-capture platforms, has become essential for the identification of both canonical and noncanonical gene fusions.

The undifferentiated small round sarcomas of soft tissue and bone tumors represent a morphologically related but molecularly heterogeneous group that exemplifies fusion-driven transcriptional activation. Despite sharing cytologic features of primitive round cells with minimal architectural complexity, these entities differ fundamentally in their molecular drivers, immunophenotypes, and clinical behaviors [207].

Ewing sarcoma represents the most extensively characterized member of this group. In approximately 85% of cases, the driving alteration is an *EWSR1::FLI1* fusion, which joins the N-terminal transactivation domain of *EWSR1* with the *ETS* DNA-binding domain of FLI1 [63]. The resulting fusion protein engages GGAA-microsatellite regions within the genome, converting them into de novo enhancers that drive aberrant transcriptional activity [88]. Chromatin remodeling by SWI/SNF and p300 is essential for sustaining the fusion-driven transcriptional program. These complexes modify chromatin architecture to establish a gene expression program favoring growth and impaired differentiation. The fusion also suppresses differentiation, in part by altering chromatin accessibility at lineage-specific loci [176]. Less frequent *ETS* partner genes, *ERG* (10%), *ETV1*, *ETV4*, and *FEV*, have been reported. Rarely, *FUS*, another FET family member, can substitute *for EWSR1*. All these fusions produce similar clinical phenotypes [184]. Ewing sarcomas exhibit strong membranous CD99 positivity, a sensitive but nonspecific finding.

CIC-rearranged sarcomas, most commonly harboring *CIC::DUX4* fusions, represent an aggressive subset of round cell tumors that upregulate PEA3 family transcription factors and show characteristic nuclear ETV4 expression by immunohistochemistry [18, 103, 162, 213]. While diffuse ETV4 staining is highly sensitive and specific for *CIC::DUX4* fusion-positive tumors, variant fusions with other partner genes such as *NUTM1*, *FOXO4*, and *LEUTX* lack DUX4 expression, requiring comprehensive molecular testing [103]. These tumors exhibit poor prognosis, with median overall survival below 12 months in metastatic cases and minimal response to standard Ewing-based chemotherapy [54].

BCOR-rearranged sarcomas constitute another important category of undifferentiated round cell tumors. These neoplasms most commonly harbor *BCOR::CCNB3* fusions resulting from cryptic paracentric inversions at Xp11.4, though *BCOR* internal tandem duplications and rare fusions with other gene partners such as *MAML3*, *ZC3H7B*, and *KMT2D* have been described [120]. The *BCOR::CCNB3* fusion juxtaposes the BCL6 corepressor with cyclin B3, creating a chimeric protein that disrupts normal cell-cycle regulation and transcriptional control. Nuclear BCOR expression characterizes these tumors, with variable SATB2 staining [18]. Clinically, BCOR-rearranged sarcomas demonstrate intermediate behavior between Ewing sarcoma and *CIC*-rearranged sarcomas, with better outcomes than the latter when treated with intensive chemotherapy regimens [54].

EWSR1::ATF1 and *EWSR1::CREB1* fusions demonstrate how identical molecular alterations produce divergent tumors depending on cellular context. These fusions activate MITF-driven melanocytic programs in clear cell sarcoma, resulting in S100 and melanoma marker expression, while the same fusions in angiomatoid fibrous histiocytoma produce different outcomes without melanocytic differentiation. The epigenetic landscape fundamentally shapes how these fusion proteins function in different cellular environments. Rare variants include *EWSR1::CREM* fusions in both entities [199].

A mechanistically distinct group of fusion-driven sarcomas operates through transcriptional repression rather than activation. Myxoid liposarcoma, characterized by *FUS::DDIT3* fusion or less commonly *EWSR1::DDIT3*, blocks adipocytic differentiation by inhibiting C/EBP and PPARγ activity [57]. The fusion protein maintains cells in an undifferentiated state through both direct transcriptional repression and chromatin remodeling via recruitment of BRD4 and SWI/SNF components [114].

Desmoplastic small round cell tumor is defined by the pathognomonic t(11;22)(p13;q12) translocation, associated to *EWSR1::WT1* fusion [207]. This fusion transforms WT1 from a developmental regulator into a constitutive transcriptional activator, driving expression of IGF2, PDGFA, and FGFR4 [133]. The tumor's characteristic co-expression of epithelial, mesenchymal, and muscle markers reflects this dysregulated developmental program [207].

Alveolar rhabdomyosarcoma represents an example of fusion-mediated amplification of lineage-specific programs while blocking terminal differentiation. The most common fusions, *PAX3::FOXO1* and *PAX7::FOXO1*, link myogenic transcriptional regulators to constitutively active FOXO1 domains, promoting persistent myogenic gene expression in cells that fail to complete differentiation [70]. Less common fusion gene variants include the fusion of *PAX3* to *FOXO4*, *NCOA1*, or *INO80D* and the fusion of *FOXO1::FGFR1*. The distinction between fusion-positive and fusion-negative rhabdomyosarcoma has major clinical implications, as fusion-positive tumors require intensified therapy and carry significantly worse prognosis [209].

Synovial sarcoma is the prototypical example of fusion-mediated epigenetic dysregulation. The *SS18::SSX* fusion, most frequently *SS18::SSX1* or *SS18::SSX2*, rarely *SS18::SSX4*, defines this entity through displacement of wild-type SS18 from the BAF complex, causing SMARCB1 eviction and profound chromatin remodeling. This altered complex cannot maintain normal enhancer function, resulting in widespread transcriptional dysregulation that locks cells in an undifferentiated state [191]. Recent studies have shown that the SSX C-terminus not only depends on H2AK119ub1 for localization but also further increases it by promoting PRC1.1 complex stability *SYT-SSX* gene fusion as a determinant of morphology and prognosis in synovial sarcoma [123].

Low-grade fibromyxoid sarcoma and extraskeletal myxoid chondrosarcoma further illustrate repression-based oncogenesis. Low-grade fibromyxoid sarcoma harbors *FUS::CREB3L2* or *EWSR1::CREB3L1* fusions that block fibroblastic maturation at the transcriptional level [69]. This differentiation blockade produces bland fibromyxoid morphology but clinically with metastatic potential. Extraskeletal myxoid chondrosarcoma, driven by *NR4A3*fusions, more commonly with *EWSR1*, less with other partner genes *TAF15T*, *CF12*, or *TFG*, blocks chondrocytic differentiation through recruitment of corepressor complexes to NR4A3 target genes [146]. Both entities illustrate that fusion-mediated differentiation blockade can produce indolent-appearing tumors with unpredictable clinical behavior.

Other fusion-driven sarcomas operate through diverse mechanisms. Solitary fibrous tumor is characterized by the *NAB2::STAT6* fusion, which results in aberrant nuclear localization and overexpression of STAT6 [177]. Multiple fusion variants exist, with different combinations of *NAB2* and *STAT6* exons, though all result in nuclear STAT6 accumulation [24]. In contrast, alveolar soft part sarcoma harbors the *ASPSCR1::TFE3* fusion, generated by a der(17)t(X;17)(p11;q25) [130]. The resulting chimeric protein leads to nuclear accumulation of TFE3, a member of the MiT family of transcription factors, which activates gene networks involved in angiogenesis and proliferation [203]. Alveolar soft part sarcoma displays a unique molecular profile and lacks clear lineage differentiation, consistent with an origin from an undifferentiated progenitor without a normal cellular counterpart [72].

Additional examples include epithelioid hemangioendothelioma, which comprises two molecular subtypes: the more common *WWTR1::CAMTA1* fusion and the less frequent *YAP1::TFE3* fusion [14]. *YAP1::TFE3*-positive cases tend to occur in younger patients and show more solid growth patterns with nuclear TFE3 expression [64].

IHC remains fundamental in the diagnostic evaluation of fusion-driven sarcomas, capturing downstream transcriptional effects that serve as surrogate markers for specific genetic alterations. However, the phenomenon of gene promiscuity, where single genes participate in fusions with multiple partners across different tumor types, significantly complicates interpretation. This complexity, first recognized with *EWSR1* rearrangements in the 1980s, has expanded dramatically with RNA sequencing. *EWSR1* alone participates in fusions with over 30 different partners, also of different lineages, producing vastly different sarcoma: EWSR1::ATF1 in both clear cell sarcoma and angiomatoid fibrous histiocytoma, *EWSR1::WT1* in desmoplastic small round cell tumor, *EWSR1::FLI1* in Ewing sarcoma, and many others. This promiscuity means detecting an *EWSR1* rearrangement by FISH provides limited diagnostic specificity without partner identification, necessitating comprehensive molecular profiling [202].

The FET gene family (EWSR1, FUS, TAF15) demonstrates particular versatility, with members forming functionally equivalent fusions, *FUS::ERG* in Ewing-like sarcomas, *FUS::CREB3L2* in low-grade fibromyxoid sarcoma, and *FUS::DDIT3* in myxoid liposarcoma. *TAF15* can substitute in several contexts, including *TAF15::NR4A3* in extraskeletal myxoid chondrosarcoma [102]. This redundancy means *EWSR1*-negative cases may harbor pathogenetically equivalent *FUS* or *TAF15* fusions, necessitating comprehensive molecular screening [199].

RNA sequencing has emerged as an indispensable tool for detecting complex gene fusions that often evade conventional cytogenetic methods. Unlike DNA-based approaches, RNA sequencing directly captures expressed fusion transcripts, bypassing the limitations of cryptic breakpoints and alternative splicing events [40]. This proves particularly valuable in settings where standard FISH may yield false-negative results. Examples include solitary fibrous tumor where the close proximity of NAB2 and STAT6 on chromosome 12 complicates detection of *NAB2::STAT6* fusions [177]; extraskeletal myxoid chondrosarcoma in which variant partners other than *EWSR1::NR4A3* may be missed [3] and Ewing sarcoma with *EWSR1::ERG* fusion, where complex inversions between oppositely oriented genes lead to FISH failure in a subset of cases [46].

The biological context profoundly influences fusion protein function. Identical fusions produce divergent tumors depending on the cell of origin and epigenetic landscape. The *EWSR1::ATF1* fusion activates melanocytic programs in clear cell sarcoma but not in angiomatoid fibrous histiocytoma. Similarly, *FUS::CREB3L2* and *FUS::CREB3L1* fusions occur in both low-grade fibromyxoid sarcoma and sclerosing epithelioid fibrosarcoma, entities with markedly different clinical behaviors. Conversely, morphologically similar round cell sarcomas harbor distinct fusions with different therapeutic responses. Ewing sarcoma responds to intensive chemotherapy while *CIC*-rearranged tumors show poor outcomes, with *BCOR*-rearranged sarcomas demonstrating intermediate behavior (Table 7.1).

Table 7.1 Molecular classification of fusion-driven soft tissue sarcomas

Classification	WHO category	Gene	Fusion partners
Myxoid liposarcoma	Adipocytic tumors	*FUS*	*DDIT3*
		EWSR1	*DDIT3*
Solitary fibrous tumor	Fibroblastic/ myofibroblastic tumors	*NAB2*	*STAT6*
Sclerosing epithelioid fibrosarcoma		*EWSR1*	*CREB3L1, CREB3L2*
		FUS	*CREB3L2*
Superficial CD34+ fibroblastic tumor		*PRDM10*	*MED12, CITED2*
Myxoinflammatory fibroblastic sarcoma		*TGFBR3*	*MGEA5*
Ewing sarcoma	Undifferentiated small round cell sarcomas	*EWSR1*	*FLI1, ERG, ETV1, ETV4*
		FUS	*ERG, FEV*
BCOR-altered sarcoma		*BCOR*	*CCNB3, MAML3, ZC3H7B, KMT2D, CIITA, CHD9, RGAG1, CLGN*
CIC-rearranged sarcoma		*CIC*	*DUX4, FOXO4, LEUTX, NUTM1, NUTM2B, CITED1, AXL, SYK*
Alveolar rhabdomyosarcoma	Skeletal muscle tumors	*PAX3/7*	*FOXO1*
Fusion-associated spindle cell rhabdomyosarcoma	Skeletal muscle tumors	*VGLL2*	*NCOA2, CITED2*
		TEAD1	*NCOA2, CITED2*
Angiomatoid fibrous histiocytoma	Tumors of uncertain differentiation	*EWSR1*	*CREB1, ATF1*
		FUS	*ATF1*
Ossifying fibromyxoid tumor		*EP400, MEAF6, PHF1*	*PHF1, other partners*
Myoepithelial carcinoma (soft tissue)		*EWSR1*	*POU5F1, PBX1, PBX3, ZNF444*
Myoepithelial tumors		*PLAG1*	*TRPS1, RAD51B, TRIM13, MIR143HG*
Synovial sarcoma		*SS18*	*SSX1, SSX2, SSX4*
Alveolar soft part sarcoma		*ASPSCR1*	*TFE3*
Clear cell sarcoma		*EWSR1*	*ATF1, CREB1*
Extraskeletal myxoid chondrosarcoma		*EWSR1, TAF15, TCF12*	*NR4A3*
Desmoplastic small round cell tumor		*EWSR1*	*WT1*
PEComa (TFE3-rearranged)		*TFE3*	*SFPQ (PSF), NONO, DVL2, MED15*
Epithelioid hemangioendothelioma	Vascular tumors	*WWTR1*	*CAMTA1*
YAP1-TFE3 hemangioendothelioma		*YAP1*	*TFE3*
Pseudomyogenic hemangioendothelioma		*SERPINE1, ACTB*	*FOSB*

Entities are organized by WHO category with corresponding gene fusions organized by WHO categories. The table demonstrates the promiscuity of FET family genes (*EWSR1*, *FUS*, *TAF15*) across multiple sarcoma subtypes and illustrates the functional redundancy among fusion partners with shared mechanisms of transcriptional dysregulation

RTK Fusion-Driven Sarcomas

Receptor tyrosine kinases constitute a large family of transmembrane proteins that control fundamental cellular processes, including proliferation, differentiation, survival, and motility through ligand-dependent activation of intracellular signaling cascades [201]. These proteins share a conserved structural architecture comprising an extracellular ligand-binding domain, a single transmembrane helix, and a cytoplasmic tyrosine kinase domain [67, 135].

In soft tissue neoplasms, RTK gene fusions define a molecularly distinct subset characterized by simple karyotypes and profound oncogenic dependence on the chimeric kinase. These rearrangements involve retention of the RTK kinase domain fused to a 5′ partner gene providing dimerization motifs, altered localization signals, or transcriptional regulatory elements. The resulting fusion proteins are constitutively active, bypassing normal ligand-dependent regulation and sustaining continuous downstream signaling [12, 17].

Among RTK fusions in sarcomas, the most extensively studied involve *ALK* and *NTRK1–3*, each associated with a broad morphological spectrum [60, 160].

RTK fusion activation occurs via three principal mechanisms. The first and most frequent involves partner-mediated dimerization, typically through coiled-coil or oligomerization domains, as seen in *TPM3::NTRK1* and *TPM3::ALK* [76, 92]. These alterations force receptor dimerization independent of ligand binding, resulting in trans-autophosphorylation and persistent kinase activation. This mechanism underlies the majority of therapeutically targetable RTK fusions in sarcomas.

ALK exhibits marked promiscuity across mesenchymal neoplasms, and tumors of other lineages, forming fusions with over 30 different partner genes. In inflammatory myofibroblastic tumors (IMTs), *ALK* fusions, found in 50% of cases, involve partners including *EML4*, *TPM3*, *TPM4*, *CLTC*, *FN1*, *SEC31A*, *ATIC*, *CARS*, *LMNA*, and *PPFIBP1*. The specific partner sometime influences anatomic distribution and clinical behavior: *FN1::ALK* predominates in bladder and genitourinary IMTs, while *RANBP2::ALK* defines the aggressive epithelioid inflammatory myofibroblastic sarcoma variant [2].

Beyond IMTs, *ALK* rearrangements also occur in other mesenchymal tumors with distinct fusion partners. *TIMP3::ALK* is characteristic of laryngeal myxoid sarcomas, while epithelioid and round cell sarcomas may harbor *EML4*, *HMBOX1*, *PRRC2B*, *VCL*, *MYH10*, *STRN*, and *PLEKHH2* as *ALK* partner genes. Some rearrangements, particularly *FLNA::ALK*, *VCL::ALK*, and *SQSTM1::ALK*, are associated with low-grade or indolent behavior, indicating some prognostic relevance of the fusion partner [2].

The *NTRK1*, *NTRK2*, and *NTRK3* genes display comparable promiscuity, with rearrangements identified in diverse histologic entities [1, 141]. Infantile fibrosarcoma typically harbors *ETV6::NTRK3* fusion in the majority of cases arising within the first year of life. However, a subset of morphologically similar but *ETV6*-negative spindle cell sarcomas harbor alternative kinase fusions involving *ALK*, *BRAF*, *NTRK1/2*, *RET*, *ROS1*, or *MET* [126, 193].

Lipofibromatosis-like neural tumors (LPF-NTs), affecting children and young adults, are histologically bland but consistently harbor *NTRK1* fusions, most commonly a cryptic *LMNA::NTRK1* and less frequently *TPR::NTRK1* or *TPM3::NTRK1*[5]. Cases lacking NTRK rearrangements may instead harbor *RET* or *ALK* fusions, particularly in infants and young children [16, 139].

In adult sarcomas, *NTRK* fusions can occur across diverse histologies, often producing high-grade tumors with pleomorphic morphology. These alterations confer constitutive kinase activity and uncontrolled proliferation, reflecting a growth pattern disconnected from lineage differentiation. While pan-TRK immunohistochemistry (IHC) serves as a useful screening tool with ~82% overall sensitivity, it has variable sensitivity by subtype (27% for *NTRK3* versus 14% for *NTRK2* and 6% for *NTRK1*). Interpretation can be difficult by nonspecific staining in neural and muscular tissue, and cryptic rearrangements, especially involving *NTRK1*, necessitate molecular confirmation [97].

Beyond *ALK* and *NTRK* rearrangements, the involvement of other RTKs expands the spectrum of kinase-driven sarcomas. *ROS1* fusions with partner genes such as *TFG*, *YWHAE*, and *TPD52L2* have been described in IMTs, often presenting in deep soft tissues or visceral sites [15, 137]. These tumors frequently lack diffuse inflammatory infiltrates and are ALK-negative by

IHC, making molecular testing essential for diagnosis [98]. *RET* fusions, notably with *CCDC6* and *NCOA4* partner genes, are found in pediatric spindle cell sarcomas that morphologically and immunophenotypically resemble *NTRK*-rearranged tumors [59].

FGFR1fusions with *FN1*, *TACC1*, *EBF2*, and *PARD6B* as partner genes have been identified in rare mesenchymal tumors with variable morphology. These fusions retain the *FGFR*1 kinase domain and achieve constitutive activation through dimerization domains provided by the fusion partner, following a pattern analogous to other RTK fusions.

MET rearrangements are exceedingly rare in sarcomas. The *TFG::MET* fusion was initially described in infantile hemangioendothelioma and subsequently in rare pediatric spindle cell sarcomas, leading to MET overexpression at mRNA level and MET protein overexpression. This represents one of the first examples of *MET* activation via chromosomal translocation in mesenchymal tumors. Although *MET* fusions involving various partners have been identified in epithelial malignancies, their role in sarcomas remains poorly characterized and limited to isolated case reports [59].

The identification of receptor tyrosine kinase (RTK) fusions has redefined sarcoma classification, moving from a morphology-based system to molecularly defined categories. *NTRK* rearrangements predict response to larotrectinib and entrectinib [100], while ALK fusions respond to crizotinib and alectinib [154].

The second mechanism involves altered subcellular localization that modifies signaling context and downstream pathway engagement. The *RANBP2::ALK* fusion in epithelioid inflammatory myofibroblastic sarcoma exemplifies this, with ALK being sequestered to the nuclear envelope via RANBP2, a nuclear pore complex protein [144]. This compartmentalization correlates with aggressive clinical behavior and reduced sensitivity to first-generation ALK inhibitors, suggesting that subcellular context influences both tumor biology and therapeutic response.

The third mechanism involves promoter-swapping events, in which the fusion partner contributes transcriptional regulatory elements that drive overexpression of a structurally intact receptor or its ligand. *COL1A1::PDGFB* in dermatofibrosarcoma protuberans operates through this mechanism; the *COL1A1* promoter drives aberrant PDGFB production, activating PDGFRB through autocrine signaling. Similar mechanisms occur in tenosynovial giant cell tumor with *COL6A3::CSF1* fusion and in phosphaturic mesenchymal tumors with *FN1::FGFR1* or *BAG4::FGFR1* fusions [115, 159] (Table 7.2).

Non-fusion Dependent Kinase Pathway-Activated Sarcomas

A subset of malignant mesenchymal neoplasms is not characterized by gene fusions, but by activating point mutations, oncogene amplifications, or biallelic inactivation of tumor suppressor genes. These alterations disrupt intracellular signaling cascades, most commonly the RTK-PI3K-AKT-mTOR, RAS-RAF-MAPK, and JAK-STAT pathways, promoting proliferative and survival advantages through sustained kinase activity [68, 153].

Non-fusion kinase-activated sarcomas operate through three principal mechanisms. Activating mutations in receptor tyrosine kinases including *KIT*, *PDGFRA*, and *FGFR4* cause ligand-independent signaling [116]. High-level oncogene amplifications of *MYC* and *FLT4* drive transcriptional and angiogenic dysregulation [11]. Biallelic tumor suppressor loss, particularly *TSC1/TSC2*, results in unchecked pathway activation.

Gastrointestinal stromal tumor (GIST) is defined by specific activating mutations in *KIT* (75–80% of cases) or *PDGFRA* (10–15% of cases) that determine both biological behavior and therapeutic response [52].

KIT mutations most frequently involve exon 11, which encodes the juxtamembrane domain. These alterations disrupt autoinhibitory regulation and result in constitutive activation of the kinase. Exon 9 duplications affect the extracellular domain and require higher imatinib doses for optimal control, whereas mutations in exons 13

Table 7.3 Non-fusion dependent kinase pathway-activated sarcomas

Classification	WHO category	Driver gene(s)	Alterations	Alteration type
Desmoid fibromatosis	Fibroblastic/ myofibroblastic tumors	*CTNNB1, APC*	*CTNNB1 (T41A, S45F, S45P), APC* mutations	Point mutations
Embryonal rhabdomyosarcoma (ERMS)	Skeletal muscle tumor	*FGFR4, RAS* family *(NRAS, KRAS, HRAS), PIK3CA*	*FGFR4 hotspots (N535K/D, V550E/L), RAS/PIK3CA* mutations	Point mutations
MYOD1-mutant spindle cell/sclerosing RMS		*MYOD1, PIK3CA*	*MYOD1 L122R ± PIK3CA* mutations	Point mutations
Angiosarcoma	Vascular tumors	*KDR (VEGFR2), PIK3CA, PLCG1*	*KDR* hotspots, *PIK3CA* (H1047R, E545K), *PLCG1* (R707Q)	Point mutations
PEComa (non-TFE3)	Perivascular tumors	*TSC1, TSC2*	Inactivating mutations	Mutation/ deletion
GIST—KIT mutant	Gastrointestinal stromal tumor	*KIT*	Exon 11, Exon 9, Exon 13, Exon 17, Exon 8 (rare)	Point mutations
GIST—PDGFRA mutant		*PDGFRA*	D842V (resistant), D842Y, DI842-843M, Exon 12, Exon 14	Point mutations

Molecular alterations that primarily affect RTK-PI3K-AKT-mTOR and RAS-RAF-MAPK pathways through point mutations rather than structural rearrangements

Sarcomas with Complex Genomic Profiles

Sarcomas with complex genomic profiles exhibit extensive genomic instability, characterized by chromosomal gains and losses, structural rearrangements, and polyplodization typically accumulating multiple alterations that disrupt core regulatory pathways [41, 48, 143, 151, 197].

They can be broadly grouped into two partially overlapping categories. The first includes tumors that, despite genomic disorganization, harbor recurrent genetic alterations with diagnostic or prognostic utility, such as *MDM2* and *CDK4* amplification in dedifferentiated liposarcoma and intimal sarcoma, or inactivating mutations in *TP53* and *RB1* in leiomyosarcoma [41, 174]. The second comprises tumors exhibiting extensive chromosomal complexity without consistent or targetable alterations, as seen in undifferentiated pleomorphic sarcoma, myxofibrosarcoma, and pleomorphic liposarcoma [41].

Some sarcomas, e.g., high-grade leiomyosarcoma and dedifferentiated liposarcoma, straddle both categories, exhibiting recurrent alterations alongside extensive genomic complexity [8, 41, 119, 178]. These tumors represent a genomic continuum rather than distinct molecular categories. Additionally, many of these tumors exhibit aberrant epigenetic regulation, including global methylation shifts and chromatin remodeling defects, which influence phenotype and clinical behavior [134].

Complex Genomic Profiles with Recurrent Drivers

These sarcomas exhibiting widespread chromosomal instability harbor recurrent molecular alterations that, while not pathognomonic, occur with sufficient regularity to support diagnostic recognition and biological stratification. These tumors often show polyploidization, widespread copy number variation, structural rearrangements, and chromothripsis-like patterns.

Well-differentiated liposarcomas (WD-LPS) are characterized by supernumerary ring or giant marker chromosomes derived from chromosome 12 [166]. These structures, which vary in size between cells due to chromosomal breakage-fusion-bridge events, contain recurrent amplification of the 12q13-q15 region involving multiple genes including *DDIT3*, *HMGA2*, *MDM2*, *CDK4*, *CPM*, and *DNM3OS* [8, 107, 195]. Amplification of *MDM2* and *CDK4* is consistently present and constitutes the defining molecular hallmark of this tumor type. As *MDM2* functions as the primary negative regulator of p53, *MDM2* amplification and *TP53* alterations are mutually exclusive in malignant adipose tissue tumors [189].

Dedifferentiated liposarcoma (DD-LPS) shares the characteristic 12q13–q15 amplification of WD-LPS, which includes canonical drivers such as MDM2 and CDK4 together with co-amplified genes on the same amplicon, including *HMGA2*, *CPM*, *TSPAN31*, *YEATS4*, and *FRS2* [166]. In addition, DD-LPS frequently acquires further copy number alterations that are uncommon in WD-LPS, most notably focal 1p32 amplification of *JUN* and, in a partially overlapping subset of cases, 6q23 amplification of *MAP 3 K5* [187] [95]. These events are associated with tumor progression and dedifferentiation rather than being exclusive to the dedifferentiated phenotype. Additional alterations in *RB1*, *TP53*, and *CDKN2A* are observed in a subset of cases, consistent with disruption of cell-cycle control mechanisms. While *MDM2* amplification is highly characteristic, it is not entirely specific to liposarcoma. It has been reported in intimal sarcoma and low-grade osteosarcoma and occasionally in myxofibrosarcoma, malignant peripheral nerve sheath tumors (MPNST), and undifferentiated sarcomas, requiring meticulous histopathologic correlation [207].

Intimal sarcoma, arising within large blood vessels, is biologically and clinically distinct from dedifferentiated liposarcoma but shares high-level *MDM2* amplification at 12q15, frequently accompanied by co-amplification of *CDK4*, *HMGA2*, and *PDGFRA* at 4q12 [156]. Management is challenging due to frequent local recurrence, distant metastasis, and anatomically critical locations.

Leiomyosarcoma is a high-grade sarcoma of smooth muscle differentiation that may originate in the uterus, retroperitoneum, or extremities [78]. While lacking a unifying molecular driver, it shows cumulative tumor suppressor disruption [23, 41, 51, 207]. Biallelic TP53 loss occurs in 40–60% of cases, causing widespread chromosomal instability [19], while *RB1* disruption through deletion or mutation at 13q14 is equally common. Combined *TP53/RB1* inactivation drives cell-cycle dysregulation in most high-grade tumors. *PTEN* loss occurs in approximately 40–45% of all leiomyosarcomas, resulting in PI3K-AKT-mTOR pathway activation [80].

Comprehensive genomic profiling reveals complex structural variation, including chromothripsis-like events and focal amplifications of *MYC*, *CCNE1*, and *VEGFA*, supporting a tumorigenesis model driven by cumulative tumor suppressor disruption rather than dominant oncogene activation [9, 48]. Whole-exome sequencing of matched primary and metastatic leiomyosarcoma samples shows that most driver alterations, including *TP53* mutations, are retained in metastases, indicating linear evolutionary progression that contrasts with the divergent clonal evolution seen in liposarcomas [27, 108].

Transcriptomic profiling identifies three clinically relevant molecular subtypes despite shared genomic alterations [27, 90].

The differentiated smooth muscle subtype expresses ACTG2, MYH11, and CNN1, retains functional RB1, and maintains myogenic differentiation features. The dedifferentiated proliferative subtype demonstrates upregulation of mitotic regulators AURKA and PLK1, near-universal TP53/RB1 co-inactivation, and aggressive clinical behavior. The immune-infiltrated subtype shows enrichment of immune-related transcripts and variable checkpoint molecule expression, suggesting potential immunotherapy responsiveness [4, 90].

This molecular stratification identifies therapeutic vulnerabilities: CDK4/6 inhibitors for RB1-intact tumors, AURKA/PLK1 inhibitors for proliferative subtypes, PI3K inhibitors for PTEN-deficient cases, and checkpoint blockade for immune-infiltrated tumors, though prospective validation remains necessary [78, 90].

Malignant peripheral nerve sheath tumor (MPNST) is a biologically aggressive sarcoma accounting for approximately 5–10% of soft tissue sarcomas [56]. While MPNST often arises in the setting of neurofibromatosis type 1, it may also develop sporadically or after radiation therapy [122]. The initiating event in both NF1-associated and a significant subset of sporadic MPNST tumors exhibits *NF1* biallelic inactivation of the leading to constitutive activation of the RAS-MAPK signaling pathway [167]. However, *NF1* loss alone is insufficient for malignant transformation. A near-universal early event in MPNST development is homozygous deletion or epigenetic silencing of *CDKN2A/B*, which disrupts both the p53 and RB tumor suppressor pathways via loss of *p16INK4a* and *p14ARF* [157].

Progression to high-grade malignancy often involves inactivation of the Polycomb Repressive Complex 2 through mutations in SUZ12 or *EED*, resulting in global reduction of H3K27me3 detectable by IHC [61]. While H3K27me3 loss is not exclusive to MPNST, also seen in synovial sarcoma and fibrosarcomatous dermatofibrosarcoma protuberans, it remains a useful diagnostic marker in the appropriate clinical and morphologic context [53].

Angiosarcomas are vascular sarcomas defined by a heterogeneous array of genomic alterations that converge on dysregulated angiogenic signaling [214]. Secondary angiosarcomas, particularly those arising post-radiotherapy or in the setting of chronic lymphedema, frequently harbor *MYC* amplification [142]. *FLT4* co-amplification occurs in a subset and is associated with poor prognosis [13]. Somatic mutations in *KDR*, *PTPRB*, and *PLCG1* have been described in both primary and secondary cases, particularly in tumors of the breast, bone, and visceral organs [28]. *CIC* alterations are enriched in younger patients with primary angiosarcoma and may carry diagnostic implications [101]. These molecular features offer potential biomarkers and therapeutic targets, indicating the importance of integrated histopathology, IHC, and comprehensive molecular profiling (Table 7.4).

Complex Genomic Profiles with Nonrecurrent Driver Sarcomas

These high-grade sarcomas exhibit extensive genomic complexity without identifiable recurrent or defining driver alterations, creating substantial diagnostic and therapeutic challenges [71].

Pleomorphic liposarcoma is an uncommon but clinically aggressive form of lipogenic sarcoma, accounting for approximately 5–10% of liposarcoma cases [77]. The diagnosis requires identification of pleomorphic lipoblasts and molecular exclusion of *MDM2/CDK4* amplification and *DDIT3* rearrangements to distinguish it from dedifferentiated and myxoid liposarcoma, respectively [79]. From a molecular standpoint, pleomorphic liposarcoma lacks a unifying genetic driver, instead exhibiting a highly complex karyotype with extensive chromosomal rear-

Table 7.4 Recurrent molecular alterations in complex genomic sarcomas

Classification	WHO category	Recurrent genes/alterations
Well-differentiated liposarcoma (WD-LPS)	Adipocytic	*MDM2*, *CDK4*, *HMGA2* amplification (12q13–q15)
Dedifferentiated liposarcoma (DD-LPS)	Adipocytic	*MDM2*, *CDK4* amplification; secondary *JUN*, *MAP3K5*, *RB1*, *ARID1A*, *RUNX3* alterations
Intimal sarcoma	Fibroblastic/myofibroblastic	*MDM2*, *CDK4*, *HMGA2*, *PDGFRA* amplification
Leiomyosarcoma (LMS)	Smooth muscle	*TP53*, *RB1*, *PTEN*, *ATRX* mutations; *MYC*, *CCNE1*, *VEGFA* amplifications
Malignant peripheral nerve sheath tumor (MPNST)	Peripheral nerve sheath	*NF1*, *CDKN2A/B* loss; *SUZ12*, *EED* inactivation (PRC2 complex)
Angiosarcoma (sporadic/secondary)	Vascular	*MYC*, *FLT4* amplification; *KDR*, *PLCG1*, *PTPRB* mutations; *CIC* (rare)

Key driver events distinguishing specific entities within the spectrum of chromosomally unstable sarcomas

Table 7.5 Complex genomic sarcomas lacking recurrent drivers

Classification	WHO category	Genomic alteration
Pleomorphic liposarcoma (PLPS)	Adipocytic tumors	*TP53*, *RB1*, *CDKN2A* mutations; PI3K/AKT/mTOR and RAS/MAPK activation
Myxofibrosarcoma (MFS)	Fibroblastic/ myofibroblastic tumors	*TP53*, *RB1*, *NF1*, and *CDKN2A* mutations; focal amplifications of *CCND1*, *CCNE1*, *EGFR*, *FGFR1*, *RET*, and *JUN*
Undifferentiated pleomorphic sarcoma (UPS)	Tumors of uncertain differentiation	*TP53*, *RB1*, *ATRX*, *CDKN2A*, and *NF1* mutations; recurrent deletions affecting *RB1* and *CDKN2A*

High mutational burden entities characterized by nonspecific alterations in tumor suppressors and cell-cycle regulators

rangements, aneuploidy, and structural instability [23]. NGS has consistently identified inactivation of key tumor suppressors, notably *TP53* and *RB1*, often in association with homozygous deletion of *CDKN2A* [79, 106]. These lesions suggest disruption of cell-cycle checkpoints as an early and fundamental feature of tumorigenesis in pleomorphic liposarcoma. Additional alterations affecting PI3K/AKT/mTOR and RAS/MAPK pathways occur variably, lacking specificity and uniform distribution across cases [73].

Myxofibrosarcoma similarly lacks a defining alteration and instead exhibits pronounced genomic complexity with widespread copy number aberrations [147]. Recurrent losses affect tumor suppressor loci including *CDKN2A*, *RB1*, *TP53*, *NF1*, and ATRX, while high-grade tumors frequently acquire focal amplifications of *CCND1*, *CCNE1*, *EGFR*, *FGFR1*, *RET*, and *JUN* [161, 208]. *TP53* alterations represent the most prevalent somatic mutations, often associated with loss of 17p13.1, and appear to represent early clonal events that precede histologic progression. Intratumoral comparison reveals identical *TP53* mutations in both low- and high-grade areas, supporting a model of early driver acquisition followed by secondary genomic derangements during dedifferentiation. Recent integrative analyses also identify deregulated DNA methylation programs, with disruption of pathways linked to genome stability, cell-cycle control, and senescence, indicating that combined genetic and epigenetic alterations drive tumor evolution [161].

Undifferentiated pleomorphic sarcoma (UPS), as described in the [207] classification, is a diagnosis of exclusion for pleomorphic neoplasms lacking lineage-specific differentiation by morphology, immunophenotype, or molecular testing [83]. These tumors show aneuploid karyotypes with multiple chromosomal aberrations and heterogeneous mutational patterns [168]. The molecular landscape reflects accumulated genomic damage characterized by recurrent inactivation of tumor suppressors, including *TP53*, *RB1*, *ATRX*, *CDKN2A*, *PTEN*, and *NF1*, yet no single mutation consistently defines the category. NGS reveals a high burden of mutations, many of which are likely passenger events secondary to genomic instability [44].

These genomically complex sarcomas lacking recurrent drivers pose significant therapeutic challenges. Unlike entities with targetable alterations, undifferentiated pleomorphic sarcoma, myxofibrosarcoma, and pleomorphic liposarcoma lack actionable molecular targets. Their high mutational burden may confer immunotherapy sensitivity, representing the most promising therapeutic avenue currently under investigation [171] (Table 7.5).

Epigenetically Deregulated Sarcomas (Oncometabolite-Related and Chromatin Remodeling-Deficient)

Epigenetically deregulated sarcomas constitute a functionally defined subset of mesenchymal malignancies in which oncogenic transformation arises primarily from disruption of chromatin and transcriptional control rather than from classical genetic drivers. Unlike sarcomas with complex karyotypes, these tumors often exhibit relatively simple genomes; however, a single initiating alteration, such as mutation of metabolic enzymes like *SDH* genes or loss of a core SWI/SNF subunit, induces widespread transcriptional reprogramming that drives aggressive clinical behavior [128, 152].

The epigenetically deregulated sarcomas discussed here fall into two main molecular categories based on their primary mechanism of chromatin disruption. First, mutations in metabolic enzymes produce oncometabolites that alter chromatin-modifying enzymes. Second is inactivation of chromatin remodeling complexes that maintain normal differentiation programs [181, 210].

This biologically distinct group includes tumors with mutations affecting mainly chromatin remodeling complexes, including SMARCB1 and SMARCA4, or metabolic enzymes such as SDH [182].

Furthermore, certain fusion-positive sarcomas, including synovial sarcoma and epithelioid hemangioendothelioma, depend on downstream epigenetic reprogramming for oncogenesis [22, 145]. The *SS18::SSX* fusion in synovial sarcoma disrupts BAF complex function and alters chromatin accessibility, while *WWTR1::CAMTA1* in hemangioendothelioma modulates transcriptional programs through chromatin remodeling [34, 198].

Unlike fusion-driven tumors with direct oncogenic drivers, epigenetically deregulated sarcomas achieve transformation through indirect mechanisms that alter the transcriptional landscape [175]. In contrast to complex karyotype sarcomas with widespread genomic instability, they maintain relatively stable genomes while exhibiting marked epigenetic instability. This distinction has critical therapeutic implications, as these tumors often respond to epigenetic modulators rather than conventional targeted therapies.

NGS panels that include epigenetic regulators or RNA-based transcriptomic profiling have become essential for identifying pathognomonic alterations. This molecular characterization has refined diagnostic classification and identified therapeutic targets, including EZH2 inhibitors, histone deacetylase inhibitors, and super-enhancer targeting agents [127].

One of the best characterized examples of sarcomas driven by mutations in metabolic enzymes that generate oncometabolites is succinate dehydrogenase (SDH)-deficient GIST [109]. These metabolites inhibit α-ketoglutarate-dependent dioxygenases, including histone demethylases and TET enzymes, causing global DNA and histone hypermethylation [211].

SDH-deficient sarcomas extend beyond GISTs, discussed previously in Sect. 2.3, to include rare mesenchymal neoplasms of the uterus, kidney, and retroperitoneum [81, 164]. These share the same mechanism of succinate accumulation inhibiting α-ketoglutarate-dependent enzymes, with SDHB loss serving as a universal immunohistochemical marker regardless of which *SDH* subunit is affected.

The second category involves loss of SWI/SNF chromatin remodeling complex components. This ATP-dependent complex maintains open chromatin at enhancers and opposes PRC2-mediated repression [117]. Biallelic inactivation of subunits including *SMARCB1*, *SMARCA4*, or *ARID1A* prevents proper differentiation and creates PRC2-dependent tumors that rely on epigenetic silencing for survival [117].

SMARCB1-deficient tumors include malignant rhabdoid tumors, atypical teratoid/rhabdoid tumors, and epithelioid sarcomas [96]. Loss of *SMARCB1(INI1)* permits unchecked PRC2 activity and H3K27me3 accumulation [206]. These aggressive tumors show complete INI1 loss by IHC and characteristic rhabdoid morphology with eccentric nuclei, prominent nucleoli, and eosinophilic cytoplasm [31].

SMARCA4-deficient tumors include thoracic sarcomas and small cell carcinoma of the ovary hypercalcemic type. Loss of *SMARCA4 (BRG1)*, often with concurrent *SMARCA2* loss, eliminates all SWI/SNF ATPase activity [169, 212]. These undifferentiated epithelioid to rhabdoid tumors show *SMARCA4/BRG1* loss with retained INI1 and positive SOX2 staining [212]. Prognosis is extremely poor with minimal chemotherapy benefit. Transcriptomic analyses reveal close clustering between SMARCA4-deficient thoracic sarcoma [10], small cell carcinoma of the ovary hypercalcemic type, and malignant rhabdoid tumors, reinforcing their shared epigenetic basis despite different anatomical origins [20] (Table 7.6).

Table 7.6 Epigenetically deregulated sarcomas

WHO histology	WHO category	Driver gene(s)	Alterations	Alteration type
Malignant peripheral nerve sheath tumor	Peripheral nerve sheath tumors	*SUZ12, EED (PRC2 components)*	H3K27me3 loss, epigenetic dysregulation	Deletion
	Peripheral nerve sheath tumors	*NF1, CDKN2A/B*	RAS activation + cell-cycle dysregulation	Deletion
Epithelioid MPNST	Peripheral nerve sheath tumors	*SMARCB1 (INI1)*	SWI/SNF complex inactivation	Deletion mutation
Epithelioid sarcoma	Tumors of uncertain differentiation	*SMARCB1 (INI1)*	SWI/SNF complex inactivation, EZH2 activation	Deletion mutation
Extrarenal rhabdoid tumor	Tumors of uncertain differentiation	SMARCB1 (INI1), SMARCA4 (rare)	SWI/SNF complex inactivation	Deletion mutation
SDH-deficient GIST (epigenetic subset)	Gastrointestinal stromal tumor	SDHC	Epigenetic silencing, pseudohypoxia	Promoter hypermethylation

These entities demonstrate a relatively simple karyotypes but profound transcriptional dysregulation through SWI/SNF complex inactivation or metabolic enzyme mutations affecting α-ketoglutarate-dependent dioxygenases

Table 7.7 Emerging molecular entities in soft tissue sarcomas identified since [207] classification

Entity	WHO category	Driver gene	Partner genes/ alteration	Molecular mechanism	Clinical behavior
PRDM10-rearranged soft tissue tumors	Fibroblastic/ myofibroblastic tumors	*PRDM10*	*MED12, CITED2*	Transcriptional regulation	Variable; superficial forms more indolent
Near-haploid rhabdomyosarcoma	Skeletal muscle tumors (embryonal RMS subset)	*Not fusion-driven*	*N/A*	Near-haploid karyotype; TP53, NF1, RAS mutations	Poor prognosis; therapy-resistant
GLI1-altered mesenchymal tumors	Tumors of uncertain differentiation	*GLI1*	*ACTB, MALAT1, PTCH1, FOXO4, APOD, FUS,* or amplification	Hedgehog pathway activation	Unpredictable; some indolent despite concerning histology
NUTM1-rearranged sarcomas		*NUTM1*	*BRD4, NSD3, CIC, MGA, MXD1, MXD4, BCORL1, ZNF532*	Chromatin reader dysfunction, p300 sequestration	Aggressive behavior
PATZ1-rearranged sarcomas		*PATZ1*	*EWSR1*	Zinc finger transcriptional dysregulation	Limited data; appears aggressive
Pseudoendocrine sarcoma		*CTNNB1*	*N/A (mutations)*	Wnt/β-catenin pathway activation	~20% with distant metastases; moderate malignant potential
FET::CREB epithelioid mesenchymal tumors		*ATF1, CREB1, CREM*	*EWSR1, FUS*	CREB/ATF pathway activation	Intermediate malignant potential
NFATC2-rearranged sarcomas	Undifferentiated small round cell sarcomas	*NFATC2*	*EWSR1, FUS*	NFAT transcriptional dysregulation	Intermediate aggressiveness

Novel fusions and molecular alterations with provisional diagnostic categories pending additional clinical validation

Emerging Entities After [207]

Since the 2020 WHO classification, several new emerging entities, identified through comprehensive genomic profiling, have been reported. These entities demonstrate recurrent genetic alterations defining distinct biological subgroups, though their formal recognition awaits accumulation of additional clinical and molecular data. Table 7.7 includes some of the emerging sarcoma entities and clinical relevance. With ongoing technical advances and decreasing costs, comprehensive molecular profiling is expected to become more progressively more accessible. Integration of NGS with liquid biopsy, artificial intelligence, and spatial biology offers powerful opportunities for precise diagnosis and treatment. Achieving the full potential of molecularly guided care in sarcomas will depend on long-term investment in diagnostic infrastructure, specialized expertise, and equitable access to novel diagnostic and targeted therapies.

Bone Tumors

Elena Bellan

Introduction

Primary bone tumors (PBTs) represent a heterogeneous group of neoplasms ranging from benign to rare but highly aggressive malignancies [50]. While most PBTs are benign, malignant forms—with an incidence of 0.9 per 100,000 persons per year according to the SEER database [99]—primarily affect adolescents and young adults and present significant challenges in both the management and the development of effective therapies. Approximately 80% of malignant PBTs consist of osteosarcoma, Ewing sarcoma, chondrosarcoma, and chordomas, which are generally treated with surgical resection, often combined with chemotherapy [172]. Although some entities occur exclusively as primary bone neoplasms, certain tumors may also involve both bone and soft tissue, and in rare instances, bone involvement may represent an exceptional presentation.

Because therapeutic strategies and patient outcomes vary markedly by tumor type, accurate diagnosis is critical. Traditionally, diagnosis has relied on clinical presentation, radiologic imaging, and histopathological assessment. However, overlapping histological features among different tumor entities often complicate the process. In recent decades, molecular assays have emerged as essential tools in musculoskeletal pathology. Advances in cytogenetics, next-generation sequencing (NGS), and other extensive genetic profiling techniques have substantially clarified the molecular underpinnings of benign, intermediate (locally aggressive and/or rarely metastasizing), and malignant bone tumors [25]. Many of these entities exhibit recurrent, tumor-defining genetic alterations that can aid in the diagnostic workup and, in some cases, provide potential therapeutic targets.

Molecular Basis of Bone Tumors

As previously mentioned for soft tissue tumors, bone tumors can be classified into four main types of genetic abnormalities: recurrent single nucleotide variants (SNVs), gene rearrangements such as chromosomal translocations, copy number changes (particularly amplifications), and complex genomic alterations. The mechanisms by which these alterations drive tumorigenesis are diverse, ranging from transcriptional dysregulation and epigenetic modification to altered protein function and overexpression. This molecular heterogeneity of these tumors makes selecting the most appropriate molecular analysis—when clinically indicated—essential.

For research purposes, whole-exome sequencing or even genome-wide panels may be employed. Following the updated classification of CNS tumors, bone tumors are increasingly being investigated and characterized based on DNA methylation profiling, although this approach is not yet widely accessible or routinely implemented in diagnostic laboratories [129, 136, 138]. Comparative genomic hybridization (CGH) and single-nucleotide polymorphism (SNP) arrays, while less commonly applied in routine practice, have been instrumental in defining the genomic complexity of primary bone tumors and their progression.

For diagnostic purposes, molecular testing can range from targeted single-gene assays (e.g., RT-PCR for *GNAS* mutations in fibrous dysplasia; FISH for *MDM2* amplification in low-grade central osteosarcoma) to more comprehensive approaches. Single-gene assays are generally straightforward to implement and interpret, without the need for advanced bioinformatics. When such assays are inconclusive or when the differential diagnosis is broad, larger commercial or custom DNA- or RNA-based panels covering over 50 genes may be employed. Importantly, NGS has transformed molecular diagnostics by enabling the parallel detection of point mutations, structural variants, and copy number changes in a single assay, even in small biopsy samples with limited nucleic acid quality. However, broader panels are often associated with longer turnaround times and higher costs [26] (PMID: 38231260).

Regardless of the method used, the reliability of such molecular techniques depends heavily on the quality, integrity, and quantity of nucleic acids, which can be significantly compromised in bone tumor samples by decalcification.

Decalcification

Among the critical routine pre-analytical steps in preparing tissue blocks from bone surgical specimens, decalcification has a significant impact on the performance of molecular assays. Strong acid-based decalcifying agents, such as hydrochloric or nitric acid, can cause extensive nucleic acid degradation and fragmentation, reducing DNA/RNA yield and compromising downstream tests such as PCR, RT-PCR, and NGS. Similarly, protein cross-linking induced by certain decalcification protocols can impair immunohistochemistry and fluorescence in situ hybridization (FISH).

To mitigate these issues, decalcification with weak acids (formic, picric, or acetic acid) or chelating agents such as ethylenediaminetetraacetic acid (EDTA) is preferred. Although slower, these methods better preserve nucleic acid integrity and are more compatible with molecular techniques [42, 150, 155, 165, 180]. Careful selection of decalcification methods, along with close communication between pathologists and molecular laboratories, is therefore essential for reliable diagnostics in PBTs.

Some centers have explored "partial decalcification" protocols, in which only a portion of the specimen undergoes decalcification for histology, while other portions are preserved fresh or frozen for molecular studies. This approach can be applied to both biopsy and resection specimens, provided sufficient tissue is available [82]. These strategies highlight the importance of pre-analytical handling in optimizing the success of molecular assays.

Molecular Analysis of Bone Tumors: Diagnostic Applications

Primary bone tumors represent a heterogeneous group of tumors with a wide spectrum of differentiation that includes osteogenic, chondrogenic, fibrogenic, vascular, myogenic, and notochordal, among others. They may, however, also be broadly subdivided by molecular underpinnings in the aforementioned groups (overview summarized in Table 7.9). Some primary bone tumors may not show recurrent genetic aberrations or show epigenetic pathogenetic processes that are not always readily identifiable by NGS techniques.

- Recurrent single nucleotide variants: SNVs are relatively uncommon in PBTs, reflecting their generally low mutational burden compared to many soft tissue sarcomas or carcinomas. Examples are found across a spectrum of benign and intermediate lesions, including osteochondroma, enchondroma, chondroblastoma, fibrous dysplasia, giant cell tumor of bone, non-ossifying fibroma, and, rarely, desmoplastic fibroma. In these tumors, SNVs frequently involve genes critical for bone development, signaling pathways, cell cycle regulation, chromatin remodeling, or tumorigenesis.

  For instance, *GNAS* mutations, which lead to constitutive activation of cell signaling pathways, are characteristic of fibrous dysplasia. Similarly, IDH1 and *IDH2 mutations* acquire an oncometabolite function, producing D-2-hydroxyglutarate and are frequently observed in enchondromas and chondrosarcomas. In the malignant spectrum, recurrent SNVs are exceedingly uncommon, though they can occasionally be detected in primary or second-

Table 7.9 Recurrent molecular alterations in primary bone tumors: overview by differentiation

Differentiation	Tumor type	Molecular alteration	Additional alterations
Chondrogenic	Osteochondroma	*EXT1/EXT2* loss of function/LOH	N/A
	Enchondroma	*IDH1/2* SNV	N/A
	Chondroblastoma	*H3F3B* epigenetic SNV: p.Lys36Met (K36M) in over 95% of cases; less frequently *H3F3A* epigenetic SNV	N/A
	Chondromyxoid fibroma	*GRM1* upregulation through promoter swapping (fusion partners include *TBL1XR1*, *COL12A1*, *BCLAF1*, *FRMD6*, *MYO1E*, and *MEF2A*)	N/A
	Central chondrosarcoma	*IDH1/2* SNV	Dedifferentiated chondrosarcoma also show additional mutations in *TP53*, *RB1*, *CDKN2A/2B*, *TERT*, SUZ12, and *EED*
	Peripheral chondrosarcoma	*EXT1/EXT2* SNV	N/A
	Mesenchymal chondrosarcoma	*HEY::NCOA2*and *IRF2BP2::CDX1* translocation	N/A
Osteogenic	Osteoid osteoma	*FOS* rearrangements	N/A
	Osteoblastoma	*FOS* and rarely *FOSB* rearrangements	N/A
	Low-grade central osteosarcoma and parosteal osteosarcoma	*MDM2* amplification	Supernumerary ring and giant chromosome markers with amplification of 12q13–15
	Conventional and high-grade surface osteosarcoma	Mutations across over 100 genes (e.g., *RB1* and *TP53*)	Complex karyotypes sometimes displaying chromothripsis and kataegis
Fibrogenic	Desmoplastic fibroma	Isolated case reports of *CTNNB1* SNV	Trisomy 8, trisomy 20, 11q13 alterations have been reported
Osteoclastic giant cell rich tumors	Aneurysmal bone cyst	*USP6* fusions with various partner genes (*CDH11*, *THRAP3*, *CNBP*, *OMD*, *COL1A1*, *CTNNB1*, *STAT3*, *FOSL2*, *EIF1*, *SPARC*, *PAFAH1B1*, *USP9X*, and *RUNX2*	N/A
	Gant cell tumor of bone	*H3F3A* epigenetic SNV: p.Gly34Trp (G34W)	N/A
	Non-ossifying fibroma	*KRAS*, *FGFR1*, and *NF1* alterations	N/A
Undifferentiated small round cell sarcomas	Ewing sarcoma	*EWSR1::FLI1* and rarely *EWRS1::ERG* translocation (other ETS genes may be involved)	Mutations in *STAG2*, *CDKN2A*, and *TP53* have been described
	Round cell sarcoma with EWSR1-non-ETS fusion	*EWSR1::NFATC2*, *FUS::NFATC2*, and *EWSR1::PATZ1*	N/A
	CIC-rearranged sarcoma	*CIC::DUX4* and alternative non-DUX4 translocations (*FOXO4*, *LEUTX*, *NUTM1*, and *NUTM2A*)	Trisomy 8 and *MYC* amplification
	BCOR-altered sarcoma	*BCOR::CCNB3 translocation* and *BCOR* ITD	N/A

(continued)

Table 7.9 (continued)

Differentiation	Tumor type	Molecular alteration	Additional alterations
Other mesenchymal primary bone tumors	Simple bone cyst	Rare *EWSR1::NFATC2* fusions	N/A
	Fibrous dysplasia	*GNAS* activating mutations	Trisomy 2 and structural aberrations of 12p13
	Adamantinoma of long bones	Recurrent pattern of numerical abnormalities of chromosomes 7, 8, 12, 19, and/or 21	*KMT2D* alterations and rare gene fusions
	Conventional chordoma	Germline tandem duplication of *TBXT*	PI3K signaling and *LYST* mutations and rarely germline loss-of-function mutations in *TSC1* or *TSC2*
	Poorly differentiated chordoma	Homozygous *SMARCB1* (INI1) gene deletion	May be associated to *EWSR1* co-deletion (complex FISH pattern)
	Epithelioid hemangioma	*FOS* translocations with *MBNL1*, *VIM*, and *LMNA* alternative *FOSB* translocations involving *ZFP36*, *WWTR1*, and *ACTB*	N/A

ary chondrosarcomas and, more rarely, in malignant giant cell tumor of bones.

- Gene rearrangements and chromosomal translocations: The molecular subgroup defined by recurrent gene rearrangements represents the largest and most clinically relevant category of primary bone tumors. Among these, undifferentiated round cell sarcomas—including *BCOR*-altered and *CIC*-rearranged tumors—and *NTRK*-rearranged spindle cell tumors have emerged as distinct entities [62].

One of the most significant advances in recent decades is the reclassification of undifferentiated small round cell sarcomas. In the 2020 WHO classification, these tumors were separated into specific molecularly defined groups, facilitated by the wider availability of molecular diagnostics. Ewing sarcoma remains the prototypical entity, defined by *EWSR1* fusions with any of the ETS family genes, but molecular profiling has revealed biologically distinct subsets, including *EWSR1/FUS::NFATC2*, *EWSR1::PATZ1*, CIC-rearranged and BCOR-altered sarcomas, which were previously grouped under undifferentiated small round cell tumors.

In addition, NTRK-rearranged spindle cell tumors, although rare in bone, represent an emerging entity of clinical importance. These tumors harbor gene fusions involving *NTRK1/2/3*, leading to constitutive activation of TRK signaling pathways. Their recognition is critical not only for diagnosis but also because they represent one of the few bone tumor types for which targeted therapies—TRK inhibitors—are clinically available and effective [158]. This highlights the growing therapeutic relevance of molecular diagnostics in bone pathology.

Molecular testing has also clarified the classification of benign and intermediate bone tumors. For example, simple bone cysts have been reported to harbor *EWSR1::NFATC2* fusions, which are more commonly associated with NFATC2-rearranged undifferentiated round cell sarcomas and intraosseous vascular tumors [104]. Similarly, *USP6* gene rearrangements are useful in differentiating aneurysmal bone cysts (ABCs) from other tumors that may display ABC-like secondary changes, such as chondroblastoma, giant cell tumor of bone, non-ossifying fibroma, and simple bone cysts.

Integrating morphologic, immunohistochemical, and molecular findings is therefore essential, as many soft tissue and bone tumors can share similar gene rearrangements, and molecular results may be misleading if interpreted in isolation.

- Copy number changes: Copy number changes in primary bone tumors typically involve recurrent amplifications or segmental chromosomal alterations and, less frequently, whole chromosome gains or losses.

  A well-studied example is *MDM2* amplification, characteristic of low-grade central and parosteal osteosarcomas. *MDM2*, a negative regulator of the p53 pathway, is amplified in nearly all cases, frequently alongside co-amplification of *CDK4 on* 12q13–15. These alterations not only contribute to tumorigenesis but also serve as robust diagnostic markers, particularly in differentiating low-grade osteosarcomas from benign fibro-osseous lesions such as fibrous dysplasia or osteofibrous dysplasia. When immunohistochemistry for MDM2 or CDK4 is inconclusive, molecular assays—including FISH, RT-PCR, or RNA in situ hybridization—can provide definitive confirmation [47].

  Chordomas also illustrate the role of copy number gains, as recurrent duplication of the *TBXT* gene (encoding brachyury, a lineage-defining transcription factor) is a common finding. This alteration reinforces TBXT's central role in notochordal development and underscores its utility as both a diagnostic and lineage-specific marker.

  In addition to gene-specific amplifications, numerical chromosomal abnormalities have been observed in several bone tumors. For example, adamantinomas frequently display recurrent whole chromosome gains and losses, reflecting broader genomic instability. While these changes are generally of limited diagnostic specificity, they contribute to a more comprehensive understanding of tumor biology and may provide supportive evidence in diagnostically challenging cases.
- Complex genomic alterations: Some of the most aggressive primary bone sarcomas, including conventional high-grade osteosarcoma, surface osteosarcoma, periosteal osteosarcoma, leiomyosarcoma, and undifferentiated pleomorphic sarcoma, are characterized by highly complex genomic landscapes. Unlike tumors defined by recurrent single-gene alterations, these sarcomas typically exhibit extensive chromosomal instability, with features such as aneuploidy, chromothripsis, kataegis, and multiple structural rearrangements.

  In conventional osteosarcoma, for example, over 100 genes may harbor mutations, yet few alterations are consistently recurrent. Instead, the hallmark is widespread genomic chaos, with alterations in key tumor suppressor pathways, most notably *TP53* and *RB1*. Loss-of-function mutations in these genes disrupt cell cycle regulation and DNA damage response, creating a permissive environment for genomic instability and tumor progression [170]. Additional recurrent events include amplifications of *MYC*, *CDK4*, and *MDM2*, although these occur less consistently than in low-grade osteosarcomas.

  Similarly, leiomyosarcomas and undifferentiated pleomorphic sarcomas demonstrate broad genomic complexity rather than signature single-gene events. Diagnosis in these cases continues to rely heavily on histomorphology and clinicoradiological correlation. For example, leiomyosarcomas are defined morphologically by atypical spindle cells with smooth muscle differentiation, whereas undifferentiated pleomorphic sarcomas are characterized by pleomorphic spindle or epithelioid cells in the absence of definitive matrix production or recognizable lineages.

Molecular Analysis of Bone Tumors: Prognostic and Predictive Applications

Although traditional clinicopathological parameters—such as tumor histology, grade, size, and histological response to chemotherapy—remain central to the prognostication of sarcomas, molecular analysis is increasingly recognized as a valuable adjunct in refining prognosis and guiding therapeutic decisions in selected cases of primary bone sarcomas.

At present, no universally accepted molecularly defined criteria directly inform standard-of-care management in bone tumors. However, the growing relevance of targeted therapies highlights the importance of molecular characterization. For instance, inhibitors of mutant *IDH1/2* are under active investigation in chondrosarcoma. Cote et al. [196] reported durable disease control with ivosidenib, an IDH1 inhibitor, in patients with IDH1-mutant chondrosarcoma, illustrating how molecularly targeted therapies may expand future treatment options.

Another clinically significant example is the identification of *NTRK* fusions in spindle cell tumors of bone and soft tissue. These alterations are therapeutically actionable, as patients may benefit from TRK inhibitors such as larotrectinib and entrectinib, which have demonstrated marked and durable responses in this setting [131, 163].

Beyond tissue-based assays, liquid biopsy approaches—including detection of circulating tumor DNA (ctDNA) and fusion transcripts—are emerging as promising tools for real-time disease monitoring. In Ewing sarcoma, for example, the presence of circulating *EWSR1::FLI1* fusion transcripts has been shown to correlate with tumor burden and relapse risk, suggesting potential utility in surveillance and early detection of recurrence [7, 74].

Taken together, molecular analysis provides a framework for advancing precision oncology in primary bone sarcomas. While morphology, histology, and clinicoradiological features remain the cornerstone of diagnosis and prognostication, molecular assays offer important complementary insights that may refine risk stratification, identify potential therapeutic targets, and facilitate individualized treatment strategies.

References

1. Aepala MR, Peiris MN, Jiang Z, Yang W, Meyer AN, Donoghue DJ. Nefarious NTRK oncogenic fusions in pediatric sarcomas: too many to Trk. Cytokine Growth Factor Rev. 2022;68:93–106.
2. Agaimy A. The expanding family of ALK-rearranged mesenchymal neoplasms. Semin Diagn Pathol. 2025;42:150947.
3. Agaram NP, Zhang L, Sung YS, Singer S, Antonescu CR. Extraskeletal myxoid chondrosarcoma with non-EWSR1-NR4A3 variant fusions correlate with rhabdoid phenotype and high-grade morphology. Hum Pathol. 2014;45(5):1084–91.
4. Agaram NP, Zhang L, LeLoarer F, Silk T, Sung YS, Scott SN, Kuk D, Qin LX, Berger MF, Antonescu CR, Singer S. Targeted exome sequencing profiles genetic alterations in leiomyosarcoma. Genes Chromosom Cancer. 2016a;55(2):124–30.
5. Agaram NP, Zhang L, Sung YS, Chen CL, Chung CT, Antonescu CR, Fletcher CD. Recurrent NTRK1 gene fusions define a novel subset of locally aggressive Lipofibromatosis-like neural tumors. Am J Surg Pathol. 2016b;40(10):1407–16.
6. Agnoletto C, Pignochino Y, Caruso C, Garofalo C. Exosome-based liquid biopsy approaches in bone and soft tissue sarcomas: review of the literature, prospectives, and hopes for clinical application. Int J Mol Sci. 2023;24(6):5159.
7. Allegretti M, Casini B, Mandoj C, Benini S, Alberti L, Novello M, Melucci E, Conti L, Covello R, Pescarmona E, Milano GM, Annovazzi A, Anelli V, Ferraresi V, Biagini R, Giacomini P. Precision diagnostics of Ewing's sarcoma by liquid biopsy: circulating EWS-FLI1 fusion transcripts. Ther Adv in Med Oncol. 2018;10:1758835918774337. https://doi.org/10.1177/1758835918774337.
8. Amin-Mansour A, George S, Sioletic S, Carter SL, Rosenberg M, Taylor-Weiner A, Stewart C, Chevalier A, Seepo S, Tracy A, Getz G, Hornick JL, Nucci MR, Quade B, Demetri GD, Raut CP, Garraway LA, Van Allen EM, Wagner AJ. Genomic evolutionary patterns of Leiomyosarcoma and Liposarcoma. Clin Cancer Res. 2019;25(16):5135–42.
9. Anderson ND, Babichev Y, Fuligni F, Comitani F, Layeghifard M, Venier RE, Dentro SC, Maheshwari A, Guram S, Wunker C, Thompson JD, Yuki KE, Hou H, Zatzman M, Light N, Bernardini MQ, Wunder JS, Andrulis IL, Ferguson P, Razak ARA, Swallow CJ, Dowling JJ, Al-Awar RS, Marcellus R, Rouzbahman M, Gerstung M, Durocher D, Alexandrov LB, Dickson BC, Gladdy RA, Shlien A. Lineage-defined leiomyosarcoma subtypes emerge years before diagnosis and determine patient survival. Nat Commun. 2021;12(1):4496.
10. Andrianteranagna M, Cyrta J, Masliah-Planchon J, Nemes K, Corsia A, Leruste A, Holdhof D, Kordes U, Orbach D, Corradini N, Entz-Werle N, Pierron G, Castex MP, Brouchet A, Weingertner N, Ranchère D, Fréneaux P, Delattre O, Bush J, Leary A, Frühwald MC, Schüller U, Servant N, Bourdeaut F. SMARCA4-deficient rhabdoid tumours show intermediate molecular features between SMARCB1-deficient rhabdoid tumours and small cell carcinomas of the ovary, hypercalcaemic type. J Pathol. 2021;255(1):1–15.
11. Antonescu CR. Targeted therapy of cancer: new roles for pathologists in identifying GISTs and other sarcomas. Mod Pathol. 2008;21(Suppl 2):S31–6.
12. Antonescu CR. Emerging soft tissue tumors with kinase fusions: an overview of the recent litera-

ture with an emphasis on diagnostic criteria. Genes Chromosom Cancer. 2020;59(8):437–44.
13. Antonescu CR, Yoshida A, Guo T, Chang NE, Zhang L, Agaram NP, Qin LX, Brennan MF, Singer S, Maki RG. KDR activating mutations in human angiosarcomas are sensitive to specific kinase inhibitors. Cancer Res. 2009;69(18):7175–9.
14. Antonescu CR, Le Loarer F, Mosquera JM, Sboner A, Zhang L, Chen CL, Chen HW, Pathan N, Krausz T, Dickson BC, Weinreb I, Rubin MA, Hameed M, Fletcher CD. Novel YAP1-TFE3 fusion defines a distinct subset of epithelioid hemangioendothelioma. Genes Chromosom Cancer. 2013;52(8):775–84.
15. Antonescu CR, Suurmeijer AJ, Zhang L, Sung YS, Jungbluth AA, Travis WD, Al-Ahmadie H, Fletcher CD, Alaggio R. Molecular characterization of inflammatory myofibroblastic tumors with frequent ALK and ROS1 gene fusions and rare novel RET rearrangement. Am J Surg Pathol. 2015;39(7):957–67.
16. Antonescu CR, Dickson BC, Swanson D, Zhang L, Sung YS, Kao YC, Chang WC, Ran L, Pappo A, Bahrami A, Chi P, Fletcher CD. Spindle cell tumors with RET gene fusions exhibit a morphologic Spectrum akin to tumors with NTRK gene fusions. Am J Surg Pathol. 2019;43(10):1384–91.
17. Assi T, Rassy E, Nassereddine H, Farhat F, Karak FE, Kattan J, Ghosn M. TRK inhibition in soft tissue sarcomas: a comprehensive review. Semin Oncol. 2020;47(1):73–84.
18. Astolfi A, Fiore M, Melchionda F, Indio V, Bertuccio SN, Pession A. BCOR involvement in cancer. Epigenomics. 2019;11(7):835–55.
19. Astolfi A, Nannini M, Indio V, Schipani A, Rizzo A, Perrone AM, De Iaco P, Pirini MG, De Leo A, Urbini M, Secchiero P, Pantaleo MA. Genomic database analysis of uterine leiomyosarcoma mutational profile. Cancers (Basel). 2020;12(8):2126.
20. Auguste A, Blanc-Durand F, Deloger M, Le Formal A, Bareja R, Wilkes DC, Richon C, Brunn B, Caron O, Devouassoux-Shisheboran M, Gouy S, Morice P, Bentivegna E, Sboner A, Elemento O, Rubin MA, Pautier P, Genestie C, Cyrta J, Leary A. Small cell carcinoma of the ovary, hypercalcemic type (SCCOHT) beyond SMARCA4 mutations: a comprehensive genomic analysis. Cells. 2020;9(6):1496.
21. Baelen J, Dewaele B, Debiec-Rychter M, Sciot R, Schöffski P, Hompes D, Sinnaeve F, Wafa H, Vanden Bempt I. Optical genome mapping for comprehensive cytogenetic analysis of soft-tissue and bone tumors for diagnostic purposes. J Mol Diagn. 2024;26(5):374–86.
22. Banito A, Li X, Laporte AN, Roe JS, Sanchez-Vega F, Huang CH, Dancsok AR, Hatzi K, Chen CC, Tschaharganeh DF, Chandwani R, Tasdemir N, Jones KB, Capecchi MR, Vakoc CR, Schultz N, Ladanyi M, Nielsen TO, Lowe SW. The SS18-SSX oncoprotein hijacks KDM2B-PRC1.1 to drive synovial sarcoma. Cancer Cell. 2018;33(3):527–541.e8. https://doi.org/10.1016/j.ccell.2018.01.018. Epub. Erratum In: Cancer Cell. 2018; 34(2):346–348. https://doi.org/10.1016/j.ccell.2018.07.006. PMID: 29502955; PMCID: PMC5881394
23. Barretina J, Taylor BS, Banerji S, Ramos AH, Lagos-Quintana M, Decarolis PL, Shah K, Socci ND, Weir BA, Ho A, Chiang DY, Reva B, Mermel CH, Getz G, Antipin Y, Beroukhim R, Major JE, Hatton C, Nicoletti R, Hanna M, Sharpe T, Fennell TJ, Cibulskis K, Onofrio RC, Saito T, Shukla N, Lau C, Nelander S, Silver SJ, Sougnez C, Viale A, Winckler W, Maki RG, Garraway LA, Lash A, Greulich H, Root DE, Sellers WR, Schwartz GK, Antonescu CR, Lander ES, Varmus HE, Ladanyi M, Sander C, Meyerson M, Singer S. Subtype-specific genomic alterations define new targets for soft-tissue sarcoma therapy. Nat Genet. 2010;42(8):715–21.
24. Barthelmeß S, Geddert H, Boltze C, Moskalev EA, Bieg M, Sirbu H, Brors B, Wiemann S, Hartmann A, Agaimy A, Haller F. Solitary fibrous tumors/hemangiopericytomas with different variants of the NAB2-STAT6 gene fusion are characterized by specific histomorphology and distinct clinicopathological features. Am J Pathol. 2014;184(4):1209–18.
25. Baumhoer D, Amary F, Flanagan AM. An update of molecular pathology of bone tumors. Lessons learned from investigating samples by next generation sequencing. Genes Chromosomes Cancer. 2019;58(2):88–99. https://doi.org/10.1002/gcc.22699.
26. Baumhoer D, Hench J, Amary F. Recent advances in molecular profiling of bone and soft tissue tumors. Skeletal Radiol. 2024;53(9):1925–36. https://doi.org/10.1007/s00256-024-04584-9.
27. Beck AH, Lee CH, Witten DM, Gleason BC, Edris B, Espinosa I, Zhu S, Li R, Montgomery KD, Marinelli RJ, Tibshirani R, Hastie T, Jablons DM, Rubin BP, Fletcher CD, West RB, van de Rijn M. Discovery of molecular subtypes in leiomyosarcoma through integrative molecular profiling. Oncogene. 2010;29(6):845–54.
28. Behjati S, Tarpey PS, Sheldon H, Martincorena I, Van Loo P, Gundem G, Wedge DC, Ramakrishna M, Cooke SL, Pillay N, Vollan HKM, Papaemmanuil E, Koss H, Bunney TD, Hardy C, Joseph OR, Martin S, Mudie L, Butler A, Teague JW, Patil M, Steers G, Cao Y, Gumbs C, Ingram D, Lazar AJ, Little L, Mahadeshwar H, Protopopov A, Al Sannaa GA, Seth S, Song X, Tang J, Zhang J, Ravi V, Torres KE, Khatri B, Halai D, Roxanis I, Baumhoer D, Tirabosco R, Amary MF, Boshoff C, McDermott U, Katan M, Stratton MR, Futreal PA, Flanagan AM, Harris A, Campbell PJ. Recurrent PTPRB and PLCG1 mutations in angiosarcoma. Nat Genet. 2014;46(4):376–9.
29. Benayed R, Offin M, Mullaney K, Sukhadia P, Rios K, Desmeules P, Ptashkin R, Won H, Chang J, Halpenny D, Schram AM, Rudin CM, Hyman DM, Arcila ME, Berger MF, Zehir A, Kris MG, Drilon A, Ladanyi M. High yield of RNA sequencing for targetable kinase fusions in lung adenocarcinomas

with no mitogenic driver alteration detected by DNA sequencing and low tumor mutation burden. Clin Cancer Res. 2019;25(15):4712–22.
30. Berenguer-Rubio A, Such E, Hernández NT, González-Rojo P, Díaz-González Á, Avetisyan G, Gil-Aparicio C, González-López J, Pantoja-Borja N, Rubio-Martínez LA, Hernández-Girón S, Valera-Cuesta MS, Ramírez-Fuentes C, Simonet-Redondo M, Díaz-Beveridge R, de la Calva C, Amaya-Valero JV, Ballester-Ibáñez C, Liquori A, Giner F, Mayordomo-Aranda E. Exploring the potential of optical genome mapping in the diagnosis and prognosis of soft tissue and bone tumors. Int J Mol Sci. 2025;26(6):2820.
31. Biegel JA, Zhou JY, Rorke LB, Stenstrom C, Wainwright LM, Fogelgren B. Germ-line and acquired mutations of INI1 in atypical teratoid and rhabdoid tumors. Cancer Res. 1999;59(1):74–9.
32. Blay JY, Kang YK, Nishida T, von Mehren M. Gastrointestinal stromal tumours. Nat Rev Dis Primers. 2021;7(1):22.
33. Boikos SA, Pappo AS, Killian JK, LaQuaglia MP, Weldon CB, George S, Trent JC, von Mehren M, Wright JA, Schiffman JD, Raygada M, Pacak K, Meltzer PS, Miettinen MM, Stratakis C, Janeway KA, Helman LJ. Molecular subtypes of KIT/PDGFRA wild-type gastrointestinal stromal tumors: a report from the National Institutes of Health gastrointestinal stromal tumor clinic. JAMA Oncol. 2016;2(7):922–8.
34. Boulay G, Cironi L, Garcia SP, Rengarajan S, Xing YH, Lee L, Awad ME, Naigles B, Iyer S, Broye LC, Keskin T, Cauderay A, Fusco C, Letovanec I, Chebib I, Nielsen PG, Tercier S, Cherix S, Nguyen-Ngoc T, Cote G, Choy E, Provero P, Suvà ML, Rivera MN, Stamenkovic I, Riggi N. The chromatin landscape of primary synovial sarcoma organoids is linked to specific epigenetic mechanisms and dependencies. Life Sci Alliance. 2020;4(2):e202000808. https://doi.org/10.26508/lsa.202000808. PMID: 33361335; PMCID: PMC7768195.
35. Brennan MF, Antonescu CR, Moraco N, Singer S. Lessons learned from the study of 10,000 patients with soft tissue sarcoma. Ann Surg. 2014;260(3):416–21. discussion 421-412.
36. Bridge JA, Cushman-Vokoun AM. Molecular diagnostics of soft tissue tumors. Arch Pathol Lab Med. 2011;135(5):588–601.
37. Bridge JA, Sumegi J, Druta M, Bui MM, Henderson-Jackson E, Linos K, Baker M, Walko CM, Millis S, Brohl AS. Clinical, pathological, and genomic features of EWSR1-PATZ1 fusion sarcoma. Mod Pathol. 2019;32(11):1593–604.
38. Burningham Z, Hashibe M, Spector L, Schiffman JD. The epidemiology of sarcoma. Clin Sarcoma Res. 2012;2(1):14.
39. Butrynski JE, D'Adamo DR, Hornick JL, Dal Cin P, Antonescu CR, Jhanwar SC, Ladanyi M, Capelletti M, Rodig SJ, Ramaiya N, Kwak EL, Clark JW, Wilner KD, Christensen JG, Jänne PA, Maki RG, Demetri GD, Shapiro GI. Crizotinib in ALK-rearranged inflammatory myofibroblastic tumor. N Engl J Med. 2010;363(18):1727–33.
40. Byron SA, Van Keuren-Jensen KR, Engelthaler DM, Carpten JD, Craig DW. Translating RNA sequencing into clinical diagnostics: opportunities and challenges. Nat Rev Genet. 2016;17(5):257–71.
41. Cancer Genome Atlas Research Network. Electronic address, e. d. s. c. and N. Cancer Genome Atlas Research. Comprehensive and integrated genomic characterization of adult soft tissue sarcomas. Cell. 2017;171(4):950–965 e928.
42. Cappello F, Angerilli V, Munari G, Ceccon C, Sabbadin M, Pagni F, Fusco N, Malapelle U, Fassan M. FFPE-based NGS approaches into clinical practice: the limits of glory from a pathologist viewpoint. J Pers Med. 2022;12(5):750. https://doi.org/10.3390/jpm12050750.
43. Chadha M, Huang PH. Proteomic and Metabolomic profiling in soft tissue sarcomas. Curr Treat Options in Oncol. 2022;23(1):78–88.
44. Chalmers ZR, Connelly CF, Fabrizio D, Gay L, Ali SM, Ennis R, Schrock A, Campbell B, Shlien A, Chmielecki J, Huang F, He Y, Sun J, Tabori U, Kennedy M, Lieber DS, Roels S, White J, Otto GA, Ross JS, Garraway L, Miller VA, Stephens PJ, Frampton GM. Analysis of 100,000 human cancer genomes reveals the landscape of tumor mutational burden. Genome Med. 2017;9(1):34.
45. Chang KTE, Goytain A, Tucker T, Karsan A, Lee C-H, Nielsen TO, Ng TL. Development and evaluation of a pan-sarcoma fusion gene detection assay using the NanoString nCounter platform. J Mol Diagn. 2018;20(1):63–77.
46. Chen S, Deniz K, Sung YS, Zhang L, Dry S, Antonescu CR. Ewing sarcoma with ERG gene rearrangements: a molecular study focusing on the prevalence of FUS-ERG and common pitfalls in detecting EWSR1-ERG fusions by FISH. Genes Chromosom Cancer. 2016;55(4):340–9.
47. Chen C, He X, Chen M, Du T, Qin W, Jing W, Zhang H. Diagnostic value of MDM2 RNA in situ hybridization for low-grade osteosarcoma: consistency comparison of RNA in situ hybridization, fluorescence in situ hybridization, and immunohistochemistry. VirchowsArchiv: Int J Pathol. 2023;482(6):999–1010. https://doi.org/10.1007/s00428-023-03530-9.
48. Chibon F, Lagarde P, Salas S, Pérot G, Brouste V, Tirode F, Lucchesi C, de Reynies A, Kauffmann A, Bui B, Terrier P, Bonvalot S, Le Cesne A, Vince-Ranchère D, Blay J-Y, Collin F, Guillou L, Leroux A, Coindre J-M, Aurias A. Validated prediction of clinical outcome in sarcomas and multiple types of cancer on the basis of a gene expression signature related to genome complexity. Nat Med. 2010;16(7):781–7.
49. Choi JH, Ro JY. The 2020 WHO classification of tumors of soft tissue: selected changes and new entities. Adv Anat Pathol. 2020;28(1):44–58.

50. Choi JH, Ro JY. The 2020 WHO classification of tumors of bone: an updated review. Adv Anat Pathol. 2021;28(3):119–38. https://doi.org/10.1097/PAP.0000000000000293.
51. Chudasama P, Mughal SS, Sanders MA, Hübschmann D, Chung I, Deeg KI, Wong S-H, Rabe S, Hlevnjak M, Zapatka M, Ernst A, Kleinheinz K, Schlesner M, Sieverling L, Klink B, Schröck E, Hoogenboezem RM, Kasper B, Heilig CE, Egerer G, Wolf S, von Kalle C, Eils R, Stenzinger A, Weichert W, Glimm H, Gröschel S, Kopp H-G, Omlor G, Lehner B, Bauer S, Schimmack S, Ulrich A, Mechtersheimer G, Rippe K, Brors B, Hutter B, Renner M, Hohenberger P, Scholl C, Fröhling S. Integrative genomic and transcriptomic analysis of leiomyosarcoma. Nat Commun. 2018;9(1):144.
52. Cicala CM, Olivares-Rivas I, Aguirre-Carrillo JA, Serrano C. KIT/PDGFRA inhibitors for the treatment of gastrointestinal stromal tumors: getting to the gist of the problem. Expert Opin Investig Drugs. 2024;33(3):159–70.
53. Cleven AH, Sannaa GA, Briaire-de Bruijn I, Ingram DR, van de Rijn M, Rubin BP, de Vries MW, Watson KL, Torres KE, Wang WL, van Duinen SG, Hogendoorn PC, Lazar AJ, Bovée JV. Loss of H3K27 tri-methylation is a diagnostic marker for malignant peripheral nerve sheath tumors and an indicator for an inferior survival. Mod Pathol. 2016;29(6):582–90.
54. Cohen-Gogo S, Cellier C, Coindre JM, Mosseri V, Pierron G, Guillemet C, Italiano A, Brugières L, Orbach D, Laurence V, Delattre O, Michon J. Ewing-like sarcomas with BCOR-CCNB3 fusion transcript: a clinical, radiological and pathological retrospective study from the Société Française des cancers de L'Enfant. Pediatr Blood Cancer. 2014;61(12):2191–8.
55. Corless CL, Schroeder A, Griffith D, Town A, McGreevey L, Harrell P, Shiraga S, Bainbridge T, Morich J, Heinrich MC. PDGFRA mutations in gastrointestinal stromal tumors: frequency, spectrum and in vitro sensitivity to imatinib. J Clin Oncol. 2005;23(23):5357–64.
56. Crago AM, Socci ND, DeCarolis P, O'Connor R, Taylor BS, Qin LX, Antonescu CR, Singer S. Copy number losses define subgroups of dedifferentiated liposarcoma with poor prognosis and genomic instability. Clin Cancer Res. 2012;18(5):1334–40.
57. Crozat A, Aman P, Mandahl N, Ron D. Fusion of CHOP to a novel RNA-binding protein in human myxoid liposarcoma. Nature. 1993;363(6430):640–4.
58. Damerell V, Pepper MS, Prince S. Molecular mechanisms underpinning sarcomas and implications for current and future therapy. Signal Transduct Target Ther. 2021;6(1):246.
59. Davis JL, Vargas SO, Rudzinski ER, López Marti JM, Janeway K, Forrest S, Winsnes K, Pinto N, Yang SE, VanSandt M, Boyd TK, Corless CL, Liu YJ, Surrey LF, Harris MH, Church A, Al-Ibraheemi A. Recurrent RET gene fusions in paediatric spindle mesenchymal neoplasms. Histopathology. 2020;76(7):1032–41.
60. Davis JL, Al-Ibraheemi A, Rudzinski ER, Surrey LF. Mesenchymal neoplasms with NTRK and other kinase gene alterations. Histopathology. 2022;80(1):4–18.
61. De Raedt T, Beert E, Pasmant E, Luscan A, Brems H, Ortonne N, Helin K, Hornick JL, Mautner V, Kehrer-Sawatzki H, Clapp W, Bradner J, Vidaud M, Upadhyaya M, Legius E, Cichowski K. PRC2 loss amplifies Ras-driven transcription and confers sensitivity to BRD4-based therapies. Nature. 2014;514(7521):247–51.
62. Dehner CA, Rudzinski ER, Davis JL. Rhabdomyosarcoma: updates on classification and the necessity of molecular testing beyond immunohistochemistry. Hum Pathol. 2024;147:72–81. https://doi.org/10.1016/j.humpath.2023.12.004.
63. Delattre O, Zucman J, Plougastel B, Desmaze C, Melot T, Peter M, Kovar H, Joubert I, de Jong P, Rouleau G, Aurias A, Thomas G. Gene fusion with an ETS DNA-binding domain caused by chromosome translocation in human tumours. Nature. 1992;359(6391):162–5.
64. Dermawan JK, Azzato EM, Billings SD, Fritchie KJ, Aubert S, Bahrami A, Barisella M, Baumhoer D, Blum V, Bode B, Aesif SW, Bovée JVMG, Dickson BC, van den Hout M, Lucas DR, Moch H, Oaxaca G, Righi A, Sciot R, Sumathi V, Yoshida A, Rubin BP. YAP1-TFE3-fused hemangioendothelioma: a multi-institutional clinicopathologic study of 24 genetically-confirmed cases. Mod Pathol. 2021;34(12):2211–21.
65. Doebele RC, Drilon A, Paz-Ares L, Siena S, Shaw AT, Farago AF, Blakely CM, Seto T, Cho BC, Tosi D, Besse B, Chawla SP, Bazhenova L, Krauss JC, Chae YK, Barve M, Garrido-Laguna I, Liu SV, Conkling P, John T, Fakih M, Sigal D, Loong HH, Buchschacher GL, Garrido P, Nieva J, Steuer C, Overbeck TR, Bowles DW, Fox E, Riehl T, Chow-Maneval E, Simmons B, Cui N, Johnson A, Eng S, Wilson TR, Demetri GD. Entrectinib in patients with advanced or metastatic NTRK fusion-positive solid tumours: integrated analysis of three phase 1–2 trials. Lancet Oncol. 2020;21(2):271–82.
66. Drilon A, Laetsch TW, Kummar S, DuBois SG, Lassen UN, Demetri GD, Nathenson M, Doebele RC, Farago AF, Pappo AS, Turpin B, Dowlati A, Brose MS, Mascarenhas L, Federman N, Berlin J, El-Deiry WS, Baik C, Deeken J, Boni V, Nagasubramanian R, Taylor M, Rudzinski ER, Meric-Bernstam F, Sohal DPS, Ma PC, Raez LE, Hechtman JF, Benayed R, Ladanyi M, Tuch BB, Ebata K, Cruickshank S, Ku NC, Cox MC, Hawkins DS, Hong DS, Hyman DM. Efficacy of larotrectinib in TRK fusion-positive cancers in adults and children. N Engl J Med. 2018;378(8):731–9.

67. Du Z, Lovly CM. Mechanisms of receptor tyrosine kinase activation in cancer. Mol Cancer. 2018;17(1):58.
68. Duensing A, Medeiros F, McConarty B, Joseph NE, Panigrahy D, Singer S, Fletcher CD, Demetri GD, Fletcher JA. Mechanisms of oncogenic KIT signal transduction in primary gastrointestinal stromal tumors (GISTs). Oncogene. 2004;23(22):3999–4006.
69. Evans HL. Low-grade fibromyxoid sarcoma: a clinicopathologic study of 33 cases with long-term follow-up. Am J Surg Pathol. 2011;35(10):1450–62.
70. Fan R, Parham DM, Wang LL. An integrative morphologic and molecular approach for diagnosis and subclassification of rhabdomyosarcoma. Arch Pathol Lab Med. 2022;146(8):953–9.
71. Fletcher CD. The evolving classification of soft tissue tumours – an update based on the new 2013 WHO classification. Histopathology. 2014;64(1):2–11.
72. Folpe AL, Deyrup AT. Alveolar soft-part sarcoma: a review and update. J Clin Pathol. 2006;59(11):1127–32.
73. Fritz B, Schubert F, Wrobel G, Schwaenen C, Wessendorf S, Nessling M, Korz C, Rieker RJ, Montgomery K, Kucherlapati R, Mechtersheimer G, Eils R, Joos S, Lichter P. Microarray-based copy number and expression profiling in dedifferentiated and pleomorphic liposarcoma. Cancer Res. 2002;62(11):2993–8.
74. Furukawa N, Hasegawa N, Kubota D, Nakamura Y, Tanaka H, Iwata S, Kawai A, Saito T, Takagi T, Kohsaka S, Ishijima M. Prognostic potential of fusion gene analysis using plasma cell-free RNA in malignant bone and soft tissue tumours. BMC Cancer. 2025;25(1):587. https://doi.org/10.1186/s12885-025-13950-2.
75. Gamboa AC, Gronchi A, Cardona K. Soft-tissue sarcoma in adults: an update on the current state of histiotype-specific management in an era of personalized medicine. CA Cancer J Clin. 2020;70(3):200–29.
76. Gatalica Z, Xiu J, Swensen J, Vranic S. Molecular characterization of cancers with NTRK gene fusions. Mod Pathol. 2019;32(1):147–53.
77. Gebhard S, Coindre JM, Michels JJ, Terrier P, Bertrand G, Trassard M, Taylor S, Chateau MC, Marques B, Picot V, Guillou L. Pleomorphic liposarcoma: clinicopathologic, immunohistochemical, and follow-up analysis of 63 cases: a study from the French Federation of Cancer Centers Sarcoma Group. Am J Surg Pathol. 2002;26(5):601–16.
78. George S, Serrano C, Hensley ML, Ray-Coquard I. Soft tissue and uterine leiomyosarcoma. J Clin Oncol. 2018;36(2):144–50.
79. Ghadimi MP, Liu P, Peng T, Bolshakov S, Young ED, Torres KE, Colombo C, Hoffman A, Broccoli D, Hornick JL, Lazar AJ, Pisters P, Pollock RE, Lev D. Pleomorphic liposarcoma: clinical observations and molecular variables. Cancer. 2011;117(23):5359–69.
80. Gibault L, Ferreira C, Perot G, Audebourg A, Chibon F, Bonnin S, Lagarde P, Vacher-Lavenu MC, Terrier P, Coindre JM, Aurias A. From PTEN loss of expression to RICTOR role in smooth muscle differentiation: complex involvement of the mTOR pathway in leiomyosarcomas and pleomorphic sarcomas. Mod Pathol. 2012;25(2):197–211.
81. Gill AJ, Hes O, Papathomas T, Šedivcová M, Tan PH, Agaimy A, Andresen PA, Kedziora A, Clarkson A, Toon CW, Sioson L, Watson N, Chou A, Paik J, Clifton-Bligh RJ, Robinson BG, Benn DE, Hills K, Maclean F, Niemeijer ND, Vlatkovic L, Hartmann A, Corssmit EPM, van Leenders GJLH, Przybycin C, McKenney JK, Magi-Galluzzi C, Yilmaz A, Yu D, Nicoll KD, Yong JL, Sibony M, Yakirevich E, Fleming S, Chow CW, Miettinen M, Michal M, Trpkov K. Succinate dehydrogenase (SDH)-deficient renal carcinoma: a morphologically distinct entity: a clinicopathologic series of 36 tumors from 27 patients. Am J Surg Pathol. 2014;38(12):1588–602.
82. Gokgoz N, Wunder JS, Mousses S, Eskandarian S, Bell RS, Andrulis IL. Comparison of p53 mutations in patients with localized osteosarcoma and metastatic osteosarcoma. Cancer. 2001;92(8):2181–9. https://doi.org/10.1002/1097-0142(20011015)92:8<2181::aid-cncr1561>3.0.co;2-3.
83. Goldblum JR. An approach to pleomorphic sarcomas: can we subclassify, and does it matter? Mod Pathol. 2014;27(Suppl 1):S39–46.
84. Gounder MM, Agaram NP, Trabucco SE, Robinson V, Ferraro R, Millis SZ, Krishnan A, Lee J, Attia S, Abida W, Drilon A, Chi P, Angelo SPD, Dickson MA, Keohan ML, Kelly CM, Agulnik M, Chawla SP, Choy E, Chugh R, Meyer CF, Myer PA, Moore JL, Okimoto RA, Pollock RE, Ravi V, Singh AS, Somaiah N, Wagner AJ, Healey JH, Frampton GM, Venstrom JM, Ross JS, Ladanyi M, Singer S, Brennan MF, Schwartz GK, Lazar AJ, Thomas DM, Maki RG, Tap WD, Ali SM, Jin DX. Clinical genomic profiling in the management of patients with soft tissue and bone sarcoma. Nat Commun. 2022;13(1):3406.
85. Grasso D, Marzocchi B, Scoccianti G, Palchetti I, Campanacci DA, Antonuzzo L, Scolari F, Pillozzi S, Bernini A. Untargeted metabolomics and liquid biopsy investigation of circulating biomarkers in soft tissue sarcoma. Cancer. 2025;17(3):553.
86. Gronchi A, Miah AB, Dei Tos AP, Abecassis N, Bajpai J, Bauer S, Biagini R, Bielack S, Blay JY, Bolle S, Bonvalot S, Boukovinas I, Bovee J, Boye K, Brennan B, Brodowicz T, Buonadonna A, De Álava E, Del Muro XG, Dufresne A, Eriksson M, Fagioli F, Fedenko A, Ferraresi V, Ferrari A, Frezza AM, Gasperoni S, Gelderblom H, Gouin F, Grignani G, Haas R, Hassan AB, Hecker-Nolting S, Hindi N, Hohenberger P, Joensuu H, Jones RL, Jungels C, Jutte P, Kager L, Kasper B, Kawai A, Kopeckova K, Krákorová DA, Le Cesne A, Le Grange F, Legius E, Leithner A, Lopez-Pousa A,

Martin-Broto J, Merimsky O, Messiou C, Mir O, Montemurro M, Morland B, Morosi C, Palmerini E, Pantaleo MA, Piana R, Piperno-Neumann S, Reichardt P, Rutkowski P, Safwat AA, Sangalli C, Sbaraglia M, Scheipl S, Schöffski P, Sleijfer S, Strauss D, Strauss S, Sundby Hall K, Trama A, Unk M, van de Sande MAJ, van der Graaf WTA, van Houdt WJ, Frebourg T, Casali PG, Stacchiotti S. Soft tissue and visceral sarcomas: ESMO-EURACAN-GENTURIS clinical practice guidelines for diagnosis, treatment and follow-up(☆). Ann Oncol. 2021;32(11):1348–65.
87. Gruel N, Quignot C, Lesage L, El Zein S, Bonvalot S, Tzanis D, Ait Rais K, Quinquis F, Manciot B, Vibert J, El Tannir N, Dahmani A, Derrien H, Decaudin D, Bièche I, Courtois L, Mariani O, Linares LK, Gayte L, Baulande S, Waterfall JJ, Delattre O, Pierron G, Watson S. Cellular origin and clonal evolution of human dedifferentiated liposarcoma. Nat Commun. 2024;15(1):7941.
88. Grünewald TG, Bernard V, Gilardi-Hebenstreit P, Raynal V, Surdez D, Aynaud MM, Mirabeau O, Cidre-Aranaz F, Tirode F, Zaidi S, Perot G, Jonker AH, Lucchesi C, Le Deley MC, Oberlin O, Marec-Bérard P, Véron AS, Reynaud S, Lapouble E, Boeva V, Rio Frio T, Alonso J, Bhatia S, Pierron G, Cancel-Tassin G, Cussenot O, Cox DG, Morton LM, Machiela MJ, Chanock SJ, Charnay P, Delattre O. Chimeric EWSR1-FLI1 regulates the Ewing sarcoma susceptibility gene EGR2 via a GGAA microsatellite. Nat Genet. 2015;47(9):1073–8.
89. Guillou L, Aurias A. Soft tissue sarcomas with complex genomic profiles. Virchows Arch. 2010;456(2):201–17.
90. Guo X, Jo VY, Mills AM, Zhu SX, Lee CH, Espinosa I, Nucci MR, Varma S, Forgo E, Hastie T, Anderson S, Ganjoo K, Beck AH, West RB, Fletcher CD, van de Rijn M. Clinically relevant molecular subtypes in leiomyosarcoma. Clin Cancer Res. 2015;21(15):3501–11.
91. Hasegawa N, Hayashi T, Niizuma H, Kikuta K, Imanishi J, Endo M, Ikeuchi H, Sasa K, Sano K, Hirabayashi K. Detection of novel tyrosine kinase fusion genes as potential therapeutic targets in bone and soft tissue sarcomas using DNA/RNA-based clinical sequencing. Clin Orthop Relat Res. 2024;482(3):549–63.
92. Hechtman JF. NTRK insights: best practices for pathologists. Mod Pathol. 2022;35(3):298–305.
93. Heinrich MC, Corless CL, Demetri GD, Blanke CD, von Mehren M, Joensuu H, McGreevey LS, Chen C-J, Van den Abbeele AD, Druker BJ, Kiese B, Eisenberg B, Roberts PJ, Singer S, Fletcher CDM, Silberman S, Dimitrijevic S, Fletcher JA. Kinase mutations and imatinib response in patients with metastatic gastrointestinal stromal tumor. J Clin Oncol. 2003;21(23):4342–9.
94. Heyer EE, Deveson IW, Wooi D, Selinger CI, Lyons RJ, Hayes VM, O'Toole SA, Ballinger ML, Gill D, Thomas DM, Mercer TR, Blackburn J. Diagnosis of fusion genes using targeted RNA sequencing. Nat Commun. 2019;10(1):1388.
95. Hirata M, Asano N, Katayama K, Yoshida A, Tsuda Y, Sekimizu M, Mitani S, Kobayashi E, Komiyama M, Fujimoto H, Goto T, Iwamoto Y, Naka N, Iwata S, Nishida Y, Hiruma T, Hiraga H, Kawano H, Motoi T, Oda Y, Matsubara D, Fujita M, Shibata T, Nakagawa H, Nakayama R, Kondo T, Imoto S, Miyano S, Kawai A, Yamaguchi R, Ichikawa H, Matsuda K. Integrated exome and RNA sequencing of dedifferentiated liposarcoma. Nat Commun. 2019;10(1):5683.
96. Hollmann TJ, Hornick JL. INI1-deficient tumors: diagnostic features and molecular genetics. Am J Surg Pathol. 2011;35(10):e47–63.
97. Hondelink LM, Schrader AMR, Asri Aghmuni G, Solleveld-Westerink N, Cleton-Jansen AM, van Egmond D, Boot A, Ouahoud S, Khalifa MN, Wai Lam S, Morreau H, Bovee J, van Wezel T, Cohen D. The sensitivity of pan-TRK immunohistochemistry in solid tumours: a meta-analysis. Eur J Cancer. 2022;173:229–37.
98. Hornick JL, Sholl LM, Dal Cin P, Childress MA, Lovly CM. Expression of ROS1 predicts ROS1 gene rearrangement in inflammatory myofibroblastic tumors. Mod Pathol. 2015;28(5):732–9.
99. Hosseini H, Heydari S, Hushmandi K, Daneshi S, Raesi R. Bone tumors: a systematic review of prevalence, risk determinants, and survival patterns. BMC Cancer. 2025;25(1):321. https://doi.org/10.1186/s12885-025-13720-0.
100. Hsiao SJ, Zehir A, Sireci AN, Aisner DL. Detection of tumor NTRK gene fusions to identify patients who may benefit from tyrosine kinase (TRK) inhibitor therapy. J Mol Diagn. 2019;21(4):553–71.
101. Huang SC, Zhang L, Sung YS, Chen CL, Kao YC, Agaram NP, Singer S, Tap WD, D'Angelo S, Antonescu CR. Recurrent CIC gene abnormalities in angiosarcomas: a molecular study of 120 cases with concurrent investigation of PLCG1, KDR, MYC, and FLT4 gene alterations. Am J Surg Pathol. 2016;40(5):645–55.
102. Huang SC, Lee JC, Hsu YC, Tsai JW, Kao YC, Hsieh TH, Chang YM, Chang KC, Wu PS, Chen PC, Chen CH, Chang CD, Lee PH, Tai HC, Liu TT, Wen MC, Li WS, Yu SC, Wang JC, Huang HY. Extraskeletal Myxoid chondrosarcomas: the uncommon Clinicopathologic manifestations and significance of TAF15::NR4A3 fusion. Mod Pathol. 2023;36(7):100161.
103. Hung YP, Fletcher CDM, Hornick JL. Evaluation of ETV4 and WT1 expression in CIC-rearranged sarcomas and histologic mimics. Mod Pathol. 2016;29(11):1324–34.
104. Hung YP, Fisch AS, Diaz-Perez JA, Iafrate AJ, Lennerz JK, Nardi V, Bredella MA, Raskin KA, Lozano-Calderon SA, Rosenberg AE, Nielsen GP. Identification of EWSR1-NFATC2 fusion in simple bone cysts. Histopathology. 2021;78(6):849–56. https://doi.org/10.1111/his.14314.

105. Huss S, Pasternack H, Ihle MA, Merkelbach-Bruse S, Heitkötter B, Hartmann W, Trautmann M, Gevensleben H, Büttner R, Schildhaus HU, Wardelmann E. Clinicopathological and molecular features of a large cohort of gastrointestinal stromal tumors (GISTs) and review of the literature: BRAF mutations in KIT/PDGFRA wild-type GISTs are rare events. Hum Pathol. 2017;62:206–14.
106. Idbaih A, Coindre JM, Derre J, Mariani O, Terrier P, Ranchere D, Mairal A, Aurias A. Myxoid malignant fibrous histiocytoma and pleomorphic liposarcoma share very similar genomic imbalances. Lab Investig. 2005;85(2):176–81.
107. Italiano A, Bianchini L, Keslair F, Bonnafous S, Cardot-Leccia N, Coindre JM, Dumollard JM, Hofman P, Leroux A, Mainguene C, Peyrottes I, Ranchere-Vince D, Terrier P, Tran A, Gual P, Pedeutour F. HMGA2 is the partner of MDM2 in well-differentiated and dedifferentiated liposarcomas whereas CDK4 belongs to a distinct inconsistent amplicon. Int J Cancer. 2008;122(10):2233–41.
108. Italiano A, Lagarde P, Brulard C, Terrier P, Lae M, Marques B, Ranchere-Vince D, Michels JJ, Trassard M, Cioffi A, Piperno-Neumann S, Chevreau C, Blay JY, Delcambre C, Isambert N, Penel N, Bay JO, Bonvalot S, Le Cesne A, Coindre JM, Chibon F. Genetic profiling identifies two classes of soft-tissue leiomyosarcomas with distinct clinical characteristics. Clin Cancer Res. 2013;19(5):1190–6.
109. Janeway KA, Kim SY, Lodish M, Nosé V, Rustin P, Gaal J, Dahia PL, Liegl B, Ball ER, Raygada M, Lai AH, Kelly L, Hornick JL, O'Sullivan M, de Krijger RR, Dinjens WN, Demetri GD, Antonescu CR, Fletcher JA, Helman L, Stratakis CA. Defects in succinate dehydrogenase in gastrointestinal stromal tumors lacking KIT and PDGFRA mutations. Proc Natl Acad Sci USA. 2011;108(1):314–8.
110. Jin G, Zhao D, Wang B, Liu X, Yang Q, Liu Z, Yang Q, Zhu J, Zhang J, Li W. Superiority of targeted RNA sequencing for fusion detection and subtype diagnosis in Chinese sarcoma patients: a multicenter study. Exp Hematol Oncol. 2025;14(1):70.
111. Jo VY. EWSR1 fusions: Ewing sarcoma and beyond. Cancer Cytopathol. 2020;128(4):229–31.
112. Joensuu H. KIT and PDGFRA variants and the survival of patients with gastrointestinal stromal tumor treated with adjuvant imatinib. Cancers. 2023;15(15):3879.
113. Jones RL, Serrano C, von Mehren M, George S, Heinrich MC, Kang YK, Schöffski P, Cassier PA, Mir O, Chawla SP, Eskens F, Rutkowski P, Tap WD, Zhou T, Roche M, Bauer S. Avapritinib in unresectable or metastatic PDGFRA D842V-mutant gastrointestinal stromal tumours: long-term efficacy and safety data from the NAVIGATOR phase I trial. Eur J Cancer. 2021;145:132–42.
114. Joseph CG, Hwang H, Jiao Y, Wood LD, Kinde I, Wu J, Mandahl N, Luo J, Hruban RH, Diaz LA Jr, He TC, Vogelstein B, Kinzler KW, Mertens F, Papadopoulos N. Exomic analysis of myxoid liposarcomas, synovial sarcomas, and osteosarcomas. Genes Chromosom Cancer. 2014;53(1):15–24.
115. Jozwik M, Bednarczuk K, Osierda Z. Dermatofibrosarcoma protuberans: an updated review of the literature. Cancer. 2024;16(18):3124.
116. Judson I, Demetri G. Advances in the treatment of gastrointestinal stromal tumours. Ann Oncol. 2007;18(Suppl 10):x20–4.
117. Kadoch C, Hargreaves DC, Hodges C, Elias L, Ho L, Ranish J, Crabtree GR. Proteomic and bioinformatic analysis of mammalian SWI/SNF complexes identifies extensive roles in human malignancy. Nat Genet. 2013;45(6):592–601.
118. Kang GH, Srivastava A, Kim YE, Park HJ, Park CK, Sohn TS, Kim S, Kang DY, Kim KM. DOG1 and PKC-**θ** are useful in the diagnosis of KIT-negative gastrointestinal stromal tumors. Mod Pathol. 2011;24(6):866–75.
119. Kanojia D, Nagata Y, Garg M, Lee DH, Sato A, Yoshida K, Sato Y, Sanada M, Mayakonda A, Bartenhagen C, Klein HU, Doan NB, Said JW, Mohith S, Gunasekar S, Shiraishi Y, Chiba K, Tanaka H, Miyano S, Myklebost O, Yang H, Dugas M, Meza-Zepeda LA, Silberman AW, Forscher C, Tyner JW, Ogawa S, Koeffler HP. Genomic landscape of liposarcoma. Oncotarget. 2015;6(40):42429–44.
120. Kao Y-C, Owosho AA, Sung Y-S, Zhang L, Fujisawa Y, Lee J-C, Wexler L, Argani P, Swanson D, Dickson BC, Fletcher CDM, Antonescu CR. BCOR-CCNB3 fusion positive sarcomas. Am J Surg Pathol. 2018;42(5):604–15.
121. Karakousis CP. Chromosomal changes in soft-tissue sarcomas. Arch Surg. 1987;122(11):1257.
122. Kaushal A, Citrin D. The role of radiation therapy in the management of sarcomas. Surg Clin North Am. 2008;88(3):629–46. viii
123. Kawai A, Woodruff J, Healey JH, Brennan MF, Antonescu CR, Ladanyi M. SYT-SSX gene fusion as a determinant of morphology and prognosis in synovial sarcoma. N Engl J Med. 1998;338(3):153–60.
124. Kenerson H, Folpe AL, Takayama TK, Yeung RS. Activation of the mTOR pathway in sporadic angiomyolipomas and other perivascular epithelioid cell neoplasms. Hum Pathol. 2007;38(9):1361–71.
125. Killian JK, Kim SY, Miettinen M, Smith C, Merino M, Tsokos M, Quezado M, Smith WI Jr, Jahromi MS, Xekouki P, Szarek E, Walker RL, Lasota J, Raffeld M, Klotzle B, Wang Z, Jones L, Zhu Y, Wang Y, Waterfall JJ, O'Sullivan MJ, Bibikova M, Pacak K, Stratakis C, Janeway KA, Schiffman JD, Fan JB, Helman L, Meltzer PS. Succinate dehydrogenase mutation underlies global epigenomic divergence in gastrointestinal stromal tumor. Cancer Discov. 2013;3(6):648–57.
126. Kinnunen M, Liu X, Niemelä E, Öhman T, Gawriyski L, Salokas K, Keskitalo S, Varjosalo M. The impact of ETV6-NTRK3 oncogenic gene fusions on molecular and signaling pathway alterations. Cancers (Basel). 2023;15(17):4246.

127. Knutson SK, Warholic NM, Wigle TJ, Klaus CR, Allain CJ, Raimondi A, Porter Scott M, Chesworth R, Moyer MP, Copeland RA, Richon VM, Pollock RM, Kuntz KW, Keilhack H. Durable tumor regression in genetically altered malignant rhabdoid tumors by inhibition of methyltransferase EZH2. Proc Natl Acad Sci USA. 2013;110(19):7922–7.
128. Koelsche C, Hartmann W, Schrimpf D, Stichel D, Jabar S, Ranft A, Reuss DE, Sahm F, Jones DTW, Bewerunge-Hudler M, Trautmann M, Klingebiel T, Vokuhl C, Gessler M, Wardelmann E, Petersen I, Baumhoer D, Flucke U, Antonescu C, Esteller M, Fröhling S, Kool M, Pfister SM, Mechtersheimer G, Dirksen U, von Deimling A. Array-based DNA-methylation profiling in sarcomas with small blue round cell histology provides valuable diagnostic information. Mod Pathol. 2018;31(8):1246–56.
129. Koelsche C, Schrimpf D, Stichel D, Sill M, Sahm F, Reuss DE, Blattner M, Worst B, Heilig CE, Beck K, Horak P, Kreutzfeldt S, Paff E, Stark S, Johann P, Selt F, Ecker J, Sturm D, Pajtler KW, Reinhardt A, et al. Sarcoma classification by DNA methylation profiling. Nat Commun. 2021;12(1):498. https://doi.org/10.1038/s41467-020-20603-4.
130. Ladanyi M, Lui MY, Antonescu CR, Krause-Boehm A, Meindl A, Argani P, Healey JH, Ueda T, Yoshikawa H, Meloni-Ehrig A, Sorensen PH, Mertens F, Mandahl N, van den Berghe H, Sciot R, Dal Cin P, Bridge J. The der(17)t(X;17)(p11;q25) of human alveolar soft part sarcoma fuses the TFE3 transcription factor gene to ASPL, a novel gene at 17q25. Oncogene. 2001;20(1):48–57.
131. Lam SW, Briaire-de Bruijn IH, van Wezel T, Cleven AHG, Hogendoorn PCW, Cleton-Jansen AM, Bovée JVMG. NTRK fusions are extremely rare in bone tumours. Histopathology. 2021;79(5):880–5. https://doi.org/10.1111/his.14432.
132. Lanic MD, Le Loarer F, Rainville V, Sater V, Viennot M, Beaussire L, Viailly PJ, Angot E, Hostein I, Jardin F, Ruminy P, Laé M. Detection of sarcoma fusions by a next-generation sequencing based-ligation-dependent multiplex RT-PCR assay. Mod Pathol. 2022;35(5):649–63.
133. Lee SB, Kolquist KA, Nichols K, Englert C, Maheswaran S, Ladanyi M, Gerald WL, Haber DA. The EWS-WT1 translocation product induces PDGFA in desmoplastic small round-cell tumour. Nat Genet. 1997;17(3):309–13.
134. Lee W, Teckie S, Wiesner T, Ran L, Prieto Granada CN, Lin M, Zhu S, Cao Z, Liang Y, Sboner A, Tap WD, Fletcher JA, Huberman KH, Qin L-X, Viale A, Singer S, Zheng D, Berger MF, Chen Y, Antonescu CR, Chi P. PRC2 is recurrently inactivated through EED or SUZ12 loss in malignant peripheral nerve sheath tumors. Nat Genet. 2014;46(11):1227–32.
135. Lemmon MA, Schlessinger J. Cell signaling by receptor tyrosine kinases. Cell. 2010;141(7):1117–34.
136. Lietz CE, Newman ET, Kelly AD, Xiang DH, Zhang Z, Luscko CA, Lozano-Calderon SA, Ebb DH, Raskin KA, Cote GM, Choy E, Nielsen GP, Haibe-Kains B, Aryee MJ, Spentzos D. Genome-wide DNA methylation patterns reveal clinically relevant predictive and prognostic subtypes in human osteosarcoma. Commun Biol. 2022;5(1):213. https://doi.org/10.1038/s42003-022-03117-1.
137. Lim JJ, Chen EY, Schaub SK, Wagner MJ. Reclassification of a spindle cell sarcoma after identification of a TFG-ROS1 fusion: a case demonstrating the clinical benefit of next-generation sequencing in sarcoma. Mol Genet Genomic Med. 2024;12(4):e2423.
138. Lyskjaer I, De Noon S, Tirabosco R, Rocha AM, Lindsay D, Amary F, Ye H, Schrimpf D, Stichel D, Sill M, Koelsche C, Pillay N, Von Deimling A, Beck S, Flanagan AM. DNA methylation-based profiling of bone and soft tissue tumours: a validation study of the 'DKFZ sarcoma classifier'. J Pathol Clin Res. 2021;7(4):350–60. https://doi.org/10.1002/cjp2.215.
139. Malik F, Santiago T, Newman S, McCarville B, Pappo AS, Clay MR. An addition to the evolving spectrum of lipofibromatosis and lipofibromatosis-like neural tumor: molecular findings in an unusual phenotype aid in accurate classification. Pathol Res Pract. 2020;216(6):152942.
140. Mandahl N, Mertens F, Willén H, Rydholm A, Kreicbergs A, Mitelman F. Nonrandom pattern of telomeric associations in atypical lipomatous tumors with ring and giant marker chromosomes. Cancer Genet Cytogenet. 1998;103(1):25–34.
141. Manea CA, Badiu DC, Ploscaru IC, Zgura A, Bacinschi X, Smarandache CG, Serban D, Popescu CG, Grigorean VT, Botnarciuc V. A review of NTRK fusions in cancer. Ann Med Surg (Lond). 2022;79:103893.
142. Manner J, Radlwimmer B, Hohenberger P, Mössinger K, Küffer S, Sauer C, Belharazem D, Zettl A, Coindre JM, Hallermann C, Hartmann JT, Katenkamp D, Katenkamp K, Schöffski P, Sciot R, Wozniak A, Lichter P, Marx A, Ströbel P. MYC high level gene amplification is a distinctive feature of angiosarcomas after irradiation or chronic lymphedema. Am J Pathol. 2010;176(1):34–9.
143. Marino-Enriquez A, Bovee JV. Molecular pathogenesis and diagnostic, prognostic and predictive molecular markers in sarcoma. Surg Pathol Clin. 2016;9(3):457–73.
144. Mariño-Enríquez A, Wang WL, Roy A, Lopez-Terrada D, Lazar AJ, Fletcher CD, Coffin CM, Hornick JL. Epithelioid inflammatory myofibroblastic sarcoma: an aggressive intra-abdominal variant of inflammatory myofibroblastic tumor with nuclear membrane or perinuclear ALK. Am J Surg Pathol. 2011;35(1):135–44.
145. McBride MJ, Pulice JL, Beird HC, Ingram DR, D'Avino AR, Shern JF, Charville GW, Hornick JL, Nakayama RT, Garcia-Rivera EM, Araujo DM, Wang WL, Tsai JW, Yeagley M, Wagner AJ, Futreal PA, Khan J, Lazar AJ, Kadoch C. The SS18-SSX fusion oncoprotein hijacks BAF complex targeting and function to drive synovial sarcoma. Cancer Cell.

2018;33(6):1128–1141.e7. https://doi.org/10.1016/j.ccell.2018.05.002. Epub 2018 May 31. PMID: 29861296; PMCID: PMC6791822
146. Meis-Kindblom JM, Bergh P, Gunterberg B, Kindblom LG. Extraskeletal myxoid chondrosarcoma: a reappraisal of its morphologic spectrum and prognostic factors based on 117 cases. Am J Surg Pathol. 1999;23(6):636–50.
147. Mentzel T, Calonje E, Wadden C, Camplejohn RS, Beham A, Smith MA, Fletcher CD. Myxofibrosarcoma. clinicopathologic analysis of 75 cases with emphasis on the low-grade variant. Am J Surg Pathol. 1996;20(4):391–405.
148. Mertens F, Antonescu CR, Mitelman F. Gene fusions in soft tissue tumors: recurrent and overlapping pathogenetic themes. Genes Chromosom Cancer. 2015;55(4):291–310.
149. Miettinen M, Wang ZF, Sarlomo-Rikala M, Osuch C, Rutkowski P, Lasota J. Succinate dehydrogenase-deficient GISTs: a clinicopathologic, immunohistochemical, and molecular genetic study of 66 gastric GISTs with predilection to young age. Am J Surg Pathol. 2011;35(11):1712–21.
150. Miquelestorena-Standley E, Jourdan ML, Collin C, Bouvier C, Larousserie F, Aubert S, Gomez-Brouchet A, Guinebretière JM, Tallegas M, Brulin B, Le Nail LR, Tallet A, Le Loarer F, Massiere J, Galant C, de Pinieux G. Effect of decalcification protocols on immunohistochemistry and molecular analyses of bone samples. Mod Pathol: Off J United States Canadian Acad Pathol, Inc. 2020;33(8):1505–17. https://doi.org/10.1038/s41379-020-0503-6.
151. Movva S, Wen W, Chen W, Millis SZ, Gatalica Z, Reddy S, von Mehren M, Van Tine BA. Multi-platform profiling of over 2000 sarcomas: identification of biomarkers and novel therapeutic targets. Oncotarget. 2015;6(14):12234–47.
152. Nacev BA, Jones KB, Intlekofer AM, Yu JSE, Allis CD, Tap WD, Ladanyi M, Nielsen TO. The epigenomics of sarcoma. Nat Rev Cancer. 2020;20(10):608–23.
153. Nacev BA, Sanchez-Vega F, Smith SA, Antonescu CR, Rosenbaum E, Shi H, Tang C, Socci ND, Rana S, Gularte-Mérida R, Zehir A, Gounder MM, Bowler TG, Luthra A, Jadeja B, Okada A, Strong JA, Stoller J, Chan JE, Chi P, D'Angelo SP, Dickson MA, Kelly CM, Keohan ML, Movva S, Thornton K, Meyers PA, Wexler LH, Slotkin EK, Glade Bender JL, Shukla NN, Hensley ML, Healey JH, La Quaglia MP, Alektiar KM, Crago AM, Yoon SS, Untch BR, Chiang S, Agaram NP, Hameed MR, Berger MF, Solit DB, Schultz N, Ladanyi M, Singer S, Tap WD. Clinical sequencing of soft tissue and bone sarcomas delineates diverse genomic landscapes and potential therapeutic targets. Nat Commun. 2022;13(1):3405.
154. Nakano K. Inflammatory myofibroblastic tumors: recent progress and future of targeted therapy. Jpn J Clin Oncol. 2023;53(10):885–92.
155. Nam SK, Im J, Kwak Y, Han N, Nam KH, Seo AN, Lee HS. Effects of fixation and storage of human tissue samples on nucleic acid preservation. Korean J Path. 2014;48(1):36–42. https://doi.org/10.4132/KoreanJPathol.2014.48.1.36.
156. Neuville A, Collin F, Bruneval P, Parrens M, Thivolet F, Gomez-Brouchet A, Terrier P, de Montpreville VT, Le Gall F, Hostein I, Lagarde P, Chibon F, Coindre JM. Intimal sarcoma is the most frequent primary cardiac sarcoma: clinicopathologic and molecular retrospective analysis of 100 primary cardiac sarcomas. Am J Surg Pathol. 2014;38(4):461–9.
157. Nielsen GP, Stemmer-Rachamimov AO, Ino Y, Møller MB, Rosenberg AE, Louis DN. Malignant transformation of neurofibromas in neurofibromatosis 1 is associated with CDKN2A/p16 inactivation. Am J Pathol. 1999;155(6):1879–84.
158. Nissim S, Leshchiner I, Mancias JD, Greenblatt MB, Maertens O, Cassa CA, Rosenfeld JA, Cox AG, Hedgepeth J, Wucherpfennig JI, Kim AJ, Henderson JE, Gonyo P, Brandt A, Lorimer E, Unger B, Prokop JW, Heidel JR, Wang XX, Ukaegbu CI, et al. Mutations in RABL3 alter KRAS prenylation and are associated with hereditary pancreatic cancer. Nat Genet. 2019;51(9):1308–14. https://doi.org/10.1038/s41588-019-0475-y.
159. O'Brien KP, Seroussi E, Dal Cin P, Sciot R, Mandahl N, Fletcher JA, Turc-Carel C, Dumanski JP. Various regions within the alpha-helical domain of the COL1A1 gene are fused to the second exon of the PDGFB gene in dermatofibrosarcomas and giant-cell fibroblastomas. Genes Chromosom Cancer. 1998;23(2):187–93.
160. O'Haire S, Franchini F, Kang Y-J, Steinberg J, Canfell K, Desai J, Fox S, Ijzerman M. Systematic review of NTRK 1/2/3 fusion prevalence pan-cancer and across solid tumours. Sci Rep. 2023;13(1):4116.
161. Ogura K, Hosoda F, Arai Y, Nakamura H, Hama N, Totoki Y, Yoshida A, Nagai M, Kato M, Arakawa E, Mukai W, Rokutan H, Kawai A, Tanaka S, Shibata T. Integrated genetic and epigenetic analysis of myxofibrosarcoma. Nat Commun. 2018;9(1):2765.
162. Okimoto RA, Wu W, Nanjo S, Olivas V, Lin YK, Ponce RK, Oyama R, Kondo T, Bivona TG. CIC-DUX4 oncoprotein drives sarcoma metastasis and tumorigenesis via distinct regulatory programs. J Clin Invest. 2019;129(8):3401–6.
163. Palmerini E, Frega G, Gambarotti M, Frisoni T, Cesari M, Bazzocchi A, Miceli M, Donati DM, Fanti S, Nanni C, Benini S, Longhi A, Paioli A, Marrari A, Hakim R, Righi A, Ibrahim T. NTRK rearranged sarcoma of the bone. Role for larotrectinib in the neoadjuvant setting of an ultra-rare tumor: a case report. Front Oncol. 2023;13:1252359. https://doi.org/10.3389/fonc.2023.1252359.
164. Papathomas TG, Gaal J, Corssmit EP, Oudijk L, Korpershoek E, Heimdal K, Bayley JP, Morreau H, van Dooren M, Papaspyrou K, Schreiner T, Hansen T, Andresen PA, Restuccia DF, van Kessel I, van Leenders GJ, Kros JM, Looijenga LH, Hofland LJ,

Mann W, van Nederveen FH, Mete O, Asa SL, de Krijger RR, Dinjens WN. Non-pheochromocytoma (PCC)/paraganglioma (PGL) tumors in patients with succinate dehydrogenase-related PCC-PGL syndromes: a clinicopathological and molecular analysis. Eur J Endocrinol. 2014;170(1):1–12.
165. Paudice M, Gambella A, Pigozzi S, Campora M, Pitto F, Bozzano S, Mastracci L, Grillo F. One protocol to rule them all: a pilot study to identify the best fixation and decalcification approach for bone marrow biopsy immunohistochemistry. Pathologica. 2025;117(2):145–52. https://doi.org/10.32074/1591-951X-1065.
166. Pedeutour F, Forus A, Coindre J-M, Berner J-M, Nicolo G, Michiels JF, Terrier P, Ranchere-Vince D, Collin F, Myklebost O, Turc-Carel C. Structure of the supernumerary ring and giant rod chromosomes in adipose tissue tumors. Genes Chromosom Cancer. 1999;24(1):30–41.
167. Pemov A, Li H, Patidar R, Hansen NF, Sindiri S, Hartley SW, Wei JS, Elkahloun A, Chandrasekharappa SC, Boland JF, Bass S, Mullikin JC, Khan J, Widemann BC, Wallace MR, Stewart DR. The primacy of NF1 loss as the driver of tumorigenesis in neurofibromatosis type 1-associated plexiform neurofibromas. Oncogene. 2017;36(22):3168–77.
168. Pérot G, Chibon F, Montero A, Lagarde P, de Thé H, Terrier P, Guillou L, Ranchère D, Coindre JM, Aurias A. Constant p53 pathway inactivation in a large series of soft tissue sarcomas with complex genetics. Am J Pathol. 2010;177(4):2080–90.
169. Perret R, Chalabreysse L, Watson S, Serre I, Garcia S, Forest F, Yvorel V, Pissaloux D, Thomas de Montpreville V, Masliah-Planchon J, Lantuejoul S, Brevet M, Blay JY, Coindre JM, Tirode F, Le Loarer F. SMARCA4-deficient thoracic sarcomas: clinicopathologic study of 30 cases with an emphasis on their nosology and differential diagnoses. Am J Surg Pathol. 2019;43(4):455–65.
170. Perry JA, Kiezun A, Tonzi P, Van Allen EM, Carter SL, Baca SC, Cowley GS, Bhatt AS, Rheinbay E, Pedamallu CS, Helman E, Taylor-Weiner A, McKenna A, DeLuca DS, Lawrence MS, Ambrogio L, Sougnez C, Sivachenko A, Walensky LD, Wagle N, et al. Complementary genomic approaches highlight the PI3K/mTOR pathway as a common vulnerability in osteosarcoma. Proc Natl Acad Sci USA. 2014;111(51):E5564–73. https://doi.org/10.1073/pnas.1419260111.
171. Petitprez F, de Reyniès A, Keung EZ, Chen TW, Sun CM, Calderaro J, Jeng YM, Hsiao LP, Lacroix L, Bougoüin A, Moreira M, Lacroix G, Natario I, Adam J, Lucchesi C, Laizet YH, Toulmonde M, Burgess MA, Bolejack V, Reinke D, Wani KM, Wang WL, Lazar AJ, Roland CL, Wargo JA, Italiano A, Sautès-Fridman C, Tawbi HA, Fridman WH. B cells are associated with survival and immunotherapy response in sarcoma. Nature. 2020;577(7791):556–60.
172. Picci P. Epidemiology of bone lesions. In: Picci P, et al., editors. Diagnosis of musculoskeletal tumors and tumor-like conditions. Cham: Springer; 2020.
173. Racanelli D, Brenca M, Baldazzi D, Goeman F, Casini B, De Angelis B, Guercio M, Milano GM, Tamborini E, Busico A, Dagrada G, Garofalo C, Caruso C, Brunello A, Pignochino Y, Berrino E, Grignani G, Scotlandi K, Parra A, Hattinger CM, Ibrahim T, Mercatali L, De Vita A, Carriero MV, Pallocca M, Loria R, Covello R, Sbaraglia M, Dei Tos AP, Falcioni R, Maestro R. next-generation sequencing approaches for the identification of pathognomonic fusion transcripts in sarcomas: the experience of the Italian ACC sarcoma working group. Front Oncol. 2020;10:**489**.
174. Ricciotti RW, Baraff AJ, Jour G, Kyriss M, Wu Y, Liu Y, Li SC, Hoch B, Liu YJ. High amplification levels of MDM2 and CDK4 correlate with poor outcome in patients with dedifferentiated liposarcoma: a cytogenomic microarray analysis of 47 cases. Cancer Genet. 2017;218-219:69–80.
175. Richarson AD, Scott DA, Zagnitko O, Aza-Blanc P, Chang CC, Russler-Germain DA. Registered report: IDH mutation impairs histone demethylation and results in a block to cell differentiation. elife. 2016;5:e10860.
176. Riggi N, Knoechel B, Gillespie SM, Rheinbay E, Boulay G, Suvà ML, Rossetti NE, Boonseng WE, Oksuz O, Cook EB, Formey A, Patel A, Gymrek M, Thapar V, Deshpande V, Ting DT, Hornicek FJ, Nielsen GP, Stamenkovic I, Aryee MJ, Bernstein BE, Rivera MN. EWS-FLI1 utilizes divergent chromatin remodeling mechanisms to directly activate or repress enhancer elements in Ewing sarcoma. Cancer Cell. 2014;26(5):668–81.
177. Robinson DR, Wu YM, Kalyana-Sundaram S, Cao X, Lonigro RJ, Sung YS, Chen CL, Zhang L, Wang R, Su F, Iyer MK, Roychowdhury S, Siddiqui J, Pienta KJ, Kunju LP, Talpaz M, Mosquera JM, Singer S, Schuetze SM, Antonescu CR, Chinnaiyan AM. Identification of recurrent NAB2-STAT6 gene fusions in solitary fibrous tumor by integrative sequencing. Nat Genet. 2013;45(2):180–5.
178. Rosenbaum E, Jonsson P, Seier K, Qin L-X, Chi P, Dickson M, Gounder M, Kelly C, Keohan ML, Nacev B, Donoghue MTA, Chiang S, Singer S, Ladanyi M, Antonescu CR, Hensley ML, Movva S, D'Angelo SP, Tap WD. Clinical outcome of Leiomyosarcomas with somatic alteration in homologous recombination pathway genes. JCO Precis Oncol. 2020;4:1350–60.
179. Sandberg AA. Updates on the cytogenetics and molecular genetics of bone and soft tissue tumors: liposarcoma. Cancer Genet Cytogenet. 2004;155:1–24.
180. Savi FM, Brierly GI, Baldwin J, Theodoropoulos C, Woodruff MA. Comparison of different decalcification methods using rat mandibles as a model. J Histochem Cytochem: Off J

Histochem Soc. 2017;65(12):705–22. https://doi.org/10.1369/0022155417733708.
181. Schaefer IM, Hornick JL. SWI/SNF complex-deficient soft tissue neoplasms: an update. Semin Diagn Pathol. 2021;38(3):222–31.
182. Schaefer I-M, Cote GM, Hornick JL. Contemporary sarcoma diagnosis, genetics, and genomics. J Clin Oncol. 2018;36(2):101–10.
183. Shi E, Chmielecki J, Tang CM, Wang K, Heinrich MC, Kang G, Corless CL, Hong D, Fero KE, Murphy JD, Fanta PT, Ali SM, De Siena M, Burgoyne AM, Movva S, Madlensky L, Heestand GM, Trent JC, Kurzrock R, Morosini D, Ross JS, Harismendy O, Sicklick JK. FGFR1 and NTRK3 actionable alterations in "wild-type" gastrointestinal stromal tumors. J Transl Med. 2016;14(1):339.
184. Shing DC, McMullan DJ, Roberts P, Smith K, Chin SF, Nicholson J, Tillman RM, Ramani P, Cullinane C, Coleman N. FUS/ERG gene fusions in Ewing's tumors. Cancer Res. 2003;63(15):4568–76.
185. Shukla N, Ameur N, Yilmaz I, Nafa K, Lau CY, Marchetti A, Borsu L, Barr FG, Ladanyi M. Oncogene mutation profiling of pediatric solid tumors reveals significant subsets of embryonal rhabdomyosarcoma and neuroblastoma with mutated genes in growth signaling pathways. Clin Cancer Res. 2011;18(3):748–57.
186. Simeone N, Frezza AM, Zaffaroni N, Stacchiotti S. Tazemetostat for advanced epithelioid sarcoma: current status and future perspectives. Future Oncol. 2021;17(10):1253–63.
187. Sioletic S, Czaplinski J, Hu L, Fletcher JA, Fletcher CD, Wagner AJ, Loda M, Demetri GD, Sicinska ET, Snyder EL. C-Jun promotes cell migration and drives expression of the motility factor ENPP2 in soft tissue sarcomas. J Pathol. 2014;234(2):190–202.
188. Smolle MA, Seidel MG, Kashofer K, Liegl-Atzwanger B, Sadoghi P, Müller DA, Leithner A. Precision medicine in diagnosis, prognosis, and disease monitoring of bone and soft tissue sarcomas using liquid biopsy: a systematic review. Arch Orthop Trauma Surg. 2025;145(1):121.
189. Somaiah N, Tap W. MDM2-p53 in liposarcoma: the need for targeted therapies with novel mechanisms of action. Cancer Treat Rev. 2024;122:102668.
190. Stacchiotti S, Frezza AM, Blay JY, Baldini EH, Bonvalot S, Bovée J, Callegaro D, Casali PG, Chiang RC, Demetri GD, Demicco EG, Desai J, Eriksson M, Gelderblom H, George S, Gounder MM, Gronchi A, Gupta A, Haas RL, Hayes-Jardon A, Hohenberger P, Jones KB, Jones RL, Kasper B, Kawai A, Kirsch DG, Kleinerman ES, Le Cesne A, Lim J, Chirlaque López MD, Maestro R, Marcos-Gragera R, Martin Broto J, Matsuda T, Mir O, Patel SR, Raut CP, Razak ARA, Reed DR, Rutkowski P, Sanfilippo RG, Sbaraglia M, Schaefer IM, Strauss DC, Sundby Hall K, Tap WD, Thomas DM, van der Graaf WTA, van Houdt WJ, Visser O, von Mehren M, Wagner AJ, Wilky BA, Won YJ, Fletcher CDM, Dei Tos AP, Trama A. Ultra-rare sarcomas: a consensus paper from the connective tissue oncology society community of experts on the incidence threshold and the list of entities. Cancer. 2021;127(16):2934–42.
191. Su L, Sampaio AV, Jones KB, Pacheco M, Goytain A, Lin S, Poulin N, Yi L, Rossi FM, Kast J, Capecchi MR, Underhill TM, Nielsen TO. Deconstruction of the SS18-SSX fusion oncoprotein complex: insights into disease etiology and therapeutics. Cancer Cell. 2012;21(3):333–47.
192. Sultan I, Rodriguez-Galindo C, Saab R, Yasir S, Casanova M, Ferrari A. Comparing children and adults with synovial sarcoma in the surveillance, epidemiology, and end results program, 1983 to 2005. Cancer. 2009;115(15):3537–47.
193. Tan SY, Al-Ibraheemi A, Ahrens WA, Oesterheld JE, Fanburg-Smith JC, Liu YJ, Spunt SL, Rudzinski ER, Coffin C, Davis JL. ALK rearrangements in infantile fibrosarcoma-like spindle cell tumours of soft tissue and kidney. Histopathology. 2022;80(4):698–707.
194. Tang YJ, Huang J, Tsushima H, Ban GI, Zhang H, Oristian KM, Puviindran V, Williams N, Ding X, Ou J, Jung S-H, Lee C-L, Jiao Y, Chen BJ, Kirsch DG, Alman BA. Tracing tumor evolution in sarcoma reveals clonal origin of advanced metastasis. Cell Rep. 2019;28(11):2837–2850.e2835.
195. Tap WD, Eilber FC, Ginther C, Dry SM, Reese N, Barzan-Smith K, Chen HW, Wu H, Eilber FR, Slamon DJ, Anderson L. Evaluation of well-differentiated/de-differentiated liposarcomas by high-resolution oligonucleotide array-based comparative genomic hybridization. Genes Chromosom Cancer. 2011;50(2):95–112.
196. Tap WD, Villalobos VM, Cote GM, Burris H, Janku F, Mir O, Beeram M, Wagner AJ, Jiang L, Wu B, Choe S, Yen K, Gliser C, Fan B, Agresta S, Pandya SS, Trent JC. Phase I study of the mutant IDH1 inhibitor Ivosidenib: safety and clinical activity in patients with advanced chondrosarcoma. J Clin Oncol Off J Am Soc Clin Oncol. 2020;38(15):1693–701. https://doi.org/10.1200/JCO.19.02492.
197. Taylor BS, Barretina J, Maki RG, Antonescu CR, Singer S, Ladanyi M. Advances in sarcoma genomics and new therapeutic targets. Nat Rev Cancer. 2011;11(9):685.
198. Thaete C, Brett D, Monaghan P, Whitehouse S, Rennie G, Rayner E, Cooper CS, Goodwin G. Functional domains of the SYT and SYT-SSX synovial sarcoma translocation proteins and co-localization with the SNF protein BRM in the nucleus. Hum Mol Genet. 1999;8(4):585–91. https://doi.org/10.1093/hmg/8.4.585. PMID: 10072425
199. Thway K, Fisher C. Tumors with EWSR1-CREB1 and EWSR1-ATF1 fusions. Am J Surg Pathol. 2012;36(7):e1–e11.
200. Thway K, Fisher C. PEComa: morphology and genetics of a complex tumor family. Ann Diagn Pathol. 2015;19(5):359–68.
201. Tomuleasa C, Tigu A-B, Munteanu R, Moldovan C-S, Kegyes D, Onaciu A, Gulei D, Ghiaur G, Einsele H, Croce CM. Therapeutic advances of tar-

geting receptor tyrosine kinases in cancer. Signal Transduct Target Ther. 2024;9(1):201.
202. Towery EA, Papke DJ. EWSR1: the promiscuous king of mesenchymal neoplasia. J Clin Pathol. 2024;77(11):721–5.
203. Tsuda M, Davis IJ, Argani P, Shukla N, McGill GG, Nagai M, Saito T, Laé M, Fisher DE, Ladanyi M. TFE3 fusions activate MET signaling by transcriptional up-regulation, defining another class of tumors as candidates for therapeutic MET inhibition. Cancer Res. 2007;67(3):919–29.
204. Vibert J, Watson S. The molecular biology of soft tissue sarcomas: current knowledge and future perspectives. Cancer. 2022;14(10):2548.
205. Wachtel M, Surdez D, Grünewald TGP, Schäfer BW. Functional classification of fusion proteins in sarcoma. Cancer. 2024;16(7):1355.
206. Wang X, Haswell JR, Roberts CW. Molecular pathways: SWI/SNF (BAF) complexes are frequently mutated in cancer--mechanisms and potential therapeutic insights. Clin Cancer Res. 2014;20(1):21–7.
207. WHO. Soft tissue and bone tumours. Lyon: International Agency for Research on Cancer (IARC Press); 2020.
208. Willems SM, Debiec-Rychter M, Szuhai K, Hogendoorn PCW, Sciot R. Local recurrence of myxofibrosarcoma is associated with increase in tumour grade and cytogenetic aberrations, suggesting a multistep tumour progression model. Mod Pathol. 2006;19(3):407–16.
209. Williamson D, Missiaglia E, de Reyniès A, Pierron G, Thuille B, Palenzuela G, Thway K, Orbach D, Laé M, Fréneaux P, Pritchard-Jones K, Oberlin O, Shipley J, Delattre O. Fusion gene-negative alveolar rhabdomyosarcoma is clinically and molecularly indistinguishable from embryonal rhabdomyosarcoma. J Clin Oncol. 2010;28(13):2151–8.
210. Wilson BG, Roberts CWM. SWI/SNF nucleosome remodellers and cancer. Nat Rev Cancer. 2011;11(7):481–92.
211. Xiao M, Yang H, Xu W, Ma S, Lin H, Zhu H, Liu L, Liu Y, Yang C, Xu Y, Zhao S, Ye D, Xiong Y, Guan KL. Inhibition of α-KG-dependent histone and DNA demethylases by fumarate and succinate that are accumulated in mutations of FH and SDH tumor suppressors. Genes Dev. 2012;26(12):1326–38.
212. Yoshida A, Kobayashi E, Kubo T, Kodaira M, Motoi T, Motoi N, Yonemori K, Ohe Y, Watanabe SI, Kawai A, Kohno T, Kishimoto H, Ichikawa H, Hiraoka N. Clinicopathological and molecular characterization of SMARCA4-deficient thoracic sarcomas with comparison to potentially related entities. Mod Pathol. 2017;30(6):797–809.
213. Yoshimoto T, Tanaka M, Homme M, Yamazaki Y, Takazawa Y, Antonescu CR, Nakamura T. CIC-DUX4 induces small round cell sarcomas distinct from Ewing sarcoma. Cancer Res. 2017;77(11):2927–37.
214. Young RJ, Brown NJ, Reed MW, Hughes D, Woll PJ. Angiosarcoma. Lancet Oncol. 2010;11(10):983–91.

Next-Generation Sequencing in Pediatric Soft Tissue Tumors: Pediatric Malignancies

8

Sabina Barresi, Emma Rullo, Damiano Arciuolo, and Rita Alaggio

Introduction

Pediatric neoplasms exhibit distinct characteristics compared to those found in adults. Although their overall incidence is low, affecting roughly 1 in 400,000 children, they are the leading cause of disease-related death in the pediatric population. According to the 2025 AACR report, leukemia and lymphomas comprise 38.6% of all pediatric cancers, while central nervous system (CNS) tumors (16.5%) and soft tissue and bone tumors (11%) are the most common solid tumors in children [1]. Embryonal tumors such as neuroblastoma, hepatoblastoma, and Wilms tumor frequently arise in infancy and early childhood and recapitulate developmental stages of the affected organ, as underscored in the historical paper by Willis—"The Borderland of Embryology and Pathology" [2].

Identification of the molecular features of pediatric neoplasms has been crucial for the development of tailored therapeutic protocols and improved survival rates. Over the past 40 years, the 5 year survival rate for all pediatric cancers in the United States has increased from 63% in the 1970s to 87% in 2015–2021 (Research [3]). Unlike adult tumors, which commonly result from the progressive accumulation of point mutations, copy number alterations, and epigenetic changes, pediatric tumors typically originate from a single genomic event, frequently a chromosomal rearrangement. The high specificity of these alterations for individual tumor types defines molecularly homogeneous groups providing a potential diagnostic tool, which is also a potential therapeutic target in a subset of tumors.

The "Copernican revolution" started by the discovery of recurrent gene fusions and structural alterations is an ongoing process changing the classification approach from a morphology based to an integrated molecular and morphologic taxonomy of pediatric malignancies. Furthermore, advances in understanding the molecular pathogenesis of these tumors have facilitated the introduction of over 20 molecularly targeted therapies and 10 immunotherapies, now approved by the FDA for pediatric cancers. The following section reviews

S. Barresi · E. Rullo
Pathology Unit, Department of Laboratories, Bambino Gesù Children's Hospital, IRCCS, Rome, Italy
e-mail: Sabina.barresi@opbg.net; Emma.rullo@opbg.net

D. Arciuolo
Anatomical Pathology Operative Research Unit, Fondazione Policlinico Università Campus Bio-Medico, Rome, Italy

R. Alaggio (✉)
Pathology Unit, Department of Laboratories, Bambino Gesù Children's Hospital, IRCCS, Rome, Italy

Department of Medical and Surgical Sciences and Biotechnologies, Sapienza University of Rome, Polo Pontino, Rome, Italy
e-mail: rita.alaggio@opbg.net

© The Author(s), under exclusive license to Springer Nature Switzerland AG 2026
S. Sioletic, L. Coppola (eds.), *Next-Generation Sequencing in Solid Tumor Histopathology*, Current Clinical Pathology, https://doi.org/10.1007/978-3-032-18790-1_8

studies show no association with worse survival [8]. Other receptor tyrosine kinase pathways are involved as well such as those of the FGFR family [12]. Mutations in TP53 are associated with a more aggressive clinical behavior and may be associated with histologic anaplasia [8].

Spindle Cell/Sclerosing RMS are clinically and molecularly heterogeneous. In fact, MYOD1 L122R defines a group of spindle cell RMS occurring most frequently in older children and associated with highly aggressive behavior [13].

The molecular pathogenetic mechanism of MYOD1L122R is still object of investigation; however, two possible mechanisms responsible for the aggressive behavior have been hypothesized. MYOD1L122R blocks normal MYOD1 and binds to MYOD1-responsive promoters but fails to transactivate these myogenic genes, with consequent block of differentiation, and maintains a proliferating state. Alternatively, MYOD1L122R can bind to MYC-responsive genes [13–15].

Other mutations are frequently associated to mutant MYOD1 RMS and are probably required for the development of the tumorigenicity, particularly PIK3CA and other genes belonging to PIK3CA or RAS pathway.

In contrast, spindle cell RMS in children under 2 years frequently harbor *NCOA2* or *VGLL2* rearrangements and are associated with favorable outcomes [16]. Lastly, a separate molecular subgroup of SSRMS is defined by *TFCP2* fusions, most often involving *FUS* o1r *EWSR1*, and typically affects young adults with tumors of bone or soft tissue showing aggressive clinical behavior [17]. These *TFCP2* rearranged RMS show immunohistochemical expression of ALK, related to intragenic deletions and aberrant splicing which result in oncogenic *ALK* variants. Recurrent *CDKN2A/MTAP* co-deletions which are potentially targetable have been reported. The pathogenetic mechanism of *TFCP2* fusions has been explored in functional studies, which show a block myogenic differentiation and induction of transcription of ALK and truncated TERT, with inhibition of DNA repair. DNA methylation profiling demonstrates a close relationship of these sarcomas with undifferentiated sarcomas.

Novel molecular alterations, mostly fusions, are being identified in spindle cell rhabdomyosarcomas, especially those occurring in adults. Their rarity and lack of a long clinical follow-up do not allow to clearly define their biological aggressivity (Table 8.2).

Table 8.2 Novel molecular alterations in spindle cell rhabdomyosarcoma

Bone	Soft tissue
FUS::TFCP2[a,b]	*FUS/EWSR::TFCP2*[d]
EWSR::TFCP2[a]	*ZFP64::NCOA2/3*[e,f]
ERSR/FUS::TCFP2[c]	*TCF12::VGLL3*[g]
EWSR r, FUS r[a,b]	*PPARGC1A::VGLL3*[g]
MEIS::NCOA 2[c]	*EP300:VGLL3*[h]
	DCTN1::ALK[i]
	MEIS::NCOA2[j]
	MEIS::FOXO1[k]
	EWSR::ZBTB41[l]
	PLOD2::RBM6[l]
	SRF::NCOA1[m]
	SRF::FOXO1[m]
	NCOA2::CITED/SRF[n]
	TEAD::NCOA2[o]
	VGLL2::CITED[p]
	VGLL2::NCOA2[p]
	EWSR1::NF2[q]

[a]Agaram et al. [18]
[b]Dashti et al. [19]
[c]Duan et al. [20]
[d]Smith et al. [21]
[e]Xu et al. [22]
[f]Han et al. [23]
[g]Dehner et al. [24]
[h]Agaimy et al. [25]
[i]Yoshida et al. [26]
[j]Fung et al. [27]
[k]Kao et al. [28]
[l]Dehner et al. [29]
[m]Bradová et al. [30]
[n]Karanian et al. [31]
[o]Mosquera et al. [32]
[p]Tan et al. [33]
[q]Alaggio et al. [34]
[r]Saoud et al. [35]

Undifferentiated Small Round Cell Sarcomas of the Bone and Soft Tissue

The group of undifferentiated small round cell sarcomas of the bone and soft tissue is described extensively in Chapter 7. This section summarizes the diagnostic approach in pediatric patients and highlights features specific to this age group.

Ewing Sarcoma and the Ewing-Like Sarcoma Family

EWSR1 is the most commonly rearranged gene in primitive small round cell tumors (PSRTs) and is frequently fused with members of the ETS transcription factor family, characterized by C-terminal DNA-binding ETS domains. Most ETS family proteins act as nuclear targets of the Ras-MAP kinase signaling pathway and influence cell proliferation by regulating immediate early response genes and other growth-related genes [36, 37]. Ewing sarcoma (ES) is an aggressive tumor of the bone and soft tissue affecting children and adolescents. It is defined in >85% of cases by the *EWSR1::FLI1* fusion and, less commonly, by alternative *FET::ETS* fusions such as *EWSR1::ERG*, *FUS::FLI1*, *FUS::ERG*, *EWSR1::ETV4*, and others. These chimeric proteins act as aberrant transcription factors, reprogramming chromatin accessibility and enhancer landscapes. A distinct group is composed of *EWSR1-non-ETS* round cell sarcomas, in which the fusion partner is not an ETS family transcription factor. These include undifferentiated round cell sarcomas with fusions such as *EWSR1::PATZ1* [38], *EWSR1::NFATC2* [39], and other emerging partners. These tumors are epigenetically distinct from classic ES [40]. In the pediatric population, *EWSR1::PATZ1* sarcomas are exceptionally rare, while *EWSR1::NFATC2* sarcomas are more common. Their morphology ranges from cystic bone lesions to neoplasms composed of small round cells in nests or sheets admixed with variable spindle cell and stromal components. In ~90% of cases, FISH demonstrates an unbalanced translocation with 5' probe gain [39, 41, 42]. Notably, *NFATC2* fusions lacking partner-gene amplification have also been identified in simple bone cysts and in vascular malformations/hemangiomas [43]. *EWSR1::FLI1* and other *FET::ETS* fusions have recently been reported in superficial neurocristic tumors. These small lesions occur in adolescents and adults and have a favorable prognosis. Histologically, neurocristic tumors show nests of bland round cells with areas of elongated/spindled cells. They demonstrate a characteristic immunophenotype, including S100 and SOX10 positivity and NKX2.2 expression [44, 45]. Diagnostic testing for EWSR1-rearranged small round cell sarcomas typically begins with break-apart FISH, although the inability to identify the partner gene may lead to diagnostic pitfalls. RT-PCR detects most *EWSR1::FLI1* and *EWSR1::ERG* transcript types with high specificity and sensitivity but requires prior knowledge of breakpoint variants. Targeted RNA-seq/anchored multiplex PCR can detect rare, cryptic, or complex fusion variants. When RNA is unavailable or degraded, targeted DNA panels or whole-genome sequencing (WGS) may identify structural variants involving EWSR1, FUS, or ETS genes.

CIC-Rearranged Sarcomas

CIC-rearranged sarcomas represent a distinct subset of undifferentiated small round cell sarcomas, most commonly driven by the CIC::DUX4 fusion. These tumors are rare in children and typically arise in the soft tissue, with occasional visceral involvement. Additional CIC fusion variants—including *CIC::NUTM1* [46] and *CIC::FOXO4* [47]—occur in the soft tissue, bone, and visceral sites. Although rare, these variants share the molecular hallmarks of *CIC::DUX4* sarcoma, including dysregulation of downstream transcriptional programs and uniformly high-grade behavior.

BCOR-Altered Sarcomas

BCOR-altered sarcomas include tumors with BCOR internal tandem duplication (BCOR-ITD) or.

YWHAE fusions and sarcomas with BCOR rearrangements, most commonly BCOR::CCNB3 and less frequently ZC3H7B::BCOR.

BCOR-ITD- and YWHAE-rearranged tumors were first described in clear cell sarcoma of the kidney (CCSK), typically arising in the first years of life. These alterations were subsequently identified in a subgroup of undifferentiated infantile soft tissue tumors, including primitive myxoid mesenchymal tumor of infancy (PMMTI) and undifferentiated round cell sarcoma (URCS), and in a subset of high-grade neuroepithelial tumors (HG-NETs) of the central nervous system. The same alterations have also been reported in high-grade endometrial stromal sarcoma (ESS-HG). All these tumors share similar histology and transcriptional signatures but display distinct methylation profiles, which separate HG-NETs from kidney and soft tissue sarcomas [48].

BCOR::CCNB3 sarcomas usually arise in the bone and less commonly in soft tissue or visceral organs, including the kidney. Prognostically, *BCOR::CCNB3*-rearranged sarcomas have a more favorable outcome compared with *CIC*-rearranged sarcomas, whereas infantile *BCOR-ITD* sarcomas behave aggressively [49].

Histology and immunophenotype may raise suspicion for CIC or BCOR rearrangements. Break-apart FISH can support detection; however, the structural complexity of CIC rearrangements can lead to false-negative results. Dual-fusion FISH for CIC and DUX4 (4q35 and 10q26) can detect CIC::DUX4 but may fail in the presence of telomeric deletions or atypical fusion partners. Breakpoint variability is also a limitation of RT-PCR, although RT-PCR reliably detects BCOR::CCNB3.

Targeted RNA-seq is the most robust diagnostic method, allowing detection of expected and novel fusion transcripts even without specific histologic suspicion. A negative RNA-seq result does not exclude the diagnosis, as BCOR-ITD sarcomas and some CIC-rearranged tumors may be missed due to current algorithmic limitations.

DNA methylation profiling is highly accurate for small round cell sarcomas with CIC or BCOR alterations and is particularly helpful when RNA quality is poor; however, methylation profiling is not universally recognized as a diagnostic standard for sarcomas.

Fibroblastic and Myofibroblastic Tumors

Fibroblastic and myofibroblastic neoplasms represent approximately 12% of all pediatric soft tissue tumors. Most lesions in this category are benign or locally aggressive with rare metastatic potential; truly malignant tumors are uncommon [50]. A large subset is driven by kinase-gene fusions, which represent a distinct oncogenic mechanism. These fusions result in constitutive or upregulated activation of receptor tyrosine kinases (RTKs) or downstream signaling pathways, including PI3K-AKT, MAPK, and transcription factors such as STAT and NF-κB. Unlike transcription factor-related fusions, kinase rearrangements produce directly targetable proteins, and therefore prompt and precise molecular characterization has immediate therapeutic relevance.

Infantile Fibrosarcoma (IFS)

Infantile fibrosarcoma is one of the most common sarcomas of infancy, typically presenting within the first year of life. It shows a broad morphologic spectrum, ranging from loosely arranged primitive ovoid cells to densely packed spindle cells forming fascicles within a variably collagenized stroma, often with a prominent hemangiopericytoma-like vascular pattern. Myxoid areas may also be present. Most IFS harbor the *ETV6::NTRK3* fusion generated by the t (12;15) (p13;q25) translocation. Less commonly, tumors show alternative *NTRK3* partners (e.g., *EML4::NTRK3*) or *NTRK1* fusions (e.g.,

TPM3::NTRK1, *LMNA::NTRK1*, *TPR::NTRK1*). Other fusions involve RTKs such as *RET* [51] and *ALK* [52] or downstream kinases including *RAF1* [53] and *BRAF* [54]. Rare cases exhibit *EGFR* kinase-domain duplications (KDD/ITD). Despite this molecular diversity, clinical behavior is generally consistent across genetic subgroups: locally aggressive growth, a 25–40% risk of local recurrence, and rare metastasis.

TRK-Rearranged Spindle Cell Mesenchymal Tumors

TRK-rearranged spindle cell tumors comprise a heterogeneous group of pediatric mesenchymal neoplasms. In the pediatric WHO classification, they are categorized as myofibroblastic neoplasms, whereas in the WHO classification of soft tissue and bone tumors, they are considered of uncertain differentiation. They show strong pediatric predominance, with most patients diagnosed within the first two decades and over half within the first year.

Morphology is variable and includes lipofibromatosis-like neural tumors, lesions resembling inflammatory myofibroblastic tumor or infantile fibrosarcoma, and less frequently higher-grade tumors mimicking malignant peripheral nerve sheath tumors. Perivascular hyalinosis is common. Immunophenotypically, **S100 and CD34 positivity with SOX10 negativity** is frequent and useful for differential diagnosis [55].

Although initially described as "NTRK-rearranged," the genetic spectrum now includes fusions involving ***NTRK1*** **(most common)**, ***NTRK2***, ***NTRK3***, ***RAF1***, ***BRAF***, ***RET***, ***MET***, ***ALK***, and ***ROS1***. These tumors typically follow an indolent clinical course, with a propensity for late local recurrence and rare metastasis. In contrast to adult cases, morphologic parameters such as cellularity, mitotic rate, or necrosis do not consistently correlate with outcome. Long-term follow-up is essential.

Inflammatory Myofibroblastic Tumor (IMT)

IMT is an RTK-driven myofibroblastic neoplasm of intermediate biologic potential, seen mainly in children and young adults. Pediatric cases commonly arise in the abdominal cavity, including the omentum, mesentery, retroperitoneum, pelvis, and intra-abdominal organs. Histology ranges from fasciitis-like myofibroblastic proliferations with myxoid stroma and mixed inflammation to more cellular spindle cell tumors forming fascicles within collagenized stroma [56].

Over 90% of pediatric IMTs contain an RTK fusion. Approximately 60% demonstrate *ALK* rearrangements with numerous partners (e.g., *TPM3*, *TPM4*, *CLTC*, *CARS*, *ATIC*, *SEC31L1*, *PPFIBP1*, *DCTN1*, *EML4*, *PRKAR1A*, *LMNA*, *TFG*, *FN1*, *MYH9*, *HNRNPA1*, *RANBP1*), producing variable ALK immunostaining patterns depending on the fusion partner [57]. About 30% harbor fusions in *ROS1*, *ETV6::NTRK3*, or rarely *PDGFRB* or *RET*.

Pediatric IMTs generally have a good prognosis, with local recurrence in ~25% and metastasis in <5%. Histologic features such as cellularity or necrosis do not reliably predict outcome.

Epithelioid IMT (EIMS) is a more aggressive variant [58], most often intra-abdominal and typically seen in adults, though pediatric cases occur. Tumors consist of epithelioid cells with myxoid stroma and frequent neutrophils, sometimes with necrosis and high mitotic activity. EIMS is strongly associated with *RANBP2::ALK* [59] and less commonly *RRBP1::ALK* fusions [60].

ALK-Rearranged Mesenchymal Neoplasms (ALK-r MN)

Newly recognized ALK-rearranged mesenchymal tumors span a broad morphologic and clinical spectrum:

1. *ALK-r* tumors resembling NTRK-rearranged spindle cell tumors are mostly observed in

adults. These are histologically indistinguishable from TRK-rearranged tumors and frequently CD34-/S100-positive and SOX10-negative [61, 62].

2. ALK-r neoplasms resembling dermatofibrosarcoma protuberans (DFSP) or plaque-like dermal fibroma (PLDF) are superficial lesions [63]. ALK partners include *DCTN1*, *PLEKHH2*, *CLIP2* (DFSP-like), and *FLNA* (PLDF-like).
3. ALK-positive dermal/superficial myxoid neoplasms (DSMN) are mostly seen in adults, but lesions with similar histologic features have been reported in some infantile IMTs [55]. These lesions are characterized by spindle/oval cells in myxoid stroma with whorled architecture. ALK partners include *FLNA*, *MYH10*, and *HMBOX1*. The follow-up is limited; however, a favorable outcome has been reported in all cases.
4. ALK-r epithelioid mesenchymal neoplasms are extremely rare lesions, occurring both in children and adults, histologically characterized by epithelioid cells in sheets within a myxohyaline stroma. ALK partners include *HMBOX1*, *PRRC2B*, *MYH10*, *STRN*, and *EML4 [64]*.

Neuroblastoma

Neuroblastoma is the most common cancer diagnosed in infancy (25–50 cases per million). About 90% occur before age 10, with a median diagnosis at 18 months. The tumor arises from the sympathetic nervous system, originating from neural crest cells, most often in the adrenal medulla or sympathetic ganglia. Familial cases account for 1–2%, usually due to germline ALK or PHOX2B mutations [65].

Histologically neuroblastic tumors are composed of neuroblasts in various differentiative stages and a schwannian stromal component. The histologic prognostic classification is based on the percentage of schwannian component, differentiation of neuroblasts, and mitotic-karyorrhectic index (MKI) (Table 8.3).

However, with the exception of ganglioneuromas and ganglioneuroblastomas intermixed (GNB-I) in neuroblastoma and nodular neuroblastoma, molecular features are crucial in therapeutic stratification and prognosis. The key molecular features include *MYCN* amplification, *ALK* alterations, and segmental chromosomal alterations.

Table 8.3 Histologic classification and prognostic categorization of neuroblastoma

Schwannian component	Histotype	Neuroblastic component	Age	MKI	Prognostic category
Stroma dominant	Ganglioneuroma	Maturing, mature	Any	–	Favorable
Stroma-rich	GNB intermixed	Mature, immature	Any	–	Favorable
Stroma-rich/ stroma-poor	Ganglioneuroblastoma, nodular*	Evaluated in the nodule(s) like in NB	See NB	See NB	According to the nodule with worst prognostic features
Stroma-poor	Neuroblastoma	Undifferentiated	Any	Any	Unfavorable
		Poorly differentiated	< 1.5y	Low	Favorable
				Intermediate	Favorable
				High	Unfavorable
			> 1.5–5y	Any	Unfavorable
			>5y	Any	Unfavorable
		Differentiating	<1.5y	Low	Favorable
				Intermediate	Favorable
				High	Unfavorable
			>1.5–5y	Low	Favorable
				Intermediate	Unfavorable
				High	Unfavorable
			>5y	Any	Unfavorable

[a]The nodular component is classified with the same criteria as neuroblastoma

ALK (anaplastic lymphoma kinase) gene, located on chromosome 2p23, is an oncogene codifying for a receptor tyrosine kinase frequently mutated or, less frequently, amplified in neuroblastoma. Germline gain-of-function ALK mutations predispose to familial neuroblastoma, while somatic mutations occur in approximately 8–14% of high-risk sporadic cases. ALK mutations at hotspots such as p. R1275 *(mostly in familial neuroblastoma)*, p.F1174, and p.F1245 *(mostly in sporadic neuroblastoma)* activate PI3K/AKT, RAS/MAPK, and RET pathways, leading to stabilization of N-MYC and promotion of proliferation [66]. Co-amplification of ALK and MYCN on 2p24 is observed in a subset of tumors, resulting in enhanced tumorigenic potential [67].

LIN28B is associated with high-risk neuroblastoma. Polymorphic variants of LIN28B, as well as overexpression (even without amplification), enhance *N-MYC* levels and promote tumorigenesis through miRNA deregulation, particularly depletion of the let-7 family and modulation of RAN and AURKA stability. This signaling axis (LIN28B-RAN-AURKA) represents a crucial pathway for tumor cell proliferation and survival [68].

High-risk neuroblastomas frequently harbor alterations in chromatin remodeling genes, including *ATRX*, *ARID1A*, and *ARID1B*. *ATRX* loss-of-function/mutations occur in approximately 10% of tumors, particularly in older children with indolent but progressive disease, and are mutually exclusive with *MYCN* amplification. *ATRX* deficiency is associated with alternative lengthening of telomeres (ALT), providing a telomere maintenance mechanism independent of TERT [69].

TERT promoter rearrangements, present in roughly 25% of tumors, activate telomerase via enhancer hijacking and are typically mutually exclusive with MYCN amplification.

Segmental copy number alterations are pervasive in neuroblastoma and serve as robust prognostic markers. Common recurrent alterations include the following:

- Gain of 17q (>50% of cases).
- Loss of 1p (~33% of cases), encompassing candidate tumor suppressors such as *CHD5*, *CAMTA1*, *KIF1B*, *CASZ1*, and *miR-34A*.
- Loss of 11q (~33% of high-risk tumors), associated with poor prognosis, inversely correlated with MYCN amplification, and involving multiple candidate tumor suppressor loci.

These structural alterations often occur early in tumor evolution, suggesting that dosage effects on oncogenes and tumor suppressors drive tumorigenesis. Numerical chromosomal alterations (whole-chromosome gains or losses) are generally observed in favorable-risk, spontaneously regressing tumors, such as stage 4S.

In neuroblastoma, ploidy is an important prognostic marker: hyperdiploid neuroblastoma is associated with a favorable outcome, especially in infants, and a good response to chemotherapy. Diploid tumors are frequently linked to *MYCN* amplification and have an aggressive behavior.

Risk-grouping in NB is based on the COG system in the USA, while the INRG system is internationally applied to make risk-based clinical trials comparable in different parts of the world. Both systems combine histology, age, stage, and molecular/cytogenetic features, with identification of different risk categories: low, intermediate, and high risk in COG; very low, low, intermediate, or high risk in the INRG system.

The molecular/cytogenetic analyses required for prognostic stratification of patients include the following:

1. FISH, qPCR, or NGS copy number analysis for the detection of *MYCN* amplification (defined as >4 copies).
2. Array CGH, SNP array, or NGS for 1p/11q loss, 17q gain; especially 11q LOH in MYCN-non-amplified cases.
3. Flow cytometry or genomic profiling to identify hyperdiploidy (near-triploid), which is associated with a better outcome.
4. Targeted NGS (DNA/RNA) to identify targetable ALK mutations and ATRX/TERT alterations.

Hepatoblastoma

Hepatoblastoma is the most common primary malignant liver tumor in childhood, with a minority occurring in children affected by familial adenomatous polyposis or associated with congenital anomalies, such as the Beckwith-Wiedemann syndrome.

Over time, the classification of hepatoblastoma has evolved substantially. Following the initial definition of the fundamental epithelial (fetal, embryonal) and mixed epithelial-mesenchymal categories [70], several morphologic variants with clinical relevance were described. This progressive refinement culminated in the current Pediatric Liver Tumors Consensus Classification, which incorporates epithelial (fetal, embryonal, pleomorphic), mesenchymal, blastemal, and undifferentiated components, as well as specific growth patterns such as the macrotrabecular subtype [71]. A provisional category of hepatocellular malignant neoplasm not otherwise specified (HCN-NOS) has been created to incorporate hepatocellular neoplasms characterized by mixed features of hepatoblastoma and hepatocellular carcinoma or showing an intermediate cytologic appearance between these two entities.

Recent genomic studies have considerably expanded the understanding of hepatoblastoma biology. Hepatoblastoma show a low mutational burden (2.9–3.9 mutations per tumor) among the lowest reported in pediatric and adult cancers. *CTNNB1* mutations occur in up to 89% of cases, indicating constitutive Wnt pathway activation.

HCN-NOS shows frequent additional recurrent alterations including NFE2L2 mutations (~5%), associated with cisplatin resistance, TERT promoter mutations, and alterations at the 11p15.5 locus involving IGF2, including copy-neutral LOH and methylation defects. Mosaic premalignant clonal expansions with 11p15.5 alterations have been described in young children, with associated histologic heterogeneity. Additional variants *include APC*, *KEAP1*, *ARID1A*, *ARID1B*, *MET*, *MAPK1*, *PIK3CA*, *RPS6KA3*, *KMT2C*, *BRCA1*, *BRCA2*, and *CDK12 and* pluripotency-signaling and developmental pathway mutations in *FGFR3*, *FGFR4*, *HRAS*, *NOTCH1*, and *EP300 MDM4*; *SALL4*, *FGF19*, and *CCND1* gains; and *CDKN2A* losses. These molecular alterations also shared with HCC suggest that HCN-NOS might represent hepatoblastomas with HCC-like features.

Transcriptional profiling carried on post-chemotherapy HB initially identified two expression groups, C1 and C2, defined by a 16-gene signature [72]. C1 tumors corresponded largely to well-differentiated fetal histology, whereas C2 tumors were enriched in embryonal or crowded fetal features and showed higher proliferation, MYC target enrichment, and poorer prognosis. A C2B subgroup with epithelial-mesenchymal transition markers, including vimentin, was later described. More recent analyses of chemo-naïve tumors proposed three molecular subtypes—HB1, HB2, HB3—distinguished by differential expression of hepatic progenitor, hepatobiliary, metabolic, and cancer-related pathways including p53 and TERT [73]. These subtypes overlap with C1/C2 subtyping, with C2 aligning to HB2 and C1 to HB1/HB3. Subgroups Epi-CA and Epi-CB, defined by epigenetic analyses, differ in patterns of hypomethylation and CpG island hypermethylation and reflect the molecular subtypes, with Epi-CA being enriched in C1/C2B and Epi-CB in C2 tumors. Overexpression of the DLK1-DIO3 locus (14q23) was also observed. Integration of methylation groups and 14q23 expression yielded three molecular risk categories (MRS-1, MRS-2, MRS-3), associated with distinct 3 year event-free survival rates (91%, 82%, and 52%) [74]. Together, these genomic, transcriptomic, and epigenetic studies highlight key biological factors that may refine risk stratification and guide future treatment protocols. Ongoing efforts, including single-cell RNA sequencing, are expected to further characterize tumor heterogeneity and underlying transcriptional programs [75].

Wilms Tumor (WT)

Wilms tumor is the most frequent malignant tumor of the kidney representing approximately 90% of all pediatric renal malignancies. It is an embryonal tumor, deriving from nephrogenic rests which may be found in 40% and 90% of unilateral and bilateral forms, respectively. Histologically it shows blastemal, stromal, and epithelial components, in variable amounts [76–78]. Evidence of anaplasia indicates a worse prognosis. Anaplasia is defined by the contemporary presence of hyperchromatic nuclei, nuclear enlargement with a nuclear diameter three times larger than the adjacent nonneoplastic cells, and atypical mitoses.

The molecular landscape of Wilms tumor is heterogeneous and involves both genetic mutations and epigenetic dysregulation.

WT1 mutations on chromosome 11p13 are considered an early event and identified in about 10–20% of case, generally associated with stromal histology. *WT1* mutations disrupt normal nephrogenesis and are associated with predisposition syndromes such as WAGR (Wilms tumor, aniridia, genitourinary anomalies, and mental retardation) and Denys-Drash syndrome. Alterations in IGF2 on chromosome 3p22 (~15%) are also an early event, being detected in nephrogenic rests. The constitutional alterations and tumor predisposition syndromes associated to risk of developing Wilms tumor are listed in Table 8.4, according to the risk categories proposed by Scott et al. [79]. Recently identified pathogenic germline variants associated with increased risk of developing Wilms tumors include CTR9 (component of the Polymerase-Associated Factor 1—PAF1 complex), DIS3L2 heterozygous pathogenetic variants (coding for an exoribonuclease), *REST* (RE1-silencing transcription factor), TRIM-28 (Tripartite motif containing 28), and *FBXW7*, *NYNRIN*, and *KDM3B* [80]. Wnt pathway activation is a recurrent oncogenic mechanism in WT.

Activating mutations in *CTNNB1* on chromosome 3p22 encountered in about ~15% of cases are considered a late event, not associated with nephrogenic rests. *CTNNB1*, which encodes β-catenin, and AMER1 (also known as WTX) lead to aberrant stabilization of β-catenin and transcriptional activation of Wnt target genes, promoting proliferation and blocking differentiation [81]. TP53 mutations, typically observed in Wilms tumors with anaplasia, are associated with poor prognosis and chemoresistance [82].

Alterations in 11p15 methylation patterns, as well as chromosomal abnormalities such as 1q gain, 1p loss, and 16q loss, have been shown to serve as biomarkers for poor prognosis [83].

In the current COG studies, loss of heterozygosity at chromosomes 1p and 16q is considered prognostic criteria, together with age, histology, tumor weight, and response to presurgery therapy, and is incorporated in the diagnostic workup. The SIOP studies besides stage, histology, tumor volume, and therapeutic response do not include molecular alterations among the prognostic parameters for further therapeutic stratification.

Recent whole-exome and genome-wide sequencing studies have expanded the spectrum of WT-associated genes. Mutations have been identified in genes involved in microRNA processing, renal developmental transcription factors

Table 8.4 Conditions associated with risk to develop Wilms tumor, according to risk categories proposed by Scott et al.

High risk (>20%)	Moderate risk (5–20%)	Low risk < 5%
WT1 deletions (WAGR syndrome)	WT1 intron 9 splice mutations (Frasier syndrome)	LFS,
Truncating and missense mutations (Denys-Drash), familial Wilms	Beckwith-Wiedemann syndrome caused by 11p15 uniparental disomy	Hereditary hyperparathyroidism jaw tumor syndrome,
Perlman syndrome	Isolated H19 hypermethylation	Mulibrey nanism
Mosaic variegated aneuploidy	Simpson-Golabi-Behmel syndrome (*GPC3* mutations)	Trisomy 18
Fanconi anemia		Trisomy 13
Biallelic BRCA2 mutations carry greater than 20% risk of developing Wilms tumor		2q37 deletions

(SIX1, SIX2), and oncogenes such as MYCN. Disruptions of chromatin remodeling and histone modification machinery are also recurrent, including BCOR, BCORL1, MAP3K4, BRD7, CREBBP, HDAC4, SMARCA4, and ARID1A, affecting transcriptional regulation, differentiation, and epigenetic control. These findings highlight the convergence of developmental, epigenetic, and oncogenic pathways in WT pathogenesis [84].

Cancer-Predisposing Germline Variants in Pediatric Malignancies

The identification of hereditary predisposition variants in pediatric has been challenging, as the rarity of these tumors, combined with reduced reproductive fitness in affected individuals, limited the feasibility of familial aggregation studies. A number of genes responsible for TPS are detectable by tumor-specific sequencing panels; thus, the percentage of malignancies associated to a TPS is increasing with the extensive use of molecular characterization of tumors, and current estimates suggest that up to 17% of children with cancer may carry a germline pathogenic variant associated with increased tumor risk [85–87].

Some tumor types are associated with a specific TPS or show peculiar features leading the pathologist to suspect an underlying TPS. Occasionally a neoplastic lesion occurring in a child may represent the sentinel event for the family and lead to extend the surveillance to the whole family.

The detailed analysis of the TPS in pediatric age is out of the scope of this section.

Classic TPS associated with insurgence of malignancies in pediatric age include Li-Fraumeni syndrome (*TP53* gene), hereditary retinoblastoma syndrome (*RB1* gene), Beckwith-Wiedemann syndrome (alteration of 11p15.5; *CDKN1C* mutation), RASopathies such as Costello syndrome (*HRAS* p.G12V/S), and neurofibromatosis type 1 (*NF1*).

Several studies have described germline mutations, which have been generally associated with malignancies in adult, in pediatric tumors, especially those arising in CNS. Examples are MLH1, MSH2, MSH6, and PMS2 genes associated with constitutional mismatch repair deficiency, predisposing individuals to Wilms tumor, osteosarcoma, and rhabdomyosarcoma [87]. Ewing sarcoma has been recently associated with germline pathogenic variants in genes involved in DNA damage repair, such as *FANCC*, *CHEK2*, *BRCA1*, and *BRCA2*.

DICER syndrome is caused by pathogenic germline DICER1 mutations and is associated with a hereditary tumor predisposition syndrome characterized by a broad spectrum of benign and malignant neoplasms. DICER1 encodes a member of the ribonuclease III (RNaseIII) family required for microRNA (miRNA) processing and is often associated with CNS sarcomas. DICER1-associated mesenchymal tumors encompass multiple well-established clinicopathological tumor entities and can be further divided into three clinically meaningful classes designated "low-grade mesenchymal tumor with DICER1 alteration" (LGMT DICER1), "sarcoma with DICER1 alteration" (SARC DICER1), and primary intracranial sarcoma with DICER1 alteration (PIS DICER1).

Given these associations, genetic counseling and targeted germline testing should be strongly considered for patients with a suggestive personal or family history.

Conclusions

Over the past two decades, the molecular landscape of pediatric malignancies has been mapped with increasing precision. Advances in next-generation sequencing, transcriptomic profiling, and epigenetic characterization have deepened our understanding of tumorigenic mechanisms and uncovered multiple targetable alterations and pathways. At the same time, the contribution of tumor predisposition syndromes to childhood cancers—historically underestimated—has become clearer, with several syndromes previously linked primarily to adult-onset cancers now recognized as relevant to pediatric tumorigenesis.

Molecular stratification for both therapeutic decision-making and prognostic assessment has already entered routine clinical practice, particularly within large international trials for embryonal tumors such as neuroblastoma. Furthermore, specific molecular markers diagnostic of defined histotypes—such as ***FOXO1*** rearrangements in rhabdomyosarcoma—are beginning to complement or even supersede traditional morphology in risk classification.

Ongoing large-scale genomic, epigenomic, and integrated multi-omic studies are poised to reshape the diagnostic framework for these rare tumors, ultimately accelerating the adoption of precision medicine and enabling more individualized, biology-driven care for children with cancer.

References

1. Sansbury BM, Blackman E, Primm KM, Zaidi SK, Sengupta R. AACR Cancer Progress Report 2025: unifying cancer science and medicine: a continuum of innovation for impact. Clin Cancer Res Off J Amer Assoc Cancer Res. 2025;31(20):4239–43. https://doi.org/10.1158/1078-0432.CCR-25-3366.
2. Willis RA. The borderland of embryology and pathology. Bull N Y Acad Med. 1950;26(7):440–60.
3. Research, A. A. f. C. "AACR Pediatric Cancer Progress Report 2025: Contents." from https://cancerprogressreport.aacr.org/pediatric/pcpr25-contents/ (2025).
4. Alaggio R, Hill DA, TS J, Jarzembowski JA, López-Terrada DH, Pfister SM, et al. WHO classification of tumors: pediatric tumors. Lyon, France; 2021.
5. Loeb DM, Thornton K, Shokek O. Pediatric soft tissue sarcomas. Surg Clin N Am. 2008;88(3):615–27.
6. Ferrari A, Miceli R, Rey A, Oberlin O, Orbach D, Brennan B, Mariani L, Carli M, Bisogno G, Cecchetto G, Salvo GLD, Casanova M, Vannoesel MM, Kelsey A, Stevens MC, Devidas M, Pappo AS, Spunt SL. Non-metastatic unresected paediatric non-rhabdomyosarcoma soft tissue sarcomas: results of a pooled analysis from United States and European groups. Eur J Cancer. 2011;47(5):724–31.
7. Davicioni E, Anderson MJ, Finckenstein FG, Lynch JC, Qualman SJ, Shimada H, Schofield DE, Buckley JD, Meyer WH, Sorensen PH, Triche TJ. Molecular classification of rhabdomyosarcoma–genotypic and phenotypic determinants of diagnosis: a report from the Children's Oncology Group. Am J Pathol. 2009;174(2):550–64.
8. Shern JF, Selfe J, Izquierdo E, Patidar R, Chou HC, Song YK, Yohe ME, Sindiri S, Wei J, Wen X, Rudzinski ER, Barkauskas DA, Lo T, Hall D, Linardic CM, Hughes D, Jamal S, Jenney M, Chisholm J, Brown R, Jones K, Hicks B, Angelini P, George S, Chesler L, Hubank M, Kelsey A, Gatz SA, Skapek SX, Hawkins DS, Shipley JM, Khan J. Genomic classification and clinical outcome in rhabdomyosarcoma: a report from an international consortium. J Clin Oncol. 2021;39(26):2859–71.
9. Williamson D, Lu YJ, Gordon T, Sciot R, Kelsey A, Fisher C, Poremba C, Anderson J, Pritchard-Jones K, Shipley J. Relationship between MYCN copy number and expression in rhabdomyosarcomas and correlation with adverse prognosis in the alveolar subtype. J Clin Oncol. 2005;23(4):880–8.
10. Skapek SX, Ferrari A, Gupta AA, Lupo PJ, Butler E, Shipley J, Barr FG, Hawkins DS. Rhabdomyosarcoma. Nat Rev Dis Primers. 2019;5(1):1.
11. Shern JF, Chen L, Chmielecki J, Wei JS, Patidar R, Rosenberg M, Ambrogio L, Auclair D, Wang J, Song YK, Tolman C, Hurd L, Liao H, Zhang S, Bogen D, Brohl AS, Sindiri S, Catchpoole D, Badgett T, Getz G, Mora J, Anderson JR, Skapek SX, Barr FG, Meyerson M, Hawkins DS, Khan J. Comprehensive genomic analysis of rhabdomyosarcoma reveals a landscape of alterations affecting a common genetic axis in fusion-positive and fusion-negative tumors. Cancer Discov. 2014;4(2):216–31.
12. de Traux De Wardin H, Cyrta J, Dermawan JK, Guillemot D, Orbach D, Aerts I, Pierron G, Antonescu CR. FGFR1 fusions as a novel molecular driver in rhabdomyosarcoma. Genes Chromosomes Cancer. 2024;63(4):e23232.
13. Di Carlo D, Chisholm J, Kelsey A, Alaggio R, Bisogno G, Minard-Colin V, Jenney M, Dávila Fajardo R, Merks JHM, Shipley JM, Selfe JL. Biological role and clinical implications of MYOD1(L122R) mutation in rhabdomyosarcoma. Cancers (Basel). 2023;15(6):1644.
14. Agaram NP, Chen CL, Zhang L, LaQuaglia MP, Wexler L, Antonescu CR. Recurrent MYOD1 mutations in pediatric and adult sclerosing and spindle cell rhabdomyosarcomas: evidence for a common pathogenesis. Genes Chromosomes Cancer. 2014;53(9):779–87.
15. Agaram NP, LaQuaglia MP, Alaggio R, Zhang L, Fujisawa Y, Ladanyi M, Wexler LH, Antonescu CR. MYOD1-mutant spindle cell and sclerosing rhabdomyosarcoma: an aggressive subtype irrespective of age. A reappraisal for molecular classification and risk stratification. Mod Pathol. 2019a;32(1):27–36.
16. Alaggio R, Zhang L, Sung YS, Huang SC, Chen CL, Bisogno G, Zin A, Agaram NP, LaQuaglia MP, Wexler LH, Antonescu CR. A molecular study of pediatric spindle and Sclerosing rhabdomyosarcoma: identification of novel and recurrent VGLL2-related fusions in infantile cases. Am J Surg Pathol. 2016a;40(2):224–35.
17. Le Loarer F, Cleven AHG, Bouvier C, Castex MP, Romagosa C, Moreau A, Salas S, Bonhomme B, Gomez-Brouchet A, Laurent C, Le Guellec S, Audard V, Giraud A, Ramos-Oliver I, Cleton-Jansen AM, Savci-Heijink DC, Kroon HM, Baud J, Pissaloux D, Pierron G, Sherwood A,

Coindre JM, Bovée J, Larousserie F, Tirode F. A subset of epithelioid and spindle cell rhabdomyosarcomas is associated with TFCP2 fusions and common ALK upregulation. Mod Pathol. 2020;33(3):404–19.
18. Agaram NP, Zhang L, Sung YS, Cavalcanti MS, Torrence D, Wexler L, Francis G, Sommerville S, Swanson D, Dickson BC, Suurmeijer AJH, Williamson R, Antonescu CR. Expanding the Spectrum of intraosseous rhabdomyosarcoma: correlation between 2 distinct gene fusions and phenotype. Am J Surg Pathol. 2019b;43(5):695–702. https://doi.org/10.1097/PAS.0000000000001227. PMID: 30720533; PMCID: PMC6613942
19. Dashti NK, Wehrs RN, Thomas BC, Nair A, Davila J, Buckner JC, Martinez AP, Sukov WR, Halling KC, Howe BM, Folpe AL. Spindle cell rhabdomyosarcoma of bone with FUS-TFCP2 fusion: confirmation of a very recently described rhabdomyosarcoma subtype. Histopathology. 2018;73(3):514–20. https://doi.org/10.1111/his.13649. Epub 2018 Jun 29. PMID: 29758589
20. Duan FL, Yang H, Gong X, Zuo Z, Qin S, Ji J, Zhou C, Dai J, Guo P, Liu Y. Clinicopathological features of rhabdomyosarcoma with novel FET::TFCP2 and TIMP3::ALK fusion: report of two cases and literature review. Histopathology. 2023;82(3):478–84. https://doi.org/10.1111/his.14833.
21. Smith BF, Doung YC, Beckett B, Corless CL, Davis LE, Davis JL. Intraosseous spindle cell Rhabdomyosarcoma with MEIS1::NCOA2 fusion – case report with substantial clinical follow-up and review of the literature. Cancer Invest. 2023;41(8):704–12. https://doi.org/10.1080/07357907.2023.2255668. Epub 2023 Sep 6. Erratum in: 2023 Sep;41(8):750. https://doi:10.1080/07357907.2023.2259655
22. Xu B, Suurmeijer AJH, Agaram NP, Zhang L, Antonescu CR. Head and neck rhabdomyosarcoma with TFCP2 fusions and ALK overexpression: a clinicopathological and molecular analysis of 11 cases. Histopathology. 2021;79(3):347–57. https://doi.org/10.1111/his.14323. Epub 2021 May 19. PMID: 33382123; PMCID: PMC8243398
23. Han R, Dermawan JK, Demicco EG, Ferguson PC, Griffin AM, Swanson D, Antonescu CR, Dickson BC. ZFP64::NCOA3 gene fusion defines a novel subset of spindle cell rhabdomyosarcoma. Genes Chromosomes Cancer. 2022;61(11):645–52. https://doi.org/10.1002/gcc.23052. Epub 2022 May 20. PMID: 35521817; PMCID: PMC9811222
24. Dehner CA, Ameline B, Amary F, Gross JM, Zou Y, Michal M, Kinkor Z, Torres-Mora J, Malik F, Kao EY, Ricciotti RW, Din NU, John I, Dickson BC, Demicco EG, Agaimy A, Linos K, Hameed MR, Folpe AL, Baumhoer D. Clinicopathologic and molecular genetic features of spindle cell rhabdomyosarcoma harboring ZFP64::NCOA2/3 fusions: a series of 14 cases. Mod Pathol. 2025b;38(12):100906. https://doi.org/10.1016/j.modpat.2025.100906. Epub ahead of print
25. Agaimy A, Dermawan JK, Leong I, Stoehr R, Swanson D, Weinreb I, Zhang L, Antonescu CR, Dickson BC. Recurrent VGLL3 fusions define a distinctive subset of spindle cell rhabdomyosarcoma with an indolent clinical course and striking predilection for the head and neck. Genes Chromosomes Cancer. 2022;61(12):701–9. https://doi.org/10.1002/gcc.23083. Epub 2022 Aug 1. PMID: 35766997; PMCID: PMC10243299
26. Yoshida KI, Kukita Y, Nakamura H, et al. A case of spindle cell rhabdomyosarcoma with an EP300::VGLL3 fusion. Genes Chromosomes Cancer. 2023 Mar;62(3):184–6.
27. Fung CK, Chow C, Chan WK, Choi EWK, To KF, Chan JKC, Cheuk W. Spindle cell/sclerosing rhabdomyosarcoma with DCTN1::ALK fusion: broadening the molecular spectrum with potential therapeutic implications. Virchows Arch. 2022;480(4):927–32. https://doi.org/10.1007/s00428-022-03305-8. Epub 2022 Mar 1
28. Kao YC, Bennett JA, Suurmeijer AJH, Dickson BC, Swanson D, Wanjari P, Zhang L, Lee JC, Antonescu CR. Recurrent MEIS1-NCOA2/1 fusions in a subset of low-grade spindle cell sarcomas frequently involving the genitourinary and gynecologic tracts. Mod Pathol. 2021;34(6):1203–12. https://doi.org/10.1038/s41379-021-00744-7. Epub 2021 Feb 11. PMID: 33574497; PMCID: PMC8207504
29. Dehner CA, Broski SM, Meis JM, Murugan P, Chrisinger JSA, Sosa C, Petersen M, Halling KC, Gupta S, Folpe AL. Fusion-driven spindle cell rhabdomyosarcomas of bone and soft tissue: a clinicopathologic and molecular genetic study of 25 cases. Mod Pathol. 2023;36(10):100271. https://doi.org/10.1016/j.modpat.2023.100271. Epub 2023 Jul 7
30. Bradová M, Mosaieby E, Michal M, Vaněček T, Ing SK, Grossmann P, Koshyk O, Kinkor Z, Laciok Š, Nemcová A, Straka Ľ, Farkas M, Michal M, Švajdler M. Spindle cell rhabdomyosarcomas: with TFCP2 rearrangements, and novel EWSR1::ZBTB41 and PLOD2::RBM6 gene fusions. A study of five cases and review of the literature. Histopathology. 2024;84(5):776–93. https://doi.org/10.1111/his.15121. Epub 2023 Dec 19. PMID: 38114270
31. Karanian M, Pissaloux D, Gomez-Brouchet A, Chevenet C, Le Loarer F, Fernandez C, Minard V, Corradini N, Castex MP, Duc-Gallet A, Blay JY, Tirode F. SRF-FOXO1 and SRF-NCOA1 fusion genes delineate a distinctive subset of well-differentiated rhabdomyosarcoma. Am J Surg Pathol. 2020;44(5):607–16. https://doi.org/10.1097/PAS.0000000000001464. PMID: 32187044
32. Mosquera JM, Sboner A, Zhang L, Kitabayashi N, Chen CL, Sung YS, Wexler LH, LaQuaglia MP, Edelman M, Sreekantaiah C, Rubin MA, Antonescu CR. Recurrent NCOA2 gene rearrangements in congenital/infantile spindle cell rhabdomyosarcoma.

Genes Chromosomes Cancer. 2013;52(6):538–50. https://doi.org/10.1002/gcc.22050. Epub 2013 Mar 5. PMID: 23463663; PMCID: PMC3734530
33. Tan GZL, Saminathan SN, Chang KTE, Odoño EG, Kuick CH, Chen H, Lee VKM. A rare case of congenital spindle cell rhabdomyosarcoma with TEAD1-NCOA2 fusion: a subset of spindle cell rhabdomyosarcoma with indolent behavior. Pathol Int. 2020;70(4):234–6. https://doi.org/10.1111/pin.12908. Epub 2020 Jan 30. PMID: 31999033
34. Alaggio R, Zhang L, Sung YS, Huang SC, Chen CL, Bisogno G, Zin A, Agaram NP, LaQuaglia MP, Wexler LH, Antonescu CR. A molecular study of pediatric spindle and Sclerosing rhabdomyosarcoma: identification of novel and recurrent VGLL2-related fusions in infantile cases. Am J Surg Pathol. 2016b;40(2):224–35. https://doi.org/10.1097/PAS.0000000000000538. PMID: 26501226; PMCID: PMC4712098
35. Saoud C, Gundem G, Domenico D, Arango-Ossa JE, Reed D, Vaynrub M, Papaemmanouil E, Bale TA, Linos K. Rhabdomyosarcoma with EWSR1::NF2 gene fusion: a case report potentially expanding its genetic Spectrum. Genes Chromosomes Cancer. 2025;64(1):e70025. https://doi.org/10.1002/gcc.70025. PMID: 39873201; PMCID: PMC12558371
36. Delattre O, Zucman J, Melot T, Garau XS, Zucker JM, Lenoir GM, Ambros PF, Sheer D, Turc-Carel C, Triche TJ. The Ewing family of tumorsDOUBLE-HYPHENa subgroup of small-round-cell tumors defined by specific chimeric transcripts. N Engl J Med. 1994;331(5):294–9. https://doi.org/10.1056/NEJM199408043310503.
37. Oikawa T, Yamada T. Molecular biology of the Ets family of transcription factors. Gene. 2003 Jan;16(303):11–34. https://doi.org/10.1016/s0378-1119(02)01156-3.
38. Chougule A, Taylor MS, Nardi V, Chebib I, Cote GM, Choy E, Nielsen GP, Deshpande V. Spindle and round cell sarcoma with EWSR1-PATZ1 gene fusion: a sarcoma with polyphenotypic differentiation. Am J Surg Pathol. 2019;43(2):220–8. https://doi.org/10.1097/PAS.0000000000001183.
39. Diaz-Perez JA, Nielsen GP, Antonescu C, Taylor MS, Lozano-Calderon SA, Rosenberg AE. EWSR1/FUS-NFATc2 rearranged round cell sarcoma: clinicopathological series of 4 cases and literature review. Hum Pathol. 2019;90:45–53. https://doi.org/10.1016/j.humpath.2019.05.001.
40. Koelsche C, Kriegsmann M, Kommoss FKF, Stichel D, Kriegsmann K, Vokuhl C, Grünewald TGP, Romero-Pérez L, Kirchner T, de Alava E, Diaz-Martin J, Hartmann W, Baumhoer D, Antonescu CR, Szuhai K, Flucke U, Dirksen U, Pfister SM, Jones DTW, Mechtersheimer G, von Deimling A. DNA methylation profiling distinguishes Ewing-like sarcoma with EWSR1-NFATc2 fusion from Ewing sarcoma. J Cancer Res Clin Oncol. 2019;145(5):1273–81. https://doi.org/10.1007/s00432-019-02895-2.
41. Brcic I, Scheipl S, Bergovec M, Leithner A, Szkandera J, Sotlar K, Suda AJ, Smolle MA, Kraus T, Rosenberg AE, Liegl-Atzwanger B, Igrec J. Implementation of copy number variations-based diagnostics in morphologically challenging EWSR1/FUS::NFATC2 neoplasms of the bone and soft tissue. Int J Mol Sci. 2022;23(24):16196.
42. Liu L, Li L, Ding Y, Kong F, Mo W, Ye H, Shen D. Report and literature review of four cases of EWSR1::NFATC2 round cell sarcoma. Diagn Pathol. 2024;19(1):19.
43. Machado I, Llombart-Bosch A, Charville GW, Navarro S, Domínguez Franjo MP, Bridge JA, Linos K. Sarcomas with EWSR1::Non-ETS Fusion (EWSR1::NFATC2 and EWSR1::PATZ1). Surg Pathol Clin. 2024;17(1):31–55. https://doi.org/10.1016/j.path.2023.07.001. Epub 2023 Aug 7. PMID: 38278606; PMCID: PMC12439224
44. Dehner CA, Warmke LM, Umphress B, Malik F, Cloutier JM, Dermawan JK, Fritz M, Que SKT, Ameline B, Fritchie KJ, Kerr DA, Linos K, Baumhoer D, Billings SD, Folpe AL. Superficial Neurocristic FET::ETS fusion tumor: expanding the clinicopathological and molecular genetic spectrum of a recently described entity. Mod Pathol. 2025a;38(2):100656. https://doi.org/10.1016/j.modpat.2024.100656.
45. Folpe AL, Tetzlaff MT, Billings SD, Torres-Mora J, Borowsky AD, Santiago TC, Ameline B, Baumhoer D. Superficial neurocristic EWSR1::FLI1 fusion tumor: a distinctive, clinically indolent, S100 protein/SOX10-positive neoplasm. Mod Pathol. 2024;37(8):100537. https://doi.org/10.1016/j.modpat.2024.100537.
46. Schaefer IM, Dal Cin P, Landry LM, Fletcher CDM, Hanna GJ, French CA. CIC-NUTM1 fusion: a case which expands the spectrum of NUT-rearranged epithelioid malignancies. Genes Chromosomes Cancer. 2018;57(9):446–51. https://doi.org/10.1002/gcc.3.
47. Sugita S, Arai Y, Tonooka A, Hama N, Totoki Y, Fujii T, Aoyama T, Asanuma H, Tsukahara T, Kaya M, Shibata T, Hasegawa T. A novel CIC-FOXO4 gene fusion in undifferentiated small round cell sarcoma: a genetically distinct variant of Ewing-like sarcoma. Am J Surg Pathol. 2014;38(11):1571–6. https://doi.org/10.1097/PAS.0000000000000286.
48. Salgado CM, Alaggio R, Ciolfi A, Zin A, Diomedi Camassei F, Pedace L, Milano GM, Serra A, Di Giannatale A, Mastronuzzi A, Gianatti A, Bisogno G, Ferrari A, Tartaglia M, Reyes-Múgica M, Locatelli F, Miele E. Pediatric BCOR-altered tumors from soft tissue/kidney display specific DNA methylation profiles. Mod Pathol. 2023;36(2):100039. https://doi.org/10.1016/j.modpat.2022.100039.
49. Palmerini E, Gambarotti M, Italiano A, Nathenson MJ, Ratan R, Dileo P, Provenzano S, Jones RL, DuBois SG, Martin-Broto J, de Alava E, Baldi GG, Grignani G, Ferraresi V, Brunello A, Paoluzzi L,

Bertulli R, Hindi N, Montemurro M, Rothermundt C, Vincenzi B. A global collaboRAtive study of CIC-rearranged, BCOR::CCNB3-rearranged and other ultra-rare unclassified undifferentiated small round cell sarcomas (GRACefUl). Eur J Cancer. (Oxford, England: 1990. 2023;183:11–23. https://doi.org/10.1016/j.ejca.2023.01.003.
50. Howlader N, Noone AM, Krapcho M, et al., editors. SEER cancer statistics review, 1975–2016. Bethesda, MD: National Cancer Institute; 2021. Based on November 2018 SEER data submission, posted to the SEER website, April 2019. Updated Apr 2020; Accessed Aug 2020
51. Davis JL, Vargas SO, Rudzinski ER, López Marti JM, Janeway K, Forrest S, Winsnes K, Pinto N, Yang SE, VanSandt M, Boyd TK, Corless CL, Liu YJ, Surrey LF, Harris MH, Church A, Al-Ibraheemi A. Recurrent RET gene fusions in paediatric spindle mesenchymal neoplasms. Histopathology. 2020;76(7):1032–41.
52. Tan SY, Al-Ibraheemi A, Ahrens WA, Oesterheld JE, Fanburg-Smith JC, Liu YJ, Spunt SL, Rudzinski ER, Coffin C, Davis JL. ALK rearrangements in infantile fibrosarcoma-like spindle cell tumours of soft tissue and kidney. Histopathology. 2022;80(4):698–707.
53. Motta M, Barresi S, Pizzi S, Bifano D, Lopez Marti J, Garrido-Pontnou M, Flex E, Bruselles A, Giovannoni I, Rotundo G, Fragale A, Tirelli V, Vallese S, Ciolfi A, Bisogno G, Alaggio R, Tartaglia M. RAF1 gene fusions are recurrent driver events in infantile fibrosarcoma-like mesenchymal tumors. J Pathol. 2024;263(2):166–77.
54. Wegert J, Vokuhl C, Collord G, Del Castillo Velasco-Herrera M, Farndon SJ, Guzzo C, Jorgensen M, Anderson J, Slater O, Duncan C, Bausenwein S, Streitenberger H, Ziegler B, Furtwängler R, Graf N, Stratton MR, Campbell PJ, Jones DT, Koelsche C, Pfister SM, Mifsud W, Sebire N, Sparber-Sauer M, Koscielniak E, Rosenwald A, Gessler M, Behjati S. Recurrent intragenic rearrangements of EGFR and BRAF in soft tissue tumors of infants. Nat Commun. 2018;9(1):2378.
55. Lopez-Nunez O, John I, Panasiti RN, Ranganathan S, Santoro L, Grélaud D, Wu T, Buccoliero AM, Casanova M, Alaggio R, Surrey LF. Infantile inflammatory myofibroblastic tumors: clinicopathological and molecular characterization of 12 cases. Mod Pathol. 2020;33(4):576–90.
56. Antonescu CR, Suurmeijer AJ, Zhang L, Sung YS, Jungbluth AA, Travis WD, Al-Ahmadie H, Fletcher CD, Alaggio R. Molecular characterization of inflammatory myofibroblastic tumors with frequent ALK and ROS1 gene fusions and rare novel RET rearrangement. Am J Surg Pathol. 2015;39(7):957–67. https://doi.org/10.1097/PAS.0000000000000404.
57. Cook JR, Dehner LP, Collins MH, Ma Z, Morris SW, Coffin CM, Hill DA. Anaplastic lymphoma kinase (ALK) expression in the inflammatory myofibroblastic tumor: a comparative immunohistochemical study. Am J Surg Pathol. 2001;25(11):1364–71. https://doi.org/10.1097/00000478-200111000-00003.
58. Mariño-Enríquez A, Wang WL, Roy A, Lopez-Terrada D, Lazar AJ, Fletcher CD, Coffin CM, Hornick JL. Epithelioid inflammatory myofibroblastic sarcoma: an aggressive intra-abdominal variant of inflammatory myofibroblastic tumor with nuclear membrane or perinuclear ALK. Am J Surg Pathol. 2011;35(1):135–44. https://doi.org/10.1097/PAS.0b013e318200cfd5.
59. Chen ST, Lee JC. An inflammatory myofibroblastic tumor in liver with ALK and RANBP2 gene rearrangement: combination of distinct morphologic, immunohistochemical, and genetic features. Hum Pathol. 2008;39(12):1854–8. https://doi.org/10.1016/j.humpath.2008.04.016.
60. Lee JC, Li CF, Huang HY, Zhu MJ, Mariño-Enríquez A, Lee CT, Ou WB, Hornick JL, Fletcher JA. ALK oncoproteins in atypical inflammatory myofibroblastic tumours: novel RRBP1-ALK fusions in epithelioid inflammatory myofibroblastic sarcoma. J Pathol. 2017;241(3):316–23. https://doi.org/10.1002/path.4836.
61. Davis JL, Lockwood CM, Stohr B, Boecking C, Al-Ibraheemi A, DuBois SG, Vargas SO, Black JO, Cox MC, Luquette M, Turpin B, Szabo S, Laetsch TW, Albert CM, Parham DM, Hawkins DS, Rudzinski ER. Expanding the spectrum of pediatric NTRK-rearranged mesenchymal tumors. Am J Surg Pathol. 2019;43(4):435–45.
62. Suurmeijer AJH, Dickson BC, Swanson D, Zhang L, Sung YS, Cotzia P, Fletcher CDM, Antonescu CR. A novel group of spindle cell tumors defined by S100 and CD34 co-expression shows recurrent fusions involving RAF1, BRAF, and NTRK1/2 genes. Genes Chromosom Cancer. 2018;57(12):611–21.
63. Agrawal S, Ameline B, Folpe AL, Azzato E, Astbury C, Mentzel T, Knapp C, Rütten A, Creytens D, Sukov W, Baumhoer D, Billings SD, Fritchie KJ. ALK-rearranged, CD34-positive spindle cell neoplasms resembling dermatofibrosarcoma protuberans: a study of seven cases. Histopathology. 2024;85(4):649–59.
64. Gestrich CK, Davis JL, Biederman L, John I, Alaggio R, Giovannoni I, Arnold MA, Shenoy A, Tchakarov A, Al-Ibraheemi A. ALK-rearranged epithelioid mesenchymal neoplasm: expanding the spectrum of tyrosine kinase-altered mesenchymal tumors. Mod Pathol. 2023;36(12):100334.
65. Ritenour LE, Randall MP, Bosse KR, Diskin SJ. Genetic susceptibility to neuroblastoma: current knowledge and future directions. Cell Tissue Res. 2018;372(2):287–307.
66. Carpenter EL, Mossé YP. Targeting ALK in neuroblastomaDOUBLEHYPHENpreclinical and clinical advancements. Nat Rev Clin Oncol. 2012;9(7):391–9.
67. Maris JM. Recent advances in neuroblastoma. N Engl J Med. 2010;362(23):2202–11.

68. Hennchen M, Stubbusch J, Abarchan-El Makhfi I, Kramer M, Deller T, Pierre-Eugene C, Janoueix-Lerosey I, Delattre O, Ernsberger U, Schulte JB, Rohrer H. Lin28B and Let-7 in the control of sympathetic neurogenesis and neuroblastoma development. J Neurosci. 2015;35(50):16531–44.
69. Matthay KK, Maris JM, Schleiermacher G, Nakagawara A, Mackall CL, Diller L, Weiss WA. Neuroblastoma. Nat Rev Dis Primers. 2016;2:16078.
70. Ishak KG, Glunz PR. Hepatoblastoma and hepatocarcinoma in infancy and childhood. Report of 47 cases. Cancer. 1967;20(3):396–422.
71. López-Terrada D, Alaggio R, de Dávila MT, Czauderna P, Hiyama E, Katzenstein H, Leuschner I, Malogolowkin M, Meyers R, Ranganathan S, Tanaka Y, Tomlinson G, Fabrè M, Zimmermann A, Finegold MJ. Towards an international pediatric liver tumor consensus classification: proceedings of the Los Angeles COG liver tumors symposium. Mod Pathol. 2014;27(3):472–91.
72. Cairo S, Armengol C, De Reyniès A, Wei Y, Thomas E, Renard CA, Goga A, Balakrishnan A, Semeraro M, Gresh L, Pontoglio M, Strick-Marchand H, Levillayer F, Nouet Y, Rickman D, Gauthier F, Branchereau S, Brugières L, Laithier V, Bouvier R, Boman F, Basso G, Michiels JF, Hofman P, Arbez-Gindre F, Jouan H, Rousselet-Chapeau MC, Berrebi D, Marcellin L, Plenat F, Zachar D, Joubert M, Selves J, Pasquier D, Bioulac-Sage P, Grotzer M, Childs M, Fabre M, Buendia MA. Hepatic stem-like phenotype and interplay of Wnt/beta-catenin and Myc signaling in aggressive childhood liver cancer. Cancer Cell. 2008;14(6):471–84.
73. Sumazin P, Chen Y, Treviño LR, Sarabia SF, Hampton OA, Patel K, Mistretta TA, Zorman B, Thompson P, Heczey A, Comerford S, Wheeler DA, Chintagumpala M, Meyers R, Rakheja D, Finegold MJ, Tomlinson G, Parsons DW, López-Terrada D. Genomic analysis of hepatoblastoma identifies distinct molecular and prognostic subgroups. Hepatology. 2017;65(1):104–21.
74. Carrillo-Reixach J, Torrens L, Simon-Coma M, Royo L, Domingo-Sàbat M, Abril-Fornaguera J, Akers N, Sala M, Ragull S, Arnal M, Villalmanzo N, Cairo S, Villanueva A, Kappler R, Garrido M, Guerra L, Sábado C, Guillén G, Mallo M, Piñeyro D, Vázquez-Vitali M, Kuchuk O, Mateos ME, Ramírez G, Santamaría ML, Mozo Y, Soriano A, Grotzer M, Branchereau S, de Andoin NG, López-Ibor B, López-Almaraz R, Salinas JA, Torres B, Hernández F, Uriz JJ, Fabre M, Blanco J, Paris C, Bajčiová V, Laureys G, Masnou H, Clos A, Belendez C, Guettier C, Sumoy L, Planas R, Jordà M, Nonell L, Czauderna P, Morland B, Sia D, Losic B, Buendia MA, Sarrias MR, Llovet JM, Armengol C. Epigenetic footprint enables molecular risk stratification of hepatoblastoma with clinical implications. J Hepatol. 2020;73(2):328–41.
75. Bondoc A, Glaser K, Jin K, Lake C, Cairo S, Geller J, Tiao G, Aronow B. Identification of distinct tumor cell populations and key genetic mechanisms through single cell sequencing in hepatoblastoma. Commun Biol. 2021;4(1):1049.
76. Beckwith JB. Nephrogenic rests and the pathogenesis of Wilms tumor: developmental and clinical considerations. Am J Med Genet. 1998;79(4):268–73.
77. Reddy R. Multifocal unilateral Wilms' tumor: Radiopathological correlation. J Microsc Ultrastr. 2022;11(3):190–2.
78. Vujanić GM, Apps JR, Moroz V, Ceroni F, Williams RD, Sebire NJ, Pritchard-Jones K. Nephrogenic rests in Wilms tumors treated with preoperative chemotherapy: the UK SIOP Wilms tumor 2001 trial experience. Pediatr Blood Cancer. 2017;64(11):e26547.
79. Scott RH, Walker L, Olsen Ø E, Levitt G, Kenney I, Maher E, Owens CM, Pritchard-Jones K, Craft A, Rahman N. Surveillance for Wilms tumour in at-risk children: pragmatic recommendations for best practice. Arch Dis Child. 2006;91(12):995–9.
80. Brzezinski JJ, Becktell KD, Bougeard G, Brodeur GM, Diller LR, Doria AS, Hansford JR, Kohlmann WK, Kratz CP, MacFarland SP, Pajtler KW, Rednam SP, Schienda J, States LJ, Villani A, Weksberg R, Zelley K, Tomlinson GE, Kalish JM. Update on surveillance guidelines in emerging Wilms tumor predisposition syndromes. Clin Cancer Res. 2025;31(1):18–24.
81. Ruteshouser EC, Robinson SM, Huff V. Wilms tumor genetics: mutations in WT1, WTX, and CTNNB1 account for only about one-third of tumors. Genes Chromosomes Cancer. 2008;47(6):461–70.
82. Maschietto M, Williams RD, Chagtai T, Popov SD, Sebire NJ, Vujanic G, Perlman E, Anderson JR, Grundy P, Dome JS, Pritchard-Jones K. TP53 mutational status is a potential marker for risk stratification in Wilms tumour with diffuse anaplasia. PLoS One. 2014;9(10):e109924.
83. Phelps HM, Kaviany S, Borinstein SC, Lovvorn HN 3rd. Biological drivers of Wilms tumor prognosis and treatment. Children (Basel). 2018;5(11):145.
84. Gadd S, Huff V, Walz AL, Ooms A, Armstrong AE, Gerhard DS, Smith MA, Guidry Auvil JM, Meerzaman D, Chen QR, Hsu CH, Yan C, Nguyen C, Hu Y, Hermida LC, Davidsen T, Gesuwan P, Ma Y, Zong Z, Mungall AJ, Moore RA, Marra MA, Dome JS, Mullighan CG, Ma J, Wheeler DA, Hampton OA, Ross N, Gastier-Foster JM, Arold ST, Perlman EJ. A children's oncology group and TARGET initiative exploring the genetic landscape of Wilms tumor. Nat Genet. 2017;49(10):1487–94.
85. Fiala EM, Jayakumaran G, Mauguen A, Kennedy JA, Bouvier N, Kemel Y, Fleischut MH, Maio A, Salo-Mullen EE, Sheehan M, Arnold AG, Latham A, Carlo MI, Cadoo K, Murkherjee S, Slotkin EK, Trippett T, Glade Bender J, Meyers PA, Wexler L, Dela Cruz FS, Cheung N-K, Basu E, Kentsis A, Ortiz M, Francis JH, Dunkel IJ, Khakoo Y, Gilheeney S, Farouk Sait S, Forlenza CJ, Sulis M, Karajannis M, Modak S, Gerstle JT, Heaton TE, Roberts S, Yang C, Jairam S, Vijai J, Topka S, Friedman DN, Stadler ZK, Robson M, Berger MF, Schultz N, Ladanyi

M, O'Reilly RJ, Abramson DH, Ceyhan-Birsoy O, Zhang L, Mandelker D, Shukla NN, Kung AL, Offit K, Zehir A, Walsh MF. Prospective pan-cancer germline testing using MSK-IMPACT informs clinical translation in 751 patients with pediatric solid tumors. Nature Cancer. 2021;2(3):357–65.

86. Kratz CP, Jongmans MC, Cavé H, Wimmer K, Behjati S, Guerrini-Rousseau L, Milde T, Pajtler KW, Golmard L, Gauthier-Villars M, Jewell R, Duncan C, Maher ER, Brugieres L, Pritchard-Jones K, Bourdeaut F. Predisposition to cancer in children and adolescents. Lancet Child Adolesc Health. 2021;5(2):142–54.

87. Villani A, Davidson S, Kanwar N, Lo WW, Li Y, Cohen-Gogo S, Fuligni F, Edward L-M, Light N, Layeghifard M, Harripaul R, Waldman L, Gallinger B, Comitani F, Brunga L, Hayes R, Anderson ND, Ramani AK, Yuki KE, Blay S, Johnstone B, Inglese C, Hammad R, Goudie C, Shuen A, Wasserman JD, Venier RE, Eliou M, Lorenti M, Ryan CA, Braga M, Gloven-Brown M, Han J, Montero M, Spatare F, Whitlock JA, Scherer SW, Chun K, Somerville MJ, Hawkins C, Abdelhaleem M, Ramaswamy V, Somers GR, Kyriakopoulou L, Hitzler J, Shago M, Morgenstern DA, Tabori U, Meyn S, Irwin MS, Malkin D, Shlien A. The clinical utility of integrative genomics in childhood cancer extends beyond targetable mutations. Nature Cancer. 2023;4(2):203–21.

9

From Biopsy to Biology: Next-Generation Sequencing in Endometrial, Ovarian, and Cervical Carcinoma

Valerio Gaetano Vellone, Gabriele Gaggero, and Michele Paudice

Abbreviations

AI	Artificial Intelligence
AMA	American Medical Association
ARID1A	AT-Rich Interaction Domain 1A
BRCA1/2	Breast Cancer Susceptibility Gene 1 and 2
cfDNA	Cell-free DNA
CNV	Copy Number Variation
ctDNA	Circulating Tumor DNA
CTCs	Circulating Tumor Cells
ESGO	European Society of Gynaecological Oncology
ESTRO	European Society for Radiotherapy and Oncology
ESP	European Society of Pathology
FFPE	Formalin-Fixed Paraffin-Embedded
FIGO	International Federation of Gynecology and Obstetrics
GI	Gastrointestinal
HRD	Homologous Recombination Deficiency
HBOC	Hereditary Breast and Ovarian Cancer
IHC	Immunohistochemistry
LS	Lynch Syndrome
MLH1, MSH2, MSH6, PMS2	Mismatch Repair Genes
MSI	Microsatellite Instability
MSI-H	Microsatellite Instability–High
MRD	Minimal Residual Disease
NCCN	National Comprehensive Cancer Network
NGS	Next-Generation Sequencing
POLE	DNA Polymerase Epsilon
ProMisE	Proactive Molecular Risk Classifier for Endometrial Cancer
SNV	Single Nucleotide Variant
TCGA	The Cancer Genome Atlas
TIL	Tumor-Infiltrating Lymphocytes
TMB	Tumor Mutational Burden
TP53	Tumor Protein p53
VUS	Variant of Uncertain Significance
WES	Whole-Exome Sequencing
WGS	Whole-Genome Sequencing
WSI	Whole Slide Imaging

V. G. Vellone (✉)
Department of Integrated Surgical and Diagnostic Sciences (DISC), University of Genoa, Genoa, Italy

Pathology Unit, IRCCS Istituto Giannina Gaslini, Genoa, Italy
e-mail: Valerio.vellone@unige.it; valeriovellone@gaslini.org

G. Gaggero
Pathology Unit, IRCCS Istituto Giannina Gaslini, Genoa, Italy
e-mail: gabrielegaggero@gaslini.org

M. Paudice
Department of Integrated Surgical and Diagnostic Sciences (DISC), University of Genoa, Genoa, Italy

Pathology University Unit, IRCCS Ospedale Policlinico San Martino, Genoa, Italy
e-mail: michele.paudice@unige.it

© The Author(s), under exclusive license to Springer Nature Switzerland AG 2026
S. Sioletic, L. Coppola (eds.), *Next-Generation Sequencing in Solid Tumor Histopathology*, Current Clinical Pathology, https://doi.org/10.1007/978-3-032-18790-1_9

Introduction

Overview of NGS Technology

NGS, also known as massively parallel sequencing, comprises a suite of high-throughput technologies that enable the rapid and simultaneous sequencing of millions of DNA or RNA fragments. In contrast to traditional Sanger sequencing, which processes one DNA fragment at a time, NGS allows comprehensive genomic profiling across targeted regions, exomes, or entire genomes within a single assay. The workflow includes key steps such as library preparation, clonal amplification, sequencing by synthesis, and bioinformatic analysis, all of which have been increasingly optimized for routine use in diagnostic pathology laboratories. Platforms like Illumina's sequencing-by-synthesis and Thermo Fisher's Ion Torrent have gained widespread clinical adoption due to their scalability, turnaround time, and cost-efficiency. These technologies support diverse applications ranging from somatic mutation detection to transcriptome analysis and fusion gene discovery. Ultimately, NGS has transformed molecular diagnostics by enabling more accurate tumor classification, refined prognostication, and personalized therapeutic strategies especially in oncology, including gynecologic malignancies [1–3].

Rationale for Applying NGS in Gynecologic Pathology

The growing application of NGS in gynecologic pathology reflects an increased understanding that many gynecologic tumors harbor recurrent, clinically relevant molecular alterations. While traditional histopathologic evaluation remains fundamental, it often proves insufficient for resolving diagnostically ambiguous cases or identifying actionable targets. NGS enables the simultaneous detection of point mutations, copy number variations, gene fusions, and microsatellite instability yielding a comprehensive molecular profile from minimal tissue input.

For example, endometrial carcinomas can now be stratified into four molecular subtypes with distinct prognostic and therapeutic implications: POLE-ultramutated, microsatellite instability-high (MSI-H), copy number-low (NSMP), and copy number-high/p53-abnormal based on high-throughput sequencing data, as first introduced by The Cancer Genome Atlas (TCGA) project [4]. Similarly, high-grade serous ovarian carcinomas, which commonly harbor TP53 mutations and may involve BRCA1/2 loss, benefit from NGS-based profiling to guide the use of PARP inhibitors [5].

Integration of Molecular Diagnostics in Modern Pathology Workflows

The integration of molecular diagnostics into contemporary pathology practice marks a transformative shift from traditional morphology-centered assessment to a multimodal approach that incorporates histologic, immunophenotypic, and genomic data for precision diagnosis and therapy selection. Next-generation sequencing (NGS) has been instrumental in this transition, enabling comprehensive molecular profiling directly from formalin-fixed, paraffin-embedded (FFPE) tissue an established cornerstone of surgical pathology workflows.

This advancement allows pathologists to refine diagnoses, especially in histologically ambiguous or rare tumors, and to deliver clinically actionable insights, including predictive biomarkers for targeted therapies and immune checkpoint inhibitors [3, 6]. For instance, incorporating NGS into diagnostic algorithms has enhanced the subclassification of gynecologic malignancies by detecting key mutations (e.g., TP53, PTEN, ARID1A) and identifying molecular signatures such as POLE mutations and microsatellite instability (MSI), both of which carry prognostic and therapeutic relevance [4].

Molecular findings are now routinely included in pathology reports, requiring close collaboration among pathologists, molecular biologists, and bioinformaticians, and reinforcing the inherently multidisciplinary nature of modern oncologic care [7]. Additionally, advances in automation, digital pathology platforms, and laboratory information systems have streamlined the reporting and integration of molecular data, reducing turnaround times and enhancing clinical applicability. Recent editorial work has further emphasized the synergistic integration of molecular diagnostics, digital pathology, and biobanking in modern gynecologic pathology. These domains are no longer parallel developments but converging technologies that collectively enhance diagnostic precision, enable personalized treatment strategies, and support translational research. In particular, molecular profiling is increasingly complemented by digital workflows and well-curated biobanked specimens, fostering a new era of data-rich, patient-centered pathology practice [8].

NGS Platforms and Methodologies

Overview of Main NGS Platforms Used in Clinical Practice

Over the past decade, several NGS platforms have become integral to clinical molecular diagnostics, each offering unique chemistries, throughput capacities, and data outputs that align with different diagnostic objectives. Broadly, NGS technologies are categorized into short-read and long-read sequencing systems, each with distinct advantages and limitations.

Illumina, currently the most widely adopted platform in clinical settings, utilizes sequencing-by-synthesis technology with cyclic reversible terminators. It offers high base-call accuracy, scalability, and throughput, making it suitable for a wide range of applications, including targeted gene panels, whole-exome sequencing (WES), and transcriptome analysis. Its widespread use in clinical oncology and genetic testing is underpinned by robust bioinformatics support and well-validated assay pipelines [2].

Ion Torrent (Thermo Fisher Scientific) employs a semiconductor-based sequencing approach that detects pH changes specifically hydrogen ions released during nucleotide incorporation. Although it has a slightly lower base-call accuracy compared to Illumina, its faster run times and lower capital investment make it an appealing option for smaller laboratories or focused applications such as hotspot mutation analysis [1].

Historically significant platforms such as Roche 454 and SOLiD (Applied Biosystems) contributed to early clinical sequencing efforts but have since been phased out due to high operating costs, complex workflows, and limited scalability [9].

In recent years, long-read sequencing technologies have gained momentum for their ability to resolve complex genomic regions that short-read systems cannot effectively characterize. Pacific Biosciences (PacBio) uses single-molecule real-time (SMRT) sequencing to generate long, high-fidelity reads (HiFi reads), facilitating the detection of structural variants, repetitive sequences, and phasing of alleles. Oxford Nanopore Technologies (ONT) offers an alternative long-read approach based on nanopore conductance, enabling ultra-long read lengths and real-time sequencing with portable devices such as the MinION. These features are increasingly applied in constitutional genomics, infectious disease diagnostics, and cancer genomics, where structural complexity is critical [10].

While short-read platforms remain dominant in routine clinical practice due to their maturity, standardization, and compatibility with FFPE-derived DNA, the integration of long-read sequencing is expected to expand, particularly in contexts requiring comprehensive structural variant detection, methylation profiling, and de novo assembly [11].

In summary, the selection of an NGS platform must consider multiple factors: the clinical question, required resolution, sample type, throughput needs, turnaround time, and available infrastructure. As technology advances and costs continue to decline, a hybrid use of short- and long-read platforms is likely to define the next phase of clinical genomics.

Targeted Panels vs Whole-Exome and Whole-Genome Sequencing

In clinical molecular diagnostics, the selection among targeted gene panels, WES, and whole-genome sequencing (WGS) is guided by the clinical indication, urgency, cost-effectiveness, and the depth and breadth of genomic information required for diagnosis or therapeutic decision-making.

Targeted gene panels focus on a curated subset of genes with well-established clinical relevance in specific diseases, particularly cancer. These panels offer high sequencing depth, allowing for sensitive detection of low-frequency variants in heterogeneous samples such as FFPE tumor tissue. Their design enables rapid turnaround times, lower costs, and simplified bioinformatic analysis compared to broader approaches. As such, they are the first-line choice in routine oncologic diagnostics, particularly for identifying actionable mutations that guide targeted therapies (e.g., TP53, BRCA1/2, PTEN, PIK3CA). Furthermore, panels can be dynamically updated to incorporate new biomarkers as clinical guidelines evolve, enhancing their adaptability in precision medicine workflows [6].

WES captures approximately 1–2% of the genome, focusing on protein-coding regions where the majority of disease-associated variants reside. WES is particularly valuable when the phenotype is unclear, when targeted testing yields negative results, or in genetically heterogeneous diseases. It allows the identification of rare, novel, or atypical mutations beyond known hotspots. In oncology, WES may uncover mutations with emerging therapeutic or prognostic significance, as well as tumor mutational burden (TMB), a biomarker for immunotherapy response [12]. However, the broader scope of analysis introduces interpretive complexity and a higher likelihood of detecting variants of uncertain significance (VUS), requiring robust annotation and multidisciplinary review.

WGS offers the most comprehensive genomic view by sequencing both coding and non-coding regions, allowing detection of structural rearrangements, copy number alterations, non-coding regulatory mutations, and mutational signatures across the entire genome. WGS excels in identifying intronic splice-site variants, promoter mutations, enhancer alterations, and complex rearrangements often missed by WES or targeted panels. Despite its unparalleled resolution, WGS remains limited in clinical settings due to its higher cost, longer analysis time, and the need for advanced bioinformatic infrastructure and expertise [13]. Nonetheless, its use is expanding in complex cases, especially in pediatric and undiagnosed diseases, hematologic malignancies, and research-driven precision oncology trials [2].

As sequencing costs continue to decrease and computational pipelines improve in speed and clinical-grade validation, the integration of WES and WGS into mainstream diagnostics is expected to increase, especially where comprehensive molecular profiling is essential for patient stratification and personalized therapy.

Sample Requirements and Quality Control (FFPE, Cytological Samples)

The success of NGS in clinical pathology critically depends on the quality, integrity, and quantity of input nucleic acids, which are intrinsically linked to the nature and handling of the specimen. Two primary types of specimens are commonly utilized in diagnostic NGS workflows: FFPE tissue and cytological samples. Each presents distinct challenges and requirements for optimal performance.

FFPE tissue is the standard material in routine anatomic pathology due to its widespread availability and preservation of histomorphological context. However, formalin fixation introduces chemical cross-linking and nucleic acid fragmentation, which can lead to sequencing artifacts, reduced library complexity, and dropout of target regions [2]. These degradation effects are particularly pronounced in older blocks or poorly fixed specimens. To mitigate these limitations, improved nucleic acid extraction kits tailored for FFPE, along with optimized protocols for DNA repair and fragmentation control, have significantly enhanced the reliability of NGS from these samples [14]. Today, FFPE-derived DNA and RNA are compatible with both targeted panel sequencing and, in many cases, whole-exome applications provided that input quality is rigorously assessed.

Cytological specimens, including fine-needle aspiration (FNA) smears, cell blocks, and fluid samples (e.g., pleural effusions, ascitic fluid), are increasingly recognized as valuable sources for molecular testing. These samples often represent the only available diagnostic material in inoperable tumors or metastatic disease. When properly processed and selected for adequate tumor cellularity, cytology-derived material can yield nucleic acids of comparable quality to FFPE tissue. Emerging data confirm high concordance in mutation profiles between cytologic and matched tissue samples, supporting their integration into NGS pipelines [15, 16].

To ensure analytical validity and minimize false-positive or false-negative results, stringent quality control (QC) measures must be implemented throughout the NGS workflow. Key preanalytical and analytical QC parameters include [17–19]:

(a) Nucleic acid quantification, typically via fluorometric methods (e.g., Qubit).
(b) Integrity assessment, using DNA Integrity Number (DIN) or RNA Integrity Number (RIN), where DIN > 2 or RIN > 5 is generally considered acceptable for most applications.
(c) Tumor cellularity estimation, often requiring a minimum of 10–20% neoplastic cells for reliable somatic mutation detection.
(d) Library complexity and fragment size distribution, assessed via bioanalyzer or equivalent systems.
(e) Coverage uniformity and read depth, particularly critical for detecting low-frequency variants in heterogeneous samples.

Standardization of QC thresholds and harmonization across platforms and laboratories is a crucial next step for ensuring interlaboratory reproducibility and clinical-grade reliability. Ongoing efforts by professional societies and working groups aim to establish consensus guidelines for tissue handling, extraction protocols, and reporting standards to support widespread adoption of NGS in routine diagnostics [1].

Molecular Landscape of Gynecologic Tumors

Gynecologic tumors comprise a diverse group of neoplasms arising from the female reproductive tract, encompassing malignancies of the endometrium, ovary, cervix, vulva, vagina, and placenta. Although traditionally classified based on histologic and morphologic criteria, these tumors are now increasingly understood through the lens of molecular pathology. Advances in high-throughput sequencing, particularly through initiatives such as TCGA, have profoundly reshaped our knowledge of their genomic landscapes [4].

Over the past decade, large-scale molecular profiling has uncovered recurrent driver mutations, copy number alterations, epigenetic changes, and pathway-level dysregulations that underpin tumor initiation, progression, and therapeutic vulnerability. These findings have enabled the stratification of tumors into molecular subtypes with distinct prognostic and predictive significance, extending well beyond conventional histopathologic boundaries [20].

The clinical integration of NGS, as discussed in previous sections, is accelerating the shift toward precision oncology in gynecologic pathology. Molecular features such have emerged as critical biomarkers that inform both diagnosis and therapeutic decision-making [21]. In parallel, rare and histologically ambiguous entities are being increasingly resolved through the identification of pathognomonic fusions and mutational signatures, expanding the diagnostic reach of the pathologist and enabling personalized treatment strategies. This section provides an overview of the molecular hallmarks of major gynecologic tumor types, organized by anatomic site. Each of the following paragraphs will detail the key genomic alterations, classification systems, and clinically actionable targets associated with tumors of the endometrium, ovary, and cervix highlighting the growing relevance of molecular profiling in contemporary gynecologic oncology.

Molecular Characteristics of Endometrial Carcinoma

From Dualism to Genomics

Endometrial carcinoma (EC) was historically framed by Bokhman's dualistic model, which distinguished between estrogen-dependent, low-grade endometrioid tumors (type I) and estrogen-independent, high-grade non-endometrioid tumors (type II). Although widely adopted, this morphologic paradigm has demonstrated limited prognostic value due to overlapping histologic features and substantial interobserver variability [22, 23]. A major conceptual shift occurred with the advent of large-scale genomic profiling, most notably through TCGA, which identified four robust molecular subtypes: POLE-ultramutated, microsatellite instability-high (MSI-H), copy-number low (NSMP), and copy-number high (serous-like) that transcend traditional histologic boundaries and carry significant clinical implications [4].

Subsequent studies have expanded on these findings, showing that high-grade endometrioid carcinomas often exhibit molecular alterations and clinical behavior more consistent with serous carcinomas than with low-grade endometrioid tumors. The incorporation of immunohistochemical surrogates such as mismatch repair (MMR) proteins, p53, and hormone receptors has proven effective in approximating molecular subtypes in routine diagnostic settings. These biomarkers not only aid in subtype classification but also provide prognostic information and guide therapeutic decisions [24].

Emerging evidence also supports the integration of hormone receptor expression into risk stratification algorithms. The presence or absence of estrogen and progesterone receptor expression has been correlated with tumor behavior, response to hormonal therapies, and overall prognosis [25].

Recent investigations have also highlighted the role of the androgen receptor (AR) in modulating tumor aggressiveness. AR expression, variably present across EC subtypes, may serve as a prognostic marker and potential therapeutic target, particularly in tumors lacking classical hormone receptors. Collectively, these developments emphasize the need for an integrated molecular approach in endometrial cancer classification, offering improved diagnostic precision and facilitating personalized therapeutic strategies.

The Four Genomic Subgroups

TCGA class	Cardinal genomic features	Approx. prevalence	Prognosis
POLE-ultramutated	Exonuclease-domain POLE hotspots (P286R / V411L), mutation rate ~ 10^2/Mb, few copy-number changes	7–10%	Excellent—even in high-grade tumors
MMRd / MSI-hypermutated	MLH1 promoter methylation or germline/ somatic MMR loss; frameshift-rich mutational signatures	25–30%	Intermediate; responsive to immune-checkpoint blockade
Copy-number-low (NSMP)	MSS, low SCNAs, PTEN/ PIK3CA/CTNNB1 mutations	30–40%	Intermediate; outcome modulated by grade & hormone-receptor status
Copy-number-high / p53-abnormal	TP53 mutation, widespread SCNAs, ERBB2/CCNE1 amplifications; serous "look-alike"	10–15%	Poor

These classes explain why some FIGO grade 3 endometrioid tumors behave like serous carcinoma, while others are unexpectedly indolent (POLE-mutant) [4, 23, 26].

Histotype–Molecular Correlations

Histotype–molecular correlations in endometrial carcinoma reveal significant, yet not absolute, associations between traditional morphologic classification and underlying genomic alterations. Most low-grade endometrioid carcinomas are enriched in the no specific molecular profile (NSMP) group or show microsatellite instability (MMRd), both of which are generally associated with a favorable to intermediate prognosis and retained expression of hormone receptors. By contrast, approximately 25% of grade 3 endometrioid tumors fall into the p53-abnormal (p53abn) molecular category, displaying more aggressive clinical behavior and overlapping features with serous carcinoma.

Uterine serous carcinomas align almost uniformly with the copy-number high/p53-abnormal group, regardless of morphologic heterogeneity, and often exhibit extensive chromosomal instability and TP53 mutations. These tumors typically lack hormone receptor expression and are associated with poor outcomes, making molecular classification especially valuable when morphology is ambiguous.

Clear cell carcinomas, carcinosarcomas, and undifferentiated/dedifferentiated carcinomas show a more heterogeneous molecular distribution, frequently mapping to either the p53-abnormal or MMRd classes [24]. Their classification can therefore benefit substantially from ancillary immunohistochemistry and molecular profiling, especially in diagnostically challenging cases or when biopsy material is limited.

Importantly, expression patterns of steroid hormone receptors, including estrogen (ER), progesterone (PR), and androgen receptor (AR), correlate with molecular subtypes. Tumors belonging to the NSMP and POLE-ultramutated (POLEmut) groups typically retain AR, ER, and PR expression, reflecting hormone dependence and potential sensitivity to endocrine therapies. Conversely, loss of receptor expression, particularly AR and PR, is characteristic of p53-abnormal tumors, which tend to exhibit hormone independence and more aggressive phenotypes [25].

Understanding these correlations is essential for diagnostic accuracy, risk stratification, and therapeutic guidance. While histotype remains a valuable first-tier classification, molecular subclassification provides critical refinement, particularly in high-grade or non-endometrioid tumors.

Why Molecular Classification Matters

The incorporation of molecular classification into the clinical management of endometrial carcinoma has revolutionized diagnostic precision, risk assessment, and therapeutic decision-making. Traditional histopathologic parameters such as grade, stage, and histotype while still valuable, often fail to capture the biological heterogeneity of these tumors. In contrast, the integration of key molecular markers, namely POLE exonuclease domain mutations, MMR status, and p53 abnormalities, has allowed for a deeper understanding of tumor behavior and prognostic trajectory.

From a prognostic standpoint, molecular classification substantially refines risk stratification. For example, POLE-ultramutated tumors, despite often presenting with high-grade morphology, exhibit an excellent prognosis and minimal risk of recurrence. On the other end of the spectrum, p53-abnormal tumors, typically associated with serous histology, display aggressive clinical behavior even when confined to the uterus. Meanwhile, MMR-deficient tumors occupy an intermediate prognostic space but are clinically relevant for their susceptibility to immune-based therapies. The ability to place tumors into one of these well-defined molecular categories improves clinical counseling and enables more personalized surveillance and management strategies.

Importantly, therapeutic choices are increasingly being guided by molecular subtype. POLE-mutated tumors, particularly in early stages, may be managed conservatively, with omission of adjuvant therapy now considered safe due to their indolent course. In contrast, p53-abnormal tumors benefit from aggressive adjuvant approaches, including combined chemotherapy and radiation, even at low stage, given their propensity for recurrence. MMR-deficient tumors are responsive to immune checkpoint inhibitors such as PD-1 blockade, a finding that has opened new horizons in the treatment of advanced or recurrent disease. Moreover, a subset of p53-abnormal carcinomas harbor ERBB2 (HER2) amplification, rendering them eligible for trastuzumab-based targeted therapy, further underscoring the predictive value of molecular profiling.

Reflecting the growing importance of these biomarkers, the 2023 revision of the FIGO staging system now includes molecular features as official modifiers. Tumors with POLE mutations are staged downward to acknowledge their excellent outcomes, while p53-abnormal tumors are staged upward to reflect their poor prognosis, regardless of anatomical confinement. This evolution marks a critical shift: staging is no longer purely anatomic but biologically contextualized.

Altogether, molecular classification is not a theoretical construct or research tool confined to academic centers, it is now an indispensable element of routine pathology reporting and oncologic decision-making. It bridges morphology and biology, enabling a truly personalized approach to endometrial cancer care.

Practical Barriers to Implementation

Despite the clear and growing clinical value of molecular classification, its universal implementation in routine practice still faces several significant challenges. First, cost and infrastructure remain limiting factors. Even streamlined NGS panels require dedicated capital investment, robust laboratory infrastructure, and access to reliable bioinformatics support. These prerequisites may be out of reach for many centers, particularly in resource-limited settings [26].

Second, sample quality can compromise molecular testing outcomes. FFPE tissue, though the standard in diagnostic pathology, introduces DNA fragmentation and cross-linking, which negatively impact nucleic acid integrity. As a result, a non-negligible proportion of samples, estimated at approximately 5%, fail to meet quality control thresholds, thus precluding reliable analysis.

Third, there are interpretive complexities that demand specialized expertise. For example, distinguishing pathogenic POLE mutations from variants of uncertain significance (VUS) can be challenging and may require complementary functional or clinical data. Similarly, standardizing p53 immunohistochemistry (IHC) interpretation, particularly the identification of aberrant versus wild-type expression patterns, calls for experience in gynecologic pathology and familiarity with established scoring criteria [27].

Lastly, the readiness of healthcare systems to incorporate molecular testing into routine workflows varies widely. The rapid inclusion of molecular parameters into the 2023 FIGO staging system has raised concerns that many institutions, especially outside of tertiary referral centers, may not yet be adequately equipped to perform or interpret the required tests. Without coordinated investment and education, there is a risk that such disparities could widen existing gaps in care.

Future Directions

Hybrid algorithms (e.g., ProMisE) that combine hot-spot sequencing with p53/MMR immunostaining already achieve >90% concordance with full TCGA typing. Long-read and single-cell sequencing will refine structural-variant detection and clonal architecture, while AR-directed trials may benefit receptor-positive NSMP cancers [28]. As multi-omic data flow seamlessly into digital pathology platforms, molecular subclassification is poised to become as routine and indispensable as grade and stage [29].

FIGO 2023 Classification of Endometrial Carcinoma and Its Limitations

Introduction: From Anatomy to Biology

Historically, EC staging was based on the 1988 and 2009 FIGO systems, which relied entirely on anatomic and histopathologic parameters such as depth of myometrial invasion, cervical involvement, and spread beyond the uterus. However, with the genomic revolution initiated by TCGA, it became clear that biology, not anatomy alone, drives prognosis and treatment response in EC. The 2023 revision of the FIGO staging system for endometrial carcinoma marks a pivotal shift toward integrated staging, incorporating molecular biomarkers, specifically POLE mutations and TP53 abnormalities, into conventional surgical staging criteria to enhance prognostic accuracy and guide management decisions [26, 30, 31].

The FIGO 2023 Staging System: Key Changes

The 2023 FIGO classification maintains the four-stage architecture but introduces molecular modifiers to stratify risk more accurately within each anatomic category. The most notable updates include:

(a) Incorporation of Molecular Subgroups

POLE ultramutated tumors, despite high-grade histology or deep invasion, are now acknowledged to have exceptionally good prognosis, justifying downstaging in selected cases.

TP53-abnormal tumors (typically associated with serous or serous-like carcinomas) are recognized as high-risk, even if early-stage or small in size, allowing for upstaging to reflect their aggressive biology.

(b) Refinement of Stage I and II

Stage I is subdivided not only by depth of myometrial invasion (IA: <50%; IB: ≥50%) but also by molecular class, allowing for nuanced risk stratification.

Involvement of the lower uterine segment or endocervical glands alone, without stromal invasion, does not upstage to stage II.

(c) Clarification of Extrauterine Disease

Stage IIIA no longer includes only serosal or adnexal involvement but recognizes the potential of isolated peritoneal implants and their molecular background.

Omental metastases, even microscopic, define stage IV disease, particularly in the context of serous carcinoma or TP53 mutation.

Clinical Implications of the New System

(a) Personalized Prognostication

By embedding POLE and TP53 status into staging, FIGO 2023 better aligns with outcome data: patients with POLE-mutated EC, previously overtreated based on morphology alone, can now be safely spared adjuvant therapy; conversely, TP53-abnormal tumors, even with superficial invasion, are flagged for systemic treatment.

(b) Streamlining of Clinical Trials and Risk Models

The molecularly integrated FIGO system harmonizes with existing ESGO/ESTRO/ESP guidelines, enabling standardized patient stratification in trials and improving the accuracy of tools such as ProMisE and MSI/TP53 IHC-based algorithms.

Limitations and Controversies

While conceptually powerful, the 2023 FIGO classification raises practical, technical, and equity-related concerns [32]:

(a) Access and Infrastructure

As previously mentioned, molecular testing (POLE sequencing, MMR/MSI analysis, and TP53 evaluation) is not yet universally available. Many centers, especially in low- and middle-income countries, lack NGS platforms, trained personnel, or reimbursement for these assays. This could widen disparities in staging quality and treatment outcomes.

(b) Interpretation Challenges

- POLE variants of uncertain significance (VUS) can lead to misclassification, requiring molecular pathology expertise to differentiate true pathogenic drivers from benign polymorphisms.
- p53 IHC scoring is not always straightforward: aberrant ("mutant-like") expression patterns may be subtle or heterogeneous, especially in biopsy specimens, risking under- or over-interpretation.

(c) Incomplete Molecular Subclassification

FIGO 2023 incorporates only two of the four TCGA subtypes (POLEmut and TP53abn), omitting MMRd and NSMP, which also carry important prognostic and therapeutic implications. This decision was likely made to balance practicality and evidence strength, but it renders the system incomplete from a biological perspective.

(d) Grey Zones in Histotype–Genotype Alignment

Morphologically ambiguous tumors (e.g., high-grade endometrioid vs serous carcinoma) may show conflicting features, complicating classification and management. Additionally, rare histotypes like clear cell carcinoma and undifferentiated carcinoma are heterogeneous at the molecular level and not yet fully integrated into staging pathways.

(e) Transitional Burden

Pathologists and clinicians must adapt reporting formats, multidisciplinary workflows, and patient communication practices to reflect FIGO 2023. This requires education, standardization, and audit systems that are not yet uniformly implemented across institutions.

The Way Forward

Despite its limitations, the 2023 FIGO classification represents a major step toward precision gynecologic oncology. As molecular testing becomes more accessible, the staging system will become more robust and equitable. Future updates will likely incorporate all four TCGA classes, possibly with integrated biomarker panels (e.g., ProMisE) and support from digital pathology and AI. In parallel, continued investment in training, quality assurance, and international collaboration will be essential to translate the promise of molecular staging into better outcomes for all patients with endometrial cancer.

Performing Molecular Classification of Endometrial Carcinoma with NGS in Clinical Practice

Introduction

The shift toward precision oncology in gynecologic pathology has placed molecular classification at the forefront of endometrial carcinoma (EC) management. Integrating genomics into diagnostic workflows not only improves prognostication but also guides adjuvant therapy and eligibility for targeted treatments. The four molecular subgroups: POLE-ultramutated, MMR-deficient (MMRd), copy-number low (NSMP), and copy-number high/p53-abnormal (p53abn) are now essential for risk stratification. NGS offers a scalable platform for implementing these classifications in routine diagnostics, enabling simultaneous assessment of multiple genomic alterations from minimal tissue input.

Pre-analytical Requirements

(a) Sample Selection

The success of NGS begins with adequate tissue quality and quantity. FFPE blocks from hysterectomy specimens or representative biopsies are commonly used. Tumor cellularity should ideally be >30%, and macrodissection may be employed to enrich neoplastic content.

(b) Nucleic Acid Extraction

High-quality DNA is essential for reliable variant detection. Degradation, crosslinking, and fragmentation from fixation can impair sequencing. QC metrics such as DNA Integrity Number (DIN) and Qubit concentration are typically required before proceeding to library preparation [2].

NGS Panel Design and Strategy

(a) Gene Targets and Technical Setup

In a diagnostic setting, a targeted gene panel is preferred over whole-exome or genome sequencing, due to cost, depth of coverage, and clinical relevance [26]. The panel should include:

- POLE (exons 9–14): Hotspots P286R and V411L are key for ultramutated classification.
- MMR genes (MLH1, MSH2, MSH6, PMS2): Mutations suggest MMRd subtype; may complement IHC.
- TP53: Mutations or LOF variants define p53abn tumors.
- PTEN, PIK3CA, CTNNB1: Useful for NSMP assignment and prognostic refinement.
- Microsatellite markers or MSI sensors may be included for automated MSI scoring.

Platforms used include Illumina MiSeq, NextSeq, or Thermo Ion Torrent instruments, with validated pipelines for variant calling, copy number alterations (CNAs), and microsatellite instability.

(b) Library Preparation and Sequencing

Library preparation includes DNA fragmentation, adapter ligation, PCR amplification, and indexing. Coverage depth should exceed 500x to ensure detection of subclonal variants, especially in mixed or low-input samples [1, 26].

Post-analytical Interpretation

(a) Bioinformatics and Variant Calling

Analysis pipelines must differentiate pathogenic mutations from VUS. Databases such as ClinVar, COSMIC, and gnomAD are used alongside in-house curated libraries. Variant allele frequency (VAF), co-mutation patterns, and context (e.g., known POLE driver mutations) guide interpretation.

(b) Assigning Molecular Class

The hierarchy generally used for classification is:

1. POLE-ultramutated: Defined by hotspot exonuclease mutations. Even if TP53 or MMRd alterations are present, POLE status supersedes.
2. MMRd: Confirmed by pathogenic mutations or high MSI score, often corroborated with IHC loss.
3. p53-abnormal: Pathogenic TP53 mutations or concordant aberrant IHC staining pattern.
4. NSMP: No defining alterations; often harbor PTEN, CTNNB1, or PIK3CA mutations.

This approach aligns with the ESGO/ESTRO/ESP guidelines and has been validated against TCGA classifications in multiple studies [33].

Reporting Standards

Molecular classification results must be clearly integrated into the pathology report, using standardized nomenclature and interpretation. Reports should state:

- Molecular subgroup (e.g., "p53-abnormal endometrial carcinoma, stage IB").
- Detected mutations, VAFs, and potential therapeutic implications.
- Any limitations (e.g., low tumor content, failed targets).

Clinical interpretation should be multidisciplinary, with input from molecular pathologists, oncologists, and genetic counselors when germline testing is indicated (e.g., in MMRd tumors).

Complementary Testing and Validation

While NGS can serve as a standalone approach, it is often used in conjunction with:

- IHC for MMR proteins and p53.
- MLH1 promoter methylation analysis to distinguish sporadic from germline MMR loss.
- HER2 IHC/FISH in TP53-abnormal tumors with serous morphology.

IHC remains a cost-effective triage tool, but discordant cases may benefit from molecular confirmation via NGS.

Challenges in Implementation

- Turnaround time (TAT): Although optimized workflows can deliver results within 7–10 days, delays can affect treatment initiation.
- Cost and reimbursement: NGS panels require institutional investment and third-party payer alignment.
- Assay failure rates: Degraded FFPE or low-input samples can produce inadequate coverage, particularly in small biopsies.
- Interpretive complexity: VUS in POLE or TP53 genes, or ambiguous IHC/NGS discordance, demand subspecialist input.

Conclusions

NGS-based molecular classification of endometrial carcinoma is now a clinical imperative, delivering meaningful prognostic and predictive information that surpasses conventional morphology. With validated workflows, cost-effective targeted panels, and integrated reporting, molecular profiling can be seamlessly incorporated into routine diagnostic practice. Continuous quality control, interdisciplinary collaboration, and adherence to evolving guidelines will be critical to optimize its clinical impact [34–36].

Molecular Landscape of Ovarian Cancer

Introduction

Ovarian cancer remains the most lethal gynecologic malignancy, with a five-year survival rate of less than 50%, primarily due to late-stage diagnosis and frequent recurrence. High-grade serous carcinoma (HGSC) accounts for ~70% of epithelial ovarian cancers (EOCs) and is the primary driver of morbidity and mortality in this disease. The advent of large-scale genomic profiling, particularly through TCGA and related international efforts, has revealed the underlying molecular complexity and heterogeneity of ovarian cancer, opening the door for personalized therapy and biomarker-driven management [20].

Major Histologic Subtypes and Their Molecular Profiles

(a) High-Grade Serous Carcinoma (HGSC)
    HGSC is characterized by:
    - TP53 mutations in >95% of cases.
    - Frequent BRCA1/BRCA2 mutations (germline or somatic) in ~22%.
    - Homologous recombination deficiency (HRD) in ~50%.
    - Extensive copy number alterations and structural genomic instability.
    - Universal p53 overexpression or null phenotype by IHC.

The TCGA integrated genomic analysis of over 300 HGSCs identified a mutationally sparse but copy-number-rich genome, with BRCA loss-of-function driving sensitivity to platinum and PARP inhibitors. Additionally, TCGA delineated four transcriptional subtypes (immunoreactive, differentiated, proliferative, mesenchymal), although these lacked prognostic independence in subsequent validations [20].

(b) Low-Grade Serous Carcinoma (LGSC)

In contrast to HGSC, LGSC is:

- TP53 wild-type
- Frequently harbors mutations in KRAS, BRAF, and NRAS
- Shows relative genomic stability
- Often hormone receptor-positive (ER+, PR+)

These tumors are typically chemoresistant but indolent and may benefit from MEK inhibitors (e.g., trametinib), as shown in randomized trials [37, 38].

(c) Endometrioid and Clear Cell Carcinomas (ECC, CCC)

These subtypes share common origins with endometrial cancer and show:

- PIK3CA, ARID1A, and PTEN mutations
- Mismatch repair deficiency (especially in ECC)
- Low TP53 mutation rates
- Clear cell carcinomas may harbor HNF1B expression and AT-rich interactive domain (ARID1A) loss

Clear cell and endometrioid tumors may arise in the setting of endometriosis, and unlike HGSC, tend to have a more indolent course, but are resistant to platinum-based chemotherapy in advanced stages [39–41].

(d) Mucinous Carcinoma

This rare subtype mimics gastrointestinal tumors and is defined by:

- KRAS mutations in up to 60%
- Frequent HER2 amplification
- Rare TP53 mutations
- Lack of BRCA or HRD features

Mucinous carcinomas are typically chemoresistant, and differentiation from metastases of GI origin is essential [42].

BRCA Genes: Biology and Clinical Use in Ovarian Cancer

Introduction to BRCA Genes

The BRCA1 (Breast Cancer gene 1) and BRCA2 (Breast Cancer gene 2) genes are tumor suppressor genes involved in the repair of double-stranded DNA breaks via homologous recombination (HR). Mutations in these genes lead to impaired DNA repair and genomic instability, contributing to cancer development, particularly in breast and ovarian cancers [43].

- BRCA1 is located on chromosome 17q21 and encodes a protein involved in cell cycle checkpoint control and DNA repair.
- BRCA2 is located on chromosome 13q13.1 and plays a key role in recruiting RAD51 to sites of DNA damage.

BRCA Mutations and Ovarian Cancer

Up to 15–20% of high-grade serous ovarian carcinomas (HGSOC) harbor germline mutations in BRCA1/2, and another 5–10% carry somatic mutations [44].

These mutations are associated with:

- Increased lifetime risk of ovarian cancer (up to 44% for BRCA1 and 17% for BRCA2).
- Better initial response to platinum-based chemotherapy.
- Improved overall survival compared to non-BRCA-mutated counterparts.

Beyond germline and somatic mutations, the pathological characteristics of ovarian cancer can also provide valuable insight into the likelihood of BRCA1/2 pathogenic variants. A recent analysis demonstrated that histopathologic features, particularly high-grade serous histology, are strong predictors of BRCA mutation status, and incorporating morphologic data into variant interpretation frameworks can improve classification of variants of uncertain significance. This underscores the importance of integrating pathology review with genetic testing to optimize identification of BRCA-driven disease and refine patient selection for targeted therapies [45].

Clinical Testing and Risk Assessment

BRCA1 and BRCA2 testing represents a cornerstone of personalized oncology in gynecologic malignancies, particularly in the context of epithelial ovarian cancer. Current guidelines recommend that all women diagnosed with epithelial ovarian, fallopian tube, or primary peritoneal carcinoma undergo germline BRCA testing, irrespective of age at diagnosis or family history. This universal approach stems from the recognition that a significant proportion of pathogenic BRCA mutations occur in individuals without a suggestive family pedigree, and that identifying such mutations has profound therapeutic and preventive implications.

In addition to patients with ovarian cancer, BRCA testing is indicated for individuals with a strong personal or family history of breast and/or ovarian cancer, especially when involving early-onset cases, bilateral tumors, male breast cancer, or known hereditary cancer syndromes. The identification of a germline BRCA mutation may not only inform the individual's management, such as eligibility for PARP inhibitor therapy, but also prompt cascade testing among at-risk relatives, enabling timely surveillance or preventive measures.

Moreover, BRCA testing plays a pivotal role in reproductive planning and risk-reducing strategies. Women who are carriers may consider options such as preimplantation genetic diagnosis or risk-reducing salpingo-oophorectomy (RRSO), depending on age and reproductive status. Such interventions have been shown to reduce cancer risk and improve long-term outcomes significantly.

Given the medical, psychological, and familial ramifications of BRCA results, genetic counseling is essential both before and after testing. Pre-test counseling ensures informed consent and helps the patient understand potential outcomes, including the possibility of variants of uncertain significance. Post-test counseling supports interpretation of the results, guides next steps in clinical management, and facilitates communication with family members who may also be affected.

Incorporating BRCA testing into routine gynecologic oncology care reflects the broader shift toward integrated, genomics-driven medicine, where molecular information not only guides therapy but also empowers preventive strategies across generations [46].

Impact on Treatment: PARP Inhibitors

BRCA-deficient tumors, including a substantial subset of high-grade serous ovarian carcinomas, display a characteristic phenotype known as "BRCAness." This term refers to a functional deficiency in the homologous recombination (HR) DNA repair pathway, not limited to BRCA1 or BRCA2 mutations alone, but also encompassing tumors with epigenetic silencing or defects in other genes involved in HR. Such homologous recombination deficiency (HRD) renders tumor cells particularly vulnerable to PARP (poly[ADP-ribose] polymerase) inhibition, a therapeutic strategy that exploits the principle of synthetic lethality. Mechanistically, PARP inhibitors (PARPi) block the repair of single-strand DNA breaks by inhibiting the PARP enzyme. In cells already deficient in homologous recombination such as those harboring BRCA mutations, this leads to the accumulation of DNA damage, replication fork collapse, and ultimately cell death. This dual failure of DNA repair creates a lethal environment selectively for tumor cells, while sparing normal tissues with intact HR repair machinery.

Several PARPi have received regulatory approval for the treatment of ovarian cancer, particularly in the maintenance setting following response to platinum-based chemotherapy. Among them, olaparib, niraparib, and rucaparib are the most clinically established agents, each supported by large randomized trials.

The SOLO1 trial was a pivotal phase III study that assessed olaparib as maintenance therapy in patients with newly diagnosed, advanced BRCA-mutated ovarian cancer who had achieved a complete or partial response to first-line platinum-based chemotherapy. The results demonstrated a dramatic improvement in progression-free survival (PFS), with the median PFS not reached in the olaparib arm versus 13.8 months in the placebo group at the time of analysis, translating into a 70% risk reduction in disease progression or death. These findings established olaparib as a new standard of care in this molecularly defined population.

Subsequent trials, such as ARIEL3 and NOVA, extended the benefits of PARP inhibition to broader patient populations. The ARIEL3 study evaluated rucaparib as maintenance therapy in patients with recurrent ovarian cancer and showed significant PFS benefit in patients with BRCA mutations and those with broader HRD-positive profiles. Similarly, the NOVA trial demonstrated the efficacy of niraparib as maintenance therapy not only in patients with germline BRCA mutations but also in those without mutations but with HRD-positive tumors, indicating that PARPi sensitivity is not exclusively limited to BRCA-mutant cases.

Together, these data support the use of PARP inhibitors as a targeted maintenance strategy in BRCA-mutated and HRD-positive ovarian cancers, significantly altering the therapeutic landscape. Ongoing research continues to explore predictive biomarkers beyond BRCA and refine the selection of patients most likely to benefit from this class of agents, including combinations with immune checkpoint inhibitors or anti-angiogenic therapies [47, 48].

Surgical and Preventive Implications

In women carrying pathogenic mutations in BRCA1 or BRCA2, risk-reducing salpingo-oophorectomy (RRSO) represents a cornerstone of cancer prevention. This surgical intervention, involving the removal of both fallopian tubes and ovaries, has been shown to reduce the risk of developing ovarian, fallopian tube, or primary peritoneal carcinoma by approximately 85–90%, and may also confer a modest reduction in breast cancer risk when performed premenopausally.

Current guidelines recommend that women with BRCA1 mutations undergo RRSO between the ages of 35 and 40, or upon completion of childbearing, due to the earlier median age of ovarian cancer onset in this group. For women with BRCA2 mutations, who tend to develop ovarian cancer at a later age, RRSO may be safely postponed to between 40 and 45 years, although individualized counseling is essential to balance oncologic risk with reproductive planning and menopausal implications.

In addition to risk reduction, the timing and extent of surgery must consider patient preferences, family planning, menopausal status, and comorbidities. Whenever possible, the surgical specimen should be thoroughly examined using the SEE-FIM protocol (Sectioning and Extensively Examining the FIMbriated end), to maximize the detection of occult carcinomas in high-risk women. Furthermore, RRSO offers an opportunity to engage patients in broader preventive strategies, including hormone replacement therapy, breast surveillance, and cascade genetic testing for at-risk family members [49, 50].

Emerging Concepts and Future Directions

The concept of HRD extends far beyond BRCA1 and BRCA2 mutations. A growing body of research has identified several other genes such as PALB2, RAD51C, RAD51D, and BRIP1 that play critical roles in the homologous recombination repair pathway and may confer a similar "BRCAness" phenotype when inactivated. Alterations in these genes are currently under investigation as potential biomarkers of sensitivity to PARP inhibitors, particularly in patients who lack canonical BRCA mutations.

As a result, HRD testing is rapidly expanding in clinical practice. The goal is to identify a broader population of patients who may benefit from PARP inhibition, beyond those with germline or somatic BRCA mutations. Assays designed to detect genomic scarring, such as loss of heterozygosity (LOH), telomeric allelic imbalance, and large-scale transitions, are being incorporated into clinical trials and, in some contexts, into routine care. These tests offer a functional readout of homologous recombination proficiency and hold promise for refining therapeutic selection in ovarian and other HR-deficient cancers.

However, the emergence of resistance to PARP inhibitors remains a critical challenge. Mechanisms of acquired resistance are diverse and include secondary or "reversion" mutations in BRCA genes, which restore the open reading frame and functional HR activity, as well as epigenetic reactivation of silenced HR pathway components and alterations in replication fork stability. Understanding and anticipating these resistance pathways is vital to improving long-term outcomes and developing rational combination therapies.

Given its central role in both therapeutic vulnerability and resistance, homologous recombination deficiency will be examined extensively in the following sections. The discussion will include not only its molecular underpinnings, but also its implications for patient selection, treatment monitoring, and future directions in precision oncology [51].

Recent work has also highlighted the importance of epigenetic alterations, particularly BRCA1 promoter methylation, as a potential determinant of homologous recombination deficiency. In a multicenter cross-validation study, pyrosequencing proved to be a robust and reproducible method for detecting BRCA1 methylation in epithelial ovarian cancers, with high concordance across laboratories and clear correlation with downregulation of BRCA1 transcripts. Importantly, promoter methylation appears to be a dynamic process, capable of being lost or reversed during treatment, suggesting that methylation testing may provide a more real-time predictor of PARP inhibitor sensitivity than static genomic scar assays [52].

Conclusions

The discovery of BRCA1 and BRCA2 mutations has revolutionized ovarian cancer management. Their role extends from risk assessment and prevention to precision therapeutics with PARP inhibitors. As testing becomes more widespread and integrated into routine care, understanding BRCA biology is essential for personalized oncologic strategies.

Homologous Recombination Deficiency in Ovarian Cancer

Introduction

Ovarian cancer remains the most lethal gynecological malignancy worldwide, largely due to its asymptomatic progression and diagnosis at advanced stages. Among EOCs, HGSOC is the most prevalent and aggressive histological subtype. Molecular profiling has identified HRD as a pivotal feature in a substantial proportion of HGSOC, profoundly influencing tumor biology, prognosis, and therapeutic response particularly to platinum-based chemotherapy and PARP inhibitors.

The Homologous Recombination Repair Pathway

Homologous recombination repair (HRR) is a critical, high-fidelity DNA damage response pathway that preserves genomic stability by accurately repairing DNA double-strand breaks (DSBs). Unlike error-prone repair mechanisms such as non-homologous end joining, HRR utilizes the sister chromatid as a template to guide the repair process, ensuring the faithful restoration of genetic information. This function is particularly vital during the S and G2 phases of the cell cycle, when sister chromatids are available as templates.

The HRR pathway is orchestrated by a network of highly conserved genes, including BRCA1, BRCA2, RAD51, PALB2, ATM, ATR, and the RAD51 paralogs (RAD51C and RAD51D), among others. These proteins operate in a coordinated manner to sense DNA damage, mediate end resection, facilitate strand invasion, and resolve recombination intermediates. Any disruption of this pathway can impair the cell's ability to repair DSBs accurately, leading to genomic instability, chromosomal rearrangements, and ultimately tumorigenesis.

The loss of HRR function, referred to as HRD, can arise from a variety of genetic and epigenetic mechanisms. The most well-characterized causes are germline or somatic mutations in BRCA1 or

BRCA2, which confer a classical HRD phenotype. However, an increasing number of non-BRCA genes involved in HRR are being implicated in HRD, expanding the landscape of tumors susceptible to DNA-damaging therapies such as PARP inhibitors.

In particular, mutations or promoter hypermethylation of genes such as RAD51C and RAD51D, as well as PALB2, have been associated with impaired HRR function. Moreover, large genomic rearrangements, copy number variations, and loss of heterozygosity (LOH) involving HRR-related loci can further compromise the repair machinery. These alterations may occur independently of BRCA status, underscoring the need for comprehensive HRD testing beyond BRCA screening alone.

It is currently estimated that up to 50% of HGSOCs harbor some form of HRD, making this phenotype one of the most clinically relevant biomarkers in gynecologic oncology. The identification of HRD not only informs prognosis but also predicts sensitivity to platinum-based chemotherapy and PARP inhibitors, reinforcing the importance of systematic molecular profiling in this tumor type.

As will be explored in greater detail in the following sections, understanding the mechanistic basis of HRD and its diverse genetic and epigenetic drivers is fundamental to advancing personalized treatment strategies and overcoming resistance in ovarian and related cancers [20, 53, 54].

Clinical Implications of HRD in Ovarian Cancer

(a) Prognostic Value

HRD-positive tumors, especially those with BRCA mutations, generally exhibit better initial responses to platinum-based chemotherapy and improved overall survival. However, this benefit may diminish over time due to resistance mechanisms such as BRCA reversion mutations [55].

(b) Predictive Value: PARP Inhibitors

PARPi exploit synthetic lethality in HRD cells. Tumors deficient in HRR are unable to repair single-strand breaks that become double-strand breaks during replication. Inhibition of PARP leads to accumulation of DNA damage and cell death in HRD tumors. Several PARPi (olaparib, niraparib, rucaparib) have been approved for use in ovarian cancer, with stratification often based on HRD status [47, 48, 56].

HRD Testing

Several complementary testing methodologies have been developed and are currently in clinical use HRD testing. One approach involves NGS panels designed to detect mutations in key homologous recombination repair (HRR) genes, including BRCA1, BRCA2, PALB2, RAD51C, RAD51D, and others. These panels can identify both germline and somatic alterations and are widely used due to their integration into comprehensive genomic profiling workflows [57].

In parallel, genomic scar assays have been developed to provide a functional readout of HRD by quantifying specific patterns of genomic instability that result from defective HRR. These include LOH, telomeric allelic imbalance (TAI), and large-scale transitions (LST). Together, these three metrics are integrated into a composite HRD score, which can reflect a historical footprint of HRR deficiency, even in the absence of an identifiable pathogenic mutation [58].

Several commercial assays have been validated and approved as companion diagnostics in this setting. The most widely adopted is Myriad's myChoice® CDx, which combines BRCA1/2 mutation analysis with a quantitative HRD score based on LOH, TAI, and LST. Tumors that exceed a predefined score threshold are classified as HRD-positive and may be eligible for PARP inhibitor treatment. Similarly, FoundationOne® CDx offers a hybrid capture-based assay that reports mutations in HRR genes and genomic instability parameters, often as part of broader next-generation sequencing reports [59, 60].

These testing strategies have been instrumental in the design and regulatory approval of landmark clinical trials such as ARIEL2, NOVA, and PRIMA continuing to guide treatment decisions in both newly diagnosed and recurrent disease. However, it is important to note that while genomic scar assays reflect past HRD, they may not always predict current PARPi sensitivity, particularly in tumors that have acquired reversion mutations or alternative resistance mechanisms. Therefore, ongoing refinement of HRD testing algorithms, including the integration of functional assays and real-time indicators, remains an area of active research.

Resistance Mechanisms

Although PARPi have significantly improved outcomes in patients with BRCA-mutated or homologous recombination-deficient tumors, a major clinical challenge is the emergence of acquired resistance, which limits the durability of therapeutic responses. Resistance mechanisms are multifactorial and can arise through both genetic and adaptive changes within the tumor, leading to restoration of DNA repair capacity, drug inactivation, or evasion of PARPi-induced cytotoxicity.

One of the most extensively characterized mechanisms is the development of secondary or "reversion" mutations in BRCA1 or BRCA2. These alterations restore the open reading frame of the mutated gene, leading to the production of functional BRCA protein and reactivation of HRR. As a result, tumor cells regain the ability to repair DNA double-strand breaks accurately, rendering them less susceptible to synthetic lethality induced by PARP inhibition.

Another key resistance mechanism involves loss of 53BP1, a DNA damage response mediator that normally acts as a barrier to end resection in the absence of BRCA1. When 53BP1 is lost or downregulated, end resection is restored even in BRCA1-deficient cells, effectively bypassing the need for BRCA1 in homologous recombination and conferring resistance to PARPi. This phenomenon underscores the complexity and redundancy of the DNA repair network.

Additional adaptive responses include the upregulation of drug efflux pumps, such as MDR1 (ABCB1), which reduce intracellular concentrations of PARPi and thereby diminish their cytotoxic effect. Overexpression of MDR1 has been observed particularly in models of long-term PARPi exposure and may represent a mechanism of cross-resistance with other chemotherapeutics.

Finally, alterations in the PARP1 protein itself either through point mutations affecting its catalytic domain or changes in PARylation dynamics can attenuate the trapping of PARP1 on DNA, a critical component of PARPi-induced cytotoxicity. Mutations that impair PARP1's ability to bind DNA or become hyper-PARylated may reduce the efficacy of inhibitors that rely on this mechanism of action.

These resistance pathways highlight the plasticity of tumor cells under therapeutic pressure and emphasize the need for dynamic biomarkers that can monitor evolving molecular profiles. Understanding the interplay among resistance mechanisms is crucial for the development of next-generation PARP inhibitors, rational combination therapies (e.g., with ATR inhibitors or immune checkpoint blockade), and adaptive treatment strategies to prolong clinical benefit [61, 62].

Future Directions

The future of HRD-directed therapy in ovarian cancer is moving well beyond the traditional focus on BRCA1/2 mutations and platinum sensitivity. Current research aims to refine the biological definition of HRD, improve patient selection, and overcome mechanisms of resistance to targeted therapies.

One key area of investigation is the rational combination of PARP inhibitors with other therapeutic modalities. Preclinical and early clinical studies suggest that synergy may be achieved by pairing PARP inhibition with anti-angiogenic agents, which can induce hypoxia and downregulate homologous recombination repair, thereby sensitizing tumors to DNA damage. Similarly, combinations with immune checkpoint inhibitors are being explored, based on the premise that PARP inhibition increases tumor mutational burden and neoantigen exposure, potentially augmenting anti-tumor immunity. Other combinations under active study include PARP inhibitors with ATR, CHK1, or WEE1 inhibitors, aiming to exploit vulnerabilities in cell cycle checkpoint and replication stress pathways.

Parallel efforts are underway to expand the spectrum of biomarkers used to identify HRD beyond BRCA1/2 mutations and genomic scarring assays. This includes the evaluation of RAD51 foci formation assays as dynamic functional readouts of homologous recombination activity, as well as the incorporation of epigenetic alterations (e.g., BRCA1 promoter methylation) and mutations in additional DNA damage response (DDR) genes such as PALB2, RAD51C, and RAD51D. The ultimate goal is to refine stratification and capture a broader population of patients who may benefit from DNA repair–targeted therapies.

Finally, the concept of synthetic lethality is expanding to other DDR pathways. Beyond PARP inhibition, therapeutic strategies are being designed to target vulnerabilities in mismatch repair, Fanconi anemia, or replication fork protection mechanisms. As our understanding of DDR network complexity grows, novel synthetic lethal interactions are likely to emerge, offering opportunities for precision drug development and personalized therapy.

Conclusions

HRD is a cornerstone of ovarian cancer biology, especially in HGSOC. Its presence not only informs prognosis but also guides precision therapy with PARP inhibitors. Understanding the intricacies of HRD testing, resistance development, and future combinatorial strategies is essential for optimizing outcomes in ovarian cancer patients.

Next-Generation Sequencing in Uterine Cervix Cancer

Introduction

Cervical cancer remains a significant global health challenge, ranking as the fourth most common malignancy among women worldwide. Persistent infection with high-risk human papillomavirus (HPV) is a well-established etiological factor, particularly in squamous cell carcinoma (SCC) and adenocarcinoma (ADC) of the cervix. While the HPV-centric paradigm has guided preventive strategies, including vaccination and screening, advancements in NGS have unraveled the complex genomic landscape of cervical cancer. NGS enables high-throughput, parallel analysis of multiple genomic regions, transforming our understanding of tumor biology and therapeutic opportunities.

Genomic Landscape of Cervical Cancer

Recent large-scale NGS studies, most notably from TCGA, have significantly advanced our understanding of the molecular landscape of cervical cancer, uncovering a complex pattern of somatic mutations, copy number variations, and epigenetic alterations that vary across histological subtypes. This molecular heterogeneity has potential implications for both classification and targeted therapy.

In SCC, the most common histotype of cervical cancer, recurrent somatic mutations are frequently observed in genes associated with PI3K/AKT signaling, including PIK3CA, which is mutated in over 40% of cases. Additional recurrent alterations include mutations in EP300 (a chromatin remodeling factor), FBXW7 (a ubiquitin ligase component), and PTEN, as well as amplifications in genes such as YAP1 and SOX2, which are implicated in oncogenic transcriptional regulation and stemness phenotypes.

In contrast, ADCs exhibit a distinct mutational profile, more commonly involving KRAS, ERBB2 (HER2), and STK11 mutations. These alterations suggest activation of RAS/MAPK signaling and mTOR pathways, which may offer opportunities for subtype-specific therapeutic targeting. ADCs also tend to harbor fewer PIK3CA mutations compared to SCCs and display distinct patterns of methylation and gene expression.

A hallmark of virtually all cervical cancers is persistent infection with high-risk HPV, with integration of viral DNA into the host genome representing a critical oncogenic event. This integration leads to constitutive expression of the E6 and E7 oncoproteins, which inactivate key tumor suppressors TP53 and RB1, respectively. The loss of p53- and Rb-mediated checkpoint control promotes genomic instability, accelerates the accumulation of additional somatic mutations, and supports malignant transformation. Moreover, HPV integration can result in local structural rearrangements, transcriptional dysregulation, and upregulation of adjacent oncogenes, further contributing to tumor progression.

Cervical tumors can be molecularly classified into keratin-low and keratin-high SCC subtypes and endometrioid-like and gastric-type ADCs, each with unique mutational and transcriptional signatures. This stratification may help refine prognosis and support biomarker-driven therapeutic strategies in the future.

As our understanding of the genomic underpinnings of cervical cancer deepens, integrating this information into routine diagnostics may allow for more precise classification and improved personalization of treatment, especially in histologically ambiguous or therapy-refractory cases [21].

Applications of NGS in Cervical Cancer

(a) Molecular Subtyping and Biomarker Discovery

NGS has facilitated subclassification of cervical tumors based on mutation profiles, transcriptional patterns, and HPV integration status. This stratification can inform prognosis and therapy [63].

- PIK3CA mutations (~40%) are associated with poor prognosis.
- KMT2D, ARID1A, and EP300 mutations suggest chromatin remodeling defects.
- HPV-negative tumors often show TP53 mutations and worse outcomes.

(b) HPV Integration Analysis.

NGS allows detection of HPV integration sites in the host genome, which often occur near oncogenes such as MYC, RAD51B, and ERBB2. Integration is more frequent in SCC and is associated with genomic instability and worse outcomes [64].

(c) Therapeutic Target Identification.

In cervical carcinoma, NGS is increasingly recognized as a valuable tool for uncovering clinically actionable genomic alterations that may guide the use of targeted therapies. Although the majority of cervical cancers are driven by persistent HPV infection and its downstream molecular consequences, a subset of tumors harbor additional somatic alterations that create therapeutic vulnerabilities.

One of the most frequently altered pathways in cervical carcinoma is the PI3K/AKT/mTOR axis, with PIK3CA mutations reported in up to 25–30% of cases. These alterations provide a rationale for therapeutic strategies involving PI3K inhibitors or mTOR inhibitors, which are being evaluated in clinical trials and may eventually complement standard treatment.

In addition, ERBB2 (HER2) amplification or mutation has been identified in a proportion of cervical adenocarcinomas and some squamous tumors. This opens the possibility of leveraging HER2-targeted therapies, including trastuzumab, trastuzumab deruxtecan, or neratinib, agents that have already transformed outcomes in other HER2-driven cancers. Early-phase studies suggest that patients with HER2-amplified cervical cancer may derive meaningful benefit from such approaches.

Although rare, NTRK fusions have also been reported in cervical carcinoma, particularly in tumors with unusual histological features. The availability of highly selective TRK inhibitors such as larotrectinib and entrectinib—approved in a tumor-agnostic fashion—underscores the importance of broad genomic profiling, since even infrequent events can provide powerful therapeutic opportunities.

Altogether, the integration of NGS into the diagnostic work-up of cervical cancer has the potential to uncover targetable alterations beyond HPV-driven oncogenesis, facilitating access to precision medicine approaches and expanding treatment options for patients with advanced or refractory disease [65–67].

(d) Monitoring Minimal Residual Disease (MRD) and Recurrence.

NGS-based assays such as circulating tumor DNA (ctDNA) and HPV cell-free DNA analysis are being investigated for monitoring treatment response and early detection of recurrence [68].

Clinical Trials and Translational Relevance

The integration of NGS into clinical trial design has profoundly reshaped the therapeutic landscape of cervical carcinoma and other solid tumors. Rather than relying solely on histological classification, modern oncology trials increasingly employ molecularly driven eligibility criteria, enabling patients to be enrolled based on the presence of actionable genomic alterations, regardless of tumor origin.

Notably, large-scale precision oncology initiatives such as the NCI-MATCH trial and its successor NCI-ComboMATCH have included patients with cervical cancer, assigning them to targeted therapies according to specific mutations detected through NGS. For instance, alterations in PIK3CA, HER2, and BRCA1/2 have served as molecular entry points for investigational targeted agents, highlighting the feasibility of this strategy in a tumor type historically characterized by limited systemic treatment options.

In parallel, basket trials have emerged as powerful tools for studying rare molecular subsets across diverse cancers. Patients with cervical carcinoma harboring PIK3CA mutations may be eligible for studies evaluating PI3K or AKT inhibitors, while those with ERBB2 amplifications or mutations can access trials of HER2-targeted agents, including trastuzumab-deruxtecan or neratinib. Similarly, the identification of BRCA1/2 alterations or other homologous recombination repair deficiencies allows cervical cancer patients to benefit from PARP inhibitor trials, which are traditionally focused on ovarian and breast cancers but increasingly adopt tumor-agnostic frameworks.

Such trial designs exemplify the paradigm shift toward genomics-guided oncology, ensuring that patients with cervical cancer are not excluded from the therapeutic advances driven by precision medicine. As genomic profiling becomes routine, the inclusion of cervical carcinoma in tumor-agnostic, biomarker-driven clinical trials is expected to expand, offering new avenues of hope for patients with advanced or refractory disease [69–71].

Limitations and Challenges

Despite its promise, the application of NGS in cervical cancer faces challenges:

- Low tumor cellularity in some biopsies limits NGS utility.
- HPV-centric pathogenesis may limit the benefit of targeting somatic mutations.
- Cost and infrastructure constraints in low- and middle-income countries with the highest disease burden.

Additionally, not all mutations found through NGS are actionable or clinically validated, necessitating careful interpretation.

Future Perspectives

The future of precision oncology in cervical cancer is moving decisively toward a more integrated and personalized paradigm. A key priority is the integration of multi-omic approaches, combining data from genomics, transcriptomics, proteomics, and epigenomics to achieve a more comprehensive view of tumor biology. This holistic perspective promises to refine molecular subtyping, identify novel therapeutic targets, and improve the prediction of treatment response and resistance mechanisms.

Alongside this, the application of AI and machine learning (ML) algorithms is expected to transform clinical decision-making. By analyzing vast datasets generated from NGS and other molecular assays, AI-based predictive models can help stratify patients, optimize treatment selection, and anticipate patterns of recurrence or resistance with greater accuracy than conventional methods.

Another promising avenue is immunogenomic profiling, particularly relevant for cervical carcinoma, where the etiologic role of HPV provides a distinct immunologic context. High-resolution profiling of immune cell infiltrates, checkpoint molecule expression, and antigen presentation pathways may enable more precise tailoring of immunotherapies, such as checkpoint inhibitors or adoptive T-cell therapies, to individual patient profiles.

Finally, the development of personalized neoantigen vaccines represents a frontier in immunotherapy. By leveraging tumor-specific mutations identified through NGS, it becomes possible to design bespoke vaccines aimed at stimulating a robust and durable immune response against cancer cells, especially in HPV-positive tumors, where viral and host-derived antigens coexist as potential therapeutic targets.

Together, these emerging strategies highlight a future in which cervical cancer treatment is increasingly data-driven, immune-informed, and tailored at the individual patient level, pushing beyond the current boundaries of targeted therapy and immunotherapy [72, 73].

Conclusions

Next-Generation Sequencing has revolutionized the landscape of cervical cancer research and clinical care. It provides insights into tumor biology, helps identify actionable targets, and enables precision medicine approaches. While challenges remain, especially in low-resource settings, the integration of NGS into cervical cancer diagnostics and treatment planning is poised to improve outcomes through individualized care.

NGS in Hereditary Gynecologic Cancer Syndromes

Introduction

Hereditary gynecologic cancer syndromes comprise a subset of gynecologic malignancies resulting from germline mutations in cancer predisposition genes. The most recognized syndromes include Hereditary Breast and Ovarian Cancer (HBOC), primarily due to BRCA1/2 mutations, and Lynch Syndrome (LS), involving MMR genes. Advances in NGS have revolutionized the detection of these genetic alterations, enabling simultaneous analysis of multiple genes with high sensitivity, specificity, and speed [74–76].

Overview of Hereditary Gynecologic Cancer Syndromes

(a) Hereditary Breast and Ovarian Cancer

Hereditary Breast and Ovarian Cancer (HBOC) syndrome is a well-characterized genetic predisposition syndrome, most commonly caused by germline pathogenic variants in BRCA1 and BRCA2. These two high-penetrance tumor suppressor genes are integral to HRR, and their loss-of-function leads to genomic instability and an increased susceptibility to tumorigenesis. HBOC is associated with markedly elevated lifetime risks for both breast and ovarian cancers, often exceeding 70% and 40%, respectively, depending on the specific gene and mutation involved.

Cancers arising in the context of HBOC tend to exhibit a younger age at onset, bilateral or multifocal presentation, and distinct histopathologic features. In the case of ovarian cancer, HBOC is strongly associated with the HGSOC, which represents the most aggressive and genomically unstable variant of epithelial ovarian tumors. These tumors often display a "BRCAness" phenotype, characterized by genomic scars and sensitivity to DNA-damaging agents such as platinum compounds and PARPi.

Although BRCA1 and BRCA2 account for the majority of HBOC cases, a subset of patients harbor mutations in other genes involved in the homologous recombination pathway, such as PALB2, RAD51C, RAD51D, and BRIP1. These genes also confer increased cancer risk—albeit generally lower than BRCA mutations and are now routinely included in multigene panel testing. Importantly, carriers of pathogenic variants in these non-BRCA genes may also benefit from enhanced surveillance, risk-reducing strategies, and PARP inhibitor therapy, supporting their clinical relevance in the broader context of hereditary cancer predisposition.

As our understanding of HBOC continues to evolve, the use of comprehensive germline testing and personalized genetic counseling has become increasingly important for appropriate risk assessment, early detection, and the selection of preventive and therapeutic interventions tailored to each individual's genetic profile [77].

(b) Lynch Syndrome

LS, also known as hereditary non-polyposis colorectal cancer (HNPCC), is an autosomal dominant cancer predisposition syndrome caused by germline pathogenic variants in one of the DNA mismatch repair (MMR) genes: MLH1, MSH2, MSH6, or PMS2 or, less frequently, by epigenetic silencing via EPCAM gene deletions that lead to downstream inactivation of MSH2. These mutations impair the cellular ability to correct base-pair mismatches during DNA replication, resulting in accumulated replication errors and microsatellite instability (MSI), a molecular hallmark of the syndrome.

While classically associated with early-onset colorectal cancer, LS is also strongly linked to gynecologic malignancies, particularly endometrial carcinoma, which is often the sentinel neoplasm, preceding colorectal cancer in female carriers. Lynch-associated endometrial cancers typically arise at a younger age than sporadic cases and frequently display endometrioid or clear cell histology, along with high MSI and loss of MMR protein expression by immunohistochemistry. Ovarian cancers associated with LS are less common but tend to occur at an earlier age and are more often of endometrioid or clear cell subtype, distinct from the high-grade serous histotype seen in BRCA-associated disease.

Identification of LS has critical implications for cancer surveillance, risk-reducing interventions, and cascade testing among relatives. Clinical suspicion is traditionally based on family history patterns meeting Amsterdam or revised Bethesda criteria, which consider factors such as multiple affected family members, early-onset disease, and the presence of synchronous or metachronous Lynch-associated tumors.

With the advent of universal screening for MMR deficiency in endometrial and colorectal cancers, the diagnosis of LS is increasingly reliant on molecular testing, including immunohistochemistry for MMR proteins, MSI testing, and confirmatory germline sequencing. Early detection not only guides patient management but also enables implementation of risk-reducing strategies, such as prophylactic hysterectomy and bilateral salpingo-oophorectomy, which significantly reduce gynecologic cancer risk in mutation carriers [78].

Clinical Utility of NGS in Hereditary Gynecologic Cancer Syndromes

(a) Early and Accurate Diagnosis

NGS enables rapid and accurate detection of germline mutations, offering critical support for risk stratification, targeted surveillance, and preventive strategies, such as risk-reducing salpingo-oophorectomy. For example, identifying BRCA1/2 mutations not only informs hereditary cancer risk management but also determines eligibility for PARP inhibitor therapy, directly linking genetic profiling to therapeutic decision-making.

(b) Multigene Panel Testing

Compared to single-gene testing, NGS-based multigene panels offer a broader diagnostic scope, increasing the detection rate of pathogenic variants, including mutations in non-BRCA genes such as *RAD51C/D* and MMR genes. However, they also frequently identify VUS, whose clinical interpretation requires caution and expert evaluation [79, 80].

(c) Cascade Testing and Family Counseling

NGS results play a pivotal role in guiding cascade testing for at-risk relatives, enabling opportunities for early detection or preventive interventions. Genetic counseling remains essential to address the implications of a positive result, navigate the uncertainty of VUS, and support individuals in managing the psychological and reproductive impacts of hereditary cancer risk [81].

Limitations and Challenges of NGS in Clinical Practice

One of the key challenges in clinical implementation of NGS is the management of VUS, which are relatively common, particularly in underrepresented or less-studied populations. These findings can create significant ambiguity in clinical decision-making, as their pathogenicity remains unclear. Proper interpretation of NGS data requires robust bioinformatic pipelines, experienced laboratories, and strict adherence to established classification frameworks, such as the ACMG (American College of Medical Genetics and Genomics) guidelines, to ensure consistency and accuracy. Moreover, the expansion of genomic testing raises important ethical and psychosocial concerns, including the possibility of incidental findings in genes unrelated to gynecologic malignancies, as well as the broader impact of genetic results on family dynamics, personal identity, and reproductive planning. Thoughtful pre- and post-test counseling is therefore indispensable to support patients through this complex landscape [82].

Future Directions

One promising development is the use of polygenic risk scores (PRS), which integrate the cumulative effect of multiple low-penetrance genetic variants. Enabled by large-scale NGS data, PRS may enhance individualized risk prediction, particularly when combined with clinical and familial factors. Another important innovation is the integration of germline and somatic testing through tumor-normal paired sequencing, which allows for the accurate distinction between inherited and acquired mutations. This approach improves interpretation and may uncover actionable somatic alterations that guide personalized therapeutic strategies. Additionally, the application of liquid biopsy, NGS performed on cell-free DNA (cfDNA) obtained from peripheral blood or uterine lavage, is gaining traction as a minimally invasive tool for early cancer detection, monitoring treatment response, and evaluating MRD. These evolving methodologies hold considerable promise for improving patient outcomes through earlier intervention and dynamic, genome-informed management [83].

Conclusions

NGS has transformed the landscape of hereditary gynecologic oncology. It facilitates comprehensive genetic assessment, guides precision medicine, and supports risk reduction strategies. Its implementation must be accompanied by genetic counseling, standardized interpretation, and ethical safeguards to maximize benefit and minimize harm.

Challenges and Limitations of NGS in Gynecologic Cancer

NGS has become a cornerstone in the molecular profiling of gynecologic malignancies, enabling personalized treatment strategies and risk stratification. However, despite its transformative potential, several technical, biological, economic, and ethical barriers limit its optimal clinical application. This chapter outlines these challenges, with a focus on variant interpretation, tumor heterogeneity, costs and logistics, and ethical-legal considerations.

Technical Issues and Variant Interpretation

Quality and Quantity of DNA/RNA Samples

FFPE tissue remains the most widely used specimen type in routine clinical pathology due to its compatibility with histologic evaluation and long-term storage. However, the formalin fixation process introduces significant challenges for molecular analysis. It can lead to nucleic acid fragmentation, cross-linking, and chemical modifications, such as cytosine deamination, which may result in sequencing artifacts, reduced coverage, and compromised variant calling accuracy. These effects are particularly pronounced in older or poorly fixed samples.

Additionally, tumor cellularity and sample integrity critically influence the reliability of NGS. Biopsy specimens from gynecologic tumors, including endometrial and cervical cancers, may exhibit extensive necrosis, inflammation, or low neoplastic cell content, all of which can hinder the extraction of high-quality DNA or RNA. Low tumor purity may dilute somatic variants below the threshold of detection, increasing the risk of false negatives, especially for low-allele frequency mutations. Careful assessment of tissue quality, tumor content, and pre-analytical variables is therefore essential to ensure robust and clinically meaningful NGS results [14, 84].

Variant Classification and Clinical Actionability

Interpreting the clinical significance of genetic variants remains one of the most challenging aspects of NGS in gynecologic oncology. Differentiating pathogenic mutations from benign polymorphisms or VUS is particularly complex when involving less-characterized genes or novel alterations not previously described in public databases. The lack of functional validation or population frequency data for many such variants further complicates their classification and clinical interpretation [85].

In gynecologic cancers, commonly altered genes such as PIK3CA, PTEN, and ARID1A frequently yield variants whose predictive or prognostic value remains unclear. While these genes are recurrently mutated across various tumor types, the therapeutic implications of specific alterations, especially outside of known hotspots, are still under investigation. Consequently, the actionability of many detected variants is limited, often precluding their direct use in guiding treatment decisions. This underscores the importance of integrating molecular data with histopathologic context, clinical parameters, and multidisciplinary expertise to avoid overinterpretation and ensure appropriate patient management [86].

Tumor Heterogeneity and Subclonal Mutations

Intra-tumoral Heterogeneity

Gynecologic malignancies, particularly HGSOC, are characterized by marked spatial and temporal heterogeneity. This intratumoral diversity reflects the dynamic evolution of the cancer genome over time and across different anatomical sites. As a result, tumors often harbor subclonal populations with distinct mutational profiles, some of which may confer therapeutic resistance or metastatic potential.

This heterogeneity poses a major challenge for next-generation sequencing, as sampling bias can lead to incomplete genomic characterization. Biopsies obtained from a single site may fail to capture the full spectrum of genetic alterations present within the tumor mass or at metastatic loci. Furthermore, limited sequencing depth may miss low-frequency subclonal mutations that could be clinically relevant, particularly in the context of treatment resistance or disease relapse. To mitigate these limitations, strategies such as multi-regional sampling, high-depth sequencing, and longitudinal monitoring through liquid biopsy are increasingly explored to achieve a more comprehensive and dynamic view of the tumor genome [87].

Temporal Heterogeneity and Treatment Resistance

Tumor evolution under therapeutic pressure represents a critical limitation of static, single-timepoint genomic testing. In gynecologic cancers, particularly those treated with chemotherapy or PARP inhibitors, the selective pressure exerted by therapy can drive the emergence of acquired resistance mutations. A well-documented example is the development of BRCA reversion mutations, which restore homologous recombination proficiency and render tumors resistant to PARP inhibition despite an initial BRCA-deficient status.

Because standard NGS testing is typically performed at diagnosis or relapse, it may fail to capture these dynamic molecular changes, leading to a misrepresentation of the current tumor biology. This is especially relevant in the context of recurrent or refractory disease, where treatment decisions based on outdated molecular profiles may be suboptimal. Re-biopsy and longitudinal molecular monitoring, including the use of liquid biopsy to detect evolving genomic alterations in real time, are increasingly recognized as important strategies to adapt therapy to the tumor's changing molecular landscape [88].

Cost, Turnaround Time, and Reimbursement

Financial and Logistical Constraints

Despite their growing clinical utility, comprehensive NGS approaches, such as large gene panels, WES, or WGS, remain cost-intensive and are not yet universally accessible. The financial burden associated with these technologies including sequencing, data interpretation, and reporting—is substantial, and reimbursement policies vary widely across countries, healthcare systems, and insurance providers. In many settings, only limited panels targeting a small number of actionable genes are covered, restricting the broader adoption of more informative but expensive assays [89, 90].

Moreover, the TAT for comprehensive NGS testing often exceeds 2–4 weeks, especially in centralized or high-throughput laboratories. This delay can significantly impact clinical decision-making in urgent scenarios, such as rapidly progressing disease or time-sensitive surgical or therapeutic planning. Streamlining workflows, expanding in-house testing capabilities, and advocating for broader reimbursement are essential steps toward integrating NGS more seamlessly into routine clinical practice.

Inequitable Access and Resource Limitations

Access to advanced genomic testing remains uneven, with significant limitations in low-resource settings and many community-based hospitals. Infrastructure constraints, lack of specialized personnel, and limited availability of validated NGS platforms often preclude the implementation of comprehensive molecular diagnostics outside of tertiary academic centers. As a result, many patients with gynecologic malignancies do not benefit from precision oncology approaches that rely on genomic profiling for risk stratification, targeted therapy selection, or trial eligibility.

This disparity contributes to a growing inequity in cancer care, where the promise of personalized medicine is realized only for those treated in well-resourced institutions. Bridging this gap will require concerted efforts to democratize access through technological innovation, decentralized testing solutions, international collaboration, and policy changes that promote equitable delivery of molecular diagnostics across healthcare systems [91].

Ethical and Legal Considerations

Incidental and Secondary Findings

NGS can incidentally uncover germline mutations that are unrelated to the patient's current cancer diagnosis, raising important ethical and clinical considerations. For instance, BRCA1/2 mutations may be detected during sequencing performed for endometrial cancer, even if the patient has no personal or family history suggestive of hereditary breast and ovarian cancer. Such secondary or incidental findings carry potential implications not only for the patient's future cancer risk but also for at-risk relatives, necessitating comprehensive genetic counseling and informed consent protocols before testing.

The management and disclosure of incidental findings must align with institutional policies and national guidelines, such as the American College of Medical Genetics and Genomics (ACMG) recommendations, which provide a framework for reporting actionable secondary findings. Ensuring that patients understand the possibility and implications of such results is essential to uphold ethical standards, protect patient autonomy, and facilitate appropriate follow-up, including cascade testing for family members when indicated.

Informed Consent and Privacy

Informed consent is a critical component of NGS in clinical practice, as patients must clearly understand the scope of testing, including which genes will be analyzed, how results will be reported, and the possibility of identifying incidental or secondary findings. Consent discussions should also address data storage, privacy, and sharing, as genomic data may be retained for future reanalysis or research purposes. Beyond clinical implications, patients should be made aware of potential insurance and employment ramifications, particularly concerning life, long-term care, or disability insurance, where protection against genetic discrimination is often incomplete despite existing legislation.

From a regulatory perspective, data privacy and patient protection are governed by frameworks such as the General Data Protection Regulation (GDPR) in Europe and the Health Insurance Portability and Accountability Act (HIPAA) in the United States. While these laws establish standards for data security, confidentiality, and secondary use, their implementation and enforcement remain variable, and cross-border data sharing introduces additional complexity. A robust consent process, combined with institutional policies aligned to these legal frameworks, is essential to safeguard patient rights in the era of precision medicine [93].

Duty to Recontact

A growing ethical and logistical challenge in the era of NGS is the management of variant reclassification over time. VUS are frequently identified during genomic testing, and as scientific knowledge evolves, some of these may later be reclassified as pathogenic or likely pathogenic, with direct implications for patient care and familial risk assessment. This dynamic raises the question of whether clinicians or testing laboratories carry an obligation to recontact patients when such reclassifications occur [94].

Currently, clear and universally accepted policies are lacking, leaving institutions to navigate these situations on a case-by-case basis. Implementing a structured recontact strategy poses significant logistical and ethical challenges, including maintaining long-term patient traceability, allocating resources for ongoing variant surveillance, and defining the respective responsibilities of laboratories and healthcare providers. As genomic medicine continues to advance, developing standardized guidelines for variant reclassification communication will be essential to balance patient safety, ethical duty, and practical feasibility.

Conclusions

While NGS has revolutionized the diagnostic and therapeutic landscape of gynecologic oncology, its full integration into routine clinical practice remains hindered by a combination of technical, biological, economic, and ethical challenges. Technical hurdles include the need for high-quality nucleic acids, optimized sequencing platforms, and robust bioinformatic pipelines capable of managing and interpreting complex genomic data. Biological barriers, such as tumor heterogeneity, subclonality, and the evolution of resistance under therapeutic pressure, can limit the accuracy and durability of a single molecular snapshot. Economically, the high cost of comprehensive NGS testing and inconsistent insurance reimbursement restrict access for many patients, particularly in community settings or low-resource environments. Ethically, genomic testing raises questions surrounding informed consent, incidental findings, variant reclassification, data privacy, and long-term patient follow-up.

Overcoming these obstacles will require a multifaceted strategy. Central to this effort is the standardization of interpretation frameworks, including the application of ACMG and ESMO guidelines, to ensure uniform reporting and clinically meaningful classification of variants. Parallel investments in bioinformatics infrastructure and specialized training are essential to support the growing volume and complexity of genomic data. On a systemic level, policy initiatives must address access disparities, reimbursement mechanisms, and legal clarity to support equitable implementation of precision oncology. Equally important is the establishment of robust informed consent processes and pre- and post-test counseling frameworks, enabling patients to understand the implications of genomic testing for themselves and their families.

Looking ahead, the future of NGS in gynecologic oncology will likely be shaped by real-time tumor profiling, liquid biopsy applications for dynamic monitoring, and AI-driven variant interpretation, which together promise to reduce diagnostic ambiguity and enhance therapeutic precision. As technologies evolve and costs continue to decline, NGS is poised to become a fully integrated pillar of gynecologic cancer care, maximizing its clinical impact and bringing the vision of personalized oncology closer to everyday practice.

Future Directions in NGS for Gynecologic Oncology

NGS has established itself as a foundational tool in the molecular profiling of gynecologic cancers. Looking ahead, a more refined, integrated, and minimally invasive approach to cancer diagnostics and treatment is emerging. Innovations such as liquid biopsy, artificial intelligence (AI), digital pathology, and multi-omics are set to reshape personalized medicine and precision oncology in gynecology.

Liquid Biopsy and Circulating Tumor DNA

Overview and Mechanism

Liquid biopsy represents a minimally invasive approach to tumor genomic assessment through the analysis of circulating tumor-derived material in body fluids, most commonly blood. It primarily focuses on ctDNA but may also include circulating tumor cells (CTCs), exosomes, and other tumor-associated biomarkers. In gynecologic malignancies, ctDNA carries tumor-specific genetic and epigenetic alterations, providing a dynamic molecular snapshot of the disease that complements or, in certain contexts, may even substitute for traditional tissue biopsies.

The applications of liquid biopsy are diverse and clinically significant. Early detection is an area of active investigation, as ctDNA may identify neoplastic changes before they become radiologically or clinically apparent. Monitoring of MRD is another promising use, allowing clinicians to detect molecular evidence of persistence or recurrence after surgery or systemic therapy, potentially guiding adjuvant treatment decisions. Moreover, liquid biopsy can identify emerging resistance mutations, such as BRCA reversion variants in patients treated with PARP inhibitors, providing insights into mechanisms of treatment failure. Finally, by enabling real-time tracking of tumor evolution, liquid biopsy offers the possibility of longitudinal disease monitoring, capturing spatial and temporal heterogeneity that may be missed by a single-site tissue biopsy [95].

As technologies improve, liquid biopsy is expected to become an integral component of precision oncology in gynecologic cancers, offering earlier intervention opportunities and facilitating the dynamic adaptation of therapy to the evolving molecular landscape of the tumor.

Applications in Gynecologic Oncology

In ovarian cancer, ctDNA has emerged as a valuable biomarker closely correlated with tumor burden, treatment response, and risk of recurrence. Rising ctDNA levels can precede radiologic evidence of relapse, offering an opportunity for earlier detection of disease progression. Moreover, ctDNA analysis can reveal BRCA reversion mutations, which restore homologous recombination repair and confer resistance to PARP inhibitors, providing crucial information for therapeutic decision-making and trial enrolment [96].

In endometrial and cervical cancers, ctDNA similarly captures tumor-specific genomic alterations, including recurrent mutations in PIK3CA, PTEN, and TP53. The detection of these mutations in plasma or other body fluids supports the use of ctDNA as a non-invasive tool for molecular profiling, which may facilitate disease monitoring, minimal residual disease (MRD) assessment, and the identification of actionable variants when tissue availability is limited [97].

As evidence continues to accumulate, ctDNA profiling is poised to complement standard imaging and tissue-based diagnostics, enhancing real-time molecular surveillance and guiding personalized therapy across gynecologic malignancies.

Challenges and Future Directions

Despite its promise, liquid biopsy still faces several important limitations. Sensitivity remains a major challenge in early-stage disease, where the amount of ctDNA is often extremely low, increasing the risk of false-negative results and limiting its utility for early detection or MRD assessment. The field also requires standardized pre-analytical and analytical protocols, along with clinically validated assays, to ensure reproducibility, accuracy, and comparability of results across laboratories and clinical trials.

For optimal clinical impact, liquid biopsy is best integrated with tissue-based NGS, allowing for comprehensive molecular profiling that captures both the baseline genomic architecture of the tumor and its dynamic evolution under treatment pressure. This combined approach maximizes diagnostic yield, supports informed therapeutic decision-making, and lays the foundation for the routine incorporation of liquid biopsy into precision oncology workflows.

Integration with Artificial Intelligence and Digital Pathology

Digital Pathology and Whole-Slide Imaging

The adoption of digital pathology has transformed traditional histopathology by enabling the digitization, storage, and computational analysis of whole-slide images (WSI). This technological shift not only facilitates remote access and archiving but also creates the foundation for AI and ML applications in diagnostic pathology.

AI-powered algorithms can uncover subtle histomorphologic patterns that may correlate with underlying molecular alterations, such as MSI or TP53 mutation status, supporting the integration of histology with genomic insights. In addition, digital pathology enables the automation of key quantitative tasks, including tumor grading, mitotic index assessment, and the quantification of tumor-infiltrating lymphocytes (TILs), improving reproducibility and reducing interobserver variability.

As computational pathology continues to advance, the synergy between AI-driven image analysis and molecular profiling is expected to enhance diagnostic precision and support the development of fully integrated, data-driven workflows in gynecologic oncology [98, 99].

AI in Genomics and Predictive Modeling

AI is increasingly being applied to the analysis of complex NGS data, offering new opportunities to enhance precision oncology in gynecologic cancers. By leveraging advanced machine learning and deep learning algorithms, AI can predict treatment response, such as estimating sensitivity to PARPi based on integrated genomic features and HRD profiles.

Beyond predictive modeling, unsupervised learning approaches can uncover novel driver mutations and molecular signatures that may not be apparent through conventional statistical methods, expanding the understanding of tumor biology and potential therapeutic targets. AI can also stratify patients into molecularly defined subtypes with distinct prognostic and therapeutic implications, supporting personalized treatment selection and clinical trial design.

As computational models become increasingly sophisticated, the integration of AI with NGS and digital pathology holds the potential to generate multi-omic, data-driven insights, ultimately improving patient outcomes and accelerating the translation of genomic discoveries into clinical practice [100].

Future Outlook

The integration of AI into clinical workflows is poised to transform the management of gynecologic cancers by providing real-time decision support during multidisciplinary tumor boards. AI-powered platforms can rapidly synthesize genomic, radiologic, and histopathologic data, offering actionable insights to guide diagnosis, prognostication, and therapeutic selection.

Emerging hybrid models that combine digital pathology, radiomics, and genomics exemplify the next frontier of precision oncology. These multi-modal systems aim to capture the full biological complexity of tumors, correlating imaging features with molecular alterations and histologic patterns. Such integrative approaches promise to enhance diagnostic accuracy, optimize patient stratification, and accelerate the transition toward fully data-driven, personalized cancer care.

Conclusions

The integration of NGS into gynecologic oncology has fundamentally reshaped the diagnostic and therapeutic paradigms of uterine, ovarian, and cervical malignancies. From refining molecular classification and identifying actionable mutations to guiding targeted therapies and familial risk assessment, NGS enables a more personalized and precise approach to patient care. However, its full clinical potential will only be realized through the systematic resolution of technical, interpretative, economic, and ethical challenges. Future directions including liquid biopsy, artificial intelligence, digital pathology, and multi-omic integration promise to enhance the dynamic understanding of tumor evolution and therapeutic response. As the field moves toward a fully integrated precision oncology model, NGS will remain a cornerstone, guiding individualized treatment and contributing to improved outcomes for women with gynecologic cancers.

Appendix

Biomarker	Gene(s)/pathway	Tumor type(s)	Clinical relevance	Detection method
BRCA1/2	Homologous recombination repair	High-grade serous ovarian carcinoma (HGSOC)	PARP inhibitor sensitivity; familial cancer risk	NGS (germline + somatic); MLPA; sanger
HRD (homologous recombination deficiency)	BRCA1/2, RAD51C/D, PALB2, etc.	Ovarian, endometrial	Predicts response to platinum/PARP inhibitors	NGS + HRD genomic scar assays
POLE ultramutated	POLE exonuclease domain	Endometrial carcinoma (endometrioid, grade 3)	Excellent prognosis; avoids overtreatment	NGS panel (POLE hotspot mutations)
MMR deficiency (MMRd)	MLH1, MSH2, MSH6, PMS2	Endometrial, ovarian (endometrioid, clear cell)	MSI; lynch syndrome screening; immunotherapy response	IHC; MSI-PCR; NGS
TP53 mutation	TP53	HGSOC, uterine serous carcinoma	Poor prognosis; guides adjuvant therapy	NGS; IHC surrogate (p53 overexpression/null)
ARID1A loss	ARID1A	Clear cell and endometrioid carcinomas	Associated with MMRd and immune activation	IHC; NGS
PIK3CA/PTEN/AKT	PI3K pathway	Endometrial carcinoma (endometrioid)	Potential for PI3K/mTOR inhibitors	NGS hotspot panels
MSI-high	Indirect of MMRd	Endometrial, ovarian	Predicts response to immune checkpoint inhibitors	MSI-PCR; NGS-based MSI calling
CTNNB1 (β-catenin)	WNT pathway	Endometrial carcinoma (low-grade)	Favorable prognosis; low risk of recurrence	NGS; IHC (nuclear β-catenin)

References

1. Goodwin S, McPherson JD, McCombie WR. Coming of age: ten years of next-generation sequencing technologies. Nat Rev Genet. 2016;17(6):333–51. https://doi.org/10.1038/nrg.2016.49.
2. Mardis ER. Next-generation sequencing platforms. Annu Rev Anal Chem. 2013;6:287–303. https://doi.org/10.1146/annurev-anchem-062012-092628.
3. Roychowdhury S, Chinnaiyan AM. Translating genomics for precision cancer medicine. Annu Rev Genomics Hum Genet. 2014;15:395–415. https://doi.org/10.1146/annurev-genom-090413-0255121.2.
4. Cancer Genome Atlas Research Network, Kandoth C, Schultz N, et al. Integrated genomic characterization of endometrial carcinoma. Nature. 2013;497(7447):67–73. https://doi.org/10.1038/nature121135.
5. Norquist BM, Brady MF, Harrell MI, et al. Mutations in homologous recombination genes and outcomes in ovarian carcinoma patients in GOG 218: an NRG oncology/gynecologic oncology group study. Clin Cancer Res. 2018;24(4):777–83. https://doi.org/10.1158/1078-0432.CCR-17-2217.
6. Zugazagoitia J, Guedes C, Ponce S, Ferrer I, Molina-Pinelo S, Paz-Ares L. Current challenges in cancer treatment. Clin Ther. 2016;38(7):1551–66. https://doi.org/10.1016/j.clinthera.2016.03.026.
7. He J, Abdel-Wahab O, Nahas MK, et al. Integrated genomic DNA/RNA profiling of hematologic malignancies in the clinical setting. Blood. 2016;127(24):3004–14. https://doi.org/10.1182/blood-2016-01-688705.
8. Vellone VG. Advancements in gynecologic pathology: a molecular, digital, and biobanking perspective. Clin Exp Obstet Gynecol. 2024;51(6):131. https://doi.org/10.31083/j.ceog5106131.
9. Liu L, Li Y, Li S, et al. Comparison of next-generation sequencing systems. J Biomed Biotechnol. 2012;2012:251364. https://doi.org/10.1155/2012/251364.
10. Logsdon GA, Vollger MR, Eichler EE. Long-read human genome sequencing and its applications. Nat Rev Genet. 2020;21(10):597–614. https://doi.org/10.1038/s41576-020-0236-x.
11. Sović I, Križanović K, Skala K, Šikić M. Evaluation of hybrid and non-hybrid methods for de novo assembly of nanopore reads. Bioinformatics. 2016;32(17):2582–9. https://doi.org/10.1093/bioinformatics/btw237.
12. Yang Y, Muzny DM, Xia F, et al. Molecular findings among patients referred for clinical whole-exome sequencing. JAMA. 2014;312(18):1870–9. https://doi.org/10.1001/jama.2014.14601.
13. Belkadi A, Bolze A, Itan Y, et al. Whole-genome sequencing is more powerful than whole-exome sequencing for detecting exome variants. Proc Natl Acad Sci USA. 2015;112(17):5473–8. https://doi.org/10.1073/pnas.1418631112.
14. Srinivasan M, Sedmak D, Jewell S. Effect of fixatives and tissue processing on the content and integrity of nucleic acids. Am J Pathol. 2002;161(6):1961–71. https://doi.org/10.1016/S0002-9440(10)64472-0.
15. VanderLaan PA. Molecular markers: implications for cytopathology and specimen collection. Cancer Cytopathol. 2015;123(8):454–60. https://doi.org/10.1002/cncy.21560.
16. Gailey MP, Stence AA, Jensen CS, Ma D. Multiplatform comparison of molecular oncology tests performed on cytology specimens and formalin-fixed, paraffin-embedded tissue. Cancer Cytopathol. 2015;123(1):30–9. https://doi.org/10.1002/cncy.21476.
17. Jennings LJ, Arcila ME, Corless C, et al. Guidelines for validation of next-generation sequencing–based oncology panels: a joint consensus recommendation of AMP and CAP. J Mol Diagn. 2017;19(3):341–65. https://doi.org/10.1016/j.jmoldx.2017.01.011.
18. Naito Y, Aburatani H, Amano T, et al. Clinical practice guidance for next-generation sequencing in cancer diagnosis and treatment (edition 2.1). Int J Clin Oncol. 2021;26(2):233–83. https://doi.org/10.1007/s10147-020-01831-6.
19. Petrackova A, Vasinek M, Sedlarikova L, et al. Standardization of sequencing coverage depth in NGS: recommendation for detection of clonal and subclonal mutations in cancer diagnostics. Front Oncologia. 2019;9:851. Published 2019 Sep 4. https://doi.org/10.3389/fonc.2019.00851.
20. Cancer Genome Atlas Research Network. Integrated genomic analyses of ovarian carcinoma. Nature. 2011;474(7353):609–15. https://doi.org/10.1038/nature10166.
21. The Cancer Genome Atlas Research Network. Integrated genomic and molecular characterization of cervical cancer. Nature. 2017;543(7645):378–84. https://doi.org/10.1038/nature21386.
22. Zannoni GF, Vellone VG, Arena V, et al. Does high-grade endometrioid carcinoma (grade 3 FIGO) belong to type I or type II endometrial cancer? A clinical-pathological and immunohistochemical study. Virchows Arch. 2010;457(1):27–34. https://doi.org/10.1007/s00428-010-0939-z.
23. Paleari L, Pesce S, Rutigliani M, et al. New insights into endometrial cancer. Cancers (Basel). 2021;13(7):1496. Published 2021 Mar 24. https://doi.org/10.3390/cancers1307149625.
24. Paudice M, Biatta CM, Scaglione G, et al. Histopathological and immunohistochemical prognostic factors in high-grade non-Endometrioid carcinomas of the endometrium (HG-NECs): is it possible to identify subgroups at increased risk? Diagnostics (Basel). 2023;13(13):2171. Published 2023 Jun 26. https://doi.org/10.3390/diagnostics13132171.
25. Paudice M, Greppi M, Valle L, et al. The role of the androgen receptor (AR) in endometrial cancer aggressiveness: correlation with other prognostic markers and therapeutic implications. A

mutant cancers. Nature. 2018;554(7691):189–94. https://doi.org/10.1038/nature25475.
72. Abrar SS, Isa SAM, Hairon SM, Ismail MP, Kadir MNBNA. Recent advances in applications of machine learning in cervical cancer research: a focus on prediction models. Obstet Gynecol Sci. 2025;68(4):247–59. https://doi.org/10.5468/ogs.25041.
73. Zou J, Lin Z, Jiao W, et al. A multi-omics-based investigation of the prognostic and immunological impact of necroptosis-related mRNA in patients with cervical squamous carcinoma and adenocarcinoma. Sci Rep. 2022;12(1):16773. Published 2022 Oct 6. https://doi.org/10.1038/s41598-022-20566-0.
74. Vellone VG, Paudice M, Varesco L. Hereditary non-BRCA gynecological tumors. Minerva Ginecol. 2016;68(5):579–86.
75. Wang Q. Cancer predisposition genes: molecular mechanisms and clinical impact on personalized cancer care: examples of lynch and HBOC syndromes. Acta Pharmacol Sin. 2016;37(2):143–9. https://doi.org/10.1038/aps.2015.
76. LaDuca H, Polley EC, Yussuf A, et al. A clinical guide to hereditary cancer panel testing: evaluation of gene-specific cancer associations and sensitivity of genetic testing criteria in a cohort of 165,000 high-risk patients. Genet Med. 2020;22(2):407–15. https://doi.org/10.1038/s41436-019-0633.
77. Suszynska M, Ratajska M, Kozlowski P. BRIP1, RAD51C, and RAD51D mutations are associated with high susceptibility to ovarian cancer: mutation prevalence and precise risk estimates based on a pooled analysis of ~30,000 cases. J Ovarian Res. 2020;13(1):50. Published 2020 May 2. https://doi.org/10.1186/s13048-020-00654-3.
78. Trujillo-Rojas MA, Ayala-Madrigal ML, Gutiérrez-Angulo M, González-Mercado A, Moreno-Ortiz JM. Diagnosis of patients with Lynch syndrome lacking the Amsterdam II or Bethesda criteria. Hered Cancer Clin Pract. 2023;21(1):21. Published 2023 Oct 20. https://doi.org/10.1186/s13053-023-00266-0.
79. Bunnell AE, Garby CA, Pearson EJ, Walker SA, Panos LE, Blum JL. The clinical utility of next generation sequencing results in a community-based hereditary cancer risk program. J Genet Couns. 2017;26(1):105–12. https://doi.org/10.1007/s10897-016-9985-2.
80. McDevitt T, Durkie M, Arnold N, et al. EMQN best practice guidelines for genetic testing in hereditary breast and ovarian cancer. Eur J Hum Genet. 2024;32(5):479–88. https://doi.org/10.1038/s41431-023-01507.
81. Kurian AW, Ward KC, Howlader N, et al. Genetic testing and results in a population-based cohort of breast cancer patients and ovarian cancer patients. J Clin Oncol. 2019;37(15):1305–15. https://doi.org/10.1200/JCO.18.01854.
82. Burke W, Parens E, Chung WK, Berger SM, Appelbaum PS. The challenge of genetic variants of uncertain clinical significance : a narrative review. Ann Intern Med. 2022;175(7):994–1000. https://doi.org/10.7326/M21-4109.
83. Kuchenbaecker KB, Hopper JL, Barnes DR, et al. Risks of breast, ovarian, and contralateral breast cancer for BRCA1 and BRCA2 mutation carriers. JAMA. 2017;317(23):2402–16. https://doi.org/10.1001/jama.2017.7112.
84. Pisapia P, Pepe F, Iaccarino A, et al. Next generation sequencing in cytopathology: focus on non-small cell lung cancer. Front Med (Lausanne). 2021;8:633923. Published 2021 Feb 11. https://doi.org/10.3389/fmed.2021.633923.
85. Richards S, Aziz N, Bale S, et al. Standards and guidelines for the interpretation of sequence variants: a joint consensus recommendation of the American College of Medical Genetics and Genomics and the Association for Molecular Pathology. Genet Med. 2015;17(5):405–24. https://doi.org/10.1038/gim.2015.30.
86. Urick ME, Bell DW. Clinical actionability of molecular targets in endometrial cancer. Nat Rev Cancer. 2019;19(9):510–21. https://doi.org/10.1038/s41568-019-0177-x.
87. McPherson A, Roth A, Laks E, et al. Divergent modes of clonal spread and intraperitoneal mixing in high-grade serous ovarian cancer. Nat Genet. 2016;48(7):758–67. https://doi.org/10.1038/ng.3573.
88. Quigley D, Alumkal JJ, Wyatt AW, et al. Analysis of circulating cell-free DNA identifies multiclonal heterogeneity of BRCA2 reversion mutations associated with resistance to PARP inhibitors. Cancer Discov. 2017;7(9):999–1005. https://doi.org/10.1158/2159-8290.CD-17-0146.
89. Meric-Bernstam F, Brusco L, Shaw K, et al. Feasibility of large-scale genomic testing to facilitate enrollment onto genomically matched clinical trials. J Clin Oncol. 2015;33(25):2753–62. https://doi.org/10.1200/JCO.2014.60.4165.
90. Roychowdhury S, Chinnaiyan AM. Translating cancer genomes and transcriptomes for precision oncology. CA Cancer J Clin. 2016;66(1):75–88. https://doi.org/10.3322/caac.21329.
91. Ferreira-Gonzalez A, Ko G, Fusco N, et al. Barriers and facilitators to next-generation sequencing use in United States oncology settings: a systematic review. Future Oncol. 2024;20(35):2765–77. https://doi.org/10.1080/14796694.2024.2390821.
92. Kalia SS, Adelman K, Bale SJ, et al. Recommendations for reporting of secondary findings in clinical exome and genome sequencing, 2016 update (ACMG SF v2.0): a policy statement of the American College of Medical Genetics and Genomics. Genet Med. 2017;19(2):249–55. https://doi.org/10.1038/gim.2016.190.
93. Appelbaum PS, Parens E, Waldman CR, et al. Models of consent to return of incidental findings in genomic research. Hast Cent Rep. 2014;44(4):22–32. https://doi.org/10.1002/hast.328.

94. Bombard Y, Brothers KB, Fitzgerald-Butt S, et al. The responsibility to Recontact research participants after reinterpretation of genetic and genomic research results. Am J Hum Genet. 2019;104(4):578–95. https://doi.org/10.1016/j.ajhg.2019.02.025.
95. Martinelli C, Ercoli A, Vizzielli G, et al. Liquid biopsy in gynecological cancers: a translational framework from molecular insights to precision oncology and clinical practice. J Exp Clin Cancer Res. 2025;44(1):140. Published 2025 May 8. https://doi.org/10.1186/s13046-025-03371-1.
96. Parkinson CA, Gale D, Piskorz AM, et al. Exploratory analysis of TP53 Mutations in circulating tumour DNA as biomarkers of treatment response for patients with relapsed high-grade serous ovarian carcinoma: a retrospective study. PLoS Med. 2016;13(12):e1002198. Published 2016 Dec 20. https://doi.org/10.1371/journal.pmed.1002198.
97. Ju HY, Ho JY, Kang J, et al. Whole-exome sequencing reveals clinical potential of circulating tumor DNA from peritoneal fluid and plasma in endometrial cancer. Cancers (Basel). 2022;14(10):2506. Published 2022 May 19. https://doi.org/10.3390/cancers14102506.
98. Madabhushi A, Lee G. Image analysis and machine learning in digital pathology: challenges and opportunities. Med Image Anal. 2016;33:170–5. https://doi.org/10.1016/j.media.2016.06.03102.
99. Bera K, Schalper KA, Rimm DL, Velcheti V, Madabhushi A. Artificial intelligence in digital pathology – new tools for diagnosis and precision oncology. Nat Rev Clin Oncol. 2019;16(11):703–15. https://doi.org/10.1038/s41571-019-0252-y.
100. Esteva A, Robicquet A, Ramsundar B, et al. A guide to deep learning in healthcare. Nat Med. 2019;25(1):24–9. https://doi.org/10.1038/s41591-018-0316-z.

Next Generation Sequencing in Cutaneous Pathology

10

Mario Della Mura, Joana Sorino, Anna Colagrande, Lucia Lospalluti, Giuseppe Ingravallo, and Gerardo Cazzato

Abbreviations

ALM	Acral Lentiginous Melanoma
AK	Actinic keratoses
AKT	AKT Serine/Threonine Kinase 1
ALK	ALK Receptor Tyrosine Kinase
ARID1A	AT-Rich Interaction Domain 1A
ARID1B	AT-Rich Interaction Domain 1B
AST	Atypical Spitz Naevus
ATM	ATM Serine/Threonine Kinase
ATRX	ATRX Chromatin Remodeler
BAP1	BRCA1 Associated Deubiquitinase 1
BCC	Basal cell carcinoma
BRAF	V-raf Murine Sarcoma Viral Oncogene Homolog B
CLIP1	CAP-Gly Domain Containing Linker Protein 1
CTNNB1	Catenin Beta 1
CCND1	Cyclin D1
CDK4	Cyclin Dependent Kinase 4
CDKN2A	Cyclin Dependent Kinase Inhibitor 2A
CHD8	Chromodomain Helicase DNA Binding Protein 8
c-Myc	MYC Proto-Oncogene, BHLH Transcription Factor
CNA	Copy Number Alteration
CSD	Cumulative Solar Damage
CM	Cutaneous Melanoma
CYSLTR2	Cysteinyl Leukotriene Receptor 2
CTNNB1	Catenin Beta 1
DM	Desmoplastic Melanoma
DCTN1	Dynactin Subunit 1
DHH	Desert hedgehog
EGFR	Epidermal Growth Factor Receptor
EIF1AX	Eukaryotic Translation Initiation Factor 1A X-Linked
ERBB2	v-erb-b2 Avian Erythroblastic Leukemia Viral Oncogene Homolog 2
ERC1	ELKS/RAB6-Interacting/CAST Family Member 1

M. D. Mura · J. Sorino · A. Colagrande · G. Ingravallo
G. Cazzato (✉)
Section of Molecular Pathology, Department of Precision and Regenerative Medicine and Ionian Area (DiMePRe-J), University of Bari "Aldo Moro", Bari, Italy
e-mail: j.sorino@studenti.uniba.it; giuseppe.ingravallo@uniba.it; gerardo.cazzato@uniba.it

L. Lospalluti
Section of Dermatology and Venereology, Department of Precision and Regenerative Medicine and Ionian Area (DiMePRe-J), University of Bari "Aldo Moro", Policlinico of Bari, Bari, Italy
e-mail: lucia.lospalluti@policlinico.ba.it

© The Author(s), under exclusive license to Springer Nature Switzerland AG 2026
S. Sioletic, L. Coppola (eds.), *Next-Generation Sequencing in Solid Tumor Histopathology*, Current Clinical Pathology, https://doi.org/10.1007/978-3-032-18790-1_10

ERK	Extracellular Signal-Regulated Kinases
FAMMM	Familial Atypical Multiple Mole Melanoma Syndrome
EZH2	Enhancer of Zeste 2 Polycomb Repressive Complex 2 Subunit
FAMMM	Familial Atypical Multiple Mole Melanoma Syndrome
FISH	Fluorescence In Situ Hybridization
GNA11	G Protein Subunit Alpha 11
GNAQ	G Protein Subunit Alpha Q
HH	Hedgehog
HLA-A	Major Histocompatibility Complex, Class I, A
HPV	human papillomavirus
IAMPUS	Intraepidermal Atypical Melanocytic Proliferation of Uncertain Significance
IHH	Indian hedgehog
KIF5B	Kinesin Family Member 5B
laBCC	locally advanced
LMNA	Lamin A/C
LMM	Lentigo Maligna Melanoma
MIS	Mediator Complex Subunit 12Melanoma in situ
MAP2K1	Mitogen-Activated Protein Kinase Kinase
MAP3K1	Mitogen-Activated Protein Kinase Kinase Kinase 1
MAP3K8	Mitogen-Activated Protein Kinase Kinase Kinase 8
MAPK (mBCC)	Mitogen-Activated Protein Kinases
MDM2	MDM2 Proto-Oncogene
MET	MET Proto-Oncogene, Receptor Tyrosine Kinase
MiTF	Melanocyte Inducing Transcription Factor
MM	Mucosal Melanoma
MYO5A	Myosin VA
NF1	Neurofibromatosis 1
NGS	Next-Generation Sequencing
NOTCH2	Notch Receptor 2
NRAS	Neuroblastoma RAS Viral v-ras Oncogene Homolog
NTRK1	Neurotrophic Receptor Tyrosine Kinase 1
PI3K	Phosphatidylinositol-4,5-Bisphosphate 3-Kinase
PIK3CA	Phosphatidylinositol-4,5-Bisphosphate 3-Kinase Catalytic Subunit Alpha
PLCB4	Phospholipase C Beta 4
PRC	Polycomb Repressive Complex
PTEN	Phosphatase And Tensin Homolog
PWWP2A	PWWP Domain Containing 2A
RAC1	Rac Family Small GTPase 1
RAF1	Raf-1 Proto-Oncogene, Serine/Threonine Kinase
RASGRF1	Ras Protein Specific Guanine Nucleotide Releasing Factor 1
RET	Ret Proto-Oncogene
ROS	ROS Proto-Oncogene, Receptor Tyrosine Kinase
SCCIS	Squamous cell carcinoma in situ
SF3B1	Splicing Factor 3b Subunit 1
SHH	Sonic hedgehog
SM	Spitz Melanoma
SMARCA4	SWI/SNF Related BAF Chromatin Remodeling Complex Subunit ATPase 4
SN	Spitz Nevus
SOS2	SOS Ras/Rho Guanine Nucleotide Exchange Factor 2
SPRED1	Sprouty Related EVH1 Domain Containing 1
SSM	Superficial Spreading Melanoma
TAX1BP1	Tax1 Binding Protein 1
TERT	Telomerase Reverse Transcriptase
TMB	Tumor mutational burden
TPM3	Tropomyosin 3
UM	Uveal Melanoma
UVR	Ultraviolet Radiation
XP	Xeroderma Pigmentosum
WES	Whole-exome sequencing
WGS	Whole-genome sequencing

Introduction

In recent years, advances in molecular diagnostics have profoundly transformed the field of dermatopathology. The advent of next-generation sequencing (NGS) has allowed for the high-throughput and comprehensive analysis of genetic alterations underlying a wide range of cutaneous neoplasms, providing insights that were previously inaccessible with conventional techniques. Through the simultaneous assessment of multiple genes, NGS has revealed the complex molecular landscapes that drive tumor initiation, progression, and therapeutic resistance in both melanocytic and non-melanocytic skin tumors. Historically, the diagnosis of cutaneous neoplasms has relied primarily on morphological and immunohistochemical features. While these approaches remain the cornerstone of dermatopathologic practice, the integration of genomic data has refined tumor classification, uncovered novel diagnostic and prognostic biomarkers, and opened new avenues for precision medicine. Indeed, several skin tumors once defined solely by histopathology are now recognized as genetically distinct entities characterized by specific driver mutations or gene fusions. In the context of melanoma, NGS has been instrumental in delineating the molecular subtypes described by The Cancer Genome Atlas (TCGA), linking particular genetic alterations to distinct clinicopathologic and prognostic features. Similarly, in non-melanoma skin cancers such as basal cell carcinoma, squamous cell carcinoma, and Merkel cell carcinoma, NGS has clarified the pivotal roles of UV-induced mutagenesis, viral oncogenesis, and key signaling pathways—including Hedgehog, MAPK, and PI3K/AKT—in tumorigenesis. Furthermore, recent studies have extended NGS applications to the rare and heterogeneous group of adnexal neoplasms, identifying recurrent fusions and mutations that contribute to their molecular taxonomy. Beyond diagnostic and classification purposes, NGS plays an increasingly critical role in clinical decision-making. The identification of actionable mutations has enabled the development of targeted therapies and immunotherapeutic strategies, marking a shift toward individualized treatment approaches in cutaneous oncology. At the same time, the detection of germline variants has improved recognition of hereditary cancer syndromes associated with cutaneous tumors, with important implications for patient management and familial screening. This review aims to provide a comprehensive overview of the applications of NGS in cutaneous pathology, summarizing current knowledge on the molecular mechanisms, diagnostic implications, and therapeutic perspectives across major categories of skin neoplasms.

Melanocytic Tumors

Melanoma

General Features

Melanoma is a malignant tumor originating from melanocytes in the skin, mucous membranes, uvea, and, more rarely, other tissues (e.g., leptomeninges) [1]. Changing diagnostic criteria, a greater number of biopsies, and increased risk behaviors (tanning beds, etc.) are likely the major risk factors for the increased incidence [2]. According to data from [3], there are more new cases among Whites than in any other racial group, with a different overall 5-year relative survival ranging from 99.3% for localized melanoma (melanoma in situ, MIS), to 68% for regional disease and to 29.8% for metastatic disease.

Etiology and Molecular Biology

The extensive use of Next Generation Sequencing (NGS) in recent years has led to a greater understanding of the mutations underlying and determining the different melanoma subtypes, allowing for the molecular delineation of what had previously been defined solely by morphology and, subsequently, supplemented by ancillary immunohistochemistry methods [4]. It is known that melanoma is not a single disease but rather several types of neoplasms, with different molecular pathways involved, melanocyte subpopulations, clinical, histological, and mutational features [5]. Melanoma is usually sporadic (90%) with only a minority of cases linked to hereditary syndromes such as Familial Atypical Multiple

Mole Melanoma Syndrome (FAMMM), BAP1 Tumor Predisposition Syndrome and Xeroderma Pigmentosum (XP). In all cases, **ultraviolet radiation** (UVR) is of primary importance in the genesis of melanoma, and more generally of melanocytic lesions, and the molecular mechanism involves initiation through *gain-of-function* alterations generated by point mutations, gene fusions, or gene amplifications that cause a constitutive activation of growth-promoting signaling pathways [3]. This phenomenon led to the presence of partially transformed clones of melanocytes that can undergo an oncogene-induced senescence mechanism (in which case they are controlled by tumor suppressor genes giving rise to a benign nevus) rather than progressing to a further step responsible for the intermediate or frankly malignant state of the melanocytic lesion (mainly alterations such as loss of tumor suppressor genes linked to inactivating mutations, deletions, epigenetic silencing) [6].

The most important signaling pathways involved in the pathogenesis of melanoma are:

1. MAP/ERK pathway, required for melanocyte proliferation and survival, of which BRAFV600E hotspot mutation is the most common, constituting approximately 50% of cutaneous melanoma (CM) mutations, with *NRAS* and *NF1* loss also being present (25% and 10% of cases, respectively). Low-CSD melanomas are frequently associated with BRAFV600E mutations, while NRAS, NF1, and non-BRAFV600E mutations are associated with high-CSD melanomas [7]. Less than 5% of melanomas are RAS-mutated within KRAS or HRAS [8].
2. The PI3K/AKT pathway, which promotes cell proliferation, motility, metabolism and survival. PTEN is a tumor suppressor that prevents the activation of AKT, and the loss of PTEN is strongly associated with an adverse prognosis in CM [9].
3. CDK4/RB pathway (so-called CDKN2A), comprising the tumor suppressor gene p16 (INK4A) and p14 (ARF), inactivation of which is linked to progression of melanoma [3, 10].
4. Gαq pathway: mutation in GNAQ and GNA11 as well as CYSLTR2 or PLCB4 are mutually exclusive and lead to constitutive activation of the downstream signaling and are virtually present in all uveal melanomas and melanoma arising in blue nevi [3, 11].
5. TERT can be mutated in the promoter region in approximately 70% of CM, in 30–41% of acral melanoma and 8% of mucosal melanomas, with associated poor prognosis [3, 12].
6. Mutation and/or amplifications of KIT that encode the c-KIT receptor tyrosine kinase (involved in signaling pathways like MAPK/ERK, PI3K/AKT and MITF) are described in 39% of mucosal melanomas, 36% of acral melanomas and 28% of melanoma on chronically sun-damaged skin [3, 13].
7. BAP1, a deubiquitinase that acts on histone H2A and is involved in chromatin modification and transcriptional regulation, is a tumor suppressor gene of which inactivation can occur by deletions or loss of function mutations [3]. It is known that the inactivation of BAP1 is a secondary driver mutation in uveal melanoma and also in melanoma arising in blue nevi [14].
8. Chromatin remodeling complexes such as SWI/SNF and PRC play a central role in shaping gene expression and, ultimately, the behavior of cancer cells. The SWI/SNF complex, typically acting as a tumor suppressor, helps "open" chromatin to make DNA more accessible for transcription. When key subunits like ARID1A or SMARCA4 are altered, this balance is disrupted, leading to increased tumor aggressiveness and therapy resistance. On the other hand, the Polycomb Repressive Complex (PRC)—particularly PRC2—silences tumor-suppressor genes through histone modifications such as H3K27 trimethylation, reinforcing the malignant cell's ability to adapt and survive. Within this intricate network, the small GTPase Rac Family Small GTPase 1 (RAC1), frequently mutated in melanoma, not only regulates cytoskeletal dynamics and intracellular signaling but also interacts with epigenetic regulators like SWI/SNF and PRC. Together, these

systems form a subtle but powerful interplay between gene activation and repression, shaping the plasticity and invasiveness that characterize melanoma [3].

The mutational landscape of melanoma includes:

1. Point mutations, of which 70–80% are canonical UV-signature type such as C → T transitions with a preceding pyrimidine base.
2. Structural alterations, such as copy number alterations (CNA) accumulating during the progression of melanoma and that include chromosomal gains (1q, 5p, 6p, 7, 8q, 11q, 17q and 20) and losses (6q, 8p, 9p, 9q, 10q and 11q).
3. Chromosomal rearrangements and chromothripsis [3].

Genetic predisposition to melanoma involves high-penetrance genes such as CDKN2A, CDK4, BAP1 and TERT, among others. On the other hand, low-to moderate-penetrance genes confer a smaller risk, but the combination with other risk factors can be enhance the effects. Examples of these genes are Melanocortin 1 Receptor (MC1R), MiTF and others. FAMMM is a rare autosomal dominant disorder caused by germline mutation in the CDKN2A gene which encodes the tumor suppressor protein p16. This leads to aberrant activation of CDK4 and CDK6, promoting cell cycle progression and, ultimately, cell replication. The syndrome is characterized by numerous (>50) moles, often atypical/dysplastic with higher risk of pancreatic cancer. BAP1 tumor predisposition syndrome is an autosomal dominant disease caused by biallelic inactivation in BAP1 gene which encodes for a deubiquitinase with tumor suppressor activity. The syndrome is characterized by BAP1-inactivated melanocytomas, melanomas including uveal melanoma, renal cell carcinoma, mesothelioma and others.

Melanoma: TGCA Classification and Multidimensional Model

Although the first classification proposed by Clark et al. in 1973 distinguished melanoma based on histopathological and clinical criteria into four major categories—superficial spreading melanoma (SSM), lentigo maligna melanoma (LMM), nodular melanoma (NM), and acral lentiginous melanoma (ALM)—in 2015 the Cancer Genome Atlas (TCGA) Network established a genomic classification of cutaneous melanoma (CM) based on distinct combinations of mutated genes. The major subtypes, in order of frequency, include:

1. BRAF subtype, characterized by BRAF hotspot mutations, most commonly V600E, followed by V600K and V600R.
2. RAS subtype, defined by hotspot mutations in RAS genes, most frequently NRAS (Q61R, Q61K, Q61L, and Q61H), but also HRAS and KRAS.
3. NF1 subtype.
4. Triple wild-type subtype, comprising tumors lacking the above mutations but harboring alterations in genes such as GNAQ, GNA11, EZH2, KIT, and CTNNB1.

The recent fifth edition of the World Health Organization (WHO) Classification of Skin tumors integrates epidemiologic, clinical, histopathological, and molecular features into distinct "pathways," each encompassing several melanoma subtypes and their respective precursor lesions.

Melanomas Arising in Sun-Exposed Skin

Pathway I: Low-Cumulative Solar Damage (Low-CSD)/SSM

Recognized as the most common form of melanoma in Western countries, SSM is molecularly characterized by BRAFV600E mutations in 70% of cases and NRAS mutations in 15%, with a secondary oncogenic mutation that include TERT promoter (already present in the MIS and also in some dysplastic nevi), additional activating mutations in other MAPK-pathway genes and CDKN2A biallelic inactivation in the invasive melanoma. Finally, mutations in TP53 and PTEN are described in advanced melanoma [3, 15, 16]. Regarding CNA (present in intermediate/MIS and also in the invasive CM) it was described gains of chromosome 1q, 6p, 7, 8q, 17q and 20q with loss of 9p, 10 and 21q [3].

Precursor lesions are recognized to be benign melanocytic nevi, melanocytomas (BAP1-inactivated, Deep Penetrating, Epithelioid Pigmented Melanocytoma) and MIS.

Pathway II: High-CSD Melanoma/LMM

LMM uncommonly harbor BRAFV600E mutation, with initial driver including NF1, non-BRAFV600E, NRAS and KIT mutations. The secondary oncogenic drivers include CCND1, TERT, RAC1, CDKN2A, ARID2, TP53 and PTEN. Regarding CNA, there were described the copy number gain of chromosome 1q, 6p, 11q13, 17q and 20q, with loss of 6q, 8p, 9p, 13 and 21q. LMM is characterized by a high Tumor Mutational Burden (TMB) with an average of 20 mutations per Mbps of DNA [3, 17]. Precursor lesion is Lentigo Maligna-type MIS.

Pathway III: Desmoplastic Melanoma (DM)

DM is molecularly characterized by initiating driver mutations like inactivation of NF1, amplification of receptor tyrosine kinase genes EGFR, MET and ERBB2, mutations of MAP2K1, MAP3K1, non-BRAFV600E, non-canonical NRAS, RAC1 and SOS2 [3, 18]. The secondary pathogenic mutations include inactivation of CDKN2A and TP53 and this type of melanoma has a very high TMB (average 62 mutations/MB) that results in being a rational for immune checkpoint blockade therapy [18, 19]. The only recognized precursor lesion is MIS [3].

Melanomas Arising at Sun-Shielded Sites or Without Known Etiological Associations with UVR Exposure

Pathway IV: Malignant Spitz Tumor (Spitz Melanoma, SM)

More than 50% of Spitz tumors are characterized by translocations involving the receptor tyrosine kinases ALK, ROS, NTRK1/3, RET, MET, MAP3K8, BRAF or RASGRF1, in a mutually exclusive pattern. For ALK-rearranged Spitz tumor the described fusion partners include Tropomyosin 3 (TPM3) and Dynactin Subunit 1 (DCTN1), while multiple fusion partners are described for ROS-rearranged Spitz lesions such as PWWP Domain Containing 2A (PWWP2A), ELKS/RAB6-Interacting/CAST Family Member 1 (ERC1), Myosin VA (MYO5A), CAP-Gly Domain Containing Linker Protein 1 (CLIP1), Major Histocompatibility Complex, Class I, A (HLA-A), among others. Regarding NTRK1/3-rearranged Spitz tumors, the most common fusion is Lamin A/C (LMNA)::NTRK1 but recently new fusion partners were described such as Peroxiredoxin 1 (PRDX1) [3, 20–22]. Common fusion partners for RET-rearranged neoplasms are represented by Kinesin Family Member 5B (KIF5B) and Golgin A5 (GOLGA5), while BRAF fusion are detected by Fluorescence in situ Hybridization (FISH) and/or NGS and recently there were described new partner genes such as Tax1 Binding Protein 1 (TAX1BP1) [3, 23–25]. Twenty percent of Spitz tumors harbor HRAS mutations (most commonly HRASQ61K/R in exon 3) with a typical copy number gain of chromosome 11p. The secondary oncogenic event includes TERT promoter mutation and loss of CDKN2A [3].

Precursor lesions are Spitz nevus and Atypical Spitz nevus (melanocytoma).

Pathway V: Acral Melanoma
Two subtypes of melanoma originate from acral skin: BRAFV600E mutant and acral melanoma without BRAFV600E mutation. First one is similar to low-CSD/SSM (pathway I) and both have a low TMB and high incidence of copy number variations and amplifications in somatic genes such as KIT, BRAF, NRAS, NF1, KRAS, HRAS, SPRED1 and MAPK21. Uncommonly there are BRAF and RAS mutations and multiple gene amplifications including CCND1, MITF, TERT and others are described [26, 27]. Secondary driving mutations include inactivation of CDKN2A, TP53 and PTEN. Known precursor lesions are Lentigo Maligna-MIS and Intraepidermal Atypical Melanocytic Proliferation of Uncertain Significance (IAMPUS).

Pathway VI: Mucosal Melanoma
MM has a low TMB and high burden of copy number changes, including amplifications of Cyclin Dependent Kinase 4 (CDK4), MDM2 Proto-Oncogene (MDM2), MiTF, TERT, CCND1, Notch Receptor 2 (NOTCH2), deletions of PTEN, NF1, SPRED1, CDKN2A, ATM Serine/Threonine Kinase (ATM), ARID1B and structural rearrangements. Furthermore, recurrent somatic mutations involve SPRED1, Splicing Factor 3b Subunit 1 (SF3B1), NF1, KIT, NRAS or BRAF. Finally, additional mutations include Catenin Beta 1 (CTNNB1), KRAS, MAP2K1, PTEN, CDKN2A, TP53, Chromodomain Helicase DNA Binding Protein 8 (CHD8) and ATRX Chromatin Remodeler (ATRX) [28, 29]. Precursor lesion is recognized to be mucosal MIS [3, 28].

Pathway VII: Melanoma Arising in a Congenital Nevus
Molecularly, the most common oncogenic mutation is NRASQ61R, with BRAFV600E and BRAF fusions described less frequently and also rare cases of ALK and Raf-1 Proto-Oncogene, Serine/Threonine Kinase (RAF1) fusions. Sometimes TERT promoter mutation can be found [3, 30]. Precursor lesions are recognized to be congenital nevus, proliferative nodule in congenital nevus and MIS in congenital nevus.

Pathway VIII: Melanoma Arising in a Blue Nevus
There is a considerable similarity between uveal melanoma and melanoma in blue nevi with mutually exclusive driver mutations in GNAQ, GNA11, PLCB4 or CYSLTR2. Furthermore, biallelic inactivation of BAP1, point mutations of SF3B1 and Eukaryotic Translation Initiation Factor 1A X-Linked (EIF1AX) are associated with transformation [3, 31]. As in UM, loss of BAP1 on chromosome 3p21 or gains/amplifications of MYC Proto-Oncogene, BHLH Transcription Factor (c-Myc) on chromosome 8q24 indicate a worse prognosis. There is not BRAFV600E mutation. Precursor lesions are blue nevus and atypical blue nevus.

Pathway IX: Uveal Melanoma
From a molecular point of view, the initiating driving mutations (usually mutually exclusive) include GNAQ, GNA11 (>90% of cases), less frequently CYSLTR2 and PLCB4. Secondary somatic alterations include BAP1, SF3B1 and EIF1AX and, cytogenetically, there are recurrent CAN such as gains of 1q, 6p and 8q and losses of 1p, 3, 8p and 16q. Tertiary recurrent mutations involve loss of function of CDKN2A, PTEN, among others and gain of function of EZH2, PIK3CA and MED12, with also possible loss of heterozygosity in the GNAQ gain of function mutation [3, 32].

NGS in Melanoma

NGS is very useful in the diagnosis of difficult melanocytic lesions, particularly for molecular pathway classification and for prognostic purposes (Fig. 10.1).

- **Clinical Indications.**
  - **Differential diagnosis between high dysplastic nevus and early melanoma**: NGS can identify the type and the number of mutations which helps in the exact classification of the neoplasms; for example, the presence of TERT promoter mutation as well as a high TMB can strongly suggest the diagnosis of melanoma.

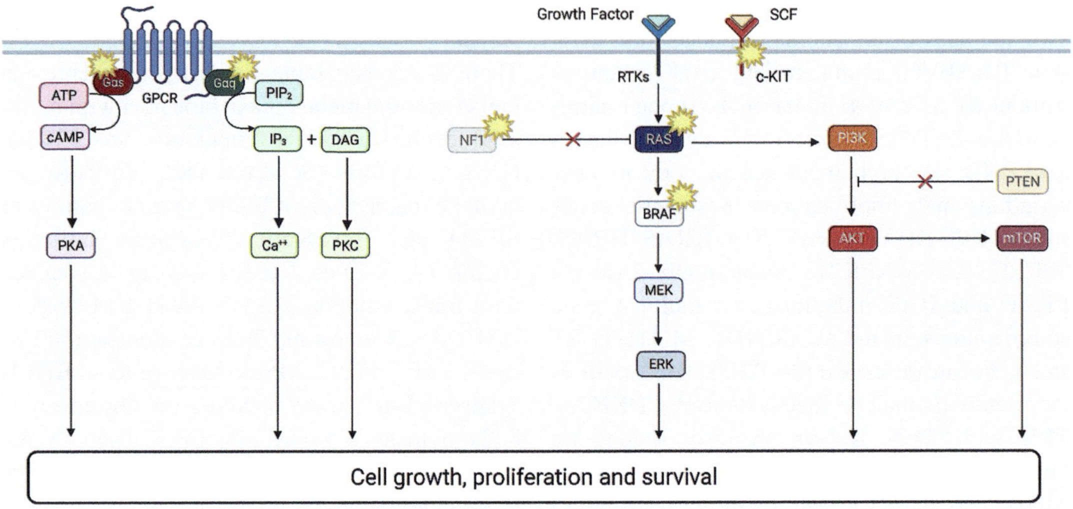

Fig. 10.1 Main molecular pathways in development of melanoma. (Created in BioRender)

- **Molecular Pathway classification**: Molecular profiling may assist in the differential diagnosis, helping to classify the melanocytic tumors into a specific pathway; for example, the recognition of kinase fusion translocations or HRAS mutation is useful to ascribe a lesion into the Spitz molecular pathway, when immunohistochemistry is not conclusive.
- **Detection of germline mutations**: NGS can identify germline alterations associated with familiar melanoma syndrome.
- **Differential diagnosis between primitive/secondary melanoma**: NGS can help to delineate the molecular background of the lesion, and, in case of metastatic disease, show an overlapping molecular pattern.
- **Therapeutic approaches**: NGS can identify the actionable molecular targets for tailored therapy as well as give information about the landscape of resistance mechanisms to the drugs. For example, a high TMB is linked to a better response to immune-checkpoint inhibitors, while c-KIT mutation is predictive to response to tyrosinase kinases inhibitors such as Imatinib.

- **Research Applications.**
  - To improve understanding of the pathogenesis and molecular landscape of melanoma.
  - To identify novel therapeutic targets and support the development of targeted therapies.

Non-melanoma Skin Cancer (NMSC)

Basal Cell Carcinoma

General Features

Basal cell carcinoma (BCC) refers to a family of epithelial malignancies arising from either the interfollicular epidermis or hair follicle stem cells. It is the most prevalent form of skin cancer worldwide, primarily affecting chronically sun-exposed areas in older individuals. Owing to its typically indolent behavior and low metastatic potential, the majority of BCCs are effectively treated with surgical excision or local therapies. However, a small subset of cases progresses to locally advanced (laBCC) or metastatic disease (mBCC), which present significant therapeutic challenges [33].

Etiology and Molecular Biology

UV radiation is the principal environmental risk factor for BCC, as evidenced by its exceptionally high mutational burden, with an average of 65 mutations per megabase (the highest among human cancers), and the presence of characteristic UV-signature mutations, including C > T and CC > TT transitions [33].

The Molecular Driver: Hedgehog (HH) Signaling Pathway Activation

The hallmark molecular event in BCC pathogenesis is the constitutive activation of the Hedgehog (HH) signaling pathway [33], which is a shared feature across lesions arising in both sun-exposed and sun-protected areas, as well as in younger patients [34, 35] (Fig. 10.2).

Virtually all hereditary BCCs (Gorlin syndrome, Bazex-Dupré-Christol syndrome) and more than 90% of sporadic cases show constitutive activation of the HH pathway. This most frequently occurs via biallelic inactivation of PTCH1 (>70% of cases) and activating mutations in SMO (10–20%); other components such as SUFU and GLI1 may also be affected.

HH pathway activation occurs in both germline and sporadic settings and has become a critical therapeutic target with the development of HH pathway inhibitors (HHIs) (e.g., vismodegib, sonidegib) [33]. Resistance to HHIs can arise

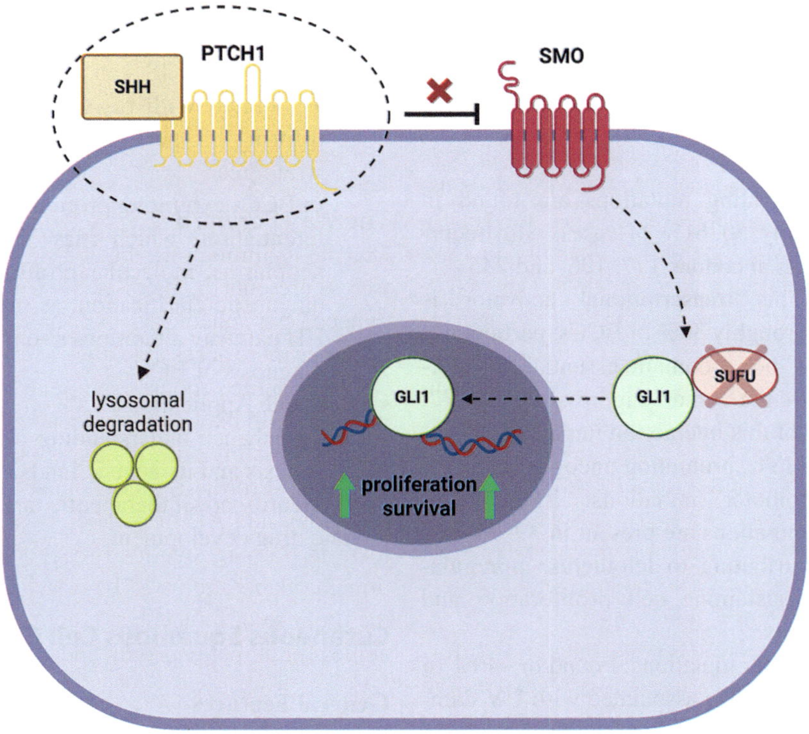

Fig. 10.2 The HH pathway is named after a family of extracellular ligands—Sonic hedgehog (SHH), Indian hedgehog (IHH), and Desert hedgehog (DHH)—which play essential roles in embryogenesis, including the development of the neural tube, musculoskeletal system, hematopoietic lineage, dentition, and skin; in contrast to embryonic development, the pathway is largely quiescent in adult tissues [36]. Under physiological conditions, its activation begins with the binding of HH ligands to the PTCH1 receptor. In the absence of ligand, PTCH1 inhibits the activity of Smoothened (SMO), a transmembrane protein responsible for propagating downstream signaling. Upon ligand binding, the HH-PTCH1 complex undergoes lysosomal degradation, thereby relieving SMO inhibition. Activated SMO initiates a signaling cascade that leads to the release of GLI transcription factors (GLI1, GLI2, GLI3) from the inhibitory complex formed with SUFU, a cytoplasmic protein that maintains GLIs in an inactive state. Once released, GLI proteins—primarily GLI1—translocate to the nucleus, where they drive the transcription of target genes involved in cell proliferation, survival, and angiogenesis [37]. (Created in BioRender)

through secondary SMO mutations or activation of parallel signaling pathways [33].

Gorlin syndrome (nevoid basal cell carcinoma syndrome) is a rare autosomal dominant disease caused by germline mutations in PTCH1 and less commonly in PTCH2 or SUFU. It presents multiple early-onset BCCs, jaw odontogenic keratocysts, skeletal anomalies, and increased risk of medulloblastoma. Tumorigenesis typically follows the "two-hit" hypothesis, whereby a second somatic mutation—often UV-induced—leads to loss of heterozygosity and malignant transformation [3, 34].

Bazex-Dupré-Christol syndrome is another rare genetic disease associated with multiple BCCs, inherited in an X-linked dominant pattern and caused by mutations in ACTRT1, resulting in increased GLI1 activity through impaired repression at the promoter level [37].

Beyond the HH pathway, several additional genes are recurrently mutated in BCC and contribute to tumorigenesis [3, 38].

- TP53: Inactivating mutations are found in approximately 50–61% of cases, with recurrent hotspots at codons 177, 196, and 245.
- MYCN: This transcriptional activator is mutated in roughly 30% of BCCs, particularly in the MYC box 1 domain, essential for interaction with the tumor suppressor FBXW7; disruption of this interaction impairs degradation of N-MYC, promoting oncogenesis.
- TERT promoter mutations: These UV-signature mutations are present in 39–74% of BCCs, contributing to telomerase upregulation, thus sustaining cell proliferation and tumorigenesis.
- DPH3 promoter mutations: Found in ~40% of cases, they are also associated with UV damage, but their functional consequences remain unclear.
- NOTCH1: Inactivating mutations in this tumor suppressor gene are found in 30–50% of BCCs, particularly in superficial subtypes, suggesting subtype-specific tumorigenic pathways and probably facilitating tumor persistence.
- DPP10: Mutations affecting this transmembrane protein, which regulates potassium channels activity involved in cell proliferation and apoptosis, were found in up to 35% of BCCs, though previous reports vary due to differences in sample size and lesion subtype.
- MAPK Pathway and Basosquamous Transformation: Secondary activating mutations in the MAPK pathway, including genes like c-FOS, may contribute to basosquamous transformation, possibly via chromatin remodeling mechanisms.

Molecular testing is not routinely required for BCC diagnosis. However, NGS may provide clinical and research value in specific settings:

- Selected Clinical Indications.
  - laBCC) or mBCC resistant to first-line therapies: NGS can uncover mutations associated with resistance to HHIs and inform personalized treatment strategies.
  - In BCCs exhibiting prominent adnexal differentiation, which may mimic adnexal neoplasms, molecular profiling can aid in diagnostic clarification, as the presence of HH pathway alterations strongly supports a diagnosis of BCC.
- Research Applications.
  - To enhance understanding of BCC pathogenesis and its genetic landscape.
- To identify novel therapeutic targets and facilitate drug development.

Cutaneous Squamous Cell Carcinoma

General Features

Cutaneous squamous cell carcinoma (cSCC) is the second most common type of non-melanoma skin cancer after BCC. It arises from keratinocytes of the epidermis, typically in chronically sun-exposed areas, and predominantly affects elderly and immunosuppressed individuals, particularly those with lighter skin pigmentation. Actinic keratoses (AKs) and squamous cell carcinoma in situ (SCCIS) are recognized precursor lesions, representing key steps in the multistage progression from photo-damaged skin to invasive carcinoma. While the majority of cases are effectively managed by surgical excision, a subset demonstrates aggressive features, including perineural invasion, local recurrence, and metastatic potential, making them worthy of attention for the identification of novel biomarkers [39].

Etiology and Pathogenesis

UV radiation (UVA and UVB) is the principal etiological factor in cSCC and accounts for its exceptionally high TMB. Characteristic UV-signature mutations, such as C > T and CC > TT transitions, are frequently observed in these tumors [40–42]. Beyond its role in inducing DNA damage, chronic UV exposure creates large areas of clinically normal skin populated by genetically altered keratinocytes, a phenomenon termed field cancerization [43]. This explains the frequent occurrence of multiple, recurrent, and clonally related lesions in sun-exposed regions.

In addition to UV exposure, other risk factors—including chronic immunosuppression (e.g., in transplant recipients), chronic inflammation, scarring, burns, topical carcinogens, arsenic, coal tar, ionizing radiation, and human papillomavirus (HPV) infection—contribute to tumorigenesis [44, 45]. Genetic predisposition further modulates susceptibility, with markedly increased risk in patients with xeroderma pigmentosum, epidermodysplasia verruciformis, oculocutaneous albinism, Bloom syndrome, and epidermolysis bullosa (Table 10.1). Patients with vitiligo also have a moderate risk of developing cSCC [42] (Table 10.1).

NGS has confirmed that sun-exposed skin exhibits a high TMB. In particular, whole-genome sequencing (WGS) of cSCC has shown an extensive mutational profile, with an average of one mutation per 30,000 base pairs [46]. These alterations frequently involve canonical driver genes such as **TP53** and **NOTCH1/2**. Although most of these mutations remain clinically silent, they provide a reservoir of precancerous clones capable of clonal expansion under selective pressures such as continued UV damage or immunosuppression. Clinically, this genetically unstable background accounts for the elevated incidence of new primary tumors in cSCC patients [47].

Molecular Biology

NGS, particularly whole-exome sequencing (WES), has revealed that cSCC harbors a highly complex genomic landscape, with multiple recurrently mutated genes contributing to tumor initiation, progression, and maintenance rather than a single dominant alteration. **TP53** is considered one of the earliest tumor suppressors functionally implicated in squamous carcinogenesis, while additional recurrent alterations involve members of the **NOTCH family (NOTCH1, NOTCH2)**, as well as **CDKN2A, FAT1**, and the **RAS family**.

Table 10.1 The main genetic syndromes associated with an increased risk of developing cSCC, with the key genes involved and the major clinical implications

Hereditary syndromes associated with cSCC		
Syndrome	Gene(s) involved	Clinical features
Xeroderma pigmentosum	NER genes (XPA–XPG, POLH)	Extreme photosensitivity, early freckling, AKs, multiple skin cancers at young age
Epidermodysplasia verruciformis	TMC6 (EVER1), TMC8 (EVER2)	Susceptibility to chronic cutaneous HPV infection, wart-like lesions, malignant transformation in sun-exposed sites
Oculocutaneous albinism	TYR, OCA2, TYRP1, SLC45A2	Hypopigmentation of skin, hair, eyes (photosensitivity and reduced UV protection)
Bloom syndrome	BLM (RecQ helicase)	Short stature, facial telangiectasias, photosensitivity, immunodeficiency, chromosomal instability
Epidermolysis bullosa	COL7A1, LAMC2, LAMB3, LAMA3	Inherited blistering disorder (chronic wounds, scarring, high risk of aggressive cSCC in recessive dystrophic form)

These genes regulate key cellular processes (cell-cycle control, keratinocyte differentiation, survival, and proliferation) and their disruption plays a critical role in carcinogenesis. In addition to these well-established molecular markers (Table 10.2), several other genes have been reported that, owing to limited evidence, are best regarded as *potential molecular markers*, requiring further studies to clarify their biological significance [39, 48–51].

- ***TP53*** is the most frequently mutated gene in cSCC, altered in 42–95% of tumors, with metastatic cSCC displaying a statistically increased prevalence of mutations relative to primary non-metastatic tumors. Mutations typically display UV-signature substitutions (C > T, CC > TT) and lead to loss of function, favoring the survival and clonal expansion of keratinocytes resistant to apoptosis [39, 46, 49, 50].
- ***NOTCH1*** and ***NOTCH2*** are also frequently inactivated, with *NOTCH1* mutations observed in up to 75% of cSCC and *NOTCH2* in 63% [48, 52]. These alterations are frequently detected in AKs and in sun-exposed skin without histological evidence of dysplasia and are considered early events in squamous carcinogenesis [53].

Table 10.2 Summary table of well-established markers associated with cSCC, with their primary functions and alteration frequencies

Established molecular markers in cSCC		
Gene	Function	Frequency (cSCC)
TP53	Tumor suppressor, regulates DNA repair, cell cycle, apoptosis	42–95%
NOTCH1, NOTCH2	Cell fate determination, keratinocyte differentiation	NOTCH1 ~75%; NOTCH2 ~63%
CDKN2A	Encodes p16^{INK4a} and p14^{ARF}; regulates RB and p53 pathways	23–45%
FAT1	Cadherin-like tumor suppressor, Hippo pathway regulation	22–60%
HRAS, KRAS, NRAS	RAS family oncogenes, MAPK pathway activation	HRAS 3–30%; KRAS 10-13%; NRAS ~5%

- ***CDKN2A***, encoding p16INK4a and p14ARF, is mutated, deleted, or inactivated in 23–45% of cSCCs. Alterations are more frequent in metastatic lesions (42%) compared to primaries (29%) [54] and play a role in the progression from AKs to invasive carcinoma [39].
- ***HRAS*** mutations, detected in 3–30% of cSCCs, represent the most common oncogenic activation in the RAS family, while ***KRAS*** (10–13%) and ***NRAS*** (~5%) occur less frequently. *HRAS* mutations are particularly enriched in cSCCs arising during **vemurafenib** therapy (60%), due to paradoxical MAPK activation under BRAF inhibition [55–57].
- ***FAT1*** encodes a cadherin-like protein belonging to the cadherin superfamily and functions as a tumor suppressor involved in keratinocyte differentiation. Mutations of *FAT1* are frequent in cSCC, with reported rates ranging from 22% to 60%, particularly involving inactivating mutations [46]. Although the precise mechanisms remain incompletely defined, data from head and neck SCC suggest that *FAT1* loss disrupts Hippo signaling by destabilizing its kinase scaffold, thereby preventing phosphorylation of of Yes-associated protein (YAP) and enabling its nuclear translocation, where YAP–TEAD complexes activate transcriptional programs that drive tumor progression [58].
- ***CARD11***, a scaffold protein for NF-κB signaling, is mutated in up to 38% of cSCCs, with many alterations driving constitutive NF-κB activity [59, 60].
- Genes involved in chromatin remodeling and histone modification, particularly ***KMT2C*** and ***KMT2D***, are frequently altered in cSCC. ***KMT2C*** exhibits inactivating mutations in ~39% of aggressive tumors, correlating with shorter recurrence-free survival, increased risk

of relapse, and bone invasion. Alterations have been reported in both primary (36%) and metastatic (43%) cSCCs. ***KMT2D*** is mutated in 69% of aggressive cases, with significantly higher mutation rates in metastatic (62%) compared to non-metastatic tumors (31%), suggesting a role in promoting aggressive disease [49, 54].

- The ***KNSTRN*** gene encodes a kinetochore-associated protein regulating anaphase onset and chromosome segregation during mitosis. UV-signature point mutations at codon 24 have been identified in 19% of cSCCs and 13% of precancerous lesions, disrupting chromatid cohesion and promoting chromosomal instability [61].
- ***RASA1***, encoding the p120-RasGAP protein, is a negative regulator of pro-oncogenic RAS signaling. Mutations have been reported in ~13% of aggressive cSCCs, with two-thirds predicted to truncate or eliminate protein function.
- ***RIPK4***, a serine/threonine kinase required for squamous epithelial differentiation [62], has been identified as a candidate tumor suppressor in cSCC, with recurrent UV-signature mutations reported in 24–28% of cases, frequently truncating or inactivating the protein [49, 52].
- ***SRCASM*** encodes a tumor suppressor platform molecule that negatively regulates Src-family kinases (SFKs) through lysosomal degradation, thereby limiting keratinocyte proliferation and promoting differentiation. Decreased *SRCASM* expression with increased SFK activity has been observed in SCCIS and cSCC compared to normal skin [63–66].

The role of NGS in cSCC is essentially related to research purposes:

- **Identification of recurrent mutations**, including key genes such as *TP53, NOTCH1/2, CDKN2A, FAT1,* and the *RAS* family, thereby establishing the molecular basis of squamous carcinogenesis.
- **Detection of potential and emerging candidates** that may contribute to tumor initiation, progression, or aggressive behavior.
- **Comparison of primary and metastatic disease**, revealing genetic differences, with certain alterations enriched in advanced cSCC.
- **Clinical translation**, allowing potentially more accurate prognostic stratification and the identification of novel biomarkers, with the future goal of developing new pathway-based therapeutic strategies.

Merkel Cell Carcinoma

General Features

Merkel cell carcinoma (MCC) is a rare but highly aggressive primary neuroendocrine carcinoma of the skin, typically arising in the dermis or subcutaneous tissue. Most cases develop on chronically sun-damaged skin and predominantly affect elderly White individuals, with a median age at diagnosis of 75 years; fewer than 5% of cases occur before the age of 50 years. Despite extensive investigation, the precise cellular origin of MCC remains unresolved. The tumor is consistently characterized by increasing incidence worldwide, aggressive clinical behavior, and poor prognosis [67, 68].

Etiology, Pathogenesis, and Molecular Biology

Advances in NGS have defined the heterogeneous pathogenesis of MCC as the interplay between UV mutagenesis and viral oncogenesis (Fig. 10.3), separating the disease into Merkel cell polyomavirus (MCPyV)-positive and MCPyV-negative tumors (Table 10.3). Finally, regardless of viral status, advanced age and immunosuppression are major predisposing risk factors [69–71].

The mutational landscape of this subtype is defined by a remarkably low TMB and the absence of a UV-induced mutational signature. Oncogenesis is primarily driven by clonal integration of the viral genome and the expression of

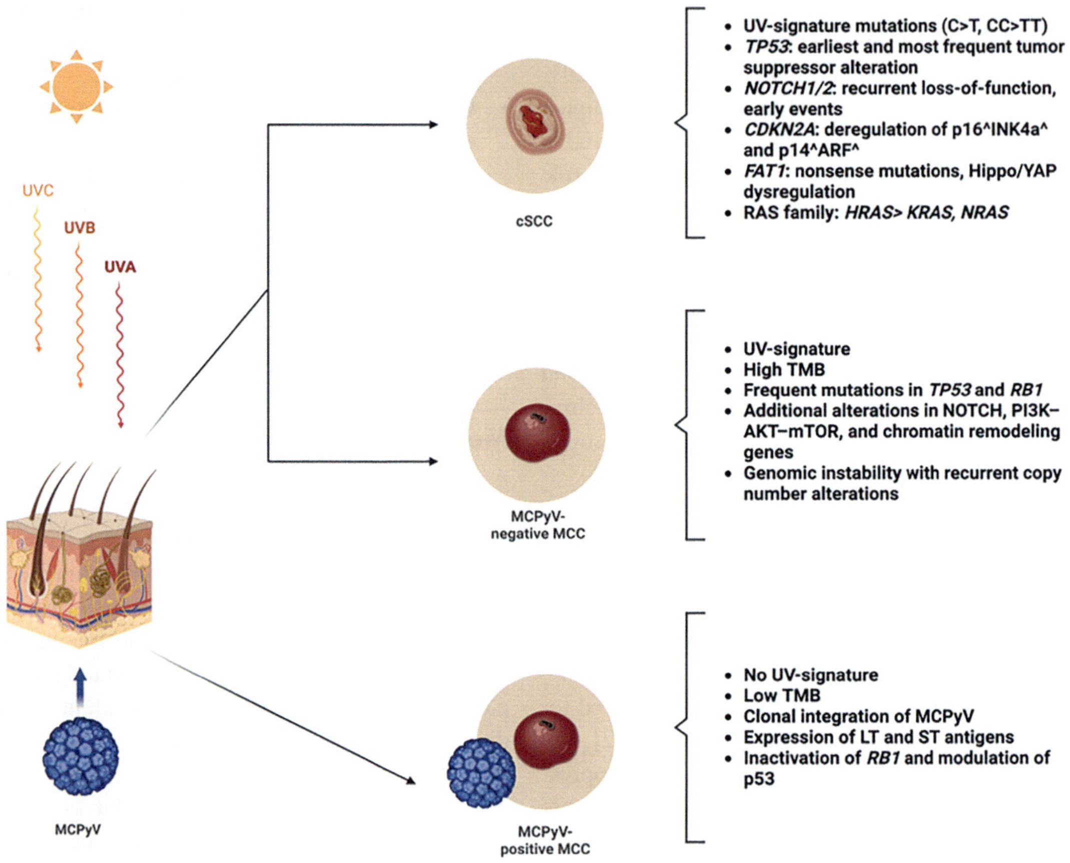

Fig. 10.3 Schematic representation of the major molecular mechanisms underlying cSCC and MCC. Chronic UV radiation induces a high TMB and UV-signature mutations in cSCC and MCPyV-negative MCC, with recurrent alterations in tumor suppressors and oncogenic pathways. In contrast, MCPyV-positive MCC is primarily driven by clonal integration of the MCPyV and expression of LT and ST antigens, leading to inactivation of RB1 and modulation of p53. (Created in BioRender (2025) https://BioRender.com/79p08hj)

the large T (LT) and small T (ST) antigens, which inactivate key tumor suppressor pathways such as RB1 and modulate p53 activity. Consistently, these tumors show low or absent RB protein expression, often resulting from RB1 copy number loss or functional inactivation of the gene. As a consequence, recurrent mutations in TP53 and RB1 are typically lacking, although occasional alterations affecting the NOTCH family or components of the PI3K–AKT pathway (e.g., KRAS, HRAS, AKT1, PIK3CA, PTEN) have been reported [70, 71].

This group presents a high TMB with a characteristic UV mutational signature dominated by C > T transitions at dipyrimidine sites. These tumors frequently harbor pathogenic alterations in *TP53* (up to 76%, including gain-of-function mutations associated with poor prognosis) and *RB1* (45–67%), along with recurrent mutations in genes involved in chromatin remodeling (*ASXL1*, *KMT2C*, *KMT2D*), stress response pathways (e.g., *MAP3K1*, *TRAF7*), and DNA damage repair (*ATM*, *MSH2*, *BRCA1*). In addition, widespread copy number alterations, particularly deletions

Table 10.3 Comparative summary of the main molecular and clinical features of MCPyV-positive and MCPyV-negative MCCs, including etiology, TMB and key genetic alterations

Comparative features of MCPyV-positive and MCPyV-negative MCCs		
	MCPyV-positive MCC	MCPyV-negative MCC
Etiology	Driven by clonal integration of MCPyV; oncogenesis via large T (LT) and small T (ST) antigens	Primarily driven by UV-induced mutagenesis
Tumor mutational burden (TMB)	Low TMB, absence of UV signature mutations	High TMB, characteristic UV signature (C > T transitions at dipyrimidine sites)
Key genetic alterations	Inactivation of RB1 through binding of LT antigen; modulation of p53 activity; occasional mutations in NOTCH, PI3K–AKT–mTOR pathway genes	Frequent mutations in TP53 (up to 76%) and RB1 (45–67%); recurrent alterations in NOTCH, chromatin remodeling genes (KMT2C, KMT2D, ASXL1), DNA repair genes (ATM, MSH2, BRCA1)

involving the 3p, 7q, and 13q regions, further contribute to genomic instability (Table 10.3).

Despite the distinct pathogenetic mechanisms that characterize MCPyV-positive and MCPyV-negative MCCs, several molecular alterations are shared across both groups. **PI3K–AKT–mTOR pathway** is frequently hyperactivated in MCC, where it sustains cellular survival and proliferation. Loss of **PTEN**, an essential tumor suppressor and negative regulator of PI3K, often results from allelic deletions at 10q23, leading to uncontrolled proliferation. Additional activating mutations in ***AKT1***, ***HRAS***, ***KRAS***, and ***PREX2***—a PTEN inhibitor—have also been reported [70, 72, 73].

The role of NGS in MCC is strictly related to research purposes:

- **Molecular classification**: distinguishes MCPyV-positive tumors from MCPyV-negative tumors.
- **Pathway analysis**: identifies alterations in PI3K–AKT–mTOR pathway and chromatin remodeling genes (*KMT2C, KMT2D, ASXL1*).
- **Copy number profiling**: reveals widespread chromosomal gains and losses, particularly enriched in virus-negative MCCs.
- **Clinical implications**: enables biomarker discovery, prognostic stratification, and identification of potential therapeutic targets.

Adnexal Neoplasm

Follicular-Derived Neoplasms

Introduction

Follicular-derived neoplasms comprise a heterogeneous group of tumors originating from hair follicle, with potential differentiation toward one or more of the epithelial and stromal components of the latter. These tumors typically exhibit benign behavior, only rarely displaying malignant features. To date, molecular data remain limited for many tumor types, often restricted to case reports or small series; no recurrent mutations have yet been identified in the majority of sporadic forms, with few exceptions [3, 74].

Trichoblastoma (Including Trichoepithelioma) and Trichoblastic Carcinoma/Carcinosarcoma

General Features

Trichoblastoma recapitulates features of the primitive hair follicle (hair germ) and follicular mesenchyme. It typically presents as a solitary nodule on the head and neck, or in association with a naevus sebaceous.

Its malignant counterpart includes trichoblastic carcinoma and trichoblastic carcinosarcoma.

Etiology and Molecular Biology

Activating *HRAS* mutations have been identified in approximately 11% of trichoblastomas. *PTCH1* mutations, commonly found in BCC, are generally absent in conventional trichoblastoma.

The trichoepithelioma subtype may arise sporadically or in association with Brooke–Spiegler syndrome. The dominant genetic driver in sporadic trichoepithelioma remains unclear. Molecular profiling of two trichoblastic carcinosarcomas has revealed inactivating mutations in tumor suppressor genes (*TP53*, *CDKN2A*), as well as oncogenic alterations (e.g., *TERT* promoter mutation, subclonal *CTNNB1* mutation).

> **Brooke–Spiegler Syndrome** is a rare autosomal dominant disorder caused by germline mutations in the ***CYLD*** gene, which encodes a deubiquitinase. This leads to aberrant activation of the **NF-κB signaling pathway**. The syndrome is characterized by **multiple cylindromas**, **spiradenomas**, and **trichoepitheliomas**, typically arising during adolescence or early adulthood, with occasional malignant transformation.

Trichilemmoma and Trichilemmal Carcinoma

General Features

Trichilemmoma shows differentiation toward the outer root sheath of the hair follicle. It typically appears as a solitary lesion, often located on the central face or within a naevus sebaceous.

Trichilemmal carcinoma is its malignant counterpart and usually has a favorable prognosis.

Etiology and Molecular Biology

Sporadic trichilemmomas and those arising within a naevus sebaceous may harbor ***HRAS*** mutations, while generally lacking PTEN alterations. By contrast, hereditary cases are associated with **Cowden syndrome**.

NGS profiling of four trichilemmal carcinomas has shown frequent *TP53* mutations and a range of additional alterations. Except for *TP53*, these mutations differ significantly from those commonly observed in squamous cell carcinoma (SCC).

> **Cowden syndrome (CS)** is a rare hereditary autosomal dominant disorder caused by germline mutations in the *PTEN* tumor suppressor gene, leading to **proteins loss** and consequent disinhibition of the **PI3K pathway. Mucocutaneous lesions** are the most common early signs, including oral papillomas, trichilemmomas, acral keratoses, followed by multisystem **hamartomas** and an increased **risk of malignancies**, particularly of the breast, thyroid, kidneys, and uterus [75].

Fibrofolliculoma / Trichodiscoma

General Features

Fibrofolliculoma/trichodiscoma demonstrates differentiation toward the hair follicle and its stromal components.

Etiology and Molecular Biology

These lesions may occur sporadically or in association with **Birt–Hogg–Dubé syndrome**. While the molecular features of sporadic lesions remain poorly characterized, syndromic cases are associated with *FLCN* mutations. The **spindle cell–predominant variant of trichodiscoma (SCPT)** is typically sporadic and may mimic spindle cell lipoma, but unlike the latter it does not show *RB1* deletion.

> **Birt–Hogg–Dubé Syndrome** is a rare inherited autosomal dominant disorder caused by mutations in the ***FLCN*** gene, which encodes the protein **folliculin** that negatively regulates the **mTORC1 signaling cascade**. The syndrome presents with **skin tumors** (fibrofolliculomas/trichodiscomas and acrochordons), **lung cysts** and increased risk of **kidney neoplasms**.

Pilomatricoma and Pilomatrical Carcinoma

General Features

Pilomatricoma and its malignant counterpart, pilomatrical carcinoma, show differentiation toward the hair matrix. Pilomatricoma is relatively common, whereas pilomatrical carcinoma is rare.

Etiology and Molecular Biology

These tumors may be hereditary or sporadic. Two key molecular mechanisms underlie pilomatrical neoplasms:

- Constitutive activation of the Wnt/β-catenin pathway: This is the most frequently observed event, present in the majority of pilomatricomas and virtually all pilomatrical carcinomas. Hereditary forms are associated with Familial Adenomatous Polyposis, whereas sporadic forms typically harbor *CTNNB1* mutations.
- Germline gain-of-function mutations in *PLCD1:* These are responsible for a minority of hereditary pilomatricomas occurring in the setting of familial pilomatricoma syndrome.

Importantly, pilomatrical carcinomas usually arise de novo, rather than from pre-existing pilomatricomas. To date, the genetic events driving progression from pilomatricoma to carcinoma remain unknown.

Familial Adenomatous Polyposis (FAP) is a hereditary cancer syndrome caused by mutations in the *APC* gene, a tumor suppressor involved in Wnt/β-catenin signaling, following an autosomal dominant inheritance pattern. Affected individuals develop hundreds to thousands of colorectal adenomatous polyps, typically in adolescence or early adulthood, and colorectal cancer, often occurring before age 40. FAP can also be associated with other tumors, including pilomatricomas.

Familial Pilomatricoma Syndrome is a rare inherited disorder characterized by multiple pilomatricomas, associated with germline mutations in the *PLCD1* gene, affecting the PKC/MAPK signaling pathway.

Other Follicular Tumors

As of this writing, the molecular genetics of several follicular tumors remain largely uncharacterized (Table 10.4). These include:

- **Trichofolliculoma.**
- **Proliferating trichilemmal tumor.**
- **Pilar sheath acanthoma.**
- **Melanocytic matricoma.**
- **Tumor of the follicular infundibulum.**

Table 10.4 Summary: molecular taxonomy of follicular-derived tumors

Neoplasm	Key molecular alterations
Trichoblastoma / Trichoepithelioma	**Hereditary**: *CYLD* mutations (Brooke–Spiegler syndrome) **Sporadic**: *HRAS* mutations (~11%)
Trichilemmoma	**Hereditary**: *PTEN* loss (Cowden syndrome) **Sporadic**: *HRAS* mutations
Trichilemmal Carcinoma	*TP53* mutations Additional variable alterations
Fibrofolliculoma / Trichodiscoma	**Hereditary**: *FLCN* mutation (Birt–Hogg–Dubé syndrome) **Sporadic**: Variable—no *RB1* deletion
Pilomatricoma	**Hereditary**: *APC* mutation (FAP syndrome; Wnt/β-catenin pathway); *PLCD1* mutations (familial pilomatricoma syndrome; PKC pathway) **Sporadic**: *CTNNB1* mutation (Wnt/β-catenin pathway)
Pilomatrical Carcinoma	**Hereditary**: *APC* mutation (FAP syndrome; Wnt/β-catenin pathway) **Sporadic**: *CTNNB1* mutation (Wnt/β-catenin pathway)

Sebaceous Neoplasms

General Features

Sebaceous neoplasm comprises an uncommon group of neoplasms arising from sebaceous glands, represented by sebaceous adenoma, sebaceoma, and sebaceous carcinoma. Recent advances in molecular profiling have revealed that these entities encompass genetically and clinically heterogeneous lesions, which differ according to anatomical site, mutational mechanisms, and histopathologic features.

Sebaceous adenoma and **sebaceoma** are purely benign neoplasms. There are few studies regarding the molecular alterations of these tumors, but it appears they are similar to sebaceous carcinoma.

Sebaceous carcinoma (SC), on the other hand, is an aggressive malignancy whose molecular landscape has been elucidated in recent years. SC is broadly classified into two major anatomical subtypes: **ocular SC**, arising from sebaceous glands in the eyelid and conjunctiva; and **cutaneous (extraocular) SC**, occurring elsewhere on the skin, particularly the head, neck, trunk, and extremities. These two subtypes differ significantly in their genetic drivers, tumor mutation burdens, and association with hereditary syndromes.

Despite advances in genomics, distinguishing between benign sebaceous adenomas/sebaceomas and SCs remains challenging due to overlapping mutations. Therefore, the differential diagnosis still relies primarily on morphology [74, 76].

Etiology and Molecular Biology

Etiologically, sebaceous neoplasms can be hereditary (**Muir-Torre syndrome**) or sporadic. A significant proportion of them, especially extraocular SCs, belongs to the first group.

SC is the most studied sebaceous neoplasm, due to its malignant behavior. Recent genomic studies have defined **three major mutational subtypes of SC** based on whole-exome sequencing and mutation signature analysis: MMR/MSI-associated SC, UV-associated SC, and paucimutational SC (Table 10.5). The first two groups include only extraocular neoplasms, while the third group includes both ocular and extraocular SC.

- **MMR/MSI-Associated SC**: This subtype comprises virtually all SCs resulting from germline (Muir-Torre syndrome) or somatic mutations in **MMR genes** (*MLH1*, *MSH2*, and *MSH6)*, which are the driver mutation, responsible for high rate of replicative errors in areas of repetitive DNA sequences (MSI) due to inability to repair mismatches, which is characteristic of this SC type, and a high proportion of insertions/deletions (indels). Frequently associated mutations include *HRAS*, *KRAS*, *RREB1*, and *KMT2D*. These tumors often arise

Table 10.5 Summary: molecular taxonomy of SC

Subtype	Mutation profile	Location	Histology	Etiology
MMR/MSI SC	*MLH1, MSH2, MSH6*	Extraocular	Well/moderately differentiated, circumscribed	Hereditary (Muir-Torre syndrome) Sporadic
UV-signature SC	*TP53, NOTCH1/2, FAT3, RREB1* and *KMT2D* with C > T and CC > TT transitions	Extraocular, sun-exposed areas (face, scalp)	Poorly differentiated, infiltrative, squamoid features	Sporadic
Paucimutational SC	*ZNF750, TP53, RB1*, PI3K pathway *PCDH15* correlates with metastasis	Ocular or Extraocular	Moderate differentiated	Sporadic - a subset is possibly HPV-related

in younger patients, are extraocular in location and histologically appear well to moderately differentiated, with circumscribed tumor borders. Immunohistochemical loss of MMR protein expression may assist in identification.

- **UV-Associated SC**: This group is characterized by a **high tumor mutation burden** (15–586 mutations/Mb) and a **UV mutational signature** (C > T and CC > TT transitions). There are frequent mutations in *TP53*, *NOTCH1/2*, *FAT3*, *RREB1* and *KMT2D*. They arise in elderly individuals in sun-exposed areas (e.g., face, scalp) and histology are poorly differentiated, infiltrative tumors, sometimes with squamous differentiation.
- **Paucimutational SC**: This subtype is characterized by a **low tumor mutational burden** (1–5 mutations/Mb) and lacks a dominant mutational signature. Frequent mutations involve ***ZNF750***, ***TP53***, ***RB1***, and the **PI3K pathway**, with occasional alterations in *NOTCH1* and ***PCDH15***—the latter associated with increased metastatic potential. *ZNF750* is a tumor suppressor gene; its mutations are typically truncating and are frequently associated with ocular localization (up to 73% of ocular SC cases). Occasional *HER2* amplifications (7–57% across studies) have also been reported, particularly in ocular SCs. Overall, this group includes all ocular SCs and a subset of extraocular SCs. These tumors tend to be moderately differentiated and are less commonly associated with sun exposure.

This class can be further subclassified into two groups:

- **HPV-associated tumors**: These tumors carry HPV DNA, raising the hypothesis that they may be HPV-related tumors, in which wild-type *TP53* and *RB1* are present, but viral E6/E7 proteins disable tumor suppressors. More common in younger patients.
- **HPV-non associated tumors:** presence of mutations in *TP53* and *RB1*.

Muir-Torre Syndrome is a phenotypic variant of Lynch syndrome characterized by germline mutations in **MMR genes** with autosomal dominant inheritance, most commonly *MSH2* (70–90%), followed by *MLH1* (10–20%), and less frequently *MSH6*. The syndrome is defined by the occurrence of **at least one sebaceous tumor and one visceral malignancy** (including colorectal, pancreatic, endometrial, urogenital cancer), characterized by microsatellite instability (MSI), a genomic hallmark resulting from replication errors in repetitive DNA sequences due to defective DNA mismatch repair.

Recommendations for Muir-Torre Syndrome Screening in Sebaceous Neoplasms.

Routine immunostaining for MMR proteins is not recommended in all sebaceous neoplasm cases. American Society of Dermatopathology indicated that immunostaining to screen for Muir-Torre syndrome should be considered in the following situations:

- Patients <60 years of age with a sebaceous neoplasm.
- Individuals with multiple sebaceous tumors and/or keratoacanthomas.
- Sebaceous neoplasm with extraocular location.
- Cystic sebaceous neoplasms.
- Patients with a history of Muir-Torre–associated internal malignancies.

breast secretory carcinomas. This fusion is targetable with TRK inhibitors (e.g., larotrectinib, entrectinib). These tumors typically exhibit a low mutation burden and a genomically simple profile.

Tubular Adenoma and Syringocystadenoma Papilliferum

General Features

Benign tumors with tubulo-papillary architecture, composed of epithelial and myoepithelial cells, commonly associated with nevus sebaceus.

Etiology and Molecular Biology

These tumors may arise sporadically or in the context of cutaneous mosaic RASopathies, particularly nevus sebaceus of Jadassohn. Both tumor types are characterized by activating mutations in the **MAPK signaling pathway**, such as BRAF p.V600E (50–66%), HRAS p.G13R (7–26%) and KRAS p.G12D (rare). Additionally, HPV types 16 and 68 have been identified in some perianal cases of syringocystadenoma papilliferum.

Tumors with Unknown or Limited Molecular Characterization

Several sweat gland tumors currently lack well-defined molecular alterations (Table 10.6):

- **Microcystic adnexal carcinoma (MAC)**: lacks a recurrent driver mutation, but shows a certain frequence of *TP53* mutations (22%), *JAK1* insertions (17%) and copy number changes; despite occurring in sun-exposed

Table 10.6 Summary: molecular taxonomy of sweat glands tumors

Neoplasm	Key molecular alterations	Frequency (%)
Poroma / Porocarcinoma	*YAP1* fusion *NUT* fusion *TP53, RB1, CDKN2A, EGFR, ERBB2, PIK3CA, RAS* mutations (in porocarcinoma)	88% 17–55%
Cylindroma / Cylindrocarcinoma	*CYLD* mutation	~100% (sporadic or Brooke–Spiegler synd.)
Spiradenoma / Spiradenocarcinoma	*CYLD* mutation ALPK1 p.V1092A *TP53* mutation (in carcinoma)	Variable
Adenoid Cystic Carcinoma	*MYB::NFIB* *MYBL1::NFIB*	73–83% 20–23%
Hidradenoma / Hidradenocarcinoma	*CRTC1::MAML2, CRTC3::MAML2* *TP53, AKT1, PIK3CA* mutation, *ERBB2* amplification (in carcinoma)	>50–75%
Cutaneous Mixed Tumor	*PLAG1* rearrangement *HMGA2* rearrangement	33% Variable
Myoepithelioma	*EWSR1* fusion (e.g., *EWSR1::PBX3*) *FUS* fusion	EWSR1: 82% FUS: 18%
Secretory Carcinoma	*ETV6::NTRK3* fusion	~100%
Tubular Adenoma / SCAP	BRAF p.V600E HRAS p.G13R KRAS p.G12D	50–64% 7–26% Rare
PCAC	*RARA::NPEPPS* fusion	Unknown (emerging evidence)
Others *(e.g., MAC, EMPSGC, Histiocytoid carcinoma, Papillary digital adenocarcinoma, Mucinous carcinoma, etc.)*	No recurrent alterations	N/A

areas, it lacks UV-associated mutational signatures.

- **Primary cutaneous apocrine carcinoma (PCAC):** one study identified a *RARA::NPEPPS* fusion, possibly defining a novel molecular subset.
- **Endocrine Mucin-Producing Sweat Gland Carcinoma (EMPSGC).**
- **Histiocytoid carcinoma.**
- **Papillary digital adenocarcinoma.**
- **Polymorphous sweat gland carcinoma.**
- **Squamoid eccrine ductal carcinoma.**
- **Mucinous carcinoma.**
- **Adnexal adenocarcinomas, NOS.**

NGS in Adnexal Neoplasms

Molecular testing is not routinely required for the diagnosis of adnexal neoplasms. However, **next-generation sequencing (NGS)** can offer clinical and research value in selected contexts:

- **Selected Clinical Indications.**
  - **Locally advanced or metastatic malignant neoplasms**: NGS can identify actionable mutations, guiding personalized treatment strategies.
  - **Morphologically overlapping or borderline neoplasms**: Molecular profiling may assist in the differential diagnosis, particularly in sweat gland tumors, some of which harbor recurrent genetic alterations. In limited cases, it can also help distinguish benign from malignant entities (e.g. carcinomatous transformation of spiradenoma).
  - **Detection of germline mutations**: NGS can identify germline alterations associated with certain adnexal neoplasms, aiding in the diagnosis of underlying genetic syndromes.
- **Research Applications.**
  - To improve understanding of the pathogenesis and molecular landscape of adnexal neoplasms.
  - To identify novel therapeutic targets and support the development of targeted therapies.

References

1. Arnold M, Singh D, Laversanne M, Vignat J, Vaccarella S, Meheus F, Cust AE, de Vries E, Whiteman DC, Bray F. Global burden of cutaneous melanoma in 2020 and projections to 2040. JAMA Dermatol. 2022;158(5):495–503. https://doi.org/10.1001/jamadermatol.2022.0160. PMID: 35353115; PMCID: PMC8968696
2. Whiteman DC, Olsen CM, MacGregor S, Law MH, Thompson B, Dusingize JC, Green AC, Neale RE, Pandeya N, QSkin Study. The effect of screening on melanoma incidence and biopsy rates. Br J Dermatol. 2022;187(4):515–22. https://doi.org/10.1111/bjd.21649. Epub 2022 Jun 28. PMID: 35531668; PMCID: PMC9796145
3. Cheng L, Netto GJ, Eble JN, editors. Molecular pathology. 2nd ed. Springer: Cham; 2018.
4. Ahmed B, Qadir MI, Ghafoor S. Malignant melanoma: skin cancer-diagnosis, prevention, and treatment. Crit Rev Eukaryot Gene Expr. 2020;30(4):291–7. https://doi.org/10.1615/CritRevEukaryotGeneExpr.2020028454.
5. Tímár J, Ladányi A. Molecular pathology of skin melanoma: epidemiology, differential diagnostics, prognosis and therapy prediction. Int J Mol Sci. 2022;23(10):5384. https://doi.org/10.3390/ijms23105384. PMID: 35628196; PMCID: PMC9140388
6. Elder DE, Massi D, Scolyer RA, Willemze R, editors. WHO Classification of Skin Tumours, WHO Classification of Tumours Series, vol. 12. 5th ed. Lyon: International Agency for Research on Cancer (IARC); 2023.
7. Rashid S, Shaughnessy M, Tsao H. Melanoma classification and management in the era of molecular medicine. Dermatol Clin. 2023;41(1):49–63. https://doi.org/10.1016/j.det.2022.07.017. Epub 2022 Oct 28
8. Randic T, Kozar I, Margue C, Utikal J, Kreis S. NRAS mutant melanoma: towards better therapies. Cancer Treat Rev. 2021;99:102238. https://doi.org/10.1016/j.ctrv.2021.102238. Epub 2021 May 29
9. Dankort D, Curley DP, Cartlidge RA, Nelson B, Karnezis AN, Damsky WE Jr, You MJ, DePinho RA, McMahon M, Bosenberg M. Braf(V600E) cooperates with Pten loss to induce metastatic melanoma. Nat Genet. 2009;41(5):544–52. https://doi.org/10.1038/ng.356. Epub 2009 Mar 12. PMID: 19282848; PMCID: PMC2705918
10. Koh SS, Cassarino DS. Immunohistochemical expression of p16 in melanocytic lesions: an updated review and meta-analysis. Arch Pathol Lab Med. 2018;142(7):815–28. https://doi.org/10.5858/arpa.2017-0435-RA.
11. Silva-Rodríguez P, Fernández-Díaz D, Bande M, Pardo M, Loidi L, Blanco-Teijeiro MJ. GNAQ and GNA11 genes: a comprehensive review on oncogenesis, prognosis and therapeutic opportunities in uveal melanoma. Cancers (Basel). 2022;14(13):3066.

https://doi.org/10.3390/cancers14133066. PMID: 35804836; PMCID: PMC9264989
12. Gandini S, Zanna I, De Angelis S, Palli D, Raimondi S, Ribero S, Masala G, Suppa M, Bellerba F, Corso F, Nezi L, Nagore E, Caini S. TERT promoter mutations and melanoma survival: a comprehensive literature review and meta-analysis. Crit Rev Oncol Hematol. 2021;160:103288. https://doi.org/10.1016/j.critrevonc.2021.103288. Epub 2021 Mar 3
13. Sergi MC, Filoni E, Triggiano G, Cazzato G, Internò V, Porta C, Tucci M. Mucosal melanoma: epidemiology, clinical features, and treatment. Curr Oncol Rep. 2023;25(11):1247–58. https://doi.org/10.1007/s11912-023-01453-x. Epub 2023 Sep 29. PMID: 37773078; PMCID: PMC10640506
14. Djulbegovic MB, Taylor DJ, Uversky VN, Galor A, Shields CL, Karp CL. Intrinsic disorder in BAP1 and its association with uveal melanoma. Genes (Basel). 2022;13(10):1703. https://doi.org/10.3390/genes13101703. PMID: 36292588; PMCID: PMC9601668
15. Horn S, Figl A, Rachakonda PS, Fischer C, Sucker A, Gast A, Kadel S, Moll I, Nagore E, Hemminki K, Schadendorf D, Kumar R. TERT promoter mutations in familial and sporadic melanoma. Science. 2013;339(6122):959–61. https://doi.org/10.1126/science.1230062. Epub 2013 Jan 24
16. Nurla LA, Aşchie M, Cozaru GC, Boşoteanu M. Multiple primary melanoma associated with CDKN2A mutation-case report and review of the literature. Medicina (Kaunas). 2024;60(5):763. https://doi.org/10.3390/medicina60050763. PMID: 38792946; PMCID: PMC11122717
17. Qasim H, Abu Shugaer M, Khattab K, Leoni MLG, Varrassi G. Histopathological subtypes of cutaneous melanoma: prognostic and molecular implications. Cureus. 2025;17(8):e90670. https://doi.org/10.7759/cureus.90670. PMID: 40984902; PMCID: PMC12450496
18. Teixido C, Castillo P, Martinez-Vila C, Arance A, Alos L. Molecular markers and targets in melanoma. Cells. 2021;10(9):2320. https://doi.org/10.3390/cells10092320. PMID: 34571969; PMCID: PMC8469294
19. Shafique N, Ertmann E, Tortorello G, Karakousis GC, Miura JT. Desmoplastic melanoma in the era of immune checkpoint blockade. J Am Acad Dermatol. 2025;92(4):890–1. https://doi.org/10.1016/j.jaad.2024.10.101. Epub 2024 Nov 26
20. Cazzato G, Colagrande A, Resta L, Trilli I, Lupo C, Ingravallo G, Caporusso C, Giovannoni I, Barresi S. LMNA::NTRK1 and PRDX1::NTRK1 atypical spitz tumor: a report of two additional cases with histological, immunohistochemical, and molecular insights. Am J Dermatopathol. 2025;47(1):22–4. https://doi.org/10.1097/DAD.0000000000002865. Epub 2024 Oct 15
21. Daruish M, Ambrogio F, Colagrande A, Marzullo A, Alaggio R, Trilli I, Ingravallo G, Cazzato G. Kinase fusions in spitz melanocytic tumors: the past, the present, and the future. Dermatopathology (Basel). 2024;11(1):112–23. https://doi.org/10.3390/dermatopathology11010010. PMID: 38390852; PMCID: PMC10885070
22. Della Mura M, Sorino J, Colagrande A, Ingravallo G, Giubellino A, Fortarezza F, Yang RK, Cho WC, Cazzato G. Atypical spitz tumor/spitz melanocytoma revealing a VIM::NTRK3 gene fusion: clinicopathological correlation of a unique molecular finding. Am J Dermatopathol. 2025; https://doi.org/10.1097/DAD.0000000000003051. Epub ahead of print
23. Donati M, Goutas D, Pissaloux D, Olivares S, Kervarrec T, Nosek D, Goto K, Lemahieu J, Loontiens S, Van der Meulen J, Mansour B, Perrone G, Macagno N, Gerami P, Kazakov DV, De la Fouchardiere A. Clinical, morphologic, and genomic findings in Spitz tumors with RET fusion: a series of 31 cases. Mod Pathol. 2025;38(5):100740. https://doi.org/10.1016/j.modpat.2025.100740. Epub 2025 Feb 20
24. Cappellesso R, Nozzoli F, Zito Marino F, Simi S, Castiglione F, De Giorgi V, Cota C, Senetta R, Scognamiglio G, Anniciello AM, Cesinaro AM, Mandalà M, Gianatti A, Valente MG, Valeri B, Sementa AR, Ricci C, Corti B, Roviello G, Dei Tos AP, Franco R, Massi D. NTRK gene fusion detection in atypical spitz tumors. Int J Mol Sci. 2021;22(22):12332. https://doi.org/10.3390/ijms222212332. PMID: 34830218; PMCID: PMC8619835
25. Sorino J, Della Mura M, Ingravallo G, Colagrande A, Cazzato G. TAX1BP1::BRAF fusion in BRAF-mutated atypical spitz tumor/spitz melanocytoma: a novel molecular finding with histopathological insights. Am J Dermatopathol. 2025;47(7):568–9. https://doi.org/10.1097/DAD.0000000000002973.
26. Gui J, Guo Z, Wu D. Clinical features, molecular pathology, and immune microenvironmental characteristics of acral melanoma. J Transl Med. 2022;20(1):367. https://doi.org/10.1186/s12967-022-03532-2. PMID: 35974375; PMCID: PMC9382740
27. Desai A, Ugorji R, Khachemoune A. Acral melanoma foot lesions. Part 1: epidemiology, aetiology, and molecular pathology. Clin Exp Dermatol. 2017;42(8):845–8. https://doi.org/10.1111/ced.13243. Epub 2017 Sep 22
28. Yip HM, Cameron A, Sheppard K, Fasanmade A, Garg M. Oral mucosal melanoma in situ: a case report and review of the literature. Int J Oral Maxillofac Surg. 2023;52(12):1230–4. https://doi.org/10.1016/j.ijom.2023.04.002. Epub 2023 May 11
29. Elder DE, Bastian BC, Cree IA, Massi D, Scolyer RA. The 2018 world health organization classification of cutaneous, mucosal, and uveal melanoma: detailed analysis of 9 distinct subtypes defined by their evolutionary pathway. Arch Pathol Lab Med. 2020;144(4):500–22. https://doi.org/10.5858/arpa.2019-0561-RA. Epub 2020 Feb 14
30. Alos L, Carrasco A, Teixidó C, Szumera-Ciećkiewicz A, Vicente A, Massi D, Carrera C. Melanoma on congenital melanocytic nevi. Pathol Res Pract.

2024;256:155262. https://doi.org/10.1016/j.prp.2024.155262. Epub 2024 Mar 11
31. Kaku Y, de la Fouchardière A. Malignant blue melanoma. Clin Dermatol. 2025;43(3):334–40. https://doi.org/10.1016/j.clindermatol.2024.09.002. Epub 2024 Sep 10
32. Iavarone L, Franco R, Zito Marino F, D'Abbronzo G, Argenziano G, Scharf C, Nucci G, Ronchi A, Cazzato G. Ocular melanoma: a comprehensive review with a focus on molecular biology. Int J Mol Sci. 2025;26:9799. https://doi.org/10.3390/ijms26199799.
33. Sergi MC, Ambrogio F, Della Mura M, Sorino J, Cazzato G. Basal cell carcinoma: an old friend with multiple faces. Cancer. 2025;17:993. https://doi.org/10.3390/cancers17060993.
34. Draper E, Li YY, Mahadevan NR, Laga AC, Hanna J, Russell-Goldman E. Clinicopathologic and molecular characterization of basal cell carcinoma arising at sun-protected sites. Am J Surg Pathol. 2025;49(4):328–35. https://doi.org/10.1097/PAS.0000000000002366. Epub 2025 Jan 14. PMID: 39807820; PMCID: PMC12271870
35. Abi Karam M, Kourie HR, Jalkh N, Mehawej C, Kesrouani C, Haddad FG, Feghaly I, Chouery E, Tomb R. Molecular profiling of basal cell carcinomas in young patients. BMC Med Genet. 2021;14(1):187. https://doi.org/10.1186/s12920-021-01030-w. PMID: 34284772; PMCID: PMC8293576
36. Iwasaki JK, Srivastava D, Moy RL, Lin HJ, Kouba DJ. The molecular genetics underlying basal cell carcinoma pathogenesis and links to targeted therapeutics. J Am Acad Dermatol. 2012;66(5):e167–78. https://doi.org/10.1016/j.jaad.2010.06.054. Epub 2010 Aug 30
37. Kilgour JM, Jia JL, Sarin KY. Review of the molecular genetics of basal cell carcinoma; inherited susceptibility, somatic mutations, and targeted therapeutics. Cancer. 2021;13:3870. https://doi.org/10.3390/cancers13153870.
38. Di Nardo L, Pellegrini C, Di Stefani A, Ricci F, Fossati B, Del Regno L, Carbone C, Piro G, Corbo V, Delfino P, De Summa S, Maturo MG, Rocco T, Tortora G, Fargnoli MC, Peris K. Molecular alterations in basal cell carcinoma subtypes. Sci Rep. 2021;11(1):13206. https://doi.org/10.1038/s41598-021-92592-3. PMID: 34168209; PMCID: PMC8225846
39. Lazar AD, Dinescu S, Costache M. Deciphering the molecular landscape of cutaneous squamous cell carcinoma for better diagnosis and treatment. J Clin Med. 2020;9:2228. https://doi.org/10.3390/jcm9072228.
40. Martincorena I, Campbell PJ. Somatic mutation in cancer and normal cells. Science. 2015;349(6255):1483–9. https://doi.org/10.1126/science.aab4082. Epub 2015 Sep 24. Erratum in: Science. 2016 Mar 4;351(6277):aaf5401. doi:10.1126/science.aaf5401
41. Brash DE. UV signature mutations. Photochem Photobiol. 2015;91(1):15–26. https://doi.org/10.1111/php.12377. Epub 2014 Nov 28. PMID: 25354245; PMCID: PMC4294947
42. Chitsazzadeh V, Coarfa C, Drummond JA, Nguyen T, Joseph A, Chilukuri S, Charpiot E, Adelmann CH, Ching G, Nguyen TN, Nicholas C, Thomas VD, Migden M, MacFarlane D, Thompson E, Shen J, Takata Y, McNiece K, Polansky MA, Abbas HA, Rajapakshe K, Gower A, Spira A, Covington KR, Xiao W, Gunaratne P, Pickering C, Frederick M, Myers JN, Shen L, Yao H, Su X, Rapini RP, Wheeler DA, Hawk ET, Flores ER, Tsai KY. Cross-species identification of genomic drivers of squamous cell carcinoma development across preneoplastic intermediates. Nat Commun. 2016;7:12601. https://doi.org/10.1038/ncomms12601. PMID: 27574101; PMCID: PMC5013636
43. Cornejo CM, Jambusaria-Pahlajani A, Willenbrink TJ, Schmults CD, Arron ST, Ruiz ES. Field cancerization: treatment. J Am Acad Dermatol. 2020;83(3):719–30. https://doi.org/10.1016/j.jaad.2020.03.127. Epub 2020 May 6
44. Kim Y, He YY. Ultraviolet radiation-induced non-melanoma skin cancer: regulation of DNA damage repair and inflammation. Genes Dis. 2014;1(2):188–98. https://doi.org/10.1016/j.gendis.2014.08.005. PMID: 25642450; PMCID: PMC4307792
45. Cozma E-C, Banciu LM, Soare C, Cretoiu S-M. Update on the molecular pathology of cutaneous squamous cell carcinoma. Int J Mol Sci. 2023;24:6646. https://doi.org/10.3390/ijms24076646.
46. Durinck S, Ho C, Wang NJ, Liao W, Jakkula LR, Collisson EA, Pons J, Chan SW, Lam ET, Chu C, Park K, Hong SW, Hur JS, Huh N, Neuhaus IM, Yu SS, Grekin RC, Mauro TM, Cleaver JE, Kwok PY, LeBoit PE, Getz G, Cibulskis K, Aster JC, Huang H, Purdom E, Li J, Bolund L, Arron ST, Gray JW, Spellman PT, Cho RJ. Temporal dissection of tumorigenesis in primary cancers. Cancer Discov. 2011;1(2):137–43. https://doi.org/10.1158/2159-8290.CD-11-0028. Epub 2011 Jun 29. PMID: 21984974; PMCID: PMC3187561
47. Hedberg ML, Berry CT, Moshiri AS, Xiang Y, Yeh CJ, Attilasoy C, Capell BC, Seykora JT. Molecular mechanisms of cutaneous squamous cell carcinoma. Int J Mol Sci. 2022;23(7):3478. https://doi.org/10.3390/ijms23073478. PMID: 35408839; PMCID: PMC8998533
48. South AP, Purdie KJ, Watt SA, Haldenby S, den Breems N, Dimon M, Arron ST, Kluk MJ, Aster JC, McHugh A, Xue DJ, Dayal JH, Robinson KS, Rizvi SH, Proby CM, Harwood CA, Leigh IM. NOTCH1 mutations occur early during cutaneous squamous cell carcinogenesis. J Invest Dermatol. 2014;134(10):2630–8. https://doi.org/10.1038/jid.2014.154. Epub 2014 Mar 24. PMID: 24662767; PMCID: PMC4753672
49. Pickering CR, Zhou JH, Lee JJ, Drummond JA, Peng SA, Saade RE, Tsai KY, Curry JL, Tetzlaff MT, Lai SY, Yu J, Muzny DM, Doddapaneni H, Shinbrot E,

Covington KR, Zhang J, Seth S, Caulin C, Clayman GL, El-Naggar AK, Gibbs RA, Weber RS, Myers JN, Wheeler DA, Frederick MJ. Mutational landscape of aggressive cutaneous squamous cell carcinoma. Clin Cancer Res. 2014;20(24):6582–92. https://doi.org/10.1158/1078-0432.CCR-14-1768. Epub 2014 Oct 10. PMID: 25303977; PMCID: PMC4367811

50. Li YY, Hanna GJ, Laga AC, Haddad RI, Lorch JH, Hammerman PS. Genomic analysis of metastatic cutaneous squamous cell carcinoma. Clin Cancer Res. 2015;21(6):1447–56. https://doi.org/10.1158/1078-0432.CCR-14-1773. Epub 2015 Jan 14. PMID: 25589618; PMCID: PMC4359951
51. Chang D, Shain AH. The landscape of driver mutations in cutaneous squamous cell carcinoma. NPJ Genom Med. 2021;6(1):61. https://doi.org/10.1038/s41525-021-00226-4. PMID: 34272401; PMCID: PMC8285521
52. Inman GJ, Wang J, Nagano A, Alexandrov LB, Purdie KJ, Taylor RG, Sherwood V, Thomson J, Hogan S, Spender LC, South AP, Stratton M, Chelala C, Harwood CA, Proby CM, Leigh IM. The genomic landscape of cutaneous SCC reveals drivers and a novel azathioprine associated mutational signature. Nat Commun. 2018;9(1):3667. https://doi.org/10.1038/s41467-018-06027-1. PMID: 30202019; PMCID: PMC6131170
53. Thomson J, Bewicke-Copley F, Anene CA, Gulati A, Nagano A, Purdie K, Inman GJ, Proby CM, Leigh IM, Harwood CA, Wang J. The genomic landscape of actinic keratosis. J Invest Dermatol. 2021;141(7):1664–1674.e7. https://doi.org/10.1016/j.jid.2020.12.024. Epub 2021 Jan 19. PMID: 33482222; PMCID: PMC8221374
54. Yilmaz AS, Ozer HG, Gillespie JL, Allain DC, Bernhardt MN, Furlan KC, Castro LT, Peters SB, Nagarajan P, Kang SY, Iwenofu OH, Olencki T, Teknos TN, Toland AE. Differential mutation frequencies in metastatic cutaneous squamous cell carcinomas versus primary tumors. Cancer. 2017;123(7):1184–93. https://doi.org/10.1002/cncr.30459. Epub 2016 Dec 1. PMID: 27906449; PMCID: PMC5360561
55. van der Schroeff JG, Evers LM, Boot AJ, Bos JL. Ras oncogene mutations in basal cell carcinomas and squamous cell carcinomas of human skin. J Invest Dermatol. 1990;94(4):423–5. https://doi.org/10.1111/1523-1747.ep12874504.
56. Pierceall WE, Goldberg LH, Tainsky MA, Mukhopadhyay T, Ananthaswamy HN. Ras gene mutation and amplification in human nonmelanoma skin cancers. Mol Carcinog. 1991;4(3):196–202. https://doi.org/10.1002/mc.2940040306.
57. Su F, Viros A, Milagre C, Trunzer K, Bollag G, Spleiss O, Reis-Filho JS, Kong X, Koya RC, Flaherty KT, Chapman PB, Kim MJ, Hayward R, Martin M, Yang H, Wang Q, Hilton H, Hang JS, Noe J, Lambros M, Geyer F, Dhomen N, Niculescu-Duvaz I, Zambon A, Niculescu-Duvaz D, Preece N, Robert L, Otte NJ, Mok S, Kee D, Ma Y, Zhang C, Habets G, Burton EA, Wong B, Nguyen H, Kockx M, Andries L, Lestini B, Nolop KB, Lee RJ, Joe AK, Troy JL, Gonzalez R, Hutson TE, Puzanov I, Chmielowski B, Springer CJ, McArthur GA, Sosman JA, Lo RS, Ribas A, Marais R. RAS mutations in cutaneous squamous-cell carcinomas in patients treated with BRAF inhibitors. N Engl J Med. 2012;366(3):207–15. https://doi.org/10.1056/NEJMoa1105358. PMID: 22256804; PMCID: PMC3724537
58. Santos-de-Frutos K, Segrelles C, Lorz C. Hippo pathway and YAP signaling alterations in squamous cancer of the head and neck. J Clin Med. 2019;8(12):2131. https://doi.org/10.3390/jcm8122131. PMID: 31817001; PMCID: PMC6947155
59. Bertin J, Wang L, Guo Y, Jacobson MD, Poyet JL, Srinivasula SM, Merriam S, DiStefano PS, Alnemri ES. CARD11 and CARD14 are novel caspase recruitment domain (CARD)/membrane-associated guanylate kinase (MAGUK) family members that interact with BCL10 and activate NF-kappa B. J Biol Chem. 2001;276(15):11877–82. https://doi.org/10.1074/jbc.M010512200. Epub 2001 Jan 12
60. Watt SA, Purdie KJ, den Breems NY, Dimon M, Arron ST, McHugh AT, Xue DJ, Dayal JH, Proby CM, Harwood CA, Leigh IM, South AP. Novel CARD11 mutations in human cutaneous squamous cell carcinoma lead to aberrant NF-κB regulation. Am J Pathol. 2015;185(9):2354–63. https://doi.org/10.1016/j.ajpath.2015.05.018. Epub 2015 Jul 26. PMID: 26212909; PMCID: PMC4597276
61. Lee CS, Bhaduri A, Mah A, Johnson WL, Ungewickell A, Aros CJ, Nguyen CB, Rios EJ, Siprashvili Z, Straight A, Kim J, Aasi SZ, Khavari PA. Recurrent point mutations in the kinetochore gene KNSTRN in cutaneous squamous cell carcinoma. Nat Genet. 2014;46(10):1060–2. https://doi.org/10.1038/ng.3091. Epub 2014 Sep 7. PMID: 25194279; PMCID: PMC4324615
62. Holland P, Willis C, Kanaly S, Glaccum M, Warren A, Charrier K, Murison J, Derry J, Virca G, Bird T, Peschon J. RIP4 is an ankyrin repeat-containing kinase essential for keratinocyte differentiation. Curr Biol. 2002;12(16):1424–8. https://doi.org/10.1016/s0960-9822(02)01075-8.
63. Kolev V, Mandinova A, Guinea-Viniegra J, Hu B, Lefort K, Lambertini C, Neel V, Dummer R, Wagner EF, Dotto GP. EGFR signalling as a negative regulator of Notch1 gene transcription and function in proliferating keratinocytes and cancer. Nat Cell Biol. 2008;10(8):902–11. https://doi.org/10.1038/ncb1750. Epub 2008 Jul 6. Erratum in: Nat Cell Biol. 2013 Jan;15(1):124. PMID: 18604200; PMCID: PMC2747621
64. Seykora JT, Mei L, Dotto GP, Stein PL. Srcasm: a novel Src activating and signaling molecule. J Biol Chem. 2002;277(4):2812–22. https://doi.org/10.1074/jbc.M106813200. Epub 2001 Nov 15
65. Li W, Marshall C, Mei L, Gelfand J, Seykora JT. Srcasm corrects Fyn-induced epidermal hyperplasia by kinase down-regulation. J Biol Chem. 2007;282(2):1161–9. https://doi.org/10.1074/jbc.

M606583200. Epub 2006 Oct 16. PMID: 17046829; PMCID: PMC3099404
66. Li W, Marshall C, Mei L, Dzubow L, Schmults C, Dans M, Seykora J. Srcasm modulates EGF and Src-kinase signaling in keratinocytes. J Biol Chem. 2005;280(7):6036–46. https://doi.org/10.1074/jbc.M406546200. Epub 2004 Dec 3
67. Liu W, MacDonald M, You J. Merkel cell polyomavirus infection and Merkel cell carcinoma. Curr Opin Virol. 2016;20:20–7. https://doi.org/10.1016/j.coviro.2016.07.011.
68. Albores-Saavedra J, Batich K, Chable-Montero F, Sagy N, Schwartz AM, Henson DE. Merkel cell carcinoma demographics, morphology, and survival based on 3870 cases: a population based study. J Cutan Pathol. 2010;37(1):20–7. https://doi.org/10.1111/j.1600-0560.2009.01370.x.
69. Pulitzer MP, Brannon AR, Berger MF, et al. Cutaneous squamous and neuroendocrine carcinoma: genetically and immunohistochemically different from Merkel cell carcinoma. Mod Pathol. 2015;28(8):1023–32. https://doi.org/10.1038/modpathol.2015.60.
70. Goh G, Walradt T, Markarov V, et al. Mutational landscape of MCPyV-positive and MCPyV-negative Merkel cell carcinomas with implications for immunotherapy. Oncotarget. 2016;7(3):3403–15. https://doi.org/10.18632/oncotarget.6494.
71. Stachyra K, Dudzisz-Śledź M, Bylina E, et al. Merkel cell carcinoma from molecular pathology to novel therapies. Int J Mol Sci. 2021;22(12):6305. Published 2021 Jun 11. https://doi.org/10.3390/ijms22126305.
72. Harms PW, Vats P, Verhaegen ME, et al. The distinctive mutational spectra of polyomavirus-negative merkel cell carcinoma. Cancer Res. 2015;75(18):3720–7. https://doi.org/10.1158/0008-5472.CAN-15-0702.
73. Van Gele M, Leonard JH, Van Roy N, Cook AL, De Paepe A, Speleman F. Frequent allelic loss at 10q23 but low incidence of PTEN mutations in Merkel cell carcinoma. Int J Cancer. 2001;92(3):409–13. https://doi.org/10.1002/ijc.1209.
74. Plotzke JM, Adams DJ, Harms PW. Molecular pathology of skin adnexal tumours. Histopathology. 2022;80(1):166–83. https://doi.org/10.1111/his.14441.
75. Dragoo DD, Taher A, Wong VK, et al. PTEN hamartoma tumor syndrome/Cowden syndrome: genomics, oncogenesis, and imaging review for associated lesions and malignancy. Cancers (Basel). 2021;13(13):3120. Published 2021 Jun 22. https://doi.org/10.3390/cancers13133120.
76. North JP. Molecular genetics of sebaceous neoplasia. Surg Pathol Clin. 2021;14(2):273–84. https://doi.org/10.1016/j.path.2021.03.005.
77. Cazzato G, Daruish M, Fortarezza F, et al. Gene fusion-driven cutaneous adnexal neoplasms: an updated review emphasizing molecular characteristics. Am J Dermatopathol. 2025;47(6):453–61. https://doi.org/10.1097/DAD.0000000000002933.
78. Macagno N, Sohier P, Kervarrec T, et al. Recent advances on immunohistochemistry and molecular biology for the diagnosis of adnexal sweat gland tumors. Cancers (Basel). 2022;14(3):476. Published 2022 Jan 18. https://doi.org/10.3390/cancers14030476.

(PR), HER2, and the Ki-67 proliferative index [7]. BC is clinically divided into four intrinsic molecular subtypes using these markers: Luminal A, Luminal B, HER2-enriched, and Triple-Negative/Basal-like [8]. These IHC-based subtypes must integrate with histopathological features such as morphological type and tumor grade. The evaluation of these biomarkers is only an initial step in understanding the complex molecular alterations driving breast cancer development, progression, and treatment response [9].

Luminal Breast Cancer: Phenotype and Genomic Assays

The molecular subtype called luminal is defined by the expression of estrogen receptor (ER) and/or progesterone receptor (PgR), assessed through immunohistochemistry (IHC), and represents the most common subtype of BC. Luminal cancers are divided into two groups (A and B), and the distinction between Luminal A and Luminal B is based on the evaluation of the proliferative index called Ki-67. Luminal A typically shows Ki-67 $\leq$ 20%, and Luminal B Ki-67 > 20%. Luminal B tumors may also show HER2 overexpression or amplification [3]. According to the 2010 ASCO/CAP guidelines, updated in 2019, hormone receptor status must be determined using IHC, and a cut-off of 1% nuclear staining in tumor cells is considered enough to confirm the positivity to ER or PgR, permitting patients access to endocrine therapy [10]. Luminal tumors are often diagnosed at an early stage, and molecular testing can refine risk stratification and guide therapeutic decision-making [11]. Gene expression profiling assays allow clinicians to predict prognosis, estimate the risk of distant recurrence, and assess potential benefits from adjuvant chemotherapy and endocrine therapy. In the context of early-stage, hormone receptor-positive breast cancer, genomic tests help stratify a patient's prognosis and guide decisions about adjuvant chemotherapy, particularly when standard clinical-pathological factors are inconclusive.

Oncotype DX® analyzes 21 genes using RT-PCR on tumor tissue to produce a Recurrence Score (RS). This score predicts the risk of distant recurrence and whether the patient will likely benefit from chemotherapy. It is instrumental in node-negative or minimally node-positive ER+/HER2– cases and is validated by major trials like TAILORx [12].

MammaPrint®, based on microarray analysis of 70 genes, categorizes patients as low or high risk for recurrence within 5–10 years. It is indicated for early-stage tumors, helping to avoid unnecessary chemotherapy, and its clinical utility has been confirmed in studies like MINDACT [13].

Prosigna® (PAM50) is designed to profile the expressions of 50 genes and assign intrinsic molecular subtypes and a Risk of Recurrence (ROR) score. Based on NanoString technology, it is meant for postmenopausal women with up to three positive lymph nodes and offers substantial prognostic value, though predictive data are still growing [14].

EndoPredict® evaluates 12 genes and integrates clinical features to produce the EPclin Score, stratifying patients by metastatic risk over 10 years. It is a valuable tool for deciding on chemotherapy and extended endocrine therapy in ER+/HER2– patients [15].

Gene expression profiling has redesigned the management of hormone receptor-positive BC, allowing for personalized therapy based on both molecular and clinical data. These assays are essential in precision oncology pathways, such as determining the need for adjuvant chemotherapy in early-stage disease. They are endorsed by major clinical guidelines, including ESMO and ASCO, even though IHC remains the foundation of routine pathology practice.

HER2-Positive Breast Cancer

The human epidermal growth factor receptor 2 (HER2) is a transmembrane tyrosine kinase receptor encoded by the ERBB2 gene (also known as C-erbB-2) located on chromosome 17 [16]. Amplification of the ERBB2 gene or overexpression of the HER2 protein represents the prototype for targeted therapy in breast cancer. Since 1998, the monoclonal antibody trastuzumab (Herceptin) has revolutionized the treatment of HER2-positive (HER2+) BC. HER2 positivity has paved the way for a new predictive marker for response to anti-HER2 therapies [17]. Starting in 2007 and with further updates in 2013, 2018, and 2023, the American Society of Clinical Oncology (ASCO) and the College of American Pathologists (CAP) have drawn up the guidelines recommending the assessment of HER2 status in all newly diagnosed cases of primary invasive BC and the re-evaluation should be done in cases of recurrence or metastasis, mainly when treatment decisions may be influenced. HER2 protein expression is routinely evaluated by immunohistochemistry (IHC), using a scoring system (0, 1+, 2+, 3+) based on the presence of the presence, localization, intensity, and the percentage of tumor cells stained. A score of 3+ is considered positive, while a score of 2+ is considered equivocal and requires confirmation by in situ hybridization (ISH) techniques. These techniques include many different methods, such as fluorescence ISH (FISH), chromogenic ISH (CISH), and silver-enhanced ISH (SISH), each with specific reporting criteria for single- and dual-probe assays [18].

Furthermore, a new category called "HER2-low" BC includes tumors with IHC scores of 1+ or 2+ without gene amplification by FISH [17]. HER2-low targeting therapies are being explored primarily in patients with metastatic or locally advanced disease and are currently under clinical evaluation [19]. Moreover, HER2 overexpression can result from activating mutations in cases lacking gene amplification. These mutations may offer an alternative route for HER2-targeted therapies, especially with small-molecule tyrosine kinase inhibitors like neratinib [20].

Triple-Negative Breast Cancer (TNBC)

Triple-negative breast cancers (TNBCs) are a heterogeneous group of tumors characterized by the complete negativity of estrogen receptor (ER), progesterone receptor (PgR), and HER2 expression first assessed by IHC [3]. Recognized as a distinct clinical entity in the mid-2000s, TNBCs are generally associated with aggressive clinical behavior, high histologic grade, elevated Ki-67, and significant genomic instability [9]. Histologically, most TNBCs fall under invasive carcinoma of no special type (NST). However, TNBC may also include several special histologic subtypes, such as metaplastic carcinoma, NST with medullary features, and in some cases, apocrine carcinoma and tall cell carcinoma with reversed polarity. Despite their aggressive biology, TNBCs are more likely than other breast cancer subtypes to achieve a pathological complete response (pCR) following neoadjuvant chemotherapy [21].

However, the TNBC spectrum also includes rare, low-grade tumors with more indolent clinical behavior, like salivary gland-like tumors of the breast, such as secretory carcinoma, adenoid cystic carcinoma, and mucoepidermoid carcinoma [3].

From a molecular perspective, TNBCs are characterized by highly complex genomes. TP53 is the most frequently mutated driver gene, followed by PIK3CA. In some cases, these mutations are subclonal, further supporting the view that TNBCs are a molecularly heterogeneous group of tumors driven by different oncogenic pathways [22]. TNBCs also tend to have a high tumor mutational burden (TMB) or occurred germline mutations or/and be a part of familiar syndromes. Notably, BRCA1 mutations are closely linked with the basal-like TNBC phenotype. Even without BRCA1/2 germline mutations, many TNBCs exhibit a "BRCAness" phenotype, reflecting similar defects in homologous recombination repair [23]. Over time, different classifications of TNBCs have been proposed, and initial gene expression profiling has divided TNBCs into basal-like and non-basal-like subtypes. A specific subgroup known as claudin-low was also identified, characterized by stem-like features and epithelial-to-mesenchymal transition (EMT), often included within the basal-like spectrum [24]. Lehmann et al. proposed a more detailed classification based on transcriptomic analysis, identifying six distinct molecular subtypes: Basal-like 1 (BL1), Basal-like 2 (BL2) Immunomodulatory (IM), Mesenchymal (M), Mesenchymal Stem-like (MSL), Luminal Androgen Receptor (LAR) [25]. Subsequent refinements led to excluding the MSL subtype, which was found to reflect stromal contamination rather than intrinsic tumor features. The IM subtype was reinterpreted as primarily driven by tumor-infiltrating lymphocytes (TILs), now recognized as key prognostic and predictive markers, especially in immunotherapy. In the updated classification, BL1 tumors exhibit high proliferative activity and DNA damage response pathways, correlating with excellent response to chemotherapy and favorable overall survival (OS) and disease-free survival (DFS). BL2 tumors are enriched for growth factor signaling and tend to have poor responses to neoadjuvant chemotherapy and worse clinical outcomes. LAR tumors express androgen receptor-related gene signatures and may be candidates for anti-androgen therapies. Mesenchymal (MES) tumors show activation of EMT and cell motility pathways [26]. An alternative classification proposed by Burstein et al. (2015) identified four TNBC subtypes: LAR (Luminal Androgen Receptor), MES (Mesenchymal), BLIS (Basal-like Immunosuppressed), BLIA (Basal-like Immune-Activated).

Among these, BLIA tumors have the most favorable prognosis due to high immune infiltration, whereas BLIS tumors, which are characterized by low immune activity, present the poorest outcomes. These findings underscore the tumor immune microenvironment's critical role in determining prognosis and response to emerging therapeutic strategies, including immune checkpoint inhibitors [27].

NGS in Breast Cancer

The molecular or intrinsic classification of breast cancer (BC) is a powerful tool in first-line disease management, laying the foundation for personalized therapeutic strategies and providing essential prognostic information [28]. In this context, the advent of precision medicine, which aims to identify specific, druggable molecular targets for each patient, has highlighted the need for high-throughput sequencing technologies such as Next-Generation Sequencing (NGS), enabling the sequencing of extensive portions of the genome, even up to the entire genome, and are also pivotal in therapy monitoring through liquid biopsy [29, 30].

In this landscape, NGS panels have become indispensable in clinical and research settings, allowing for the massive parallel analysis of multiple cancer-related genes. These panels vary in size, composition, and intended use, ranging from commercially available assays to custom-designed research platforms based on clinical or investigative needs. Beyond therapeutic target identification, molecular tools are crucial in detecting hereditary cancer syndromes and resolving complex diagnostic cases, like challenging diagnoses. Furthermore, molecular profiling improves the detection of druggable alterations such as gene fusions, pathway-specific mutations, and immunotherapy-related biomarkers, thereby supporting more precise and effective treatment decisions. These tools significantly contribute to a deeper understanding of BC biology, including its initiation, progression, and behavior (Table 11.1) [31].

The European Society for Medical Oncology (ESMO), in collaboration with the Precision Medicine Working Group (PMWG), updated in 2024 its guidelines for the clinical use of NGS in patients with advanced cancer, including BC [32, 33]. Using the ESMO Scale for Clinical Actionability of Molecular Targets (ESCAT), these recommendations assess the clinical relevance of genomic alterations and help guide treatment decisions while considering cost-effectiveness and accessibility. The updated ESMO/PMWG guidelines recommend the use of NGS in the management of breast cancer in the following specific situations:

- Detection of tumor-agnostic genomic alterationsTumor-agnostic genomic alterations, such as NTRK fusions, high tumor mutational burden (TMBTumor Mutation Burden (TMB)-H), and microsatellite instability (MSI), can inform targeted therapies regardless of cancer type.
- Detection of ESR1 mutations in patients with hormone receptor-positive and HER2-negative advanced breast cancer (ABC). This mutation was recently upgraded to ESCAT level I based

Table 11.1 Applications of next-generation sequencing (NGS) in breast cancer

Biomarker	Alteration	Indications	Significance
BRCA1/2	Inactivating variants	Germline testing Therapeutic	Hereditary BC Sensitivity to PARP-inhibitors
PALB2	Inactivating variants	Germline testing Therapeutic	Hereditary BC Sensitivity to PARP-inhibitors
ATM	Inactivating variants	Germline testing	Hereditary BC
CHEK2	Inactivating variants	Germline testing	Li-Fraumeni syndrome
TP53	Inactivating variants	Germline testing Somatic testing	Li-Fraumeni syndrome Enriched in TNBC
PIK3CA	Activating variants	Therapeutic	Predicts response to capivasertib+fulvestrant
AKT	Activating variants	Therapeutic	Predicts response to capivasertib+fulvestrant
PTEN	Inactivating variants	Germline testing Therapeutic	Predicts response to capivasertib+fulvestrant; Germline variants associated with Cowden syndrome
HER2	Amplification activating variants	Therapeutic	Molecular/intrinsic subtype classification Amplification predicts response to anti-HER2 therapies Protein expression makes it possible eligibility for targeted tyrosine kinase inhibitors
ESR1	Activating variants	Therapeutic	Predicts response to elacestrant after progression on endocrine therapy
CDH1	Inactivating variants	Germline testing Diagnostic	Inactivated in lobular carcinoma (LCIS and ILC) Germline variants associated with ILC and hereditary diffuse gastric cancer
IDH2	p.Arg172 hotspot variant	Diagnostic	Tall cell carcinoma with reversed polarity
MYB::NFIB	Fusion	Diagnostic	Adenoid cystic carcinoma
ETV::NTRK3	Fusion	Diagnostic Therapeutic	Secretory carcinoma Predict response to larotrecinib and entrectinib
CTRC1::MAML2	Fusion	Diagnostic	Mucoepidermoid carcinoma
TERT	Promoter variants	Diagnostic	Presence favors Phyllodes tumor vs. Fibroadenoma
HMGA2 or PLAG1	Fusion	Diagnostic	Pleomorphic adenoma
CTNNB1	Activating variants	Diagnostic	Desmoid fibromatosis
ALK	Fusions	Diagnostic, therapeutic	Inflammatory Myofibroblastic tumor
MYC	Amplification	Diagnostic	Post-radiation Angiosarcoma
RARA	Activating variants	Diagnostic	Presence favors Fibroadenoma vs. Phyllodes tumor
MED12	Exon 2 variants	Diagnostic	Fibroepithelial lesions
TMB	SNVs and indels	Therapeutic	TMB $\geq$ 10 variants/Mb eligible for immune checkpoint inhibitor (unresectable/metastatic tumors)
MSI/MMR	Loss of MLH1, PMS2, MSH2, MSH6	Germline testing Therapeutic	Lynch syndrome Predicts response to immune checkpoint inhibitor (unresectable/metastatic tumors)

Note: *BC* breast cancer, *TNBC* triple-negative breast cancer, *ILC* invasive lobular carcinoma, *LCIS* lobular carcinoma in situ, *MSI* microsatellite instability, *TMB* = tumor mutational burden

on results from the EMERALD trial, affirming its clinical actionability and permitting patients to benefit from Elacestrant.

- Identification of germline BRCA1/2 mutations. NGS can detect many of these mutations, but approximately 7% may remain undetected. Therefore, patients at high risk of hereditary breast cancer with negative somatic results should undergo dedicated germline testing to ensure accurate risk assessment.
- Assessment of alterations in the AKT signaling pathway, including mutations in

PIK3CA, AKT1, and PTEN, in patients with hormone receptor-positive, HER2-negative ABC, guide for the use of targeted therapy with Capivasertib in combination with Fulvestrant [33].

BRCA1 and BRCA2

The BRCA gene family, which stands for BReast CAncer, comprises two well-characterized tumor suppressor genes: BRCA1, located on chromosome 17, and BRCA2, located on chromosome 13. These genes play a central role in the homologous recombination (HR) repair pathway, a crucial mechanism for repairing DNA double-strand breaks, leading to genomic instability and promoting tumorigenesis.

Today, it's estimated that 5–10% of all BCs and 25–30% of familial BCs are associated with inherited pathogenic variants in BRCA1 or BRCA2 [34, 36]. The prevalence of these mutations varies significantly across populations. BRCA mutations may be germline or, more rarely, somatic. Paul Broca first described the hereditary nature of BC in 1866 and observed the recurrence across generations. These genes were discovered in the mid-1990s (BRCA1 in 1994 and BRCA2 in 1995). Furthermore, they are the key to the diagnosis of Hereditary Breast and Ovarian Cancer Syndrome (HBOC) [35, 36].

Over 1600 variants in BRCA1 and 1800 in BRCA2 have been identified, many of which are missense, nonsense, or frameshift mutations resulting in truncated, non-functional proteins. The lifetime risk of developing breast cancer is estimated at up to 72% for BRCA1 carriers and 69% for BRCA2 carriers [37]. BRCA1-associated tumors typically occur at a young age (often <50 years), are frequently bilateral, and tend to show basal-like phenotype [34, 38]. In contrast, BRCA2-associated breast cancers are more often hormone receptor-positive and tend to have a less aggressive clinical course [39]. Histologically, BRCA1-mutated BC frequently exhibit features of basal-like carcinomas, expressing basal cytokeratins and sometimes presenting with medullary-like morphology. This phenotype is observed in 30–60% of BRCA1-mutated breast cancers but is rare in BRCA2-associated tumors [3].

Next-generation sequencing (NGS) has introduced and revolutionized the detection of germline BRCA mutations, allowing for simultaneous identification of both point mutations and larger rearrangements. Importantly, NGS-based tumor profiling also enables the detection of somatic BRCA mutations, expanding therapeutic eligibility beyond hereditary cases [40].

The identification of pathogenic variants in BRCA1, BRCA2, and other genes like PALB2, which are involved in homologous recombination repair pathways, has important therapeutic implications showing sensibility to PARP inhibitors (PARPi), such as Olaparib or Talazoparib [41]. Additionally, since clinical phenotypes associated with mutations in BRCA1/2, PALB2, ATM, and CHEK2 may overlap, comprehensive NGS panels including all these genes are recommended for eligible patients, particularly those with early-onset breast cancer or strong family history [42].

PALB2

PALB2 (Partner and Localizer of BRCA2) is another gene located on chromosome 16, involved in the homologous recombination DNA repair pathway producing the stabilization of BRCA2, leading to its nuclear accumulation [43]. Germline monoallelic mutations in PALB2 confer a higher risk of developing BC up to nine times [44]. On the contrary, somatic mutations are less frequently found [45]. Despite PALB2 mutations being less frequent than those in BRCA1/2, women carrying pathogenic PALB2 variants have an estimated 30–60% lifetime risk of developing breast cancer. In comparison, the risk for males bringing the mutation is approximately 1%. This classifies PALB2 among the high-penetrance cancer predisposition genes [44, 45].

PALB2 mutations are generally non-syndromic, though there is growing evidence of their role in a spectrum of hereditary cancer phenotypes. Most PALB2-associated breast tumors are estrogen receptor-positive, although some studies have reported enrichment of triple-negative tumors among mutation carriers falling within the phenotype called BRCAness. While the gene is still under investigation, recent research indicates that PALB2 mutation carriers tend to develop BC at a younger age compared to the general population [46]. In agreement with the ESCAT scale, PALB2 is considered level IIB for its sensibility to PARPi. The inclusion of PALB2 in both germline and somatic NGS testing panels reflects its growing recognition as a BRCA-like gene, with implications for treatment decisions and genetic counseling [33].

ATM

The AT (Ataxia-Telangiectasia) gene is localized on chromosome 11 and encodes for an oncosuppressor, a serine/threonine kinase that belongs to the phosphatidylinositol 3-kinase-related kinase (PIKK) family. The mutated form of this gene is called ATM and plays an essential role in cell cycle regulation, oxidative stress, and telomerase maintenance, providing genomic stability. ATM mutations can be germinal and sporadic, but the underlying mechanism of BC development is poorly understood.

Next-Generation Sequencing (NGS) analyses have shown that loss of heterozygosity (LOH) in the ATM locus occurs in approximately 40% of sporadic breast cancers. Among the pathogenic variants, the c.7271 T > G (p.V2424G) missense mutation is one of the most strongly associated with breast cancer risk and has been reported in both Asian and Caucasian populations [42, 47, 48]. ATM mutations are often associated with luminal phenotype BCs, which may have a more aggressive clinical course and a higher propensity for distant metastases. Because ATM is involved in DNA repair, tumors with ATM deficiency may be treated with PARP inhibitors. However, BC arising from ATM mutations shows biallelic inactivation of ATM without mutation signatures of homologous recombination deficiency [49]. Nevertheless, ATM mutation testing is included in panels that value genetic counseling and familial risk assessment [50].

CHEK2

CHEK2 (Checkpoint Kinase 2), located on chromosome 22, is another gene that belongs to the pathway involved in DNA damage response. It functions downstream of ATM, mediating cell cycle arrest and apoptosis in response to genomic stress. CHEK2 plays a tumor suppressor role and is implicated in both hereditary and sporadic forms of BC. The most studied pathogenic variant is c.1100delC, a frameshift mutation that confers a moderate risk of developing BC, mainly belonging to the luminal intrinsic class [51]. The BC risk is notably increased in women who carry this mutation and have a strong family history of breast cancer. BC panels testing germline mutations include high-risk or high-penetrance genes like BRCA1/2, CDH1, PALB2, and TP53. CHEK2 germline mutation is associated with Li-Fraumeni syndrome [3]. Like ATM mutations, CHEK2 is inherited in an autosomal dominant manner but with moderate penetrance, and they are both routinely included in multigene germline testing panels via NGS for individuals who meet clinical criteria for hereditary BC screening.

TP53

TP53, called "guardian of the genome," is a gene on the short arm of chromosome 17 that encodes the p53 protein, a central tumor suppressor involved in cell cycle arrest, DNA repair, apoptosis, and senescence. Mutations in TP53 are among the most common alterations in human cancers, found in over 50% of all malignancies. In BC, germline TP53 mutations, such as CHEK2 mutations, are associated with Li-Fraumeni syndrome, a hereditary cancer predisposition syndrome characterized by early-onset BC and other multiple carcinomas. Most TP53 mutations are missense variants occurring in the DNA-binding domain, resulting in loss of transcriptional activity, aggressive tumor biology, high histologic grade, poor prognosis, and resistance to standard therapies. In BC, ~26% of mutations of TP53 are found in luminal tumors, ~55% in HER2-enriched tumors, and up to 88% in basal-like/triple-negative breast cancers (TNBCs) [52].

In luminal cancers, TP53 mutations are frequently accompanied by MDM2 or MDM4 amplifications or co-alterations in genes like ATM or CHEK2, contributing to hormone therapy resistance and more aggressive behavior [53]. In basal-like TP53 regulates epithelial-mesenchymal transition (EMT) and cancer stem cell traits. These tumors often carry complex mutations, including insertions and deletions, and are frequently found in BRCA1-mutated backgrounds [4, 9, 22].

Although not yet actionable in routine clinical practice, TP53 is emerging as a relevant biomarker in precision oncology. TP53 mutation status germline or somatic can now be directly detected through NGS-based multigene panels, providing important prognostic information and, in specific investigational contexts, helping to select patients for clinical trials involving targeted agents such as WEE1 inhibitors or MDM2 antagonists [54, 55].

PIK3CA

Phosphatidylinositol-4,5-bisphosphate 3-kinase catalytic subunit alpha (PIK3CA) is the second most common somatic mutation in BC after TP53, particularly within the luminal subtype, where mutations occur in approximately 40% of cases [56]. Gene PIK3CA lies on chromosome 3 and encodes for the catalytic subunit of the class I PI3K enzyme, a critical component of the PI3K/AKT/mTOR signaling pathway, which regulates cell proliferation, metabolism, survival, and resistance to therapy. Activating mutations in the PIK3CA cluster in specific hotspot regions, primarily in exon 9 (E542K, E545K) and exon 20 (H1047R), leading to constitutive activation of downstream signaling [57].

The availability of Next-Generation Sequencing (NGS) allows the precise identification of these mutations, enabling a specific therapeutic approach for postmenopausal patients with estrogen receptor (ER)-positive and HER2-negative and locally advanced or metastatic BC who show progression or resistance to endocrine therapy [33].

The presence of PIK3CA mutation represents a prototype of precision oncology. Based on the results of the SOLAR-1 trial, FDA-approved patients harboring this alteration can benefit from Alpelisib, a PI3Kα-specific inhibitor plus fulvestrant [58].

AKT

AKT (Protein Kinase B) is a serine/threonine kinase that participates in the PIK3/AKT/PTEN pathway as an effector downstream of PI3K. There are three isoforms of this gene (AKT1, AKT2, AKT3) involved in tumorigenesis, growth, or metastasis, but the most recurrent in BC is AKT1. Mutations in AKT1, particularly the E17K substitution, promote tumor initiation, increasing cell proliferation. Whereas AKT2 is responsible for tumor progression and metastasis, the role of AKT3 is still poorly clarified [59]. All AKT isoforms are implicated in resistance to endocrine therapy, and the clinical utility of AKT testing is still under investigation. Capivasertib, an orally bioavailable pan-AKT inhibitor that can inhibit all three isoforms, has been approved for use with fulvestrant after phase 3, randomized trial CAPItello-291 [60].

According to the ESMO Scale for Clinical Actionability of Molecular Targets (ESCAT), AKT1 and PTEN mutations are classified as Level I/II, supporting their inclusion in routine NGS panels for advanced breast cancer. These mutations may co-occur with PIK3CA alterations, contributing to the observed therapeutic benefit from inhibitors targeting the PI3K/AKT axis [33].

PTEN

PTEN (Phosphatase and Tensin Homolog) is a tumor suppressor gene that negatively regulates the PI3K/AKT/mTOR pathway. Inactivation of the second gene copy leads to loss of function in PTEN. Alterations found include mutations, deletions, or promoter methylation, which determines pathway hyperactivation, contributing to tumorigenesis, therapeutic resistance, and poor prognosis [61]. PTEN alterations are particularly observed in triple-negative breast cancers (TNBCs), especially the basal-like subtype [22]. In addition to somatic alterations, germline PTEN mutations are associated with Cowden Syndrome (also known as PTEN Hamartoma Tumor Syndrome), which confers a significantly increased lifetime risk of developing breast cancer. Early reports described a moderate risk of developing BC in PTEN carriers. Still, more recent studies suggest that individuals with germline PTEN mutations may face an up to 80% lifetime risk of developing breast cancer [3, 61]. Today, according to the ESCAT scale, PTEN is considered level I/II, is involved in investigational NGS panels, and is regarded as an emerging biomarker for future targeted therapies. NGS enables the detection of inactivating mutation or deletion of PTEN, which results in hyperactivation of the PI3K-AKT-PTEN pathway and the hypothetical co-occurring alterations in other genes (e.g., PIK3CA, AKT1), providing a comprehensive view of pathway dysregulation and enhancing molecular profiling strategies for personalized treatment [33, 62].

HER2 (ERBB2)

HER2 (human epidermal growth factor receptor 2) is a well-established molecular biomarker in BC and represents one of the primary axes of molecular classification alongside hormone receptor status. HER2 status is crucial for determining prognosis and guiding anti-HER2 therapies like trastuzumab, pertuzumab, and trastuzumab-emtansine (T-DM1) [20, 63, 64].

While most HER2-positive tumors are identified by protein overexpression or gene amplification by classic methods such as IHC or ISH, Next-Generation Sequencing (NGS) has expanded the ability to detect ERBB2 activating point mutations, particularly in ER-positive, HER2-negative tumors in patients with advanced BC (ESCAT level II). HER2 somatic mutations are less prevalent than amplification, occurring only in 2.7 of BC; rarely, they can harbor gene amplification [65, 66].

To the best of knowledge, most HER2 mutations are localized into exon 19–20, codifying for the tyrosine kinase domain and the other for the extracellular domain. The most relevant mutations are L755S, V777L, and D769H/Y [66]. These mutations are not detectable by IHC/ISH, may respond to Neratinib, an irreversible pan-HER tyrosine kinase inhibitor, and can be a potential acquired method to the resistance of classic HER2 targeted therapies [67, 68].

Furthermore, NGS may enhance the precision in defining the emerging HER2-low category, which includes tumors with IHC 1+ or 2+ without amplification. This subgroup is now eligible for trastuzumab deruxtecan (T-DXd), a HER2-targeting antibody-drug conjugate, in the second-line setting for inoperable or metastatic breast cancer [69].

This reclassification highlights the therapeutic importance of subtle HER2 expression levels, even without classic overexpression. Today, IHC/ISH can't be replaced for the first molecular assessment of BC because NGS doesn't directly quantify the amount of HER2 protein expressed on the surface of the tumor. Nevertheless, massive parallel sequencing can used when there is a discordance between IHC and ISH or in advanced BC/translational research.

ESR1

ESR1 gene encodes for the estrogen receptor alpha (ERα), a central player in hormone receptor-positive (HR+) breast cancer. Acquired ESR1 mutations were discovered in BC in 1997, but until 2013, their role was poorly understood. Today, they represent a key mechanism of resistance to endocrine therapy, especially following prolonged treatment with aromatase inhibitors or CDK4/6 inhibitors [32, 33]. Approximately 30% of patients with ER+/HER2− advanced BC who progress after endocrine therapy harbor ESR1 mutations, most frequently in the ligand-binding domain (e.g., Y537S, D538G). These mutations confer ligand-independent receptor activation, making tumors resistant to standard hormone therapies such as tamoxifen or aromatase inhibitors [70].

Based on the Phase-3 EMERALD Trial from 2023, patients harboring these alterations may benefit from elacestrant, a selective estrogen receptor degrader (SERD) that remains effective in the presence of activating ESR1 mutations. This drug has been approved by both the U.S. FDA and the European Medicines Agency (EMA) for postmenopausal women and adult men with ER+/HER2− advanced breast cancer with an ESR1 mutation and prior endocrine therapy resistance, including CDK4/6 inhibitor [58].

Previously included in ESCAT level II, ESR1 assessment is included in level I, and evaluation of its mutations is now incorporated into clinical guidelines. There are many technologies for detecting ESR1 mutation like droplet digital PCR (ddPCR) and NGS-based assays, mediated use of liquid biopsy to detect circulating tumor DNA (ctDNA) offering a minimally invasive method to capture real-time genomic alterations, especially valuable when tumor tissue is inaccessible or to monitor for emerging resistance mechanisms during therapy [33].

NGS in Diagnostic BC

Comprehensive molecular profiling through next-generation sequencing (NGS) is also utilized as a diagnostic tool, particularly in challenging or ambiguous breast cancer cases or when there is a need for precise tumor biomarkers. While immunohistochemistry (IHC) remains a reliable surrogate for assigning tumors to molecular subtypes, NGS can confirm and uncover subtype-specific genetic alterations, enhancing diagnostic accuracy and offering therapeutic insight. For example, in triple-negative breast cancer (TNBC), particularly the basal-like subtype, mutations or overexpression of EGFR are found in 50–70% of cases. Although not universally present, EGFR alterations represent potential experimental therapeutic targets [71].

CDH1 and Invasive Lobular Carcinoma

CDH1 is a gene on chromosome 16 encoding for E-cadherin, a transmembrane glycoprotein involved in cell-cell adhesion and epithelial tissue integrity. Loss of E-cadherin function leads to tissue discohesion, promotes epithelial-mesenchymal transition (EMT), and facilitates tumor invasion and metastasis [72]. CDH1 mutations in breast cancer may be germline or somatic and are primarily associated with invasive lobular carcinoma (ILC), the second most common histologic subtype after IDC [3].

Germline CDH1 mutations are also linked to Hereditary Diffuse Gastric Cancer (HDGC), inherited in an autosomal dominant pattern. In ILC, CDH1 mutations are often truncating mutations or large deletions, leading to absent or aberrant E-cadherin expression [73].

While IHC assessment of E-cadherin is routine in pathology by immunohistochemistry, interpretation can be challenging in some cases due to CDH1 gene mutation or aberrant/loss of the expression of the catenin binding proteins of loss of heterozygosity or partial protein expression [74]. Given its diagnostic, prognostic, prognostic, and potential therapeutic relevance, NGS panels now routinely include CDH1 for hereditary cancer screening and tumor molecular profiling [74]. Current research also explores the role of PI3K/AKT/mTOR pathway inhibitors in lobular carcinoma, as these are often co-altered alongside CDH1 loss [75].

Tall Cell Carcinoma with Reverse Polarity (TCCRP)

TCCRP, formerly known as solid papillary carcinoma with reverse polarity, is a rare triple-negative breast cancer (TNBC) variant that histologically resembles the tall cell variant of papillary thyroid carcinoma. It is molecularly characterized by IDH2 R172 hotspot mutations (77–100% of cases), frequently accompanied by TET2 truncating mutations and PIK3CA mutations, but notably lacking BRAF and RET/PTC rearrangements, which help distinguish it from metastatic thyroid carcinomas [76].

Salivary Gland–Like Tumors of the Breast

Several special subtypes of TNBC share histopathologic features with salivary gland tumors. NGS can help resolve differential diagnoses and provide critical information for prognosis and treatment:

- Adenoid Cystic Carcinoma (AdCCAdenoid Cystic Carcinoma (AdCC)): Generally indolent with low recurrence/metastasis rates, AdCCAdenoid Cystic Carcinoma (AdCC) of the breast often harbors the MYB::NFIB gene fusion or, more rarely, MYBL1 rearrangements or MYB amplification. In solid vari-

ants, NOTCH1 and CREBBP mutations may also be seen.
- Secretory Carcinoma (SC): A rare TNBC subtype with characteristic morphology and typically indolent clinical course associated with the ETV6::NTRK3 fusion, shared with its salivary gland counterpart.
- Mucoepidermoid Carcinoma (MEC): Usually low-grade with a favorable prognosis, though high-grade forms may metastasize. The tumor often carries a t(11;19)(q21;p13) translocation, resulting in the CRTC1::MAML2 fusion—a diagnostic hallmark.
- Acinic Cell Carcinoma (AciCC): Though morphologically like its salivary counterpart, AciCC of the breast typically lacks NR4A3 expression and instead shows alterations commonly seen in TNBC, such as TP53 or PIK3CA mutations.
- Pleomorphic Adenoma (PA): A benign lesion of the breast that may recur if not entirely excised. These tumors are associated with PLAG1 or HMGA2 rearrangements [77, 78].

Spindle Cell Lesions and Fibroepithelial Neoplasms

NGS can aid diagnosis in morphologically challenging cases, especially when IHC is inconclusive:

- When fibromatosis is suspected, but the evaluation of β-catenin by IHC is negative, a CTNNB1 mutation (seen in ~70% of cases) supports the diagnosis of fibromatosis-like metaplastic carcinoma [79].
- Inflammatory Myofibroblastic Tumors (IMT) can be confirmed by ALK rearrangements, particularly when there is a cytokeratin-positive spindle cell lesion.
- Post-radiation angiosarcoma typically shows high-level MYC amplification (>90%), in contrast to primary breast angiosarcomas, which rarely exhibit MYC amplification [80].

Fibroepithelial Lesions: FA vs. Phyllodes Tumor

Distinguishing between fibroadenomas (FA) and phyllodes tumors (PT) can be difficult, particularly on biopsy. NGS offers helpful molecular clues:

- RARA (retinoic acid receptor alpha) mutations are frequently found in FA than in PT.
- MED12 exon 2 codon 44 mutations are common in FA (excluding myxoid subtypes) and low-grade PT. Higher-grade PTs often harbor mutations in NF1, RB1, PIK3CA, EGFR, TP53, ERBB4, and overexpression or promoter mutations of TERT.
- Recurrent MED12 and TERT hotspot mutations are central to fibroepithelial lesion pathogenesis and aid in differential diagnosis.
- In malignant PT, TPM4::NTRK1 fusion has been identified in recent studies, highlighting the value of RNA-based NGS in detecting targetable gene fusions [81–83].

NGS-based comprehensive molecular profiling is becoming indispensable in the diagnostic and prognostic evaluation of breast cancer, particularly in rare histologic subtypes and morphologically ambiguous cases. By revealing actionable mutations, gene fusions, or co-alterations not evident through routine methods, it paves the way for precision diagnostics, targeted therapy, and improved risk stratification across a spectrum of breast malignancies [84].

Tumor Agnostic-Molecular Marker

Tumor Mutation Burden (TMB) is defined as the number of somatic mutations per megabase (mut/Mb) of the coding genome sequenced. In recent years, TMB has emerged as a potential predictive biomarker for the efficacy of immune checkpoint inhibitors (ICIs) in various solid tumors [85]. The role of TMB has been considered as ESCAT level IC, but the clinical role in BC remains obscure and less understood. This is partly due to BC's biological complexity and molecular heterogeneity, which causes lower TMB than other malignancies. About 5% of BC had a high tumor burden, especially in metastatic TNBC, compared to hormone receptor-positive or HER2-positive [33, 86, 87].

Following KEYNOTE-355 and KEYNOTE-522 trial results, the Food and Drug Administration (FDA) approved anti-PD-1 pembrolizumab for metastatic and early-stage TNBC. Still, the clinical use of immune checkpoint blockades (ICBs) in TNBC is inconsistent [88]. In this regard, the FDA proved high TMB as a biomarker for predicting the response to ICBs [89]. Combining TMB with other biomarkers may be a powerful tool in the landscape of the personalized management of BC, especially for patients with limited treatment options.

High TMB has been found to arise among triple-negative breast cancers (TNBC, especially in cancer associated with underlying defects in DNA repair mechanisms, such as homologous recombination repair (HRR) or with high microsatellite instability (MSI-H). MSI-H and mismatch repair deficiency (MMRd) are very rare in breast cancer, with a prevalence of less than 2% [90]. Nonetheless, epidemiological data suggest that women with Lynch syndrome, an inherited cancer predisposition syndrome caused by germline mutations in MMR genes, may have an increased risk of developing BC. However, this association remains under investigation [91].

The accurate quantification of TMB requires high-throughput genomic technologies, specifically next-generation sequencing (NGS), using large, targeted gene panels or whole-exome sequencing (WES), representing the gold standard for evaluating TMB. Commercially available NGS-based platforms, such as FoundationOne CDx (Foundation Medicine, Inc.) and Memorial Sloan Kettering-Integrated Mutation Profiling of Actionable Cancer Targets MSK-IMPACT, are approved by U.S. FDA and are utilized in clinical practice for the molecular characterization of advanced or metastatic breast cancers. By their own bioinformatic workflow, these platforms assess TMB and provide a detailed analysis of somatic mutations, copy number alterations, gene rearrangements, and MSI status. Significantly, they normalized TMB values (expressed in mut/Mb), detecting somatic coding mutations per megabase of the tumor genome examined, including point mutations, frameshift, small insertions, and deletions [87].

In conclusion, although the routine use of TMB in breast cancer management is still evolving, current evidence suggests that in specific subgroups, particularly metastatic TNBC, TMB may serve as a valuable biomarker for guiding immunotherapeutic strategies. As NGS technologies become more integrated into clinical workflows, TMB assessment is expected to play a growing role in advancing precision oncology in breast cancer.

Conclusions and Features Perspectives

Integrating Next-Generation Sequencing (NGS) into BC management is poised to revolutionize clinical practice and research approaches. While traditional intrinsic classification based on ER, PR, HER2, and Ki-67 remains a milestone for diagnosis and treatment, the availability of comprehensive genomic profiling (CGP) is expanding the horizons of precision oncology [9]. The application of NGS, through targeted panels or whole-exome sequencing, will be hypothetical but expected to become standard practice in the diagnostic work-up of advanced BC, enabling the identification of actionable somatic and germline mutations, tumor mutational burden (TMB) and novel biomarkers [87].

Emerging technologies such as liquid biopsy, through the analysis of circulating tumor DNA (ctDNA) or cell-free DNA (cfDNA), permit a real-time monitoring of clonal evolution, early detection of resistance mechanisms, and identification of minimal residual disease (MRD) following curative treatments. These advancements facilitate earlier therapeutic interventions and improve patient outcomes by anticipating disease progression before clinical manifestation [92]. Currently, NGS is primarily recommended for advanced BC cases, focusing on specific alterations such as ESR1 mutations, PIK3CA-AKT-PTEN pathway disruptions, and germline BRCA1/2 mutations [33, 78]. Nevertheless, its role is expected to broaden significantly, encompassing hereditary risk assessment with expanded germline panels and including polygenic risk scores [93]. Furthermore, molecular screening programs based on NGS will enhance patient access to clinical trials investigating targeted therapies against specific genomic alterations classified under the ESCAT Level II evidence scale [33]. Beyond its clinical applications, NGS is an invaluable research tool, offering comprehensive insights into the spatial and temporal heterogeneity of BC through the integration of multi-omics approaches, including transcriptomics, proteomics, metabolomics, and radiogenomics [31, 94]. This deeper molecular understanding will address several critical unresolved questions, such as the progression from ductal carcinoma in situ (DCIS) to invasive disease, the relationship between the primary and metastatic sites, or between atypical/micro glandular adenosis and triple-negative BC, the malignant potential of lesions such as radial scars and the landscape under papillary lesions [95–98]. In conclusion, NGS promises to redefine the future of breast cancer management, from diagnosis and treatment selection to disease monitoring and prognostication. Its progressive implementation will drive the realization of precision oncology, offering personalized therapeutic strategies and ultimately improving outcomes for a broader population of patients [99, 100].

References

1. Kim J, Harper A, McCormack V, Sung H, Houssami N, Morgan E, Mutebi M, Garvey G, Soerjomataram I, Fidler-Benaoudia MM. Global patterns and trends in breast cancer incidence and mortality across 185 countries. Nat Med. 2025;31(4):1154–62. https://doi.org/10.1038/s41591-025-03502-3. PMID: 39994475
2. Yalaza M, İnan A, Bozer M. Male breast cancer. J Breast Health. 2016;12(1):1–8. https://doi.org/10.5152/tjbh.2015.2711. PMID: 28331724; PMCID: PMC5351429
3. Ellis IO, Schnitt SJ, Sastre-Garau X, et al. WHO classification of tumours of the breast. 5th ed. Lyon: International Agency for Research on Cancer (IARC); 2019.
4. Cancer Genome Atlas Network. Comprehensive molecular portraits of human breast tumours. Nature. 2012;490(7418):61–70. https://doi.org/10.1038/nature11412. PMID: 23000897; PMCID: PMC3465532
5. Perou CM, Sørlie T, Eisen MB, van de Rijn M, Jeffrey SS, Rees CA, Pollack JR, Ross DT, Johnsen H, Akslen LA, Fluge O, Pergamenschikov A, Williams C, Zhu SX, Lønning PE, Børresen-Dale AL, Brown PO, Botstein D. Molecular portraits of human breast tumours. Nature. 2000;406(6797):747–52. https://doi.org/10.1038/35021093. PMID: 10963602
6. Sorlie T, Perou CM, Tibshirani R, et al. Gene expression patterns of breast carcinomas distinguish tumor subclasses with clinical implications. Proc Natl Acad Sci USA. 2001;98(19):10869–74.
7. Untch M, Gerber B, Harbeck N, Jackisch C, Marschner N, Möbus V, von Minckwitz G, Loibl S, Beckmann MW, Blohmer JU, Costa SD, Decker T, Diel I, Dimpfl T, Eiermann W, Fehm T, Friese K, Jänicke F, Janni W, Jonat W, Kiechle M, Köhler U, Lück HJ, Maass N, Possinger K, Rody A, Scharl A, Schneeweiss A, Thomssen C, Wallwiener D, Welt A. 13th st. Gallen international breast cancer conference 2013: primary therapy of early breast cancer evidence, controversies, consensus – opinion of a German team of experts (Zurich 2013). Breast Care (Basel). 2013;8(3):221–9. https://doi.org/10.1159/000351692. PMID: 24415975; PMCID: PMC3728634
8. Sorlie T, Tibshirani R, Parker J, Hastie T, Marron JS, Nobel A, Deng S, Johnsen H, Pesich R, Geisler S, Demeter J, Perou CM, Lønning PE, Brown PO, Børresen-Dale AL, Botstein D. Repeated observation of breast tumor subtypes in independent gene expression data sets. Proc Natl Acad Sci USA. 2003;100(14):8418–23. https://doi.org/10.1073/pnas.0932692100. PMID: 12829800; PMCID: PMC166244
9. Zhang X. Molecular classification of breast cancer: relevance and challenges. Arch Pathol Lab Med. 2023;147(1):46–51. https://doi.org/10.5858/arpa.2022-0070-RA. PMID: 36136295
10. Allison KH, Hammond MEH, Dowsett M, McKernin SE, Carey LA, Fitzgibbons PL, Hayes DF, Lakhani SR, Chavez-MacGregor M, Perlmutter J, Perou CM, Regan MM, Rimm DL, Symmans WF, Torlakovic EE, Varella L, Viale G, Weisberg TF, McShane LM, Wolff AC. Estrogen and progesterone receptor testing in breast cancer: ASCO/CAP guideline update. J Clin Oncol. 2020;38(12):1346–66. https://doi.org/10.1200/JCO.19.02309. PMID: 31928404
11. Loibl S, André F, Bachelot T, Barrios CH, Bergh J, Burstein HJ, Cardoso MJ, Carey LA, Dawood S, Del Mastro L, Denkert C, Fallenberg EM, Francis PA, Gamal-Eldin H, Gelmon K, Geyer CE, Gnant M, Guarneri V, Gupta S, Kim SB, Krug D, Martin M, Meattini I, Morrow M, Janni W, Paluch-Shimon S, Partridge A, Poortmans P, Pusztai L, Regan MM, Sparano J, Spanic T, Swain S, Tjulandin S, Toi M, Trapani D, Tutt A, Xu B, Curigliano G, Harbeck N. ESMO guidelines committee. Electronic address: clinicalguidelines@esmo.org. Early breast cancer: ESMO clinical practice guideline for diagnosis, treatment and follow-up. Ann Oncol.

2024;35(2):159–82. https://doi.org/10.1016/j.annonc.2023.11.016. PMID: 38101773
12. Paik S, Shak S, Tang G, Kim C, Baker J, Cronin M, Baehner FL, Walker MG, Watson D, Park T, Hiller W, Fisher ER, Wickerham DL, Bryant J, Wolmark N. A multigene assay to predict recurrence of tamoxifen-treated, node-negative breast cancer. N Engl J Med. 2004;351(27):2817–26. https://doi.org/10.1056/NEJMoa041588. PMID: 15591335
13. Cardoso F, van't Veer LJ, Bogaerts J, Slaets L, Viale G, Delaloge S, Pierga JY, Brain E, Causeret S, DeLorenzi M, Glas AM, Golfinopoulos V, Goulioti T, Knox S, Matos E, Meulemans B, Neijenhuis PA, Nitz U, Passalacqua R, Ravdin P, Rubio IT, Saghatchian M, Smilde TJ, Sotiriou C, Stork L, Straehle C, Thomas G, Thompson AM, van der Hoeven JM, Vuylsteke P, Bernards R, Tryfonidis K, Rutgers E, Piccart M, MINDACT Investigators. 70-Gene signature as an aid to treatment decisions in early-stage breast cancer. N Engl J Med. 2016;375(8):717–29. https://doi.org/10.1056/NEJMoa1602253. PMID: 27557300
14. Parker JS, Mullins M, Cheang MC, Leung S, Voduc D, Vickery T, Davies S, Fauron C, He X, Hu Z, Quackenbush JF, Stijleman IJ, Palazzo J, Marron JS, Nobel AB, Mardis E, Nielsen TO, Ellis MJ, Perou CM, Bernard PS. Supervised risk predictor of breast cancer based on intrinsic subtypes. J Clin Oncol. 2009;27(8):1160–7. https://doi.org/10.1200/JCO.2008.18.1370. PMID: 19204204; PMCID: PMC2667820
15. Dubsky P, Filipits M, Jakesz R, Rudas M, Singer CF, Greil R, Dietze O, Luisser I, Klug E, Sedivy R, Bachner M, Mayr D, Schmidt M, Gehrmann MC, Petry C, Weber KE, Kronenwett R, Brase JC, Gnant M, Austrian Breast and Colorectal Cancer Study Group (ABCSG). EndoPredict improves the prognostic classification derived from common clinical guidelines in ER-positive, HER2-negative early breast cancer. Ann Oncol. 2013;24(3):640–7. https://doi.org/10.1093/annonc/mds334. PMID: 23035151; PMCID: PMC3574544
16. Ross JS, Fletcher JA. The HER-2/neu oncogene: prognostic factor, predictive factor and target for therapy. Semin Cancer Biol. 1999;9(2):125–38. https://doi.org/10.1006/scbi.1998.0083. PMID: 10202134
17. Marchiò C, Annaratone L, Marques A, Casorzo L, Berrino E, Sapino A. Evolving concepts in HER2 evaluation in breast cancer: heterogeneity, HER2-low carcinomas and beyond. Semin Cancer Biol. 2021;72:123–35. https://doi.org/10.1016/j.semcancer.2020.02.016. PMID: 32112814
18. Wolff AC, Somerfield MR, Dowsett M, Hammond MEH, Hayes DF, McShane LM, Saphner TJ, Spears PA, Allison KH. Human epidermal growth factor receptor 2 testing in breast cancer: ASCO-College of American pathologists guideline update. J Clin Oncol. 2023;41(22):3867–72. https://doi.org/10.1200/JCO.22.02864. PMID: 37284804
19. Guarneri V, Passos Coelho JL, Duhoux FP, Egle D, García-Sáenz JÁ, Penault-Llorca F, Selander K, Wildiers H, Zaman K, Laeis P, Lucerna M, Pierga JY. Study design for DESTINY-breast respond HER2-low Europe: T-DXd in patients with HER2-low advanced breast cancer. Future Oncol. 2024;20(18):1237–50. https://doi.org/10.2217/fon-2024-0015. PMID: 38592002; PMCID: PMC11318675
20. Cheng X. A comprehensive review of HER2 in cancer biology and therapeutics. Genes (Basel). 2024;15(7):903. https://doi.org/10.3390/genes15070903. PMID: 39062682; PMCID: PMC11275319
21. Denkert C, Liedtke C, Tutt A, von Minckwitz G. Molecular alterations in triple-negative breast cancer-the road to new treatment strategies. Lancet. 2017;389(10087):2430–42. https://doi.org/10.1016/S0140-6736(16)32454-0. PMID: 27939063
22. Derakhshan F, Reis-Filho JS. Pathogenesis of triple-negative breast cancer. Annu Rev Pathol. 2022;17:181–204. https://doi.org/10.1146/annurev--pathol-042420-093238. PMID: 35073169; PMCID: PMC9231507
23. Turner N, Tutt A, Ashworth A. Hallmarks of 'BRCAness' in sporadic cancers. Nat Rev Cancer. 2004;4(10):814–9. https://doi.org/10.1038/nrc1457. PMID: 15510162
24. Prat A, Adamo B, Cheang MC, Anders CK, Carey LA, Perou CM. Molecular characterization of basal-like and non-basal-like triple-negative breast cancer. Oncologist. 2013;18(2):123–33. https://doi.org/10.1634/theoncologist.2012-0397. PMID: 23404817; PMCID: PMC3579595
25. Lehmann BD, Bauer JA, Chen X, Sanders ME, Chakravarthy AB, Shyr Y, Pietenpol JA. Identification of human triple-negative breast cancer subtypes and preclinical models for selection of targeted therapies. J Clin Invest. 2011;121(7):2750–67. https://doi.org/10.1172/JCI45014. PMID: 21633166; PMCID: PMC3127435
26. Lehmann BD, Jovanović B, Chen X, Estrada MV, Johnson KN, Shyr Y, Moses HL, Sanders ME, Pietenpol JA. Refinement of triple-negative breast cancer molecular subtypes: implications for neoadjuvant chemotherapy selection. PLoS One. 2016;11(6):e0157368. https://doi.org/10.1371/journal.pone.0157368. PMID: 27310713; PMCID: PMC4911051
27. Burstein MD, Tsimelzon A, Poage GM, Covington KR, Contreras A, Fuqua SA, Savage MI, Osborne CK, Hilsenbeck SG, Chang JC, Mills GB, Lau CC, Brown PH. Comprehensive genomic analysis identifies novel subtypes and targets of triple-negative breast cancer. Clin Cancer Res. 2015;21(7):1688–98. https://doi.org/10.1158/1078-0432.CCR-14-0432. PMID: 25208879; PMCID: PMC4362882
28. Colomer R, González-Farré B, Ballesteros AI, Peg V, Bermejo B, Pérez-Mies B, de la Cruz S, Rojo F, Pernas S, Palacios J. Biomarkers in breast can-

cer 2024: an updated consensus statement by the Spanish Society of Medical Oncology and the Spanish Society of Pathology. Clin Transl Oncol. 2024;26(12):2935–51. https://doi.org/10.1007/s12094-024-03541-1. PMID: 38869741; PMCID: PMC11564209

29. Desmedt C, Voet T, Sotiriou C, Campbell PJ. Next-generation sequencing in breast cancer: first take-home messages. Curr Opin Oncol. 2012;24(6):597–604. https://doi.org/10.1097/CCO.0b013e328359554e. PMID: 23014189; PMCID: PMC3713550
30. Addanki S, Meas S, Sarli VN, Singh B, Lucci A. Applications of circulating tumor cells and circulating tumor DNA in precision oncology for breast cancers. Int J Mol Sci. 2022;23(14):7843. https://doi.org/10.3390/ijms23147843. PMID: 35887191; PMCID: PMC9315812
31. Rakha EA, Pareja FG. New advances in molecular breast cancer pathology. Semin Cancer Biol. 2021;72:102–13. https://doi.org/10.1016/j.semcancer.2020.03.014. PMID: 32259641
32. Gennari A, André F, Barrios CH, Cortés J, de Azambuja E, DeMichele A, Dent R, Fenlon D, Gligorov J, Hurvitz SA, Im SA, Krug D, Kunz WG, Loi S, Penault-Llorca F, Ricke J, Robson M, Rugo HS, Saura C, Schmid P, Singer CF, Spanic T, Tolaney SM, Turner NC, Curigliano G, Loibl S, Paluch-Shimon S, Harbeck N. ESMO guidelines committee. Electronic address: clinicalguidelines@esmo.org. ESMO clinical practice guideline for the diagnosis, staging and treatment of patients with metastatic breast cancer. Ann Oncol. 2021;32(12):1475–95. https://doi.org/10.1016/j.annonc.2021.09.019. PMID: 34678411
33. Mosele MF, Westphalen CB, Stenzinger A, Barlesi F, Bayle A, Bièche I, Bonastre J, Castro E, Dienstmann R, Krämer A, Czarnecka AM, Meric-Bernstam F, Michiels S, Miller R, Normanno N, Reis-Filho J, Remon J, Robson M, Rouleau E, Scarpa A, Serrano C, Mateo J, André F. Recommendations for the use of next-generation sequencing (NGS) for patients with advanced cancer in 2024: a report from the ESMO precision medicine working group. Ann Oncol. 2024;35(7):588–606. https://doi.org/10.1016/j.annonc.2024.04.005. Erratum in: Ann Oncol. 2025 Apr; 36(4):472. 10.1016/j.annonc.2024.11.010. PMID: 38834388
34. Yoshida R. Hereditary breast and ovarian cancer (HBOC): review of its molecular characteristics, screening, treatment, and prognosis. Breast Cancer. 2021;28(6):1167–80. https://doi.org/10.1007/s12282-020-01148-2. PMID: 32862296; PMCID: PMC8514387
35. van der Groep P, van der Wall E, van Diest PJ. Pathology of hereditary breast cancer. Cell Oncol (Dordr). 2011;34(2):71–88. https://doi.org/10.1007/s13402-011-0010-3. PMID: 21336636; PMCID: PMC3063560
36. Honrado E, Benítez J, Palacios J. Histopathology of BRCA1- and BRCA2-associated breast cancer. Crit Rev Oncol Hematol. 2006;59(1):27–39. https://doi.org/10.1016/j.critrevonc.2006.01.006. PMID: 16530420
37. Petrucelli N, Daly MB, Feldman GL. Hereditary breast and ovarian cancer due to mutations in BRCA1 and BRCA2. Genet Med. 2010;12(5):245–59. https://doi.org/10.1097/GIM.0b013e3181d38f2f. PMID: 20216074
38. Petrucelli N, Daly MB, Pal T. BRCA1- and BRCA2-associated hereditary breast and ovarian cancer. 1998 [updated 2025 Mar 20]. In: Adam MP, Feldman J, Mirzaa GM, Pagon RA, Wallace SE, Amemiya A, editors. GeneReviews® [Internet]. Seattle: University of Washington, Seattle; 1993–2025. PMID: 20301425.
39. Stevens KN, Vachon CM, Couch FJ. Genetic susceptibility to triple-negative breast cancer. Cancer Res. 2013;73(7):2025–30. https://doi.org/10.1158/0008-5472.CAN-12-1699. PMID: 23536562; PMCID: PMC3654815
40. Wallace AJ. New challenges for BRCA testing: a view from the diagnostic laboratory. Eur J Hum Genet. 2016;24(Suppl 1):S10–8. https://doi.org/10.1038/ejhg.2016.94. PMID: 27514839; PMCID: PMC5141576
41. Rose M, Burgess JT, O'Byrne K, Richard DJ, Bolderson E. PARP inhibitors: clinical relevance, mechanisms of action and tumor resistance. Front Cell Dev Biol. 2020;8:564601. https://doi.org/10.3389/fcell.2020.564601. PMID: 33015058; PMCID: PMC7509090
42. Huber-Keener KJ. Cancer genetics and breast cancer. Best Pract Res Clin Obstet Gynaecol. 2022;82:3–11. https://doi.org/10.1016/j.bpobgyn.2022.01.007. PMID: 35272929
43. Rahman N, Seal S, Thompson D, Kelly P, Renwick A, Elliott A, Reid S, Spanova K, Barfoot R, Chagtai T, Jayatilake H, McGuffog L, Hanks S, Evans DG, Eccles D, Breast Cancer Susceptibility Collaboration (UK), Easton DF, Stratton MR. PALB2, which encodes a BRCA2-interacting protein, is a breast cancer susceptibility gene. Nat Genet. 2007;39(2):165–7. https://doi.org/10.1038/ng1959. PMID: 17200668; PMCID: PMC2871593
44. Antoniou AC, Foulkes WD, Tischkowitz M. Breast-cancer risk in families with mutations in PALB2. N Engl J Med. 2014;371(17):1651–2. https://doi.org/10.1056/NEJMc1410673. PMID: 25337756
45. Nik-Zainal S, Davies H, Staaf J, Ramakrishna M, Glodzik D, Zou X, Martincorena I, Alexandrov LB, Martin S, Wedge DC, Van Loo P, Ju YS, Smid M, Brinkman AB, Morganella S, Aure MR, Lingjærde OC, Langerød A, Ringnér M, Ahn SM, Boyault S, Brock JE, Broeks A, Butler A, Desmedt C, Dirix L, Dronov S, Fatima A, Foekens JA, Gerstung M, Hooijer GK, Jang SJ, Jones DR, Kim HY, King TA, Krishnamurthy S, Lee HJ, Lee JY, Li Y, McLaren

S, Menzies A, Mustonen V, O'Meara S, Pauporté I, Pivot X, Purdie CA, Raine K, Ramakrishnan K, Rodríguez-González FG, Romieu G, Sieuwerts AM, Simpson PT, Shepherd R, Stebbings L, Stefansson OA, Teague J, Tommasi S, Treilleux I, Van den Eynden GG, Vermeulen P, Vincent-Salomon A, Yates L, Caldas C, van't Veer L, Tutt A, Knappskog S, Tan BK, Jonkers J, Borg Å, Ueno NT, Sotiriou C, Viari A, Futreal PA, Campbell PJ, Span PN, Van Laere S, Lakhani SR, Eyfjord JE, Thompson AM, Birney E, Stunnenberg HG, van de Vijver MJ, Martens JW, Børresen-Dale AL, Richardson AL, Kong G, Thomas G, Stratton MR. Landscape of somatic mutations in 560 breast cancer whole-genome sequences. Nature. 2016;534(7605):47–54. https://doi.org/10.1038/nature17676. Erratum in: Nature. 2019 Feb; 566(7742):E1. 10.1038/s41586-019-0883-2. PMID: 27135926; PMCID: PMC4910866

46. Yang X, Leslie G, Doroszuk A, Schneider S, Allen J, Decker B, Dunning AM, Redman J, Scarth J, Plaskocinska I, Luccarini C, Shah M, Pooley K, Dorling L, Lee A, Adank MA, Adlard J, Aittomäki K, Andrulis IL, Ang P, Barwell J, Bernstein JL, Bobolis K, Borg Å, Blomqvist C, Claes KBM, Concannon P, Cuggia A, Culver JO, Damiola F, de Pauw A, Diez O, Dolinsky JS, Domchek SM, Engel C, Evans DG, Fostira F, Garber J, Golmard L, Goode EL, Gruber SB, Hahnen E, Hake C, Heikkinen T, Hurley JE, Janavicius R, Kleibl Z, Kleiblova P, Konstantopoulou I, Kvist A, Laduca H, Lee ASG, Lesueur F, Maher ER, Mannermaa A, Manoukian S, McFarland R, McKinnon W, Meindl A, Metcalfe K, Mohd Taib NA, Moilanen J, Nathanson KL, Neuhausen S, Ng PS, Nguyen-Dumont T, Nielsen SM, Obermair F, Offit K, Olopade OI, Ottini L, Penkert J, Pylkäs K, Radice P, Ramus SJ, Rudaitis V, Side L, Silva-Smith R, Silvestri V, Skytte AB, Slavin T, Soukupova J, Tondini C, Trainer AH, Unzeitig G, Usha L, van Overeem Hansen T, Whitworth J, Wood M, Yip CH, Yoon SY, Yussuf A, Zogopoulos G, Goldgar D, Hopper JL, Chenevix-Trench G, Pharoah P, George SHL, Balmaña J, Houdayer C, James P, El-Haffaf Z, Ehrencrona H, Janatova M, Peterlongo P, Nevanlinna H, Schmutzler R, Teo SH, Robson M, Pal T, Couch F, Weitzel JN, Elliott A, Southey M, Winqvist R, Easton DF, Foulkes WD, Antoniou AC, Tischkowitz M. Cancer risks associated with germline PALB2 pathogenic variants: an international study of 524 families. J Clin Oncol. 2020;38(7):674–85. https://doi.org/10.1200/JCO.19.01907. PMID: 31841383; PMCID: PMC7049229
47. Moslemi M, Moradi Y, Dehghanbanadaki H, Afkhami H, Khaledi M, Sedighimehr N, Fathi J, Sohrabi E. The association between ATM variants and risk of breast cancer: a systematic review and meta-analysis. BMC Cancer. 2021;21(1):27. https://doi.org/10.1186/s12885-020-07749-6. PMID: 33402103; PMCID: PMC7786920
48. Stucci LS, Internò V, Tucci M, Perrone M, Mannavola F, Palmirotta R, Porta C. The ATM gene in breast cancer: its relevance in clinical practice. Genes (Basel). 2021;12(5):727. https://doi.org/10.3390/genes12050727. PMID: 34068084; PMCID: PMC8152746
49. Weigelt B, Bi R, Kumar R, Blecua P, Mandelker DL, Geyer FC, Pareja F, James PA, kConFab Investigators, Couch FJ, Eccles DM, Blows F, Pharoah P, Li A, Selenica P, Lim RS, Jayakumaran G, Waddell N, Shen R, Norton L, Wen HY, Powell SN, Riaz N, Robson ME, Reis-Filho JS, Chenevix-Trench G. The landscape of somatic genetic alterations in breast cancers from ATM germline mutation carriers. J Natl Cancer Inst. 2018;110(9):1030–4. https://doi.org/10.1093/jnci/djy028. PMID: 29506079; PMCID: PMC6136925
50. Seca M, Narod SA. Breast cancer and ATM mutations: treatment implications. Hered Cancer Clin Pract. 2024;22(1):26. https://doi.org/10.1186/s13053-024-00300-9. PMID: 39543654; PMCID: PMC11566136
51. Nevanlinna H, Bartek J. The CHEK2 gene and inherited breast cancer susceptibility. Oncogene. 2006;25(43):5912–9. https://doi.org/10.1038/sj.onc.1209877. PMID: 16998506
52. Bertheau P, Lehmann-Che J, Varna M, Dumay A, Poirot B, Porcher R, Turpin E, Plassa LF, de Roquancourt A, Bourstyn E, de Cremoux P, Janin A, Giacchetti S, Espié M, de Thé H. p53 in breast cancer subtypes and new insights into response to chemotherapy. Breast. 2013;22(Suppl 2):S27–9. https://doi.org/10.1016/j.breast.2013.07.005. PMID: 24074787
53. Ellis MJ, Perou CM. The genomic landscape of breast cancer as a therapeutic roadmap. Cancer Discov. 2013;3(1):27–34. https://doi.org/10.1158/2159-8290.CD-12-0462. PMID: 23319768; PMCID: PMC3553590
54. Li Y, Saini P, Sriraman A, Dobbelstein M. Mdm2 inhibition confers protection of p53-proficient cells from the cytotoxic effects of Wee1 inhibitors. Oncotarget. 2015;6(32):32339–52. https://doi.org/10.18632/oncotarget.5891. PMID: 26431163; PMCID: PMC4741697
55. Fallah Y, Demas DM, Jin L, He W, Shajahan-Haq AN. Targeting WEE1 inhibits growth of breast cancer cells that are resistant to endocrine therapy and CDK4/6 inhibitors. Front Oncol. 2021;11:681530. https://doi.org/10.3389/fonc.2021.681530. PMID: 34277427; PMCID: PMC8281892
56. Nagy TR, Maistro S, Encinas G, Katayama MLH, Pereira GFL, Gaburo-Júnior N, Franco LAM, Gouvêa ACRC, Diz MDPE, Leite LAS, Folgueira MAAK. Germline and somatic mutations in postmenopausal breast cancer patients. Clinics (Sao Paulo). 2021;76:e2837. https://doi.org/10.6061/clinics/2021/e2837. PMID: 34287479; PMCID: PMC8266163
57. Fusco N, Malapelle U, Fassan M, Marchiò C, Buglioni S, Zupo S, Criscitiello C, Vigneri P, Dei Tos AP, Maiorano E, Viale G. PIK3CA mutations as a molecular target for hormone receptor-positive, HER2-negative metastatic breast cancer. Front

Oncol. 2021;11:644737. https://doi.org/10.3389/fonc.2021.644737. PMID: 33842357; PMCID: PMC8027489
58. Neill NE, Mauro LA, Pennisi A. Novel estrogen receptor—targeted therapies in hormone-receptor positive breast cancer. Curr Treat Options in Oncol. 2025;26(4):302–12.https://doi.org/10.1007/s11864--025-01310-y. PMID: 40163189
59. Hinz N, Jücker M. Distinct functions of AKT isoforms in breast cancer: a comprehensive review. Cell Commun Signal. 2019;17(1):154. https://doi.org/10.1186/s12964-019-0450-3. PMID: 31752925; PMCID: PMC6873690
60. Turner NC, Oliveira M, Howell SJ, Dalenc F, Cortes J, Gomez Moreno HL, Hu X, Jhaveri K, Krivorotko P, Loibl S, Morales Murillo S, Okera M, Park YH, Sohn J, Toi M, Tokunaga E, Yousef S, Zhukova L, de Bruin EC, Grinsted L, Schiavon G, Foxley A, Rugo HS, CAPItello-291 Study Group. Capivasertib in hormone receptor-positive advanced breast cancer. N Engl J Med. 2023;388(22):2058–70. https://doi.org/10.1056/NEJMoa2214131. PMID: 37256976; PMCID: PMC11335038
61. Mester J, Eng C. When overgrowth bumps into cancer: the PTEN-opathies. Am J Med Genet C Semin Med Genet. 2013;163C(2):114–21. https://doi.org/10.1002/ajmg.c.31364. PMID: 23613428
62. DeGraffenried LA, Fulcher L, Friedrichs WE, Grünwald V, Ray RB, Hidalgo M. Reduced PTEN expression in breast cancer cells confers susceptibility to inhibitors of the PI3 kinase/Akt pathway. Ann Oncol. 2004;15(10):1510–6. https://doi.org/10.1093/annonc/mdh388. PMID: 15367412
63. Drebin JA, Stern DF, Link VC, Weinberg RA, Greene MI. Monoclonal antibodies identify a cell-surface antigen associated with an activated cellular oncogene. Nature. 1984;312(5994):545–8. https://doi.org/10.1038/312545a0. PMID: 6504162
64. Ishii K, Morii N, Yamashiro H. Pertuzumab in the treatment of HER2-positive breast cancer: an evidence-based review of its safety, efficacy, and place in therapy. Core Evid. 2019;14:51–70. https://doi.org/10.2147/CE.S217848. PMID: 31802990; PMCID: PMC6827570
65. Petrelli F, Tomasello G, Barni S, Lonati V, Passalacqua R, Ghidini M. Clinical and pathological characterization of HER2 mutations in human breast cancer: a systematic review of the literature. Breast Cancer Res Treat. 2017;166(2):339–49. https://doi.org/10.1007/s10549-017-4419-x. PMID: 28762010
66. Ross JS, Gay LM, Wang K, Ali SM, Chumsri S, Elvin JA, Bose R, Vergilio JA, Suh J, Yelensky R, Lipson D, Chmielecki J, Waintraub S, Leyland-Jones B, Miller VA, Stephens PJ. Nonamplification ERBB2 genomic alterations in 5605 cases of recurrent and metastatic breast cancer: an emerging opportunity for anti-HER2 targeted therapies. Cancer. 2016;122(17):2654–62. https://doi.org/10.1002/cncr.30102. PMID: 27284958
67. von Minckwitz G, Huang CS, Mano MS, Loibl S, Mamounas EP, Untch M, Wolmark N, Rastogi P, Schneeweiss A, Redondo A, Fischer HH, Jacot W, Conlin AK, Arce-Salinas C, Wapnir IL, Jackisch C, DiGiovanna MP, Fasching PA, Crown JP, Wülfing P, Shao Z, Rota Caremoli E, Wu H, Lam LH, Tesarowski D, Smitt M, Douthwaite H, Singel SM, Geyer CE Jr, Katherine Investigators. Trastuzumab emtansine for residual invasive HER2-positive breast cancer. N Engl J Med. 2019;380(7):617–28. https://doi.org/10.1056/NEJMoa1814017. PMID: 30516102
68. Xu X, De Angelis C, Burke KA, Nardone A, Hu H, Qin L, Veeraraghavan J, Sethunath V, Heiser LM, Wang N, Ng CKY, Chen ES, Renwick A, Wang T, Nanda S, Shea M, Mitchell T, Rajendran M, Waters I, Zabransky DJ, Scott KL, Gutierrez C, Nagi C, Geyer FC, Chamness GC, Park BH, Shaw CA, Hilsenbeck SG, Rimawi MF, Gray JW, Weigelt B, Reis-Filho JS, Osborne CK, Schiff R. HER2 reactivation through acquisition of the HER2 L755S mutation as a mechanism of acquired resistance to HER2-targeted therapy in HER2+ breast cancer. Clin Cancer Res. 2017;23(17):5123–34. https://doi.org/10.1158/1078-0432.CCR-16-2191. PMID: 28487443; PMCID: PMC5762201
69. Santamaria S, Gagliani MC, Bellese G, Marconi S, Lechiara A, Dameri M, Aiello C, Tagliatti E, Castagnola P, Cortese K. Imaging of endocytic trafficking and extracellular vesicles released under neratinib treatment in ERBB2+ breast cancer cells. J Histochem Cytochem. 2021;69(7):461–73. https://doi.org/10.1369/00221554211026297. PMID: 34126793; PMCID: PMC8246527
70. Brett JO, Spring LM, Bardia A, Wander SA. ESR1 mutation as an emerging clinical biomarker in metastatic hormone receptor-positive breast cancer. Breast Cancer Res. 2021;23(1):85. https://doi.org/10.1186/s13058-021-01462-3. PMID: 34392831; PMCID: PMC8365900
71. Li X, Zhao L, Chen C, Nie J, Jiao B. Can EGFR be a therapeutic target in breast cancer? Biochim Biophys Acta Rev Cancer. 2022;1877(5):188789. https://doi.org/10.1016/j.bbcan.2022.188789. PMID: 36064121
72. Thomas M, Kelly ED, Abraham J, Kruse M. Invasive lobular breast cancer: a review of pathogenesis, diagnosis, management, and future directions of early stage disease. Semin Oncol. 2019;46(2):121–32. https://doi.org/10.1053/j.seminoncol.2019.03.002. PMID: 31239068
73. Corso G, Montagna G, Figueiredo J, La Vecchia C, Fumagalli Romario U, Fernandes MS, Seixas S, Roviello F, Trovato C, Guerini-Rocco E, Fusco N, Pravettoni G, Petrocchi S, Rotili A, Massari G, Magnoni F, De Lorenzi F, Bottoni M, Galimberti V, Sanches JM, Calvello M, Seruca R, Bonanni B. Hereditary gastric and breast cancer syndromes related to CDH1 germline mutation: a multidisciplinary clinical review. Cancers (Basel). 2020;12(6):1598. https://doi.org/10.3390/cancers12061598. PMID: 32560361; PMCID: PMC7352390

74. McCart Reed AE, Kutasovic JR, Lakhani SR, Simpson PT. Invasive lobular carcinoma of the breast: morphology, biomarkers and 'omics'. Breast Cancer Res. 2015;17(1):12. https://doi.org/10.1186/s13058-015-0519-x. PMID: 25849106; PMCID: PMC4310190
75. Ciriello G, Gatza ML, Beck AH, Wilkerson MD, Rhie SK, Pastore A, Zhang H, McLellan M, Yau C, Kandoth C, Bowlby R, Shen H, Hayat S, Fieldhouse R, Lester SC, Tse GM, Factor RE, Collins LC, Allison KH, Chen YY, Jensen K, Johnson NB, Oesterreich S, Mills GB, Cherniack AD, Robertson G, Benz C, Sander C, Laird PW, Hoadley KA, King TA, TCGA Research Network, Perou CM. Comprehensive molecular portraits of invasive lobular breast cancer. Cell. 2015;163(2):506–19. https://doi.org/10.1016/j.cell.2015.09.033. PMID: 26451490; PMCID: PMC4603750
76. Chiang S, Weigelt B, Wen HC, Pareja F, Raghavendra A, Martelotto LG, Burke KA, Basili T, Li A, Geyer FC, Piscuoglio S, Ng CK, Jungbluth AA, Balss J, Pusch S, Baker GM, Cole KS, von Deimling A, Batten JM, Marotti JD, Soh HC, McCalip BL, Serrano J, Lim RS, Siziopikou KP, Lu S, Liu X, Hammour T, Brogi E, Snuderl M, Iafrate AJ, Reis-Filho JS, Schnitt SJ. IDH2 mutations define a unique subtype of breast cancer with altered nuclear polarity. Cancer Res. 2016;76(24):7118–29. https://doi.org/10.1158/0008-5472.CAN-16-0298. PMID: 27913435; PMCID: PMC5502804
77. Richardson ET, Jo VY, Schnitt SJ. Salivary gland-like tumors of the breast. Arch Pathol Lab Med. 2023;147(9):1014–24. https://doi.org/10.5858/arpa.2023-0038-RA. PMID: 37651394
78. Varga Z, Maccio U. Molecular pathology in breast disease: diagnostic, prognostic, and therapeutic tools. Virchows Arch. 2024;484(2):247–61. https://doi.org/10.1007/s00428-023-03709-0. PMID: 38015260; PMCID: PMC10948467
79. Garcia-Ortega DY, Martín-Tellez KS, Cuellar-Hubbe M, Martínez-Said H, Álvarez-Cano A, Brener-Chaoul M, Alegría-Baños JA, Martínez-Tlahuel JL. Desmoid-type fibromatosis. Cancers (Basel). 2020;12(7):1851. https://doi.org/10.3390/cancers12071851. PMID: 32660036; PMCID: PMC7408653
80. Guo T, Zhang L, Chang NE, Singer S, Maki RG, Antonescu CR. Consistent MYC and FLT4 gene amplification in radiation-induced angiosarcoma but not in other radiation-associated atypical vascular lesions. Genes Chromosomes Cancer. 2011;50(1):25–33. https://doi.org/10.1002/gcc.20827. PMID: 20949568; PMCID: PMC3150534
81. Bansal R, Adeyelu T, Elliott A, Tan AR, Ribeiro JR, Meisel J, Oberley MJ, Graff SL, Sledge GW Jr, Grilley-Olson JE, Sammons SL, Rosenberger LH. Genomic landscape of malignant phyllodes tumors identifies subsets for targeted therapy. JCO Precis Oncol. 2024;8:e2400289. https://doi.org/10.1200/PO.24.00289. PMID: 39637336; PMCID: PMC11634179
82. Mon KS, Tang P. Fibroepithelial lesions of the breast: update on molecular profile with focus on pediatric population. Arch Pathol Lab Med. 2023;147(1):38–45. https://doi.org/10.5858/arpa.2022-0011-RA. PMID: 35776911
83. Tan J, Ong CK, Lim WK, Ng CC, Thike AA, Ng LM, Rajasegaran V, Myint SS, Nagarajan S, Thangaraju S, Dey S, Nasir ND, Wijaya GC, Lim JQ, Huang D, Li Z, Wong BH, Chan JY, McPherson JR, Cutcutache I, Poore G, Tay ST, Tan WJ, Putti TC, Ahmad BS, Iau P, Chan CW, Tang AP, Yong WS, Madhukumar P, Ho GH, Tan VK, Wong CY, Hartman M, Ong KW, Tan BK, Rozen SG, Tan P, Tan PH, Teh BT. Genomic landscapes of breast fibroepithelial tumors. Nat Genet. 2015;47(11):1341–5. https://doi.org/10.1038/ng.3409. PMID: 26437033
84. Gremke N, Rodepeter FR, Teply-Szymanski J, Griewing S, Boekhoff J, Stroh A, Tarawneh TS, Riera-Knorrenschild J, Balser C, Hattesohl A, Middeke M, Ross P, Litmeyer AS, Romey M, Stiewe T, Wündisch T, Neubauer A, Denkert C, Wagner U, Mack EKM. NGS-guided precision oncology in breast cancer and gynecological tumors-a retrospective molecular tumor board analysis. Cancers (Basel). 2024;16(8):1561. https://doi.org/10.3390/cancers16081561. PMID: 38672643; PMCID: PMC11048446
85. Barroso-Sousa R, Pacífico JP, Sammons S, Tolaney SM. Tumor mutational burden in breast cancer: current evidence, challenges, and opportunities. Cancers (Basel). 2023;15(15):3997. https://doi.org/10.3390/cancers15153997. PMID: 37568813; PMCID: PMC10417019
86. Barroso-Sousa R, Jain E, Cohen O, Kim D, Buendia-Buendia J, Winer E, Lin N, Tolaney SM, Wagle N. Prevalence and mutational determinants of high tumor mutation burden in breast cancer. Ann Oncol. 2020;31(3):387–94. https://doi.org/10.1016/j.annonc.2019.11.010. PMID: 32067680
87. Sha D, Jin Z, Budczies J, Kluck K, Stenzinger A, Sinicrope FA. Tumor mutational burden as a predictive biomarker in solid tumors. Cancer Discov. 2020;10(12):1808–25. https://doi.org/10.1158/2159-8290.CD-20-0522. PMID: 33139244; PMCID: PMC7710563
88. Jin M, Fang J, Peng J, Wang X, Xing P, Jia K, Hu J, Wang D, Ding Y, Wang X, Li W, Chen Z. PD-1/PD-L1 immune checkpoint blockade in breast cancer: research insights and sensitization strategies. Mol Cancer. 2024;23(1):266. https://doi.org/10.1186/s12943-024-02176-8. PMID: 39614285; PMCID: PMC11605969
89. McGrail DJ, Pilié PG, Rashid NU, Voorwerk L, Slagter M, Kok M, Jonasch E, Khasraw M, Heimberger AB, Lim B, Ueno NT, Litton JK, Ferrarotto R, Chang JT, Moulder SL, Lin SY. High tumor mutation burden fails to predict immune checkpoint blockade response across all cancer

types. Ann Oncol. 2021;32(5):661–72. https://doi.org/10.1016/j.annonc.2021.02.006. PMID: 33736924; PMCID: PMC8053682

90. Ren XY, Song Y, Wang J, Chen LY, Pang JY, Zhou LR, Shen SJ, Cao X, Wang YX, Shao MM, Liang ZY, Sun Q, Wu HW. Mismatch repair deficiency and microsatellite instability in triple-negative breast cancer: a retrospective study of 440 patients. Front Oncol. 2021;11:570623. https://doi.org/10.3389/fonc.2021.570623. PMID: 33747906; PMCID: PMC7970194
91. Stoll J, Rosenthal E, Cummings S, Willmott J, Bernhisel R, Kupfer SS. No evidence of increased risk of breast cancer in women with lynch syndrome identified by multigene panel testing. JCO Precis Oncol. 2020;4:51–60. https://doi.org/10.1200/PO.19.00271. PMID: 35050728
92. Freitas AJA, Causin RL, Varuzza MB, Calfa S, Hidalgo Filho CMT, Komoto TT, Souza CP, Marques MMC. Liquid biopsy as a tool for the diagnosis, treatment, and monitoring of breast cancer. Int J Mol Sci. 2022;23(17):9952. https://doi.org/10.3390/ijms23179952. PMID: 36077348; PMCID: PMC9456236
93. Baumann A, Ruckert C, Meier C, Hutschenreiter T, Remy R, Schnur B, Döbel M, Fankep RCN, Skowronek D, Kutz O, Arnold N, Katzke AL, Forster M, Kobiela AL, Thiedig K, Zimmer A, Ritter J, Weber BHF, Honisch E, Hackmann K, Bioinformatics Working Group of the German Consortium for Hereditary Breast & Ovarian Cancer, Schmidt G, Sturm M, Ernst C. Limitations in next-generation sequencing-based genotyping of breast cancer polygenic risk score loci. Eur J Hum Genet. 2024;32(8):987–97. https://doi.org/10.1038/s41431-024-01647-2. PMID: 38907004; PMCID: PMC11291653
94. Bergholtz H, Carter JM, Cesano A, Cheang MCU, Church SE, Divakar P, Fuhrman CA, Goel S, Gong J, Guerriero JL, Hoang ML, Hwang ES, Kuasne H, Lee J, Liang Y, Mittendorf EA, Perez J, Prat A, Pusztai L, Reeves JW, Riazalhosseini Y, Richer JK, Sahin Ö, Sato H, Schlam I, Sørlie T, Stover DG, Swain SM, Swarbrick A, Thompson EA, Tolaney SM, Warren SE, On Behalf Of The GeoMx Breast Cancer Consortium. Best practices for spatial profiling for breast cancer research with the GeoMx® digital spatial profiler. Cancers (Basel). 2021;13(17):4456. https://doi.org/10.3390/cancers13174456. PMID: 34503266; PMCID: PMC8431590
95. Kaur H, Mao S, Shah S, Gorski DH, Krawetz SA, Sloane BF, Mattingly RR. Next-generation sequencing: a powerful tool for the discovery of molecular markers in breast ductal carcinoma in situ. Expert Rev Mol Diagn. 2013;13(2):151–65. https://doi.org/10.1586/erm.13.4. PMID: 23477556; PMCID: PMC3804339
96. Schwartz CJ, Dolgalev I, Yoon E, Osman I, Heguy A, Vega-Saenz de Miera EC, Nimeh D, Jour G, Darvishian F. Microglandular adenosis is an advanced precursor breast lesion with evidence of molecular progression to matrix-producing metaplastic carcinoma. Hum Pathol. 2019;85:65–71. https://doi.org/10.1016/j.humpath.2018.10.021. PMID: 30428388
97. Liu X, Huang X, Bai Y, Zhang Z, Jin T, Wu H, Liang Z. Next-generation sequencing revealed recurrent ZFPM1 mutations in encapsulated papillary carcinoma of the breast. NPJ Precis Oncol. 2021;5(1):42. https://doi.org/10.1038/s41698-021-00180-5. PMID: 34007008; PMCID: PMC8131604
98. Kader T, Elder K, Zethoven M, Semple T, Hill P, Goode DL, Thio N, Cheasley D, Rowley SM, Byrne DJ, Pang JM, Miligy IM, Green AR, Rakha EA, Fox SB, Mann GB, Campbell IG, Gorringe KL. The genetic architecture of breast papillary lesions as a predictor of progression to carcinoma. NPJ Breast Cancer. 2020;6:9. https://doi.org/10.1038/s41523-020-0150-6. PMID: 32195332; PMCID: PMC7067788
99. Nourieh M, Vibert R, Saint-Ghislain M, Cyrta J, Vincent-Salomon A. Next-generation sequencing in breast pathology: real impact on routine practice over a decade since its introduction. Histopathology. 2023;82(1):162–9. https://doi.org/10.1111/his.14794. PMID: 36482269; PMCID: PMC10108312
100. Lee H, Cho YA, Kim DG, Cho EY. Next-generation sequencing in breast cancer patients: real-world data for precision medicine. Cancer Res Treat. 2024;56(1):149–61. https://doi.org/10.4143/crt.2023.800. PMID: 37591784; PMCID: PMC10789952

Head and Neck Pathology

12

Marc Lucas Ooft and Stefan M. Willems

Introduction

Head and neck tumors encompass a wide array of neoplasms originating from the upper aerodigestive tract, salivary glands, thyroid, sinonasal cavities, and other complex anatomical regions in the head and neck. These tumors exhibit both significant diversity and overlap in their histomorphology, molecular profiles and *in vivo* behavior, presenting considerable diagnostic and therapeutic challenges for both pathologists, surgeons and oncologists. Recent advancements in Next-Generation Sequencing (NGS), RNA sequencing, and methylation profiling have significantly deepened our understanding of the (epi)genomic landscape of head and neck tumors. These molecular ancillary tests have not only improved diagnostic classification but have also paved the way for targeted therapies and personalized treatment approaches [125].

M. L. Ooft (✉)
Pathology-DNA, Rijnstate Hospital, Arnhem, The Netherlands

Department of Histopathology, King's College Hospital, King's College, London, UK
e-mail: mooft@rijnstate.nl

S. M. Willems
Department of Pathology and Medical Biology, University Medical Center Groningen, Groningen, The Netherlands
e-mail: s.m.willems@umcg.nl

As the number of recognized head and neck entities continues to expand, often defined along molecular lines, traditional hematoxylin/eosin (H&E) slides or cytology alone, even coupled with immunohistochemistry, are frequently insufficient for providing a definitive diagnosis and guiding treatment decisions.

Molecular Landscape of Squamous Cell Carcinomas (SCC)

Squamous cell carcinoma (SCC) stands as the most prevalent malignant tumor within the head and neck region. Within the SCCs the most important distinction is between the non-viral related SCCs and viral related SCC. HPV-negative SCCs frequently show mutations in TP53, CDKN2A, and FAT1, along with higher genomic instability [28]. Viral related SCC involve Human Papillomavirus (HPV) or Epstein-Barr virus (EBV). HPV-positive SCCs often have PIK3CA mutations and fewer overall mutations [28, 36]. EBV-positive SCCs (like nasopharyngeal carcinoma) feature the EBV genome, NF-\kappaB pathway activation, and mutations in CYLD and TNFAIP3 [97]. Although not extensively studied, lymphoepithelial carcinomas (LEC) of the head and neck likely are strongly linked to EBV infection (often Epstein-Barr virus-encoded small RNAs (EBER)-positive) and share some molecular traits with NPC due to

© The Author(s), under exclusive license to Springer Nature Switzerland AG 2026

S. Sioletic, L. Coppola (eds.), *Next-Generation Sequencing in Solid Tumor Histopathology*, Current Clinical Pathology, https://doi.org/10.1007/978-3-032-18790-1_12

their common viral etiology [99]. Additionally, certain HPV-related sinonasal squamous cell carcinomas (i.e., the HPV related multiphenotypic sinonasal carcinoma) can histologically mimic other cancer types, such as salivary gland adenocarcinomas. These genomic differences are vital for tailored diagnosis, treatment, and prognostication. Thus, HPV/EBV status is critical for both treatment and classification of SCC as these require different treatment regimens compared to non-viral related SCCs. Consequently, the utility of viral PCR/ RNA testing is essential in the diagnosis of head and neck SCC. The viral PCR testing is in addition to p16 immunohistochemistry, especially for staging of oropharyngeal carcinoma in accordance with TNM staging developed by the Union for International Cancer Control (UICC) and the American Joint Committee on Cancer (AJCC).

Clonality Testing

Important to mention is clonality testing through broad NGS panels, and within the Head and Neck SCC (HNSCC) context specific focus on p53 mutational analysis. A substantial proportion of HNSCC patients have multiple risk factors (most commonly smoking and alcohol usage) [69], leading to field cancerization and the development of synchronous or metachronous SCCs [84, 106, 118, 148]. Therefore, p53 mutational analysis comparing different tumors and metastasis through NGS is frequently essential for accurate TNM staging, which subsequently informs treatment planning.

Unknown Primary SCC of the Head and Neck

When dealing with SCC metastases of unknown origin in the head and neck region, fine needle aspiration (FNA) and biopsy material should be tested for High-Risk Human Papillomavirus (HR-HPV). The presence of HR-HPV suggests an oropharyngeal origin [101]. Concurrently, testing for EBV, potentially via EBER, is recommended, as EBV positivity indicates a nasopharyngeal origin as previously indicated [120, 123, 159, 161].

Moreover, UV signature and clonality testing is also recommended in SCCs with no primary tumor, including screening by a dermatologist for skin cancers. Finding a prominent UV mutational signature (e.g., C > T transitions, CC > TT dinucleotide substitutions) in a metastatic HNSCC suggests a cutaneous (skin) primary [23]. This helps direct further investigation to the skin and can influence treatment strategies, as cutaneous SCCs behave differently from mucosal SCCs [58]. If a patient has a history of previous SCC (either mucosal or skin), then clonality testing can be useful to compare genetic alterations between the metastatic HNSCC of unknown primary and the known past primary tumor(s). This distinguishes a new primary tumor from a recurrence or metastasis of the previously known cancer, which is crucial for determining the right management plan and TNM stage.

Sinonasal and Nasopharyngeal Tumors

Rare tumors in the sinonasal and nasopharyngeal regions often benefit from molecular classification as differential diagnosis based of H&E and (immuno)histochemical stainings can still be very challanging as correct classification remains important. Highlights include SMARCB1 loss in SWI/SNF-deficient carcinomas, NUTM1 gene fusions in NUT carcinoma, IDH2 mutations seen in sinonasal undifferentiated carcinoma, EBV detection, which is essential in nasopharyngeal carcinoma, and EGFR exon 20 insertion mutations in SCCs arsing from sinonasal papillomas.

Molecular testing in sinonasal and nasopharyngeal carcinomas is crucial for precise diagnosis, especially given their varied and often challenging histological features, and increasingly influences therapeutic decisions. Plasma EBV DNA detection also serves as a critical prognostic biomarker and a tool for monitoring treatment response and recurrence [93].

For sinonasal carcinomas, molecular testing helps refine classification and identify distinct entities. EGFR exon 20 insertion mutations are highly characteristic of SCCs arising from sinonasal inverted papillomas, aiding in their definitive diagnosis and differentiation from other HNSCC subtypes [25, 163]. The presence of NUTM1 fusions (e.g., BRD4-NUTM1) confirms the diagnosis of NUT carcinoma, a highly aggressive, undifferentiated tumor often found in the sinonasal tract [7, 54–56, 142]. Loss of SMARCB1 (INI-1) expression, typically detected by immunohistochemistry [2, 18], is a key diagnostic marker for SMARCB1-deficient sinonasal carcinoma, an aggressive subtype of undifferentiated sinonasal tumors. Another specific sinonasal carcinoma is the SMARCA4 deficient carcinoma with loss of BRG1 by immunohistochemistry [1, 3]. Loss of either SMARCA4 of SMARCB1 define SWI/SNF complex–deficient sinonasal carcinomas which have no histological features allowing specific classification into a specific entity. Specific IDH2 mutations (e.g., R172 hotspot) are found in a subset of high-grade, undifferentiated sinonasal tumors, including some previously classified as sinonasal undifferentiated carcinoma (SNUC) or large cell neuroendocrine carcinoma, establishing them as a distinct entity [45, 60]. For sinonasal adenocarcinomas, fusions like ETV6-NTRK3 and mutations of CTNNB1 and BRAF have been reported in non-intestinal type adenocarcinomas [8, 14, 53, 166] while KRAS mutations are frequently seen in intestinal-type adenocarcinoma [136].

Molecular Diagnostic Approach to Undifferentiated Sinonasal Tumors and Impact on Treatment

In cases of undifferentiated sinonasal tumors where routine histology and immunohistochemistry are insufficient for a definitive diagnosis, a comprehensive molecular approach is essential. This often involves NGS panels to screen for a wide array of fusions, mutations, and copy number variations specific to sinonasal malignancies (Table 12.1).

Table 12.1 Molecular findings in head and neck carcinomas (excluding salivary gland carcinomas)

Tumor type	Key molecular features	References
Standard squamous cell carcinoma (HNSCC)	Chromosomal losses at 3p, 8p, 9p, and 17p, with gains at 3q, 5p, 8q, and 11q TP53, CDKN2A, FAT1, NOTCH1, KMT2D,CASP8, AJUBA, NSD1, HLA-A, TGFBR2, USP9X, KMT2D (MLL4), HRAS, UNC13C, ARID2, TRPM3 somatic mutations	[5, 28, 30, 77, 122, 154, 155]
NUT carcinoma	NUTM1 rearrangements	[43, 65, 142, 153]
Sinonasal undifferentiated carcinoma (SNUC)	IDH2 and IDH1 mutations	[45, 82, 104, 126]
SWI/SNF-deficient carcinomas	Loss of SMARCB1 or SMARCA4	[2, 3]
Viral carcinomas	HPV+ (e.g., oropharyngeal SCC): p16 overexpression, E6/E7 oncoproteins; EBV+ (e.g., nasopharyngeal): LMP1, NF-κB pathway activation	[26, 49, 95, 97, 160]
Intestinal-type adenocarcinoma (ITAC)	KRAS mutations	[136]
Non-intestinal-type adenocarcinoma	NTRK3-ETV6 fusions, CTNNB*1* and BRAF mutations	[8, 9, 53, 166]
Neuroendocrine carcinomas	ARID1A mutations with small cell type, LCNECs have recurrent IDH2 mutations	[35, 45, 47, 60]
Sinonasal squamous cell carcinoma	EGFR abberations	[25, 163]

Genetic Alterations in Sinonasal and Nasopharyngeal Tumors (Non-carcinomas)

Tumor type	Genetic alteration(s)	References
Sinonasal melanoma	KIT, NRAS, BRAF mutations	[34, 109, 111, 177]
Biphenotypic Sinonasal sarcoma	PAX3 fusions	[76, 89, 170, 175]

Salivary Gland Tumors

Salivary gland tumors are characterized by their histological and genetic diversity. Next-Generation Sequencing (NGS) has been instrumental in identifying several tumor-defining gene fusions, which are crucial for diagnosis. Notable examples include MYB–NFIB [103] fusions in adenoid cystic carcinoma, ETV6–NTRK3 [143] fusions in secretory carcinoma, and CRTC1–MAML2 fusions in mucoepidermoid carcinoma [116]. These molecular markers are invaluable in resolving diagnostic uncertainty, particularly in small biopsies or poorly differentiated tumors.

Molecular testing in salivary gland neoplasms serves to refine diagnosis when histology or FNA cytology are ambiguous or indeterminate, potentially avoiding unnecessary surgery [134]. For example, in a salivary gland FNA classified as Category III (Atypia of Undetermined Significance—AUS) or Category IVb (Salivary Gland Neoplasm of Uncertain Malignant Potential—SUMP) by the Milan System, detecting a CRTC1-MAML2 fusion would definitively diagnose a mucoepidermoid carcinoma, thereby upgrading the risk of malignancy and guiding management. Similarly, in histology, if a basaloid salivary gland tumor appears equivocal between a basal cell adenoma and an adenoid cystic carcinoma, the presence of a MYB-NFIB fusion confirms the diagnosis of adenoid cystic carcinoma. Ultimately, molecular discoveries have led to the reclassification of previously ambiguous salivary gland carcinomas into distinct entities with unique molecular signatures. This testing also aids in prognosis, as certain molecular alterations, including specific fusions, TP53 mutations, and HER2 amplification, can predict disease aggressiveness [140]. Furthermore, molecular testing guides targeted therapy by identifying actionable alterations like NTRK fusions, AR expression/amplification, or HER2 amplification [59, 75, 98, 124, 139, 167]. In adenoid cystic carcinomas (ACC), activating NOTCH1 mutations are particularly significant, defining a subgroup with a more aggressive phenotype, poor prognosis, and potential responsiveness to NOTCH inhibitors [51, 52] (Table 12.2).

Table 12.2 Genetic alterations in salivary gland neoplasms

Tumor type	Genetic alteration(s)	References
Acinic cell carcinoma	NR4A subfamily rearrangements	[66–68]
Adenoid cystic carcinoma	MYB-NFIB, MYBL1-NFIB, NOTCH1 signalling pathways	[57, 73]
Basal cell adenoma	CTNNB1 and CYLD (CYLD1) alterations	[81, 92, 127, 128]
Carcinoma ex pleomorphic adenoma	PLAG1, HMGA2, TP53, HRAS, PIK3CA; amplification of MYC; and/or amplification of EGFR	[33, 100, 121, 129, 169]
Epithelial-myoepithelial carcinoma	HRAS mutations, most commonly at codon 61	[31, 48, 62, 164]
Hyalinizing clear cell carcinoma	EWSR1-ATF1, EWSR1-CREM	[10, 29, 71]
Intraductal carcinoma	NCOA4-RET and rarely has STRN-ALK, TUT1-ETV5, or KIAA1217-RET, TRIM33-RET, NCOA4-RET, or BRAF p.V600, TRIM27-RET	[19, 20, 107, 133, 145, 144, 173]

(continued)

Table 12.2 (continued)

Tumor type	Genetic alteration(s)	References
Microsecretory adenocarcinoma	MEF2C-SS18, SS18-ZBTB7A	[21, 174]
Mucinous adenocarcinoma	AKT1 p.E17K, TP53	[132]
Mucoepidermoid carcinoma	CRTC1-MAML2, CRTC3-MAML2, CDKN2A, EWSR1-POU5F1	[79, 105, 116, 138, 165]
Myoepithelial carcinoma	PLAG1, HMGA2 and EWSR1 fusions	[40, 147, 176]
Pleomorphic adenoma	PLAG1, HMGA2	[152]
Polymorphous adenocarcinoma	PRKD1, PRKD2, PRKD3	[137, 171, 172, 178]
Salivary duct carcinoma	AR, TP53, HER2/ERBB2, PIK3CA, HRAS, PTEN, CDKN2A, FGFR1, PLAG1 or HMGA2 rearrangements, ALK, ETV6::NTRK3, others	[13, 32, 39, 46, 102, 108, 140, 158]
Sebaceous adenocarcinoma	MSH2	[110, 149]
Secretory carcinoma	ETV6-NTRK3, ETV6-RET, ETV6-MAML3, ETV6-MET, VIM-RET	[64, 78, 131, 146, 143]
Sialadenoma Papilliferum	BRAF V600E	[74]

Tumors of Uncertain Histogenesis and Mesenchymal Neoplasms

While the majority of head and neck malignancies fall within well-defined epithelial categories, a diverse group of rare tumors with mesenchymal differentiation or uncertain histogenesis may occasionally present in this region. Although these entities are uncommon, they are increasingly being characterized by distinct molecular alterations that can assist in diagnosis, prognostication, and, in some cases, eligibility for targeted therapy. The following table (Table 12.3) provides a brief overview of key molecular findings in selected mesenchymal tumors and neoplasms of uncertain histogenesis encountered in the head and neck, included here for completeness.

Odontogenic Tumors of the Head and Neck

Odontogenic tumors represent a diverse group of lesions originating from tooth-forming tissues. Their varied histological appearances often make diagnosis challenging. Molecular testing in odontogenic neoplasms can assist in refining diagnosis when histology is ambiguous, as specific molecular alterations can offer definitive classification.

Molecular Markers in Odontogenic Tumors

Next-generation sequencing (NGS) has identified several key molecular alterations characteristic of specific odontogenic tumors (see Table 12.4). For example, BRAF V600E mutations are identified in some ameloblastomas [24, 70]. These molecular markers are crucial for resolving diagnostic uncertainty, especially in small biopsies or ambiguous cases.

DNA Methylation Profiling in Head and Neck Pathology Diagnostics: Applications and Pitfalls

DNA methylation profiling deserves a special mention and is emerging as a powerful tool in head and neck pathology diagnostics, offering a refined approach to tumor classification and characterization, particularly in cases where conventional histology is ambiguous. This technique involves analyzing patterns of DNA methylation across the genome, which can provide a unique molecular signature for different tumor types and subtypes. In salivary gland tumors, DNA methylation profiling supports and expands conventional classification, allowing for a more precise diagnostic categorization of complex or ambigu-

Table 12.3 Molecular findings in tumors of uncertain histogenesis and mesenchymal tumors of the head and neck

A: Tumors of uncertain histogenesis		
Tumor type	Molecular alterations	References
Undifferentiated round/spindle cell sarcoma	Heterogeneous; diagnosis of exclusion; extensive and complex genetic aberrations	[63, 151]
Phosphaturic mesenchymal tumor	FN1–FGFR1 fusion	[90, 91]
Ectomesenchymal Chondromyxoid tumor (tongue)	Recurrent RREB1–MKL2 fusion.	[42]
Extraskeletal Myxoid chondrosarcoma	Classic EWSR1–NR4A3 fusion.	[12, 72, 117]
Synovial sarcoma (head/neck)	SS18–SSX1/2/4 fusion; SS18-SSX–specific IHC markers.	[112]

B: Mesenchymal tumors of the head and neck		
Tumor type	Molecular alterations	PMID
Biphenotypic Sinonasal sarcoma	PAX3 rearrangements	[83]
Alveolar rhabdomyosarcoma	PAX3-FOXO1, PAX7-FOXO1 gene fusions	[15]
Rhabdomyosarcoma with TFCP2 fusion	EWSR1/FUS–TFCP2 fusion in head/neck cases.	[180]
Adamantinoma-like Ewing sarcoma	EWSR1–FLI1 fusion	[130]
GLI1-altered mesenchymal Tumors	ACTB/PTCH1/MALAT1–GLI1 fusions; GLI1 amplification with MDM2/CDK4/STAT6.	[4, 38, 113, 179]
Nodular fasciitis / cranial fasciitis	USP6 fusions	[50]
Fibroblastic/Myofibroblastic Tumors (IMT)	ALK or ROS1 rearrangements	[11, 61]

ous cases [85, 86]. For sinonasal tumors, DNA methylation-based classification has demonstrated clinical reliability, helping to resolve diagnostic challenges posed by the heterogeneous spectrum of these tumors and reassigning previously poorly defined entities like sinonasal undifferentiated carcinomas (SNUCs) to distinct molecular classes based on their epigenetic, mutational, and proteomic profiles [85]. This reclassification aids in improving diagnostic accuracy and can alter the perception of SNUCs, indicating they are not as undifferentiated as their morphology suggests.

Table 12.4 Genetic alterations in odontogenic and maxillofacial bone tumors

Tumor type	Genetic alteration(s)	References
Ameloblastoma	BRAF V600E, MAPK (KRAS, NRAS, HRAS), SMO	[24, 70, 87, 156]
Adenomatoid odontogenic tumor (AOT)	*KRAS*	[22, 37]
Ameloblastic fibroma	BRAF V600E	[24, 27]
Ameloblastic carcinoma	BRAF V600E, TP53	[44, 114, 115]
Clear cell odontogenic carcinoma	EWSR1 rearrangements (e.g., EWSR1-ATF1)	[17, 168]
Odontogenic Keratocyst	PTCH1 (hedgehog pathway)	[94, 96]
Cementoblastoma	*FOS* rearrangement	[88]
Osteosarcoma (maxillofacial)	TP53, RB1, MDM2 amp, CDK4 amp	[135]
Ewing sarcoma	*EWSR1* or *FUS* rearrangement	[41, 80, 141, 150, 162]
Chondrosarcoma	IDH1 and IDH2 mutations	[157]

Practical Considerations and Limitations Specific to Molecular Head and Neck Cancer Diagnostics

Though the mainstay of diagnostic pathology remains H&E, additional (histo)chemical stainings and in particular molecular ancillary tests have shown to be of crucial value for classification and prognostication of head and neck tumors. Moreover, the latter provide unique clues to potential (targeted) therapies. With an increasing amount of (specific) genetic aberrations identified, molecular pathology has earned an important place in the routine histopathological work-up of many head and neck tumors over the last years. Despite the considerable benefits, the real-world implementation of Next-Generation Sequencing (NGS) in head and neck pathology encounters several challenges. Firstly, obtaining limited tumor tissue from small biopsies or fine needle aspirates (FNAs), which are common for head and neck lesions because of the complexities of head and neck anatomy, can impede successful NGS analysis due to insufficient DNA/RNA quantity or quality. Secondly, fixation artifacts from formalin-fixed paraffin-embedded (FFPE) material, the standard tissue preservation method, can introduce DNA damage (i.e., DNA fragmentation, cross-linking, base modifications/cytosine deamination), but also fixation artefacts, leading to sequencing errors, challenging variant interpretation and chemical modifications that interfere with accurate methylation analysis. A specific challenge in head and neck cancer specimens, given its frequent involvement of bone and cartilage, is the necessity of decalcification of resection specimens containing bone. This process, often employing strong acids (e.g., hydrochloric or nitric acid), can severely degrade nucleic acids (DNA and RNA), resulting in reduced yield and quality, and potentially compromising molecular testing success. Therefore, careful selection of decalcification methods (e.g., EDTA or short-term formic acid) is essential to preserve molecular integrity.

Future Directions

The future of molecular diagnostics in head and neck pathology holds immense promise, with several advancements poised to enhance precision and personalized medicine. Liquid biopsy, particularly the analysis of circulating tumor DNA (ctDNA) from blood or saliva, is gaining importance for non-invasive treatment monitoring, early detection or recurrence, and assessing minimal residual disease in head and neck cancers, especially for HPV-associated cancers [16, 119]. RNA sequencing (RNA-seq) offers a powerful tool to detect novel gene fusions and transcriptomic alterations that may serve as diagnostic markers or actionable therapeutic targets, expanding beyond DNA-centric analyses. DNA methylation profiling is an emerging area, as aberrant methylation patterns are crucial in HNSCC pathogenesis, holding potential as diagnostic, prognostic, and predictive biomarkers, and even identifying specific tumor subtypes [85, 86]. Finally, the integration with Artificial Intelligence (AI) and image analysis tools promises to revolutionize pathology by automating the analysis of whole-slide images, enhancing diagnostic accuracy and efficiency, identifying subtle or rare patterns, and integrating with molecular data for improved prognostication and personalized treatment strategies [6, 181].

Conclusion

NGS has transformed head and neck pathology from a histomorphologic and immunohistochemical field into one increasingly shaped by specific molecular profiles. As sequencing becomes more accessible, its role in diagnosis, prognostication, and therapy selection will continue to expand, necessitating close and more frequent collaboration between molecular pathology, surgical pathology, surgery, and medical- and clinical oncology.

References

1. Agaimy A, Bishop JA. SWI/SNF-deficient head and neck neoplasms: an overview. Semin Diagn Pathol. 2021;38(3):175–82. https://doi.org/10.1053/j.semdp.2021.02.002.
2. Agaimy A, Hartmann A, Antonescu CR, Chiosea SI, El-Mofty SK, Geddert H, et al. SMARCB1 (INI-1)-deficient Sinonasal carcinoma: a series of 39 cases expanding the morphologic and clinicopathologic spectrum of a recently described entity. Am J Surg Pathol. 2017;41(4):458–71. https://doi.org/10.1097/PAS.0000000000000797.
3. Agaimy A, Jain D, Uddin N, Rooper LM, Bishop JA. SMARCA4-deficient Sinonasal carcinoma: a series of 10 cases expanding the genetic spectrum of SWI/SNF-driven sinonasal malignancies. Am J Surg Pathol. 2020;44(5):703–10. https://doi.org/10.1097/PAS.0000000000001428.
4. Agaram NP, Zhang L, Sung YS, Singer S, Stevens T, Prieto-Granada CN, et al. GLI1-amplifications expand the spectrum of soft tissue neoplasms

defined by GLI1 gene fusions. Mod Pathol. 2019;32(11):1617–26. https://doi.org/10.1038/s41379-019-0293-x.
5. Agrawal N, Frederick MJ, Pickering CR, Bettegowda C, Chang K, Li RJ, et al. Exome sequencing of head and neck squamous cell carcinoma reveals inactivating mutations in NOTCH1. Science. 2011;333(6046):1154–7. https://doi.org/10.1126/science.1206923.
6. Ahuja S, Zaheer S. Advancements in pathology: digital transformation, precision medicine, and beyond. J Pathol Inform. 2025;16:100408. https://doi.org/10.1016/j.jpi.2024.100408.
7. Alekseyenko AA, Walsh EM, Zee BM, Pakozdi T, Hsi P, Lemieux ME, et al. Ectopic protein interactions within BRD4-chromatin complexes drive oncogenic megadomain formation in NUT midline carcinoma. Proc Natl Acad Sci USA. 2017;114(21):E4184–92. https://doi.org/10.1073/pnas.1702086114.
8. Andreasen S, Skalova A, Agaimy A, Bishop JA, Laco J, Leivo I, et al. ETV6 gene rearrangements characterize a morphologically distinct subset of sinonasal low-grade non-intestinal-type adenocarcinoma: a novel translocation-associated carcinoma restricted to the sinonasal tract. Am J Surg Pathol. 2017;41(11):1552–60. https://doi.org/10.1097/PAS.0000000000000912.
9. Andreasen S, Kiss K, Melchior LC, Laco J. The ETV6-RET gene fusion is found in ETV6-rearranged low-grade sinonasal adenocarcinoma without NTRK3 involvement. Am J Surg Pathol. 2018;42(7):985–8. https://doi.org/10.1097/PAS.0000000000001069.
10. Antonescu CR, Katabi N, Zhang L, Sung YS, Seethala RR, Jordan RC, et al. EWSR1-ATF1 fusion is a novel and consistent finding in hyalinizing clear-cell carcinoma of salivary gland. Genes Chromosomes Cancer. 2011;50(7):559–70. https://doi.org/10.1002/gcc.20881.
11. Antonescu CR, Suurmeijer AJ, Zhang L, Sung YS, Jungbluth AA, Travis WD, et al. Molecular characterization of inflammatory myofibroblastic tumors with frequent ALK and ROS1 gene fusions and rare novel RET rearrangement. Am J Surg Pathol. 2015;39(7):957–67. https://doi.org/10.1097/PAS.0000000000000404.
12. Attwooll C, Tariq M, Harris M, Coyne JD, Telford N, Varley JM. Identification of a novel fusion gene involving hTAFII68 and CHN from a t(9;17)(q22;q11.2) translocation in an extraskeletal myxoid chondrosarcoma. Oncogene. 1999;18(52):7599–601. https://doi.org/10.1038/sj.onc.1203156.
13. Bahrami A, Perez-Ordonez B, Dalton JD, Weinreb I. An analysis of PLAG1 and HMGA2 rearrangements in salivary duct carcinoma and examination of the role of precursor lesions. Histopathology. 2013;63(2):250–62. https://doi.org/10.1111/his.12152.
14. Baneckova M, Michal M, Laco J, Leivo I, Ptakova N, Horakova M, et al. Immunohistochemical and genetic analysis of respiratory epithelial adenomatoid hamartomas and seromucinous hamartomas: are they precursor lesions to sinonasal low-grade tubulopapillary adenocarcinomas? Hum Pathol. 2020;97:94–102. https://doi.org/10.1016/j.humpath.2019.09.018.
15. Barr FG. Gene fusions involving PAX and FOX family members in alveolar rhabdomyosarcoma. Oncogene. 2001;20(40):5736–46. https://doi.org/10.1038/sj.onc.1204599.
16. Bartolomucci A, Nobrega M, Ferrier T, Dickinson K, Kaorey N, Nadeau A, et al. Circulating tumor DNA to monitor treatment response in solid tumors and advance precision oncology. NPJ Precis Oncol. 2025;9(1):84. https://doi.org/10.1038/s41698-025-00876-y.
17. Bilodeau EA, Weinreb I, Antonescu CR, Zhang L, Dacic S, Muller S, et al. Clear cell odontogenic carcinomas show EWSR1 rearrangements: a novel finding and a biological link to salivary clear cell carcinomas. Am J Surg Pathol. 2013;37(7):1001–5. https://doi.org/10.1097/PAS.0b013e31828a6727.
18. Bishop JA, Antonescu CR, Westra WH. SMARCB1 (INI-1)-deficient carcinomas of the sinonasal tract. Am J Surg Pathol. 2014;38(9):1282–9. https://doi.org/10.1097/PAS.0000000000000285.
19. Bishop JA, Nakaguro M, Whaley RD, Ogura K, Imai H, Laklouk I, et al. Oncocytic intraductal carcinoma of salivary glands: a distinct variant with TRIM33-RET fusions and BRAF V600E mutations. Histopathology. 2021a;79(3):338–46. https://doi.org/10.1111/his.14296.
20. Bishop JA, Rooper LM, Sangoi AR, Gagan J, Thompson LDR, Inagaki H. The myoepithelial cells of salivary intercalated duct-type intraductal carcinoma are neoplastic: a study using combined whole-slide imaging, immunofluorescence, and RET fluorescence in situ hybridization. Am J Surg Pathol. 2021b;45(4):507–15. https://doi.org/10.1097/PAS.0000000000001605.
21. Bishop JA, Sajed DP, Weinreb I, Dickson BC, Bilodeau EA, Agaimy A, et al. Microsecretory adenocarcinoma of salivary glands: an expanded series of 24 cases. Head Neck Pathol. 2021c;15(4):1192–201. https://doi.org/10.1007/s12105-021-01331-7.
22. Bologna-Molina R, Ogawa I, Mosqueda-Taylor A, Takata T, Sanchez-Romero C, Villarroel-Dorrego M, et al. Detection of MAPK/ERK pathway proteins and KRAS mutations in adenomatoid odontogenic tumors. Oral Dis. 2019;25(2):481–7. https://doi.org/10.1111/odi.12989.
23. Brash DE. UV signature mutations. Photochem Photobiol. 2015;91(1):15–26. https://doi.org/10.1111/php.12377.
24. Brown NA, Rolland D, McHugh JB, Weigelin HC, Zhao L, Lim MS, et al. Activating FGFR2-RAS-BRAF mutations in ameloblastoma. Clin Cancer Res. 2014;20(21):5517–26. https://doi.org/10.1158/1078-0432.CCR-14-1069.

25. Brown NA, Plouffe KR, Yilmaz O, Weindorf SC, Betz BL, Carey TE, et al. TP53 mutations and CDKN2A mutations/deletions are highly recurrent molecular alterations in the malignant progression of sinonasal papillomas. Mod Pathol. 2021;34(6):1133–42. https://doi.org/10.1038/s41379-020-00716-3.
26. Bruce JP, To KF, Lui VWY, Chung GTY, Chan YY, Tsang CM, et al. Whole-genome profiling of nasopharyngeal carcinoma reveals viral-host co-operation in inflammatory NF-kappaB activation and immune escape. Nat Commun. 2021;12(1):4193. https://doi.org/10.1038/s41467-021-24348-6.
27. Brunner P, Bihl M, Jundt G, Baumhoer D, Hoeller S. BRAF p.V600E mutations are not unique to ameloblastoma and are shared by other odontogenic tumors with ameloblastic morphology. Oral Oncol. 2015;51(10):e77–8. https://doi.org/10.1016/j.oraloncology.2015.07.010.
28. Cancer Genome Atlas, N. Comprehensive genomic characterization of head and neck squamous cell carcinomas. Nature. 2015;517(7536):576–82. https://doi.org/10.1038/nature14129.
29. Chapman E, Skalova A, Ptakova N, Martinek P, Goytain A, Tucker T, et al. Molecular profiling of hyalinizing clear cell carcinomas revealed a subset of tumors harboring a novel EWSR1-CREM fusion: report of 3 cases. Am J Surg Pathol. 2018;42(9):1182–9. https://doi.org/10.1097/PAS.0000000000001114.
30. Chen C, Zhang Y, Loomis MM, Upton MP, Lohavanichbutr P, Houck JR, et al. Genome-wide loss of heterozygosity and DNA copy number aberration in HPV-negative oral squamous cell carcinoma and their associations with disease-specific survival. PLoS One. 2015;10(8):e0135074. https://doi.org/10.1371/journal.pone.0135074.
31. Chiosea SI, Miller M, Seethala RR. HRAS mutations in epithelial-myoepithelial carcinoma. Head Neck Pathol. 2014;8(2):146–50. https://doi.org/10.1007/s12105-013-0506-4.
32. Chiosea SI, Williams L, Griffith CC, Thompson LD, Weinreb I, Bauman JE, et al. Molecular characterization of apocrine salivary duct carcinoma. Am J Surg Pathol. 2015;39(6):744–52. https://doi.org/10.1097/PAS.0000000000000410.
33. Chiosea SI, Thompson LD, Weinreb I, Bauman JE, Mahaffey AM, Miller C, et al. Subsets of salivary duct carcinoma defined by morphologic evidence of pleomorphic adenoma, PLAG1 or HMGA2 rearrangements, and common genetic alterations. Cancer. 2016;122(20):3136–44. https://doi.org/10.1002/cncr.30179.
34. Chlopek M, Lasota J, Thompson LDR, Szczepaniak M, Kuzniacka A, Hincza K, et al. Alterations in key signaling pathways in sinonasal tract melanoma. A molecular genetics and immunohistochemical study of 90 cases and comprehensive review of the literature. Mod Pathol. 2022;35(11):1609–17. https://doi.org/10.1038/s41379-022-01122-7.
35. Classe M, Yao H, Mouawad R, Creighton CJ, Burgess A, Allanic F, et al. Integrated multi-omic analysis of esthesioneuroblastomas identifies two subgroups linked to cell ontogeny. Cell Rep. 2018;25(3):811–821 e815. https://doi.org/10.1016/j.celrep.2018.09.047.
36. Cochicho D, Esteves S, Rito M, Silva F, Martins L, Montalvao P, et al. PIK3CA gene mutations in HNSCC: systematic review and correlations with HPV status and patient survival. Cancers (Basel). 2022;14(5) https://doi.org/10.3390/cancers14051286.
37. Coura BP, Bernardes VF, de Sousa SF, Franca JA, Pereira NB, Pontes HAR, et al. KRAS mutations drive adenomatoid odontogenic tumor and are independent of clinicopathological features. Mod Pathol. 2019;32(6):799–806. https://doi.org/10.1038/s41379-018-0194-4.
38. Dahlen A, Fletcher CD, Mertens F, Fletcher JA, Perez-Atayde AR, Hicks MJ, et al. Activation of the GLI oncogene through fusion with the beta-actin gene (ACTB) in a group of distinctive pericytic neoplasms: pericytoma with t(7;12). Am J Pathol. 2004;164(5):1645–53. https://doi.org/10.1016/s0002-9440(10)63723-6.
39. Dalin MG, Desrichard A, Katabi N, Makarov V, Walsh LA, Lee KW, et al. Comprehensive molecular characterization of salivary duct carcinoma reveals actionable targets and similarity to apocrine breast cancer. Clin Cancer Res. 2016;22(18):4623–33. https://doi.org/10.1158/1078-0432.CCR-16-0637.
40. Dalin MG, Katabi N, Persson M, Lee KW, Makarov V, Desrichard A, et al. Multi-dimensional genomic analysis of myoepithelial carcinoma identifies prevalent oncogenic gene fusions. Nat Commun. 2017;8(1):1197. https://doi.org/10.1038/s41467-017-01178-z.
41. Delattre O, Zucman J, Melot T, Garau XS, Zucker JM, Lenoir GM, et al. The Ewing family of tumors–a subgroup of small-round-cell tumors defined by specific chimeric transcripts. N Engl J Med. 1994;331(5):294–9. https://doi.org/10.1056/NEJM199408043310503.
42. Dickson BC, Antonescu CR, Argyris PP, Bilodeau EA, Bullock MJ, Freedman PD, et al. Ectomesenchymal chondromyxoid tumor: a neoplasm characterized by recurrent RREB1-MKL2 fusions. Am J Surg Pathol. 2018a;42(10):1297–305. https://doi.org/10.1097/PAS.0000000000001096.
43. Dickson BC, Sung YS, Rosenblum MK, Reuter VE, Harb M, Wunder JS, et al. NUTM1 gene fusions characterize a subset of undifferentiated soft tissue and visceral tumors. Am J Surg Pathol. 2018b;42(5):636–45. https://doi.org/10.1097/PAS.0000000000001021.
44. Diniz MG, Gomes CC, Guimaraes BV, Castro WH, Lacerda JC, Cardoso SV, et al. Assessment of BRAFV600E and SMOF412E mutations in epithelial odontogenic tumours. Tumour Biol.

2015;36(7):5649–53. https://doi.org/10.1007/s13277-015-3238-0.
45. Dogan S, Chute DJ, Xu B, Ptashkin RN, Chandramohan R, Casanova-Murphy J, et al. Frequent IDH2 R172 mutations in undifferentiated and poorly-differentiated sinonasal carcinomas. J Pathol. 2017;242(4):400–8. https://doi.org/10.1002/path.4915.
46. Dogan S, Ng CKY, Xu B, Kumar R, Wang L, Edelweiss M, et al. The repertoire of genetic alterations in salivary duct carcinoma including a novel HNRNPH3-ALK rearrangement. Hum Pathol. 2019a;88:66–77. https://doi.org/10.1016/j.humpath.2019.03.004.
47. Dogan S, Vasudevaraja V, Xu B, Serrano J, Ptashkin RN, Jung HJ, et al. DNA methylation-based classification of sinonasal undifferentiated carcinoma. Mod Pathol. 2019b;32(10):1447–59. https://doi.org/10.1038/s41379-019-0285-x.
48. El Hallani S, Udager AM, Bell D, Fonseca I, Thompson LDR, Assaad A, et al. Epithelial-myoepithelial carcinoma: frequent morphologic and molecular evidence of preexisting pleomorphic adenoma, common HRAS mutations in PLAG1-intact and HMGA2-intact cases, and occasional TP53, FBXW7, and SMARCB1 alterations in high-grade cases. Am J Surg Pathol. 2018;42(1):18–27. https://doi.org/10.1097/PAS.0000000000000933.
49. El-Naggar AK, Westra WH. p16 expression as a surrogate marker for HPV-related oropharyngeal carcinoma: a guide for interpretative relevance and consistency. Head Neck. 2012;34(4):459–61. https://doi.org/10.1002/hed.21974.
50. Erickson-Johnson MR, Chou MM, Evers BR, Roth CW, Seys AR, Jin L, et al. Nodular fasciitis: a novel model of transient neoplasia induced by MYH9-USP6 gene fusion. Lab Investig. 2011;91(10):1427–33. https://doi.org/10.1038/labinvest.2011.118.
51. Even C, Lassen U, Merchan J, Le Tourneau C, Soria JC, Ferte C, et al. Safety and clinical activity of the Notch inhibitor, crenigacestat (LY3039478), in an open-label phase I trial expansion cohort of advanced or metastatic adenoid cystic carcinoma. Investig New Drugs. 2020;38(2):402–9. https://doi.org/10.1007/s10637-019-00739-x.
52. Ferrarotto R, Eckhardt G, Patnaik A, LoRusso P, Faoro L, Heymach JV, et al. A phase I dose-escalation and dose-expansion study of brontictuzumab in subjects with selected solid tumors. Ann Oncol. 2018;29(7):1561–8. https://doi.org/10.1093/annonc/mdy171.
53. Franchi A, Innocenti DR, Palomba A, Miligi L, Paiar F, Franzese C, Santucci M. Low prevalence of K-RAS, EGF-R and BRAF mutations in sinonasal adenocarcinomas. Implications for anti-EGFR treatments. Pathol Oncol Res. 2014;20(3):571–9. https://doi.org/10.1007/s12253-013-9730-1.
54. French CA, Miyoshi I, Kubonishi I, Grier HE, Perez-Atayde AR, Fletcher JA. BRD4-NUT fusion oncogene: a novel mechanism in aggressive carcinoma. Cancer Res. 2003;63(2):304–7. Retrieved from https://www.ncbi.nlm.nih.gov/pubmed/12543779
55. French CA, Ramirez CL, Kolmakova J, Hickman TT, Cameron MJ, Thyne ME, et al. BRD-NUT oncoproteins: a family of closely related nuclear proteins that block epithelial differentiation and maintain the growth of carcinoma cells. Oncogene. 2008;27(15):2237–42. https://doi.org/10.1038/sj.onc.1210852.
56. French CA, Rahman S, Walsh EM, Kuhnle S, Grayson AR, Lemieux ME, et al. NSD3-NUT fusion oncoprotein in NUT midline carcinoma: implications for a novel oncogenic mechanism. Cancer Discov. 2014;4(8):928–41. https://doi.org/10.1158/2159-8290.CD-14-0014.
57. Fujii K, Murase T, Beppu S, Saida K, Takino H, Masaki A, et al. MYB, MYBL1, MYBL2 and NFIB gene alterations and MYC overexpression in salivary gland adenoid cystic carcinoma. Histopathology. 2017;71(5):823–34. https://doi.org/10.1111/his.13281.
58. Furlan KC, Saeed-Vafa D, Mathew TM, Saller JJ, Tabbara SO, Boyle TA, et al. Utility of UV signature mutations in the diagnostic assessment of metastatic head and neck carcinomas of unknown primary. Head Neck Pathol. 2024;18(1):11. https://doi.org/10.1007/s12105-024-01620-x.
59. Fushimi C, Tada Y, Takahashi H, Nagao T, Ojiri H, Masubuchi T, et al. A prospective phase II study of combined androgen blockade in patients with androgen receptor-positive metastatic or locally advanced unresectable salivary gland carcinoma. Ann Oncol. 2018;29(4):979–84. https://doi.org/10.1093/annonc/mdx771.
60. Gloss S, Jurmeister P, Thieme A, Schmid S, Cai WY, Serrette RN, et al. IDH2 R172 mutations across poorly differentiated sinonasal tract malignancies: forty molecularly homogenous and histologically variable cases with favorable outcome. Am J Surg Pathol. 2021;45(9):1190–204. https://doi.org/10.1097/PAS.0000000000001697.
61. Griffin CA, Hawkins AL, Dvorak C, Henkle C, Ellingham T, Perlman EJ. Recurrent involvement of 2p23 in inflammatory myofibroblastic tumors. Cancer Res. 1999;59(12):2776–80. Retrieved from https://www.ncbi.nlm.nih.gov/pubmed/10383129
62. Grunewald I, Vollbrecht C, Meinrath J, Meyer MF, Heukamp LC, Drebber U, et al. Targeted next generation sequencing of parotid gland cancer uncovers genetic heterogeneity. Oncotarget. 2015;6(20):18224–37. https://doi.org/10.18632/oncotarget.4015.
63. Guillou L, Aurias A. Soft tissue sarcomas with complex genomic profiles. Virchows Arch. 2010;456(2):201–17. https://doi.org/10.1007/s00428-009-0853-4.
64. Guilmette J, Dias-Santagata D, Nose V, Lennerz JK, Sadow PM. Novel gene fusions in secretory carcinoma of the salivary glands: enlarging the ETV6

family. Hum Pathol. 2019;83:50–8. https://doi.org/10.1016/j.humpath.2018.08.011.
65. Haack H, Johnson LA, Fry CJ, Crosby K, Polakiewicz RD, Stelow EB, et al. Diagnosis of NUT midline carcinoma using a NUT-specific monoclonal antibody. Am J Surg Pathol. 2009;33(7):984–91. https://doi.org/10.1097/PAS.0b013e318198d666.
66. Haller F, Bieg M, Will R, Korner C, Weichenhan D, Bott A, et al. Enhancer hijacking activates oncogenic transcription factor NR4A3 in acinic cell carcinomas of the salivary glands. Nat Commun. 2019a;10(1):368. https://doi.org/10.1038/s41467-018-08069-x.
67. Haller F, Skalova A, Ihrler S, Markl B, Bieg M, Moskalev EA, et al. Nuclear NR4A3 immunostaining is a specific and sensitive novel marker for acinic cell carcinoma of the salivary glands. Am J Surg Pathol. 2019b;43(9):1264–72. https://doi.org/10.1097/PAS.0000000000001279.
68. Haller F, Moskalev EA, Kuck S, Bieg M, Winkelmann C, Muller SK, et al. Nuclear NR4A2 (Nurr1) immunostaining is a novel marker for acinic cell carcinoma of the salivary glands lacking the classic NR4A3 (NOR-1) upregulation. Am J Surg Pathol. 2020;44(9):1290–2. https://doi.org/10.1097/PAS.0000000000001494.
69. Hashibe M, Brennan P, Chuang SC, Boccia S, Castellsague X, Chen C, et al. Interaction between tobacco and alcohol use and the risk of head and neck cancer: pooled analysis in the international head and neck cancer epidemiology consortium. Cancer Epidemiol Biomarkers Prev. 2009;18(2):541–50. https://doi.org/10.1158/1055-9965.EPI-08-0347.
70. Heikinheimo K, Huhtala JM, Thiel A, Kurppa KJ, Heikinheimo H, Kovac M, et al. The mutational profile of unicystic ameloblastoma. J Dent Res. 2019;98(1):54–60. https://doi.org/10.1177/0022034518798810.
71. Hirose K, Usami Y, Kohara M, Sato S, Iwamoto Y, Murakami S, et al. Clear cell carcinoma of palatal minor salivary gland harboring a novel EWSR1-ATF1 fusion gene: report of a case and review of the literature. Head Neck Pathol. 2021;15(2):676–81. https://doi.org/10.1007/s12105-020-01211-6.
72. Hisaoka M, Hashimoto H. Extraskeletal myxoid chondrosarcoma: updated clinicopathological and molecular genetic characteristics. Pathol Int. 2005;55(8):453–63. https://doi.org/10.1111/j.1440-1827.2005.01853.x.
73. Ho AS, Ochoa A, Jayakumaran G, Zehir A, Valero Mayor C, Tepe J, et al. Genetic hallmarks of recurrent/metastatic adenoid cystic carcinoma. J Clin Invest. 2019;129(10):4276–89. https://doi.org/10.1172/JCI128227.
74. Hsieh MS, Bishop JA, Wang YP, Poh CF, Cheng YL, Lee YH, et al. Salivary sialadenoma papilliferum consists of two morphologically, immunophenotypically, and genetically distinct subtypes. Head Neck Pathol. 2020;14(2):489–96. https://doi.org/10.1007/s12105-019-01068-4.
75. Huang FW, Feng FY. A tumor-agnostic NTRK (TRK) inhibitor. Cell. 2019;177(1):8. https://doi.org/10.1016/j.cell.2019.02.049.
76. Huang SC, Ghossein RA, Bishop JA, Zhang L, Chen TC, Huang HY, Antonescu CR. Novel PAX3-NCOA1 fusions in biphenotypic sinonasal sarcoma with focal rhabdomyoblastic differentiation. Am J Surg Pathol. 2016;40(1):51–9. https://doi.org/10.1097/PAS.0000000000000492.
77. India Project Team of the International Cancer Genome C. Mutational landscape of gingivobuccal oral squamous cell carcinoma reveals new recurrently-mutated genes and molecular subgroups. Nat Commun. 2013;4:2873. https://doi.org/10.1038/ncomms3873.
78. Ito Y, Ishibashi K, Masaki A, Fujii K, Fujiyoshi Y, Hattori H, et al. Mammary analogue secretory carcinoma of salivary glands: a clinicopathologic and molecular study including 2 cases harboring ETV6-X fusion. Am J Surg Pathol. 2015;39(5):602–10. https://doi.org/10.1097/PAS.0000000000000392.
79. Jee KJ, Persson M, Heikinheimo K, Passador-Santos F, Aro K, Knuutila S, et al. Genomic profiles and CRTC1-MAML2 fusion distinguish different subtypes of mucoepidermoid carcinoma. Mod Pathol. 2013;26(2):213–22. https://doi.org/10.1038/modpathol.2012.154.
80. Jeon IS, Davis JN, Braun BS, Sublett JE, Roussel MF, Denny CT, Shapiro DN. A variant Ewing's sarcoma translocation (7;22) fuses the EWS gene to the ETS gene ETV1. Oncogene. 1995;10(6):1229–34. Retrieved from https://www.ncbi.nlm.nih.gov/pubmed/7700648
81. Jo VY, Sholl LM, Krane JF. Distinctive patterns of CTNNB1 (beta-catenin) alterations in salivary gland basal cell adenoma and basal cell adenocarcinoma. Am J Surg Pathol. 2016;40(8):1143–50. https://doi.org/10.1097/PAS.0000000000000669.
82. Jo VY, Chau NG, Hornick JL, Krane JF, Sholl LM. Recurrent IDH2 R172X mutations in sinonasal undifferentiated carcinoma. Mod Pathol. 2017;30(5):650–9. https://doi.org/10.1038/modpathol.2016.239.
83. Jo VY, Marino-Enriquez A, Fletcher CDM, Hornick JL. Expression of PAX3 distinguishes biphenotypic sinonasal sarcoma from histologic mimics. Am J Surg Pathol. 2018;42(10):1275–85. https://doi.org/10.1097/PAS.0000000000001092.
84. Jones AS, Morar P, Phillips DE, Field JK, Husband D, Helliwell TR. Second primary tumors in patients with head and neck squamous cell carcinoma. Cancer. 1995;75(6):1343–53. https://doi.org/10.1002/1097-0142(19950315)75:6<1343::aid-cncr2820750617>3.0.co;2-t.
85. Jurmeister P, Gloss S, Roller R, Leitheiser M, Schmid S, Mochmann LH, et al. DNA methylation-based classification of sinonasal tumors. Nat Commun. 2022;13(1):7148. https://doi.org/10.1038/s41467-022-34815-3.

86. Jurmeister P, Leitheiser M, Arnold A, Capilla EP, Mochmann LH, Zhdanovic Y, et al. DNA methylation profiling of salivary gland tumors supports and expands conventional classification. Mod Pathol. 2024;37(12):100625. https://doi.org/10.1016/j.modpat.2024.100625.
87. Kurppa KJ, Caton J, Morgan PR, Ristimaki A, Ruhin B, Kellokoski J, et al. High frequency of BRAF V600E mutations in ameloblastoma. J Pathol. 2014;232(5):492–8. https://doi.org/10.1002/path.4317.
88. Lam SW, Cleven AHG, Briaire-de Bruijn IH, Schreuder WH, Kroon HM, Savci-Heijink DC, et al. FOS rearrangement and expression in cementoblastoma. Am J Surg Pathol. 2021;45(5):690–3. https://doi.org/10.1097/PAS.0000000000001695.
89. Le Loarer F, Laffont S, Lesluyes T, Tirode F, Antonescu C, Baglin AC, et al. Clinicopathologic and molecular features of a series of 41 biphenotypic sinonasal sarcomas expanding their molecular spectrum. Am J Surg Pathol. 2019;43(6):747–54. https://doi.org/10.1097/PAS.0000000000001238.
90. Lee JC, Jeng YM, Su SY, Wu CT, Tsai KS, Lee CH, et al. Identification of a novel FN1-FGFR1 genetic fusion as a frequent event in phosphaturic mesenchymal tumour. J Pathol. 2015;235(4):539–45. https://doi.org/10.1002/path.4465.
91. Lee JC, Su SY, Changou CA, Yang RS, Tsai KS, Collins MT, et al. Characterization of FN1-FGFR1 and novel FN1-FGF1 fusion genes in a large series of phosphaturic mesenchymal tumors. Mod Pathol. 2016;29(11):1335–46. https://doi.org/10.1038/modpathol.2016.137.
92. Lee YH, Huang WC, Hsieh MS. CTNNB1 mutations in basal cell adenoma of the salivary gland. J Formos Med Assoc. 2018;117(10):894–901. https://doi.org/10.1016/j.jfma.2017.11.011.
93. Lee VH, Kwong DL, Leung TW, Choi CW, O'Sullivan B, Lam KO, et al. The addition of pretreatment plasma Epstein-Barr virus DNA into the eighth edition of nasopharyngeal cancer TNM stage classification. Int J Cancer. 2019;144(7):1713–22. https://doi.org/10.1002/ijc.31856.
94. Levanat S, Gorlin RJ, Fallet S, Johnson DR, Fantasia JE, Bale AE. A two-hit model for developmental defects in Gorlin syndrome. Nat Genet. 1996;12(1):85–7. https://doi.org/10.1038/ng0196-85.
95. Lewis JS Jr, Beadle B, Bishop JA, Chernock RD, Colasacco C, Lacchetti C, et al. Human papillomavirus testing in head and neck carcinomas: guideline from the college of american pathologists. Arch Pathol Lab Med. 2018;142(5):559–97. https://doi.org/10.5858/arpa.2017-0286-CP.
96. Li TJ. The odontogenic keratocyst: a cyst, or a cystic neoplasm? J Dent Res. 2011;90(2):133–42. https://doi.org/10.1177/0022034510379016.
97. Li YY, Chung GT, Lui VW, To, K. F, Ma BB, Chow C, et al. Exome and genome sequencing of nasopharynx cancer identifies NF-kappaB pathway activating mutations. Nat Commun. 2017;8:14121. https://doi.org/10.1038/ncomms14121.
98. Locati LD, Cavalieri S, Bergamini C, Resteghini C, Colombo E, Calareso G, et al. Abiraterone acetate in patients with castration-resistant, androgen receptor-expressing salivary gland cancer: a phase II trial. J Clin Oncol. 2021;39(36):4061–8. https://doi.org/10.1200/JCO.21.00468.
99. Low YH, Loh CJL, Peh DYY, Chu AJM, Han S, Toh HC. Pathogenesis and therapeutic implications of EBV-associated epithelial cancers. Front Oncol. 2023;13:1202117. https://doi.org/10.3389/fonc.2023.1202117.
100. Martins C, Fonseca I, Roque L, Pereira T, Ribeiro C, Bullerdiek J, Soares J. PLAG1 gene alterations in salivary gland pleomorphic adenoma and carcinoma ex-pleomorphic adenoma: a combined study using chromosome banding, in situ hybridization and immunocytochemistry. Mod Pathol. 2005;18(8):1048–55. https://doi.org/10.1038/modpathol.3800386.
101. Mashiana SS, Navale P, Khandakar B, Sobotka S, Posner MR, Miles BA, et al. Human papillomavirus genotype distribution in head and neck cancer: informing developing strategies for cancer prevention, diagnosis, treatment and surveillance. Oral Oncol. 2021;113:105109. https://doi.org/10.1016/j.oraloncology.2020.105109.
102. Mitani Y, Rao PH, Maity SN, Lee YC, Ferrarotto R, Post JC, et al. Alterations associated with androgen receptor gene activation in salivary duct carcinoma of both sexes: potential therapeutic ramifications. Clin Cancer Res. 2014;20(24):6570–81. https://doi.org/10.1158/1078-0432.CCR-14-1746.
103. Mitani Y, Liu B, Rao PH, Borra VJ, Zafereo M, Weber RS, et al. Novel MYBL1 gene rearrangements with recurrent MYBL1-NFIB fusions in salivary adenoid cystic carcinomas lacking t(6;9) translocations. Clin Cancer Res. 2016;22(3):725–33. https://doi.org/10.1158/1078-0432.CCR-15-2867-T.
104. Mito JK, Bishop JA, Sadow PM, Stelow EB, Faquin WC, Mills SE, et al. Immunohistochemical detection and molecular characterization of IDH-mutant sinonasal undifferentiated carcinomas. Am J Surg Pathol. 2018;42(8):1067–75. https://doi.org/10.1097/PAS.0000000000001064.
105. Moller E, Stenman G, Mandahl N, Hamberg H, Molne L, van den Oord JJ, et al. POU5F1, encoding a key regulator of stem cell pluripotency, is fused to EWSR1 in hidradenoma of the skin and mucoepidermoid carcinoma of the salivary glands. J Pathol. 2008;215(1):78–86. https://doi.org/10.1002/path.2327.
106. Morris LG, Sikora AG, Hayes RB, Patel SG, Ganly I. Anatomic sites at elevated risk of second primary cancer after an index head and neck cancer. Cancer Causes Control. 2011;22(5):671–9. https://doi.org/10.1007/s10552-011-9739-2.
107. Nakaguro M, Urano M, Suzuki H, Yamada K, Sakaguchi A, Ogura K, et al. Low-grade intra-

ductal carcinoma of the salivary gland with prominent oncocytic change: a newly described variant. Histopathology. 2018;73(2):314–20. https://doi.org/10.1111/his.13517.
108. Nakaguro M, Tada Y, Faquin WC, Sadow PM, Wirth LJ, Nagao T. Salivary duct carcinoma: updates in histology, cytology, molecular biology, and treatment. Cancer Cytopathol. 2020;128(10):693–703. https://doi.org/10.1002/cncy.22288.
109. Nassar KW, Tan AC. The mutational landscape of mucosal melanoma. Semin Cancer Biol. 2020;61:139–48. https://doi.org/10.1016/j.semcancer.2019.09.013.
110. Neelakantan IV, Di Palma S, Smith CE, McCoombe A. Parotid sebaceous carcinoma in patient with muir torre syndrome, caused by MSH2 mutation. Head Neck Pathol. 2016;10(3):354–61. https://doi.org/10.1007/s12105-015-0670-9.
111. Newell F, Kong Y, Wilmott JS, Johansson PA, Ferguson PM, Cui C, et al. Whole-genome landscape of mucosal melanoma reveals diverse drivers and therapeutic targets. Nat Commun. 2019;10(1):3163. https://doi.org/10.1038/s41467-019-11107-x.
112. Nielsen TO, Poulin NM, Ladanyi M. Synovial sarcoma: recent discoveries as a roadmap to new avenues for therapy. Cancer Discov. 2015;5(2):124–34. https://doi.org/10.1158/2159-8290.CD-14-1246.
113. Nitta Y, Takeda M, Fujii T, Itami H, Tsukamoto S, Honoki K, Ohbayashi C. A case of pericytic neoplasm in the shoulder with a novel DERA-GLI1 gene fusion. Histopathology. 2021;78(3):466–9. https://doi.org/10.1111/his.14280.
114. Niu Z, Li Y, Chen W, Zhao J, Zheng H, Deng Q, et al. Study on clinical and biological characteristics of ameloblastic carcinoma. Orphanet J Rare Dis. 2020;15(1):316. https://doi.org/10.1186/s13023-020-01603-5.
115. Nobusawa A, Sano T, Yokoo S, Oyama T. Ameloblastic carcinoma developing in preexisting ameloblastoma with a mutation of the p53 gene: a case report. Oral Surg Oral Med Oral Pathol Oral Radiol. 2014;118(5):e146–50. https://doi.org/10.1016/j.oooo.2014.03.021.
116. Okumura Y, Nakano S, Murase T, Ueda K, Kawakita D, Nagao T, et al. Prognostic impact of CRTC1/3-MAML2 fusions in salivary gland mucoepidermoid carcinoma: a multiinstitutional retrospective study. Cancer Sci. 2020;111(11):4195–204. https://doi.org/10.1111/cas.14632.
117. Panagopoulos I, Mertens F, Isaksson M, Domanski HA, Brosjo O, Heim S, et al. Molecular genetic characterization of the EWS/CHN and RBP56/CHN fusion genes in extraskeletal myxoid chondrosarcoma. Genes Chromosomes Cancer. 2002;35(4):340–52. https://doi.org/10.1002/gcc.10127.
118. Panosetti E, Luboinski B, Mamelle G, Richard JM. Multiple synchronous and metachronous cancers of the upper aerodigestive tract: a nine-year study. Laryngoscope. 1989;99(12):1267–73. https://doi.org/10.1288/00005537-198912000-00011.
119. Parisi FM, Lentini M, Chiesa-Estomba CM, Mayo-Yanez M, Leichen JR, White M, et al. Liquid biopsy in HPV-associated head and neck cancer: a comprehensive review. Cancers (Basel). 2025;17(6) https://doi.org/10.3390/cancers17060977.
120. Paul P, Deka H, Malakar AK, Halder B, Chakraborty S. Nasopharyngeal carcinoma: understanding its molecular biology at a fine scale. Eur J Cancer Prev. 2018;27(1):33–41. https://doi.org/10.1097/CEJ.0000000000000314.
121. Persson F, Andren Y, Winnes M, Wedell B, Nordkvist A, Gudnadottir G, et al. High-resolution genomic profiling of adenomas and carcinomas of the salivary glands reveals amplification, rearrangement, and fusion of HMGA2. Genes Chromosomes Cancer. 2009;48(1):69–82. https://doi.org/10.1002/gcc.20619.
122. Pickering CR, Zhang J, Yoo SY, Bengtsson L, Moorthy S, Neskey DM, et al. Integrative genomic characterization of oral squamous cell carcinoma identifies frequent somatic drivers. Cancer Discov. 2013;3(7):770–81. https://doi.org/10.1158/2159-8290.CD-12-0537.
123. Raab-Traub N. Nasopharyngeal carcinoma: an evolving role for the Epstein-Barr virus. Curr Top Microbiol Immunol. 2015;390(Pt 1):339–63. https://doi.org/10.1007/978-3-319-22822-8_14.
124. Rached L, Saleh K, Casiraghi O, Even C. Salivary gland carcinoma: towards a more personalised approach. Cancer Treat Rev. 2024;124:102697. https://doi.org/10.1016/j.ctrv.2024.102697.
125. Riedl JM, Moik F, Esterl T, Kostmann SM, Gerger A, Jost PJ. Molecular diagnostics tailoring personalized cancer therapy-an oncologist's view. Virchows Arch. 2024;484(2):169–79. https://doi.org/10.1007/s00428-023-03702-7.
126. Riobello C, Lopez-Hernandez A, Cabal VN, Garcia-Marin R, Suarez-Fernandez L, Sanchez-Fernandez P, et al. IDH2 mutation analysis in undifferentiated and poorly differentiated sinonasal carcinomas for diagnosis and clinical management. Am J Surg Pathol. 2020;44(3):396–405. https://doi.org/10.1097/PAS.0000000000001420.
127. Rito M, Mitani Y, Bell D, Mariano FV, Almalki ST, Pytynia KB, et al. Frequent and differential mutations of the CYLD gene in basal cell salivary neoplasms: linkage to tumor development and progression. Mod Pathol. 2018;31(7):1064–72. https://doi.org/10.1038/s41379-018-0018-6.
128. Robinson RA. Basal cell adenoma and basal cell adenocarcinoma. Surg Pathol Clin. 2021;14(1):25–42. https://doi.org/10.1016/j.path.2020.09.005.
129. Roijer E, Nordkvist A, Strom AK, Ryd W, Behrendt M, Bullerdiek J, et al. Translocation, deletion/amplification, and expression of HMGIC and MDM2 in a carcinoma ex pleomorphic adenoma. Am J Pathol.

2002;160(2):433–40. https://doi.org/10.1016/S0002-9440(10)64862-6.

130. Rooper LM, Bishop JA. Soft tissue special issue: adamantinoma-like Ewing sarcoma of the head and neck: a practical review of a challenging emerging entity. Head Neck Pathol. 2020;14(1):59–69. https://doi.org/10.1007/s12105-019-01098-y.

131. Rooper LM, Karantanos T, Ning Y, Bishop JA, Gordon SW, Kang H. Salivary secretory carcinoma with a novel ETV6-MET fusion: expanding the molecular spectrum of a recently described entity. Am J Surg Pathol. 2018;42(8):1121–6. https://doi.org/10.1097/PAS.0000000000001065.

132. Rooper LM, Argyris PP, Thompson LDR, Gagan J, Westra WH, Jordan RC, et al. Salivary mucinous adenocarcinoma is a histologically diverse single entity with recurrent AKT1 E17K mutations: clinicopathologic and molecular characterization with proposal for a unified classification. Am J Surg Pathol. 2021a;45(10):1337–47. https://doi.org/10.1097/PAS.0000000000001688.

133. Rooper LM, Thompson LDR, Gagan J, Oliai BR, Weinreb I, Bishop JA. Salivary intraductal carcinoma arising within intraparotid lymph node: a report of 4 cases with identification of a novel STRN-ALK fusion. Head Neck Pathol. 2021b;15(1):179–85. https://doi.org/10.1007/s12105-020-01198-0.

134. Rossi ED, Baloch Z, Barkan G, Foschini MP, Kurtycz D, Pusztaszeri M, et al. Second edition of the Milan system for reporting salivary gland cytopathology: refining the role of salivary gland FNA. Cytopathology. 2024;35(2):188–98. https://doi.org/10.1111/cyt.13331.

135. Salinas-Souza C, De Andrea C, Bihl M, Kovac M, Pillay N, Forshew T, et al. GNAS mutations are not detected in parosteal and low-grade central osteosarcomas. Mod Pathol. 2015;28(10):1336–42. https://doi.org/10.1038/modpathol.2015.91.

136. Sanchez-Fernandez P, Riobello C, Costales M, Vivanco B, Cabal VN, Garcia-Marin R, et al. Next-generation sequencing for identification of actionable gene mutations in intestinal-type sinonasal adenocarcinoma. Sci Rep. 2021;11(1):2247. https://doi.org/10.1038/s41598-020-80242-z.

137. Sebastiao APM, Xu B, Lozada JR, Pareja F, Geyer FC, Da Cruz Paula A, et al. Histologic spectrum of polymorphous adenocarcinoma of the salivary gland harbor genetic alterations affecting PRKD genes. Mod Pathol. 2020;33(1):65–73. https://doi.org/10.1038/s41379-019-0351-4.

138. Seethala RR, Dacic S, Cieply K, Kelly LM, Nikiforova MN. A reappraisal of the MECT1/MAML2 translocation in salivary mucoepidermoid carcinomas. Am J Surg Pathol. 2010;34(8):1106–21. https://doi.org/10.1097/PAS.0b013e3181de3021.

139. Sheng J, Chen H, Fu B, Pan H, Wang J, Han W. BPI-28592 as a novel second generation inhibitor for NTRK fusion tumors. NPJ Precis Oncol. 2024;8(1):198. https://doi.org/10.1038/s41698-024-00686-8.

140. Shimura T, Tada Y, Hirai H, Kawakita D, Kano S, Tsukahara K, et al. Prognostic and histogenetic roles of gene alteration and the expression of key potentially actionable targets in salivary duct carcinomas. Oncotarget. 2018;9(2):1852–67. https://doi.org/10.18632/oncotarget.22927.

141. Shing DC, McMullan DJ, Roberts P, Smith K, Chin SF, Nicholson J, et al. FUS/ERG gene fusions in Ewing's tumors. Cancer Res. 2003;63(15):4568–76. Retrieved from https://www.ncbi.nlm.nih.gov/pubmed/12907633

142. Shiota H, Elya JE, Alekseyenko AA, Chou PM, Gorman SA, Barbash O, et al. "Z4" complex member fusions in NUT carcinoma: implications for a novel oncogenic mechanism. Mol Cancer Res. 2018;16(12):1826–33. https://doi.org/10.1158/1541-7786.MCR-18-0474.

143. Skalova A, Vanecek T, Sima R, Laco J, Weinreb I, Perez-Ordonez B, et al. Mammary analogue secretory carcinoma of salivary glands, containing the ETV6-NTRK3 fusion gene: a hitherto undescribed salivary gland tumor entity. Am J Surg Pathol. 2010;34(5):599–608. https://doi.org/10.1097/PAS.0b013e3181d9efcc.

144. Skalova A, Vanecek T, Uro-Coste E, Bishop JA, Weinreb I, Thompson LDR, et al. Molecular profiling of salivary gland intraductal carcinoma revealed a subset of tumors harboring NCOA4-RET and novel TRIM27-RET fusions: a report of 17 cases. Am J Surg Pathol. 2018;42(11):1445–55. https://doi.org/10.1097/PAS.0000000000001133.

145. Skalova A, Ptakova N, Santana T, Agaimy A, Ihrler S, Uro-Coste E, et al. NCOA4-RET and TRIM27-RET are characteristic gene fusions in salivary intraductal carcinoma, including invasive and metastatic tumors: is "intraductal" correct? Am J Surg Pathol. 2019;43(10):1303–13. https://doi.org/10.1097/PAS.0000000000001301.

146. Skalova A, Baneckova M, Thompson LDR, Ptakova N, Stevens TM, Brcic L, et al. Expanding the molecular spectrum of secretory carcinoma of salivary glands with a novel VIM-RET fusion. Am J Surg Pathol. 2020;44(10):1295–307. https://doi.org/10.1097/PAS.0000000000001535.

147. Skalova A, Agaimy A, Vanecek T, Baneckova M, Laco J, Ptakova N, et al. Molecular profiling of clear cell myoepithelial carcinoma of salivary glands with EWSR1 rearrangement identifies frequent PLAG1 gene fusions but no EWSR1 fusion transcripts. Am J Surg Pathol. 2021;45(1):1–13. https://doi.org/10.1097/PAS.0000000000001591.

148. Slaughter DP, Southwick HW, Smejkal W. Field cancerization in oral stratified squamous epithelium; clinical implications of multicentric origin. Cancer. 1953;6(5):963–8. https://doi.org/10.1002/1097-0142(195309)6:5<963::aid-cncr2820060515>3.0.co;2-q.

149. Soares CD, Morais TML, Carlos R, Jorge J, de Almeida OP, de Carvalho MGF, Altemani AMM. Sebaceous adenocarcinomas of the major

salivary glands: a clinicopathological analysis of 10 cases. Histopathology. 2018;73(4):585–92. https://doi.org/10.1111/his.13664.

150. Sorensen PH, Lessnick SL, Lopez-Terrada D, Liu XF, Triche TJ, Denny CT. A second Ewing's sarcoma translocation, t(21;22), fuses the EWS gene to another ETS-family transcription factor. ERG Nat Genet. 1994;6(2):146–51. https://doi.org/10.1038/ng0294-146.
151. Steele CD, Tarabichi M, Oukrif D, Webster AP, Ye H, Fittall M, et al. Undifferentiated sarcomas develop through distinct evolutionary pathways. Cancer Cell. 2019;35(3):441–456 e448. https://doi.org/10.1016/j.ccell.2019.02.002.
152. Stenman G. Fusion oncogenes in salivary gland tumors: molecular and clinical consequences. Head Neck Pathol. 2013;7(Suppl 1):S12–9. https://doi.org/10.1007/s12105-013-0462-z.
153. Stevens TM, Morlote D, Xiu J, Swensen J, Brandwein-Weber M, Miettinen MM, et al. NUTM1-rearranged neoplasia: a multi-institution experience yields novel fusion partners and expands the histologic spectrum. Mod Pathol. 2019;32(6):764–73. https://doi.org/10.1038/s41379-019-0206-z.
154. Stransky N, Egloff AM, Tward AD, Kostic AD, Cibulskis K, Sivachenko A, et al. The mutational landscape of head and neck squamous cell carcinoma. Science. 2011;333(6046):1157–60. https://doi.org/10.1126/science.1208130.
155. Su SC, Lin CW, Liu YF, Fan WL, Chen MK, Yu CP, et al. Exome sequencing of oral squamous cell carcinoma reveals molecular subgroups and novel therapeutic opportunities. Theranostics. 2017;7(5):1088–99. https://doi.org/10.7150/thno.18551.
156. Sweeney RT, McClary AC, Myers BR, Biscocho J, Neahring L, Kwei KA, et al. Identification of recurrent SMO and BRAF mutations in ameloblastomas. Nat Genet. 2014;46(7):722–5. https://doi.org/10.1038/ng.2986.
157. Tallegas M, Miquelestorena-Standley E, Labit-Bouvier C, Badoual C, Francois A, Gomez-Brouchet A, et al. IDH mutation status in a series of 88 head and neck chondrosarcomas: different profile between tumors of the skull base and tumors involving the facial skeleton and the laryngotracheal tract. Hum Pathol. 2019;84:183–91. https://doi.org/10.1016/j.humpath.2018.09.015.
158. Todorovic E, Dickson BC, Weinreb I. Salivary gland cancer in the era of routine next-generation sequencing. Head Neck Pathol. 2020;14(2):311–20. https://doi.org/10.1007/s12105-020-01140-4.
159. Tsang CM, Tsao SW. The role of Epstein-Barr virus infection in the pathogenesis of nasopharyngeal carcinoma. Virol Sin. 2015;30(2):107–21. https://doi.org/10.1007/s12250-015-3592-5.
160. Tsang CM, Lui VWY, Bruce JP, Pugh TJ, Lo KW. Translational genomics of nasopharyngeal cancer. Semin Cancer Biol. 2020;61:84–100. https://doi.org/10.1016/j.semcancer.2019.09.006.
161. Tsao SW, Tsang CM, Lo KW. Epstein-Barr virus infection and nasopharyngeal carcinoma. Philos Trans R Soc Lond Ser B Biol Sci. 2017;372(1732) https://doi.org/10.1098/rstb.2016.0270.
162. Turc-Carel C, Aurias A, Mugneret F, Lizard S, Sidaner I, Volk C, et al. Chromosomes in Ewing's sarcoma. I. An evaluation of 85 cases of remarkable consistency of t(11;22)(q24;q12). Cancer Genet Cytogenet. 1988;32(2):229–38. https://doi.org/10.1016/0165-4608(88)90285-3.
163. Udager AM, Rolland DCM, McHugh JB, Betz BL, Murga-Zamalloa C, Carey TE, et al. High-frequency targetable EGFR mutations in sinonasal squamous cell carcinomas arising from inverted sinonasal papilloma. Cancer Res. 2015;75(13):2600–6. https://doi.org/10.1158/0008-5472.CAN-15-0340.
164. Urano M, Nakaguro M, Yamamoto Y, Hirai H, Tanigawa M, Saigusa N, et al. Diagnostic significance of HRAS mutations in epithelial-myoepithelial carcinomas exhibiting a broad histopathologic spectrum. Am J Surg Pathol. 2019;43(7):984–94. https://doi.org/10.1097/PAS.0000000000001258.
165. Urbano A, Babiloni C, Onorati P, Carducci F, Ambrosini A, Fattorini L, Babiloni F. Responses of human primary sensorimotor and supplementary motor areas to internally triggered unilateral and simultaneous bilateral one-digit movements. A high-resolution EEG study. Eur J Neurosci. 1998;10(2):765–70. https://doi.org/10.1046/j.1460-9568.1998.00072.x.
166. Villatoro TM, Mardekian SK. Two cases of sinonasal non-intestinal-type adenocarcinoma with squamoid morules expressing nuclear beta-catenin and CDX2: a curious morphologic finding supported by molecular analysis. Case Rep Pathol. 2018;2018:8741017. https://doi.org/10.1155/2018/8741017.
167. Viscuse PV, Price KA, Garcia JJ, Schembri-Wismayer DJ, Chintakuntlawar AV. First line androgen deprivation therapy vs. chemotherapy for patients with androgen receptor positive recurrent or metastatic salivary gland carcinoma-a retrospective study. Front Oncol. 2019;9:701. https://doi.org/10.3389/fonc.2019.00701.
168. Vogels R, Baumhoer D, van Gorp J, Eijkelenboom A, Verdijk M, van Cleef P, et al. Clear cell odontogenic carcinoma: occurrence of EWSR1-CREB1 as alternative fusion gene to EWSR1-ATF1. Head Neck Pathol. 2019;13(2):225–30. https://doi.org/10.1007/s12105-018-0953-z.
169. von Holstein SL, Fehr A, Persson M, Nickelsen M, Therkildsen MH, Prause JU, et al. Lacrimal gland pleomorphic adenoma and carcinoma ex pleomorphic adenoma: genomic profiles, gene fusions, and clinical characteristics. Ophthalmology. 2014;121(5):1125–33. https://doi.org/10.1016/j.ophtha.2013.11.037.
170. Wang X, Bledsoe KL, Graham RP, Asmann YW, Viswanatha DS, Lewis JE, et al. Recurrent PAX3-MAML3 fusion in biphenotypic sinonasal sar-

coma. Nat Genet. 2014;46(7):666–8. https://doi.org/10.1038/ng.2989.
171. Weinreb I, Piscuoglio S, Martelotto LG, Waggott D, Ng CK, Perez-Ordonez B, et al. Hotspot activating PRKD1 somatic mutations in polymorphous low-grade adenocarcinomas of the salivary glands. Nat Genet. 2014a;46(11):1166–9. https://doi.org/10.1038/ng.3096.
172. Weinreb I, Zhang L, Tirunagari LM, Sung YS, Chen CL, Perez-Ordonez B, et al. Novel PRKD gene rearrangements and variant fusions in cribriform adenocarcinoma of salivary gland origin. Genes Chromosomes Cancer. 2014b;53(10):845–56. https://doi.org/10.1002/gcc.22195.
173. Weinreb I, Bishop JA, Chiosea SI, Seethala RR, Perez-Ordonez B, Zhang L, et al. Recurrent RET gene rearrangements in intraductal carcinomas of salivary gland. Am J Surg Pathol. 2018;42(4):442–52. https://doi.org/10.1097/PAS.0000000000000952.
174. Weinreb I, Hahn E, Dickson BC, Rooper LM, Rupp NJ, Freiberger SN, et al. Microcribriform adenocarcinoma of salivary glands: a unique tumor entity characterized by an SS18::ZBTB7A fusion. Am J Surg Pathol. 2023;47(2):194–201. https://doi.org/10.1097/PAS.0000000000001980.
175. Wong WJ, Lauria A, Hornick JL, Xiao S, Fletcher JA, Marino-Enriquez A. Alternate PAX3-FOXO1 oncogenic fusion in biphenotypic sinonasal sarcoma. Genes Chromosomes Cancer. 2016;55(1):25–9. https://doi.org/10.1002/gcc.22295.
176. Xu B, Katabi N. Myoepithelial carcinoma. Surg Pathol Clin. 2021;14(1):67–73. https://doi.org/10.1016/j.path.2020.09.008.
177. Xu L, Cheng Z, Cui C, Wu X, Yu H, Guo J, Kong Y. Frequent genetic aberrations in the cell cycle related genes in mucosal melanoma indicate the potential for targeted therapy. J Transl Med. 2019;17(1):245. https://doi.org/10.1186/s12967-019-1987-z.
178. Xu B, Barbieri AL, Bishop JA, Chiosea SI, Dogan S, Di Palma S, et al. Histologic classification and molecular signature of polymorphous adenocarcinoma (PAC) and cribriform adenocarcinoma of salivary gland (CASG): an international interobserver study. Am J Surg Pathol. 2020a;44(4):545–52. https://doi.org/10.1097/PAS.0000000000001431.
179. Xu B, Chang K, Folpe AL, Kao YC, Wey SL, Huang HY, et al. Head and neck mesenchymal neoplasms with GLI1 gene alterations: a pathologic entity with distinct histologic features and potential for distant metastasis. Am J Surg Pathol. 2020b;44(6):729–37. https://doi.org/10.1097/PAS.0000000000001439.
180. Xu B, Suurmeijer AJH, Agaram NP, Zhang L, Antonescu CR. Head and neck rhabdomyosarcoma with TFCP2 fusions and ALK overexpression: a clinicopathological and molecular analysis of 11 cases. Histopathology. 2021;79(3):347–57. https://doi.org/10.1111/his.14323.
181. Zarella MD, McClintock DS, Batra H, Gullapalli RR, Valante M, Tan VO, et al. Artificial intelligence and digital pathology: clinical promise and deployment considerations. J Med Imaging (Bellingham). 2023;10(5):051802. https://doi.org/10.1117/1.JMI.10.5.051802.

Next-Generation Sequencing in Kidney, Bladder, and Prostate Pathology

13

Stefano Sioletic, Alessia Cimadamore, Elisa Melucci, and Giuseppe Simone

Renal Cell Carcinoma

Sioletic Stefano, Melucci Elisa, Simone Giuseppe.

Introduction

Renal cell carcinoma (RCC) comprises a heterogeneous group of malignancies that has undergone substantial reclassification in recent years. Traditionally, these tumors were grouped into a limited number of morphologic subtypes, primarily clear cell (ccRCC), papillary (pRCC), and chromophobe variants (ChRCC) [147]. Advances in molecular profiling have reshaped our understanding of RCC biology, leading the 2022 WHO Classification to recognize more than 20 distinct entities defined by specific genetic alterations rather than histologic appearance alone [146, 219].

Next-generation sequencing (NGS) is now becoming essential for accurate diagnosis in renal tumor pathology. Several subtypes require molecular characterization: Fumarate hydratase (FH) deficient RCC, succinate dehydrogenase (SDH) deficient RCC, ELOC-mutated RCC, anaplastic lymphoma kinase (ALK)-rearranged RCC, and tumors with constitutive mTORC1 activation [73, 86, 115, 116, 203]. Although these molecularly defined entities represent only a minority of RCC cases, their identification has significant clinical relevance. They exhibit distinct biological behavior, variable associations with hereditary cancer predisposition syndromes, and show different responses to targeted therapies [32, 35].

Hereditary RCC syndromes account for 5–8% of all cases, where molecular testing serves dual purposes: establishing the diagnosis and facilitating genetic screening for at-risk family members [130, 199]. Young patients presenting with bilateral or multifocal disease particularly benefit from molecular testing, which often reveals germline mutations in genes such as VHL, FH, FLCN, or MET, necessitating genetic counseling and familial screening [157, 174]. Furthermore, while targetable somatic alterations remain relatively uncommon in most RCC subtypes, their

S. Sioletic (✉)
Department of Pathology, San Camillo-Forlanini Hospital, Rome, Italy

A. Cimadamore
Institute of Pathological Anatomy, Department of Medicine, University of Udine, Udine, Italy

E. Melucci
Molecular Diagnostic Laboratory, Pathology Department, Advanced Diagnostics Research and Technological Innovation Department, Regina, Elena National Cancer Institute, Rome, Italy
e-mail: elisa.melucci@ifo.it

G. Simone
Department of Urology, IRCCS "Regina Elena" National Cancer Institute, Rome, Italy
e-mail: giuseppe.simone@ifo.it

© The Author(s), under exclusive license to Springer Nature Switzerland AG 2026

S. Sioletic, L. Coppola (eds.), *Next-Generation Sequencing in Solid Tumor Histopathology*, Current Clinical Pathology, https://doi.org/10.1007/978-3-032-18790-1_13

detection can significantly influence therapeutic decision-making, particularly in advanced disease where options such as MET inhibitors for MET-altered tumors or mTOR inhibitors for TSC-mutant neoplasms may provide clinical benefit [46, 231, 232].

This chapter aims to provide a framework for understanding the molecular landscape of RCC subtypes as defined by the 2022 WHO Classification.

Molecular Mechanisms in RCC Pathogenesis

A clear understanding of key molecular pathways is essential to understand how genetic alterations define RCC classification.

The VHL–HIF Hypoxia Response Pathway

VHL inactivation, present in approximately 90% of ccRCC, prevents degradation of hypoxia-inducible factor (HIF), triggering an angiogenic program through VEGF and PDGF upregulation [29]. In other RCC subtypes, HIF stabilization occurs through alternative mechanisms. ELOC mutations disrupt VHL complex assembly, while FH and SDH deficiency leads to oncometabolite accumulation that inhibits prolyl hydroxylases and stabilizes HIF [179, 215].

Chromatin Remodeling Complex Disruption

RCC frequently harbors mutations in multiple chromatin remodeling complexes, particularly within the SWI/SNF family [78]. These alterations affect chromatin architecture, transcriptional regulation, and DNA repair, with implications for both tumor behavior and therapy.

PBRM1 mutations (40–50% of ccRCC) represent one of the most frequent genomic alterations in ccRCC after VHL. PBRM1 loss disrupts chromatin accessibility and gene expression patterns, fundamentally altering the tumor-immune microenvironment [153, 165]. SETD2, which catalyzes H3K36 trimethylation (H3K36me3), is essential for DNA mismatch repair; its inactivation promotes genomic instability and facilitates tumor evolution [126]. In renal medullary carcinoma, loss of SMARCB1 (INI1) defines the tumor phenotype and causes global chromatin dysregulation [28]. Chromatin remodeler mutations define clinically distinct molecular subgroups. PBRM1 loss, particularly without concurrent BAP1 alterations, correlates with superior checkpoint inhibitor response, potentially through enhanced neoantigen presentation or altered chromatin accessibility at immune gene loci [144]. Conversely, BAP1-deficient tumors show aggressive biology independent of treatment modality, with rapid progression even in otherwise favorable-risk patients [102].

Metabolic Reprogramming Pathways

RCC metabolic phenotypes reflect both histologic origin and the molecular alterations driving tumorigenesis.

mTORC1 pathway activation defines several recently characterized eosinophilic tumors harboring MTOR or RHEB mutations, or biallelic TSC1/TSC2 loss, resulting in constitutive mTORC1 activation [231, 232]. In contrast, chromophobe RCC and oncocytoma maintain oxidative phosphorylation capacity, characterized by increased mitochondrial content and retained respiration [58]. Oncocytomas often carry mitochondrial DNA mutations in complex I subunits, which impair electron transport efficiency without complete loss of function [103]. FH- and SDH-deficient RCCs represent a distinct metabolic class where Krebs cycle disruption causes oncometabolite (fumarate and succinate) accumulation. These metabolites stabilize HIF, promote DNA hypermethylation, and impair cellular differentiation, contributing to tumorigenesis through integrated metabolic and epigenetic mechanisms [197].

Chromosomal Instability Patterns

Chromosomal instability varies across RCC subtypes and reveals distinct mechanisms of genomic disruption. Chromophobe RCC is defined by characteristic whole-chromosome losses involving chromosomes 1, 2, 6, 10, 13, 17, and 21 [36]. In contrast, ccRCC is marked by focal chromosomal deletions, most notably involving chromosome 3p, which harbors VHL, PBRM1, BAP1, and SETD2. Additional 9p and 14q deletions, along with subclonal amplifications, emerge during tumor evolution and contribute to intratumoral heterogeneity [223]. Chromosomal copy number profiles serve as important diagnostic tools, particularly in cases with overlapping morphology. Moreover, tumors with complex structural rearrangements or chromothripsis often exhibit aggressive progression, while those with stable whole-chromosome losses tend to follow a more indolent course [145].

Pathway Convergence and Therapeutic Implications

Molecular alterations in RCC rarely occur in isolation. In ccRCC, for example, VHL loss and HIF activation are frequently accompanied by mutations in chromatin remodelers such as PBRM1 or BAP1, together with metabolic reprogramming that allows tumor cells to survive in hypoxic and nutrient-poor environments [84]. Understanding how these molecular pathways converge within specific RCC subtypes provides the basis for integrated therapeutic strategies [91].

Major RCC Subtypes Metabolically Defined Entities

Clear Cell Renal Cell Carcinoma (ccRCC)

Clear cell renal cell carcinoma (ccRCC) represents the predominant histological subtype of kidney cancer, comprising approximately 75–80% of all RCC [92]. Loss of chromosome 3p, present in nearly all cases, defines its molecular signature. This deletion involves a critical genomic region containing multiple tumor-suppressor genes, most notably VHL at 3p25, as well as PBRM1, BAP1, and SETD2 [29].

The VHL gene undergoes biallelic inactivation in 85–90% of sporadic clear cell carcinomas through mutation, deletion, or promoter hypermethylation. Loss of VHL function leads to constitutive accumulation of hypoxia-inducible factor (HIF) transcription factors, independent of oxygen availability. This metabolic shift toward aerobic glycolysis and lipid accumulation produces the characteristic clear cytoplasm that defines this tumor histologically [85]. HIF-mediated VEGF upregulation also drives the marked ccRCC vascularity, explaining the clinical efficacy of anti-angiogenic therapies in this setting [45].

Additional tumor-suppressor genes on chromosome 3p contribute to molecular subtyping and have important prognostic and therapeutic implications. PBRM1 mutations are found in 40–50% of cases and are typically associated with lower tumor grade and more indolent clinical behavior [153]. These tumors show enhanced sensitivity to immune checkpoint blockade, likely through chromatin remodeling defects that enhance neoantigen presentation [144]. In contrast, BAP1 mutations, present in approximately 10–15% of tumors, are linked to a more aggressive clinical course, with features such as high-grade histology, genomic instability, sarcomatoid transformation, and early metastatic spread [165]. SETD2 mutations, also occurring in 10–15% of tumors, impair histone methylation and DNA repair processes, further contributing to genomic instability and resistance to genotoxic therapies [126]. PBRM1 and BAP1 mutations rarely co-occur, suggesting distinct evolutionary trajectories with differing therapeutic vulnerabilities [105].

Tumors evolve through branched rather than linear mutation accumulation. VHL loss typically occurs as an early, truncal event present throughout the neoplasm, while alterations in PBRM1, BAP1, and SETD2 emerge later as subclonal events restricted to specific regions [71].Tumor progression increases spatial heterogeneity. TP53 mutations often arise within sarcomatoid components, while activation of the PI3K/AKT/mTOR pathway occurs in approximately 20% of advanced tumors [91]. KEAP1 mutations, found in 5–10% of cases, enable resistance to oxidative stress via activation of the NRF2 pathway [32]. Secondary genetic events critically shape therapeutic response and resistance. However, single-region biopsies capture only 60–70% of the total mutational landscape, potentially missing clinically relevant alterations that could influence treatment selection [223].

Von Hippel–Lindau syndrome, caused by germline VHL mutations, illustrates how sporadic tumor genetics can illuminate hereditary cancer syndromes. Affected individuals are at risk for central nervous system and retinal hemangioblastomas, pheochromocytomas, pancreatic neuroendocrine tumors, and typically bilateral or multifocal ccRCC [131]. Identification of VHL mutations in patients younger than 45 years or in those presenting with bilateral renal tumors should prompt genetic counseling and cascade testing of at-risk family members[199].

Papillary Renal Cell Carcinoma

Papillary renal cell carcinoma (pRCC) accounts for approximately 15% of all kidney cancers and has undergone significant reclassification based on molecular insights. The 2022 WHO Classification eliminated the type 1 and 2 distinction, recognizing type 2 tumors as multiple molecularly distinct entities [146]. These have been reclassified as separate diseases, including FH-deficient RCC, SDH-deficient RCC, and ALK-rearranged RCC, each exhibiting unique biological behaviors and therapeutic implications.

Current "true" papillary carcinomas show both morphological uniformity and distinctive chromosomal alterations. Former type 1 tumors typically show trisomies of chromosomes 7 and 17, often accompanied by gains of chromosome 16 and loss of the Y chromosome in male patients [61]. MET tyrosine kinase mutations drive ligand-independent signaling in nearly all hereditary pRCC and in up to 20% of sporadic tumors. MET-driven carcinomas typically follow an indolent clinical course and show particular sensitivity to MET inhibitors such as cabozantinib and savolitinib [181].

The group of tumors formerly classified as type 2 pRCC reveals considerable molecular heterogeneity, with distinct profiles correlating with clinical behavior. TCGA analysis identified multiple molecular subtypes within this group [32]. One subset harbor MET alterations with low mutation burden and favorable outcomes. In contrast, a molecularly diverse subset exhibits widespread chromosomal losses involving 1p, 3p, 6p, 9p, and 14q, accompanied by inactivation of key tumor-suppressor genes including CDKN2A, SETD2, BAP1, and NF2 [162]. These tumors frequently display a CpG island methylator phenotype and associate with high-grade morphology, lymphovascular invasion, and poor prognosis. Co-occurring SETD2/BAP1 mutations and 3p loss demonstrate molecular convergence with ccRCC, suggesting overlapping evolutionary pressures. Tumors with NF2 mutations often show sarcomatoid features and mTOR pathway activation, potentially identifying candidates for mTOR inhibitor therapy [231, 232].

Integrated transcriptomic and methylation analyses provide further stratification. Activation of the NRF2-ARE pathway through mutations in NFE2L2, KEAP1, or CUL3 promotes resistance to oxidative stress and correlates with limited therapeutic response [161]. CpG island hypermethylation frequently silences tumor suppressors and associates with adverse clinical features. Common chromosomal gains (2, 6, 12, 20) and focal MYC/EGFR alterations lack functional definition.

Chromophobe Renal Cell Carcinoma and Oncocytic Neoplasms

Chromophobe renal cell carcinoma (ChRCC) represents for approximately 5% of kidney cancers and is characterized by widespread whole-chromosome losses rather than focal driver mutations, marking a fundamental distinction from other RCC subtypes [58]. The typical hypodiploid karyotype involves consistent monosomies of chromosomes 1, 2, 6, 10, 13, 17, and 21, with additional losses of chromosomes 3, 5, 8, 9, 11, and 18 observed in many cases. Despite a low mutation rate (0.4/Mb), TP53 mutations occur in one-third of cases and correlate with aggressive behavior. PTEN alterations (9–10%) and mutations in MTOR, TSC1, TSC2, and NRAS contribute to PI3K-AKT-mTOR pathway dysregulation in up to 25% of cases, suggesting potentially actionable therapeutic targets [66]. The characteristic chromosomal pattern enables diagnosis by microarray or FISH in ambiguous cases. Focal hypermethylation and CDKN2A silencing disrupt cell cycle regulation in selected cases. The metabolic phenotype of ChRCC contrasts sharply with ccRCC. Rather than shifting toward glycolysis, ChRCC maintains oxidative phosphorylation, with upregulation of mitochondrial biogenesis regulators such as PPARGC1A and elevated mitochondrial DNA content [172]. Somatic mitochondrial DNA mutations affecting complex I subunits, particularly MT-ND5, occur in about 20% of tumors, especially those with eosinophilic cytoplasm. These mutations define a subgroup maintaining oxidative metabolism despite mitochondrial alterations [120]. Transcriptomic profiling supports a lineage origin from intercalated cells of the collecting duct, reflected in the tumor's immunoprofile. Typical markers include positivity for CK7, KIT, parvalbumin, claudin-7, and EpCAM, with negativity for vimentin and CAIX [156]. Eosinophilic variants of ChRCC present diagnostic challenges in small biopsies, as they often lack consistent chromosomal losses or canonical mutations.

Renal oncocytoma, sharing an intercalated cell origin, exhibits molecular features allowing reliable distinction from ChRCC. Type 1 oncocytomas maintain a diploid genome and frequently show CCND1 rearrangements leading to cyclin D1 overexpression [103]. Type 2 oncocytomas show limited chromosomal losses, typically involving chromosomes 1, 14, 21, and sex chromosomes, and are considered potential precursors of eosinophilic variants of ChRCC. A key molecular feature is the presence of mitochondrial complex I mutations in MT-ND4, MT-ND5, or MT-COX1, which impair oxidative phosphorylation and activate AMPK-mediated growth arrest. Combined with defective autophagy, characterized by LC3 and p62 accumulation, these alterations create a metabolically quiescent state maintaining the benign phenotype.

Hereditary syndromes account for a meaningful proportion of ChRCC and hybrid oncocytic-chromophobe tumors [167]. Birt-Hogg-Dubé syndrome, caused by germline FLCN mutations, and Cowden syndrome, associated with germline PTEN mutations, often produce bilateral or multifocal tumors with overlapping morphologic and molecular features [143, 193]. These tumors are increasingly regarded as part of a biologic spectrum rather than distinct entities. In patients with FLCN mutations, associated features such as pulmonary cysts and increased risk of pneumothorax require careful clinical monitoring.

Organ-confined ChRCC follows an indolent course with >90% five-year survival. However, prognosis worsens when associated with TP53 mutations and TERT activation [70]. Unlike ccRCC, ChRCC rarely responds to VEGF-targeted agents, and mTOR inhibitor benefit is limited to cases with pathway-specific mutations. In morphologically ambiguous oncocytic tumors, NGS should prioritize chromosomal copy number analysis to detect ChRCC-defining losses, mitochondrial genome sequencing to confirm complex I mutations characteristic of oncocytoma, and targeted sequencing for TP53, PTEN, and FLCN mutations to guide assessment of malignant potential and hereditary risk.

Metabolically Defined Entities

FH-deficient RCC has emerged as a distinct entity within the pRCC spectrum, defined by biallelic fumarate hydratase inactivation [215].

FH loss causes fumarate accumulation, which stabilizes HIF transcription factorsdespite normal oxygen levels, and induces widespread protein succination that disrupts multiple cellular pathways [197]. Morphologically, these tumors show prominent eosinophilic nucleoli with perinuclear halos, a highly characteristic finding [203].

Absent FH immunostaining serves as an initial screening tool, while positive staining for 2-succinylcysteine confirms the metabolic consequences of fumarate accumulation [17]. Molecular sequencing provides definitive confirmation and distinguishes between somatic and germline mutations. This distinction is clinically relevant, as over 70% of patientswith FH-deficient RCCs, harbor germline FH mutations indicating hereditary leiomyomatosis and RCC syndrome [142]. Such patients require genetic counseling and family member testing, as well as surveillance for the syndrome's other manifestations, particularly cutaneous and uterine leiomyomas that may precede renal tumors by decades [121]. Despite early detection through syndrome screening, FH-deficient RCC follows an aggressive clinical course and often presents with metastatic disease.

SDH-deficient RCC represents another metabolically defined entity arising from loss of SDHB or SDHC function [72]. While these tumors generally have a more indolent course than their FH-deficient counterparts, documented progression cases necessitate careful long-term monitoring. SDH deficiency often indicates hereditary paraganglioma-pheochromocytoma syndrome, requiring surveillance for catecholamine-secreting tumors [178]. Diagnostic workup parallels FH-deficient RCC and includes immunohistochemistry for SDHB loss, followed by germline testing and targeted NGS analysis.

Loss of FH or SDHB on immunohistochemistry suggests a hereditary syndrome, prompting germline testing and comprehensive NGS panel analysis to confirm SDHB/C or FH mutations and guide appropriate clinical management [192].

mTORC1-Driven Eosinophilic Tumors

The landscape of eosinophilic renal tumors has expanded with the recognition of three molecularly defined entities united by constitutive mTORC1 activation. Despite morphologic overlap with ChRCC and oncocytoma, their distinct genomic profiles reveal them as distinct entities with different clinical approaches [217].

Eosinophilic solid and cystic RCC Eosinophilic solid and cystic RCC results from biallelic TSC1/TSC2 inactivation, causing constitutive mTORC1 activation without other recurrent genomic alterations [40]. These tumors lack typical ccRCC alterations (VHL, PBRM1, SETD2), showing instead distinct morphologic and immunophenotypic features reflecting mTORC1 hyperactivation. While most follow an indolent course, rare metastatic cases respond to mTOR inhibitors, validating their TSC-driven biology [82].

Low-grade oncocytic tumors activate mTORC1 through mechanisms distinct from TSC1/TSC2 inactivation. Instead, they harbor activating MTOR mutations, particularly affecting exon 53, or, less commonly, alterations in RHEB, RRAGD, or PDGFRA amplification [107]. This causes persistent mTORC1 activation without disrupting the TSC complex. Wild-type VHL and TSC1/2, intact mitochondrial genes, and chromosomal stability distinguish these from ChRCC and oncocytoma. Despite morphologic features like perinuclear clearing that might suggest metabolic reprogramming, these tumors lack mitochondrial DNA accumulation and show distinct transcriptomic profiles [218].

Eosinophilic vacuolated tumors represent another variation on the mTORC1 theme, characterized by MTOR or TSC2 mutations that converge on pathway activation [88]. These diploid tumors show large eosinophilic cells with prominent intracytoplasmic vacuoles and lack VHL, MET, or TSC1 mutations. They typically follow an indolent course, though isolated nodal or distant spread has been reported [119].

Acquired cystic disease–associated RCC (ACD-RCC) arises exclusively in end-stage renal disease with acquired cystic kidney disease. They display a characteristic molecular profile, with recurrent TSC1/TSC2 mutations in approximately 70% of cases and KMT2C mutations in up to 50% [206]. TSC1/TSC2 loss activates mTORC1, while KMT2C mutations alter histone methylation, jointly driving tumorigenesisThe presence of KMT2C mutations associate with cribriform architecture, whilewild-type KMT2C tumorsshow papillary features, indicating direct genotype-phenotype correlation [41]. Unlike other RCCs, ACD-RCC lacks VHL alterations and typically shows chromosomal gains (3, 7, 16) without 3p loss. Polarizable calcium oxalate crystals and cytoplasmic vacuoles are characteristic diagnostic features in ESRD patients [213].

Translocation-Associated RCCs

MiT family translocation RCC comprise TFE3-rearranged and TFEB-rearranged RCCs, unified by translocations involving microphthalmia transcription factor family members. These represent distinct entities in the WHO 2022 classification, occurring predominantly in younger patients but also affecting adults [9].

Fusion partner identity correlates with clinical outcomes, independent of morphologic features.*ASPSCR1-TFE3* fusions confer aggressive behavior with early metastatic potential, while *MED15-TFE3* translocations have remarkably indolent courses [10]. *PRCC, SFPQ, NONO,* and *CLTC* fusions follow intermediate prognosis with variable metastatic rates [51]. TFE3 immunohistochemistry shows variable sensitivity; FISH or RNA sequencing provides definitive diagnosis [176]. While break-apart FISH remains widely used, RNA sequencing directly identifies fusion partners and detects cryptic rearrangements [11].

TFE3-rearranged RCC results from chromosomal translocations at Xp11.23, generating multiple chimeric transcripts. Partners include *ASPSCR1, PRCC, SFPQ, NONO, MED15, RBM10, CLTC, DVL2, PARP14, KAT6A, MATR3,* and *EWSR1*, each bringing unique properties to the resulting fusion protein [246]. These neoplasms account for 40% of pediatric kidney cancers but only 1.6–4% of adult cases. The fusion proteins consistently preserve TFE3's C-terminal helix-loop-helix/leucine zipper domain, maintaining the ability to dimerize and bind DNA [107].

Break-apart FISH remains the standard approach, although cryptic intrachromosomal inversions involving partners such as RBM10 or NONO can yield false-negative results. In such cases, RNA sequencing or targeted RT-PCR is required [216].

The genomic landscape shows fewer recurrent alterations than clear cell or papillary RCC. Recurrent copy number losses (3p, 9p, 17p, 18, 22q) and gains (17q) occur in 20–40% of cases, with some correlating with poor outcomes [133]. A subset of tumors harbors mutations in CDKN2A/2B through 9p21.3 deletion, chromatin-remodeling genes including ARID1A and SMARCA4, and DNA damage response genes such as ATM, BRCA2, and WRN [135]. TERT promoter mutations remain restricted to advanced tumors, marking progression rather than initiation. Pediatric cases show lower mutational burden than adult tumors, correlating with better prognosis and suggesting age-dependent pathogenesis [27].

ALK-Rearranged RCC

ALK-rearranged RCC is one of the rarest molecularly defined RCC subtypes, characterized by translocations involving the ALK gene on chromosome 2p23. These rearrangements produce fusion proteins that constitutively activate ALK tyrosine kinase signaling [205].Despite the variety of fusion partners such as *VCL, TPM3, EML4, STRN, HOOK1, PLEKHA7, CLIP1, KIF5B,* and *KIAA1217*. ALK-rearranged RCCs uniformly retain the ALK kinase domain, resulting in constitutive activation of canonical signaling cascades, including MAPK, PI3K–AKT–mTOR, and JAK–STAT [116]. Immunohistochemistry using ALK antibodies serves as an excellent screening tool, but the definitive molecular diagnosis depends on demonstrating ALK rearrangement through FISH or sequencing approaches [117].

Aggressive Variants

Collecting duct carcinoma (CDC), comprising less than 1% of renal carcinomas, presents particular diagnostic challenges. This tumor exhibits aggressive behavior despite lacking a specific molecular signature. Diagnosis requires excluding other RCC subtypes with more distinctive molecular profiles [57]. Recurrent alterations include NF2 mutations, CDKN2A deletions, SETD2 loss, and dysregulation of Notch and BMP signaling, though none are diagnostically specific [234]. In a subset of cases, HER2 amplification occurs, offering potential for trastuzumab targeting [250].

Renal medullary (RM) carcinoma is characterized by complete loss of SMARCB1 through biallelic inactivation. This alteration results in loss of INI1 nuclear expression on immunohistochemistry, which serves as a reliable marker to distinguish it from morphologically similar CDC [28]. The epidemiology reveals a critical interplay between genetics and environment: it develops exclusively in individuals with sickle cell trait, where chronic medullary hypoxia enables SMARCB1-deficient cells to survive and transform rather than undergo apoptosis [150].

The molecular architecture extends beyond SMARCB1 loss. TP53 mutations and 8q gains (MYC overexpression) occur despite low overall mutational burden [100]. This suggests chromatin dysregulation as the primary driver, rather than mutational accumulation. *Sarcomatoid and rhabdoid transformation* represent high-grade dedifferentiation occurring in 5–8% of RCC [175]. These WHO/ISUP grade 4 transformations arise through convergent pathways. Histospecific alterations (VHL loss in ccRCC, chromosomal losses in ChRCC, FH mutations) remain constant throughout tumors, but dedifferentiated areas acquire additional mutations driving phenotypic transformation. TP53 mutations emerge in over 60% of sarcomatoid RCC, frequently accompanied by BAP1 loss in clear cell tumors, creating molecular signatures that predict rapid progression and widespread metastasis [20].

The dedifferentiation process involves epigenetic reprogramming with SWI/SNF complex alterations affecting PBRM1, ARID1A, SMARCA4, and SMARCB1 in up to 70% of sarcomatoid/rhabdoid cases [132]. These disruptions enable aberrant transcriptional programs activating epithelial mesenchymal transition (EMT) transcription factors ZEB1, SNAIL, and TWIST1 while suppressing epithelial markers including E-cadherin [235]. This molecular switch transforms adherent epithelial cells into invasive mesenchymal phenotypes capable of metastatic dissemination.

Molecular profiling reveals differential responses with high chromosomal instability and elevated neoantigen burden predicting superior immunotherapy response. Conversely, CDKN2A/B deletions may confer primary resistance [15]. NGS should focus on detecting alterations in TP53, BAP1, and chromatin-remodeling genes to support diagnosis and uncover potential therapeutic vulnerabilities, while also screening for rare but actionable events such as MET amplification or BRAF mutations [163].

Spatial heterogeneity documented through multi-region sequencing presents diagnostic challenges as focal sarcomatoid transformation may be missed on single biopsies, requiring comprehensive sampling and consideration of liquid biopsy to capture the full molecular landscape [223].

Emerging and Provisional Entities

ELOC-mutated RCC (formerly TCEB1), recently defined by biallelic ELOC inactivation on chromosome 8q21.2, represents a novel molecularly defined entity [86]. Somatic mutations affecting conserved residues in the elongin C domain disrupt VHL complex binding. These mutations are accompanied by second allele loss, typically through monosomy 8, establishing ELOC as a classical tumor suppressor [191]. Unlike VHL-deficient ccRCC, ELOC-RCC lacks chromosome 3p deletion and VHL, PBRM1, BAP1, or SETD2 alterations, displaying stable genomic architecture with minimal chromosomal complexity [233, 243, 244]. Mutational signature analysis reveals SBS1 enrichment, distinguishing ELOC-RCC from ccRCC. Linear evolutionary patterns show truncal ELOC mutations driving clonal expansion, with subclonal 8q loss emerging during progression [62].

Elongin C loss disrupts VHL E3 ubiquitin ligase assembly, impairing HIF1α degradation. While HIF1α accumulation parallels VHL-inactivated RCC, the upstream drivers and transcriptional responses differ [194]. While both express hypoxia-associated transcripts, ELOC-RCC shows distinct regulatory profiles beyond canonical VHL/HIF signaling.

These tumors often present as localized renal masses with predominantly indolent behavior, though higher-grade cases with complex alterations may show adverse features or progression. The inclusion of ELOC-mutated RCC in the 2022 WHO classification demonstrates how targeted sequencing helps classify previously unclassified renal tumors.

Clear cell papillary RCC shows discordant molecular features, exhibiting strong HIF pathway activation with HIF1α, CAIX, and GLUT-1 expression mimicking VHL-deficient ccRCC, yet consistently lacking 3p loss and VHL mutations [242]. This discordance suggests HIF activation through alternative mechanisms, including metabolic dysregulation or epigenetic VHL silencing. Comprehensive sequencing reveals absence of recurrent driver mutations, with only sporadic MET, EGFR, ASXL1, and CDKN2A alterations, indicating epigenetic rather than genetic drivers [151].

Recently recognized variants continue expanding our understanding of renal tumor biology. *Biphasic hyalinizing psammomatous RCC*, characterized by biallelic NF2 loss, and *papillary renal neoplasm with reverse polarity*, harboring KRAS mutations, both follow indolent courses despite concerning morphologic features [6].

Unclassified RCC now represents less than 5% of cases due to improved molecular diagnostics, and includes tumors that remain not classifiable despite extensive histologic, immunophenotypic, and genetic evaluation [236, 247]. These typically high-grade aggressive neoplasms contain complex genomic alterations including chromothripsis, multiple driver mutations across different pathways, or novel unrecognized gene fusions [39]. Broad molecular profiling using comprehensive panels or whole exome sequencing identifies targetable findings, including BRAF mutations amenable to targeted therapy, high tumor mutational burden suggesting immunotherapy benefit, and rare kinase fusions responsive to specific inhibitors [162]. The aggressive nature requires urgent molecular testing. Standard chemotherapy shows minimal efficacy, while targeted approaches based on genomic findings offer superior disease control [134] (Table 13.1).

Table 13.1 Molecular diagnostic algorithm for RCC classification according to WHO 2022. The flowchart illustrates histology with immunohistochemical screening and targeted molecular testing for accurate RCC subtype determination

RCC subtype	Molecular alterations	Immunophenotype
Clear cell RCC	3p loss (VHL, PBRM1, BAP1, SETD2)	CAIX+, CD10+, CK7-
Papillary RCC	Trisomy 7, 17; MET mutations (15–20%)	CK7+, AMACR+, CD10+
Chromophobe RCC	Multiple monosomies (1,2,6,10,13,17,21)	CK7+, CD117+, Claudin-7+
FH-deficient RCC	FH biallelic loss	FH loss, 2-succinylcysteine+
SDH-deficient RCC	SDHB/SDHC loss	SDHB loss
Eosinophilic solid and cystic RCC	TSC1/TSC2 biallelic loss	CK20+, CK7−
Low-grade Oncocytic tumor	MTOR mutations (exon 53)	CK7+, CD117−
TFE3-rearranged RCC	Xp11.2 translocations	TFE3+ nuclear, Cathepsin K+
ALK-rearranged RCC	ALK fusions (VCL, TPM3, EML4)	ALK+ (high specificity)
Collecting duct carcinoma	Non-specific (NF2, CDKN2A, SETD2, HER2)	PAX8+, INI1 retained
Renal medullary carcinoma	SMARCB1 biallelic loss	INI1 loss
ELOC-mutated RCC	ELOC biallelic loss + chr 8 LOH	CAIX+, CK7+
Clear cell papillary RCC	No recurrent mutations	CK7+, CAIX+ (box pattern), CD10-

Conclusion

NGS has transformed RCC classification from morphological to molecular criteria, revealing distinct therapeutic vulnerabilities. While no tissue-based biomarkers have achieved regulatory approval for treatment selection in RCC, genomic alterations provide prognostic information increasingly integrated into clinical decision-making [63].

For example, BAP1 loss predicts aggressive behavior and inferior survival even in otherwise low-risk patients, identifying candidates for early intervention or intensified surveillance independent of conventional staging [105]. Similarly, multigene transcriptomic signatures, including the ClearCode34 classifier, 16-gene recurrence score, and cell-cycle progression score, provide prognostic value beyond grade and stage [26, 180].

In metastatic disease, IMmotion150 and JAVELIN Renal 101 demonstrated that transcriptomic profiling predicts therapeutic benefit from immune checkpoint inhibitors versus anti-angiogenic agents [139, 149].

NGS helps resolve morphologically unclassifiable tumors by identifying defining alterations such as TFE3/TFEB fusions, FH mutations, or recurrent chromosomal imbalances [243, 244]. Molecular distinction proves critical in eosinophilic/oncocytic tumors to differentiate ChRCC, oncocytoma, and TSC/mTORC1-driven neoplasms [217]. Actionable alterations, while uncommon, may support targeted therapy in selected cases, such as ALK inhibitors for ALK-rearranged RCC or mTOR inhibitors in tumors with TSC1/TSC2 inactivation [119].

However, clinical implementation of NGS faces limitations. Intratumoral heterogeneity means single biopsies may miss aggressive subclones like sarcomatoid dedifferentiation [71]. Temporal evolution during metastatic progression may alter the mutational landscape, potentially obscuring or eliminating actionable targets present in the primary tumor. DNA-based panels miss gene fusions and splicing variants, requiring complementary RNA sequencing that isn't always available [216]. NGS costs significantly limit access in smaller institutions, restricting use to select cases such as specific tumor types or advanced disease. In such contexts, routine NGS for rare RCC subtypes remains difficult to implement in the absence of reimbursement or research support [34].

A tiered approach optimizes resource utilization. Initial immunohistochemical screening for FH, SDHB, TFE3, TFEB, ALK, or mTOR pathway surrogates can guide downstream molecular testing, reserving comprehensive NGS panels for metastatic, unclassified, or clinically aggressive tumors [225]. Platform selection depends on clinical context: targeted panels for histologically defined tumors, comprehensive DNA/RNA panels for metastatic/high-grade disease, and germline testing when hereditary syndromes are suspected [157]. Frequent germline alterations in FH, SDHB, TSC1/2, and MET necessitate genetic counseling and cascade testing for at-risk family members [35].Germline testing is indicated for young patients, bilateral/multifocal tumors, or positive family history, regardless of morphologic appearance [200].

Its wider use will require validated predictive biomarkers, matched targeted therapies, and reimbursement extending beyond academic centers. Until then, molecular testing should prioritize metastatic, unclassified, or hereditary cases to maximize clinical impact while containing costs (Fig. 13.1).

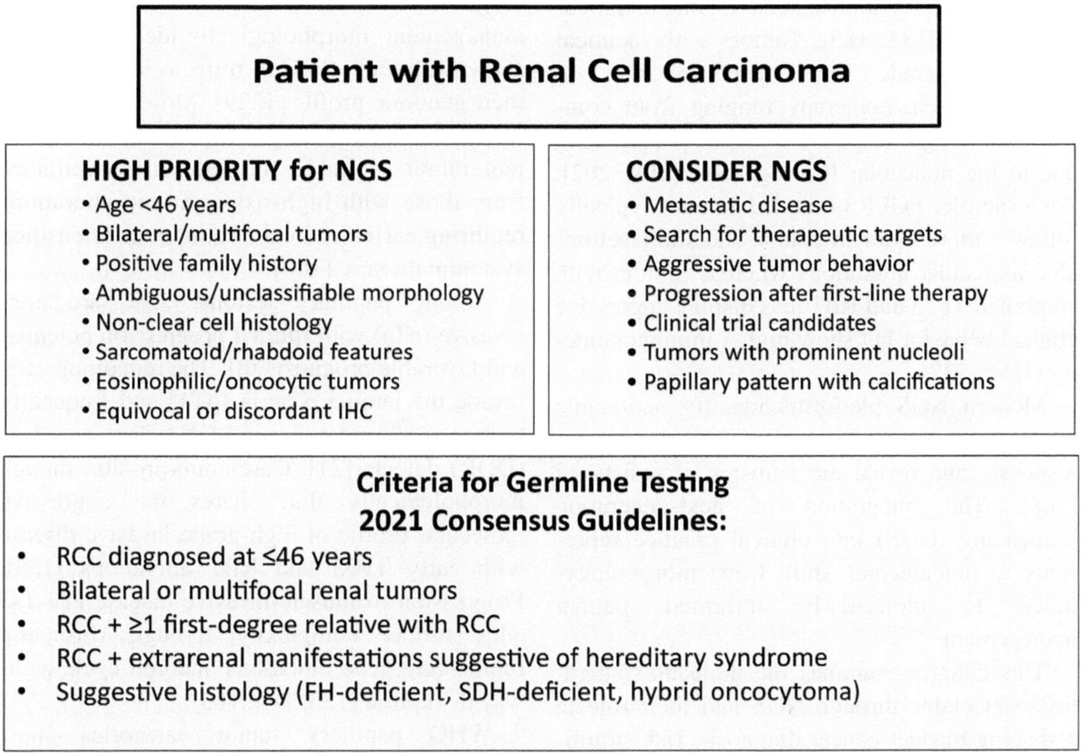

Fig. 13.1 Key molecular pathways and genetic alterations in RCC subtypes. The diagram shows the convergence of VHL-HIF pathway dysregulation, chromatin remodeling defects, metabolic reprogramming, and chromosomal instability patterns across different RCC entities

Bladder Carcinoma

Sioletic Stefano, Melucci Elisa, Simone Giuseppe.

Introduction

Bladder cancer represents a significant clinical challenge, with marked heterogeneity in molecular and histopathologic features. The current staging system relies on anatomical criteria and histopathologic assessment; this conventional approach often fails to reflect the molecular complexity that drives clinical behavior and therapeutic response [184, 185]. Tumors with identical stage and grade show response rates to neoadjuvant chemotherapy ranging from complete pathologic response to rapid progression, due to the molecular heterogeneity [104, 202]. For example, FGFR3-mutated tumors typically follow a more indolent course and show actionable molecular alterations whereas tumors with combined TP53 and RB1 loss display aggressive clinical behavior but show higher immunogenicity [1, 95, 112].

Modern NGS platforms identify actionable alterations, define biomarkers of therapeutic response, and reveal mechanisms of resistance [168]. The integration of next-generation sequencing (NGS) into clinical practice represents a fundamental shift from morphology-based to molecularly informed patient management.

This chapter examines the molecular alterations detectable through NGS and their role in reshaping bladder cancer diagnosis, risk stratification, and therapeutic selection.

Molecular Landscape of Bladder Cancer in Classical Histopathological Approach

Urothelial carcinoma, once considered a uniform pathological entity, is now recognized as a biologically and morphologically diverse group of diseases. The AJCC TNM system distinguishes non-muscle-invasive (NMIBC: Ta, T1) from muscle-invasive bladder cancer (MIBC: T2-T4) based on invasion depth, while the WHO employs a two-tiered grading scheme (low-grade/high-grade). Though clinically useful, these classifications only partially capture the underlying molecular complexity that drives disease behavior [67]. Approximately 75–80% of newly diagnosed bladder cancers are NMIBC [14]. Among these, 5-year progression to MIBC ranges from <1% in low-risk disease to >40% in very high-risk tumors, with an overall progression rate of 10–20% across all risk categories despite appropriate treatment [209]. This heterogeneity has direct implications for patient management: morphologically identical tumors show different clinical trajectories based on their genomic profiles [229]. Molecular stratification helps to distinguish patients with indolent tumors suitable for reduced surveillance from those with high-risk genomic alterations requiring earlier radical treatment or intensified systemic therapy [160].

Among papillary lesions, 75% are non-invasive (pTa) with limited progression potential and favorable prognosis [8]. The remaining 25% invade the lamina propria (pT1) and frequently harbor TP53 mutations and DNA damage repair (DDR) defects [21]. Carcinoma in situ, though morphologically flat, shares the aggressive molecular profile of high-grade invasive disease with early TP53 and RB1 alterations [152]. Progression to muscle-invasive disease (T2-T4) adds further complexity through chromatin remodeling gene mutations and cell cycle pathway disruption [125, 184, 185].

WHO papillary tumor categories show molecular-morphologic correlation. At the benign end of the spectrum, urothelial papillomas harbor activating RAS pathway mutations (predominantly HRAS/KRAS) without progression to malignancy. Low-grade papillary lesions (PUNLMP and LGPUC) demonstrate frequent recurrence but minimal progression risk, reflecting their stable genomic profiles. In contrast, high-grade papillary tumors exhibit aggressive molecular features including TP53 mutations, RB1 loss, and elevated tumor mutational burden—a profile shared by carcinoma in situ despite its non-invasive flat morphology [108].

Beyond conventional urothelial morphology, which accounts for 75% of bladder cancers, approximately 25% of cases display specific morphological patterns [33, 238]. These subtypes, including micropapillary, plasmacytoid, sarcomatoid and others, are characterized by specific genomic alterations that predict therapeutic response more accurately than morphology alone [33].

ERBB2-amplified micropapillary carcinoma (42–72% of cases) falls within the luminal-unstable subtype with concurrent TP53/RB1 alterations [93, 171, 190], Plasmacytoid variant shows CDH1 loss driving infiltrative growth and PI3K/AKT activation [177]. Sarcomatoid carcinoma exhibits EMT activation through epithelial marker loss (TP63, KRT5) and mesenchymal marker gain (VIM, ZEB1), with universal TP53/RB1 co-inactivation [80]. Small cell carcinoma requires biallelic TP53/RB1 loss with TERT and MYC alterations [90]. Pure squamous and adenocarcinoma lack typical urothelial alterations (FGFR3, KDM6A), indicating distinct pathogenesis [96, 184, 185].

Molecular Landscape of Bladder Cancer

Over the past two decades, molecular profiling has transformed our understanding of somatic alterations in urothelial carcinoma. The 2014 TCGA analysis of 131 muscle-invasive bladder cancers [124], expanded to 412 cases in 2017 [184, 185], established bladder cancer as one of the highest tumor mutational burdens among solid tumors (median 5–10 mutations/Mb), comparable to smoking-related lung cancers and surpassed only by melanoma and MSI-H tumors [122].

Key driver mutations affect multiple oncogenic pathways. Among them, FGFR3 alterations represent one of the earliest events, detected in approximately 65–70% of low-grade Ta papillary tumors, decreasing to 30% in Ta high-grade and 10–15% in T1 high-grade lesions and < 5% in CIS [184, 185]. They typically involve hotspot mutations (S249C, Y375C) that activate MAPK and PI3K signaling [214]. The mutual exclusivity with HRAS mutations suggests these represent alternative oncogenic pathways [241]. Telomerase activation via TERT promoter mutations occurs in 60–80% of both NMIBCs and MIBCs, providing replicative immortality [7]. TP53 alterations appear in approximately 48% of muscle-invasive cases, with MDM2 amplification in an additional 7%, collectively disrupting p53 pathway function in more than 65% of MIBCs.

Bladder cancer, particularly MIBCs, frequently shows widespread epigenetic dysregulation via recurrent mutations in chromatin-modifying genes. KDM6A inactivation (40% of Ta/T1 tumors) shows female predominance, suggesting sex-linked epigenetic susceptibility [123]. ARID1A mutations, present in 20–29% of NMIBCs, enhance PI3K-AKT-mTOR signaling. STAG2 mutations associate with favorable outcomes and reduced progression risk [16], while KMT2D mutations, often co-altered with EP300 and CREBBP, contribute to transcriptional deregulation and phenotypic plasticity.

DNA damage repair (DDR) pathway disruption characterizes both high-grade NMIBC and MIBC. ERCC2 mutations are present in 10–12% of MIBCs. Other recurrent DDR alterations involve ATM (12–15%), FANCC, and BRCA2 [169]. These defects coincide with elevated tumor mutational burden (TMB) and neoantigen load.

Cell cycle regulation is commonly disrupted through the RB1/CDKN2A/E2F pathway. RB1 inactivation occurs in 15–20% of cases, while CDKN2A deletion, often coupled with E2F3 amplification, appears across multiple tumor subtypes. Co-inactivation of TP53 and RB1 characterizes particularly aggressive molecular phenotypes [113].

PI3K-AKT-mTOR signaling activation is common, with PIK3CA mutations found in 25–30% of NMIBCs and 20% of MIBCs [114, 188]. These mutations frequently co-occur with other alterations. PTEN loss further promotes pathway activation.

Receptor tyrosine kinase pathway alterations include ERBB2 amplification in 9–15% of MIBCs, with an additional 5–10% harboring activating mutations [110]. EGFR amplification and mutations in oxidative stress regulators like NFE2L2 indicate additional RTK-MAPK signaling mechanisms.

Early-stage NMIBCs demonstrate tumor suppressor gene hypermethylation (RASSF1A, CDH1, TERT) that correlates with recurrence. Multi-region sequencing reveals substantial intratumoral heterogeneity, where subclones diverge through alterations in DDR, PI3K, and chromatin remodeling pathways [69, 212]. This clonal diversity contributes to resistance and complicates tissue sampling, as a single biopsy may not capture the full genomic landscape. The introduction of targeted NGS panels has enabled detailed molecular characterization even from limited biopsy tissue. Panels including TERT, FGFR3, PIK3CA, TP53, ERCC2, ARID1A, and KDM6A inform risk stratification and therapeutic response prediction. Liquid biopsy platforms analyzing cfDNA, urinary DNA, and exosomal RNA demonstrate utility for real-time monitoring, with urinary detection of driver mutations showing greater sensitivity than cytology [47, 65].

Liquid Biopsy in Bladder Cancer

Tissue-based molecular profiling has advanced bladder cancer stratification, but serial biopsies are invasive and single samples cannot capture spatial heterogeneity. These limitations particularly affect high-risk NMIBC, where flat lesions like carcinoma in situ (CIS) are difficult to sample adequately [94]. Liquid biopsy, analyzing circulating tumor DNA (ctDNA), urinary tumor DNA (utDNA), and circulating tumor cells (CTCs), allows non-invasive assessment of tumor burden and molecular evolution [53].

Bladder cancer is well-suited for liquid biopsy development. The direct tumor-urine interface allows high concentrations of tumor-derived nucleic acids in voided samples. High-depth NGS of urine specimens achieves 400× coverage and detects alterations at 2% allele frequency. This sensitivity captures point mutations, copy number variations, and gene fusions that tissue sampling often misses.

Urinary NGS panels target recurrent driver alterations including TERT promoter mutations (more than 60% frequency), FGFR3 alterations, and chromatin remodeling gene mutations (KDM6A, ARID1A, KMT2D). Platforms like UroSEEK combine mutation detection with aneuploidy analysis, achieving higher sensitivity than cytology while maintaining specificity for high-grade tumors [245]. Urinary NGS detects field cancerization and multifocal disease patterns undetectable by single tissue biopsies.

In muscle-invasive and metastatic disease, plasma ctDNA NGS quantifies systemic tumor burden and tracks molecular evolution over time. Serial sampling captures temporal molecular changes, including resistance mutations and molecular subtype transitions. Post-surgical ctDNA detection detect recurrences months before radiological imaging evidence [38].

Detection sensitivity drops in patients with minimal residual disease, while clonal hematopoiesis requires advanced filtering algorithms to distinguish tumor-derived from age-related mutations. Lack of standardization in sample collection, DNA extraction, sequencing platforms, and bioinformatic pipelines limits clinical adoption.

Emerging platforms combine ctDNA, CTCs, and exosomal RNA for detailed molecular characterization. Methylation-based classifiers may enable molecular subtyping directly from liquid specimens. With improved standardization, liquid biopsy complements tissue-based NGS in bladder cancer molecular diagnosis.

Luminal and Basal Molecular Subtypes in Bladder Cancer

Transcriptomic profiling has identified six consensus molecular subtypes, each associated with distinct biology and clinical behavior: luminal papillary (20–25%, FGFR3-driven), luminal nonspecified (8%), luminal-unstable (15%, ERBB2-amplified), stroma-rich (15%), basal/

squamous (30–35%, immune-infiltrated), and neuroendocrine-like (3–5%). This classification, derived from over 1750 tumor transcriptomes, refines traditional grading by incorporating molecular features that correlate with clinical outcomes [104].

Luminal Papillary (LumP)

Representing approximately 20–25% of muscle-invasive tumors, LumP displays papillary morphology with high expression of luminal differentiation markers such as GATA3, FOXA1, and PPARγ [104, 201, 237]. These tumors frequently harbor FGFR3 alterations and CDKN2A deletions, maintaining their luminal differentiation program [89]. LumP tumors show scant lymphocyte infiltration and low interferon-stimulated gene expression, creating an immunologically cold profile driven by mutations in chromatin remodelers (STAG2, KDM6A) that repress immune-related loci [208].

Luminal Nonspecified (LumNS)

Representing approximately 8% of MIBCs, LumNS tumors express canonical luminal markers (GATA3, PPARγ) but lack cohesive molecular identity [240]. A defining feature is dense stromal infiltrate comprising fibroblasts, myofibroblasts, and infiltrating lymphocytes, particularly B cells and CD4+/CD8+ T cells, trapped at the tumor-stroma interface rather than penetrating the tumor itself. TGF-β signaling mediates this spatial exclusion by driving stromal remodeling and immunosuppressive fibroblast activation [136].

Luminal-Unstable (LumU)

Accounting for 15% of MIBCs, LumU tumors exhibit genomic instability, high proliferative index, and frequent mutations in TP53, ERBB2, and chromatin modifier [109]. These tumors display pronounced copy number variation and APOBEC-driven mutagenesis, resulting in elevated tumor mutational burden [183]. The non-inflamed immune environment with variable CD8+ infiltration limits checkpoint inhibitor response [187].

ERBB2 amplification represents a defining feature and potential therapeutic target [77].

Stroma-Rich

This subtype (15% of MIBCs) is distinguished by its microenvironment characteristics, with overexpression of extracellular matrix remodeling and fibroblast activation genes [104]. Cancer-associated fibroblasts shape the immune landscape through secretion of immunosuppressive cytokines that prevent T-cell infiltration and impair antigen presentation [189]. Dense stromal component challenges accurate transcriptomic subtype assignment despite retained luminal markers in epithelial cells.

Basal/Squamous (Ba/Sq)

The most prevalent MIBC subtype (30–35%) exhibits basal epithelial differentiation with high expression of KRT5, KRT6, KRT14, and TP63 [80, 104]. Histologically, many display overt squamous differentiation including keratinization and occasionally sarcomatoid transformation. Frequent biallelic TP53 and RB1 inactivation characterizes these tumors genomically, with additional EGFR amplification and NFE2L2 mutations [30, 184, 185].

The T-cell-inflamed phenotype shows dense CD8+ infiltration and checkpoint molecule expression (PD-L1, CTLA-4, LAG3), though immune activation varies considerably [106]. DNA damage repair mutations (ERCC2, ATM, FANCC) occur frequently in this subtype [228].

Neuroendocrine-Like (NE-Like)

This rare aggressive variant (3–5%) morphologically resembles small-cell carcinoma with neuroendocrine marker expression, though often focal or heterogeneous [18]. The defining molecular feature is concurrent TP53 and RB1 inactivation, nearly universal in this subtype and shared with neuroendocrine carcinomas of other sites [90].

Immunohistochemistry and Molecular Subtyping

The classification of urothelial carcinoma into luminal and basal molecular subtypes refines diagnostic classification and prognostic assessment. In routine pathology practice, this categorization integrates histomorphological evaluation, immunohistochemical staining, and transcriptomic profiling when available [201].

Immunohistochemistry remains the most widely applicable ancillary technique for transcriptomic classification when RNA profiling is unavailable. Small immunopanels combining GATA3 and CK5/6 enable reliable subtype assignment in most cases [55]. GATA3 expression supports luminal differentiation, while CK5/6 positivity with or without TP63 co-expression indicates basal phenotype [81, 237]. Tumors exhibiting both markers often show phenotypic plasticity or intermediate features [44]. Tumors with double-negative expression patterns lacking both markers commonly associate with poorly differentiated histology and molecular outlier subtypes including claudin-low and neuroendocrine-like variants [106]. In diagnostically ambiguous cases, expanded panels incorporating CK14, FOXA1, UPK2, and SOX2 refine classification by detecting mixed or lineage-divergent differentiation states [19, 25].

Transcriptomic profiling resolves cases where immunohistochemistry and histopathology yield conflicting results. The BASE47 classifier, based on 47 lineage-informative genes, has demonstrated consistent reliability in categorizing urothelial tumors into basal and luminal subtypes [56, 198]. Originally derived from integrated microarray and RNA-seq datasets, BASE47 has been adapted for formalin-fixed, paraffin-embedded tissue, achieving classification concordance rates up to 93% concordance in independent validation cohorts [198].

Modern NGS platforms extract and analyze both RNA and DNA from single formalin fixed paraffin embedded (FFPE) specimens [140]. This enables comprehensive molecular characterization including gene expression profiling, identification of pathogenic alterations like FGFR3 mutations, TMB quantification, and DNA repair deficiency detection [168]. Multidimensional profiling enhances subtype precision and guides therapy, risk assessment, and disease monitoring in both localized and advanced disease settings [155] (Fig. 13.2).

Next-Generation Sequencing and Precision Medicine in Bladder Cancer

The molecular classification of bladder cancer into luminal papillary, luminal-unstable, basal/squamous, stroma-rich, and neuroendocrine-like subtypes is clinically relevant, as each exhibit distinct therapeutic response patterns.Each subtype has specific molecular signatures detectable by NGS [104, 210].

Multi-region sequencing reveals substantial intratumoral heterogeneity, with single biopsies capturing only 60–70% of the mutational landscape [212]. Field cancerization further complicates assessment, as genetically altered but histologically normal urothelium harbors malignant potential [204]. This spatial and temporal complexity necessitates comprehensive profiling strategies that capture both baseline diversity and clonal evolution [69].

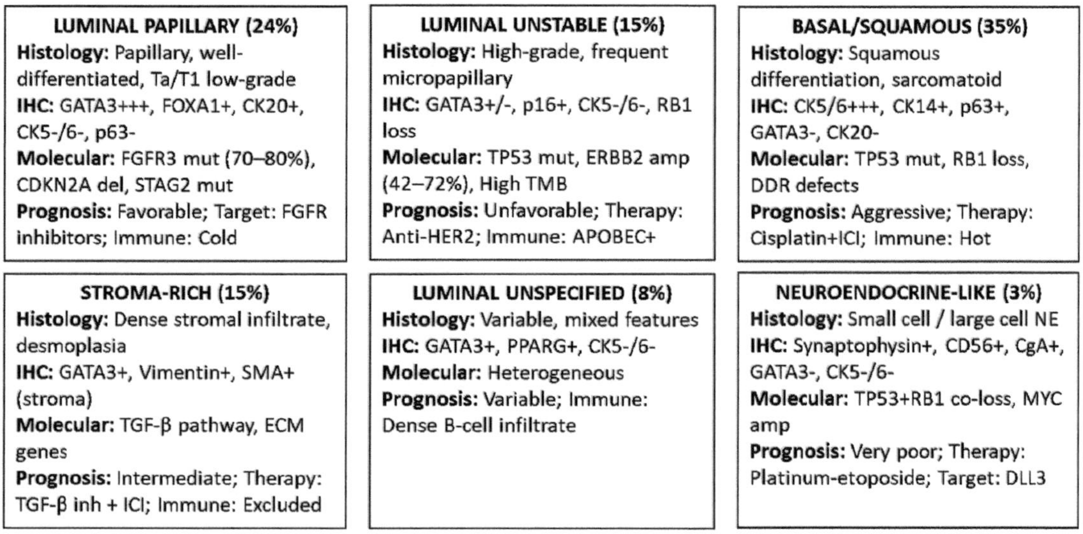

Fig. 13.2 Integrated diagnostic algorithm for molecular classification of bladder carcinoma. The flowchart illustrates the sequential approach from initial histological evaluation, through immunohistochemical (IHC) screening, to molecular characterization via NGS for identification of luminal papillary, luminal unstable, basal/squamous, and neuroendocrine-like subtypes

Within this heterogeneous landscape, certain biomarkers are now clinically validated. FGFR2/3 alterations, present in 70% of luminal papillary tumors, represent well-characterized molecular features[127]. Modern NGS panels expand beyond single-gene testing, simultaneously detecting point mutations, copy number alterations, and mutational signatures from single FFPE specimens [168]. DNA damage response alterations, particularly in ERCC2 (10–12%), ATM (12–15%), and FANCC, predict treatment sensitivity accurately enough to guide clinical management [170, 228]. Liquid biopsy helps overcome the sampling limitations of tissue-based molecular profiling. Bladder cancer's unique tumor-urine interface enables high-sensitivity molecular detection.

Implementation challenges remain despite proven diagnostic utility. High sequencing costs, variable specimen quality, and absence of standardized interpretation guidelines limit widespread adoption. Focused gene panels targeting established biomarkers reduce costs while maintaining clinical relevance. Centralized testing laboratories and validated bioinformatics pipelines make molecular profiling increasingly accessible beyond academic centers.A systematic approach to NGS implementation requires clinical algorithms that prioritize testing based on disease stage, histologic features, and treatment intent (Fig. 13.3).

Molecular profiling has redefined the pathologist's role in bladder cancer management. Contemporary practice requires integrating molecular data with histologic findings, selecting appropriate tests, assessing specimen adequacy, and translating genomic results into actionable recommendations.

NGS-informed bladder cancer diagnosis continues to evolve. The integration of transcriptomic and proteomic data is expected to improve further the diagnostic precision and prognostic stratification. Despite implementation challenges, molecular diagnostics is going to be an integral part of bladder cancer evaluation (Fig. 13.4).

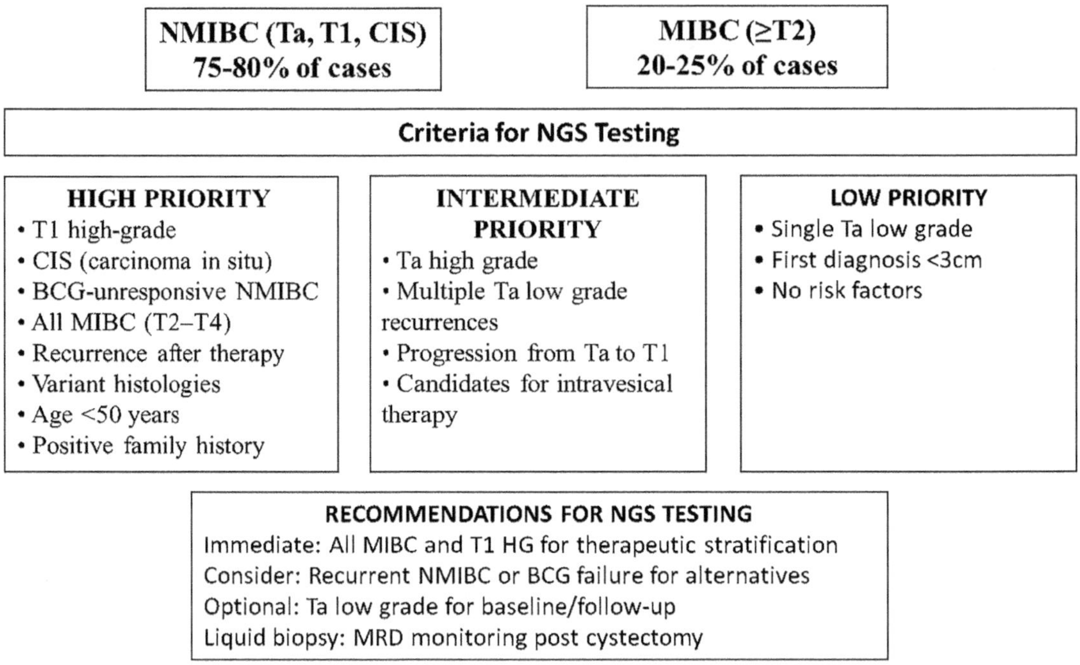

Fig. 13.3 Clinical decision algorithm for NGS implementation in urothelial carcinoma management. The flowchart stratifies patients based on initial histopathological assessment into non-muscle-invasive (NMIBC: Ta, T1, CIS) and muscle-invasive (MIBC: ≥T2) disease. NGS testing recommendations are prioritized into three tiers based on clinical utility and cost-effectiveness. High-priority indications include scenarios where molecular profiling directly impacts treatment selection or identifies aggressive disease requiring intensified management. Intermediate-priority cases represent situations where NGS may guide surveillance intensity or identify candidates for bladder-sparing approaches. Low-priority settings indicate minimal expected benefit from routine molecular testing

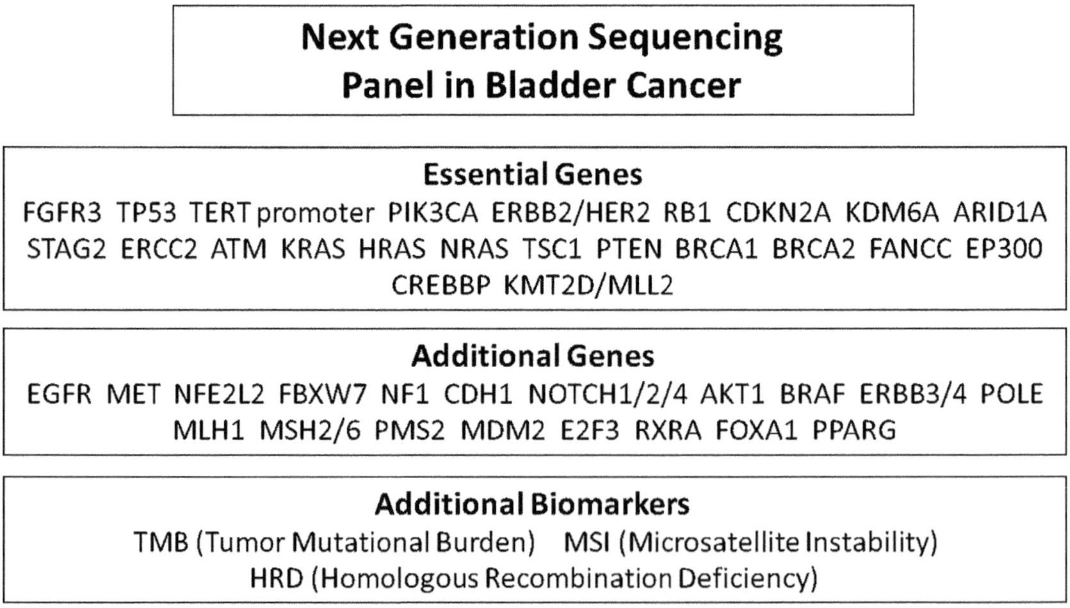

Fig. 13.4 Comprehensive NGS panel for molecular profiling of bladder cancer. The panel is stratified into three tiers based on clinical actionability and diagnostic utility

Prostate Cancer

Cimadamore Alessia

Introduction

Prostate cancer (PCa) is a heterogeneous disease ranging from indolent tumors to lethal disease. PCa is still the most frequent type of malignant neoplasia in men and represents a leading cancer-related cause of death. Next-generation sequencing (NGS) has allowed the classification of PCa at multiple strata of molecular information, incorporating data at genomic, transcriptomic, epigenetic, and proteomic levels. Due to the increased quality and decreased cost of genomic sequencing platforms, the landscape of somatic mutations in prostate cancer has rapidly changed in recent years, improving our knowledge of tumor biology and tailored therapies.

Predicting prostate cancer progression and aggressiveness at the molecular level will require continued research to determine the chronology of these genetic events and distinguish cancer-initiating lesions from later changes that may promote disease progression. Based on these concepts, a molecular definition of progression might be a very useful tool for risk-stratification of patients at intermediate risk or for patients under active surveillance. In addition to providing accurate diagnosis, grading, and staging, the pathologist plays a crucial role in directing subsequent tissue-based molecular biomarker testing in PCa [221]. This requires comprehensive knowledge of the available assays, their use in specific disease contexts, and the evidence supporting their clinical utility. A complicating factor in both molecular research and clinical handling is that about 80% of men with PCa have more than one malignant focus in their prostate with intratumoral and intertumoral genomic heterogeneity that may impact molecular classifications. Molecular heterogeneity was found between individual PCa foci especially regarding the activity of gene sets underlying the assays for risk stratification and androgen receptor activity. Caution is advised when making treatment decisions based on a single biopsy or index lesions [239]. More recently, there has been growing recognition of both androgen receptor (AR) signaling–dependent and AR signaling–independent forms of castration-resistant prostate cancer (CRPC), with the latter often corresponding to small cell neuroendocrine (NE) carcinoma. Additionally, potentially targetable CRPC subtypes, such as those with homologous recombination deficiency and mismatch repair (MMR) deficiency, along with an expanding range of treatment options—including chemotherapy, AR signaling inhibitors, targeted therapies, and immunotherapy—have spurred intensive research into diagnostic and predictive biomarkers to better guide CRPC management [48].

Mutational Landscape of Prostate Cancer

Common somatic changes in localized PCa emerged from The Cancer Genome Atlas study which performed a comprehensive molecular analysis of 333 primary PCa. Seven molecular subclasses have been defined on the basis of early genomic alterations, which are largely mutually exclusive. These included the mutually exclusive ETS-rearrangement prostate cancer (PCa with rearrangements and overexpression of ERG, ETV1, ETV4, or other ETS family transcription factors), and those negative for ETS factors. ETS negative prostate cancers show recurrent mutations in SPOP, FOXA1, and IDH1. Alterations in PI3K and TP53 signaling are common in ETS positive cancers, while deletions of CHD1 and overexpression of SPINK1 are specific to ETS negative cancers [31].

The most common ETS family rearrangement is the *TMPRSS2:ERG* fusion, which has now been identified in approximately 50% of prostate cancers. ETS rearrangements have been detected in high grade prostatic intraepithelial neoplasia (HGPIN) and in the adjacent PCa, and are thus theorized to precede other mutations and to be an early event in PCa carcinogenesis [31].

Recurrent mutations in the SPOP gene are found in 5–15% of tumors and occur exclusively in tumors without ETS rearrangement. This constitutes a unique subclass of PCa with several distinguishing molecular characteristics. The highest levels of AR transcriptional activity has been specifically observed in tumors with SPOP mutations. Crucially, it has now been shown that SPOP affects DNA double strand break (DSB) repair; it is linked to genomic instability and sensitizes to DNA damaging agents such as PARP inhibitors [24].

SPINK1 is commonly overexpressed in SPOP-mutant and other ETS-negative PCa. SPINK1 overexpression, independent of Gleason score, lymph node status, surgical margin status, seminal vesicle invasion, extracapsular extension, and preoperative PSA, has been shown to be a significant predictor of clinical recurrence [37, 166].

FOXA1-mutant prostate cancers are approximately 4% of all primary PCa, have similar molecular features to SPOP-mutant tumors including highest levels of AR transcriptional activity [101].

Novel molecular subclass of PCa is characterized by IDH1 mutations, most notably at residue R132. The prevalence of hotspot IDH1 mutations in PCa is estimated to be 0.3–2.5%. Highly recurrent hotspot IDH1 mutations have been reported in PCa with intratumoral psammomatous calcification [138, 141]. Several active clinical trials are testing a variety of IDH1 inhibitors in other solid tumors, including IDH1-mutant prostate cancer (e.g., NCT02073994, NCT02381886, NCT02481154, NCT02746081, NCT03684811, and NCT04521686).

The TCGA also reported a 25% of PCa had a presumed actionable lesion in the PI3K or MAPK signaling pathways, and 19% of alterations in DNA repair genes in localized primary tumors, with BRCA2 being the most frequent (3%). DNA repair-mutated tumors tend to exhibit higher Gleason grade and more aggressive behavior, with shorter metastasis-free and cause-specific survival [211].

Loss of PTEN, TP53 mutation, and MYC amplification are early events in tumorigenesis and their identification in early disease setting may suggest more aggressive biological behavior. Their detection could influence decisions regarding surgery, radiotherapy, or intensified systemic therapy [50, 52, 186].

- PTEN (10q23) loss is common in localized PCa and increases in frequency during disease progression. Inactivation of the PTEN gene by deletion or mutation is identified in ~20% of primary prostate tumor samples at radical prostatectomy and as many as 50% of castration resistant tumors. Loss of PTEN function leads to activation of the PI3K–AKT pathway and is strongly associated with adverse oncological outcomes, making PTEN a potentially useful genomic marker to distinguish indolent from aggressive disease in patients with clinically localized tumors [99].
- C-myc amplification is observed in around 25% of the clinically localized PCa tumors and in 46% of advanced PCa, suggesting that MYC amplification is associated with disease progression [12].
- TP53 alterations and RB1 loss are associated with disease progression and frequently enriched in advanced PCa. TP53/RB1 loss is associated with diminished responses to AR antagonists and reduced survival and are frequently lost in PCa with neuroendocrine (NE) differentiation [159].

Several tissue-based prognostic markers have been developed in the past years for clinical application and are now available commercially. These are RNA-based commercial genomic assays and are listed by the guidelines of the National Comprehensive Cancer Network (NCCN) as an option for better patient stratification.

The Oncotype® DX Genomic Prostate Score (GPS) is a quantitative real-time polymerase chain reaction (PCR) assay performed on fixed paraffin-embedded tissue from needle prostate biopsies. It assesses a 17-gene signature spanning four biological pathways: androgen signaling, cellular organization, stromal response, and cellular proliferation, along with five housekeeping genes. GPS scores range from 0 to 100, with higher values indicating greater cancer aggressiveness [111].

The Genomic Classifier (GC) Decipher® test was developed and validated through a retrospective study of 639 radical prostatectomy patients from the Mayo Clinic registry [68]. Using a microarray platform analyzing 1.4 million genomic markers, it identifies a 22-gene signature linked to various cellular functions such as cell proliferation, differentiation, immune response regulation, and androgen-signaling modulation. Decipher provides a risk score between 0 and 1, which correlates with the probability of adverse clinical outcomes like biochemical recurrence (BCR) and early metastasis after RP [68].

The Prolaris® test is a tissue-based RT-PCR assay measuring the expression of 31 cell-cycle progression (CCP) genes alongside 15 housekeeping genes. It generates a proliferative index called the CCP score, ranging from 0 to 10, which is associated with clinical outcomes [54].

Finally, the ProMark® test is an advanced, automated multiplex immunofluorescence in situ imaging technique that quantitatively assesses eight protein biomarkers and their activation states in prostate biopsy tissues. Originally featuring a panel of 12 protein biomarkers designed to predict PCa aggressiveness and lethality, it has been refined to an 8-protein panel that more accurately differentiates between favorable and unfavorable pathology at RP compared to clinical risk stratification alone [22].

Together, these prognostic assays aim to enhance tumor characterization and bridge the gap between clinical guidelines and real-world practice. There is an increasing trend toward using tissue-based genomic testing for PCa. However, these tests are currently used in fewer than 2% of PCa patients, both at initial diagnosis and following surgical treatment. While their adoption is expected to grow as more scientific evidence emerges, their precise role still needs to be better defined [23].

Despite significant advances in biomarker validation, urological societies currently do not recommend the routine use of prognostic biomarkers in prostate cancer. As a result, the choice and implementation of these tests are often determined by urologists and/or oncologists based on institutional policies [129].

Predictive Biomarkers in Advanced/ Metastatic Prostate Cancer

In the setting of metastatic castration-resistant prostate cancer (mCRPC), treatment strategy is moving from a "one-therapy fits all" to a patient-tailored approach and NGS is increasingly incorporated into clinical care. The FDA approval in 2020 of Olaparib mCRPC patients with germline or somatic homologous recombination repair (HRR) gene-mutated signed the beginning of this new biomarker-driven era [158].

Homologous Recombination Repair (HRR) Gene Mutations

The identification of homologous recombination repair (HRR) gene mutations, especially BRCA1, BRCA2, and ATM, is essential for determining eligibility for PARP inhibitors (PARPi) such as olaparib and rucaparib, now approved in multiple jurisdictions [2, 4, 59, 60, 227] and can be performed only with an NGS-based platform. In the PROfound study [59] 28% of 2792 mCRPC samples had DDR mutations—most commonly BRCA2 (8.7%), CDK12 (6.3%), and ATM (5.9%).

In aggressive histologic subtypes of primary PCa—such as ductal and intraductal carcinoma, as well as primary Gleason pattern 5 disease—recent studies have found that the prevalence of homologous recombination deficiency (HRD) mutations, both germline and somatic, matches or even surpasses that observed in metastatic disease [97, 98, 128, 182, 195].

Molecular testing for BRCA1/BRCA 2 has become of pivotal importance for patients selection. Indeed, patients harboring germline and/or somatic BRCA genes alterations proved to be the most responsive to PARPi, even when tested in combination with AR signaling inhibitors (ARSI). BRCA1 and BRCA2 genes have been reported to be altered in 0.3% and 13% at somatic level, and in 0.9% and 5.3% at germinal level, respectively, while alterations in gene involved in the HRR pathway, such as ATM, RAD51, RAD52, RAD54, DSS1, RPA1, ATR, CHK1, CHK2, NBS1, FANCD2, FANCA and

FANCC, are identified in approximately 20% of MCRPC. Notably, recent studies suggest that tumors with homozygous deletions in BRCA2 exhibit prolonged responses to PARPi compared with those harboring other types of mutations, such as frameshift insertions or missense mutations. This indicates that deeper genomic characterization, including zygosity analysis, could guide more precise treatment decisions [60, 137].

Both germinal and somatic DNA damage response gene mutations have a prognostic value, being associated with a more aggressive disease and worse survival outcomes. Concerning other DNA damage repair genes such as ATM, CDK12, or CHEK2 limited radiographic/PSA responses to PARP inhibition has been reported, while responses have been seen in patients with tumors harboring alterations in PALB2, FANCA, BRIP1, and RAD51B [2, 4].

Importantly, not all patients with HRR mutations benefit equally from PARPi, and a subset of patients without canonical DDR mutations still respond to these therapies. Ongoing studies are investigating additional genomic alterations that may confer sensitivity to PARPi. In this context, broad-panel NGS approaches covering emerging predictive markers (e.g., CDK12, PALB2, RAD51) are essential to avoid missed therapeutic opportunities [220, 251].

Moreover, further development in mCRPC therapy is represented by the recent trials'results supporting the use of PARPi in combination with AR pathway inhibitors (ARPI). The rationale behind these trials is that the co-inhibition of the androgen receptor and PARP might result in enhanced benefit with the potential to extend efficacy of PARP inhibitors to tumors regardless of HRR gene alterations. While PARPi/ARPI combinations show activity in all mCRPC patients, HRR-mutated tumors derive greatest benefit, as demonstrated in three pivotal trials (TALAPRO-2, PROPEL, MAGNITUDE). These data led recently to FDA approval of olaparib with abiraterone and talazoparib with enzalutamide for all HRR mutated mCRPC patients and niraparib plus abiraterone for BRCA1/2 mutated mCRPC patients in first-line [5, 42, 43, 248].

Recently, the results of the phase 3 AMPLITUDE trial (NCT04497844) were published. The trial was designed to assess the efficacy of niraparib plus abiraterone acetate with prednisone (AAP) in patients with metastatic castration-sensitive PCa harboring at least one HRR mutation in one of these genes: BRCA1, BRCA2, BRIP1, CDK12, CHEK2, FANCA, PALB2, RAD51B, RAD54L. The trial met its primary endpoint, demonstrating that the combination of the PARP inhibitor and AAP significantly reduced the risk of radiographic progression or death by 48% in the BRCAm group and by 37% in the broader HRRm population. These findings may change the paradigm of therapy in castration-sensitive patients as potential new treatment option for patients with BRCA or other HRR gene alterations [13] (Table 13.2).

Mismatch Repair Alterations

Defects in the mismatch repair (MMR) pathway are more commonly found in metastatic PCa compared to primary tumors. Pathogenic mutations in MMR genes occur in up to 10% of CRPC cases, whereas they are present in less than 3% of primary tumors when considering all Grade Groups together [3, 154, 173].

Similar to HRD, MMR mutations are highly enriched in primary tumors with aggressive histology, including ductal adenocarcinomas and primary Gleason pattern 5 tumors, as recently reported [79, 196]. Compared to HRD alterations, a smaller proportion of MMR mutations (around 20%) in prostate cancer are germline, although prostate cancer is increasingly recognized among patients with Lynch syndrome [64, 87]. While prostate cancer has generally shown limited response to immunotherapy in most trials, with programmed death-ligand 1 (PD-L1) expression observed in only 8% of primary tumors and 32% of CRPC cases [83], recent studies have reported anecdotal responses in patients harboring MMR defects [76].

Table 13.2 Recommendation for germline and somatic BRCA testing in metastatic and localized PCa patients

Guidelines	Germline	Somatic
ESMO [164]	**Metastatic:** All patients **Localized:** Men with pathogenic mutations in cancer-risk genes on somatic testing Patients with family history suggestive of hereditary cancer predisposition syndrome at least two close blood relatives on the same side of the family	**Metastatic:** Consider in mCRPC
EAU [226]	**Metastatic:** All patients who are candidates for targeted treatment **Localized:** Men with BRCA mutations on somatic testing Men with multiple family members diagnosed with HSPC at age < 60 years or a family member who died from prostate cancer Men with a family history of high-risk germline mutations or a family history of multiple cancers on the same side of the family	**Metastatic:** All patients (preferably before first-line mCRPC treatment is established)

PI3K/AKT/PTEN Pathway Alterations

PTEN tumor suppressor loss is observed in roughly 50% of patients with mCRPC, resulting in activation of AKT signaling and diminished response to AR blockade. Ipatasertib, an AKT small-molecule inhibitor, has shown promising activity when combined with abiraterone in patients harboring PTEN loss. However, the final results of IPATential 150, a phase III randomized trial, evaluating ipatasertib (AKT inhibitor) with abiraterone and prednisone compared with standard therapy, showed a minimal rPFS benefit (2 months) in mCRPC with PI3K/AKT activating aberrations with no OS benefit [207]. A phase III trial is currently evaluating capivasertib (another AKT inhibitor) in combination with abiraterone for patients with PTEN-deficient mHSPC (NCT04493853) with promising preliminary results [224]. Efforts to optimize biomarker strategies, such as ctDNA profiling for PI3K/AKT pathway alterations, and to elucidate the effects of co-occurring molecular events may enhance future patient selection. In addition, combination approaches are under investigation, including AKT inhibitors with DNA damage response agents, or immunotherapies, as PTEN loss contributes to resistance against these modalities [249].

Liquid Biopsy in Prostate Cancer

Roughly one-third of tissue samples are suboptimal for NGS due to insufficient/inadequate tumor tissue, low DNA quality/quantity at extraction, and/or failure after DNA extraction, particularly when archival FFPE specimens are used [49, 74, 148, 222]. According to ESMO-AIOM recommendations, the test for pathogenic variants of BRCA1/2 is first performed on tumor tissue on metastatic PCa patients. However, given the high probability of quantitatively or qualitatively inadequate tissue for molecular analysis, liquid biopsy is a valid alternative, and it has been included in the current AIOM recommendation after failure of tissue-test if FFPE tumor material is unavailable [148].

Although sensitivity may be reduced in patients with low tumor DNA burden, ctDNA analysis is increasingly used to detect HRR alterations and track clonal evolution during therapy [42, 43, 49, 74, 148, 222, 230].

Shedding of ctDNA differs between untreated patients, androgen deprivation (ADT)-treated patients, and mCRPC patients. In the study of Vandekerkhove et al. 74% of the patients had detectable ctDNA before ADT initiation, while in the patients who received ADT prior to blood collection, only 59% had detectable ctDNA. Cell-free DNA concentration changes after PARP inhibitor therapy are predictive biomarkers of response; indeed, a $\geq$ 50% fall in cfDNA concentration after 8 weeks of therapy was independently associated with longer OS [75].

The most recent and largest study on ctDNA in advanced PCa demonstrated high concordance between alterations identified by liquid and tissue biopsy and, moreover, proved the added value of liquid biopsy [222]. In 79.5% of all the patients, liquid biopsy identified at least one genomic alteration predicted to have deleterious/oncogenic effects on protein function: Tp53 (46%), AR (42%), BRCA2 (7.5%), BRCA1 (1.4%), PI3K/AKT/mTOR (14%), WNT/β-catenin pathway genes (17%), RAS/RAF/MEK (5%), MSI-H status (1.4%). Regarding BRCA mutations, concordance between tissue and ctDNA, 67 (8.0%) BRCA1/2 alterations were detected concordantly in tissue and liquid biopsy, 5 (0.6%)—exclusively in tissue biopsy, and 20 (2.4%)—exclusively in liquid biopsy. Of the five patients with BRCA alterations detected only in tissue biopsy, four had a ctDNA fraction below 1%. The 20 cases detected only in ctDNA analysis may represent alterations acquired after tissue specimen collection. However, liquid biopsy have some relevant limitations that have to be acknowledged [118]. Despite concordance between tissue and ctDNA for HRR gene mutations is excellent, exceeding 90% in most studies, at variant-subtype level, using tissue as reference, concordance proved to be high for nonsense (93%), splice (87%), and frameshift (86%) alterations but low for large rearrangements (63%) and homozygous deletions (27%), with low ctDNA fraction being a limiting factor [42, 43].

Moreover, in routine practice, US FDA-approved commercial tests (e.g., FoundationOne Liquid CDx, Guardant360 CDx) can be utilized, though their high cost may limit access for patients lacking adequate reimbursement.

Conclusions

In a scenario with rapidly growing options, treatment selection is still based on clinical features in all settings of PCa, due to the lack of molecular parameters driving the therapeutic algorithm, with the exception of BRCA ½. Therefore, besides the awaited results from the ongoing clinical trials exploring the activity of novel agents, there is a strong need for valid biomarkers that could help clinicians to decide which agent and which sequence of treatments should be administrated at any given time, in order to improve patients' clinical management. Comprehensive gene panels are required to identify interactions among genes and proteins and a single gene test will not be sufficient to predict sensitivity or resistance to a certain therapy.

Plasma DNA analysis, together with other molecular tests (i.e., circulating miRNA and tumor cells, extracellular vesicles analysis), could represent a valid tool for the clinicians for treatment selection, response prediction, and identification of treatment resistance.

References

1. Abdeltwab RM, Yacoub E, Rashad AH, Shohdy KS. Molecular basis of tumorigenesis of bladder cancer and emerging concepts in developing therapeutic targets. Bladder Cancer. 2023;9(4):313–22.
2. Abida W, Campbell D, Patnaik A, Shapiro JD, Sautois B, Vogelzang NJ, Voog EG, Bryce AH, McDermott R, Ricci F, Rowe J, Zhang J, Piulats JM, Fizazi K, Merseburger AS, Higano CS, Krieger LE, Ryan CJ, Feng FY, Simmons AD, Loehr A, Despain D, Dowson M, Green F, Watkins SP, Golsorkhi T, Chowdhury S. Non-BRCA DNA damage repair gene alterations and response to the PARP inhibitor Rucaparib in metastatic castration-resistant prostate cancer: analysis from the phase II TRITON2 study. Clin Cancer Res. 2020a;26(11):2487–96.
3. Abida W, Cheng ML, Armenia J, Middha S, Autio KA, Vargas HA, Rathkopf D, Morris MJ, Danila DC, Slovin SF, Carbone E, Barnett ES, Hullings M, Hechtman JF, Zehir A, Shia J, Jonsson P, Stadler ZK, Srinivasan P, Laudone VP, Reuter V, Wolchok JD, Socci ND, Taylor BS, Berger MF, Kantoff PW, Sawyers CL, Schultz N, Solit DB, Gopalan A, Scher HI. Analysis of the prevalence of microsatellite instability in prostate cancer and response to immune checkpoint blockade. JAMA Oncol. 2019;5(4):471.
4. Abida W, Patnaik A, Campbell D, Shapiro J, Bryce AH, McDermott R, Sautois B, Vogelzang NJ, Bambury RM, Voog E, Zhang J, Piulats JM, Ryan CJ, Merseburger AS, Daugaard G, Heidenreich A, Fizazi K, Higano CS, Krieger LE, Sternberg CN, Watkins SP, Despain D, Simmons AD, Loehr A, Dowson M, Golsorkhi T, Chowdhury S. Rucaparib in men with metastatic castration-resistant prostate

cancer harboring a BRCA1 or BRCA2 gene alteration. J Clin Oncol. 2020b;38(32):3763–72.
5. Agarwal N, Azad AA, Carles J, Fay AP, Matsubara N, Heinrich D, Szczylik C, De Giorgi U, Young Joung J, Fong PCC, Voog E, Jones RJ, Shore ND, Dunshee C, Zschäbitz S, Oldenburg J, Lin X, Healy CG, Di Santo N, Zohren F, Fizazi K. Talazoparib plus enzalutamide in men with first-line metastatic castration-resistant prostate cancer (TALAPRO-2): a randomised, placebo-controlled, phase 3 trial. Lancet. 2023;402(10398):291–303.
6. Al-Obaidy KI, Eble JN, Cheng L, Williamson SR, Sakr WA, Gupta N, Idrees MT, Grignon DJ. Papillary renal neoplasm with reverse polarity. Am J Surg Pathol. 2019;43(8):1099–111.
7. Allory Y, Beukers W, Sagrera A, Flández M, Marqués M, Márquez M, van der Keur KA, Dyrskjot L, Lurkin I, Vermeij M. Telomerase reverse transcriptase promoter mutations in bladder cancer: high frequency across stages, detection in urine, and lack of association with outcome. Eur Urol. 2014;65(2):360–6.
8. Amin MB, Comperat E, Epstein JI, True LD, Hansel D, Paner GP, Al-Ahmadie H, Baydar D, Bivalacqua T, Brimo F. The genitourinary pathology society update on classification and grading of flat and papillary urothelial neoplasia with new reporting recommendations and approach to lesions with mixed and early patterns of neoplasia. Adv Anat Pathol. 2021;28(4):179–95.
9. Argani P. MiT family translocation renal cell carcinoma. Semin Diagn Pathol. 2015;32(2):103–13.
10. Argani P, Antonescu CR, Illei PB, Lui MY, Timmons CF, Newbury R, Reuter VE, Garvin AJ, Perez-Atayde AR, Fletcher JA, Beckwith JB, Bridge JA, Ladanyi M. Primary renal neoplasms with the ASPL-TFE3 gene fusion of alveolar soft part sarcoma: a distinctive tumor entity previously included among renal cell carcinomas of children and adolescents. Am J Pathol. 2001;159(1):179–92.
11. Argani P, Zhang L, Reuter VE, Tickoo SK, Antonescu CR. RBM10-TFE3 renal cell carcinoma: a potential diagnostic pitfall due to cryptic Intrachromosomal Xp11.2 inversion resulting in false-negative TFE3 FISH. Am J Surg Pathol. 2017;41(5):655–62.
12. Armenia J, Wankowicz SAM, Liu D, Gao J, Kundra R, Reznik E, Chatila WK, Chakravarty D, Han GC, Coleman I, Montgomery B, Pritchard C, Morrissey C, Barbieri CE, Beltran H, Sboner A, Zafeiriou Z, Miranda S, Bielski CM, Penson AV, Tolonen C, Huang FW, Robinson D, Wu YM, Lonigro R, Garraway LA, Demichelis F, Kantoff PW, Taplin M-E, Abida W, Taylor BS, Scher HI, Nelson PS, de Bono JS, Rubin MA, Sawyers CL, Chinnaiyan AM, Schultz N, Van Allen EM. The long tail of oncogenic drivers in prostate cancer. Nat Genet. 2018;50(5):645–51.
13. Attard G, et al. Phase 3 AMPLITUDE trial: Niraparib (NIRA) and abiraterone acetate plus prednisone (AAP) for metastatic castration-sensitive prostate cancer (mCSPC) patients (pts) with alterations in homologous recombination repair (HRR) genes. J Clin Oncol. 2025;43(17_suppl)
14. Babjuk M, Burger M, Compérat EM, Gontero P, Mostafid AH, Palou J, van Rhijn BWG, Rouprêt M, Shariat SF, Sylvester R, Zigeuner R, Capoun O, Cohen D, Escrig JLD, Hernández V, Peyronnet B, Seisen T, Soukup V. European Association of Urology guidelines on non-muscle-invasive bladder cancer (TaT1 and carcinoma in situ) -2019 update. Eur Urol. 2019;76(5):639–57.
15. Bakouny Z, Braun DA, Shukla SA, Pan W, Gao X, Hou Y, Flaifel A, Tang S, Bosma-Moody A, He MX. Integrative molecular characterization of sarcomatoid and rhabdoid renal cell carcinoma. Nat Commun. 2021;12(1):808.
16. Balbás-Martínez C, Sagrera A, Carrillo-de-Santa-Pau E, Earl J, Márquez M, Vazquez M, Lapi E, Castro-Giner F, Beltran S, Bayés M, Carrato A, Cigudosa JC, Domínguez O, Gut M, Herranz J, Juanpere N, Kogevinas M, Langa X, López-Knowles E, Lorente JA, Lloreta J, Pisano DG, Richart L, Rico D, Salgado RN, Tardón A, Chanock S, Heath S, Valencia A, Losada A, Gut I, Malats N, Real FX. Recurrent inactivation of STAG2 in bladder cancer is not associated with aneuploidy. Nat Genet. 2013;45(12):1464–9.
17. Bardella C, El-Bahrawy M, Frizzell N, Adam J, Ternette N, Hatipoglu E, Howarth K, O'Flaherty L, Roberts I, Turner G, Taylor J, Giaslakiotis K, Macaulay VM, Harris AL, Chandra A, Lehtonen HJ, Launonen V, Aaltonen LA, Pugh CW, Mihai R, Trudgian D, Kessler B, Baynes JW, Ratcliffe PJ, Tomlinson IP, Pollard PJ. Aberrant succination of proteins in fumarate hydratase-deficient mice and HLRCC patients is a robust biomarker of mutation status. J Pathol. 2011;225(1):4–11.
18. Batista da Costa J, Gibb EA, Bivalacqua TJ, Liu Y, Oo HZ, Miyamoto DT, Alshalalfa M, Davicioni E, Wright J, Dall'Era MA, Douglas J, Boormans JL, Van der Heijden MS, Wu CL, van Rhijn BWG, Gupta S, Grivas P, Mouw KW, Murugan P, Fazli L, Ra S, Konety BR, Seiler R, Daneshmand S, Mian OY, Efstathiou JA, Lotan Y, Black PC. Molecular characterization of neuroendocrine-like bladder cancer. Clin Cancer Res. 2019;25(13):3908–20.
19. Batista R, Vinagre N, Meireles S, Vinagre J, Prazeres H, Leão R, Máximo V, Soares P. Biomarkers for bladder cancer diagnosis and surveillance: a comprehensive review. Diagnostics. 2020;10(1):39.
20. Bi M, Zhao S, Said JW, Merino MJ, Adeniran AJ, Xie Z, Nawaf CB, Choi J, Belldegrun AS, Pantuck AJ, Kluger HM, Bilguvar K, Lifton RP, Shuch B. Genomic characterization of sarcomatoid transformation in clear cell renal cell carcinoma. Proc Natl Acad Sci U S A. 2016;113(8):2170–5.
21. Billerey C, Chopin D, Aubriot-Lorton M-H, Ricol D, de Medina SGD, Van Rhijn B, Bralet M-P, Lefrere-Belda M-A, Lahaye J-B, Abbou CC. Frequent FGFR3 mutations in papillary non-invasive bladder (pTa) tumors. Am J Pathol. 2001;158(6):1955–9.

22. Blume-Jensen P, Berman DM, Rimm DL, Shipitsin M, Putzi M, Nifong TP, Small C, Choudhury S, Capela T, Coupal L, Ernst C, Hurley A, Kaprelyants A, Chang H, Giladi E, Nardone J, Dunyak J, Loda M, Klein EA, Magi-Galluzzi C, Latour M, Epstein JI, Kantoff P, Saad F. Development and clinical validation of an in situ biopsy-based multimarker assay for risk stratification in prostate cancer. Clin Cancer Res. 2015;21(11):2591–600.
23. Bologna E, Ditonno F, Licari LC, Franco A, Manfredi C, Mossack S, Pandolfo SD, De Nunzio C, Simone G, Leonardo C, Franco G. Tissue-based genomic testing in prostate cancer: 10-year analysis of National Trends on the use of Prolaris, decipher, pro mark, and Oncotype DX. Clin Practice. 2024;14(2):508–20.
24. Boysen G, Barbieri CE, Prandi D, Blattner M, Chae S-S, Dahija A, Nataraj S, Huang D, Marotz C, Xu L, Huang J, Lecca P, Chhangawala S, Liu D, Zhou P, Sboner A, de Bono JS, Demichelis F, Houvras Y, Rubin MA. SPOP mutation leads to genomic instability in prostate cancer. elife. 2015;4
25. Breyer J, Wirtz RM, Otto W, Erben P, Worst TS, Stoehr R, Eckstein M, Denzinger S, Burger M, Hartmann A. High PDL1 mRNA expression predicts better survival of stage pT1 non-muscle-invasive bladder cancer (NMIBC) patients. Cancer Immunol Immunother. 2018;67(3):403–12.
26. Brooks SA, Brannon AR, Parker JS, Fisher JC, Sen O, Kattan MW, Hakimi AA, Hsieh JJ, Choueiri TK, Tamboli P, Maranchie JK, Hinds P, Miller CR, Nielsen ME, Rathmell WK. ClearCode34: a prognostic risk predictor for localized clear cell renal cell carcinoma. Eur Urol. 2014;66(1):77–84.
27. Cajaiba MM, Jennings LJ, Rohan SM, Perez-Atayde AR, Marino-Enriquez A, Fletcher JA, Geller JI, Leuer KM, Bridge JA, Perlman EJ. ALK-rearranged renal cell carcinomas in children. Genes Chromosomes Cancer. 2016;55(5):442–51.
28. Calderaro J, Masliah-Planchon J, Richer W, Maillot L, Maille P, Mansuy L, Bastien C, de la Taille A, Boussion H, Charpy C, Jourdain A, Bléchet C, Pierron G, Gentien D, Choudat L, Tournigand C, Delattre O, Allory Y, Bourdeaut F. Balanced translocations disrupting SMARCB1 are Hallmark recurrent genetic alterations in renal medullary carcinomas. Eur Urol. 2016;69(6):1055–61.
29. Cancer Genome Atlas Research, N. Comprehensive molecular characterization of clear cell renal cell carcinoma. Nature. 2013;499(7456):43–9.
30. Cancer Genome Atlas Research, N. Comprehensive molecular characterization of urothelial bladder carcinoma. Nature. 2014;507(7492):315–22.
31. Cancer Genome Atlas Research, N. The molecular taxonomy of primary prostate cancer. Cell. 2015;163(4):1011–25.
32. Cancer Genome Atlas Research, N, et al. Comprehensive molecular characterization of papillary renal-cell carcinoma. N Engl J Med. 2016;374(2):135–45.
33. Cancer, I. A. f. R. o. WHO Classification of Tumours. Urinary and Male Genital Tumours. Lyon: International Agency for Research on Cancer; 2022.
34. Carlo MI, Manley B, Patil S, Woo KM, Coskey DT, Redzematovic A, Arcila M, Ladanyi M, Lee W, Chen YB, Lee CH, Feldman DR, Hakimi AA, Motzer RJ, Hsieh JJ, Voss MH. Genomic alterations and outcomes with VEGF-targeted therapy in patients with clear cell renal cell carcinoma. Kidney Cancer. 2017;1(1):49–56.
35. Carlo MI, Mukherjee S, Mandelker D, Vijai J, Kemel Y, Zhang L, Knezevic A, Patil S, Ceyhan-Birsoy O, Huang K-C, Redzematovic A, Coskey DT, Stewart C, Pradhan N, Arnold AG, Hakimi AA, Chen Y-B, Coleman JA, Hyman DM, Ladanyi M, Cadoo KA, Walsh MF, Stadler ZK, Lee C-H, Feldman DR, Voss MH, Robson M, Motzer RJ, Offit K. Prevalence of germline mutations in cancer susceptibility genes in patients with advanced renal cell carcinoma. JAMA Oncol. 2018;4(9):1228.
36. Casuscelli J, Weinhold N, Gundem G, Wang L, Zabor EC, Drill E, Wang PI, Nanjangud GJ, Redzematovic A, Nargund AM, Manley BJ, Arcila ME, Donin NM, Cheville JC, Thompson RH, Pantuck AJ, Russo P, Cheng EH, Lee W, Tickoo SK, Ostrovnaya I, Creighton CJ, Papaemmanuil E, Seshan VE, Hakimi AA, Hsieh JJ. Genomic landscape and evolution of metastatic chromophobe renal cell carcinoma. JCI Insight. 2017;2(12)
37. Cerveira N, Ribeiro FR, Peixoto A, Costa V, Henrique R, Jerönimo C, Teixeira MR. TMPRSS2-ERG gene fusion causing ERG overexpression precedes chromosome copy number changes in prostate carcinomas, paired HGPIN lesions. Neoplasia. 2006;8(10):826–32.
38. Chauhan PS, Chen K, Babbra RK, Feng W, Pejovic N, Nallicheri A, Harris PK, Dienstbach K, Atkocius A, Maguire L, Qaium F, Szymanski JJ, Baumann BC, Ding L, Cao D, Reimers MA, Kim EH, Smith ZL, Arora VK, Chaudhuri AA. Urine tumor DNA detection of minimal residual disease in muscle-invasive bladder cancer treated with curative-intent radical cystectomy: a cohort study. PLoS Med. 2021;18(8):e1003732.
39. Chen Y-B, Xu J, Skanderup AJ, Dong Y, Brannon AR, Wang L, Won HH, Wang PI, Nanjangud GJ, Jungbluth AA, Li W, Ojeda V, Hakimi AA, Voss MH, Schultz N, Motzer RJ, Russo P, Cheng EH, Giancotti FG, Lee W, Berger MF, Tickoo SK, Reuter VE, Hsieh JJ. Molecular analysis of aggressive renal cell carcinoma with unclassified histology reveals distinct subsets. Nat Commun. 2016;7(1)
40. Chen YB, Mirsadraei L, Jayakumaran G, Al-Ahmadie HA, Fine SW, Gopalan A, Sirintrapun SJ, Tickoo SK, Reuter VE. Somatic mutations of TSC2 or MTOR characterize a morphologically distinct subset of sporadic renal cell carcinoma with eosinophilic and vacuolated cytoplasm. Am J Surg Pathol. 2019;43(1):121–31.

41. Chen YB, Tickoo SK. Spectrum of preneoplastic and neoplastic cystic lesions of the kidney. Arch Pathol Lab Med. 2012;136(4):400–9.
42. Chi KN, Barnicle A, Sibilla C, Lai Z, Corcoran C, Barrett JC, Adelman CA, Qiu P, Easter A, Dearden S, Oxnard GR, Agarwal N, Azad A, de Bono J, Mateo J, Olmos D, Thiery-Vuillemin A, Harrington EA. Detection of BRCA1, BRCA2, and ATM alterations in matched tumor tissue and circulating tumor DNA in patients with prostate cancer screened in PROfound. Clin Cancer Res. 2023a;29(1):81–91.
43. Chi KN, Sandhu S, Smith MR, Attard G, Saad M, Olmos D, Castro E, Roubaud G, et al. Niraparib plus abiraterone acetate with prednisone in patients with metastatic castration-resistant prostate cancer and homologous recombination repair gene alterations: second interim analysis of the randomized phase III MAGNITUDE trial. Ann Oncol. 2023b;34(9):772–82.
44. Choi W, Ochoa A, McConkey DJ, Aine M, Höglund M, Kim WY, Real FX, Kiltie AE, Milsom I, Dyrskjøt L, Lerner SP. Genetic alterations in the molecular subtypes of bladder cancer: illustration in the cancer genome atlas dataset. Eur Urol. 2017;72(3):354–65.
45. Choueiri TK, Kaelin WG Jr. Targeting the HIF2-VEGF axis in renal cell carcinoma. Nat Med. 2020;26(10):1519–30.
46. Choueiri TK, Plimack E, Arkenau H-T, Jonasch E, Heng DYC, Powles T, Frigault MM, Clark EA, Handzel AA, Gardner H, Morgan S, Albiges L, Pal SK. Biomarker-based phase II trial of Savolitinib in patients with advanced papillary renal cell cancer. J Clin Oncol. 2017;35(26):2993–3001.
47. Christensen E, Birkenkamp-Demtröder K, Sethi H, Shchegrova S, Salari R, Nordentoft I, Wu H-T, Knudsen M, Lamy P, Lindskrog SV. Early detection of metastatic relapse and monitoring of therapeutic efficacy by ultra-deep sequencing of plasma cell-free DNA in patients with urothelial bladder carcinoma. J Clin Oncol. 2019;37(18):1547–57.
48. Cimadamore A, Boixareu C, Sharp A, Beltran H, de Bono JS. Novel therapeutic strategies for metastatic prostate cancer care. Eur Urol. 2025;88:437.
49. Cimadamore A, Cheng L, Massari F, Santoni M, Pepi L, Franzese C, Scarpelli M, Lopez-Beltran A, Galosi AB, Montironi R. Circulating tumor DNA testing for homology recombination repair genes in prostate cancer: from the lab to the clinic. Int J Mol Sci. 2021;22(11):5522.
50. Cimadamore A, Lopez-Beltran A, Massari F, Santoni M, Mazzucchelli R, Scarpelli M, Galosi AB, Cheng L, Montironi R. Germline and somatic mutations in prostate cancer: focus on defective DNA repair, PARP inhibitors and immunotherapy. Future Oncol. 2020;16(5):75–80.
51. Classe M, Malouf GG, Su X, Yao H, Thompson EJ, Doss DJ, Grégoire V, Lenobin J, Fantoni JC, Sudour-Bonnange H, Khayat D, Aubert S, Tannir NM, Leroy X. Incidence, clinicopathological features and fusion transcript landscape of translocation renal cell carcinomas. Histopathology. 2017;70(7):1089–97.
52. Cotter K, Rubin MA. The evolving landscape of prostate cancer somatic mutations. Prostate. 2022;82(S1)
53. Crocetto F, Amicuzi U, Musone M, Magliocchetti M, Di Lieto D, Tammaro S, Pastore AL, Fuschi A, Falabella R, Ferro M, Bianchi R, Finati M, Busetto GM, Lucarelli G, Del Giudice F, Caputo VF, Balsamo R, Terracciano D. Liquid biopsy: current advancements in clinical practice for bladder cancer. J Liq Biopsy. 2025;9:100310.
54. Cuzick J, Swanson GP, Fisher G, Brothman AR, Berney DM, Reid JE, Mesher D, Speights VO, Stankiewicz E, Foster CS, Møller H, Scardino P, Warren JD, Park J, Younus A, Flake DD, Wagner S, Gutin A, Lanchbury JS, Stone S. Prognostic value of an RNA expression signature derived from cell cycle proliferation genes in patients with prostate cancer: a retrospective study. Lancet Oncol. 2011;12(3):245–55.
55. Dadhania V, Zhang M, Zhang L, Bondaruk J, Majewski T, Siefker-Radtke A, Guo CC, Dinney C, Cogdell DE, Zhang S, Lee S, Lee JG, Weinstein JN, Baggerly K, McConkey D, Czerniak B. Meta-analysis of the luminal and basal subtypes of bladder cancer and the identification of signature Immunohistochemical markers for clinical use. EBioMedicine. 2016;12:105–17.
56. Damrauer JS, Roell KR, Smith MA, Sun X, Kirk EL, Hoadley KA, Benefield HC, Iyer G, Solit DB, Milowsky MI. Identification of a novel inflamed tumor microenvironment signature as a predictive biomarker of bacillus Calmette-Guérin immunotherapy in non–muscle-invasive bladder cancer. Clin Cancer Res. 2021;27(16):4599–609.
57. Dason S, Allard C, Sheridan-Jonah A, Gill J, Jamshaid H, Aziz T, Kajal B, Kapoor A. Management of renal collecting duct carcinoma: a systematic review and the McMaster experience. Curr Oncol. 2013;20(3):e223–32.
58. Davis CF, et al. The somatic genomic landscape of chromophobe renal cell carcinoma. Cancer Cell. 2014;26(3):319–30.
59. de Bono J, Mateo J, Fizazi K, Saad F, Shore N, Sandhu S, Chi KN, Sartor O, Agarwal N, Olmos D, Thiery-Vuillemin A, Twardowski P, Mehra N, Goessl C, Kang J, Burgents J, Wu W, Kohlmann A, Adelman CA, Hussain M. Olaparib for metastatic castration-resistant prostate cancer. N Engl J Med. 2020;382(22):2091–102.
60. De Bono JS, Matsubara N, Penel N, Mehra N, Kolinsky MP, Bompas E, Feyerabend S, Gravis G, Joung JY, Nishimura K, Gedye C, Mateo J, Saad F, Fizazi K, Shore N, Kang J, Desai C, Burgents JE, Harrington E, Hussain MHA. Exploratory gene-by-gene analysis of olaparib in patients (pts) with metastatic castration-resistant prostate cancer (mCRPC): PROfound. J Clin Oncol. 2021;39(6_suppl):126.

Pritchard CC, Eisenberger MA, Lotan TL. Molecular characterization and clinical outcomes of primary Gleason pattern 5 prostate cancer after radical prostatectomy. JCO Precis Oncol. 2019;3:1–13.
98. Isaacsson Velho P, Silberstein JL, Markowski MC, Luo J, Lotan TL, Isaacs WB, Antonarakis ES. Intraductal/ductal histology and lymphovascular invasion are associated with germline DNA-repair gene mutations in prostate cancer. Prostate. 2018;78(5):401–7.
99. Jamaspishvili T, Berman DM, Ross AE, Scher HI, De Marzo AM, Squire JA, Lotan TL. Clinical implications of PTEN loss in prostate cancer. Nat Rev Urol. 2018;15(4):222–34.
100. Jia L, Carlo MI, Khan H, Nanjangud GJ, Rana S, Cimera R, Zhang Y, Hakimi AA, Verma AK, Al-Ahmadie HA, Fine SW, Gopalan A, Sirintrapun SJ, Tickoo SK, Reuter VE, Gartrell BA, Chen YB. Distinctive mechanisms underlie the loss of SMARCB1 protein expression in renal medullary carcinoma: morphologic and molecular analysis of 20 cases. Mod Pathol. 2019;32(9):1329–43.
101. Jin H-J, Zhao JC, Ogden I, Bergan RC, Yu J. Androgen receptor-independent function of fox A1 in prostate cancer metastasis. Cancer Res. 2013;73(12):3725–36.
102. Joseph RW, Kapur P, Serie DJ, Parasramka M, Ho TH, Cheville JC, Frenkel E, Parker AS, Brugarolas J. Clear cell renal cell carcinoma subtypes identified by BAP1 and PBRM1 expression. J Urol. 2016;195(1):180–7.
103. Joshi S, Tolkunov D, Aviv H, Hakimi AA, Yao M, Hsieh JJ, Ganesan S, Chan CS, White E. The genomic landscape of renal Oncocytoma identifies a metabolic barrier to tumorigenesis. Cell Rep. 2015;13(9):1895–908.
104. Kamoun A, de Reynies A, Allory Y, Sjodahl G, Robertson AG, Seiler R, Hoadley KA, Groeneveld CS, Al-Ahmadie H, Choi W, Castro MAA, Fontugne J, Eriksson P, Mo Q, Kardos J, Zlotta A, Hartmann A, Dinney CP, Bellmunt J, Powles T, Malats N, Chan KS, Kim WY, McConkey DJ, Black PC, Dyrskjot L, Hoglund M, Lerner SP, Real FX, Radvanyi F, et al. A consensus molecular classification of muscle-invasive bladder cancer. Eur Urol. 2020;77(4):420–33.
105. Kapur P, Pena-Llopis S, Christie A, Zhrebker L, Pavia-Jimenez A, Rathmell WK, Xie XJ, Brugarolas J. Effects on survival of BAP1 and PBRM1 mutations in sporadic clear-cell renal-cell carcinoma: a retrospective analysis with independent validation. Lancet Oncol. 2013;14(2):159–67.
106. Kardos J, Chai S, Mose LE, Selitsky SR, Krishnan B, Saito R, Iglesia MD, Milowsky MI, Parker JS, Kim WY, Vincent BG. Claudin-low bladder tumors are immune infiltrated and actively immune suppressed. JCI Insight. 2016;1(3):e85902.
107. Kauffman EC, Ricketts CJ, Rais-Bahrami S, Yang Y, Merino MJ, Bottaro DP, Srinivasan R, Linehan WM. Molecular genetics and cellular features of TFE3 and TFEB fusion kidney cancers. Nat Rev Urol. 2014;11(8):465–75.
108. Kim J, Kwiatkowski D, McConkey DJ, Meeks JJ, Freeman SS, Bellmunt J, Getz G, Lerner SP. The cancer genome atlas expression subtypes stratify response to checkpoint inhibition in advanced urothelial cancer and identify a subset of patients with high survival probability. Eur Urol. 2019;75(6):961–4.
109. Kim J, Mouw KW, Polak P, Braunstein LZ, Kamburov A, Kwiatkowski DJ, Rosenberg JE, Van Allen EM, D'Andrea A, Getz G. Somatic ERCC2 mutations are associated with a distinct genomic signature in urothelial tumors. Nat Genet. 2016;48(6):600–6.
110. Kiss B, Wyatt AW, Douglas J, Skuginna V, Mo F, Anderson S, Rotzer D, Fleischmann A, Genitsch V, Hayashi T, Neuenschwander M, Buerki C, Davicioni E, Collins C, Thalmann GN, Black PC, Seiler R. Her2 alterations in muscle-invasive bladder cancer: patient selection beyond protein expression for targeted therapy. Sci Rep. 2017;7:42713.
111. Klein EA, Cooperberg MR, Magi-Galluzzi C, Simko JP, Falzarano SM, Maddala T, Chan JM, Li J, Cowan JE, Tsiatis AC, Cherbavaz DB, Pelham RJ, Tenggara-Hunter I, Baehner FL, Knezevic D, Febbo PG, Shak S, Kattan MW, Lee M, Carroll PR. A 17-gene assay to predict prostate cancer aggressiveness in the context of Gleason grade heterogeneity, tumor multifocality, and biopsy undersampling. Eur Urol. 2014;66(3):550–60.
112. Knowles MA. FGFR3–a central player in bladder cancer pathogenesis? Bladder Cancer. 2020;6(4):403–23.
113. Knowles MA, Hurst CD. Molecular biology of bladder cancer: new insights into pathogenesis and clinical diversity. Nat Rev Cancer. 2015;15(1):25–41.
114. Kompier LC, Lurkin I, van der Aa MN, van Rhijn BW, van der Kwast TH, Zwarthoff EC. FGFR3, HRAS, KRAS, NRAS and PIK3CA mutations in bladder cancer and their potential as biomarkers for surveillance and therapy. PLoS One. 2010;5(11):e13821.
115. Kuroda N, Tamura M, Hamaguchi N, Mikami S, Pan CC, Brunelli M, Martignoni G, Hes O, Michal M, Lee GH. Acquired cystic disease-associated renal cell carcinoma with sarcomatoid change and rhabdoid features. Ann Diagn Pathol. 2011;15(6):462–6.
116. Kuroda N, Trpkov K, Gao Y, Tretiakova M, Liu YJ, Ulamec M, Takeuchi K, Agaimy A, Przybycin C, Magi-Galluzzi C, Fushimi S, Kojima F, Sibony M, Hang J-F, Pan C-C, Yilmaz A, Siadat F, Sugawara E, Just P-A, Ptakova N, Hes O. ALK rearranged renal cell carcinoma (ALK-RCC): a multi-institutional study of twelve cases with identification of novel partner genes CLIP1, KIF5B and KIAA1217. Mod Pathol. 2020;33(12):2564–79.
117. Kusano H, Togashi Y, Akiba J, Moriya F, Baba K, Matsuzaki N, Yuba Y, Shiraishi Y, Kanamaru H, Kuroda N, Sakata S, Takeuchi K, Yano H. Two cases of renal cell carcinoma harboring a novel

STRN-ALK fusion gene. Am J Surg Pathol. 2016;40(6):761–9.
118. Kwan EM, Wyatt AW, Chi KN. Towards clinical implementation of circulating tumor DNA in metastatic prostate cancer: opportunities for integration and pitfalls to interpretation. Front Oncol. 2022;12
119. Kwiatkowski DJ, Choueiri TK, Fay AP, Rini BI, Thorner AR, de Velasco G, Tyburczy ME, Hamieh L, Albiges L, Agarwal N, Ho TH, Song J, Pignon JC, Barrios PM, Michaelson MD, Van Allen E, Krajewski KM, Porta C, Pal S, Bellmunt J, McDermott DF, Heng DYC, Gray KP, Signoretti S. Mutations in TSC1, TSC2, and MTOR are associated with response to Rapalogs in patients with metastatic renal cell carcinoma. Clin Cancer Res. 2016;22(10):2445–52.
120. Lang M, Vocke CD, Merino MJ, Schmidt LS, Linehan WM. Mitochondrial DNA mutations distinguish bilateral multifocal renal oncocytomas from familial Birt-Hogg-Dubé tumors. Mod Pathol. 2015;28(11):1458–69.
121. Launonen V, Vierimaa O, Kiuru M, Isola J, Roth S, Pukkala E, Sistonen P, Herva R, Aaltonen LA. Inherited susceptibility to uterine leiomyomas and renal cell cancer. Proc Natl Acad Sci USA. 2001;98(6):3387–92.
122. Lawrence MS, Stojanov P, Polak P, Kryukov GV, Cibulskis K, Sivachenko A, Carter SL, Stewart C, Mermel CH, Roberts SA, Kiezun A, Hammerman PS, McKenna A, Drier Y, Zou L, Ramos AH, Pugh TJ, Stransky N, Helman E, Kim J, Sougnez C, Ambrogio L, Nickerson E, Shefler E, Cortes ML, Auclair D, Saksena G, Voet D, Noble M, DiCara D, Lin P, Lichtenstein L, Heiman DI, Fennell T, Imielinski M, Hernandez B, Hodis E, Baca S, Dulak AM, Lohr J, Landau DA, Wu CJ, Melendez-Zajgla J, Hidalgo-Miranda A, Koren A, McCarroll SA, Mora J, Crompton B, Onofrio R, Parkin M, Winckler W, Ardlie K, Gabriel SB, Roberts CWM, Biegel JA, Stegmaier K, Bass AJ, Garraway LA, Meyerson M, Golub TR, Gordenin DA, Sunyaev S, Lander ES, Getz G. Mutational heterogeneity in cancer and the search for new cancer-associated genes. Nature. 2013;499(7457):214–8.
123. Ler LD, Ghosh S, Chai X, Thike AA, Heng HL, Siew EY, Dey S, Koh LK, Lim JQ, Lim WK. Loss of tumor suppressor KDM6A amplifies PRC2-regulated transcriptional repression in bladder cancer and can be targeted through inhibition of EZH2. Sci Transl Med. 2017;9(378):eaai8312.
124. Lerner SP, Weinstein J, Kwiatkowski D, Kim J, Robertson G, Hoadley KA, Akbani R, Creighton C. The cancer genome atlas project on muscle-invasive bladder cancer. Eur Urol Focus. 2015;1(1):94–5.
125. Li H-T, Duymich CE, Weisenberger DJ, Liang G. Genetic and epigenetic alterations in bladder cancer. Int Neurourol J. 2016;20(Suppl 2):S84.
126. Liu J, Hanavan PD, Kras K, Ruiz YW, Castle EP, Lake DF, Chen X, O'Brien D, Luo H, Robertson KD, Gu H, Ho TH. Loss of SETD2 induces a metabolic switch in renal cell carcinoma cell lines toward enhanced oxidative phosphorylation. J Proteome Res. 2019;18(1):331–40.
127. Loriot Y, Necchi A, Park SH, Garcia-Donas J, Huddart R, Burgess E, Fleming M, Rezazadeh A, Mellado B, Varlamov S. Erdafitinib in locally advanced or metastatic urothelial carcinoma. N Engl J Med. 2019;381(4):338–48.
128. Lotan TL, Kaur HB, Alharbi AM, Pritchard CC, Epstein JI. DNA damage repair alterations are frequent in prostatic adenocarcinomas with focal pleomorphic giant-cell features. Histopathology. 2019;74(6):836–43.
129. Lotan TL, Tomlins SA, Bismar TA, Van der Kwast TH, Grignon D, Egevad L, Kristiansen G, Pritchard CC, Rubin MA, Bubendorf L. Report from the International Society of Urological Pathology (ISUP) consultation conference on molecular pathology of urogenital cancers. I. Molecular biomarkers in prostate cancer. Am J Surg Pathol. 2020;44(7):e15–29.
130. Maher ER. Hereditary renal cell carcinoma syndromes: diagnosis, surveillance and management. World J Urol. 2018;36(12):1891–8.
131. Maher ER, Neumann HP, Richard S. von Hippel-Lindau disease: a clinical and scientific review. Eur J Hum Genet. 2011;19(6):617–23.
132. Malouf GG, Ali SM, Wang K, Balasubramanian S, Ross JS, Miller VA, Stephens PJ, Khayat D, Pal SK, Su X, Sircar K, Tamboli P, Jonasch E, Tannir NM, Wood CG, Karam JA. Genomic characterization of renal cell carcinoma with Sarcomatoid dedifferentiation pinpoints recurrent genomic alterations. Eur Urol. 2016;70(2):348–57.
133. Malouf GG, Camparo P, Oudard S, Schleiermacher G, Theodore C, Rustine A, Dutcher J, Billemont B, Rixe O, Bompas E, Guillot A, Boccon-Gibod L, Couturier J, Molinié V, Escudier B. Targeted agents in metastatic Xp11 translocation/TFE3 gene fusion renal cell carcinoma (RCC): a report from the juvenile RCC network. Ann Oncol. 2010;21(9):1834–8.
134. Malouf GG, Flippot R, Dong Y, Dinatale RG, Chen YB, Su X, Compérat E, Rouprêt M, Mano R, Blum KA, Yao H, Mouawad R, Spano JP, Khayat D, Karam JA, Ho TH, Tickoo SK, Russo P, Hsieh JJ, Tannir NM, Hakimi AA. Molecular characterization of sarcomatoid clear cell renal cell carcinoma unveils new candidate oncogenic drivers. Sci Rep. 2020;10(1):701.
135. Malouf GG, Monzon FA, Couturier J, Molinié V, Escudier B, Camparo P, Su X, Yao H, Tamboli P, Lopez-Terrada D, Picken M, Garcia M, Multani AS, Pathak S, Wood CG, Tannir NM. Genomic heterogeneity of translocation renal cell carcinoma. Clin Cancer Res. 2013;19(17):4673–84.
136. Mariathasan S, Turley SJ, Nickles D, Castiglioni A, Yuen K, Wang Y, Kadel Iii EE, Koeppen H, Astarita JL, Cubas R, Jhunjhunwala S, Banchereau R, Yang Y, Guan Y, Chalouni C, Ziai J, Şenbabaoğlu Y, Santoro S, Sheinson D, Hung J, Giltnane JM, Pierce

AA, Mesh K, Lianoglou S, Riegler J, Carano RAD, Eriksson P, Höglund M, Somarriba L, Halligan DL, van der Heijden MS, Loriot Y, Rosenberg JE, Fong L, Mellman I, Chen DS, Green M, Derleth C, Fine GD, Hegde PS, Bourgon R, Powles T. TGFβ attenuates tumour response to PD-L1 blockade by contributing to exclusion of T cells. Nature. 2018;554(7693):544–8.
137. Mateo J, Carreira S, Sandhu S, Miranda S, Mossop H, Perez-Lopez R, Nava Rodrigues D, Robinson D, Omlin A, Tunariu N, Boysen G, Porta N, Flohr P, Gillman A, Figueiredo I, Paulding C, Seed G, Jain S, Ralph C, Protheroe A, Hussain S, Jones R, Elliott T, McGovern U, Bianchini D, Goodall J, Zafeiriou Z, Williamson CT, Ferraldeschi R, Riisnaes R, Ebbs B, Fowler G, Roda D, Yuan W, Wu YM, Cao X, Brough R, Pemberton H, A'Hern R, Swain A, Kunju LP, Eeles R, Attard G, Lord CJ, Ashworth A, Rubin MA, Knudsen KE, Feng FY, Chinnaiyan AM, Hall E, de Bono JS. DNA-repair defects and Olaparib in metastatic prostate cancer. N Engl J Med. 2015;373(18):1697–708.
138. Mauzo SH, Lee M, Petros J, Hunter S, Chang C-M, Shu H-K, Bellail AC, Hao C, Cohen C. Immunohistochemical demonstration of Isocitrate dehydrogenase 1 (IDH1) mutation in a Small subset of prostatic carcinomas. Appl Immunohistochem Mol Morphol. 2014;22(4):284–7.
139. McDermott DF, Huseni MA, Atkins MB, Motzer RJ, Rini BI, Escudier B, Fong L, Joseph RW, Pal SK, Reeves JA, Sznol M, Hainsworth J, Rathmell WK, Stadler WM, Hutson T, Gore ME, Ravaud A, Bracarda S, Suárez C, Danielli R, Gruenwald V, Choueiri TK, Nickles D, Jhunjhunwala S, Piault-Louis E, Thobhani A, Qiu J, Chen DS, Hegde PS, Schiff C, Fine GD, Powles T. Clinical activity and molecular correlates of response to atezolizumab alone or in combination with bevacizumab versus sunitinib in renal cell carcinoma. Nat Med. 2018;24(6):749–57.
140. Meeks JJ, Al-Ahmadie H, Faltas BM, Taylor JA 3rd, Flaig TW, DeGraff DJ, Christensen E, Woolbright BL, McConkey DJ, Dyrskjøt L. Genomic heterogeneity in bladder cancer: challenges and possible solutions to improve outcomes. Nat Rev Urol. 2020;17(5):259–70.
141. Mehra R, Shah T, Liu C-J, Plouffe KR, Wang X, Mannan R, Cao X, Chinnaiyan AM, Tomlins SA, Udager AM. Highly recurrent IDH1 mutations in prostate cancer with Psammomatous calcification. Mod Pathol. 2023;36(6):100146.
142. Menko FH, Maher ER, Schmidt LS, Middelton LA, Aittomäki K, Tomlinson I, Richard S, Linehan WM. Hereditary leiomyomatosis and renal cell cancer (HLRCC): renal cancer risk, surveillance and treatment. Fam Cancer. 2014;13(4):637–44.
143. Mester J, Eng C. Cowden syndrome: recognizing and managing a not-so-rare hereditary cancer syndrome. J Surg Oncol. 2015;111(1):125–30.
144. Miao D, Margolis CA, Gao W, Voss MH, Li W, Martini DJ, Norton C, Bossé D, Wankowicz SM, Cullen D, Horak C, Wind-Rotolo M, Tracy A, Giannakis M, Hodi FS, Drake CG, Ball MW, Allaf ME, Snyder A, Hellmann MD, Ho T, Motzer RJ, Signoretti S, Kaelin WG, Choueiri TK, Van Allen EM. Genomic correlates of response to immune checkpoint therapies in clear cell renal cell carcinoma. Science. 2018;359(6377):801–6.
145. Mitchell TJ, et al. Timing the landmark events in the evolution of clear cell renal cell cancer: TRACERx renal. Cell. 2018;173(3):611–23.
146. Moch H, Amin MB, Berney DM, Compérat EM, Gill AJ, Hartmann A, Menon S, Raspollini MR, Rubin MA, Srigley JR, Hoon Tan P, Tickoo SK, Tsuzuki T, Turajlic S, Cree I, Netto GJ. The 2022 World Health Organization classification of Tumours of the urinary system and male genital organs – part a: renal, penile, and testicular Tumours. Eur Urol. 2022;82(5):458–68.
147. Moch H, Cubilla AL, Humphrey PA, Reuter VE, Ulbright TM. The 2016 WHO classification of tumours of the urinary system and male genital organs – part a: renal, penile, and testicular tumours. Eur Urol. 2016;70:93–105.
148. Mosele MF, Westphalen CB, Stenzinger A, Barlesi F, Bayle A, Bièche I, Bonastre J, Castro E, Dienstmann R, Krämer A, Czarnecka AM, Meric-Bernstam F, Michiels S, Miller R, Normanno N, Reis-Filho J, Remon J, Robson M, Rouleau E, Scarpa A, Serrano C, Mateo J, André F. Recommendations for the use of next-generation sequencing (NGS) for patients with advanced cancer in 2024: a report from the ESMO precision medicine working group. Ann Oncol. 2024;35(7):588–606.
149. Motzer RJ, Robbins PB, Powles T, Albiges L, Haanen JB, Larkin J, Mu XJ, Ching KA, Uemura M, Pal SK, Alekseev B, Gravis G, Campbell MT, Penkov K, Lee JL, Hariharan S, Wang X, Zhang W, Wang J, Chudnovsky A, di Pietro A, Donahue AC, Choueiri TK. Avelumab plus axitinib versus sunitinib in advanced renal cell carcinoma: biomarker analysis of the phase 3 JAVELIN renal 101 trial. Nat Med. 2020;26(11):1733–41.
150. Msaouel P, Tannir NM, Walker CL. A model linking sickle cell Hemoglobinopathies and SMARCB1 loss in renal medullary carcinoma. Clin Cancer Res. 2018;24(9):2044–9.
151. Munari E, Marchionni L, Chitre A, Hayashi M, Martignoni G, Brunelli M, Gobbo S, Argani P, Allaf M, Hoque MO, Netto GJ. Clear cell papillary renal cell carcinoma: micro-RNA expression profiling and comparison with clear cell renal cell carcinoma and papillary renal cell carcinoma. Hum Pathol. 2014;45(6):1130–8.
152. Musangile FY, Matsuzaki I, Iwamoto R, Sagan K, Nishikawa M, Mikasa Y, Takahashi Y, Kojima F, Hara I, Murata S-I. Targeted next-generation sequencing of flat urothelial lesions reveals puta-

tive Pathobiological pathways, potential biomarkers, and rational therapeutic targets. Mod Pathol. 2023;36(5):100120.
153. Nargund AM, Pham CG, Dong Y, Wang PI, Osmangeyoglu HU, Xie Y, Aras O, Han S, Oyama T, Takeda S, Ray CE, Dong Z, Berge M, Hakimi AA, Monette S, Lekaye CL, Koutcher JA, Leslie CS, Creighton CJ, Weinhold N, Lee W, Tickoo SK, Wang Z, Cheng EH, Hsieh JJ. The SWI/SNF protein PBRM1 restrains VHL-loss-driven clear cell renal cell carcinoma. Cell Rep. 2017;18(12):2893–906.
154. Nava Rodrigues D, Rescigno P, Liu D, Yuan W, Carreira S, Lambros MB, Seed G, Mateo J, Riisnaes R, Mullane S, Margolis C, Miao D, Miranda S, Dolling D, Clarke M, Bertan C, Crespo M, Boysen G, Ferreira A, Sharp A, Figueiredo I, Keliher D, Aldubayan S, Burke KP, Sumanasuriya S, Fontes MS, Bianchini D, Zafeiriou Z, Teixeira Mendes LS, Mouw K, Schweizer MT, Pritchard CC, Salipante S, Taplin ME, Beltran H, Rubin MA, Cieslik M, Robinson D, Heath E, Schultz N, Armenia J, Abida W, Scher H, Lord C, D'Andrea A, Sawyers CL, Chinnaiyan AM, Alimonti A, Nelson PS, Drake CG, Van Allen EM, de Bono JS. Immunogenomic analyses associate immunological alterations with mismatch repair defects in prostate cancer. J Clin Invest. 2018;128(10):4441–53.
155. Necchi A, Madison R, Raggi D, Jacob JM, Bratslavsky G, Shapiro O, Elvin JA, Vergilio J-A, Killian JK, Ngo N. Comprehensive assessment of immuno-oncology biomarkers in adenocarcinoma, urothelial carcinoma, and squamous-cell carcinoma of the bladder. Eur Urol. 2020;77(4):548–56.
156. Ng KL, Morais C, Bernard A, Saunders N, Samaratunga H, Gobe G, Wood S. A systematic review and meta-analysis of immunohistochemical biomarkers that differentiate chromophobe renal cell carcinoma from renal oncocytoma. J Clin Pathol. 2016;69(8):661–71.
157. Nguyen KA, Syed JS, Espenschied CR, LaDuca H, Bhagat AM, Suarez-Sarmiento A, O'Rourke TK, Brierley KL, Hofstatter EW, Shuch B. Advances in the diagnosis of hereditary kidney cancer: initial results of a multigene panel test. Cancer. 2017;123(22):4363–71.
158. Nuhn P, De Bono JS, Fizazi K, Freedland SJ, Grilli M, Kantoff PW, Sonpavde G, Sternberg CN, Yegnasubramanian S, Antonarakis ES. Update on systemic prostate cancer therapies: management of metastatic castration-resistant prostate cancer in the era of precision oncology. Eur Urol. 2019;75(1):88–99.
159. Nyquist MD, Corella A, Coleman I, De Sarkar N, Kaipainen A, Ha G, Gulati R, Ang L, Chatterjee P, Lucas J, Pritchard C, Risbridger G, Isaacs J, Montgomery B, Morrissey C, Corey E, Nelson PS. Combined TP53 and RB1 loss promotes prostate cancer resistance to a spectrum of therapeutics and confers vulnerability to replication stress. Cell Rep. 2020;31(8):107669.
160. Olislagers M, de Jong FC, Rutten VC, Boormans JL, Mahmoudi T, Zuiverloon TCM. Molecular biomarkers of progression in non-muscle-invasive bladder cancer – beyond conventional risk stratification. Nat Rev Urol. 2025;22(2):75–91.
161. Ooi A, Wong JC, Petillo D, Roossien D, Perrier-Trudova V, Whitten D, Min BW, Tan MH, Zhang Z, Yang XJ, Zhou M, Gardie B, Molinié V, Richard S, Tan PH, Teh BT, Furge KA. An antioxidant response phenotype shared between hereditary and sporadic type 2 papillary renal cell carcinoma. Cancer Cell. 2011;20(4):511–23.
162. Pal SK, Ali SM, Yakirevich E, Geynisman DM, Karam JA, Elvin JA, Frampton GM, Huang X, Lin DI, Rosenzweig M. Characterization of clinical cases of advanced papillary renal cell carcinoma via comprehensive genomic profiling. Eur Urol. 2018;73(1):71–8.
163. Pal SK, He M, Tong T, Wu H, Liu X, Lau C, Wang JH, Warden C, Wu X, Signoretti S, Choueiri TK, Karam JA, Jones JO. RNA-seq reveals aurora kinase-driven mTOR pathway activation in patients with sarcomatoid metastatic renal cell carcinoma. Mol Cancer Res. 2015;13(1):130–7.
164. Parker C, Castro E, Fizazi K, Heidenreich A, Ost P, Procopio G, Tombal B, Gillessen S. Prostate cancer: ESMO clinical practice guidelines for diagnosis, treatment and follow-up. Ann Oncol. 2020;31(9):1119–34.
165. Pena-Llopis S, Vega-Rubin-de-Celis S, Liao A, Leng N, Pavia-Jimenez A, Wang S, Yamasaki T, Zhrebker L, Sivanand S, Spence P, Kinch L, Hambuch T, Jain S, Lotan Y, Margulis V, Sagalowsky AI, Summerour PB, Kabbani W, Wong SW, Grishin N, Laurent M, Xie XJ, Haudenschild CD, Ross MT, Bentley DR, Kapur P, Brugarolas J. BAP1 loss defines a new class of renal cell carcinoma. Nat Genet. 2012;44(7):751–9.
166. Perner S, Mosquera J-M, Demichelis F, Hofer MD, Paris PL, Simko J, Collins C, Bismar TA, Chinnaiyan AM, De Marzo AM, Rubin MA. TMPRSS2-ERG fusion prostate cancer: an early molecular event associated with invasion. Am J Surg Pathol. 2007;31(6):882–8.
167. Petersson F, Gatalica Z, Grossmann P, Perez Montiel MD, Alvarado Cabrero I, Bulimbasic S, Swatek A, Straka L, Tichy T, Hora M, Kuroda N, Legendre B, Michal M, Hes O. Sporadic hybrid oncocytic/chromophobe tumor of the kidney: a clinicopathologic, histomorphologic, immunohistochemical, ultrastructural, and molecular cytogenetic study of 14 cases. Virchows Arch. 2010;456(4):355–65.
168. Pietzak EJ, Bagrodia A, Cha EK, Drill EN, Iyer G, Isharwal S, Ostrovnaya I, Baez P, Li Q, Berger MF, Zehir A, Schultz N, Rosenberg JE, Bajorin DF, Dalbagni G, Al-Ahmadie H, Solit DB, Bochner BH. Next-generation sequencing of nonmuscle invasive bladder cancer reveals potential biomarkers and rational therapeutic targets. Eur Urol. 2017;72(6):952–9.

169. Plimack ER, Dunbrack RL, Brennan TA, Andrake MD, Zhou Y, Serebriiskii IG, Slifker M, Alpaugh K, Dulaimi E, Palma N, Hoffman-Censits J, Bilusic M, Wong YN, Kutikov A, Viterbo R, Greenberg RE, Chen DY, Lallas CD, Trabulsi EJ, Yelensky R, McConkey DJ, Miller VA, Golemis EA, Ross EA. Defects in DNA repair genes predict response to Neoadjuvant cisplatin-based chemotherapy in muscle-invasive bladder cancer. Eur Urol. 2015;68(6):959–67.
170. Plimack ER, Tangen C, Plets M, Kokate R, Xiu J, Nabhan C, Ross EA, Grundy E, Choi W, Dinney CPN, Lee IC, Fong M, Lucia MS, Daneshmand S, Theodorescu D, Goldkorn A, Lerner SP, Flaig TW, McConkey DJ. Correlative analysis of ATM, RB1, ERCC2, and FANCC mutations and pathologic complete response after Neoadjuvant chemotherapy in patients with muscle-invasive bladder cancer: results from the SWOG S1314 trial. Eur Urol. 2024;86(4):297–300.
171. Posada JM, Yakirevich E, Kamat AM, Sood A, Jacob JM, Bratslavsky G, Grivas P, Spiess PE, Li R, Necchi A, Mega AE, Golijanin DJ, Pavlick D, Huang RSP, Lin D, Danziger N, Sokol ES, Sivakumar S, Ross JS, Cheng L. Characterizing the genomic landscape of the micropapillary subtype of urothelial carcinoma of the bladder harboring activating extracellular mutations of ERBB2. Mod Pathol. 2024;37(3):100424.
172. Priolo C, Khabibullin D, Reznik E, Filippakis H, Ogórek B, Kavanagh TR, Nijmeh J, Herbert ZT, Asara JM, Kwiatkowski DJ, Wu CL, Henske EP. Impairment of gamma-glutamyl transferase 1 activity in the metabolic pathogenesis of chromophobe renal cell carcinoma. Proc Natl Acad Sci USA. 2018;115(27):E6274–e6282.
173. Pritchard CC, Morrissey C, Kumar A, Zhang X, Smith C, Coleman I, Salipante SJ, Milbank J, Yu M, Grady WM, Tait JF, Corey E, Vessella RL, Walsh T, Shendure J, Nelson PS. Complex MSH2 and MSH6 mutations in hypermutated microsatellite unstable advanced prostate cancer. Nat Commun. 2014;5(1)
174. Przybycin CG, Magi-Galluzzi C, McKenney JK. Hereditary syndromes with associated renal neoplasia: a practical guide to histologic recognition in renal tumor resection specimens. Adv Anat Pathol. 2013;20(4):245–63.
175. Przybycin CG, McKenney JK, Reynolds JP, Campbell S, Zhou M, Karafa MT, Magi-Galluzzi C. Rhabdoid differentiation is associated with aggressive behavior in renal cell carcinoma: a clinicopathologic analysis of 76 cases with clinical follow-up. Am J Surg Pathol. 2014;38(9):1260–5.
176. Rao Q, Williamson SR, Zhang S, Eble JN, Grignon DJ, Wang M, Zhou XJ, Huang W, Tan PH, Maclennan GT, Cheng L. TFE3 break-apart FISH has a higher sensitivity for Xp11.2 translocation-associated renal cell carcinoma compared with TFE3 or cathepsin K immunohistochemical staining alone: expanding the morphologic spectrum. Am J Surg Pathol. 2013;37(6):804–15.
177. Raspollini MR, Sardi I, Giunti L, Di Lollo S, Baroni G, Stomaci N, Menghetti I, Franchi A. Plasmacytoid urothelial carcinoma of the urinary bladder: clinicopathologic, immunohistochemical, ultrastructural, and molecular analysis of a case series. Hum Pathol. 2011;42(8):1149–58.
178. Ricketts CJ, Forman JR, Rattenberry E, Bradshaw N, Lalloo F, Izatt L, Cole TR, Armstrong R, Kumar VK, Morrison PJ, Atkinson AB, Douglas F, Ball SG, Cook J, Srirangalingam U, Killick P, Kirby G, Aylwin S, Woodward ER, Evans DG, Hodgson SV, Murday V, Chew SL, Connell JM, Blundell TL, Macdonald F, Maher ER. Tumor risks and genotype-phenotype-proteotype analysis in 358 patients with germline mutations in SDHB and SDHD. Hum Mutat. 2010;31(1):41–51.
179. Ricketts CJ, Shuch B, Vocke CD, Metwalli AR, Bratslavsky G, Middelton L, Yang Y, Wei MH, Pautler SE, Peterson J, Stolle CA, Zbar B, Merino MJ, Schmidt LS, Pinto PA, Srinivasan R, Pacak K, Linehan WM. Succinate dehydrogenase kidney cancer: an aggressive example of the Warburg effect in cancer. J Urol. 2012;188(6):2063–71.
180. Rini B, Goddard A, Knezevic D, Maddala T, Zhou M, Aydin H, Campbell S, Elson P, Koscielny S, Lopatin M, Svedman C, Martini JF, Williams JA, Verkarre V, Radulescu C, Neuzillet Y, Hemmerlé I, Timsit MO, Tsiatis AC, Bonham M, Lebret T, Mejean A, Escudier B. A 16-gene assay to predict recurrence after surgery in localised renal cell carcinoma: development and validation studies. Lancet Oncol. 2015;16(6):676–85.
181. Rini BI, Plimack ER, Stus V, Gafanov R, Hawkins R, Nosov D, Pouliot F, Alekseev B, Soulières D, Melichar B, Vynnychenko I, Kryzhanivska A, Bondarenko I, Azevedo SJ, Borchiellini D, Szczylik C, Markus M, McDermott RS, Bedke J, Tartas S, Chang Y-H, Tamada S, Shou Q, Perini RF, Chen M, Atkins MB, Powles T. Pembrolizumab plus Axitinib versus Sunitinib for advanced renal-cell carcinoma. N Engl J Med. 2019;380(12):1116–27.
182. Risbridger GP, Taylor RA, Clouston D, Sliwinski A, Thorne H, Hunter S, Li J, Mitchell G, Murphy D, Frydenberg M, Pook D, Pedersen J, Toivanen R, Wang H, Papargiris M, Lawrence MG, Bolton DM. Patient-derived xenografts reveal that Intraductal carcinoma of the prostate is a prominent pathology in BRCA2 mutation carriers with prostate cancer and correlates with poor prognosis. Eur Urol. 2015;67(3):496–503.
183. Roberts SA, Lawrence MS, Klimczak LJ, Grimm SA, Fargo D, Stojanov P, Kiezun A, Kryukov GV, Carter SL, Saksena G, Harris S, Shah RR, Resnick MA, Getz G, Gordenin DA. An APOBEC cytidine deaminase mutagenesis pattern is widespread in human cancers. Nat Genet. 2013;45(9):970–6.
184. Robertson AG, Kim J, Al-Ahmadie H, Bellmunt J, Guo G, Cherniack AD, Hinoue T, Laird PW, Hoadley KA, Akbani R. Comprehensive molecular

characterization of muscle-invasive bladder cancer. Cell. 2017a;171(3):540–56. e525

185. Robertson AG, Kim J, Al-Ahmadie H, Bellmunt J, Guo G, Cherniack AD, Hinoue T, Laird PW, Hoadley KA, Akbani R, Castro MAA, Gibb EA, Kanchi RS, Gordenin DA, Shukla SA, Sanchez-Vega F, Hansel DE, Czerniak BA, Reuter VE, Su X, de Sa Carvalho B, Chagas VS, Mungall KL, Sadeghi S, Pedamallu CS, Lu Y, Klimczak LJ, Zhang J, Choo C, Ojesina AI, Bullman S, Leraas KM, Lichtenberg TM, Wu CJ, Schultz N, Getz G, Meyerson M, Mills GB, McConkey DJ, Weinstein JN, Kwiatkowski DJ, Lerner SP. Comprehensive molecular characterization of muscle-invasive bladder cancer. Cell. 2017b;171(3):540–56.
186. Robinson D, Van Allen EM, Wu YM, Schultz N, Lonigro RJ, Mosquera JM, Montgomery B, Taplin ME, Pritchard CC, Attard G, Beltran H, Abida W, Bradley RK, Vinson J, Cao X, Vats P, Kunju LP, Hussain M, Feng FY, Tomlins SA, Cooney KA, Smith DC, Brennan C, Siddiqui J, Mehra R, Chen Y, Rathkopf DE, Morris MJ, Solomon SB, Durack JC, Reuter VE, Gopalan A, Gao J, Loda M, Lis RT, Bowden M, Balk SP, Gaviola G, Sougnez C, Gupta M, Yu EY, Mostaghel EA, Cheng HH, Mulcahy H, True LD, Plymate SR, Dvinge H, Ferraldeschi R, Flohr P, Miranda S, Zafeiriou Z, Tunariu N, Mateo J, Perez-Lopez R, Demichelis F, Robinson BD, Schiffman M, Nanus DM, Tagawa ST, Sigaras A, Eng KW, Elemento O, Sboner A, Heath EI, Scher HI, Pienta KJ, Kantoff P, de Bono JS, Rubin MA, Nelson PS, Garraway LA, Sawyers CL, Chinnaiyan AM. Integrative clinical genomics of advanced prostate cancer. Cell. 2015;161(5):1215–28.
187. Rosenberg JE, Hoffman-Censits J, Powles T, van der Heijden MS, Balar AV, Necchi A, Dawson N, O'Donnell PH, Balmanoukian A, Loriot Y, Srinivas S, Retz MM, Grivas P, Joseph RW, Galsky MD, Fleming MT, Petrylak DP, Perez-Gracia JL, Burris HA, Castellano D, Canil C, Bellmunt J, Bajorin D, Nickles D, Bourgon R, Frampton GM, Cui N, Mariathasan S, Abidoye O, Fine GD, Dreicer R. Atezolizumab in patients with locally advanced and metastatic urothelial carcinoma who have progressed following treatment with platinum-based chemotherapy: a single-arm, multicentre, phase 2 trial. Lancet. 2016;387(10031):1909–20.
188. Ross RL, Askham JM, Knowles MA. PIK3CA mutation spectrum in urothelial carcinoma reflects cell context-dependent signaling and phenotypic outputs. Oncogene. 2013;32(6):768–76.
189. Sahai E, Astsaturov I, Cukierman E, DeNardo DG, Egeblad M, Evans RM, Fearon D, Greten FR, Hingorani SR, Hunter T, Hynes RO, Jain RK, Janowitz T, Jorgensen C, Kimmelman AC, Kolonin MG, Maki RG, Powers RS, Puré E, Ramirez DC, Scherz-Shouval R, Sherman MH, Stewart S, Tlsty TD, Tuveson DA, Watt FM, Weaver V, Weeraratna AT, Werb Z. A framework for advancing our understanding of cancer-associated fibroblasts. Nat Rev Cancer. 2020;20(3):174–86.
190. Sanguedolce F, Russo D, Mancini V, Selvaggio O, Calo B, Carrieri G, Cormio L. Prognostic and therapeutic role of HER2 expression in micropapillary carcinoma of the bladder. Mol Clin Oncol. 2019;10(2):205–13.
191. Sato Y. Integrated molecular analysis of clear-cell renal cell carcinoma. Nat Genet. 2013;45:860–7.
192. Schmidt L, Junker K, Nakaigawa N, Kinjerski T, Weirich G, Miller M, Lubensky I, Neumann HP, Brauch H, Decker J, Vocke C, Brown JA, Jenkins R, Richard S, Bergerheim U, Gerrard B, Dean M, Linehan WM, Zbar B. Novel mutations of the MET proto-oncogene in papillary renal carcinomas. Oncogene. 1999;18(14):2343–50.
193. Schmidt LS, Linehan WM. FLCN: the causative gene for Birt-Hogg-Dubé syndrome. Gene. 2018;640:28–42.
194. Schödel J, Mole DR, Ratcliffe PJ. Pan-genomic binding of hypoxia-inducible transcription factors. Biol Chem. 2013;394(4):507–17.
195. Schweizer MT, Antonarakis ES, Bismar TA, Guedes LB, Cheng HH, Tretiakova MS, Vakar-Lopez F, Klemfuss N, Konnick EQ, Mostaghel EA, Hsieh AC, Nelson PS, Yu EY, Montgomery RB, True LD, Epstein JI, Lotan TL, Pritchard CC. Genomic characterization of prostatic ductal adenocarcinoma identifies a high prevalence of DNA repair gene mutations. JCO Precis Oncol. 2019;3:1–9.
196. Schweizer MT, Cheng HH, Tretiakova MS, Vakar-Lopez F, Klemfuss N, Konnick EQ, Mostaghel EA, Nelson PS, Yu EY, Montgomery B, True LD, Pritchard CC. Mismatch repair deficiency may be common in ductal adenocarcinoma of the prostate. Oncotarget. 2016;7(50):82504–10.
197. Sciacovelli M, Gonçalves E, Johnson TI, Zecchini VR, da Costa ASH, Gaude E, Drubbel AV, Theobald SJ, Abbo SR, Tran MGB, Rajeeve V, Cardaci S, Foster S, Yun H, Cutillas P, Warren A, Gnanapragasam V, Gottlieb E, Franze K, Huntly B, Maher ER, Maxwell PH, Saez-Rodriguez J, Frezza C. Fumarate is an epigenetic modifier that elicits epithelial-to-mesenchymal transition. Nature. 2016;537(7621):544–7.
198. Seiler R, Gibb EA, Wang NQ, Oo HZ, Lam H-M, van Kessel KE, Voskuilen CS, Winters B, Erho N, Takhar MM. Divergent biological response to neoadjuvant chemotherapy in muscle-invasive bladder cancer. Clin Cancer Res. 2019;25(16):5082–93.
199. Shuch B. Defining early-onset kidney cancer: implications for germline and somatic mutation testing and clinical management. J Clin Oncol. 2014;32:431–7.
200. Shuch B, Vourganti S, Ricketts CJ, Middleton L, Peterson J, Merino MJ, Metwalli AR, Srinivasan R, Linehan WM. Defining early-onset kidney cancer: implications for germline and somatic mutation testing and clinical management. J Clin Oncol. 2014;32(5):431–7.

201. Sjödahl G, Eriksson P, Liedberg F, Höglund M. Molecular classification of urothelial carcinoma: global mRNA classification versus tumour-cell phenotype classification. J Pathol. 2017;242(1):113–25.
202. Sjödahl G, Lauss M, Lövgren K, Chebil G, Gudjonsson S, Veerla S, Patschan O, Aine M, Fernö M, Ringnér M, Månsson W, Liedberg F, Lindgren D, Höglund M. A molecular taxonomy for urothelial carcinoma. Clin Cancer Res. 2012;18(12):3377–86.
203. Smith SC, Trpkov K, Chen YB, Mehra R, Sirohi D, Ohe C, Cani AK, Hovelson DH, Omata K, McHugh JB, Jochum W, Colecchia M, Amin M, Divatia MK, Hes O, Menon S, Werneck da Cunha I, Tripodi S, Brimo F, Gill AJ, Osunkoya AO, Magi-Galluzzi C, Sibony M, Williamson SR, Nesi G, Picken MM, Maclean F, Agaimy A, Cheng L, Epstein JI, Reuter VE, Tickoo SK, Tomlins SA, Amin MB. Tubulocystic carcinoma of the kidney with poorly differentiated foci: a frequent morphologic pattern of fumarate hydratase-deficient renal cell carcinoma. Am J Surg Pathol. 2016;40(11):1457–72.
204. Strandgaard T, Nordentoft I, Birkenkamp-Demtröder K, Salminen L, Prip F, Rasmussen J, Andreasen TG, Lindskrog SV, Christensen E, Lamy P, Knudsen M, Steiniche T, Jensen JB, Dyrskjøt L. Field cancerization is associated with tumor development, T-cell exhaustion, and clinical outcomes in bladder cancer. Eur Urol. 2024;85(1):82–92.
205. Sugawara E, Togashi Y, Kuroda N, Sakata S, Hatano S, Asaka R, Yuasa T, Yonese J, Kitagawa M, Mano H, Ishikawa Y, Takeuchi K. Identification of anaplastic lymphoma kinase fusions in renal cancer: large-scale immunohistochemical screening by the intercalated antibody-enhanced polymer method. Cancer. 2012;118(18):4427–36.
206. Sule N, Yakupoglu U, Shen SS, Krishnan B, Yang G, Lerner S, Sheikh-Hamad D, Truong LD. Calcium oxalate deposition in renal cell carcinoma associated with acquired cystic kidney disease: a comprehensive study. Am J Surg Pathol. 2005;29(4):443–51.
207. Sweeney C, Bracarda S, Sternberg CN, Chi KN, Olmos D, Sandhu S, Massard C, Matsubara N, Alekseev B, Parnis F, Atduev V, Buchschacher GL, Gafanov R, Corrales L, Borre M, Stroyakovskiy D, Alves GV, Bournakis E, Puente J, Harle-Yge M-L, Gallo J, Chen G, Hanover J, Wongchenko MJ, Garcia J, de Bono JS. Ipatasertib plus abiraterone and prednisolone in metastatic castration-resistant prostate cancer (IPATential150): a multicentre, randomised, double-blind, phase 3 trial. Lancet. 2021;398(10295):131–42.
208. Sweis RF, Spranger S, Bao R, Paner GP, Stadler WM, Steinberg G, Gajewski TF. Molecular drivers of the non-T-cell-inflamed tumor microenvironment in urothelial bladder cancer. Cancer Immunol Res. 2016;4(7):563–8.
209. Sylvester RJ, Rodríguez O, Hernández V, Turturica D, Bauerová L, Bruins HM, Bründl J, van der Kwast TH, Brisuda A, Rubio-Briones J, Seles M, Hentschel AE, Kusuma VRM, Huebner N, Cotte J, Mertens LS, Volanis D, Cussenot O, Subiela Henríquez JD, de la Peña E, Pisano F, Pešl M, van der Heijden AG, Herdegen S, Zlotta AR, Hacek J, Calatrava A, Mannweiler S, Bosschieter J, Ashabere D, Haitel A, Côté JF, El Sheikh S, Lunelli L, Algaba F, Alemany I, Soria F, Runneboom W, Breyer J, Nieuwenhuijzen JA, Llorente C, Molinaro L, Hulsbergen-van de Kaa CA, Evert M, Kiemeney L, N'Dow J, Plass K, Čapoun O, Soukup V, Dominguez-Escrig JL, Cohen D, Palou J, Gontero P, Burger M, Zigeuner R, Mostafid AH, Shariat SF, Rouprêt M, Compérat EM, Babjuk M, van Rhijn BWG. European Association of Urology (EAU) prognostic factor risk groups for non-muscle-invasive bladder cancer (NMIBC) incorporating the WHO 2004/2016 and WHO 1973 classification systems for grade: an update from the EAU NMIBC guidelines panel. Eur Urol. 2021;79(4):480–8.
210. Taber A, Christensen E, Lamy P, Nordentoft I, Prip F, Lindskrog SV, Birkenkamp-Demtröder K, Okholm TLH, Knudsen M, Pedersen JS. Molecular correlates of cisplatin-based chemotherapy response in muscle invasive bladder cancer by integrated multi-omics analysis. Nat Commun. 2020;11(1):4858.
211. Taneja SS. Re: germline BRCA mutations are associated with higher risk of nodal involvement, distant metastasis, and poor survival outcomes in prostate cancer. J Urol. 2013;190(6):2093–4.
212. Thomsen MB, Nordentoft I, Lamy P, Høyer S, Vang S, Hedegaard J, Borre M, Jensen JB, Ørntoft TF, Dyrskjøt L. Spatial and temporal clonal evolution during development of metastatic urothelial carcinoma. Mol Oncol. 2016;10(9):1450–60.
213. Tickoo SK, de Peralta-Venturina MN, Harik LR, Worcester HD, Salama ME, Young AN, Moch H, Amin MB. Spectrum of epithelial neoplasms in end-stage renal disease: an experience from 66 tumor-bearing kidneys with emphasis on histologic patterns distinct from those in sporadic adult renal neoplasia. Am J Surg Pathol. 2006;30(2):141–53.
214. Tomlinson DC, Baldo O, Harnden P, Knowles MA. FGFR3 protein expression and its relationship to mutation status and prognostic variables in bladder cancer. J Pathol. 2007;213(1):91–8.
215. Tomlinson IP, Alam NA, Rowan AJ, Barclay E, Jaeger EE, Kelsell D, Leigh I, Gorman P, Lamlum H, Rahman S, Roylance RR, Olpin S, Bevan S, Barker K, Hearle N, Houlston RS, Kiuru M, Lehtonen R, Karhu A, Vilkki S, Laiho P, Eklund C, Vierimaa O, Aittomäki K, Hietala M, Sistonen P, Paetau A, Salovaara R, Herva R, Launonen V, Aaltonen LA. Germline mutations in FH predispose to dominantly inherited uterine fibroids, skin leiomyomata and papillary renal cell cancer. Nat Genet. 2002;30(4):406–10.
216. Tretiakova MS, Wang W, Wu Y, Tykodi SS, True L, Liu YJ. Gene fusion analysis in renal cell carcinoma by fusion Plex RNA-sequencing and correlations of molecular findings with clinicopathological features. Genes Chromosomes Cancer. 2020;59(1):40–9.

217. Trpkov K, Hes O. New and emerging renal entities: a perspective post-<scp>WHO</scp> 2016 classification. Histopathology. 2018;74(1):31–59.
218. Trpkov K, Williamson SR, Gao Y, Martinek P, Cheng L, Sangoi AR, Yilmaz A, Wang C, et al. Low-grade oncocytic tumour of kidney (CD117-negative, cytokeratin 7-positive): a distinct entity? Histopathology. 2019;75(2):174–84.
219. Trpkov K, Williamson SR, Gill AJ, Adeniran AJ, Agaimy A, Alaghehbandan R, Amin MB, Argani P, Chen Y-B, Cheng L, Epstein JI, Cheville JC, Comperat E, da Cunha IW, Gordetsky JB, Gupta S, He H, Hirsch MS, Humphrey PA, Kapur P, Kojima F, Lopez JI, Maclean F, Magi-Galluzzi C, McKenney JK, Mehra R, Menon S, Netto GJ, Przybycin CG, Rao P, Rao Q, Reuter VE, Saleeb RM, Shah RB, Smith SC, Tickoo S, Tretiakova MS, True L, Verkarre V, Wobker SE, Zhou M, Hes O. Novel, emerging and provisional renal entities: the genitourinary pathology society (GUPS) update on renal neoplasia. Mod Pathol. 2021;34(6):1167–84.
220. Tsujino T, Takai T, Hinohara K, Gui F, Tsutsumi T, Bai X, Miao C, Feng C, Gui B, Sztupinszki Z, Simoneau A, Xie N, Fazli L, Dong X, Azuma H, Choudhury AD, Mouw KW, Szallasi Z, Zou L, Kibel AS, Jia L. CRISPR screens reveal genetic determinants of PARP inhibitor sensitivity and resistance in prostate cancer. Nat Commun. 2023;14(1):252.
221. Tuffaha H, Edmunds K, Fairbairn D, Roberts MJ, Chambers S, Smith DP, Horvath L, Arora S, Scuffham P. Guidelines for genetic testing in prostate cancer: a scoping review. Prostate Cancer Prostatic Dis. 2023;27(4):594–603.
222. Tukachinsky H, Madison RW, Chung JH, Gjoerup OV, Severson EA, Dennis L, Fendler BJ, Morley S, Zhong L, Graf RP, Ross JS, Alexander BM, Abida W, Chowdhury S, Ryan CJ, Fizazi K, Golsorkhi T, Watkins SP, Simmons A, Loehr A, Venstrom JM, Oxnard GR. Genomic analysis of circulating tumor DNA in 3,334 patients with advanced prostate cancer identifies targetable BRCA alterations and AR resistance mechanisms. Clin Cancer Res. 2021;27(11):3094–105.
223. Turajlic S, et al. Tracking cancer evolution reveals constrained routes to metastases: TRACERx renal. Cell. 2018;173(3):581–94.
224. Turner NC, Oliveira M, Howell SJ, Dalenc F, Cortes J, Gomez Moreno HL, Hu X, Jhaveri K, Krivorotko P, Loibl S, Morales Murillo S, Okera M, Park YH, Sohn J, Toi M, Tokunaga E, Yousef S, Zhukova L, de Bruin EC, Grinsted L, Schiavon G, Foxley A, Rugo HS. Capivasertib in hormone receptor–positive advanced breast cancer. N Engl J Med. 2023;388(22):2058–70.
225. Udager AM, Mehra R. Morphologic, molecular, and taxonomic evolution of renal cell carcinoma: a conceptual perspective with emphasis on updates to the 2016 World Health Organization classification. Arch Pathol Lab Med. 2016;140(10):1026–37.
226. Urology, E. A. o. EAU Guidelines: Prostate Cancer. The Netherlands: Arnhem; 2025.
227. Valsecchi AA, Dionisio R, Panepinto O, Paparo J, Palicelli A, Vignani F, Di Maio M. Frequency of germline and somatic BRCA1 and BRCA2 mutations in prostate cancer: an updated systematic review and meta-analysis. Cancer. 2023;15(9):2435.
228. Van Allen EM, Mouw KW, Kim P, Iyer G, Wagle N, Al-Ahmadie H, Zhu C, Ostrovnaya I, Kryukov GV, O'Connor KW. Somatic ERCC2 mutations correlate with cisplatin sensitivity in muscle-invasive urothelial carcinoma. Cancer Discov. 2014;4(10):1140–53.
229. van Rhijn BWG, Burger M, Lotan Y, Solsona E, Stief CG, Sylvester RJ, Witjes JA, Zlotta AR. Recurrence and progression of disease in non–muscle-invasive bladder cancer: from epidemiology to treatment strategy. Eur Urol. 2009;56(3):430–42.
230. Vandekerkhove G, Struss WJ, Annala M, Kallio HML, Khalaf D, Warner EW, Herberts C, Ritch E, Beja K, Loktionova Y, Hurtado-Coll A, Fazli L, So A, Black PC, Nykter M, Tammela T, Chi KN, Gleave ME, Wyatt AW. Circulating tumor DNA abundance and potential utility in De novo metastatic prostate cancer. Eur Urol. 2019;75(4):667–75.
231. Voss MH, Hakimi AA, Pham CG, Brannon AR, Chen Y-B, Cunha LF, Akin O, Liu H, Takeda S, Scott SN, Socci ND, Viale A, Schultz N, Sander C, Reuter VE, Russo P, Cheng EH, Motzer RJ, Berger MF, Hsieh JJ. Tumor genetic analyses of patients with metastatic renal cell carcinoma and extended benefit from mTOR inhibitor therapy. Clin Cancer Res. 2014a;20(7):1955–64.
232. Voss MH, Hakimi AA, Pham CG, Brannon AR, Chen YB, Cunha LF, Akin O, Liu H, Takeda S, Scott SN, Socci ND, Viale A, Schultz N, Sander C, Reuter VE, Russo P, Cheng EH, Motzer RJ, Berger MF, Hsieh JJ. Tumor genetic analyses of patients with metastatic renal cell carcinoma and extended benefit from mTOR inhibitor therapy. Clin Cancer Res. 2014b;20(7):1955–64.
233. Wang J, Huang R, Cone B, Kang S-H, Setoodeh R, Sisk A, Sajed D, Shuch B, Sowalsky A, Ye H. ELOC-mutated renal cell carcinoma is a rare indolent tumor with distinctive genomic characteristics. Mod Pathol. 2025;38:100777.
234. Wang J, Papanicolau-Sengos A, Chintala S, Wei L, Liu B, Hu Q, Miles KM, Conroy JM, Glenn ST, Costantini M, Magi-Galluzzi C, Signoretti S, Choueiri T, Gallucci M, Sentinelli S, Fazio VM, Poeta ML, Liu S, Morrison C, Pili R. Collecting duct carcinoma of the kidney is associated with CDKN2A deletion and SLC family gene up-regulation. Oncotarget. 2016;7(21):29901–15.
235. Wang Z, Kim TB, Peng B, Karam J, Creighton C, Joon A, Kawakami F, Trevisan P, Jonasch E, Chow CW, Canales JR, Tamboli P, Tannir N, Wood C, Monzon F, Baggerly K, Varella-Garcia M, Czerniak B, Wistuba I, Mills G, Shaw K, Chen K, Sircar K. Sarcomatoid renal cell carcinoma has a distinct

molecular pathogenesis, driver mutation profile, and transcriptional landscape. Clin Cancer Res. 2017;23(21):6686–96.
236. Warren AY, Harrison D. WHO/ISUP classification, grading and pathological staging of renal cell carcinoma: standards and controversies. World J Urol. 2018;36(12):1913–26.
237. Warrick JI, Walter V, Yamashita H, Chung E, Shuman L, Amponsa VO, Zheng Z, Chan W, Whitcomb TL, Yue F. FOXA1, GATA3 and PPARɣ cooperate to drive luminal subtype in bladder cancer: a molecular analysis of established human cell lines. Sci Rep. 2016;6(1):38531.
238. Wasco MJ, Daignault S, Zhang Y, Kunju LP, Kinnaman M, Braun T, Lee CT, Shah RB. Urothelial carcinoma with divergent histologic differentiation (mixed histologic features) predicts the presence of locally advanced bladder cancer when detected at transurethral resection. Urology. 2007;70(1):69–74.
239. Wei L, Wang J, Lampert E, Schlanger S, DePriest AD, Hu Q, Gomez EC, Murakam M, Glenn ST, Conroy J, Morrison C, Azabdaftari G, Mohler JL, Liu S, Heemers HV. Intratumoral and intertumoral genomic heterogeneity of multifocal localized prostate cancer impacts molecular classifications and genomic prognosticators. Eur Urol. 2017;71(2):183–92.
240. Williams SB, Black PC, Dyrskjøt L, Seiler R, Schmitz-Dräger B, Nawroth R, Todenhöfer T, Kamat AM, et al. A consensus molecular classification of muscle-invasive bladder cancer. Eur Urol. 2020;77(4):e105–6.
241. Williams SV, Hurst CD, Knowles MA. Oncogenic FGFR3 gene fusions in bladder cancer. Hum Mol Genet. 2013;22(4):795–803.
242. Williamson SR, Eble JN, Cheng L, Grignon DJ. Clear cell papillary renal cell carcinoma: differential diagnosis and extended immunohistochemical profile. Mod Pathol. 2013;26(5):697–708.
243. Williamson SR, Gill AJ, Argani P, Chen Y-B, Egevad L, Kristiansen G, Grignon DJ, Hes O. Report from the International Society of Urological Pathology (ISUP) consultation conference on molecular pathology of urogenital cancers: III: molecular pathology of kidney cancer. Am J Surg Pathol. 2020a;44(7):e47–65.
244. Williamson SR, Gill AJ, Argani P, Chen YB, Egevad L, Kristiansen G, Grignon DJ, Hes O. Report from the International Society of Urological Pathology (ISUP) consultation conference on molecular pathology of urogenital cancers: III: molecular pathology of kidney cancer. Am J Surg Pathol. 2020b;44(7):e47–65.
245. Wu J, Lin Y, Yang K, Liu X, Wang H, Yu T, Tao R, Guo J, Chen L, Cheng H, Lou F, Cao S, Yu W, Hu H, Ye D. Clinical effectiveness of a multitarget urine DNA test for urothelial carcinoma detection: a double-blinded, multicenter, prospective trial. Mol Cancer. 2024;23(1):57.
246. Xia QY, Wang Z, Chen N, Gan HL, Teng XD, Shi SS, Wang X, Wei X, Ye SB, Li R, Ma HH, Lu ZF, Zhou XJ, Rao Q. Xp11.2 translocation renal cell carcinoma with NONO-TFE3 gene fusion: morphology, prognosis, and potential pitfall in detecting TFE3 gene rearrangement. Mod Pathol. 2017;30(3):416–26.
247. Yamamoto A, Tamada T, Higaki A, Arita Y, Ueno Y, Murakami T, Jinzaki M. Evaluation of the clinical behavior of unclassified renal cell carcinoma and its imaging findings on computed tomography and magnetic resonance imaging based on World Health Organization (WHO) 2022. Jpn J Radiol. 2024;42(1):78–86.
248. Yuan S, Chen P, Sun F, Li T. Efficacy and safety of Olaparib plus Abiraterone versus placebo plus Abiraterone in the first-line treatment of patients with asymptomatic/mildly symptomatic and symptomatic metastatic castration-resistant prostate cancer: analyses from the phase 3 PROpel trial. Eur Urol Oncol. 2025; https://doi.org/10.1016/j.euo.2024.09.013.
249. Zahraeifard S, Xiao Z, So JY, Ahad A, Montoya S, Park WY, Sornapudi T, Andohkow T, Read A, Kedei N, Koparde V, Yang H, Lee M, Wong N, Cam M, Wang K, Ruppin E, Luo J, Hollander C, Yang L. Loss of tumor suppressors promotes inflammatory tumor microenvironment and enhances LAG3+T cell mediated immune suppression. Nat Commun. 2024;15(1):5873.
250. Zhao RN, Nie LH, Gong R, Wang JZ, Wazir R, Liu LR, Song TR, Wei Q. Active targeted therapy for metastatic collecting duct carcinoma of the kidney: a case report and review of the literature. Int Urol Nephrol. 2013;45(4):1017–21.
251. Zimmermann M, Murina O, Reijns MAM, Agathanggelou A, Challis R, Tarnauskaitė Ž, Muir M, Fluteau A, Aregger M, McEwan A, Yuan W, Clarke M, Lambros MB, Paneesha S, Moss P, Chandrashekhar M, Angers S, Moffat J, Brunton VG, Hart T, de Bono J, Stankovic T, Jackson AP, Durocher D. CRISPR screens identify genomic ribonucleotides as a source of PARP-trapping lesions. Nature. 2018;559(7713):285–9.

14 Next-Generation Sequencing in Central Nervous System Tumor Diagnostics

Antonio d'Amati, Filippo Nozzoli, and Marco Gessi

Introduction

The classification of central nervous system (CNS) tumors has undergone a profound transformation over the past decade, driven by advances in molecular diagnostics and the increasing integration of molecular data into routine neuropathology practice.

The publication of the 2016 WHO Classification of Tumors of the Central Nervous System (WHO CNS 4+ 2016) marked the beginning of this paradigm shift, which culminated in the last edition (WHO CNS 5 2021), that more basically incorporated molecular criteria into the diagnostic framework for many tumor types [1]. Key examples of this evolution include the delineation of *IDH*-mutant versus *IDH*-wild-type diffuse gliomas, the identification of H3 *K27*-altered diffuse midline gliomas, and the recognition of relatively rare but diagnostically critical fusion-driven entities, such as *ZFTA*-fused ependymomas and *BCOR*-altered embryonal tumors [2–4]. In pediatric neuro-oncology, in particular, the integration of molecular markers has enabled more precise risk stratification and redefinition of tumor classes, such as the subdivision of medulloblastomas (MB) into molecular subgroups with distinct prognoses and therapeutic implications [5–7]. After the WHO CNS 5 classification, the cIMPACT-NOW consortium initiative provided and is providing continuous interim updates to CNS tumor classification, bridging the gap between WHO editions and pinpointing the most significative advances in CNS tumor biology, which may have potential significance in CNS tumor classification, or clarifying issues still present in the current WHO CNS classification. Among others, its Update 6, cIMPACT-NOW, acknowledged the utility of genome-wide DNA methylation profiling in CNS tumor diagnostics, recognizing its potential to refine tumor classification and to identify novel entities [8]. Besides WHO classification and cIMPACT-NOW publications, also the European Association of Neuro-Oncology (EANO) provided comprehensive recommendations for molecular testing in gliomas, glioneuronal, and neuronal tumors. They advocate for the assessment of predictive genetic alterations, including *BRAF, EGFR, FGFR1-3, NTRK1-3*, and *IDH1/2* mutations, to inform targeted therapy decisions. The guidelines also emphasize standardized reporting and interpretation of molecular findings, highlighting the importance of next-generation sequencing (NGS)

A. d'Amati · M. Gessi (✉)
Pathology Division, Department of Life Sciences and Public Health, Policlinico Universitario "A. Gemelli" IRCCS, Università Cattolica Sacro Cuore, Rome, Italy
e-mail: marco.gessi@policlinicogemelli.it; marco.gessi@unicatt.it

F. Nozzoli
Histopathology and Molecular Diagnostics, Careggi University Hospital, Florence, Italy
e-mail: filippo.nozzoli@unifi.it

© The Author(s), under exclusive license to Springer Nature Switzerland AG 2026

S. Sioletic, L. Coppola (eds.), *Next-Generation Sequencing in Solid Tumor Histopathology*, Current Clinical Pathology, https://doi.org/10.1007/978-3-032-18790-1_14

in identifying actionable targets and facilitating personalized treatment strategies [9, 10].

As molecular data become increasingly central to neuro-oncology, the role of neuropathologist is pivotal being uniquely positioned to reconcile molecular alterations—such as mutations, fusions, copy number variations, and methylation signatures—with histologic patterns, immunophenotypes, radiologic features, and clinical behavior. This role is particularly crucial when dealing with rare or uncertain variants, where classification may depend as much on molecular evidence as on morphologic judgment.

Next-Generation Sequencing (NGS) in CNS Tumor Diagnostics and Neuro-oncology

NGS technologies have become essential tools in modern neuropathology, enabling the simultaneous analysis of dozens to hundreds of genes with high sensitivity and specificity. NGS-based analysis plays a critical role in identifying both single-nucleotide variants (SNVs) and structural alterations, including gene fusions and CNVs. NGS usually complements other molecular platforms and methods such as DNA methylation profiling, SNP array, array CGH, multiplex ligation-dependent probe amplification (MLPA), or fluorescence in situ hybridization (FISH) and is now incorporated into routine diagnostic workflows in many tertiary centers. On the other hand, techniques like whole-genome sequencing (WGS), whole-exome sequencing (WES) or single-cell analysis remain, to date, mainly discovery tools.

From a diagnostic perspective, NGS-based analysis allows the confirmation of WHO-defined molecular criteria (e.g., presence of *IDH* mutation, *H3* K27M mutation, *1p/19q* codeletion, etc.) and the identification of specific alterations in rare entities (e.g., *MYB*-driven tumors) [11]. Furthermore, NGS may enable the correct diagnosis in "histologically ambiguous" tumors by uncovering defining genetic alterations and permits classification in accordance with WHO CNS5 classification and cIMPACT-NOW consortium recommendations [12].

Prognostically, simultaneous identification of alterations such as *CDKN2A/2B* homozygous deletion, *TERT* promoter mutations, and complex chromosomal alterations confer relevant risk stratification and may influence clinical decision-making [13, 14].

Predictively, NGS analysis may reveal potential therapeutic targets, including *BRAF* ^{V600E} mutations, *NTRK* fusions, *EGFR* amplification or exon 20 insertions, and *ALK* rearrangements, some of which are now eligible for matched targeted therapies or basket trials [15–17]. Moreover, identification of mismatch repair deficiency (MMRd) and high tumor mutational burden (TMB) through NGS may guide the use of immune checkpoint inhibitors, although their role in CNS tumors remains under investigation [18]. Beyond bulk sequencing, emerging approaches such as single-cell and spatial transcriptomics are shedding light on intratumoral heterogeneity and the tumor microenvironment, offering novel perspectives on glioma biology and therapeutic resistance.

The increasing availability of targeted panels, optimized for CNS tumors, has facilitated the implementation of NGS in formalin-fixed paraffin-embedded (FFPE) tissue samples. These neuropathology-oriented panels typically include key genes such as *IDH1, IDH2, TP53, ATRX, BRAF, H3F3A, TERT, EGFR,* and *CDKN2A/2B*, among others.

Targeted NGS panels, which sequence predefined sets of genes or hotspots, offer a practical and cost-effective alternative to WGS and WES, particularly when working with FFPE-derived DNA. Limitations include the potential to miss novel or unexpected variants, structural rearrangements, or selected methylation-defined tumor classes, which require complementary assays (e.g., DNA methylation profiling). Several commercial and institution-specific CNS tumors-focused NGS panels are available (see Table 14.1) [19–22]. Detection of potential germline alterations is becoming more frequent due to larger NGS panel sizes, and it should be managed according to local guidelines [23].

Table 14.1 Representative NGS panels and methylation platforms commonly used in CNS tumor diagnostics, with a focus on their variant coverage and clinical applications

Panel name	Platform	Variants detected	Notes
Oncomine v3	Thermo fisher	Mutations, fusions, CNVs	Used in INFORM cit. pediatric studies
TruSight oncology 500	Illumina	Mutations, CNVs, fusions	Broad panel, DNA + RNA
MSK-IMPACT	Custom (Memorial Sloan Kettering)	Mutations, CNVs	Includes CNS-specific genes
UCSF500	Custom (University of California San Francisco)	Mutations, CNVs	Includes CNS-specific genes
EPIC methylation array	Illumina	Methylation, CNVs (derived)	Used in classifier, MGMT analysis

Many platforms also allow detection, along SNV, of copy number variations (CNVs) and selected gene fusions using DNA-based or hybrid capture assays. Panels that incorporate RNA-sequencing modules can also detect clinically relevant fusions (e.g., *KIAA1549::BRAF, FGFR::TACC, NTRK* fusions), but with limited efficacy since most of these alterations involve noncoding regions which are not or partially represented in most NGS assays. NGS-based CNV detection, especially from targeted or low-pass whole-genome sequencing (lpWGS), allows for genome-wide or locus-specific assessment of chromosomal gains and losses from FFPE-derived DNA. Algorithms such as IchorCNA, CNVkit, control-FREEC, and QDNAseq are commonly used for computational analysis. Despite lower resolution compared to SNP arrays, NGS-based CNV profiling provides valuable insights and is increasingly integrated into routine diagnostics [24].

The interpretation and reporting of molecular variants in central nervous system (CNS) tumors present specific challenges that require a nuanced, integrated approach. Unlike many systemic malignancies, in which variant interpretation is mostly driven by therapeutic implications, in CNS tumors, the primary role of molecular profiling is diagnostic and prognostic.

Interpretation begins with the identification of relevant variants, typically categorized according to established classification frameworks, such as the AMP/ASCO/CAP tiered system. This system stratifies variants into categories based on clinical significance—from tier I (well-established clinical relevance) to tier IV (likely benign) [25, 26]. However, in CNS tumors, variant classification cannot be separated from the broader diagnostic context. For example, an *IDH* mutation is not only pathogenic but diagnostically defining for several glioma types; similarly, $H3^{K27M}$ and *ZFTA::RELA* fusions establish specific entities irrespective of histology.

Databases such as ClinVar, COSMIC, OncoKB, and CIViC are valuable resources, but they often lack CNS-specific granularity, particularly for rare or pediatric tumors [27]. Therefore, expert interpretation and correlation with other findings—histopathology, immunohistochemistry, DNA methylation profiling, and copy number alterations—remain essential.

The reporting of variants should follow structured principles [28]: (1) Clearly indicate the variant type, genomic coordinates, protein change, and allelic frequency; (2) assign a classification tier, and when applicable, include diagnostic or prognostic relevance; (3) contextualize the variant within the integrated diagnosis, especially when it defines or excludes a CNS tumor entity; and (4) flag variants of uncertain significance (VUS) appropriately, avoiding overinterpretation. (5) In pediatric cases or low-grade gliomas, where data may be limited, rare fusions or mutations (e.g., *FGFR1, MYB, BCOR*) may carry significant diagnostic weight despite lacking formal tier I evidence. These must be reported with clarity and awareness of their emerging relevance. Broader panel testing also raises regulatory and ethical issues, particularly regarding incidental germline findings, which require clear policies for reporting and patient counseling.

DNA Methylation Profiling

DNA methylation profiling has emerged as a powerful tool in the integrated diagnosis of CNS tumors. By capturing epigenetic signatures that reflect both developmental origin and neoplastic transformation, methylation-based classification has dramatically improved the precision of CNS tumor diagnostics. Its impact is particularly significant in cases with ambiguous morphology or limited tissue samples. The most widely adopted platform for genome-wide methylation profiling in neuropathology is the Infinium MethylationEPIC BeadChip array (850 k array, Illumina), which interrogates over 850,000 CpG sites across the genome using bisulfite-converted DNA from FFPE tissue. This approach provides high-resolution, quantitative data and is compatible with standard pathology workflows. It requires minimal input DNA (~200–250 ng), making it suitable for small biopsies. In terms of sample type, FFPE samples are usually used with similar results compared to fresh frozen tissue. More recently, nanopore-based methylation analysis, using real-time sequencing of native DNA without bisulfite conversion, has been explored as an alternative [29–32]. While still emerging in clinical practice, Nanopore technology offers the potential for faster turnaround and broader coverage, including non-CpG methylation and structural variants. However, its use in routine CNS tumor diagnostics remains investigational due to current limitations in accuracy, standardization, and computational infrastructure [32].

The most impactful application of DNA methylation profiling in neuropathology is its use for tumor classification via machine learning. The Heidelberg Brain Tumor Classifier, developed by Capper et al., assigns tumor samples to one of over 100 methylation classes based on genome-wide profiles, using a random forest algorithm trained on a large reference cohort [3]. This approach enables objective classification in diagnostically ambiguous cases, including distinguishing histologically similar entities (e.g., ependymoma subtypes, glioblastoma vs. CNS embryonal tumors), identifying novel or rare tumor classes, and refining initial histologic diagnoses when methylation profiles indicate a different lineage. The classifier outputs a calibrated score (range 0–1), with scores ≥0.9 considered highly confident matches. Copy number profiles, including chromosomal gains, losses, and focal amplifications (e.g., *EGFR, CDKN2A/2B*), are simultaneously generated from the array data and contribute further to the integrated diagnosis. The classifier and its continuously updated versions are now accessible through the new online platform: https://app.epignostix.com (Heidelberg Epignostix Research App). An additional classifier, the NCI/Bethesda from NIH, based and derived from analysis of a different tumor series, is freely available for use: https://methylscape.ccr.cancer.gov/.

DNA methylation profiling represented a cornerstone of the WHO Classification of CNS tumors. However, its role in tumor diagnostics has afterward been better redefined by cIMPACT-NOW publications. The cIMPACT-NOW Update 6 publication underscores the significant role of genome-wide DNA methylation profiling in the diagnostics of central nervous system (CNS) tumors [33]. This update advocates for its application in diagnostically challenging cases and incorporates methylation class assignment into the integrated diagnostic framework. Specifically, it highlights the utility of methylation analysis in (1) enhancing tumor classification, particularly for morphologically ambiguous cases; (2) facilitating risk stratification, exemplified by its application in posterior fossa ependymomas and medulloblastoma subgroups; and (3) identifying and delineating emerging tumor entities. The consensus emphasizes that methylation profiling should not be interpreted in isolation but rather in conjunction with histological examination, immunohistochemistry (IHC), and sequencing data to achieve a comprehensive and accurate diagnosis.

Practical Applications of NGS-Based Analysis in Routine CNS Tumor Diagnostics

Adult-Type Diffuse Gliomas

Diffuse gliomas represent the most common type of primary malignant brain tumor in adults. These neoplasms are characterized by infiltrative growth and variable combinations of nuclear atypia, mitotic activity, microvascular proliferation, and necrosis. The WHO CNS 5 2021 classification marked a turning point in glioma taxonomy, shifting from a primarily histological classification to an integrated model based on both morphological and molecular parameters [34]. According to the current WHO classification, adult-type diffuse gliomas are subdivided into three key molecular entities: astrocytoma, *IDH*-mutant; oligodendroglioma, *IDH*-mutant and chr.1p/19q-codeleted; and glioblastoma, *IDH*-wild type.

Such diagnosis requires the identification of specific genetic alterations that serve as defining criteria. Detection of *IDH, ATRX, TP53*, and *TERT* promoter mutations is fundamental to the classification of gliomas. While IHC represent the first-line method of analysis and covers the majority of cases, these alterations can be detected using different techniques (i.e., RT-based methods, pyrosequencing, MLPA, etc.) or using an NGS-based approach [35]. NGS-based analysis is now widely considered one of the most efficient and scalable methods to capture the required diagnostic and predictive markers in a single assay [34].

The most common alterations in these group of tumors are mostly included in standard NGS panels but robust results with glioma-tailored NGS panel are well documented in literature [36, 37]. In particular, evaluation of *EGFR* amplification, *TERT* promoter mutations and chromosome 7 gain/chromosome 10 loss (+7/−10), mandatory in diffuse glioma affecting adult patients without histological glioblastoma features, can be detected by NGS either through read-depth–based copy number profiling or hybrid capture panels [38]. Also, *CDKN2A/2B* homozygous deletion, marker of grade 4 in *IDH*-mutant astrocytomas and often present in aggressive oligodendroglioma, may also be assessed by copy number profiling, including via NGS-based methods. Moreover, NGS platforms permit identification of rare glioblastoma *IDH*-wt variants such as those with *FGFR3::TACC3* fusion, whose clinical behavior seems not completely overlapping to standard glioblastoma [39]. Notably, costs and TAT limitations may hinder the use of broad NGS panel in routine diagnostics, and "small panel" approach can be considered.

Identification of *IDH*-mutant glioma is pivotal also from a predictive point of view. Targeting *IDH* mutation may have a significant impact on the natural course of *IDH*-mutant gliomas. INDIGO trial demonstrated substantial improvements in progression-free survival in *IDH*-glioma patients treated with vorasidenib [40], recently approved by the Food and Drug Administration (FDA) for grade 2 *IDH*-mutant astrocytomas and oligodendrogliomas. Besides *IDH*, recent studies confirm that glioma-targeted NGS panels not only support diagnostic classification but frequently reveal additional alterations of potential clinical relevance, including *PTEN, NF1, PIK3CA*, and *BRAF* mutations [41]. Moreover, large NGS-based series have demonstrated that a subset of adult gliomas harbor actionable targets, making patients eligible for clinical trials or off-label therapies [42].

MGMT (O6-methylguanine-DNA methyltransferase) promoter methylation is an established predictive biomarker in glioblastoma, associated with improved response to alkylating agents such as temozolomide. While multiple testing methods exist, including MSP (methylation-specific PCR), pyrosequencing, MLPA, and digital PCR, DNA methylation profiling (Illumina EPIC arrays) also provide quantitative methylation data at CpG sites within the *MGMT* promoter region. Pyrosequencing remains the most commonly used and clinically validated method, with cutoffs varying across institutions. Recent studies suggest that machine-learning classifiers trained on EPIC-derived methylation data may enhance reproducibility and allow harmonization across platforms [43] (Table 14.2).

Table 14.2 Summary of key molecular alterations across CNS tumor types

Tumor type	Key mutations/ fusions	CNVs	Methylation class	Clinical relevance
IDH-mutant astrocytoma	IDH1/2, TP53, ATRX	CDKN2A/B del	Adult-type diffuse glioma	Diagnosis, grading
Oligodendroglioma	IDH1/2, TERT promoter	1p/19q co-deletion	Oligodendroglioma, IDH-mutant	Diagnosis, prognosis
Glioblastoma, IDH-wild type	TERT promoter, EGFR, PTEN, TP53	+7/−10, EGFR amp	GBM, IDH-wild type	Diagnosis, poor prognosis
ST-EPN-ZFTA	ZFTA::RELA fusion	Chromosome 1q gain	ST-EPN-ZFTA	Diagnostic
PF-EPN Group A	None recurrent	+1q, −6q	PFA	Risk stratification
Medulloblastoma SHH TP53-wt	PTCH1, SUFU	chr9q loss	MB SHH	Intermediate risk
Medulloblastoma SHH TP53-mut	TP53, MYCN	+3q, +17q	MB SHH TP53-mut	High risk
ATRT	SMARCB1 inactivation	chr22 loss	ATRT	Diagnostic, pediatric
Meningioma	NF2, KLF4, TRAF7, SMO, POLR2A	1p loss, 22q loss, 1q gain	Multiple classes	Prognostic stratification
Solitary fibrous tumor	NAB2::STAT6	Variable	SFT	Diagnostic
CIC-rearranged sarcoma	CIC::DUX4	Complex karyotype	CIC-fused	Aggressive behavior

Pediatric-Type High-Grade Diffuse Gliomas

Pediatric-type high-grade diffuse gliomas (pHGGs) comprise a heterogeneous group of aggressive central nervous system tumors that primarily affect children and adolescents. In the WHO CNS 5 2021 classification, these tumors were redefined into four distinct molecular entities: diffuse midline glioma, *H3 K27*-altered; diffuse hemispheric glioma, *H3 G34*-mutant; diffuse pediatric-type high-grade glioma, *H3*-wild type and *IDH*-wild type; and infant-type hemispheric glioma [34]. This molecular classification has replaced the previous umbrella diagnosis of "pediatric glioblastoma," underscoring the central role of genetic alterations in determining tumor classification and behavior.

The presence of mutation is usually screened by IHC (H3 K27M, H3K27me3, and H3 G34R/V antibodies), but sequencing is required for ambiguous cases or rare/unusual variants. Importantly, identification of concurrent alterations such as *TP53* mutations or *PDGFRA* amplification may influence clinical behavior [44]. The *H3*- and *IDH*-wild-type HGG group is challenging due to its lack of defining alterations. Analysis with comprehensive NGS panels along DNA methylation profiling may be useful to exclude other molecular entities and to detect alterations such as *EGFR*, *MYCN*, or *PTEN* mutations, which may guide patients' inclusion in clinical trials [45, 46].

For infant-type hemispheric gliomas, fusion detection is essential. NGS-based RNA sequencing (or DNA-based fusion panels) allows identification of oncogenic fusions involving *ALK, NTRK, ROS1*, or *MET*. These findings have immediate therapeutic implications, as TRK inhibitors (e.g., larotrectinib, entrectinib) and ALK inhibitors are approved in pediatric settings for fusion-positive tumors [47]. Moreover, CNV analysis through NGS can reveal *CDKN2A/2B* deletions, *MYCN* amplifications, or complex chromosomal alterations that may carry prognostic significance. High tumor mutational burden (TMB), rare in pediatric gliomas and observed in cMMRD patients, can be identified by whole-exome or large-panel NGS and may support immunotherapy decisions in selected cases [48].

Pediatric-Type Low-Grade Diffuse Gliomas, Circumscribed Astrocytic Gliomas, and Glioneuronal Tumors

The categories encompass a large series of tumors, which are typically slow-growing lesions, with or without infiltrating growth pattern and with/without the presence of a neuronal component. They often show favorable prognoses and relative indolent behavior.

The diagnosis relies often on characteristic histology, although it may be largely overlapping throughout several entities. Notably, the majority of these neoplasms are driven by a single genetic alteration (mutations or fusion of *NF1, FGFR1, BRAF*, etc.) resulting in upregulation of the RAS/MAPK pathway. Among the non-RAS/MAPK alterations, the most common includes those affecting *MYB* and *MYBL1* genes [49].

Given the high number of different molecular alterations and their wide distribution in several tumors, it is difficult to recommend a specific strategy of analysis. Sequential testing of specific alterations in a tier-based approach or upfront NGS panels optimized for identification of alterations of genes coding members of the RAS/MAPK pathway can be suggested. The goal is to accurately identify the molecular driver, limiting the costs and reducing TAT of analysis.

Identifying specific mutations, also in tumors with classic histopathological features (such as pilocytic astrocytoma or gangliogliomas), via NGS can help to predict behavior, support risk stratification, and expand therapeutic options, in particular in cases resistant to standard therapy or after incomplete resection. Growing attention has been given to design tailored therapies with MAPK-inhibitors in pediatric low-grade gliomas with BRAF activation, using small molecules such as dabrafenib or vemurafenib targeting *BRAF* ^{V600E} mutation, or trametinib, selumetinib, and binimetinib inhibiting MEK1/2 kinases [50].

While for uncommon tumor variants (such as HGAP, PGNT, DGONC, etc.), the diagnosis can be more practically established by DNA methylation profiling, key alterations for integrated classification and therapy selection can be detected by NGS. For instance, in HGAP, sequencing may be useful to detect MAPK pathway mutations (e.g., *BRAF, FGFR1*), *ATRX* loss, and *CDKN2A/2B* deletions, typically harbored by this tumor.

Ependymal Tumors

Ependymal tumors are glial neoplasms originating from the ependymal lining of the ventricular system and the central canal of the spinal cord. The WHO CNS 5 2021 classification emphasizes an integrated approach, combining histopathological features with molecular characteristics and anatomical location. This framework defines ependymomas based on localization (supratentorial, infratentorial end spinal), histopathological and molecular data, delineating several distinct subtypes [34].

Supratentorial ependymomas (ST-EPN) include ST-EPN, ZFTA fusion-positive (formerly known as RELA fusion-positive ependymomas), and ST-EPN, YAP1 fusion-positive (characterized by fusions involving the *YAP1* gene, often with *MAMLD1* or other partners). Recently identified as a distinct methylation class, neuroepithelial tumors with PLAGL1 fusion (NET-PLAGL1) are supratentorial pediatric tumors exhibiting ependymal differentiation and recurrent fusions of the *PLAGL1* gene with partners such as *EWSR1*, *FOXO1*, and *MAML2*.

Posterior fossa ependymomas (PF-EPN) are mainly classified according to their epigenomic profile and include PF-EPN, group A (PFA), and PF-EPN, group B (PFB). Specific CNV alterations and *TERT* promoter mutation have been identified as prognostic parameter in PFA and PFB, respectively.

While in posterior fossa ependymomas, DNA methylation profiling may be recommended to differentiate PFA from PFB, in supratentorial ependymomas, NGS could be used to detect gene fusions involving *ZFTA* (formerly C11orf95) and *YAP1*. In cases suspected to represent NET-PLAGL1, fusion detection is crucial to identify rearrangements involving *PLAGL1* with partner genes. These fusions may be detected via targeted RNA-sequencing or hybrid-capture panels and are critical for an integrated diagnosis [51].

In spinal ependymomas (SP-EPN), analysis of *MYCN* status (i.e., via targeted analysis using FISH, MLPA, etc.) is mandatory for identification of the rare SP-EPN with MYCN amplification which shows a more aggressive clinical course [52].

Embryonal Tumors

Embryonal tumors are a heterogeneous group of malignant, mostly pediatric, CNS neoplasms. According to the WHO CNS 5 2021 classification, they include [34] MB, atypical teratoid/rhabdoid tumor (AT/RT), cribriform neuroepithelial tumor (CRINET), CNS neuroblastoma, FOXR2-activated, CNS tumor with BCOR internal tandem duplication, and embryonal tumor with multilayered rosettes (ETMR). Several emerging entities (such as CNS tumor with *EP300::BCOR* fusion, CNS embryonal tumor with PLAGL amplification, and CNS embryonal tumor with BRD4::LEUTX fusion) have been described [53].

MB represents the most common neoplasm in this group accounting for 20% of all brain tumors in pediatric age. Because MB represents a heterogeneous disease, subtyping is mandatory. Several methods can be used to confirm the subgrouping (SHH activated, WNT activated, and non-SHH/non-WNT including Group 3 and 4) FFPE samples. The simplest and fastest way is the use of IHC. However, DNA methylation profiling reliably distinguish the four core subgroups and can further identify subtypes with distinct clinical features. Expression profiling or DNA methylation profiling permits molecular grouping and subclassification, but none of these methods identifies the molecular alteration (mutations) responsible for the activation of a specific pathway and may become specific target therapy (such as in SHH MB) [54]. MB-tailored NGS panels may permit enables classification into WNT, SHH, Group 3, and Group 4 subtypes with identification of *CTNNB1* mutations (WNT pathway), *PTCH1/SMO/SUFU* alterations (SHH pathway), and *TP53* mutations, with *TP53*-mutant cases having markedly worse outcomes in SHH-MB.

Additional alterations like *MYC* amplification (Group 3) and *MYCN* or *CDK6* amplifications (Group 4), associated with poor outcome, can be identified using NGS panels.

Despite advances in the molecular classification of these subgroups, treatment of medulloblastoma has historically been defined by histopathological and clinical radiological findings. Mutational targets are being investigated in this population but are limited by the relatively silent mutational landscape, particularly in Group 3, which shows the lowest overall survival [55].

Although some entities, like ETMR, CRINET, or ATRT, can be identified by histopathology, RNA-seq or DNA-based approach may be useful besides DNA methylation profiling to detect *FOXR2* activation or *BCOR* internal tandem duplication in CNS neuroblastoma, FOXR2-activated, and CNS tumor with BCOR Internal Tandem Duplication, respectively.

Meningiomas and Other Meningeal Mesenchymal Tumors

Meningiomas are the most frequent primary intracranial tumors in adults, originating from the meningothelial cells of the arachnoid layer. Importantly, the WHO CNS 5 2021 classification introduces molecular criteria that can in some cases override histologic grade. Specifically, the presence of *TERT* promoter mutations, and/or homozygous deletions of *CDKN2A* or *CDKN2B*, is now sufficient to upgrade a meningioma to CNS WHO grade 3, regardless of its histologic appearance, due to their strong correlation with early recurrence and poor prognosis [1].

Recently, cIMPACT-NOW consortium proposed the evaluation of some CNV alterations (including 22q loss, 1p loss) for a more accurate meningioma classification and precise risk assessment. Scenarios where additional molecular testing may be useful include brain-invasive, otherwise benign meningiomas; tumors with borderline histopathological features between CNS

WHO grade 1 and 2; CNS WHO grade 1 meningiomas with unexpectedly rapid growth on serial imaging or recurrence; CNS WHO grade 2 (confirmation, distinguishing from CNS WHO grade 1/3); and chordoid, clear cell, rhabdoid, or papillary histology [56].

Targeted NGS panels can detect *TERT* promoter mutations, *CDKN2A/B* deletions, and other mutations in *NF2, TRAF7, AKT1, KLF4*, or *SMARCB1*, which help delineate meningioma subgroups associated with specific histology or prognosis and potential therapeutic targets [57]. In particular, based on the prominent biological differences between NF2 and non-NF2 driver alterations, dividing meningiomas into NF2 (harboring NF2 variants), TRAKLS (with TRAF7, AKT1, KLF4, and SMO alterations), and not otherwise classified (NOS) molecular tumor types, have been suggested [58].

Primary mesenchymal tumors of the CNS are rare and histologically diverse. Many correspond to their systemic counterparts, while others show unique molecular or epigenetic features when arising intracranially. The WHO CNS 5 2021 classification recognizes several defined entities and encourages molecular subclassification where relevant [34], such as solitary fibrous tumor (SFT), CIC-rearranged sarcomas, and tumors with *FET::CREB* Fusions.

SFT is characterized, as its systemic counterpart, by the presence of the *NAB2::STAT6* fusion, resulting from a paracentric inversion at chromosome 12q13. This genetic alteration leads to the nuclear expression of STAT6, which serves as a highly sensitive and specific diagnostic marker for SFTs. In SFTs, NGS or RNA-based assays are used to detect the *NAB2::STAT6* fusion, which is diagnostic. Fusion variant analysis (e.g., *NAB2* exon 6/7—*STAT6* exon 16/17/18) may also provide prognostic insights, as certain variants are associated with increased metastatic risk and worse clinical outcomes [59].

NGS is useful to identify *CIC::DUX4* fusions or rearrangements involving *FET::CREB* family genes (e.g., *EWSR1::ATF1, EWSR1::CREB1*), which define specific entities not distinguishable by morphology alone.

In tumors with ambiguous morphology and immunophenotype, especially when negative for lineage-defining markers, DNA methylation profiling as well as NGS analysis is highly recommended.

Conclusions

The incorporation of NGS analysis, together with complementary molecular platforms like DNA methylation profiling and CNV analysis, has redefined tumor taxonomies, enabled risk-adapted patient stratification, and opened the door to targeted therapies even in historical treatment-refractory diseases. This is not merely a technical necessity but a conceptual evolution: The molecular signature of a tumor is often more defining than its morphologic appearance, and only through a multidisciplinary lens can diagnostic precision and clinical relevance be ensured. WHO CNS5, cIMPACT-NOW updates, and EANO guidelines all converge on this principle, and the neuropathologist's role is central in making this synthesis clinically actionable.

References

1. Louis DN, Perry A, Wesseling P, Brat DJ, Cree IA, Figarella-Branger D, et al. The 2021 WHO classification of tumors of the central nervous system: a summary. Neuro-Oncology. 2021;23:1231–51.
2. Eckel-Passow JE, Lachance DH, Molinaro AM, Walsh KM, Decker PA, Sicotte H, et al. Glioma groups based on 1p/19q, IDH, and TERT promoter mutations in tumors. N Engl J Med. 2015;372:2499–508.
3. Capper D, Jones DTW, Sill M, Hovestadt V, Schrimpf D, Sturm D, et al. DNA methylation-based classification of central nervous system tumours. Nature. 2018;555:469–74.
4. Korshunov A, Ryzhova M, Hovestadt V, Bender S, Sturm D, Capper D, et al. Integrated analysis of pediatric glioblastoma reveals a subset of biologically favorable tumors with associated molecular prognostic markers. Acta Neuropathol. 2015;129:669–78.
5. d'Amati A, Bargiacchi L, Rossi S, Carai A, Bertero L, Barresi V, et al. Pediatric CNS tumors and 2021 WHO classification: what do oncologists need from pathologists? Front Mol Neurosci. 2024;17:1268038.

6. d'Amati A, Nicolussi A, Miele E, Mastronuzzi A, Rossi S, Gianno F, et al. NSD1 mutations and pediatric high-grade gliomas: a comparative genomic study in primary and recurrent tumors. Diagnostics (Basel). 2022;13:78.
7. Northcott PA, Buchhalter I, Morrissy AS, Hovestadt V, Weischenfeldt J, Ehrenberger T, et al. The whole-genome landscape of medulloblastoma subtypes. Nature. 2017;547:311–7.
8. Louis DN, Wesseling P, Aldape K, Brat DJ, Capper D, Cree IA, et al. cIMPACT-NOW update 6: new entity and diagnostic principle recommendations of the cIMPACT-Utrecht meeting on future CNS tumor classification and grading. Brain Pathol. 2020;30:844–56.
9. Capper D, Reifenberger G, French PJ, Schweizer L, Weller M, Touat M, et al. EANO guideline on rational molecular testing of gliomas, glioneuronal, and neuronal tumors in adults for targeted therapy selection. Neuro-Oncology. 2023;25:813–26.
10. van den Bent MJ, Franceschi E, Touat M, French PJ, Idbaih A, Lombardi G, et al. Updated EANO guideline on rational molecular testing of gliomas, glioneuronal, and neuronal tumors in adults for targeted therapy selection—update 1. Neuro-Oncology. 2025;27:331–7.
11. Sturm D, Orr BA, Toprak UH, Hovestadt V, Jones DTW, Capper D, et al. New brain tumor entities emerge from molecular classification of CNS-PNETs. Cell. 2016;164:1060–72.
12. Louis DN, Wesseling P, Paulus W, Giannini C, Batchelor TT, Cairncross JG, et al. cIMPACT-NOW update 1: not otherwise specified (NOS) and not elsewhere classified (NEC). Acta Neuropathol. 2018;135:481–4.
13. Yokoda RT, Cobb WS, Yong RL, Crary JF, Viapiano MS, Walker JM, et al. CDKN2A mutations have equivalent prognostic significance to homozygous deletion in IDH-mutant astrocytoma. J Neuropathol Exp Neurol. 2023;82:845–52.
14. Fortin Ensign SP, Jenkins RB, Giannini C, Sarkaria JN, Galanis E, Kizilbash SH. Translational significance of CDKN2A/B homozygous deletion in isocitrate dehydrogenase-mutant astrocytoma. Neuro-Oncology. 2023;25:28–36.
15. Solomon JP, Hechtman JF. Detection of NTRK fusions: merits and limitations of current diagnostic platforms. Cancer Res. 2019;79:3163–8.
16. Wen PY, Stein A, van den Bent M, De Greve J, Wick A, FYFL d V, et al. Dabrafenib plus trametinib in patients with BRAFV600E-mutant low-grade and high-grade glioma (ROAR): a multicentre, open-label, single-arm, phase 2, basket trial. Lancet Oncol. 2022;23:53–64.
17. Bouffet E, Hansford JR, Garrè ML, Hara J, Plant-Fox A, Aerts I, et al. Dabrafenib plus Trametinib in pediatric glioma with BRAF V600 mutations. N Engl J Med. 2023;389:1108–20.
18. Bouffet E, Larouche V, Campbell BB, Merico D, de Borja R, Aronson M, et al. Immune checkpoint inhibition for Hypermutant glioblastoma Multiforme resulting from germline Biallelic mismatch repair deficiency. J Clin Oncol. 2016;34:2206–11.
19. van Tilburg CM, Pfaff E, Pajtler KW, Langenberg KPS, Fiesel P, Jones BC, et al. The pediatric precision oncology INFORM registry: clinical outcome and benefit for patients with very high-evidence targets. Cancer Discov. 2021;11:2764–79.
20. Sharaf R, Pavlick DC, Frampton GM, Cooper M, Jenkins J, Danziger N, et al. FoundationOne CDx testing accurately determines whole arm 1p19q codeletion status in gliomas. Neurooncol Adv. 2021;3:vdab017.
21. Al-Kateb H, Knight SM, Sivasankaran G, Voss JS, Pitel BA, Blommel JH, et al. Clinical validation of the TruSight oncology 500 assay for the detection and reporting of Pan-cancer biomarkers. J Mol Diagn. 2025;27:292–305.
22. Kuehn JC, Metzger P, Neidert N, Matysiak U, Gräßel L, Philipp U, et al. Comprehensive genetic profiling and molecularly guided treatment for patients with primary CNS tumors. NPJ Precis Oncol. 2024;8:1–11.
23. Bertero L, Mangherini L, Ricci AA, Cassoni P, Sahm F. Molecular neuropathology: an essential and evolving toolbox for the diagnosis and clinical management of central nervous system tumors. Virchows Arch. 2024;484:181–94.
24. Singh AK, Olsen MF, Lavik LAS, Vold T, Drabløs F, Sjursen W. Detecting copy number variation in next generation sequencing data from diagnostic gene panels. BMC Med Genet. 2021;14:214.
25. Richards S, Aziz N, Bale S, Bick D, Das S, Gastier-Foster J, et al. Standards and guidelines for the interpretation of sequence variants: a joint consensus recommendation of the American College of Medical Genetics and Genomics and the Association for Molecular Pathology. Genet Med. 2015;17:405–24.
26. Li MM, Cottrell CE, Pullambhatla M, Roy S, Temple-Smolkin RL, Turner SA, et al. Assessments of somatic variant classification using the Association for Molecular Pathology/American Society of Clinical Oncology/College of American Pathologists Guidelines: a report from the Association for Molecular Pathology. J Mol Diagn. 2023;25:69–86.
27. Gudmundsson S, Singer-Berk M, Watts NA, Phu W, Goodrich JK, Solomonson M, et al. Variant interpretation using population databases: lessons from gnomAD. Hum Mutat. 2022;43:1012–30.
28. Tack V, Dufraing K, Deans ZC, van Krieken HJ, Dequeker EMC. The ins and outs of molecular pathology reporting. Virchows Arch. 2017;471:199–207.
29. Liu Y, Rosikiewicz W, Pan Z, Jillette N, Wang P, Taghbalout A, et al. DNA methylation-calling tools for Oxford Nanopore sequencing: a survey and human epigenome-wide evaluation. Genome Biol. 2021;22:295.
30. Deacon S, Cahyani I, Holmes N, Fox G, Munro R, Wibowo S, et al. ROBIN: a unified nanopore-based assay integrating intraoperative methylome classification and next-day comprehensive profiling for ultra-rapid tumor diagnosis. Neuro-oncol. 2025;27:noaf103.

31. Patel A, Dogan H, Payne A, Krause E, Sievers P, Schoebe N, et al. Rapid-CNS2: rapid comprehensive adaptive nanopore-sequencing of CNS tumors, a proof-of-concept study. Acta Neuropathol. 2022;143:609–12.
32. Patel A, Göbel K, Ille S, Hinz F, Schoebe N, Bogumil H, et al. Prospective, multicenter validation of a platform for rapid molecular profiling of central nervous system tumors. Nat Med. 2025;31(5):1567–77.
33. Aldape K, Capper D, von Deimling A, Giannini C, Gilbert MR, Hawkins C, et al. cIMPACT-NOW update 9: recommendations on utilization of genome-wide DNA methylation profiling for central nervous system tumor diagnostics. Neuro-oncol Adv. 2025;7:vdae228.
34. WHO Classification of Tumours Editorial Board. Central nervous system tumours. Lyon: International Agency for Research on Cancer; 2021. (WHO classification of tumours series, 5th ed.; vol. 6). https://publications.iarc.fr/601
35. Visani M, Acquaviva G, Marucci G, Paccapelo A, Mura A, Franceschi E, et al. Non-canonical IDH1 and IDH2 mutations: a clonal and relevant event in an Italian cohort of gliomas classified according to the 2016 World Health Organization (WHO) criteria. J Neuro-Oncol. 2017;135:245–54.
36. Synhaeve NE, van den Bent MJ, French PJ, Dinjens WNM, Atmodimedjo PN, Kros JM, et al. Clinical evaluation of a dedicated next generation sequencing panel for routine glioma diagnostics. Acta Neuropathol Commun. 2018;6:126.
37. Zacher A, Kaulich K, Stepanow S, Wolter M, Köhrer K, Felsberg J, et al. Molecular diagnostics of gliomas using next generation sequencing of a glioma-tailored gene panel. Brain Pathol. 2016;27:146–59.
38. Lim-Fat MJ, Youssef GC, Touat M, Iorgulescu JB, Whorral S, Allen M, et al. Clinical utility of targeted next-generation sequencing assay in IDH-wildtype glioblastoma for therapy decision-making. Neuro-Oncol. 2021;24:1140–9.
39. Bielle F, Di Stefano A-L, Meyronet D, Picca A, Villa C, Bernier M, et al. Diffuse gliomas with FGFR3-TACC3 fusion have characteristic histopathological and molecular features. Brain Pathol. 2018;28:674–83.
40. Pan Z, Bao J, Wei S. Vorasidenib for IDH-mutant grade 2 gliomas: clinical advances and future directions. Front Oncol. 2025;15:1628195.
41. Padovan M, Maccari M, Bosio A, De Toni C, Vizzaccaro S, Cestonaro I, et al. Actionable molecular alterations in newly diagnosed and recurrent *IDH1/2* wild-type glioblastoma patients and therapeutic implications: a large mono-institutional experience using extensive next-generation sequencing analysis. Eur J Cancer. 2023;191:112959.
42. Vivancos Sánchez C, Esteban Rodríguez MI, Peláez García A, Taravilla-Loma M, Rodríguez-Domínguez V, Rodríguez-Antolín C, et al. Clinical impact of a next-generation sequencing approach for glioblastoma patients. Cancers (Basel). 2025;17:744.
43. Wojewodzic MW, Lavender JP. Diagnostic classification based on DNA methylation profiles using sequential machine learning approaches. PLoS One. 2024;19:e0307912.
44. Karremann M, Gielen GH, Hoffmann M, Wiese M, Colditz N, Warmuth-Metz M, et al. Diffuse high-grade gliomas with H3 K27M mutations carry a dismal prognosis independent of tumor location. Neuro-Oncology. 2018;20:123–31.
45. Das A, Nobre L. Genomics in pediatric high-grade gliomas: Hope or hype: practical implications for resource-limited settings. Pediatr Hematol Oncol J. 2023;8:90–6.
46. Sturm D, Capper D, Andreiuolo F, Gessi M, Kölsche C, Reinhardt A, et al. Multiomic neuropathology improves diagnostic accuracy in pediatric neuro-oncology. Nat Med. 2023;29:917–26.
47. Hong DS, DuBois SG, Kummar S, Farago AF, Albert CM, Rohrberg KS, et al. Larotrectinib in patients with TRK fusion-positive solid tumours: a pooled analysis of three phase 1/2 clinical trials. Lancet Oncol. 2020;21:531–40.
48. Johnson A, Severson E, Gay L, Vergilio J, Elvin J, Suh J, et al. Comprehensive genomic profiling of 282 pediatric low- and high-grade gliomas reveals genomic drivers, tumor mutational burden, and Hypermutation signatures. Oncologist. 2017;22:1478–90.
49. Ryall S, Tabori U, Hawkins C. Pediatric low-grade glioma in the era of molecular diagnostics. Acta Neuropathol Commun. 2020;8:30.
50. Bruno F, Pellerino A, Bertero L, Soffietti R, Rudà R. Targeted therapies in rare brain tumours. Int J Mol Sci. 2021;22:7949.
51. Pajtler KW, Mack SC, Ramaswamy V, Smith CA, Witt H, Smith A, et al. The current consensus on the clinical management of intracranial ependymoma and its distinct molecular variants. Acta Neuropathol. 2017;133:5–12.
52. Raffeld M, Abdullaev Z, Pack SD, Xi L, Nagaraj S, Briceno N, et al. High level MYCN amplification and distinct methylation signature define an aggressive subtype of spinal cord ependymoma. Acta Neuropathol Commun. 2020;8:101.
53. Andreiuolo F, Ferrone CK, Rajan S, Perry A, Guney E, Cham E, et al. Molecular and clinicopathologic characteristics of CNS embryonal tumors with BRD4::LEUTX fusion. Acta Neuropathol Commun. 2024;12:42.
54. Frappaz D, Barritault M, Montané L, Laigle-Donadey F, Chinot O, Le Rhun E, et al. MEVITEM-a phase I/II trial of vismodegib + temozolomide vs temozolomide in patients with recurrent/refractory medulloblastoma with sonic hedgehog pathway activation. Neuro-Oncology. 2021;23:1949–60.
55. Haltom AR, Toll SA, Cheng D, Maegawa S, Gopalakrishnan V, Khatua S. Medulloblastoma epigenetics and the path to clinical innovation. J Neuro-Oncol. 2020;150:35–46.
56. Sahm F, Aldape KD, Brastianos PK, Brat DJ, Dahiya S, von Deimling A, et al. cIMPACT-NOW update 8:

clarifications on molecular risk parameters and recommendations for WHO grading of meningiomas. Neuro-Oncology. 2025;27:319–30.

57. Mawrin C, Koch R, Waldt N, Sandalcioglu IE, Braunsdorf WEK, Warnke J-P, et al. A new amplicon-based gene panel for next generation sequencing characterization of meningiomas. Brain Pathol. 2022;32:e13046.
58. Yuzawa S, Nishihara H, Yamaguchi S, Mohri H, Wang L, Kimura T, Tsuda M, Tanino M, Kobayashi H, Terasaka S, Houkin K, Sato N, Tanaka S. Clinical impact of targeted amplicon sequencing for meningioma as a practical clinical-sequencing system. Mod Pathol. 2016;29(7):708–16. https://doi.org/10.1038/modpathol.2016.81. Epub 2016 Apr 22
59. Eschbacher KL, Tran QT, Moskalev EA, Jenkins S, Fritchie K, Stoehr R, et al. NAB2::STAT6 fusions and genome-wide DNA methylation profiling: predictors of patient outcomes in meningeal solitary fibrous tumors. Brain Pathol. 2024;34:e13256.

Molecular Pathology of the Endocrine System

15

Vincenzo Fiorentino, Maurizio Martini, and Guido Fadda

Introduction

The diagnosis and management of endocrine neoplasms are undergoing a profound transformation, driven by the convergence of morphology on one side and high-throughput sequencing (HTS) on the other. For over a century, the microscopic examination of tissue has represented the basis of diagnosis, providing a structural and contextual understanding of disease. However, the advent of massively parallel sequencing has opened a window into the fundamental genomic and transcriptomic alterations that drive tumorigenesis. Today, HTS technologies can sequence an entire human genome for a few hundred dollars in a matter of days. This exponential decrease in cost and increase in speed has moved molecular analysis from the research laboratory to the forefront of clinical diagnostics. HTS allows for the simultaneous analysis of millions of DNA or RNA sequences, transforming molecular pathology from a slow, single-gene, hypothesis-driven endeavor to a broad, discovery-oriented, hypothesis-generating process. The integration of this powerful genomic data with traditional histopathology is forging a new, synergistic paradigm: morpho-molecular pathology. This is not a replacement of old techniques with new ones, but a synthesis. Morphology provides the essential, irreplaceable context, while genomics provides the deep mechanistic basis. This fusion of disciplines is the cornerstone of modern precision endocrine oncology, an approach that aims to tailor diagnosis, prognosis, and therapy to the specific molecular characteristics of each individual patient's tumor. This chapter will explore this paradigm shift in detail, from its foundational principles to its most advanced clinical applications across the spectrum of endocrine neoplasms.

V. Fiorentino · M. Martini · G. Fadda (✉)
Department of Human Pathology, of the Adulthood and of the Developing Age "Gaetano Barresi", "Gaetano Martino" University Hospital, University of Messina, Messina, Italy
e-mail: vincenzo.fiorentino@unime.it; maurizio.martini@unime.it; guido.fadda@unime.it

Histopathology and High-Throughput Sequencing

The Primacy of Histopathology in a Molecular World

In an era increasingly captivated by the allure of complex molecular data and the promise of "big data" analytics, it is imperative to reaffirm that histopathology is not becoming obsolete. On the contrary, its role is becoming even more critical, serving as the essential and nonnegotiable scaffold upon which all genomic data must be interpreted. The pathologist's expert assessment of H&E-stained slides and adjunctive studies like

© The Author(s), under exclusive license to Springer Nature Switzerland AG 2026

S. Sioletic, L. Coppola (eds.), *Next-Generation Sequencing in Solid Tumor Histopathology*, Current Clinical Pathology, https://doi.org/10.1007/978-3-032-18790-1_15

immunohistochemistry provides a rich tapestry of information that no sequencing assay, however powerful, can currently replicate.

Context, Localization, and Tumor Purity The diagnostic process begins with the pathologist. Before any sample is sent for molecular testing, a pathologist must identify the tumor, confirm the histopathological diagnosis, and, critically, assess the specimen's adequacy. This involves delineating the area of highest tumor cellularity for DNA/RNA extraction while avoiding areas of extensive necrosis, inflammation, or desmoplasia. A key parameter is **tumor purity**, the percentage of tumor cells relative to normal tissue, stromal cells, and infiltrating lymphocytes. A sample with low tumor purity (e.g., <20%) may yield a false-negative molecular result, because the mutant DNA from the cancer cells is diluted below the assay's limit of detection. Only a trained pathologist can accurately assess and enrich for tumor content, ensuring the validity of the downstream molecular analysis.

The Indispensable Role of Architectural and Invasive Features Many of the most critical, management-altering determinations in endocrine oncology are based purely on the interpretation of tissue architecture and invasive properties.

- **Thyroid Cancer:** The definitive distinction between a benign, encapsulated follicular adenoma and a malignant, encapsulated follicular thyroid carcinoma is not based on the nuclear features of the cells (which can be identical), but on the pathologist's unequivocal microscopic identification of transcapsular invasion (tumor breaking completely through the surrounding fibrous capsule) or angiolymphatic invasion (tumor cells unequivocally within the lumen of a vessel outside the capsule). Similarly, recognizing aggressive histological variants of papillary thyroid carcinoma (PTC), such as the tall cell variant (cells twice as tall as they are wide, with eosinophilic cytoplasm), the hobnail variant (cells with apical nuclei and a "tombstone" appearance), or the columnar cell variant, has direct and significant prognostic implications and is a purely morphological diagnosis that elevates the tumor's risk profile [1].
- **Adrenocortical Tumors:** The diagnosis of adrenocortical carcinoma (ACC) relies on a constellation of histological features, formalized in the widely used **Weiss scoring system**. This system assigns points for features such as a high mitotic rate (>5 per 50 high-power fields), the presence of atypical mitoses, extensive necrosis, and invasion of sinusoidal or capsular structures. A score of ≥3 is diagnostic of carcinoma. This determination is entirely dependent on meticulous histological examination [2].
- **Neuroendocrine Neoplasms (NENs):** The grading of gastroenteropancreatic NENs (GEP-NENs) is one of the single most powerful predictors of clinical outcome and is the primary determinant of therapeutic strategy. The WHO classification grades these tumors as G1, G2, or G3 based on the pathologist's meticulous counting of mitoses per unit area and the estimation of the Ki-67 labeling index, an immunohistochemical marker of cellular proliferation. This grade separates indolent tumors (G1) from more aggressive ones (G2/G3) and dictates whether a patient is a candidate for somatostatin analogues versus more aggressive chemotherapy [3].

Immunohistochemistry as a Morpho-molecular Bridge Immunohistochemistry (IHC) remains a vital ancillary technique. It provides protein-level information within a preserved morphological context. In endocrine pathology, IHC is used to determine cell lineage (e.g., TTF-1 and thyroglobulin for thyroid origin; synaptophysin and chromogranin for neuroendocrine differentiation), to assess hormone production (e.g., ACTH, GH in pituitary tumors), and to evaluate prognostic markers like the Ki-67 index. A crucial application has emerged in the context of PPGL, where IHC for the **SDHB** protein serves as a highly effective and inexpensive surrogate marker for the presence of a mutation in any of the *SDHx* complex genes. Loss of SDHB staining is a strong indicator of a Cluster 1 (pseudohypoxia) tumor and flags the patient for germline genetic testing [4].

The Inherent Limitations of Morphology Despite its power, morphology has well-defined and clinically significant limits. The classic and most vexing example is the follicular-patterned thyroid lesion, where the cells of a benign adenoma, a minimally invasive carcinoma, and the now-reclassified nonmalignant entity NIFTP can appear absolutely identical on FNA cytology, leading to the diagnostically ambiguous "indeterminate" categories. In pituitary tumors, routine histology is a notoriously poor predictor of which tumors will recur or behave aggressively. In pheochromocytomas, there are no reliable histological features to distinguish a benign from a malignant tumor at the time of initial diagnosis; malignancy is still, by definition, established only by the presence of metastases in non-neuroendocrine tissues. It is precisely within these well-delineated zones of morphological uncertainty and prognostic ambiguity that molecular pathology provides its greatest and most transformative clinical utility.

The Genomic Revolution: A Deep Dive into High-Throughput Sequencing (HTS/NGS)

HTS represents a quantum leap in the technology of DNA and RNA sequencing, fundamentally altering the scale and scope of genomic analysis in medicine. Understanding its core principles, the nuances of different clinical methodologies, and the complexities of its data analysis pipeline is essential for any modern practitioner in oncology.

Core Principles: From Sanger to Sequencing by Synthesis

The predecessor to HTS was the **Sanger sequencing** method, which, while revolutionary in its time and still used for single-gene confirmation, is an analog technology in a digital world. It interrogates one DNA fragment at a time in a slow, laborious process. HTS platforms, in contrast, are digital, employing massive parallelism. The most widely used HTS technology, pioneered and commercialized by Illumina, is based on the principle of **sequencing by synthesis**. The clinical workflow, from the moment a tissue block or slide arrives in the molecular lab, proceeds as follows:

1. **Nucleic Acid Extraction:** The process begins with the extraction of high-quality DNA and/or RNA from the clinical specimen. For many solid endocrine tumors, the starting material is formalin-fixed, paraffin-embedded (FFPE) tissue. This preservation method is excellent for morphology but is notoriously harsh on nucleic acids, causing chemical cross-linking and significant DNA/RNA fragmentation. This necessitates the use of specialized, robust extraction protocols designed to reverse cross-links and purify the often-degraded nucleic acids. The quantity and quality (e.g., fragment size distribution) of the extracted material are meticulously assessed before proceeding [5].
2. **Library Preparation:** This multistep enzymatic process converts the extracted nucleic acids into a format, or "library," that is readable by the sequencer. The DNA is first fragmented into smaller, more uniform pieces (typically 200–500 base pairs). A series of enzymatic reactions are then used to repair the ends of these fragments and to ligate synthetic, double-stranded DNA sequences known as **adapters** to both ends. These adapters are sophisticated molecules with several critical functions: They contain sequences that allow the fragments to bind to the sequencing flow cell; they include universal priming sites for the sequencing reaction; and they harbor unique molecular identifiers or "barcodes." **Index barcodes** are short, unique sequences that are specific to each patient sample. This allows multiple patient libraries to be pooled (multiplexed) and sequenced in the same run, dramatically increasing throughput and reducing cost [6].

3. **Clonal Amplification:** To generate a strong enough fluorescent signal for reliable detection during sequencing, each individual DNA fragment in the library must be clonally amplified. On Illumina platforms, this is achieved via **bridge amplification** on a proprietary glass slide called a flow cell. The flow cell surface is coated with a dense lawn of millions of short oligonucleotides that are complementary to the library adapters. The prepared library is washed over the flow cell, where each fragment binds to a complementary oligo. A polymerase then creates a copy of the bound fragment. The original strand is washed away, and the newly synthesized strand "bridges" over to a nearby oligo, where it is copied again. This process is repeated for ~35 cycles, creating a dense, localized cluster containing thousands of identical copies of the original DNA fragment [7].
4. **Sequencing by Synthesis:** The flow cell, now covered in millions of distinct clonal clusters, is placed in the sequencer. The process of sequencing involves the cyclical addition of fluorescently labeled nucleotides. In each cycle, a cocktail of reagents, including DNA polymerase and all four nucleotides (A, C, G, T), is flushed over the flow cell. Each nucleotide has a unique fluorescent dye attached and a reversible terminator that ensures only one base is added per cycle. The polymerase adds the one complementary, fluorescently labeled nucleotide to the growing strand within each cluster. After this incorporation step, a laser scans the flow cell, exciting the fluorophores, and a high-resolution camera captures the emitted light from every cluster. The color of the light identifies which base was added at that position in that cluster. The fluorescent tag and the reversible terminator are then chemically cleaved, and the cycle repeats for the next base. This process is repeated for 75–150 cycles, building up the sequence read one base at a time for every cluster on the flow cell [8].
5. **Data Generation:** The instrument performs millions of these reactions in parallel across all clusters, generating a massive output of data—typically billions of short sequence "reads" (each 75–150 bases long)—in a single run [9].

Key HTS Methodologies in Clinical Endocrine Oncology

While the core technology is the same, it can be strategically applied in several ways, each with its own advantages and disadvantages for clinical practice:

- **Whole-Genome Sequencing (WGS):** This method sequences the entire ~3 billion base pair human genome, including both coding and noncoding regions. It provides the most comprehensive and unbiased view of all types of genomic alterations. However, it is expensive, generates enormous and computationally demanding data files, and often yields a large number of variants in noncoding regions whose clinical significance is unknown. For these reasons, WGS remains primarily a research tool, though its use in rare and undiagnosed diseases is growing [10].
- **Whole-Exome Sequencing (WES):** This method uses a capture-based approach to selectively sequence only the protein-coding regions of the genome (the exome). The exome constitutes only about 1–2% of the total genome but is where approximately 85% of known disease-causing mutations reside. WES is significantly more cost-effective and generates a more manageable dataset than WGS, making it a powerful tool for discovering novel cancer genes in research settings and for diagnosing rare hereditary cancer syndromes [11].
- **Targeted Gene Panels:** This is the undisputed workhorse of clinical molecular oncology today. These panels use either a capture-based or amplicon-based approach to selectively sequence a predefined set of genes (ranging from a few dozen to over 500) that are known to be clinically relevant for a particular cancer type or for cancer in general. The advantages of this approach for routine diagnostics are numerous [12]:

  - **Cost-Effectiveness:** It is far cheaper than WES or WGS.
  - **High Depth of Coverage:** By focusing the sequencing power on a small portion of the genome, each base in the target region can be sequenced hundreds or even thousands of times. This high "depth" is crucial for sensitively detecting mutations that may be present in only a small fraction of the cells in a heterogeneous tumor sample (i.e., mutations with a low variant allele frequency).
  - **Manageable Data:** The data output is much smaller and easier to analyze and interpret.
  - **Clinically Focused:** The results are enriched for potentially actionable findings, minimizing the ethical and clinical dilemma of discovering variants of unknown significance in medically irrelevant genes.
- **RNA Sequencing (RNA-Seq):** This method sequences the transcriptome (the RNA molecules, or transcripts, in a cell) rather than the genome. This provides a wealth of information, including quantitative gene expression levels. However, in the context of clinical oncology, its primary and most powerful use is for the robust and sensitive detection of **gene fusions**. Gene fusions are created by chromosomal translocations that join parts of two different genes. RNA-seq is superior to DNA-based methods for this purpose, because it directly sequences the resulting chimeric mRNA transcript, providing definitive evidence of the fusion's existence and its potential to be translated into an oncogenic protein [13].
- **Methylation Profiling:** This involves specialized techniques (e.g., methylation arrays or whole-genome bisulfite sequencing) to map the patterns of DNA methylation across the genome. As will be discussed for pituitary tumors, this epigenetic information can be a more powerful tool for tumor classification and prognostication than DNA sequence information alone [14].

The Bioinformatics Bottleneck: The Crucial Path from Raw Data to Actionable Report

Generating the terabytes of raw sequence data is now the relatively easy part. The most significant challenge, or "bottleneck," in clinical HTS is the complex, multistep bioinformatics pipeline required to process this raw data into a clinically meaningful and actionable report.

- **Quality Control (QC) and Alignment:** The pipeline begins with rigorous QC checks of the raw sequencing reads. The reads that pass QC are then mapped, or "aligned," to their correct chromosomal position on the reference human genome build (e.g., GRCh38/hg38) [15].
- **Variant Calling:** Once aligned, specialized software tools compare the patient's aligned sequence to the reference genome to identify all differences, or "variants." A robust pipeline uses multiple algorithms to call different types of variants:
  - **Single-Nucleotide Variants (SNVs):** e.g., *BRAF* c.1799 T > A (p.V600E).
  - **Small Insertions and Deletions (Indels):** The insertion or deletion of one or more nucleotides.
  - **Copy Number Variations (CNVs):** Gains (amplifications) or losses (deletions) of large segments of DNA.
  - **Structural Variants (SVs):** Large-scale rearrangements like chromosomal translocations, which are the basis of gene fusions. These are called from both DNA and RNA data [16].
- **Annotation, Filtering, and Interpretation:** Each identified variant is then **annotated** with a vast amount of information from various public and proprietary databases (e.g., its population frequency in gnomAD, its presence in the COSMIC database of somatic mutations in cancer, its classification in ClinVar for germline variants, and predictions of its functional impact from tools like SIFT and PolyPhen). The final, and most intellectually demanding, step is **interpretation**. A board-

certified pathologist or molecular geneticist must carefully review all the evidence and classify each variant according to the established guidelines from the Association for Molecular Pathology (AMP), American Society of Clinical oncology (ASCO), and College of American Pathologists (CAP). These guidelines establish a four-tier system for somatic variants based on their clinical significance:

- **Tier I: Variants with Strong Clinical Significance.** These are typically predictive biomarkers for response or resistance to FDA-approved therapies (e.g., *BRAF* V600E in thyroid cancer predicts response to BRAF/MEK inhibitors).
- **Tier II: Variants with Potential Clinical Significance.** These are variants that may have prognostic value or make a patient eligible for a clinical trial of a targeted agent.
- **Tier III: Variants of Unknown Significance (VUS).** This is a major challenge. A VUS is a genetic change whose impact on protein function or clinical outcome is not yet known. Reporting these can cause significant clinical confusion and patient anxiety. It is a fundamental principle that therapeutic decisions should not be based on a VUS outside the context of a clinical trial.
- **Tier IV: Benign or Likely Benign Variants.** These are common polymorphisms with no known clinical impact.

The culmination of this entire process is the creation of a clear, concise, and integrated morpho-molecular report that is delivered to the treating clinician, providing the foundation for precision medicine [17].

Morpho-molecular Integration in Thyroid Carcinoma

The clinical management of thyroid nodules and thyroid cancer stands as the most mature, extensively validated, and clinically impactful application of HTS in the entire field of endocrine oncology. It has served as a powerful and instructive blueprint for how to rationally incorporate molecular data into every step of the patient care pathway, from the initial diagnostic workup of a common clinical problem to the selection of life-saving therapies in advanced, metastatic disease.

The Preoperative Challenge

Thyroid nodules are a rampant clinical entity, detected in up to 65% of the general population by high-resolution ultrasound. While the overwhelming majority (>90%) are benign, the core clinical challenge is to accurately, efficiently, and cost-effectively identify the small subset that are malignant while avoiding unnecessary intervention for the benign majority. Fine-needle aspiration (FNA) cytology is the primary diagnostic tool for this purpose. The Bethesda System for Reporting Thyroid Cytopathology (TBSRTC) provides a standardized, tiered reporting framework that links cytomorphological findings to a specific Risk of Malignancy (ROM), thereby guiding clinical management [18].

The Bethesda System's six categories are:

I. **Nondiagnostic or Unsatisfactory** (ROM, 5–10%; recommendation, repeat FNA with ultrasound guidance).
II. **Benign** (ROM, 0–3%; recommendation, clinical follow-up).
III. **Atypia of Undetermined Significance (AUS) or Follicular Lesion of Undetermined Significance (FLUS)** (ROM, 10–30% in the latest revision; recommendation, repeat FNA, molecular testing, or diagnostic surgery).
IV. **Follicular Neoplasm (FN) or Suspicious for a Follicular Neoplasm (SFN)** (ROM, 25–40%; recommendation, molecular testing or diagnostic surgery).
V. **Suspicious for Malignancy** (ROM, 45–75%; recommendation, (near) total thyroidectomy).
VI. **Malignant** (ROM, 97–99%; recommendation, (near) total thyroidectomy).

While this system provides excellent clarity for categories II, V, and VI, the indeterminate categories III and IV represent a major diagnostic and clinical "gray zone." Together, they account for a substantial proportion, up to 30%, of all thyroid FNAs performed. The cytomorphological features of the cells in these categories are inherently ambiguous. They often show a microfollicular architecture, cellular crowding, or mild nuclear atypia but lack the definitive features of PTC or other malignancies. Critically, these features do not allow for a reliable distinction between a benign follicular adenoma and a follicular carcinoma, as that distinction requires the histological assessment of invasion. The historical management for many of these patients, particularly those with Bethesda IV nodules, was a **diagnostic hemithyroidectomy**. This strategy, while safe, resulted in a definitive benign diagnosis on final pathology in a staggering 60–80% of cases. This represented a massive burden of unnecessary operations, with their attendant surgical risks (recurrent laryngeal nerve injury, hypoparathyroidism), financial costs to the healthcare system, and the frequent need for lifelong thyroid hormone replacement for the patient. This clear and pressing unmet clinical need for better preoperative risk-stratification tools was the primary impetus for the development and clinical validation of molecular testing in thyroid cytopathology.

Molecular Cytopathology

HTS-based testing performed on residual material from the FNA needle rinse has fundamentally and permanently altered the management of these indeterminate nodules. The two most prominent and extensively validated commercial assays in the United States, ThyroSeq® and Afirma®, exemplify the two major molecular strategies that have proven successful.

The Comprehensive "Rule-In/Rule-Out" Approach: Targeted NGS Panels (ThyroSeq®)

The ThyroSeq platform is a targeted NGS assay designed to provide a comprehensive genomic profile of the thyroid nodule by simultaneously analyzing for a wide array of DNA and RNA alterations known to be implicated in thyroid tumorigenesis. Its development has been iterative, with the current version (ThyroSeq v3) covering 112 genes and reporting on the following:

- **Point mutations and indels** in key driver genes like *BRAF*, *RAS* (*NRAS, HRAS, KRAS*), the *TERT* promoter, *TP53*, and genes in the PI3K pathway.
- **Gene fusions**, detected via RNA sequencing, involving critical kinases like *RET*, *NTRK1/2/3*, *ALK*, and *BRAF*.
- **Copy number alterations**, such as amplification of *PIK3CA*.
- **Gene expression alterations** of specific markers.

The clinical philosophy of ThyroSeq is to function as both a powerful "rule-in" and an effective "rule-out" test. The detection of a known or likely pathogenic alteration provides strong positive evidence for malignancy, "ruling in" the need for surgery and even informing the extent of that surgery. Conversely, a completely negative result provides high confidence that the nodule is benign, "ruling out" the immediate need for surgery and justifying a strategy of conservative clinical observation [19]. The performance of ThyroSeq v3 was established in a large, prospective, blinded, multicenter validation study published in *JAMA Oncology*:

- **Negative Predictive Value (NPV):** 97%. This is arguably its most impactful clinical metric. For a Bethesda III or IV nodule with a negative ThyroSeq result, the residual risk of

malignancy is only ~3%. This risk is comparable to the risk associated with a benign (Bethesda II) FNA diagnosis, providing a robust, evidence-based rationale for managing these patients with clinical and sonographic follow-up rather than immediate surgery.
- **Positive Predictive Value (PPV):** 38% for Bethesda III nodules and 66% for Bethesda IV nodules. While numerically lower than the NPV, the PPV provides significant risk stratification. It is highly dependent on the specific alteration found. The detection of a *BRAF* V600E mutation carries a PPV for malignancy that approaches 100%. The detection of a *RAS* mutation carries a lower PPV for malignancy (~50–60%), because this alteration can also be found in benign adenomas and the low-risk NIFTP entity, but it still significantly elevates the risk over the baseline and provides crucial information for the surgeon and patient.
- **Sensitivity:** 94% (the ability to correctly identify malignancy).
- **Specificity:** 82% (the ability to correctly identify a benign nodule).

The "Rule-Out" Focused Approach: Gene Expression Classifiers (Afirma®)

The Afirma platform initially gained prominence as a Gene Expression Classifier (GEC), an assay based on microarray technology. The GEC analyzed the expression levels of 167 genes to generate a binary classification: "Benign" or "Suspicious." Its primary design and clinical validation were as a "rule-out" test. A "Benign" GEC result had a very high NPV (>95%), providing a safe and effective rationale to avoid surgery for a large number of patients. However, its specificity was relatively low, meaning a significant number of benign nodules were classified as "Suspicious," limiting its "rule-in" utility.

The platform has since evolved into the **Afirma Genomic Sequencing Classifier (GSC)**, which leverages the power of RNA sequencing. The GSC analyzes the expression patterns of over 1000 genes and simultaneously incorporates an analysis of DNA variants and fusions derived from the RNA sequence data. While its core strength remains its "rule-out" capability, the addition of these genomic components provides significantly more "rule-in" information.

- When an Afirma GSC result is **"Benign,"** the NPV remains exceptionally high at >96%, confidently guiding a conservative management approach.
- When the result is **"Suspicious,"** the GSC report now provides additional information, including the estimated risk of malignancy and the presence of specific alterations like *BRAF* V600E, *RET/PTC* fusions, or *TERT* promoter mutations. The detection of these specific markers can elevate the risk of malignancy to >90%, effectively ruling in the need for surgery.

The widespread clinical adoption of both ThyroSeq and Afirma, along with other similar validated tests, is now explicitly incorporated into the management guidelines of the American Thyroid Association (ATA). Their routine use has led to a dramatic and safe reduction in the number of nontherapeutic diagnostic surgeries for indeterminate thyroid nodules, representing a landmark achievement for morpho-molecular pathology and a clear win for patients and the healthcare system.

Molecular Histopathology

While molecular testing has transformed preoperative cytology, its role extends powerfully into the postoperative setting, where it is used to refine risk stratification and guide adjuvant therapy decisions based on the analysis of the surgically resected tumor (the histological specimen). The 2015 ATA management guidelines, in a paradigm-shifting move, were among the first major cancer guidelines to formally incorporate specific molecular markers into their initial risk stratification framework.

Refining the ATA Risk Stratification System

The ATA guidelines stratify patients with differentiated thyroid cancer (DTC) into low, intermediate, and high-risk categories for structural disease recurrence based on clinicopathological features. Molecular data serves as a critical additional layer to this framework. A patient with a small, intrathyroidal PTC might be classified as ATA low risk based on histology alone. However, if molecular testing of the tumor reveals the co-occurrence of *BRAF* V600E and *TERT* promoter mutations, their true biological risk of recurrence is significantly higher, and they may be "upstaged" to ATA intermediate or even high risk, justifying more aggressive management (e.g., consideration of radioactive iodine ablation) and more intensive long-term surveillance [20].

The Prognostic Power of Key Genetic Alterations in Histology

- ***BRAF* V600E Mutation:** In the histological specimen, the *BRAF* V600E mutation continues to be a robust marker of increased risk. It results in the constitutive, ligand-independent activation of the downstream MEK-ERK signaling cascade of the MAPK pathway, a cellular program that promotes proliferation, survival, and dedifferentiation. This molecular event translates clinically to a strong association with aggressive histological subtypes (e.g., tall cell, hobnail), a significantly higher propensity for developing extrathyroidal extension and lymph node metastasis, and a reduced avidity for radioactive iodine (RAI) due to the mutation's effect of downregulating the expression of the sodium-iodide symporter (NIS, gene *SLC5A5*). This latter effect contributes to its association with a higher rate of RAI-refractory disease and poorer long-term outcomes.
- ***RAS* Mutations (*NRAS, HRAS, KRAS*):** In resected specimens, *RAS* mutations are the hallmark of follicular-patterned lesions. They are the defining molecular feature of follicular thyroid carcinoma and the encapsulated/infiltrative follicular variants of PTC. Generally, *RAS*-mutated cancers are associated with a more indolent clinical course than *BRAF* V600E-mutated cancers, with a lower risk of lymph node metastasis. However, they have a distinct and higher propensity for developing distant hematogenous metastases (to lung and bone), a critical consideration for long-term surveillance.
- ***TERT* Promoter Mutations: The Most Powerful Prognostic Marker** – The mutations in the promoter region of the telomerase reverse transcriptase (*TERT*) gene (most commonly C228T and C250T) lead to the creation of a new transcription factor-binding site, resulting in increased TERT expression. TERT is the catalytic subunit of telomerase, an enzyme that maintains telomere length, thus allowing cancer cells to bypass replicative senescence and achieve cellular immortality. In histological series of DTC, *TERT* promoter mutations are found in ~10–20% of cases, but their prevalence increases dramatically with tumor aggressiveness, reaching up to 70% in poorly differentiated (PDTC) and anaplastic (ATC) thyroid cancers. A *TERT* promoter mutation is arguably the single most powerful negative prognostic marker in thyroid cancer. While it confers a significantly worse prognosis as a standalone event, its impact is most profound and synergistic when it co-occurs with a MAPK pathway driver mutation. Numerous large-scale studies have definitively shown that the combination of ***BRAF* V600E + *TERT* promoter mutation** or ***RAS* + *TERT* promoter mutation** identifies a subset of tumors with a very high risk of aggressive behavior, rapid progression, distant metastasis, and a five- to tenfold increase in disease-specific mortality. The identification of this combination on a histological specimen is a major red flag that warrants consideration of the most aggressive available therapies and the most intensive surveillance protocols [21].
- **Tumor Suppressor Gene Mutations (*TP53, PTEN*, etc.):** The progression from well-differentiated thyroid cancer to the highly lethal anaplastic thyroid cancer (ATC) is a multistep process driven by the sequential accumulation of additional mutations, particularly in critical tumor suppressor genes. Somatic mutations in *TP53*, the "guardian of

the genome," are rare in DTC (<5%) but are found in over 70% of ATCs, often representing a late event that drives dedifferentiation. Similarly, mutations in genes of the PI3K/AKT/mTOR pathway (*PIK3CA*, *PTEN*) are more common in advanced and aggressive cancers. An ATC genome is typically a complex and chaotic landscape, often built upon a foundation of a driver mutation (*BRAF* or *RAS*) and a *TERT* promoter mutation, with the subsequent addition of *TP53* inactivation and other tumor suppressor gene hits [22].

Predictive Molecular Histopathology

For the subset of patients who develop progressive, recurrent, or metastatic disease that is refractory to standard therapies (surgery and radioactive iodine), systemic therapy is required. HTS-based profiling of the metastatic tumor tissue is now the mandatory standard of care to guide the selection of these therapies.

- **BRAF/MEK Inhibitors:** For patients with *BRAF* V600E-mutant RAI-refractory DTC, the combination of a BRAF inhibitor (dabrafenib) and a MEK inhibitor (trametinib) is an FDA-approved standard of care, showing significant improvements in response rates and progression-free survival compared to single-agent BRAF inhibition.
- **RET Inhibitors:** For patients with advanced thyroid cancer driven by a *RET* gene fusion (in PTC) or a *RET* point mutation (in MTC), the highly selective RET inhibitors selpercatinib and pralsetinib have demonstrated remarkable efficacy. The LIBRETTO-001 trial, for example, showed an overall response rate of 79% in previously treated *RET* fusion-positive PTC patients [23].
- **TRK Inhibitors:** The "tumor-agnostic" TRK inhibitors larotrectinib and entrectinib are approved for any solid tumor harboring an *NTRK* gene fusion. In the small subset of thyroid cancer patients with these fusions, these drugs have produced dramatic, rapid, and durable responses [24].
- **Multi-kinase Inhibitors (MKIs):** Before the advent of highly selective inhibitors, broad-spectrum MKIs like lenvatinib and sorafenib were the standard of care for RAI-refractory DTC, regardless of mutational status. They remain an important option, particularly for *RAS*-mutated or non-mutated tumors. Lenvatinib demonstrated a significant improvement in progression-free survival in the pivotal SELECT trial [25].

This landscape makes it imperative that any patient with advanced DTC undergo comprehensive molecular profiling via HTS to ensure they have the opportunity to receive the most effective, targeted therapy available for their specific tumor biology.

Medullary Thyroid Carcinoma (MTC)

Medullary thyroid carcinoma, a neuroendocrine tumor arising from the calcitonin-producing parafollicular C-cells, is a genetically distinct and simpler entity compared to follicular cell-derived cancers. Its pathogenesis is overwhelmingly dominated by activating alterations in a single gene: the ***RET* proto-oncogene** [26].

- **Hereditary MTC:** Approximately 25% of all MTC cases are hereditary, caused by a germline (hereditary) activating mutation in the *RET* gene. This occurs in the context of the autosomal dominant multiple endocrine neoplasia type 2 (MEN2) syndromes.
  - **MEN2A:** The most common form, characterized by MTC, pheochromocytoma, and primary hyperparathyroidism. It is most often caused by germline mutations in one of the cysteine codons in exon 10 or 11 of the *RET* gene.
  - **MEN2B:** The most aggressive form, characterized by MTC with a very early onset, pheochromocytoma, and a characteristic phenotype (marfanoid habitus, mucosal neuromas). MEN2B is almost exclusively caused by a single point mutation, the M918T mutation in exon 16.
  - **Familial MTC (FMTC):** A variant of MEN2A where MTC is the only clinical manifestation.

- **Sporadic MTC:** Approximately 75% of MTC cases are sporadic (nonhereditary). However, the majority of these are still driven by somatic (acquired, tumor-specific) mutations in the *RET* gene. The M918T mutation is the most common somatic event, found in ~50% of sporadic cases.

Clinical Integration of *RET* Testing Genetic testing is an absolute cornerstone of MTC management.

- **Diagnostic and Germline Testing:** Every patient diagnosed with MTC, whether on cytology or histology, should undergo *RET* gene testing. This typically involves sequencing the relevant exons from peripheral blood DNA. If a germline mutation is found, it confirms a diagnosis of MEN2, which mandates lifelong screening for associated tumors (annual biochemical screening for pheochromocytoma and hyperparathyroidism). It also has profound implications for the family, necessitating genetic counseling and cascade genetic testing for all first-degree relatives.
- **Prophylactic Surgery:** For individuals who are found to carry a germline *RET* mutation before they develop cancer (e.g., through family screening), prophylactic thyroidectomy in childhood is the standard of care. The timing of the surgery is risk-stratified based on the specific *RET* mutation, with carriers of the high-risk M918T mutation often undergoing surgery in the first year of life to prevent the near-certain development of aggressive, metastatic MTC.
- **Therapeutic Guidance:** As mentioned, for patients with advanced, progressive, or metastatic MTC, the selective RET inhibitors selpercatinib and pralsetinib are now the standard first-line systemic therapy, having demonstrated superior efficacy and lower toxicity compared to older MKIs like vandetanib and cabozantinib. Molecular testing of the tumor is therefore essential to guide treatment.

Anaplastic Thyroid Carcinoma (ATC)

Anaplastic thyroid carcinoma is one of the most aggressive and lethal of all human cancers, with a median survival of only 5–6 months. Histologically, it is an undifferentiated carcinoma composed of pleomorphic, spindled, or giant cells. Its genomic landscape reflects its aggressive biology, representing a state of genomic catastrophe. Most ATCs arise from a preexisting DTC through the process of dedifferentiation, driven by the sequential accumulation of additional mutations. The typical ATC genome is built upon a foundation of an initial driver mutation (*BRAF* V600E in ~40% or a *RAS* mutation in ~20%) and a *TERT* promoter mutation (~70%), with the subsequent acquisition of inactivating mutations in critical tumor suppressor genes, most commonly *TP53* (>70%) and others such as *CDKN2A* and members of the SWI/SNF chromatin remodeling complex [27].

Given the rapid and aggressive nature of ATC, the 2021 ATA guidelines recommend that **comprehensive molecular profiling via HTS should be performed for all patients with ATC at the time of diagnosis**. This is because the results can directly inform the choice of therapy in a disease where time is of the essence. Patients with *BRAF* V600E-mutant ATC are candidates for the combination of dabrafenib and trametinib, which has been shown in clinical trials to produce response rates of nearly 70%, a dramatic improvement over traditional cytotoxic chemotherapy. Patients with rare *RET* or *NTRK* fusions may be eligible for their respective targeted inhibitors. For others, immunotherapy with checkpoint inhibitors is being actively investigated, particularly for tumors with high TMB or PD-L1 expression. Upfront molecular testing is therefore no longer an academic exercise but a critical component of modern, evidence-based management for this devastating disease.

Pheochromocytoma and Paraganglioma (PPGL)

Pheochromocytomas (PCC) are neuroendocrine tumors arising from the chromaffin cells of the adrenal medulla, while paragangliomas (PGL) arise from sympathetic or parasympathetic ganglia outside the adrenal gland. Collectively termed PPGL, these tumors hold the remarkable distinction of being the most hereditary of all human tumors. The old clinical axiom, the "rule of 10s" (10% bilateral, 10% extra-adrenal, 10% malignant, 10% hereditary), has been rendered completely obsolete by the findings of HTS. It is now known that a germline mutation in one of at least 20 known susceptibility genes can be identified in 30–40% of all patients presenting with a PPGL. When somatic mutations in these same genes are included, a clear genetic driver can be identified in up to 70% of all cases. This profound genetic basis has led to a paradigm-shifting recommendation in clinical guidelines: **universal genetic testing should be considered for all patients diagnosed with a pheochromocytoma or paraganglioma**.

The Molecular Clusters: A Functional Classification of PPGL Pathogenesis

HTS has been instrumental in defining a robust and clinically relevant molecular-driven classification system for PPGL. This system categorizes tumors into three main clusters based on the underlying signaling pathways that are disrupted. This classification has powerful correlations with the tumor's location, biochemical phenotype, and, most importantly, its risk of malignancy.

Cluster 1: The Pseudohypoxia Cluster

This is the largest and most complex cluster, accounting for approximately 30% of all PPGLs. It includes tumors with mutations in genes whose normal function is intricately related to the cellular oxygen-sensing and metabolic pathways. The unifying molecular consequence of these mutations is the stabilization of **hypoxia-inducible factors (HIFs)**, particularly HIF-2α. This leads to a transcriptional state of **"pseudohypoxia,"** where the cell behaves as if it is chronically starved of oxygen, even in normoxic conditions. This drives the expression of genes involved in angiogenesis (like VEGF), erythropoiesis, and anaerobic glycolysis, promoting tumor growth and survival. The key genes in this cluster are the following:

- **Succinate Dehydrogenase (SDH) Subunit Genes (*SDHA, SDHB, SDHC, SDHD, SDHAF2*):** The SDH complex (mitochondrial complex II) is a critical enzyme in both the Krebs cycle and the electron transport chain. Germline mutations in any of these genes impair the enzyme's function, leading to a massive accumulation of its substrate, **succinate**. Succinate acts as an "oncometabolite," competitively inhibiting 2-oxoglutarate-dependent dioxygenases, including the prolyl hydroxylases that normally target HIF-α for degradation. The result is constitutive HIF stabilization.
- ***Von Hippel-Lindau (VHL)*:** The VHL protein is the substrate recognition component of an E3 ubiquitin ligase complex that is responsible for degrading HIF-α under normoxic conditions. Germline inactivating mutations in *VHL* cause VHL disease, which includes a high risk of PPGL, clear cell renal cell carcinoma, and hemangioblastomas. Loss of VHL function leads directly to HIF stabilization.
- ***Endothelial PAS domain-containing protein 1 (EPAS1)*:** This gene encodes the HIF-2α protein itself. Somatic gain-of-function mutations in *EPAS1* create a form of HIF-2α that is resistant to degradation, leading to its accumulation.

Cluster 2: The Kinase Signaling Cluster

This cluster accounts for ~40% of PPGLs and includes tumors with mutations that lead to the activation of kinase signaling pathways, primarily the PI3K/AKT/mTOR and RAS/MAPK pathways. These pathways are central regulators of cell growth, proliferation, and survival. The key genes are the following:

- ***REarranged during Transfection (RET)*:** Germline activating mutations in this receptor tyrosine kinase cause the MEN2 syndromes, with PPGL being a cardinal feature.
- ***Neurofibromin 1 (NF1)*:** Germline inactivating mutations in this tumor suppressor gene cause neurofibromatosis type 1. NF1 is a GTPase-activating protein that negatively regulates RAS signaling. Loss of NF1 leads to hyperactive RAS/MAPK signaling.
- ***Transmembrane Protein 127 (TMEM127)*:** A tumor suppressor gene that negatively regulates mTOR signaling.
- ***MYC-Associated Factor X (MAX)*:** A transcription factor that forms a complex with MYC. Germline mutations in *MAX* lead to a hereditary PPGL syndrome [28].

Cluster 3: The Wnt Signaling and Other Pathways
This is a more recently described and still evolving cluster. It includes tumors with alterations that activate the Wnt signaling pathway, such as somatic fusions involving the *MAML3* gene. Other rare drivers are continuously being discovered, further populating the genetic landscape of PPGL.

Powerful Genotype-Phenotype Correlations: From Bench to Bedside

The clinical power of this molecular classification lies in its strong and predictable correlations with clinical features, which directly impact patient management.

Molecular cluster	Key genes	Typical location	Biochemical phenotype	Metastatic risk	Clinical implications
Cluster 1 (pseudohypoxia)	*SDHB*, *SDHD*, *SDHA*, *SDHC*, *VHL*, *EPAS1*, *FH*	Extra-adrenal (especially head/neck PGL for *SDHD*, abdominal PGL for *SDHB*), bilateral PCC (*VHL*)	Noradrenergic (norepinephrine only) or dopaminergic	**Very high (35–75%) for *SDHB***; moderate for *SDHA*, low for others	**Universal germline testing.** *SDHB* mutation mandates intensive, lifelong surveillance. SDHB IHC is a crucial screening tool
Cluster 2 (kinase signaling)	*RET*, *NF1*, *MAX*, *TMEM127*	Adrenal (PCC), often bilateral (*RET*, *NF1*)	Adrenergic (epinephrine + norepinephrine)	Low to moderate	Screen for MEN2/NF1 syndrome features. Family screening is crucial

The Critical Role of *SDHB* The single most important clinical correlation is the link between germline mutations in the ***SDHB* gene and a very high risk of malignancy** (i.e., metastatic disease). Patients with germline *SDHB* mutations have a lifetime risk of developing metastatic PPGL that can range from 35% to as high as 75%. This is a profound and life-altering risk. The identification of an *SDHB* mutation at the time of initial diagnosis, even for a seemingly benign and localized tumor, completely changes the patient's management trajectory. It immediately stratifies them into a high-risk category, mandating intensive, lifelong surveillance with annual biochemical testing and alternating full-body MRI and CT/PET scans to detect metastatic disease at its earliest and most treatable stage. This has transformed the management of these patients from a reactive approach (treating metastases when they become clinically apparent) to a proactive, risk-stratified surveillance model [29].

The Role of Histology and Immunohistochemistry in the Molecular Era

While the molecular genotype is the most powerful predictor of behavior, histology remains important. The **PASS score (Pheochromocytoma of the Adrenal gland Scaled Score)** is a histological algorithm that attempts to predict metastatic potential, but it has significant interobserver variability and is not reliably predictive. Its primary utility is in identifying tumors with atypical features that warrant closer follow-up [30].

Of greater importance is the use of **SDHB immunohistochemistry** on the resected tumor specimen. Because all the SDH subunit proteins are required to form a stable mitochondrial complex, a pathogenic mutation in *any* of the *SDHx* genes (*SDHA*, *SDHB*, *SDHC*, *SDHD*) typically leads to the degradation of the entire complex, including the SDHB protein. Therefore, loss of SDHB protein expression by IHC (i.e., a negative stain in tumor cells with a positive internal control in normal cells) serves as a highly sensitive and specific surrogate marker for the presence of an *SDHx* mutation. Any tumor with negative SDHB staining should prompt immediate referral for germline genetic testing, as it is a strong indicator of a Cluster 1 tumor.

Adrenal Cortex and Pituitary Gland

Adrenocortical Carcinoma (ACC)

Adrenocortical carcinoma is a rare but exceptionally aggressive malignancy with a 5-year survival rate of less than 50%. The histological diagnosis, which relies on the multifactorial Weiss scoring system, can be challenging in borderline cases, and distinguishing ACC from an atypical adenoma can be difficult. HTS has revealed that ACC is a disease characterized by profound genomic instability, widespread aneuploidy, and a high mutational burden, reflecting its aggressive biology.

The Genomic Landscape of ACC Comprehensive genomic analyses, including those from The Cancer Genome Atlas (TCGA), have identified recurrent somatic alterations in several key pathways:

- **Wnt/β-catenin Signaling:** This pathway is activated in 30–40% of ACCs, most commonly through activating mutations in the *CTNNB1* gene (encoding β-catenin) or inactivating mutations in its negative regulator, *ZNRF3*.
- ***TP53* and Li-Fraumeni Syndrome:** Somatic mutations in the *TP53* tumor suppressor gene are found in ~30% of sporadic ACCs and are associated with a poorer prognosis. Critically, germline mutations in *TP53* cause **Li-Fraumeni syndrome**, a highly penetrant hereditary cancer syndrome. ACC is one of the cardinal tumors of this syndrome, particularly in children. Therefore, any child, and many adults, diagnosed with ACC should be considered for germline *TP53* testing.
- **Cell Cycle Regulation:** Alterations in genes that control the cell cycle, such as homozygous deletion of *CDKN2A* and amplification of *CDK4*, are common and drive proliferation.
- **Copy Number Alterations:** ACCs are characterized by massive numbers of CNVs and frequent whole-genome doubling, a hallmark of genomic instability [31].

Molecular Prognostication and Therapeutic Implications Beyond identifying drivers, molecular profiling has powerful prognostic utility. Gene expression profiling (using RNA-seq or microarrays) has robustly demonstrated the ability to not only distinguish malignant ACC from benign adenomas but also to stratify ACCs into at least two major prognostic molecular subtypes (often termed C1A and C1B). The C1A subtype is characterized by the upregulation of proliferation genes and is associated with a significantly worse survival outcome, providing prognostic information that is independent of and complementary to traditional tumor staging. While targeted therapies for ACC have been challenging, the identification of recurrent alterations is opening doors for clinical trials of agents targeting the Wnt pathway, cell cycle regulators (e.g., CDK4/6 inhibitors), and DNA damage repair pathways [32].

Pituitary Neuroendocrine Tumors (PitNETs)

The molecular landscape of PitNETs presents a fascinating and instructive contrast to most other solid tumors. For decades, researchers were frustrated by the fact that PitNETs are remarkably "quiet" at the point mutation level. HTS has confirmed this, revealing a very low somatic mutation burden across all subtypes [33]. With the notable exceptions of the following:

- Activating mutations in the G-protein alpha subunit gene, *GNAS*, found in approximately 40% of somatotroph (GH-secreting) tumors causing acromegaly.
- Activating mutations in the deubiquitinase gene, *USP8*, present in about 40–60% of a subset of corticotroph (ACTH-secreting) tumors causing Cushing's disease [34].

Recurrent, druggable driver mutations are virtually absent in the majority of PitNETs. This makes standard targeted DNA sequencing panels of very limited clinical utility for diagnosis or therapy selection [35].

The key to unlocking the molecular biology and prognostication of PitNETs lies in looking beyond simple DNA sequence mutations:

- **Copy Number Variations (CNVs):** Large-scale genomic alterations are much more informative. Approximately one-third of PitNETs are classified as "genomically disrupted," characterized by widespread, chromosome arm-level CNVs (aneuploidy). This chromosomal instability is a key driver of tumorigenesis in this subset and is strongly correlated with more aggressive clinical behavior, invasion, and recurrence. Assessing the copy number profile can therefore provide valuable prognostic information that is not apparent from histology.
- **Epigenomics, Specifically DNA Methylation Profiling:** This has emerged as the single most powerful and revolutionary molecular tool for PitNETs. DNA methylation is a chemical modification (the addition of a methyl group) to DNA, primarily at CpG dinucleotides, that regulates gene expression without changing the underlying DNA sequence itself. It is a fundamental component of the "epigenome." Genome-wide DNA methylation profiling (using techniques like methylation arrays) has demonstrated two remarkable capabilities:

1. **Robust Classification:** Unsupervised clustering of methylation data can robustly and accurately classify PitNETs according to their cell of origin and transcription factor lineage (e.g., PIT1-lineage [somatotroph, lactotroph, thyrotroph], TPIT-lineage [corticotroph], and SF1-lineage [gonadotroph]). The accuracy of this molecular classification meets or even exceeds that of the standard panel of immunohistochemical stains for transcription factors. It can resolve the classification of the ~15% of tumors that are "null cell" or negative by IHC.
2. **Powerful Prognostication:** Most critically, distinct and reproducible methylation signatures have been identified that can reliably differentiate typical, indolent PitNETs from the small subset of "atypical" tumors that will behave aggressively, recur multiple times, or even metastasize (pituitary carcinomas). This holds immense and imminent promise for developing the first truly reliable molecular prognostic biomarkers for these tumors, allowing for the prospective identification of high-risk patients who may benefit from adjuvant radiation or more intensive surveillance.

Gastroenteropancreatic Neuroendocrine Neoplasms (GEP-NENs)

GEP-NENs are a heterogeneous group of tumors arising from the neuroendocrine cells of the digestive system. The cornerstone of their management, from a pathological perspective, is the crucial distinction between **well-differentiated neuroendocrine tumors (NETs)** and **poorly differentiated neuroendocrine carcinomas (NECs)**. This distinction is based on morphology (NETs have an "organoid" architecture with uniform cells, while NECs are high-grade carcinomas with sheet-like growth and necrosis) and is quantified by the **Ki-67 proliferation index**, which forms the basis of the WHO grading system (G1, G2, G3). HTS has provided a robust and unequivocal genetic validation of this fundamental histological dichotomy, proving that NETs and NECs are not merely points on a single continuum of aggressiveness but are, in fact, fundamentally distinct biological and genetic entities [36, 37].

The Molecular Landscape of Well-Differentiated NETs (G1/G2/some G3)

Well-differentiated NETs, particularly those arising in the pancreas (PanNETs), have a relatively low mutational burden compared to common adenocarcinomas. Their genomic landscape is characterized by recurrent alterations in three key genetic pathways:

1. ***MEN1* Gene:** Inactivating mutations in the *MEN1* tumor suppressor gene are the most common genetic event in PanNETs. Germline mutations cause the hereditary MEN1 syndrome (characterized by tumors of the parathyroid, pituitary, and pancreas). Somatic mutations in *MEN1* are found in ~40% of sporadic PanNETs.
2. ***DAXX* and *ATRX* Genes:** Inactivating mutations in these two genes, which encode chromatin remodeling proteins involved in telomere maintenance, are mutually exclusive and are found in a combined ~40% of PanNETs. Loss of DAXX or ATRX function leads to a specific molecular phenotype called the Alternative Lengthening of Telomeres (ALT), and these mutations are strongly associated with the development of chromosomal instability.
3. **mTOR Pathway Genes:** Mutations in genes of the PI3K/AKT/mTOR signaling pathway (e.g., *PTEN*, *TSC2*, *PIK3CA*) are found in ~15% of PanNETs. This provides a direct molecular rationale for the use of mTOR inhibitors in this disease [38].

The Molecular Landscape of Poorly Differentiated NECs (Always G3)

Poorly differentiated NECs are genetically completely different from NETs. Their genomes are often chaotic and characterized by a high mutational burden. Crucially, they are defined by the near-universal biallelic inactivation of two critical tumor suppressor genes:

- ***TP53***
- ***RB1*** (Retinoblastoma gene)

  This molecular signature (*TP53* + *RB1* loss) is the hallmark of NECs and is very rarely, if ever, seen in well-differentiated NETs. This genetic profile is much more similar to that of other aggressive, poorly differentiated carcinomas, particularly small cell lung carcinoma. This provides a clear and powerful biological rationale for why NECs have such an aggressive clinical course and why they are treated with platinum-based cytotoxic chemotherapy, similar to small cell lung cancer, rather than the therapies used for NETs.

Clinical and Therapeutic Implications of Molecular Profiling in GEP-NENs

- **Differential Diagnosis:** In rare, challenging biopsy cases, molecular testing can help distinguish a high-grade G3 NET from a true NEC. The presence of *TP53*/*RB1* mutations strongly favors NEC.
- **Hereditary Syndrome Identification:** HTS can identify germline mutations in genes like

MEN1, *VHL* (associated with PanNETs), and *NF1*, establishing a hereditary syndrome diagnosis with implications for patient screening and family management.

- **Guiding Targeted Therapy:** The presence of mTOR pathway mutations provides a rationale for the use of mTOR inhibitors like everolimus in advanced PanNETs.
- **Identifying Candidates for Immunotherapy:** While most NETs are "immunologically cold" with a low TMB, a subset of high-grade NECs can have a high tumor mutational burden (TMB) or may exhibit mismatch repair deficiency (dMMR/MSI-H). The identification of these biomarkers by HTS can make these patients candidates for immunotherapy with immune checkpoint inhibitors, offering a novel and potentially effective therapeutic option for this otherwise difficult-to-treat disease.

The Future Horizon: Integrating Multi-omics and Artificial Intelligence

The morpho-molecular revolution in endocrine pathology is still in its early stages. The current paradigm, largely based on bulk sequencing of DNA from tissue samples, is already being enhanced and will eventually be complemented by a new wave of technologies that provide an even more granular, dynamic, and holistic picture of each patient's cancer.

Deconstructing Heterogeneity: The Power of Single-Cell and Spatial "Omics"

A major limitation of bulk HTS is that it provides an averaged genomic or transcriptomic profile from the millions of different cells present in a tissue biopsy. However, tumors are not monolithic entities; they are complex, evolving ecosystems composed of multiple distinct subclones of cancer cells, as well as a diverse array of noncancerous cells—including fibroblasts, endothelial cells, and various immune cells—that collectively form the **tumor microenvironment (TME)**. The intricate cross talk between cancer cells and the TME profoundly influences tumor growth, invasion, and response to therapy.

- **Single-Cell Sequencing (scRNA-seq, scDNA-seq):** This powerful suite of technologies allows for the genomic or transcriptomic profiling of thousands of individual cells from a dissociated tumor sample. This provides a high-resolution map of the tumor's cellular composition, allowing researchers to identify rare therapy-resistant cell populations, reconstruct clonal evolutionary trajectories, and perform a detailed census of the specific immune cell types that are infiltrating (or being excluded from) the tumor.
- **Spatial Transcriptomics:** This revolutionary technology bridges the gap between single-cell resolution and histological context. It performs RNA sequencing directly on an intact tissue slide, preserving the two-dimensional spatial coordinates of the transcriptomic data. The result is a molecular map of the tumor that can be directly overlaid onto the H&E image. This allows for the in situ investigation of the molecular underpinnings of morphological features. For example, one could specifically analyze the gene expression programs of cancer cells located at the invasive front versus those in the tumor core to precisely identify the molecular pathways driving metastasis. Spatial transcriptomics represents the ultimate convergence of genomics and histology, allowing us to see the molecular biology of the tumor in its native habitat.

Noninvasive Longitudinal Monitoring: The Promise of Liquid Biopsies

The characterization of tumors has traditionally relied on an invasive solid tissue biopsy, which provides only a static snapshot of the tumor at a single point in time. **Liquid biopsy**, the analysis of tumor-derived material from a blood sample or other body fluid, offers the potential for a minimally invasive, dynamic, and longitudinal monitoring of a patient's cancer [39].

- **Circulating Tumor DNA (ctDNA):** As tumor cells die, they release small fragments of their DNA into the bloodstream. This ctDNA carries the same mutations as the tumor itself. Because ctDNA has a very short half-life in the blood (often less than two hours), its analysis provides a real-time reflection of the tumor's current genomic state. The potential clinical applications are vast:
  - **Early Detection of Recurrence:** Detecting a rise in the level of a known tumor mutation in the blood after surgery could identify **minimal residual disease (MRD)** and predict clinical relapse months before it becomes visible on imaging scans.
  - **Tracking Therapeutic Response and Resistance:** A rapid decrease in the allele frequency of a driver mutation can serve as an early indicator of response to targeted therapy. Conversely, the emergence of a new, known resistance mutation in the ctDNA can signal the development of therapeutic resistance, prompting a change in treatment before the patient develops overt clinical progression.

  While the utility of ctDNA is currently most established in high-shedding cancers, and can be challenging in indolent, low-volume endocrine tumors, it is an area of intense investigation and holds immense promise, particularly for the management of advanced, aggressive endocrine cancers like ATC, NECs, and metastatic MTC.

Artificial Intelligence (AI) in Integrated Diagnostics

The ultimate challenge and opportunity in modern pathology lie in the synthesis of the vast and disparate streams of high-dimensional data being generated for each patient: digital pathology (giga-pixel whole-slide images), genomics (HTS data), radiology (CT, MRI, PET scans), and clinical records. The human mind is not equipped to process and integrate this level of complexity. **Artificial intelligence**, particularly the subfields of machine learning and deep learning, is the essential computational engine required to unlock the full potential of this multimodal data.

- **AI in Computational Pathology:** AI algorithms are already being deployed to assist with and automate tasks in digital pathology. This includes the precise quantification of IHC biomarkers like Ki-67, the objective grading of tumors, and the detection of micrometastases in lymph nodes [40].
- **The Predictive Power of Histology-to-Genomics Mapping:** A truly transformative application is the training of deep learning models on large, paired datasets of whole-slide images and HTS data from the same tumors. These models can learn the subtle and often subvisual morphological patterns that are correlated with specific underlying genomic alterations. AI models are already being developed that can predict, with high accuracy, the presence of specific mutations, like *BRAF* V600E in thyroid cancer or *TP53* status in various cancers, directly from the routine H&E image alone. This "virtual molecular pathology" could serve as a powerful and inexpensive screening tool to prioritize which cases require definitive and expensive molecular testing, optimizing resource allocation [41].
- **Integrated Prognostic and Predictive Modeling:** The true power of AI will be realized in its ability to integrate all available data modalities—morphological features, the full genomic landscape, spatial transcriptomic maps, and clinical variables—to create powerful and highly accurate prognostic and predictive models that far surpass the performance of any single data type alone.

The logical endpoint and ultimate goal of this technological and analytical convergence is the creation of a **"digital twin"** for each patient's cancer. This would be a dynamic, multi-scale, computational model of the tumor, constructed from all of its patient-specific data. This model would be used to simulate the tumor's likely behavior and to predict its response to various therapeutic options. This would allow clinicians to test and optimize treatment strategies in silico before administering them to the patient, representing the pinnacle of personalized, predictive, and proactive medicine [42].

Conclusion

The integration of high-throughput sequencing into the daily practice of endocrine pathology has catalyzed a paradigm shift that is deeper and more rapid than any in the last century. This morpho-molecular revolution is not a future concept; it is the current, dynamic, and rapidly evolving standard of care. What began as a novel research tool to resolve a specific diagnostic dilemma in thyroid cytology has evolved into an essential and indispensable component of patient care across the entire spectrum of endocrine oncology. It provides diagnostic clarity, powerful prognostic stratification, and the essential predictive biomarkers that enable the use of life-saving targeted therapies.

In this new era, the role of the pathologist is expanding and becoming more critical than ever. The pathologist is no longer solely a morphological diagnostician but rather the central integrator and interpreter of complex, multimodal data. The modern endocrine pathologist must be fluent in the languages of both classic histopathology and clinical genomics, expertly weaving together the information from the microscope slide, the HTS report, the clinical history, and the radiological findings to generate a single, coherent, and clinically actionable diagnosis. As the technologies of genomics, spatial-omics, liquid biopsy, and artificial intelligence continue to mature and converge, the field is poised to move ever closer to the ultimate goal of precision oncology: delivering the right treatment, to the right patient, at the right time, based on a deep and holistic understanding of their individual tumor's biology.

References

1. Al-Hakami HA, Alqahtani R, Alahmadi A, Almutairi D, Algarni M, Alandejani T. Thyroid nodule size and prediction of cancer: a study at tertiary care hospital in Saudi Arabia. Cureus. 2020;12(3):e7478. https://doi.org/10.7759/cureus.7478. PMID: 32351856; PMCID: PMC7188016
2. Papotti M, Libè R, Duregon E, Volante M, Bertherat J, Tissier F. The Weiss score and beyond--histopathology for adrenocortical carcinoma. Horm Cancer. 2011;2(6):333–40. https://doi.org/10.1007/s12672-011-0088-0. PMID: 21997290; PMCID: PMC10358021
3. Fang JM, Li J, Shi J. An update on the diagnosis of gastroenteropancreatic neuroendocrine neoplasms. World J Gastroenterol. 2022;28(10):1009–23. https://doi.org/10.3748/wjg.v28.i10.1009. PMID: 35431496; PMCID: PMC8968521
4. Rosai J. Immunohistochemical markers of thyroid tumors: significance and diagnostic applications. Tumori. 2003;89(5):517–9. https://doi.org/10.1177/030089160308900511. PMID: 14870775
5. Shin JH. Nucleic acid extraction techniques. In: Advanced techniques in diagnostic microbiology; 2012. p. 209–25. https://doi.org/10.1007/978-1-4614-3970-7_11. PMCID: PMC7122149.
6. van Dijk EL, Jaszczyszyn Y, Thermes C. Library preparation methods for next-generation sequencing: tone down the bias. Exp Cell Res. 2014;322(1):12–20. https://doi.org/10.1016/j.yexcr.2014.01.008. Epub 2014 Jan 15. PMID: 24440557.
7. Abil Z, Restrepo Sierra AM, Danelon C. Clonal amplification-enhanced gene expression in synthetic vesicles. ACS Synth Biol. 2023;12(4):1187–203. https://doi.org/10.1021/acssynbio.2c00668. Epub 2023 Apr 4. PMID: 37014369; PMCID: PMC10127449
8. Ju J, Kim DH, Bi L, Meng Q, Bai X, Li Z, Li X, Marma MS, Shi S, Wu J, Edwards JR, Romu A, Turro NJ. Four-color DNA sequencing by synthesis using cleavable fluorescent nucleotide reversible terminators. Proc Natl Acad Sci USA. 2006;103(52):19635–40. https://doi.org/10.1073/pnas.0609513103. Epub 2006 Dec 14. PMID: 17170132; PMCID: PMC1702316
9. Pezoulas VC, Zaridis DI, Mylona E, Androutsos C, Apostolidis K, Tachos NS, Fotiadis DI. Synthetic data generation methods in healthcare: a review on open-source tools and methods. Comput Struct Biotechnol J. 2024;23:2892–910. https://doi.org/10.1016/j.csbj.2024.07.005. PMID: 39108677; PMCID: PMC11301073
10. Bagger FO, Borgwardt L, Jespersen AS, Hansen AR, Bertelsen B, Kodama M, Nielsen FC. Whole genome sequencing in clinical practice. BMC Med Genet.

2024;17(1):39. https://doi.org/10.1186/s12920-024-01795-w. PMID: 38287327; PMCID: PMC10823711
11. Daud D, Griffin H, Douroudis K, Kleinle S, Eglon G, Pyle A, Chinnery PF, Horvath R. Whole exome sequencing and the clinician: we need clinical skills and functional validation in variant filtering. J Neurol. 2015;262(7):1673–7. https://doi.org/10.1007/s00415-015-7755-y. Epub 2015 May 10. PMID: 25957632; PMCID: PMC4503877
12. Quaio CRDC, Obando MJR, Perazzio SF, Dutra AP, Chung CH, Moreira CM, Novo Filho GM, Sacramento-Bobotis PR, Penna MG, Souza RRF, Cintra VP, Carnavalli JEP, Silva RAD, Santos MNP, Paixão D, Baratela WADR, Olivati C, Spolador GM, Pintao MC, Fornari ARDS, Burger M, Ramalho RF, Pereira OJE, Ferreira ENE, Mitne-Neto M, Kim CA. Exome sequencing and targeted gene panels: a simulated comparison of diagnostic yield using data from 158 patients with rare diseases. Genet Mol Biol. 2021;44(4):20210061. https://doi.org/10.1590/1678-4685-GMB-2021-0061. PMID: 34609444; PMCID: PMC8485181
13. Kukurba KR, Montgomery SB. RNA sequencing and analysis. Cold Spring Harb Protoc. 2015;2015(11):951–69. https://doi.org/10.1101/pdb.top084970. PMID: 25870306; PMCID: PMC4863231
14. Huang J, Wang L. Cell-free DNA methylation profiling analysis-technologies and bioinformatics. Cancers (Basel). 2019;11(11):1741. https://doi.org/10.3390/cancers11111741. PMID: 31698791; PMCID: PMC6896050
15. Hadfield J, Eldridge MD. Multi-genome alignment for quality control and contamination screening of next-generation sequencing data. Front Genet. 2014;5:31. https://doi.org/10.3389/fgene.2014.00031. PMID: 24600470; PMCID: PMC3930033
16. Zverinova S, Guryev V. Variant calling: considerations, practices, and developments. Hum Mutat. 2022;43(8):976–85. https://doi.org/10.1002/humu.24311. Epub 2021 Dec 16. PMID: 34882898; PMCID: PMC9545713
17. Yang H, Wang K. Genomic variant annotation and prioritization with ANNOVAR and wANNOVAR. Nat Protoc. 2015;10(10):1556–66. https://doi.org/10.1038/nprot.2015.105. Epub 2015 Sep 17. PMID: 26379229; PMCID: PMC4718734
18. Nikiforov YE, Carty SE, Chiosea SI, Coyne C, Duvvuri U, Ferris RL, Gooding WE, LeBeau SO, Ohori NP, Seethala RR, Tublin ME, Yip L, Nikiforova MN. Impact of the multi-gene ThyroSeq next-generation sequencing assay on cancer diagnosis in thyroid nodules with atypia of undetermined significance/follicular lesion of undetermined significance cytology. Thyroid. 2015;25(11):1217–23. https://doi.org/10.1089/thy.2015.0305. Epub 2015 Sep 10. PMID: 26356635; PMCID: PMC4652198
19. Cibas ES, Ali SZ. The 2017 Bethesda system for reporting thyroid cytopathology. Thyroid. 2017;27(11):1341–6. https://doi.org/10.1089/thy.2017.0500. PMID: 29091573
20. Haugen BR, Alexander EK, Bible KC, Doherty GM, Mandel SJ, Nikiforov YE, Pacini F, Randolph GW, Sawka AM, Schlumberger M, Schuff KG, Sherman SI, Sosa JA, Steward DL, Tuttle RM, Wartofsky L. 2015 American Thyroid Association management guidelines for adult patients with thyroid nodules and differentiated thyroid cancer: the American Thyroid Association guidelines task force on thyroid nodules and differentiated thyroid cancer. Thyroid. 2016;26(1):1–133. https://doi.org/10.1089/thy.2015.0020. PMID: 26462967; PMCID: PMC4739132
21. Xing M, Liu R, Liu X, Murugan AK, Zhu G, Zeiger MA, Pai S, Bishop J. BRAF V600E and TERT promoter mutations cooperatively identify the most aggressive papillary thyroid cancer with highest recurrence. J Clin Oncol. 2014;32(25):2718–26. https://doi.org/10.1200/JCO.2014.55.5094. Epub 2014 July 14. PMID: 25024077; PMCID: PMC4145183
22. Steward DL, Carty SE, Sippel RS, Yang SP, Sosa JA, Sipos JA, Figge JJ, Mandel S, Haugen BR, Burman KD, Baloch ZW, Lloyd RV, Seethala RR, Gooding WE, Chiosea SI, Gomes-Lima C, Ferris RL, Folek JM, Khawaja RA, Kundra P, Loh KS, Marshall CB, Mayson S, McCoy KL, Nga ME, Ngiam KY, Nikiforova MN, Poehls JL, Ringel MD, Yang H, Yip L, Nikiforov YE. Performance of a multigene genomic classifier in thyroid nodules with indeterminate cytology: a prospective blinded Multicenter study. JAMA Oncol. 2019;5(2):204–12. https://doi.org/10.1001/jamaoncol.2018.4616. Erratum in: JAMA Oncol. ;5(2):271. doi:10.1001/jamaoncol.2018.6413. PMID: 30419129; PMCID: PMC6439562
23. Wirth LJ, Sherman E, Robinson B, et al. Efficacy of Selpercatinib in RET-altered thyroid cancers. N Engl J Med. 2020;383(9):825–35.
24. Drilon A, Laetsch TW, Kummar S, DuBois SG, Lassen UN, Demetri GD, Nathenson M, Doebele RC, Farago AF, Pappo AS, Turpin B, Dowlati A, Brose MS, Mascarenhas L, Federman N, Berlin J, El-Deiry WS, Baik C, Deeken J, Boni V, Nagasubramanian R, Taylor M, Rudzinski ER, Meric-Bernstam F, Sohal DPS, Ma PC, Raez LE, Hechtman JF, Benayed R, Ladanyi M, Tuch BB, Ebata K, Cruickshank S, Ku NC, Cox MC, Hawkins DS, Hong DS, Hyman DM. Efficacy of Larotrectinib in TRK fusion-positive cancers in adults and children. N Engl J Med. 2018;378(8):731–9. https://doi.org/10.1056/NEJMoa1714448. PMID: 29466156; PMCID: PMC5857389
25. Kiyota N, Robinson B, Shah M, Hoff AO, Taylor MH, Li D, Dutcus CE, Lee EK, Kim SB, Tahara M. Defining radioiodine-refractory differentiated thyroid cancer: efficacy and safety of lenvatinib by radioiodine-refractory criteria in the SELECT trial. Thyroid. 2017;27(9):1135–41. https://doi.org/10.1089/thy.2016.0549. Epub 2017 Aug 14. PMID: 28665259; PMCID: PMC5646742
26. Wells SA Jr, Asa SL, Dralle H, Elisei R, Evans DB, Gagel RF, Lee N, Machens A, Moley JF, Pacini

F, Raue F, Frank-Raue K, Robinson B, Rosenthal MS, Santoro M, Schlumberger M, Shah M, Waguespack SG. American Thyroid Association guidelines task force on medullary thyroid carcinoma. Revised American Thyroid Association guidelines for the management of medullary thyroid carcinoma. Thyroid. 2015;25(6):567–610. https://doi.org/10.1089/thy.2014.0335. PMID: 25810047; PMCID: PMC4490627

27. Hamidi S, Dadu R, Zafereo ME, Ferrarotto R, Wang JR, Maniakas A, Gunn GB, Lee A, Spiotto MT, Iyer PC, Sousa LG, Akhave NS, Ahmed S, Learned KO, Lu C, Lai SY, Williams M, Hosseini SM, Busaidy NL, Cabanillas ME. Initial management of BRAF V600E-variant anaplastic thyroid cancer: the FAST multidisciplinary group consensus statement. JAMA Oncol. 2024;10(9):1264–71. https://doi.org/10.1001/jamaoncol.2024.2133. PMID: 38990526
28. Vit O, Talacko P, Musil Z, Hartmann I, Pacak K, Petrak J. Identification of potential molecular targets for the treatment of cluster 1 human pheochromocytoma and paraganglioma via comprehensive proteomic characterization. Clin Proteomics. 2023;20(1):39. https://doi.org/10.1186/s12014-023-09428-7. PMID: 37749499; PMCID: PMC10518975
29. Rijken JA, Niemeijer ND, Leemans CR, Eijkelenkamp K, van der Horst-Schrivers ANA, van Berkel A, Timmers HJLM, Kunst HPM, Bisschop PHLT, van Dooren MF, Hes FJ, Jansen JC, Corssmit EPM, Hensen EF. Nationwide study of patients with head and neck paragangliomas carrying SDHB germline mutations. BJS Open. 2018;2(2):62–9. https://doi.org/10.1002/bjs5.39. PMID: 29951630; PMCID: PMC5952381
30. Thompson LD. Pheochromocytoma of the adrenal gland scaled score (PASS) to separate benign from malignant neoplasms: a clinicopathologic and immunophenotypic study of 100 cases. Am J Surg Pathol. 2002;26(5):551–66. https://doi.org/10.1097/00000478-200205000-00002. PMID: 11979086
31. Sun-Zhang A, Juhlin CC, Carling T, Scholl U, Schott M, Larsson C, Bajalica-Lagercrantz S. Comprehensive genomic analysis of adrenocortical carcinoma reveals genetic profiles associated with patient survival. ESMO Open. 2024;9(7):103617. https://doi.org/10.1016/j.esmoop.2024.103617. Epub 2024 Jun 26. PMID: 38935991; PMCID: PMC11260375
32. Fishbein L, Leshchiner I, Walter V, Danilova L, Robertson AG, Johnson AR, Lichtenberg TM, Murray BA, Ghayee HK, Else T, Ling S, Jefferys SR, de Cubas AA, Wenz B, Korpershoek E, Amelio AL, Makowski L, Rathmell WK, Gimenez-Roqueplo AP, Giordano TJ, Asa SL, Tischler AS; Cancer Genome Atlas Research Network; Pacak K, Nathanson KL, Wilkerson MD. Comprehensive molecular characterization of Pheochromocytoma and Paraganglioma. Cancer Cell 2017; 31(2):181–193. doi:https://doi.org/10.1016/j.ccell.2017.01.001. Epub 2017 Feb 2. PMID: 28162975; PMCID: PMC5643159.
33. Lenders JW, Duh QY, Eisenhofer G, Gimenez-Roqueplo AP, Grebe SK, Murad MH, Naruse M, Pacak K, Young WF, Endocrine Society. Pheochromocytoma and paraganglioma: an endocrine society clinical practice guideline. J Clin Endocrinol Metab. 2014;99(6):1915–42. https://doi.org/10.1210/jc.2014-1498. Erratum in: J Clin Endocrinol Metab. 2023 Apr 13;108(5):e200. doi:10.1210/clinem/dgad064. PMID: 24893135.
34. Reincke M, Sbiera S, Hayakawa A, Theodoropoulou M, Osswald A, Beuschlein F, Meitinger T, Mizuno-Yamasaki E, Kawaguchi K, Saeki Y, Tanaka K, Wieland T, Graf E, Saeger W, Ronchi CL, Allolio B, Buchfelder M, Strom TM, Fassnacht M, Komada M. Mutations in the deubiquitinase gene USP8 cause Cushing's disease. Nat Genet. 2015;47(1):31–8. https://doi.org/10.1038/ng.3166. Epub 2014 Dec 8. PMID: 25485838
35. Neumann HPH, Young WF Jr, Eng C. Pheochromocytoma and Paraganglioma. N Engl J Med. 2019;381(6):552–65. https://doi.org/10.1056/NEJMra1806651. PMID: 31390501
36. Prisciandaro M, Antista M, Raimondi A, Corti F, Morano F, Centonze G, Sabella G, Mangogna A, Randon G, Pagani F, Prinzi N, Niger M, Corallo S, Castiglioni di Caronno E, Massafra M, Bartolomeo MD, de Braud F, Milione M, Pusceddu S. Biomarker landscape in neuroendocrine tumors with high-grade features: current knowledge and future perspective. Front Oncol. 2022;4(12):780716. https://doi.org/10.3389/fonc.2022.780716. PMID: 35186729; PMCID: PMC8856722
37. Jiao Y, Shi C, Edil BH, de Wilde RF, Klimstra DS, Maitra A, Schulick RD, Tang LH, Wolfgang CL, Choti MA, Velculescu VE, Diaz LA Jr, Vogelstein B, Kinzler KW, Hruban RH, Papadopoulos N. DAXX/ATRX, MEN1, and mTOR pathway genes are frequently altered in pancreatic neuroendocrine tumors. Science. 2011;331(6021):1199–203. https://doi.org/10.1126/science.1200609. Epub 2011 Jan 20. PMID: 21252315; PMCID: PMC3144496
38. Yachida S, Vakiani E, White CM, Zhong Y, Saunders T, Morgan R, de Wilde RF, Maitra A, Hicks J, Demarzo AM, Shi C, Sharma R, Laheru D, Edil BH, Wolfgang CL, Schulick RD, Hruban RH, Tang LH, Klimstra DS, Iacobuzio-Donahue CA. Small cell and large cell neuroendocrine carcinomas of the pancreas are genetically similar and distinct from well-differentiated pancreatic neuroendocrine tumors. Am J Surg Pathol. 2012;36(2):173–84. https://doi.org/10.1097/PAS.0b013e3182417d36. PMID: 22251937; PMCID: PMC3261427
39. Wan JCM, Massie C, Garcia-Corbacho J, Mouliere F, Brenton JD, Caldas C, Pacey S, Baird R, Rosenfeld N. Liquid biopsies come of age: towards implementation of circulating tumour DNA. Nat Rev Cancer. 2017;17(4):223–38. https://doi.org/10.1038/nrc.2017.7. Epub 2017 Feb 24. PMID: 28233803

40. Ludwig M, Ludwig B, Mikuła A, Biernat S, Rudnicki J, Kaliszewski K. The use of artificial intelligence in the diagnosis and classification of thyroid nodules: an update. Cancers (Basel). 2023;15(3):708. https://doi.org/10.3390/cancers15030708. PMID: 36765671; PMCID: PMC9913834
41. Gröschel S, Bommer M, Hutter B, Budczies J, Bonekamp D, Heining C, Horak P, Fröhlich M, Uhrig S, Hübschmann D, Geörg C, Richter D, Pfarr N, Pfütze K, Wolf S, Schirmacher P, Jäger D, von Kalle C, Brors B, Glimm H, Weichert W, Stenzinger A, Fröhling S. Integration of genomics and histology revises diagnosis and enables effective therapy of refractory cancer of unknown primary with PDL1 amplification. Cold Spring Harb Mol Case Stud. 2016;2(6):a001180. https://doi.org/10.1101/mcs.a001180. PMID: 27900363; PMCID: PMC5111004
42. AlOsaimi HM, Alshilash AM, Al-Saif LK, Bosbait JM, Albeladi RS, Almutairi DR, Alhazzaa AA, Alluqmani TA, Al Qahtani SM, Almohammadi SA, Alamri RA, Alkurdi AA, Aljohani WK, Alraddadi RH, Alshammari MK. AI models for the identification of prognostic and predictive biomarkers in lung cancer: a systematic review and meta-analysis. Front Oncol. 2025;15:1424647. https://doi.org/10.3389/fonc.2025.1424647. PMID: 40078179; PMCID: PMC11896857

NGS in Cytopathology

16

Giuseppa Zannini, Marco Montella,
Renato Franco, and Federica Zito Marino

Introduction

The advent of precision medicine has underlined the critical importance of molecular profiling in the management of oncological patients. As therapeutic decisions increasingly depend on the identification of specific genomic alterations, ensuring the availability of adequate biological material for both morphological assessment and molecular testing have become essential. However, obtaining sufficient tissue can be particularly challenging in patients with advanced-stage malignancies, where anatomical inaccessibility, comorbidities, or poor clinical condition may limit the feasibility of conventional biopsy procedures [49, 60]. In this context, where surgical biopsies often involve invasive and sometimes impracticable procedures, cytological samples frequently represent the only accessible material for integrated morphological and molecular analyses [50, 60].

Cytological sampling plays a crucial diagnostic role in assessing of both superficial and deep-seated lesions, as well as in malignancy risk stratification, particularly in cases classified as atypical or of undetermined significance. In this setting, nucleic acids extracted from cytological preparations can yield crucial molecular insights that enhance diagnostic accuracy and inform clinical decision-making [77]. The use of next-generation sequencing (NGS) has greatly enhanced the role of cytological specimens in molecular diagnostics, since it allows the concurrent analysis of numerous genomic targets even from samples with low tumor cellularity or minimal input material [33, 64]. This advancement is particularly relevant given that, although cytological specimens often provide nucleic acids of sufficient quality, the amount of DNA or RNA obtained is generally lower compared to small biopsies or histological specimens [40, 53, 60, 72]. The high analytical sensitivity of NGS technologies has overcome the critical issues associated with the biomaterial, improving the feasibility of using cytological samples for comprehensive molecular profiling [63]. Consequently, the implementation of NGS analysis on cytological samples offers both promising opportunities and notable challenges in the clinical and research settings [54].

G. Zannini · M. Montella · R. Franco (✉)
F. Zito Marino
Pathology Unit, Department of Mental and Physical Health and Preventive Medicine, University of Campania "Luigi Vanvitelli", Naples, Italy
e-mail: giuseppa.zannini@unicampania.it;
marco.montella@unicampania.it;
renato.franco@unicampania.it;
federica.zitomarino@unicampania.it

© The Author(s), under exclusive license to Springer Nature Switzerland AG 2026

S. Sioletic, L. Coppola (eds.), *Next-Generation Sequencing in Solid Tumor Histopathology*, Current Clinical Pathology, https://doi.org/10.1007/978-3-032-18790-1_16

Cytological Sample Types Used for NGS

Cytological specimens are recognized as valuable sources of nucleic acids for NGS, particularly in cases where conventional tissue biopsies are unavailable or insufficient. Various cytological preparations vary in terms of cellularity, processing methods, fixation protocols, and nucleic acid preservation, all of which can significantly impact the quality and quantity of DNA and RNA extracted (Table 16.1) [64, 66].

Understanding the characteristics, advantages, and limitations of each cytological sample type is essential for optimizing molecular testing workflows and ensuring reliable NGS results. Multiple studies have evaluated different types of cytological samples, each reporting specific success rates for both DNA-based and RNA-based NGS analyses [1–4, 12, 23, 27, 30, 31, 35, 37, 38, 44, 46–48, 51, 52, 57, 59, 67, 70, 80, 82–87, 89] (Table 16.2).

The following sections provide a detailed overview of the main cytological sample types used for molecular analysis, including direct smears, liquid-based cytology (LBC), cytospin preparations, cell blocks, and supernatants derived from cytological processing [6, 54, 68, 77].

Direct Cytological Smears

Direct cytological smears, generally obtained through fine-needle aspiration (FNA), are among the most commonly used cytological samples for NGS analysis. The most commonly employed cytological staining techniques are the Diff-Quik and Papanicolaou stains, both offering high-resolution cytomorphological detail essential for diagnostic assessment [77].

The Diff-Quik stain is widely used in cytology, especially for FNA specimens, body fluids, and other non-gynecological samples. It is a rapid and efficient staining technique that provides excellent cytoplasmic detail, making it especially useful for the identification of inflammatory, infectious, and neoplastic processes. The protocol comprises a three-step procedure: initial methanol fixation, followed by staining with an eosinophilic solution that stains cytoplasmic components in pink/orange, and subsequent application of a basophilic solution that stains nucleic acids and certain cytoplasmic structures blue to purple [71].

The Papanicolaou stain is a polychromatic staining technique commonly used for the cytological evaluation of gynecological specimens, particularly for cervical cancer screening, as well as other exfoliative cytology specimens. Its application extends to non-gynecological specimens derived from diverse bodily fluids and fine-needle aspiration of organs and tissues [77]. The staining protocol includes ethanol fixation, nuclear staining with hematoxylin, and two cytoplasmic stains that lead to cellular differentiation based on cytoplasmic keratinization and cell origin: the Orange G selectively stains keratinized cells with an orange coloration, while the Eosin Azure stains the cytoplasm in varying shades of pink, green, or blue depending on the cell type. This staining enables for excellent differentiation between various cell types, allowing the identification of cytological abnormalities such as precancerous or malignant lesions. Compared to Diff-Quik, the Papanicolaou stain is more time-consuming and requires additional reagents and preparation steps, but it yields a more permanent and diagnostically precise result, particularly in the assessment of nuclear atypia [71].

Different studies have shown that direct cytological smears are capable of yielding high-quality DNA, with a high degree of concordance between molecular results and those obtained from histological specimens. This is likely attributable to the preservation of intact cells and well-preserved nuclei. Both alcohol-fixed and air-dried smears have been shown to be suitable for the extraction of high-quality nucleic acids [32, 68, 69]. The fixative adopted for the preparation of the cytological smear is one of the most critical pre-analytical factors that can significantly influence the quality and reliability of NGS results. Notably, methanol-fixed FNA smears have been reported to yield higher average DNA concentrations and improved nucleic acid quality compared to ethanol-fixed smears, indicating

Table 16.1 Advantages and limitations of cytology specimens for NGS analysis

Sample type	Source/specimen	Preparation/ fixation	Advantages	Limitations/ challenges	NGS suitability
Direct cytological smears	FNA, body fluids	Methanol (diff-Quik stain), ethanol (Papanicolaou stain)	Rapid, good cellular detail; high DNA quality from methanol-fixed smears; excellent nuclear detail; the presence of intact cells and nuclei; possibility of executing the ROSE	RNA degradation with alcohol fixation; limited slides available; slide type affects cell retention; Slide sacrificing; Delay due to sample digitalizing and coverslip removal	High-quality Nucleic acids; additional unstained slides recommended
Liquid-based cytology (LBC)	Bodily fluids (pleural effusion, ascitic fluid, bronchoalveolar lavage)	Sample collected in a preservation solution; alcohol-based fixatives preferred over formaldehyde	Aspirated material rapidly collected and preserved; clean background, evenly distributed cells; high nucleic acid quality; the presence of intact cells and nuclei; improved diagnostic sensitivity	Dependent on fixative choice; formaldehyde may reduce nucleic acid quality; impossibility of executing the ROSE	Suitable for NGS, high concordance with tissue testing; variable quality of nucleic acids depending on fixatives used
Cytospin preparations	Low-cellularity fluids (CSF, urine, BAL, serous effusions)	Ethanol or methanol fixation	Concentrates cells in small area; enhances sensitivity in low cellularity samples	Morphological alterations from centrifugation; RNA quality sensitive to processing conditions; impossibility of executing the ROSE	DNA suitable for NGS; RNA quality variable depending on fixation, staining protocol, handling and storage
Cell blocks	Liquid specimens (pleural/ascitic effusion, urine, BAL, FNA)	Formalin fixation; paraffin embedding	Preserves morphology; allows multiple tests; long-term archival; Multiple sections	Lower nucleic acid yield; fixation artifacts (e.g., C > T transitions); impossibility of executing the ROSE	Suitable if tumor content adequate; may need multiple sections to increase nucleic acid input; time-dependent negative effects on the overall integrity of RNA
Supernatants from cytological preparations	FNA needle rinses, supernatants after centrifugation	Usually refrigerated or frozen if not immediately processed	Additional source of nucleic acids; useful when cellular material is limited; preservation of diagnostic material	No morphologic evaluation, impossibility of executing the ROSE; Low nucleic acid yield and quality; nucleic acids fragmented; RNA degradation risk	High-quality Nucleic acids; potentially informative for NGS when cellular samples insufficient; processing delay affects acid nucleic quality

Abbreviations: *FNA* fine-needle aspiration, *LBC* liquid-based cytology, *CSF* cerebrospinal fluid, *BAL* bronchoalveolar lavage, *ROSE* rapid on-site evaluation

Table 16.2 Overview of the main studies that used NGS approach on cytological samples

Cytological sample type	Number of analyzed samples	Adequate sample rate for DNA-based NGS	Adequate sample rate for RNA-based NGS	References
Direct cytological smears	180	91.1%	NP	Pepe et al. [51]
	8	100%	92%	Velizheva et al. [80]
	5	100%	NP	Karnes et al. [38]
	32	100%	NP	Yamamoto et al. [86]
	11	100%	NP	Fumagalli et al. [27]
	56	89.3%	89.3%	Ramani et al. [57]
	8	100%	NP	Fielding et al. [23]
Liquid-based cytology	49	77.5%	NP	Reynolds et al. [59]
	37	70.3%	NP	Yamaguchi et al. [85]
	10	100%	NP	Akahane et al. [2]
	37	100%	NP	Akahane et al. [1]
	357	100%	NP	Xiao et al. [84]
	25	83.3%	NP	Iwaya et al. [35]
	20	100%	100%	Akahane et al. [3]
Cytospin preparations	41	100%	NP	Scott et al. [70]
	31	100%	NP	Miceska et al. [44]
Cell blocks	180	91.1%	NP	Pepe et al. [51]
	16	93.8%	NP	Zhang et al. [89]
	35	100%	NP	Roy-Chowdhuri et al. [67]
	129	100%	93.8%	Wei et al. [83]
	120	97.5%	97.5%	Vormittag-Nocito et al. [82]
	12	100%	NP	Balitzer and Greenland [4]
	78	92.3%	92.3%	Ramani et al. [57]
	30	80%	NP	Perrone et al. [52]
Supernatants from cytological preparations	465	100%	NP	Nikiforov et al. [46]
	175	100%	100%	Nikiforova et al. [47]
	33	97%	NP	Carrara et al. [12]
	35	100%	NP	Roy-Chowdhuri et al. [67]
	30	100%	100%	Janaki et al. [37]
	116	89.7%	NP	Hannigan et al. [31]
	17	100%	NP	Guibert et al. [30]
	156	83%	NP	Ye et al. [87]
	30	90%	NP	Perrone et al. [52]
	15	100%	NP	Patel et al. [48]

Abbreviation: *NP* not performed

enhanced DNA recovery from methanol-based preparations [20, 55, 73].

RNA extracted from cytological smears is often of suboptimal quality due to nucleic acid degradation occurring during alcohol-based fixation, which does not fully inactivate RNases.

Consequently, RNA extracted from these samples is frequently of low quality and highly fragmented, making it unsuitable for RNA-based NGS analysis. However, recent advancements in sequencing technologies, particularly those optimized for the analysis of degraded RNA, have enabled the yield of informative data from such samples [33, 73]. One potential strategy to improve the success rate of RNA-based NGS from cytological smears involves the preparation of an additional unstained slide dedicated exclusively to nucleic acid extraction, thereby minimizing exposure to fixation-related degradation.

Another critical pre-analytical factor influencing nucleic acid quality in cytological samples is the type of slide used for smear preparation. Various slide types are commercially available, with fully frosted slides offering the highest cell retention and minimal cell loss during fixation in alcohol-based solutions. Previous studies have shown that fully frosted slides provide superior cell adhesion compared to positively charged slides and standard uncoated slides. In particular, the positively charged slides retain cells via electrostatic interaction, while the standard uncoated slides, lacking surface modifications, may be more suitable for samples with high cellularity due to their ease of cell recovery. Despite their enhanced adhesive properties, fully frosted slides present significant challenges for molecular applications, as the recovery of tumor cells, whether through scraping or cell-lifting techniques, can be technically difficult and inefficient. Consequently, the use of fully frosted slides for nucleic acid extraction is generally limited [54, 65, 77].

Another challenge in the molecular analysis of cytological smears is that the diagnostic slide is irreversibly consumed for nucleic acid extraction, and since typically only a few slides available for each patient, the sample preservation represents a critical issue. As these diagnostic slides are non-replicable, it is essential to implement appropriate strategies to preserve diagnostic material before proceeding with the extraction process. A widely adopted approach involves whole-slide digitizing through digital scanner, enabling permanent storage and ensuring that the diagnostic material remains available for review or reevaluation if necessary (Fig. 16.1).

Moreover, a preliminary assessment of factors that may influence the success rate of NGS analysis on cytological smears is essential. Among these, adequate tumor cellularity is paramount to satisfy the analytical sensitivity thresholds of the molecular assay employed. Although no universally accepted minimum threshold for tumor cell content in NGS analysis has been established, low tumor content remains a key limiting factor. In the case of poorly cellular cytological samples that fail quality control, additional cytological smears can be employed to perform NGS analysis, if they are available [6, 63].

Liquid-Based Cytology (LBC)

LBC specimens obtained from bodily fluids, such as pleural effusion, ascitic fluid, or bronchoalveolar lavage, represent a valuable source of genetic

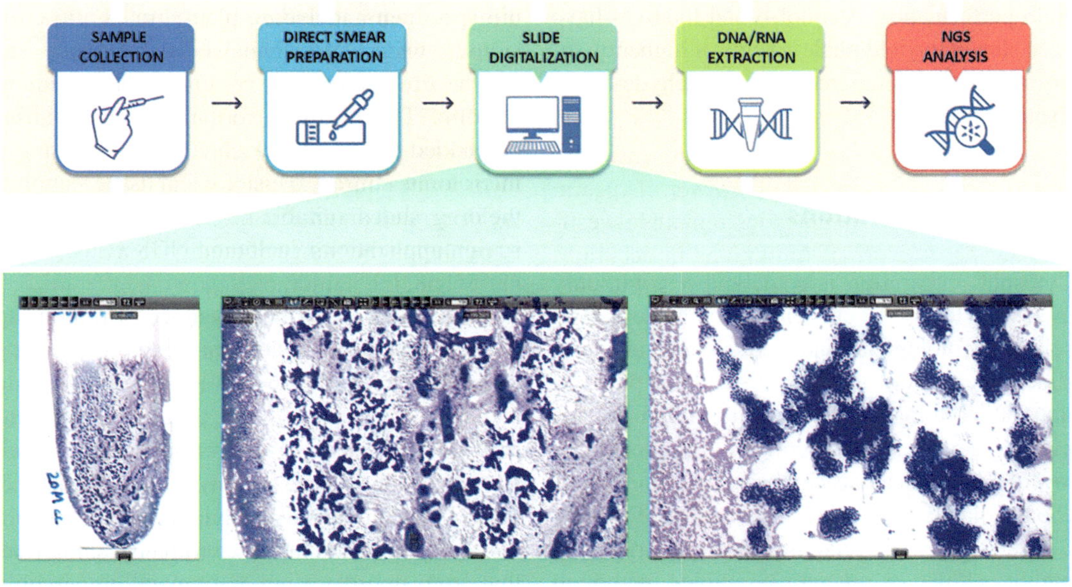

Fig. 16.1 Adequate workflow for smear samples management: integration of digital pathology and molecular profiling through NGS approach

material when tissue specimens are unavailable. These samples are collected in a preservation solution and subsequently processed in the laboratory to concentrate and evenly distribute the cells on a slide. In contrast to direct smears, which often result in an irregular cellular layer, LBC preparations are characterized by a clean background, free of debris, and with well-distributed cells exhibiting minimal overlapping, thereby enhancing diagnostic sensitivity [6]. Molecular analysis can be performed either by scraping cells from the monolayer slide or by utilizing the cellular material suspended in the fixative solution [62]. Although laser capture or manual microdissection is technically feasible, it is more challenging on monolayer slides than on direct smears, due to the limited area of cell deposition [18].

NGS performed on LBC samples has demonstrated high concordance with tissue-based molecular testing in the detection of clinically relevant oncogenic mutations [1, 2]. Similar to direct cytological smears, LBC samples offer a significant advantage in terms of nucleic acid quality due to the presence of intact cells and nuclei, which enable the extraction of high-quality DNA and RNA. In this context, the choice of fixative remains a critical factor in determining NGS performance: Alcohol-based fixatives have been shown to yield nucleic acids of higher quantity and quality compared to formaldehyde-based fixatives [22].

Cytospin Preparations

Cytospin preparation is a technique commonly used in cytology to concentrate cells from low-cellularity biological fluids on a defined area of a slide, resulting in high-density cellular preparations suitable for morphological evaluation. This method is particularly useful for specimens with low cellularity, such as cerebrospinal fluid, bronchoalveolar lavage, urine, and serous effusions. Conversely, it is generally not preferred for highly cellular or mucinous samples. Although cytospin enhances diagnostic sensitivity concentrating the limited number of cells present, the process may cause morphological alterations due to centrifugal forces and the cellular distribution on the slide does not replicate the native tissue architecture [5, 16, 56]. These preparations are generally fixed in ethanol or methanol, which may adversely affect the quality and reliability of NGS results. Despite these limitations, several studies have demonstrated that these samples can be successfully employed for NGS analysis in some tumor types, such as lung cancer, providing reliable results even in cases of low cellularity [11, 14, 36, 63].

DNA extracted from cytospin preparations is generally of sufficient quantity and quality for NGS analysis, especially when slides are either unstained and properly fixed. Conversely, RNA quality is more variable and is significantly affected by pre-analytical factors, including the time interval between sample collection and fixation, the staining protocol employed, and the handling and storage conditions of the slides [17, 33].

Cell Blocks

Cell blocks are cytological preparations that enable the processing of cells obtained from liquid specimens, including pleural or ascitic effusions, urine, bronchoalveolar lavage, or fine-needle aspirations, by embedding them in paraffin. The resulting formalin-fixed paraffin-embedded (FFPE) blocks are sectioned using a microtome, similar to histological tissue samples, yielding slides suitable for a variety of downstream applications, including NGS assay [9, 32, 43, 54, 58, 69, 81, 88].

Cell blocks offer the advantage of preserving cellular morphology and enable more accurate diagnoses through the application of multiple ancillary techniques. In addition, paraffin-embedded material allows for long-term archival. However, the overall quality of the sample is largely dependent on the initial cellularity, and the yield of nucleic acids is typically lower than that from non-paraffinized preparations, mainly for RNA which is more susceptible to degradation process [22, 32, 76]. Formalin fixation introduces DNA-protein crosslinks that can compromise the integrity of extracted nucleic acids. For example, prolonged fixation may lead to sequencing artifacts, such as cytosine-to-thymine (C > T) transitions [21, 62]. Moreover, RNA integrity is particularly susceptible to the duration of formalin exposure, exhibiting a time-dependent decline. Prior to initiating NGS analysis, the cytopathologist should evaluate whether the tumor cell content of the sample is sufficient for molecular testing, in cases of limited cellularity additional sections from the cell block may be employed to increase input material [69].

Supernatants from Cytological Preparations

Supernatants generated during cytological specimen processing, often considered waste, may contain nucleic acids released from apoptotic or necrotic cells. These supernatants are typically obtained from FNA needle rinses or from the supernatant remaining after cell pellet collection and centrifugation during cytology sample preparation [32, 54].

Recent studies have shown that NGS performed on cytological supernatants can yield informative molecular data, highlighting their potential as a source of good-quality nucleic acids suitable for genomic profiling. The use of supernatant material may be particularly advantageous in cases where cellular material is limited or when diagnostic cytological slides are inadequate or insufficient for molecular testing due to low tumor cell content [10, 19, 24, 25, 30, 32, 67].

However, a key limitation of supernatant-derived material is that nucleic acids in supernatants often derive from apoptotic or necrotic cells, resulting in fragmented or partially degraded DNA and RNA. The overall yield and integrity of nucleic acids from these preparations are generally lower than those obtained from cellular components. RNA quality, in particular, is highly susceptible to degradation, which can be enhanced by delays in sample processing. Therefore, immediate processing or storage at low temperatures, preferably refrigeration or freezing at −20 °C to −80 °C, is recommended to preserve nucleic acid integrity [79].

Advantages, Disadvantages, and Challenges of NGS on Cytological Specimens

Benefits and Potential of Cytological Samples in NGS Workflow

One of the main advantages of using cytological samples is associated with the minimally invasive nature of sampling techniques, such as FNA, bronchial brushings, or effusion fluid collection. These procedures are generally well-tolerated by patients and can be performed repeatedly, making them particularly useful in clinical scenario where traditional surgical biopsies are contraindicated or not feasible due to anatomical or clinical ineligibility [15].

Additionally, cytological samples can often be obtained more quickly and at lower cost, which facilitates faster diagnostic turnaround and enables timely initiation of targeted therapies. From a molecular perspective, cytological specimens can yield nucleic acids of adequate quality for NGS, particularly when careful handling and optimized extraction protocols are applied. In some cases, these samples may contain a higher proportion of tumor cells compared to FFPE tissue biopsies, potentially enhancing the sensitivity of mutation detection. Furthermore, the use of residual material from cytology slides, cell blocks, or liquid-based cytology preparations allows for an optimization of the biomaterial, especially in settings where tissue is scarce [28].

Limitations and Challenges of Cytological Samples in NGS Workflow

Several technical challenges must be addressed to ensure the reliable implementation of NGS on cytological specimens in routine clinical practice. A principal limitation is the frequently low quantity of cellular material in cytological samples, which determines a poor yield of DNA and RNA available for sequencing, particularly when comprehensive genomic profiling or large-panel NGS assays are required. In this context, cytopathologists play a pivotal role in evaluating stained slides to identify those with optimal cellular preservation and maximal tumor cell content, while minimizing potential contaminants, such as blood, necrotic debris, or inflammatory cells, that may interfere with the quality of the extracted nucleic acids.

Particular attention should be paid to selecting samples with limited necrosis (<20%), as higher degrees of necrosis have been associated with reduced nucleic acid quality and impaired polymerase chain reaction (PCR) amplification efficiency [26, 64]. Furthermore, the tumor cell fraction should be carefully assessed to determine whether it meets the analytical sensitivity threshold of the intended molecular assay. As a general guideline, the neoplastic cell content should exceed at least twice the limit of detection (LOD) specified by the assay to ensure reliable variant detection [42].

An additional limitation intrinsic to cytological specimens is the absence of preserved tissue architecture. Unlike histological tissue, cytology does not preserve the spatial arrangement of cells, making it more difficult to assess tumor heterogeneity, invasiveness, or the tumor microenvironment factors that may influence treatment decisions or prognostic evaluation. Furthermore, cytological specimens do not allow for precise microdissection of neoplastic areas and may contain a heterogeneous mixture of neoplastic and nonneoplastic cells, leading to a dilution of tumor DNA reducing the sensitivity of variant detection, particularly for low-frequency oncogenic variants [60, 72].

A major limitation of cytological samples in NGS analysis is the potential underestimation of variant allele frequency (VAF), which can compromise the detection of clinically relevant mutations. The VAF of an oncogenic mutation typically reflects the proportion of neoplastic cells within the sample, and it should correspond to approximately half the tumor cell content. However, in cytological specimens, especially those with significant contamination by nonneoplastic cells (e.g., inflammatory or blood-derived cells), the VAF can be markedly diluted. This dilution effect increases the risk of false-negative results, particularly for low-frequency driver mutations, thereby representing a substantial challenge in the molecular profiling of tumors using cytology-based NGS approach [45]. Therefore, performing NGS testing on cytological specimens with the highest available tumor cellularity minimizes the risk of obtaining false-negative results [42, 77]. Different methods for nucleic acid extraction are available, all aiming to efficiently isolate DNA and/or RNA removing contaminants, such as proteins and lipids, that may interfere with amplification techniques [7]. The selection of an appropriate extraction method largely depends on the available instrumentation, testing throughput, and the specific types of nucleic acids required for analysis. DNA-only extraction methods are typically employed for the detection of single-nucleotide variants (SNVs), insertions and deletions (indels), and copy number variations (CNVs), whereas RNA extraction is required for the identification of gene fusions and transcriptomic alterations. For more comprehensive analysis, such as those involving many NGS panels, both DNA and RNA are required. In this regard, the simultaneous co-extraction of DNA/RNA is increasingly favored, particularly for cytological samples, to maximize molecular data output [77]. In addition, pre-analytical variables, such as fixative method, staining method, storage conditions, and preparation format, can impact nucleic acid integrity and yield affecting the NGS results [74].

Furthermore, the standardization and validation of NGS workflows for cytology remain ongoing challenges. Cytological samples have demonstrated compatibility with NGS workflows; however, protocols originally developed for FFPE tissue require careful adaptation and validation to be effectively used for non-FFPE cytological samples.

Current Clinical Application of NGS to Cytological Samples

In recent years, NGS has increasingly been integrated into routine clinical practice for the molecular characterization of solid tumors. Although NGS is typically performed on FFPE tissue samples, it is now being successfully applied to cytological specimens as well, expanding diagnostic and predictive possibilities, especially in cases where tissue is limited or unobtainable. This approach has shown increasing clinical utility in lung cancer, particularly in cases where cytological samples are the only material available for molecular testing. Advances in molecular diagnostics now make it possible to have a comprehensive lung cancer biomarker profile from even a small number of cells. By simultaneously extracting DNA and RNA from cytological samples, a full molecular characterization of key predictive biomarkers can be obtained, including mutations in *EGFR*, *BRAF*, and *KRAS*, as well as gene fusions involving *ALK*, *ROS1*, *RET*, and *NTRK*. Different studies have demonstrated a high concordance between NGS analysis performed on cytological and histological samples from the same patients, with mutations consistently detected in genes such as *EGFR*, *KRAS*, *BRAF*, and *PIK3CA*. Moreover, DNA quality index assessments have shown that DNA extracted from pleural fluid cell blocks is comparable in quality to that obtained from FFPE tissue blocks [45, 89]. However, one of the main challenges is that the VAF can differ significantly between cytological and FFPE samples, which may lead to underestimation or overestimation of the patient's potential response to a specific targeted therapy [45].

Numerous studies have evaluated the NGS on cytological samples in various other solid tumors, including urothelial, pancreatic, breast cancers and melanoma, highlighting a promising application that could expand future diagnostic and therapeutic strategies and potentially be integrated into routine clinical practice. In urothelial carcinoma, a high concordance of NGS results has been observed between urine cytology samples and corresponding bladder tumor biopsies/resections [39, 75]. Similar results have been reported in pancreatic cancer, particularly molecular results on cytological samples have shown high concordance with surgical tissue for many key mutations, proving to be a valuable alternative or complement to histological analysis and a useful tool in clinical practice [29, 41]. In breast cancer patients, cytological samples have been shown to be suitable for detecting predictive mutations affecting oncogenes, such as *PIK3CA*, *ESR1*, and *BRCA1/2* [49, 78].

Moreover, numerous studies have demonstrated high concordance for *BRAF* mutation identified on FNA samples with those on surgical tissue, supporting the reliability of cytology samples for molecular testing. Therefore, molecular profiling on FNA material constitute an alternative approach for selecting appropriate targeted therapies in melanoma patients [8, 13, 34, 61].

Conclusions

Cytological specimens represent a minimally invasive resource of biomaterial for molecular testing in oncological patients, particularly in clinical scenarios where conventional tissue biopsy is contraindicated or not feasible. The integration of NGS into cytopathology has significantly expanded the clinical utility of these samples, enabling comprehensive genomic profiling even in cases with limited tumor content. The successful implementation of NGS on cytological material, however, required a careful optimization of pre-analytical workflows and methodological standardization. Finally, to fully harness the potential of cytology-based NGS within the framework of precision oncology, coordinated efforts are essential to refine pre-analytical handling procedures, harmonize molecular testing protocols, and validate cytology-specific workflows that ensure analytical reproducibility and clinical relevance.

References

1. Akahane T, Yamaguchi T, Kato Y, et al. Comprehensive validation of liquid-based cytology specimens for next-generation sequencing in cancer genome analysis. PLoS One. 2019;14(6):e0217724. https://doi.org/10.1371/journal.pone.0217724.
2. Akahane T, Kitazono I, Yanazume S, et al. Next-generation sequencing analysis of endometrial screening liquid-based cytology specimens: a comparative study to tissue specimens. BMC Med Genet. 2020;13(1):101. https://doi.org/10.1186/s12920-020-00753-6.
3. Akahane T, Isochi-Yamaguchi T, Hashiba-Ohnuki N, et al. Cancer gene analysis of liquid-based cytology specimens using next-generation sequencing: a technical report of bimodal DNA- and RNA-based panel application. Diagn Cytopathol. 2023;51(8):493–500. https://doi.org/10.1002/dc.25149.
4. Balitzer DJ, Greenland NY. The utility of next-generation sequencing in challenging liver FNA biopsies. Cancer Cytopathol. 2024;132(11):714–22. https://doi.org/10.1002/cncy.22893.
5. Baykus N, Özekinci S, Erdem ZB, et al. Comparison of morphological similarities and differences between liquid-based cytology and conventional techniques of serous effusion cytology specimens. Acta Cytol. 2022;66(2):159–64. https://doi.org/10.1159/000521052.
6. Bellevicine C, Malapelle U, Vigliar E, et al. How to prepare cytological samples for molecular testing. J Clin Pathol. 2017;70(10):819–26. https://doi.org/10.1136/jclinpath-2017-204561.
7. Berensmeier S. Magnetic particles for the separation and purification of nucleic acids. Appl Microbiol Biotechnol. 2006;73(3):495–504. https://doi.org/10.1007/s00253-006-0675-0.
8. Bernacki KD, Betz BL, Weigelin HC, et al. Molecular diagnostics of melanoma fine-needle aspirates: a cytology-histology correlation study. Am J Clin Pathol. 2012;138(5):670–7. https://doi.org/10.1309/AJCPEQJW3PLOOZTC.
9. Billah S, Stewart J, Staerkel G, et al. EGFR and KRAS mutations in lung carcinoma: molecular testing by using cytology specimens. Cancer Cytopathol. 2011;119(2):111–7. https://doi.org/10.1002/cncy.20151.
10. Brown AE, Lim KS, Corpus G, et al. Detection of BRAF mutation in the cytocentrifugation supernatant fluid from fine-needle aspiration of thyroid lesions may enhance the diagnostic yield. Cytojournal. 2017;14:4. https://doi.org/10.4103/1742-6413.200935.
11. Bubendorf L, Lantuejoul S, de Langen AJ, et al. Nonsmall cell lung carcinoma: diagnostic difficulties in small biopsies and cytological specimens: number 2 in the series "pathology for the clinician" edited by Peter Dorfmüller and Alberto Cavazza. Eur Respir Rev. 2017;26(144):170007. https://doi.org/10.1183/16000617.0007-2017.
12. Carrara S, Soldà G, Di Leo M, et al. Side-by-side comparison of next-generation sequencing, cytology, and histology in diagnosing locally advanced pancreatic adenocarcinoma. Gastrointest Endosc. 2021;93(3):597–604.e5. https://doi.org/10.1016/j.gie.2020.06.069.
13. Chen S, Randolph M, Cramer HM, et al. Detection of BRAF mutation in metastatic melanoma utilizing cell-transferred cytological smears. Acta Cytol. 2014;58(5):478–82. https://doi.org/10.1159/000368273.
14. Chen H, Luthra R, Goswami RS, et al. Analysis of pre-analytic factors affecting the success of clinical next-generation sequencing of solid organ malignancies. Cancers (Basel). 2015;7(3):1699–715. https://doi.org/10.3390/cancers7030859.
15. Cibas ES, Ali SZ. The Bethesda system for reporting thyroid cytopathology. Am J Clin Pathol. 2009;132(5):658–65. https://doi.org/10.1309/AJCPPHLWMI3JV4LA.
16. Collins L. Examination of body fluids: preparation of slides and cell morphology. Clin Lab Sci. 2009;22(1):49–53.
17. da Cunha SG, Saieg MA. Preanalytic specimen triage: smears, cell blocks, cytospin preparations, transport media, and cytobanking. Cancer Cytopathol. 2017;125(S6):455–64. https://doi.org/10.1002/cncy.21850.
18. da Cunha Santos G, Saieg MA, Troncone G, et al. Cytological preparations for molecular analysis: a review of technical procedures, advantages and limitations for referring samples for testing. Cytopathology. 2018;29(2):125–32. https://doi.org/10.1111/cyt.12534.
19. Deftereos G, Finkelstein SD, Jackson SA, et al. The value of mutational profiling of the cytocentrifugation supernatant fluid from fine-needle aspiration of pancreatic solid mass lesions. Mod Pathol. 2014;27(4):594–601. https://doi.org/10.1038/modpathol.2013.147.
20. Dejmek A, Zendehrokh N, Tomaszewska M, et al. Preparation of DNA from cytological material: effects of fixation, staining, and mounting medium on DNA yield and quality. Cancer Cytopathol. 2013;121(7):344–53. https://doi.org/10.1002/cncy.21276.
21. Dotti I, Bonin S, Basili G, et al. Effects of formalin, methacarn, and fineFIX fixatives on RNA preservation. Diagn Mol Pathol. 2010;19(2):112–22. https://doi.org/10.1097/PDM.0b013e3181b520f8.
22. Evers DL, Fowler CB, Cunningham BR, et al. The effect of formaldehyde fixation on RNA: optimization of formaldehyde adduct removal. J Mol Diagn. 2011;13(3):282–8. https://doi.org/10.1016/j.jmoldx.2011.01.010.

23. Fielding D, Dalley AJ, Singh M, et al. Whole genome sequencing in advanced lung cancer can be performed using Diff-Quik cytology smears derived from endobronchial ultrasound, transbronchial needle aspiration (EBUS TBNA). Lung. 2023;201(4):407–13. https://doi.org/10.1007/s00408-023-00631-9.
24. Finkelstein SD, Bibbo M, Loren DE, et al. Molecular analysis of centrifugation supernatant fluid from pancreaticobiliary duct samples can improve cancer detection. Acta Cytol. 2012;56(4):439–47. https://doi.org/10.1159/000339638.
25. Finkelstein SD, Bibbo M, Kowalski TE, et al. Mutational analysis of cytocentrifugation supernatant fluid from pancreatic solid mass lesions. Diagn Cytopathol. 2014;42(8):719–25. https://doi.org/10.1002/dc.23048.
26. Fujii S, Yoshino T, Yamazaki K, et al. Histopathological factors affecting the extraction of high quality genomic DNA from tissue sections for next-generation sequencing. Biomed Rep. 2019;11(4):171–80. https://doi.org/10.3892/br.2019.1235.
27. Fumagalli C, Rappa A, Casadio C, et al. Next-generation sequencing-based BRCA testing on cytological specimens from ovarian cancer ascites reveals high concordance with tumour tissue analysis. J Clin Pathol. 2020;73(3):168–71. https://doi.org/10.1136/jclinpath-2019-206127.
28. Gailey MP, Stence AA, Jensen CS, et al. Multiplatform comparison of molecular oncology tests performed on cytology specimens and formalin-fixed, paraffin-embedded tissue. Cancer Cytopathol. 2015;123(1):30–9. https://doi.org/10.1002/cncy.21476.
29. Gleeson FC, Kerr SE, Kipp BR, et al. Targeted next generation sequencing of endoscopic ultrasound acquired cytology from ampullary and pancreatic adenocarcinoma has the potential to aid patient stratification for optimal therapy selection. Oncotarget. 2016;7(34):54526–36. https://doi.org/10.18632/oncotarget.9440.
30. Guibert N, Tsukada H, Hwang DH, et al. Liquid biopsy of fine-needle aspiration supernatant for lung cancer genotyping. Lung Cancer. 2018;122:72–5. https://doi.org/10.1016/j.lungcan.2018.05.024.
31. Hannigan B, Ye W, Mehrotra M, et al. Liquid biopsy assay for lung carcinoma using centrifuged supernatants from fine-needle aspiration specimens. Ann Oncol. 2019;30(6):963–9. https://doi.org/10.1093/annonc/mdz102.
32. Huang M, Wei S. Overview of molecular testing of cytology specimens. Acta Cytol. 2020;64(1–2):136–46. https://doi.org/10.1159/000497187.
33. Hwang DH, Garcia EP, Ducar MD, et al. Next-generation sequencing of cytologic preparations: an analysis of quality metrics. Cancer Cytopathol. 2017;125(10):786–94. https://doi.org/10.1002/cncy.21897.
34. Iaccarino A, Nacchio M, Acanfora G, et al. Multiple predictive biomarker testing in melanoma: another challenge in identifying the optimal approach on cytological samples. Cytopathology. 2023;34(3):198–203. https://doi.org/10.1111/cyt.13211.
35. Iwaya H, Tanimoto A, Toyodome K, et al. Next-generation sequencing analysis of pancreatic cancer using residual liquid cytology specimens from endoscopic ultrasound-guided fine-needle biopsy: a prospective comparative study with tissue specimens. Diagnostics (Basel). 2023;13(6):1078. https://doi.org/10.3390/diagnostics13061078.
36. Jain D, Roy-Chowdhuri S. Molecular pathology of lung cancer cytology specimens: a concise review. Arch Pathol Lab Med. 2018;142(9):1127–33. https://doi.org/10.5858/arpa.2017-0444-RA.
37. Janaki N, Harbhajanka A, Michael CW, et al. Comparison of cytocentrifugation supernatant fluid and formalin-fixed paraffin-embedded tissue for targeted next-generation sequencing. Cancer Cytopathol. 2019;127(5):297–305. https://doi.org/10.1002/cncy.22126.
38. Karnes HE, Duncavage EJ, Bernadt CT. Targeted next-generation sequencing using fine-needle aspirates from adenocarcinomas of the lung. Cancer Cytopathol. 2014;122(2):104–13. https://doi.org/10.1002/cncy.21361.
39. Katims AB, Gaffney C, Firouzi S, et al. Feasibility and tissue concordance of genomic sequencing of urinary cytology in upper tract urothelial carcinoma. Urol Oncol. 2023;41(10):433.e19–24. https://doi.org/10.1016/j.urolonc.2023.07.007.
40. Kim D, Vanderbilt CM, Yang SR, et al. Maximizing the clinical utility and performance of cytology samples for comprehensive genetic profiling. Nat Commun. 2025;16(1):116. https://doi.org/10.1038/s41467-024-55456-8.
41. Laquière AE, Lagarde A, Napoléon B, et al. Genomic profile concordance between pancreatic cyst fluid and neoplastic tissue. World J Gastroenterol. 2019;25(36):5530–42. https://doi.org/10.3748/wjg.v25.i36.5530.
42. Li MM, Datto M, Duncavage EJ, et al. Standards and guidelines for the interpretation and reporting of sequence variants in cancer: a joint consensus recommendation of the Association for Molecular Pathology, American Society of Clinical Oncology, and College of American Pathologists. J Mol Diagn. 2017;19(1):4–23. https://doi.org/10.1016/j.jmoldx.2016.10.002.
43. Magnini D, Fuso L, Varone F, et al. Molecular testing in EBUS-TBNA specimens of lung adenocarcinoma: a study of concordance between cell block method and liquid-based cytology in appraising sample cellularity and EGFR mutations. Mol Diagn Ther. 2018;22(6):723–8. https://doi.org/10.1007/s40291-018-0359-3.
44. Miceska S, Škof E, Novaković S, et al. Cytopathological assessment is an accurate method for identifying immunophenotypic features and BRCA1/2 mutations of high-grade serous carcinoma from ascites. Cancer Cytopathol.

2023;131(3):188–97. https://doi.org/10.1002/cncy.22664.
45. Morikawa K, Kida H, Handa H, et al. A prospective validation study of lung cancer gene panel testing using cytological specimens. Cancers (Basel). 2022;14(15):3784. https://doi.org/10.3390/cancers14153784.
46. Nikiforov YE, Carty SE, Chiosea SI, et al. Impact of the multi-gene ThyroSeq next-generation sequencing assay on cancer diagnosis in thyroid nodules with atypia of undetermined significance/follicular lesion of undetermined significance cytology. Thyroid. 2015;25(11):1217–23. https://doi.org/10.1089/thy.2015.0305.
47. Nikiforova MN, Mercurio S, Wald AI, et al. Analytical performance of the ThyroSeq v3 genomic classifier for cancer diagnosis in thyroid nodules. Cancer. 2018;124(8):1682–90. https://doi.org/10.1002/cncr.31245.
48. Patel A, Hissong E, Rosado L, et al. Next-generation sequencing of cell-free DNA extracted from pleural effusion supernatant: applications and challenges. Front Med (Lausanne). 2021;8:662312. https://doi.org/10.3389/fmed.2021.662312.
49. Peña KB, Riu F, Hernandez A, et al. Study of liquid-based cytology using next-generation sequencing as a liquid biopsy application in patients with advanced oncological disease. Biomedicine. 2023;11(6):1578. https://doi.org/10.3390/biomedicines11061578.
50. Penault-Llorca F, Kerr KM, Garrido P, et al. Expert opinion on NSCLC small specimen biomarker testing - part 1: tissue collection and management. Virchows Arch. 2022;481(3):335–50. https://doi.org/10.1007/s00428-022-03343-2.
51. Pepe F, De Luca C, Smeraglio R, et al. Performance analysis of SiRe next-generation sequencing panel in diagnostic setting: focus on NSCLC routine samples. J Clin Pathol. 2019;72(1):38–45. https://doi.org/10.1136/jclinpath-2018-205386.
52. Perrone ME, Alvarez R, Vo TT, et al. Validating cell-free DNA from supernatant for molecular diagnostics on cytology specimens. Cancer Cytopathol. 2021;129(12):956–65. https://doi.org/10.1002/cncy.22491.
53. Pisapia P, Malapelle U, Roma G, et al. Molecular cytopathology meeting group. Consistency and reproducibility of next-generation sequencing in cytopathology: a second worldwide ring trial study on improved cytological molecular reference specimens. Cancer Cytopathol. 2019;127(5):285–96. https://doi.org/10.1002/cncy.22134.
54. Pisapia P, Pepe F, Sgariglia R, et al. Next generation sequencing in cytology. Cytopathology. 2021;32(5):588–95. https://doi.org/10.1111/cyt.12974.
55. Piskorz AM, Ennis D, Macintyre G, et al. Methanol-based fixation is superior to buffered formalin for next-generation sequencing of DNA from clinical cancer samples. Ann Oncol. 2016;27(3):532–9. https://doi.org/10.1093/annonc/mdv613.
56. Qamar I, Rehman S, Mehdi G, et al. Utility of cytospin and cell block technology in evaluation of body fluids and urine samples: a comparative study. J Cytol. 2018;35(2):79–82. https://doi.org/10.4103/JOC.JOC_240_16.
57. Ramani NS, Chen H, Broaddus RR, et al. Utilization of cytology smears improves success rates of RNA-based next-generation sequencing gene fusion assays for clinically relevant predictive biomarkers. Cancer Cytopathol. 2021;129(5):374–82. https://doi.org/10.1002/cncy.22381.
58. Rekhtman N, Roy-Chowdhuri S. Cytology specimens: a goldmine for molecular testing. Arch Pathol Lab Med. 2016;140(11):1189–90. https://doi.org/10.5858/arpa.2016-0379-ED.
59. Reynolds JP, Zhou Y, Jakubowski MA, et al. Next-generation sequencing of liquid-based cytology non-small cell lung cancer samples. Cancer Cytopathol. 2017;125(3):178–87. https://doi.org/10.1002/cncy.21812.
60. Roh MH. The utilization of cytologic and small biopsy samples for ancillary molecular testing. Mod Pathol. 2019;32(Suppl 1):77–85. https://doi.org/10.1038/s41379-018-0138-z.
61. Ronchi A, Montella M, Carraturo E, et al. To get the Most out of the least: BRAF molecular evaluation in melanoma metastases on cell suspension from fine needle aspiration cytology needle rinses. Acta Cytol. 2023;67(4):357–64. https://doi.org/10.1159/000529769.
62. Roy-Chowdhuri S. Molecular testing of residual cytology samples: rethink, reclaim, repurpose. Cancer Cytopathol. 2019;127(1):15–7. https://doi.org/10.1002/cncy.22076.
63. Roy-Chowdhuri S, Stewart J. Preanalytic variables in cytology: lessons learned from next-generation sequencing-the MD Anderson experience. Arch Pathol Lab Med. 2016;140(11):1191–9. https://doi.org/10.5858/arpa.2016-0117-RA.
64. Roy-Chowdhuri S, Goswami RS, Chen H, et al. Factors affecting the success of next-generation sequencing in cytology specimens. Cancer Cytopathol. 2015;123(11):659–68. https://doi.org/10.1002/cncy.21597.
65. Roy-Chowdhuri S, Chow CW, Kane MK, et al. Optimizing the DNA yield for molecular analysis from cytologic preparations. Cancer Cytopathol. 2016;124(4):254–60. https://doi.org/10.1002/cncy.21664.
66. Roy-Chowdhuri S, Roy S, Monaco SE, et al. Big data from small samples: informatics of next-generation sequencing in cytopathology. Cancer Cytopathol. 2017;125(4):236–44. https://doi.org/10.1002/cncy.21805.
67. Roy-Chowdhuri S, Mehrotra M, Bolivar AM, et al. Salvaging the supernatant: next generation cytopathology for solid tumor mutation profiling. Mod Pathol. 2018;31(7):1036–45. https://doi.org/10.1038/s41379-018-0006-x.

68. Roy-Chowdhuri S, Pisapia P, Salto-Tellez M, et al. Invited review-next-generation sequencing: a modern tool in cytopathology. Virchows Arch. 2019;475(1):3–11. https://doi.org/10.1007/s00428-019-02559-z.
69. Sanchez A, Bocklage T. Precision cytopathology: expanding opportunities for biomarker testing in cytopathology. J Am Soc Cytopathol. 2019;8(2):95–115. https://doi.org/10.1016/j.jasc.2018.12.003.
70. Scott SN, Ostrovnaya I, Lin CM, et al. Next-generation sequencing of urine specimens: a novel platform for genomic analysis in patients with non-muscle-invasive urothelial carcinoma treated with bacille Calmette-Guérin. Cancer Cytopathol. 2017;125(6):416–26. https://doi.org/10.1002/cncy.21847.
71. Shiratori Y, Ikeya T, Nakamura K. Comparison of Papanicolaou and Diff-Quick staining in pancreatic endoscopic ultrasound-fine needle aspiration biopsy with rapid on-site cytologic evaluation. Dig Endosc. 2020;32(3):434. https://doi.org/10.1111/den.13604.
72. Silva RSD, Schmitt F. Next step of molecular pathology: next-generation sequencing in cytology. J Pathol Transl Med. 2024;58(6):291–8. https://doi.org/10.4132/jptm.2024.10.22.
73. Sorber L, Claes B, Zwaenepoel K, et al. Evaluation of cytologic sample preparations for compatibility with nucleic acid analysis. Am J Clin Pathol. 2022;157(2):293–304. https://doi.org/10.1093/ajcp/aqab121.
74. Souza da Silva R, Pinto R, Cirnes L. Tissue management in precision medicine: what the pathologist needs to know in the molecular era. Front Mol Biosci. 2022;9:983102. https://doi.org/10.3389/fmolb.2022.983102.
75. Sun T, Hutchinson L, Tomaszewicz K, et al. Diagnostic value of a comprehensive, urothelial carcinoma-specific next-generation sequencing panel in urine cytology and bladder tumor specimens. Cancer Cytopathol. 2021;129(7):537–47. https://doi.org/10.1002/cncy.22410.
76. Tian SK, Killian JK, Rekhtman N, et al. Optimizing workflows and processing of cytologic samples for comprehensive analysis by next-generation sequencing: memorial sloan kettering cancer center experience. Arch Pathol Lab Med. 2016;140(11):1200–5. https://doi.org/10.5858/arpa.2016-0108-RA.
77. Turner SA, Abou Shaar R, Yang Z. The basics of commonly used molecular techniques for diagnosis, and application of molecular testing in cytology. Diagn Cytopathol. 2023;51(1):83–94. https://doi.org/10.1002/dc.25067.
78. Uzan C, Andre F, Scott V, et al. Fine-needle aspiration for nucleic acid-ased molecular analyses in breast cancer. Cancer. 2009;117(1):32–9. https://doi.org/10.1002/cncy.20008.
79. van Maldegem F, de Wit M, Morsink F, et al. Effects of processing delay, formalin fixation, and immunohistochemistry on RNA recovery from formalin-fixed paraffin-embedded tissue sections. Diagn Mol Pathol. 2008;17(1):51–8. https://doi.org/10.1097/PDM.0b013e31814b8866.
80. Velizheva NP, Rechsteiner MP, Wong CE, et al. Cytology smears as excellent starting material for next-generation sequencing-based molecular testing of patients with adenocarcinoma of the lung. Cancer Cytopathol. 2017;125(1):30–40. https://doi.org/10.1002/cncy.21771.
81. Vishnubhotla PS. Molecular testing of cytology specimens: are we ready for the new era? Cancer Cytopathol. 2016;124(1):9–10. https://doi.org/10.1002/cncy.21665.
82. Vormittag-Nocito E, Kumar R, Narayan KD, et al. Utilization of cytologic cell blocks for targeted sequencing of solid tumors. Cancer Med. 2023;12(4):4042–63. https://doi.org/10.1002/cam4.5261.
83. Wei S, Talarchek JN, Huang M, et al. Cell block-based RNA next generation sequencing for detection of gene fusions in lung adenocarcinoma: an institutional experience. Cytopathology. 2023;34(1):28–34. https://doi.org/10.1111/cyt.13175.
84. Xiao X, Sun Z, Liang S, et al. Liquid-based cytology specimens for next-generation sequencing in lung adenocarcinoma: challenges and evaluation of targeted therapy. BMC Cancer. 2024;24(1):749. https://doi.org/10.1186/s12885-024-12520-2.
85. Yamaguchi T, Akahane T, Harada O, et al. Next-generation sequencing in residual liquid-based cytology specimens for cancer genome analysis. Diagn Cytopathol. 2020;48(11):965–71. https://doi.org/10.1002/dc.24511.
86. Yamamoto S, Sakamoto Y, Nakano S, et al. Next-generation sequencing assay in salivary gland cytology: a pilot study. J Oral Pathol Med. 2020;49(10):1037–43. https://doi.org/10.1111/jop.13109.
87. Ye W, Hannigan B, Zalles S, et al. Centrifuged supernatants from FNA provide a liquid biopsy option for clinical next-generation sequencing of thyroid nodules. Cancer Cytopathol. 2019;127(3):146–60. https://doi.org/10.1002/cncy.22098.
88. Zhang M, Lin O. Molecular testing of thyroid nodules: a review of current available tests for fine-needle aspiration specimens. Arch Pathol Lab Med. 2016;140(12):1338–44. https://doi.org/10.5858/arpa.2016-0100-RA.
89. Zhang Y, Li J, Hua P, et al. Targeted next-generation sequencing in cytology specimens for molecular profiling of lung adenocarcinoma. Int J Clin Exp Pathol. 2018;11(7):3647–55.

Molecular Testing in Neuroendocrine Tumours

17

Theodore Evan, Raj Srirajaskanthan, and Debashis Sarker

Introduction

Neuroendocrine neoplasms (NENs) are a diverse, heterogenous group of cancers with wide variation in clinical presentation and outcome [1, 2]. They arise from neuroendocrine cells, subpopulations of hormonally active cells which are distributed ubiquitously around the body. The most frequent sites of origin include the bowel, pancreas, and lung, and cancers may occur as part of an inherited syndrome, such as multiple endocrine neoplasia type 1 (MEN-1) [3]. Traditional classification systems for NENs depend on their site of origin and histological features, primarily differentiation status and indices for cellular proliferation [4]. Treatment varies depending on where a given tumour sits along this spectrum. Well-differentiated tumours with lower rates of proliferation are often treated with systemic therapies such as somatostatin analogues, small molecule inhibitors, and peptide radionucleotide receptor therapy (PRRT). Conversely, conventional cytotoxic chemotherapy is typically reserved for higher-grade tumours or to reduce the burden of large-volume disease [5].

Nevertheless, many NENs defy simplistic classification, exhibiting features of both more aggressive and more indolent disease simultaneously [6]. This heterogeneity renders management decisions complex, often requiring highly varied approaches for individual patients. The increasing role of genomic testing in routine oncological practice has led to a more nuanced understanding of the biology of NENs, extending beyond routine clinical and histological classification. This chapter will first discuss the current classification of NENs, before addressing the growing role of molecular testing in determining the diagnosis, prognosis, and subsequent treatment of these cancers.

Classification of NENs

NENs are diagnosed through clinical, radiological, and histological assessment. Although NENs are overall rare cancers, clinical suspicion may be increased due to unique radiological appearances or the presence of functional symptoms. Aspects of classification vary dependent on site of origin, as described below.

T. Evan · D. Sarker
School of Cancer and Pharmaceutical Sciences, King's College London, Department of Medical Oncology, Guy's Hospital, London, UK
e-mail: theodore.evan@nhs.net; Debashis.sarker@kcl.ac.uk

R. Srirajaskanthan (✉)
Neuroendocrine Tumour Unit, ENETS Centre of Excellence, Kings College Hospital, London, UK
e-mail: r.srirajaskanthan@nhs.net

© The Author(s), under exclusive license to Springer Nature Switzerland AG 2026

S. Sioletic, L. Coppola (eds.), *Next-Generation Sequencing in Solid Tumor Histopathology*, Current Clinical Pathology, https://doi.org/10.1007/978-3-032-18790-1_17

Gastroenteropancreatic (GEP) NENs

GEP-NENs are classified into two broad categories based on differentiation status, according to the World Health Organisation (WHO) 2022 Classification system [4] (Table 17.1). Well-differentiated tumours, regardless of proliferation rate, are termed neuroendocrine tumours (NETs), which vary considerably in prognosis and presentation. Conversely, poorly differentiated tumours, the neuroendocrine carcinomas (NECs), are highly proliferative by definition and exhibit distinct molecular aberrations from NETs, as discussed further later this chapter.

NENs exhibit distinct morphological features and express specific markers identified on immunohistochemistry (IHC), including synaptophysin and chromogranin A [7]. Marker expression is typically abundant in low-grade, well-differentiated NETs, while staining may be more heterogeneous or faint in poorly differentiated NECs. Small bowel, pancreatic and most other NETs are then further classified further according to their Ki67 index, which is measured as a per cent proportion of tumour cells.

Pulmonary and Other NENs

Pulmonary NENs are classified differently from GEP-NENs, and the WHO classification as above does not apply in their case. Lung NETs are sometimes known as “carcinoid tumours”. Proliferation is measured in terms of number of mitotic index (MI), the number of mitotic figures per high-power field, instead of Ki67 IHC. In addition, classification takes the presence or absence of necrosis into account (Table 17.2). Recent attempts have been made to better unify definitions [4, 8], but differences in histological classification remain significant between these subtypes in routine clinical practice.

Table 17.1 Summary of the 2022 World Health Organisation (WHO) classification of neuroendocrine neoplasms

Category	Differentiation	Ki67 index (%)
Neuroendocrine tumours (NETS)		
NET grade 1	Well-differentiated	<3
NET grade 2	Well-differentiated	3–20
NET grade 3	Well-differentiated	>20
Neuroendocrine carcinomas (NECS)		
Small-cell type	Poorly differentiated	>20
Large-cell type		
Others		
Mixed neuroendocrine non-neuroendocrine neoplasms		

Limitations of Histological Classification

Both differentiation status and proliferative indices are imperfect measures of tumour biology in large part due to tumour heterogeneity. For example, Ki67 index can vary significantly within and between different biopsies, sometimes to the point of effecting overall grading and classification [10]. In such cases, the highest index is typically preferred. A further Ki67 subcategory beyond the WHO classification has been proposed to account for further prognostic impact for highly proliferative tumours: Tumours with a Ki67 index of >55% have notably worse outcomes than those between 20% and 55% [11]. Finally, NENs typically become more aggressive over time, which frequently correspond with an increase in proliferation indices if repeat biopsies are performed [12].

Molecular Classification of NENs

Although the current histological classification system has considerable diagnostic and prognostic utility, NENs are increasingly recognized as distinct molecular entities, with unique driver mutations, prognostic biomarkers, and therapeutic targets. Recent large-scale genomic studies have attempted to refine the classification of NENs in molecular terms. Cross-species analyses of human and murine pancreatic neuroendocrine tumours have revealed the presence of at least three distinct transcriptomic subtypes: an “islet-like” phenotype defined by elevated expression of pancreatic islet genes, a “metastasis-like primary” subtype with poorly differentiated features shared between primary and metastatic

Table 17.2 Classification of pulmonary NENs

	Typical carcinoid	Atypical carcinoid	Carcinoid with high MI/PI	Small cell carcinoma	Large cell NEC
Histological features					
Morphology	Organoid, trabecular, rosette formation, nested	Organoid, trabecular, rosette formation, nested	Organoid, trabecular, rosette formation, nested	Sheet-like, diffuse	Organoid, trabecular, palisading
Mitotic count/HPF	0–2	2–10	>10	>10 (typically >60)	>10 (typically >50)
Necrosis	Absent	Focal, punctate	Focal, punctate	Geographic	Extensive
Cell size	Variable	Variable	Variable	Small	Large

Adapted from Trucco et al. [9]

sites, and a mutationally enriched subgroup [13]. Further data have demonstrated subgroups of panNETs driven by distinct mutations, including germline mutations in BRCA2 [14]. Although such testing is not currently routine in clinical practice, it is likely to have increasing relevance going forward, as such mutations may predict sensitivity to targeted therapies (see "Molecularly Targeted Treatment in NENs").

The growing application of molecular diagnostics is rapidly altering the diagnostic and treatment landscape for NENs. The remainder of this chapter will discuss the growing role of molecular testing technologies in NEN diagnosis, prognosis, and treatment, with an emphasis on emerging clinically relevant prognostic biomarkers and therapeutic targets.

Diagnostic and Prognostic Biomarkers in NENs

Pancreatic Neuroendocrine Tumours (PanNETs)

Of the major subtypes of NENs, prognostic biomarkers for PanNETs remain the best characterized, and several coding and non-coding variants have been linked closely with clinical outcomes.

ATRX, DAXX, and MEN1

Landmark genomic studies in the 2010s identified common inactivating mutations in *MEN1*, *ATRX*, and *DAXX* in PanNETs, with an overall frequency of approximately 43% combined [15]. Loss of function of *ATRX* or *DAXX* activates the alternative lengthening of telomeres pathway (ALT) [16], an aberrant biological pathway active in many cancers, which serves to facilitate limitless replicative potential. ATRX and DAXX function as tumour suppressors by regulating histone H3.3 [17], which frequently localizes to telomeres but is also involved in gene silencing elsewhere in the genome. In addition, ATRX and DAXX interact with other notable tumour suppressor genes, including TP53, to facilitate appropriate DNA damage responses [18]. Loss-of-function mutations in *ATRX* and *DAXX* are typically mutually exclusive, bolstering that they act in the same biological pathway [15].

ATRX/DAXX mutations can be detected directly by NGS, or indirectly through loss of staining on IHC [19]. In early PanNETs, mutations are strongly associated with shorter progression-free survival and higher rates of metastatic recurrence [20–23]. In the advanced context, the data are more mixed, with some studies suggesting better prognosis in overt metastatic disease [15, 24]. This distinction remains unresolved but may relate to patient population differences in the relevant studies. The prognostic significance of MEN1 itself is comparably less clear, in large part due to ambiguity in outcomes between somatic versus germline loss of gene function [25].

Alternative Lengthening of Telomeres (ALT)

The alternative lengthening of telomeres (ALT) pathway is an alternative mechanism for preserving telomere length independent of the canonical telomerase pathway. ALT differs in its use of a DNA rather than RNA template, which extends telomeres using those found on sister chromatids or other chromosomes [26]. ALT activation is intimately linked to ATRX/DAXX function and, indeed, classically emerges when ATRX/DAXX are mutated [27]. ALT is typically identified by telomere-specific FISH assays, though these are not currently used in routine clinical practice [26]. Activation of the pathway is detected in approximately 30% of PanNETs. Akin to ATRX/DAXX, ALT is strongly linked to survival and metastatic recurrence in localised PanNETs [28], while the data are more ambiguous in metastatic disease [29, 30].

Other Mutations

Activating mutations in the mitogen-activated protein kinase (MAPK) pathway, including *KRAS* and *BRAF*, is associated with worse prognosis and decreased overall survival [24], a finding consistent with other gastrointestinal malignancies such as colorectal cancer. Loss-of-function variants in the *CDKN2A/B* genes are enriched in metastatic PanNETS relative to primary tumours, suggesting these mutations may also be drivers of disease progression [20]. CDKN2A mutations are frequent in many cancer types and are readily identified in common NGS gene panels and are likely to have greater prognostic significance in the future.

Other Epigenetic Markers

Non-coding genomic variants also have prognostic significance in PanNETs. Hypermethylation of certain genes, including *ATRX*, *DAXX* [31], and methylated-DNA-protein-cysteine methyltransferase (MGMT), has all been associated with lower long-term survival [32]. Although methylation testing is not routinely available in clinical practice, resultant low protein expression can be inferred clinically by loss of staining on IHC. miRNAs involved in regulation of histone deacetylases have also been linked with poor outcomes [33].

Small Intestinal NETs (SI-NETs)

Prognostic somatic mutations in SI-NETs are considerably less well characterised [25], and unlike PanNETs, there is limited evidence for prognostically significant somatic mutations that are shared widely across populations. In contrast, structural and transcriptomic variants have greater significance in these cancers.

Copy Number Variants (CNVs)

Copy number variants (CNVs) are more common genomic aberrations in SI-NETs [34], though patterns vary with tumour grade. CNVs closely associated with poor prognosis include gains of chromosome 14 and the *SRC* locus on chromosome 20, a non-receptor tyrosine kinase involved in cellular proliferation [35, 36]. Other CNVs more closely correlate with better outcomes, including 3p13 and chromosome 18 loss of heterozygosity [35, 37]. The case of 3p13 is particularly notable, as this deletion is a poor prognostic marker in other solid tumours, such as prostate cancer [38]. In many cases, the critical driver gene(s) at these variant loci remain yet to be fully elucidated.

Transcriptional Variants

In the absence of obvious genetic mutations of prognostic significance, several studies have sought to identify variant transcripts that correlate with outcomes in SI-NETs. Expression of miRNAs related to genes involved in apoptosis and the cell cycle correlates with worse outcomes, notably *BIRC5*, *CDCA5*, and *PTTG1* [34, 39]. *BIRC5* somatic mutations have also been identified in SI-NETs, albeit at low frequency [40]. Low mRNA expression of several tumour suppressors, including *p16* and *RASSF1A*, is also associated with poor prognosis [25, 41].

Pulmonary and Other NETs

Comparatively little is known about prognostic biomarkers for pulmonary carcinoids, and none are currently used in clinical practice beyond routine assessment of mitotic index and differentiation status. Low mRNA expression of orthopaedia homeobox protein (OTP) and CD44 have both been associated with worse long-term outcomes. Loss of nuclear staining for OTP can additionally be assessed through immunohistochemistry, though is not used in routine practice.

Methylation of the tumour suppressor p16 is associated with worse long-term survival in large bowel NETs [42]. In addition, SETD1B mutations have been associated with poor prognosis in hepatic NETs [43].

Neuroendocrine Carcinomas (NECs)

Gastrointestinal and pulmonary NECs have a distinct mutational landscape from NETs, frequently exhibiting mutations in the tumour suppressor genes TP53 and RB1 [44]. Indeed, the presence of these genomic features can clinically distinguish NECs from high-grade NETs, which can subsequently impact both treatment and overall prognosis. Efforts to identify prognostic mutations in NECs have thus far met limited success. Like PanNETs, KRAS mutations are associated with worse outcomes in PanNECs [44]. Catastrophic chromosomal shattering, termed chromothripsis, is associated with poor outcomes in a variety of solid tumours. Genomic signatures of chromothripsis have been identified in gastrointestinal NECs with moderately high frequency but are very rare in GI-NETs [45].

Current Treatment of NENs

Optimal treatment for NENs relies on a combination of clinical, radiological, and histological features. Patients who are fit and amenable to a curative resection are typically offered surgery, as this gives the best possible chance for a long-term cure. Outside of NECs, there is limited role to support the use of adjuvant therapy [8]. Those with limited metastatic disease are also offered debulking surgery in combination with locoregional treatments, such as resection or ablation of liver metastases, which can also offer the possibility of cure if adequate margins are achieved [46].

In diffuse metastatic disease, the primary factors determining treatment include the following:

1. *Somatostatin receptor (SSTR) expression*: Tumour SSTR expression is usually determined through specialised nuclear medicine imaging, although IHC for the SSTR can also be performed in resource-limited environments where functional imaging is not available. Indium-111-labelled octreotide scans have progressively been replaced by newer technologies such as SSTR-PET imaging, which is considerably more sensitive [47]. Functional assessment of SSTR expression is often paired with standard FDG-PET imaging to determine relative avidity of the two markers. SSTR-avid tumours are generally responsive to hormonal and targeted therapies, while FDG-avid tumours respond better to chemotherapy, though many patients exhibit avidity to both markers.
2. *Organ of origin*: Trials conducted in NENs have had variable patient populations, and in many notable studies, certain subgroups of patients have been excluded. A notable example of this is peptide receptor radionuclide therapy, which is only approved by the European Medicines Agency for SSTR-positive gastrointestinal NETs, as lung carcinoids were not included in the NETTER-1 study [48].
3. *Tumour grade and differentiation status*: Well-differentiated, low-grade tumours are more likely to express SSTR and respond to targeted treatments. Conversely, there is no role for SSTR-based therapy in poorly differentiated NECs, and chemotherapy remains the standard treatment of choice for these patients. Similarly, tumours with a higher pro-

liferative index tend to be more responsive to cytotoxic chemotherapy.

4. *Functional status*: Patients with functional tumours may need specific monitoring or treatment to alleviate their symptoms, at least until more definitive management such as surgery is performed. A detailed discussion of the management of carcinoid syndrome is beyond the scope of this chapter but is addressed elsewhere [8].

The main treatments used in NENs are summarised below (Table 17.3).

Choice of treatment in NENs does not depend on the mutational status of the patient in the current standard-of-care setting. However, with ever-greater proportions of patients undergoing genetic sequencing as part of their diagnostic pathway, a number of emerging targets have rapidly growing clinical relevance.

Table 17.3 Summary of current systemic treatments for NENs based on molecular target, organ of origin, and tumour subtype

Treatment	Target	Population	Notes
Somatostatin receptor analogues (SSAs)	SSTR	SSTR +ve GEP and pulmonary NETs	Validated in GEP and pulmonary NETS [49–51]
Peptide receptor radionuclide therapy (PRRT)	SSTR	SSTR +ve GEP NETs	Validated in GEP-NETs [52, 53]
Everolimus	mTOR signalling pathway	GEP and pulmonary NETs	Validated in PanNETs [54], GEP and pulmonary NETs [55]
Sunitinib	Multiple receptor tyrosine kinases (VEGFR, c-KIT, PDGFR)	Pancreatic NETs	Only validated in PanNETs [56]
Cabozantinib	Multiple receptor tyrosine kinases (VEGFR, c-KIT, PDGFR)	GEP, pulmonary and other NETs (G1-G3)	Validated in GEP, pulmonary and extrapulmonary NETs [57]
Interferon-alpha	Multiple immune targets	GEP, pancreatic and pulmonary NETs	Limited evidence as monotherapy. Used in second line [58]
Cytotoxic chemotherapy	Cell cycle, DNA replication, metabolism	High-grade NETs* (G2, G3) NECs *used in low-grade NETs on progression	Platinum-based chemotherapy favoured in NECs. 5-FU-based chemotherapy favoured in NETs [8]

SSTR somatostatin receptor, *GEP* gastroenteropancreatic, *mTOR* mammalian target of rapamycin, *VEGFR* vascular endothelial growth factor, *PDGFR* platelet-derived growth factor receptor

Molecularly Targeted Treatment in NENs

Identification of Driver Mutations in NENs

PanNETs

The earliest sequencing studies in PanNETs identified loss-of-function mutations in *MEN1*, *ATRX*, and *DAXX* as the most frequent driver events in these cancers [15]. Subsequent larger studies have also identified frequent somatic mutations in components of the mTOR signalling pathway, including *PTEN*, *TSC1/2*, and *DEPDC5* [14]. Activation of the mTOR signalling pathway is also observed at the transcriptional level in these tumours. PanNETs also exhibit somatic mutations in canonical DNA repair mediators, notably *BRCA2* and *CHEK2*. Large-scale structural variants are comparatively uncommon but are more frequent in high-grade disease [45]. Those observed often affect chromosomal regions harbouring canonical tumour suppressors, notably *CDKN2A* and *CDKN2B*, as well as chromatin modifiers, including *ARID2* and *SMARCA4*. This mutational landscape differs considerably from pancreatic adenocarcinomas, although there is greater overlap in more aggressive disease [14].

SI-NETs

Unified somatic mutations in SI-NETs are considerably less common, and in general, there is less data available in SI-NETs relative to panNETs. Targeted exome sequencing has demonstrated these cancers are often genomically stable, with an overall low somatic tumour mutational burden (TMB) relative to other solid tumours. Pathological variants have been identified in a variety of genes but at low overall frequency across populations [40], including cell cycle mediators (e.g. *CDKN1B*), signalling pathway components (ex: *FGFR2*) and chromatin modifiers (e.g. *EZH2*). A significant minority of cases appear to have unique driver mutations that are cryptic in pathogenicity and not widely shared with other patients [45].

In contrast, CNVs are more widely shared across SI-NETs. In one large cohort, greater than 50% of SI-NETs exhibited loss of chromosome 18, a region harbouring multiple known tumour suppressor genes, notably *SMAD4* and *DCC* [45, 59]. Amplifications of *AKT1* and *AKT2*, a major component of the mTOR signalling pathway, have also been observed, further implicating this pathway as a major driver in gastroenteropancreatic NENs.

Pulmonary NETs

The most frequent driver mutations in pulmonary carcinoids affect chromatin and histone modifiers, notably *MEN1*, *PSIP1*, *ARID1A*, and components of the SWI/SNF complex. Mutations in these pathways are mutually exclusive, suggesting a common convergent oncogenic mechanism involving these epigenetic regulators. Like SI-NETs, the overall TMB in lung carcinoids is low, averaging less than 1 mutation per megabase, far lower than that observed in classic smoking-related lung cancers and NECs. Pulmonary carcinoids seldom exhibit mutations in *TP53* and *RB1*, the most frequent driver mutations observed in pulmonary and other NECs. This suggests that typical and atypical carcinoids are usually distinct clinical entities rather than precursor lesions for these more aggressive cancers, although there have been rare, reported cases of direct transformation of low-grade carcinoids into high-grade NECs [60].

NECs

The genomic landscape for NECs is markedly distinct from other NENs. Both pulmonary and GI-NECs exhibit frequent inactivating mutations of the canonical tumour suppressors *TP53* and *RB1* [44] and, as a result, frequently bear the hallmarks of genomic instability. Somatic mutations are frequently observed in classical oncogenic signalling pathways, particularly the MAPK pathway (e.g. *KRAS*, *BRAF*). The TMB in NECs is considerably greater than in other NETs, and these cancers frequently show evidence of aneuploidy and large-scale structural abnormalities, including evidence of chromothripsis and kataegis. NECs, particularly pulmonary NECs, frequently show evidence of NOTCH pathway downregulation, with consequent overexpression of NOTCH inhibitory receptors, such as DLL3 [61]. NECs exhibit mutational landscapes more similar to high-grade epithelial carcinoma of their organ of origin and are less distinct than well-differentiated NETs.

Actionable Genomic Drivers

The growing role of genomic testing both at baseline and at progression in routine oncology practice has revealed that a substantial proportion of NENs have potentially actionable driver mutations. Current estimates suggest at least 25–33% of NEN patients have genetic drivers which are actionable with approved therapies [62], with other variants likely to be targetable in the future. However, access to comprehensive genomic testing for NENs is not currently uniform, leading to considerable heterogeneity of practice across centres and between different countries. Access to free testing is sometimes only available in context of clinical studies, and a large proportion of advanced assays, including NGS panels, whole-exome, and whole-genome sequencing, are funded privately either by patients themselves or through insurance, limiting access to those in lower socioeconomic groups [63].

Such inequities are amplified in rare cancers such as NENs, where large-scale characterisation efforts have been hampered by lower patient numbers and considerable intra- and inter-patient heterogeneity. Growing evidence has demonstrated the value of early genomic testing in other rare tumours. Upfront genomic testing has proven fruitful in both facilitating more accurate diagnosis and identifying molecularly targeted treatments in other rare cancers such as sarcomas [64]. Dedicated trials of molecularly targeted therapies in NENs are lacking, in large part due to their rarity. As a result, prompt referral into tumour-agnostic precision medicine studies, such as the DETERMINE trial in the UK (NCT05722886), is paramount for facilitating access to molecularly targeted therapies. [64] The available data suggest there are multitude of potentially druggable pathways in NENs outside of standard therapy, as summarised below.

Mismatch Repair Deficiency and Tumour Mutational Burden (TMB)

Mismatch repair (MMR) deficiency arises most commonly due to mutations in one of the four principal components of the MMR pathway, namely, *MLH1*, *MSH2*, *MSH6*, and *PMS2* [65]. Hereditary defects in these genes cause Lynch syndrome, a cancer predisposition syndrome associated with multiple solid tumours, particularly gastrointestinal adenocarcinomas and gynaecological malignancies [66]. Routine testing is conducted by immunohistochemistry, although microsatellite instability (MSI) can also be detected through PCR-based assays [67]. Mutations in MMR pathway components can also be identified through NGS and non-targeted sequencing modalities.

The hallmark consequence of MMR deficiency is an elevated tumour mutational burden (TMB). However, an elevated TMB may also arise by alternative mechanisms, notably environmental exposures including smoking and ultraviolet light exposure [68], as well as certain cytotoxic drugs, such as temozolomide [69]. MMR deficiency, high MSI, and an elevated TMB are all predictors of response to PD-1-based immunotherapy across a wide range of solid tumours [70, 71], though response rates are not equivalent across different cancers [72].

Genuine microsatellite instability and mismatch repair deficiency appears to be rare in spontaneous NENs. Indeed, in unselected NENs, immunotherapy has not proven efficacious. In the MMR-proficient context, the anti PD-1-inhibitor pembrolizumab has no proven benefit, with response rates less than 10% in an unselected cohort [73]. Similarly disappointing overall response rates have been observed with other anti-PD1 inhibitors in the absence of prospective biomarker-based selection [74, 75].

Nevertheless, in the presence of an elevated TMB, there are reported durable responses to immunotherapy, typically in high-grade NETs and NECs [76]. Intriguingly, treatment with the alkylating agent temozolomide can induce a hypermutated state resembling MMR deficiency in normally MMR-proficient tumours [69]. Temozolomide is commonly employed as a first-line cytotoxic chemotherapy agent in NENs in combination with capecitabine, yet at present, it remains unclear if temozolomide-induced hypermutation can generally induce responses to PD-1-based-immunotherapy, despite some positive data from case reports [77]. A combination regimen of temozolomide with the PD-1 inhibitor nivolumab has demonstrated early evidence of efficacy, with an ORR of 32% in one phase II study [78]. However, the relationship between response and TMB in this trial remains unclear, and concerningly, in some solid tumours such as gliomas, temozolomide-induced hypermutation is associated with worse long-term outcomes [79]. Such uncertainties warrant dedicated testing in context of a NEN-specific clinical trial.

mTOR Signalling Pathway

As discussed previously, mTOR signalling pathway mutations are common across gastroentero-pancreatic NENs, and the mTOR inhibitor everolimus is currently approved in this context regardless of mutational status [76]. However, there is surprisingly limited evidence that mTOR pathway mutations are strong predictors of response in NENs, a finding consistent with observations in other solid tumours [80], although there are reports of exceptional individual responses in select cases [81]. Indeed, everolimus has proven efficacy in lung NENs despite much lower frequency of mTOR pathway mutations in this subtype relative to gastrointestinal NENs. At present, despite the observed high prevalence of mTOR pathway mutations, predictors for response to these drugs remain unclear at the genomic level [82].

BRAF and MAPK Pathway Mutations

BRAF V600E mutations are routinely targeted in solid tumours such as melanoma and non-small cell lung cancer [83, 84]. Indeed, combination therapy with the BRAF inhibitor dabrafenib and MEK inhibitor trametinib now has tumour-agnostic approval from the Food and Drug Administration in the USA. BRAF mutations have also been identified in high-grade gastrointestinal NETs and NECs, with frequencies estimated at around 10% of cases [85]. Impressive responses to combined BRAF/MEK inhibition have been reported in both gastrointestinal and pancreatic NETs, most notably in large bowel NENs, where the data are particularly promising. However, these responses are not always sustained long term, a common issue observed in other BRAF-mutated malignancies [86, 87]. Routine testing for BRAF mutations is not conducted for NENs in most centres, but mutations are easily detected by the majority of commercial NGS panels. With the advent of tumour-agnostic approval for combination therapy, a larger proportion of NEN patients are likely to benefit from access to these treatments.

Other components of the MAPK signalling pathway have proven more difficult to target successfully. Although KRAS mutations are theoretically druggable, the only currently approved inhibitors target the G12C variant, which is rare in NENs despite some case reports suggesting potential efficacy [88]. Indirect, nonspecific inhibitors of KRAS, such as farnesyltransferase inhibitors, have demonstrated responses in individual cases [76], but these compounds are not widely available outside of the experimental or early phase setting. Nevertheless, the role of KRAS inhibitors in NENs is likely to grow in the future as more validated inhibitors progress through clinical trials [89].

Other DNA Repair Pathways

Targetable defects in double-stranded DNA repair are observed in a subset of NENs. For example, somatic mutations in BRCA1 and BRCA2 have been detected in a subset of NENs, typically higher-grade NETs and NECs. Poly-ADP ribose polymerase (PARP) inhibitors such as olaparib have proven efficacy in BRCA-mutant and HRD-deficient solid tumours, most prominently breast [90], ovarian [91], and prostate cancers [92]. In NENs, responses to these agents have been reported, though data are limited to case reports and small series [93]. Mutations in ataxia-telengiectasia mutated (ATM), a targetable serine-threonine kinase recruited to double-stranded breaks, also occur in a subset of small intestinal NETs, typically in the advanced and metastatic context [94]. Trials of ATR inhibitors, which are synthetic-lethal in context of ATM mutations, are underway [95, 96], though specific data in NENs remains limited.

PRMT5 Inhibitors

As described earlier, loss of the CDKN2A tumour suppressor is a frequent event in NEN evolution, particularly in pNETs [97]. In many cases, deletion of CDKN2A coincides with loss of methylthioadenosine phosphorylase (MTAP), a neighbouring gene which resides at the same locus on chromosome 9. Studies suggest loss of MTAP confers synthetic lethality in context of inhibition of protein arginine methyltransferase 5 (PRMT5). Novel inhibitors of PRMT5 are in development and progressing through clinical trials [98, 99].

Rare Gene Fusions

Oncogenic gene fusions, most notably in receptor tyrosine kinases such as NTRK, RET, and ROS1 are oncogenic drivers in a wide variety of solid tumours. Although these events are rare as a proportion of total tumours, responses to these targeted therapies are often exceptionally potent and durable, and as a result, compounds targeting these fusions have tumour-agnostic approval despite their rarity. Such fusion events are rare in NENs (less than 1%), and testing is not performed routinely. However, responses to these agents are well-documented [100, 101]. Improving access to genomic testing will be critical to facilitate access to these therapies.

Conclusions

The growing role of molecular testing in oncology is likely to upend the classification, prognostication, and treatment of NENs in the coming years. Current predictive frameworks, which rely on heterogeneous clinical and histological factors, are already being refined through the detection of diagnostically and prognostically significant mutations at baseline assessment. Greater access to NGS and other unbiased means of detecting targetable driver mutations will further influence treatment options, particularly once standard therapies have been exhausted. Access to potential targeted therapies remains a pressing issue, especially given the rarity of NENs and the absence of dedicated trials. Early and streamlined referral into tumour-agnostic studies, that facilitate access to these medicines, will be critical to maximise benefit for patients.

References

1. Oronsky B, Ma PC, Morgensztern D, Carter CA. Nothing but NET: a review of neuroendocrine tumors and carcinomas. Neoplasia. 2017;19:991–1002.
2. Kaltsas GA, Besser GM, Grossman AB. The diagnosis and medical management of advanced neuroendocrine tumors. Endocr Rev. 2004;25:458–511.
3. Taal BG, Visser O. Epidemiology of neuroendocrine tumours. Neuroendocrinology. 2004;80(Suppl 1):3–7.
4. Rindi G, et al. Overview of the 2022 WHO classification of neuroendocrine neoplasms. Endocr Pathol. 2022;33:115–54.
5. Panzuto F, et al. European Neuroendocrine Tumor Society (ENETS) 2023 guidance paper for gastroduodenal neuroendocrine tumours (NETs) G1-G3. J Neuroendocrinol. 2023;35:e13306.
6. Chan DL, et al. Dual [68Ga] DOTATATE and [18F] FDG PET/CT in patients with metastatic gastroenteropancreatic neuroendocrine neoplasms: a multicentre validation of the NETPET score. Br J Cancer. 2023;128:549–55.
7. Klimstra DS, Beltran H, Lilenbaum R, Bergsland E. The spectrum of neuroendocrine tumors: histologic classification, unique features and areas of overlap. Am Soc Clin Oncol Educ Book. 2015;35:92–103. https://doi.org/10.14694/EdBook_AM.2015.35.92.
8. Pavel M, et al. Gastroenteropancreatic neuroendocrine neoplasms: ESMO Clinical Practice Guidelines for diagnosis, treatment and follow-up. Ann Oncol. 2020;31:844–60.
9. Vocino Trucco G, Righi L, Volante M, Papotti M. Updates on lung neuroendocrine neoplasm classification. Histopathology. 2024;84:67–85.
10. Yang Z, Tang LH, Klimstra DS. Effect of tumor heterogeneity on the assessment of Ki67 labeling index in well-differentiated neuroendocrine tumors metastatic to the liver: implications for prognostic stratification. Am J Surg Pathol. 2011;35:853–60.

11. Milione M, et al. The clinicopathologic heterogeneity of grade 3 gastroenteropancreatic neuroendocrine neoplasms: morphological differentiation and proliferation identify different prognostic categories. Neuroendocrinology. 2017;104:85–93.
12. Panzuto F, et al. Impact of Ki67 re-assessment at time of disease progression in patients with pancreatic neuroendocrine neoplasms. PLoS One. 2017;12:e0179445.
13. Sadanandam A, et al. A cross-species analysis in pancreatic neuroendocrine tumors reveals molecular subtypes with distinctive clinical, metastatic, developmental, and metabolic characteristics. Cancer Discov. 2015;5:1296–313.
14. Scarpa A, et al. Whole-genome landscape of pancreatic neuroendocrine tumours. Nature. 2017;543:65–71.
15. Jiao Y, et al. DAXX/ATRX, MEN1, and mTOR pathway genes are frequently altered in pancreatic neuroendocrine tumors. Science. 2011;331:1199–203.
16. Heaphy CM, et al. Altered telomeres in tumors with ATRX and DAXX mutations. Science. 2011;333:425.
17. Elsässer SJ, et al. DAXX envelops a histone H3.3-H4 dimer for H3.3-specific recognition. Nature. 2012;491:560–5.
18. Gulve N, et al. DAXX-ATRX regulation of p 53 chromatin binding and DNA damage response. Nat Commun. 2022;13:5033.
19. Hechtman JF, et al. Performance of DAXX Immunohistochemistry as a screen for DAXX mutations in pancreatic neuroendocrine tumors. Pancreas. 2019;48:396–9.
20. Roy S, et al. Loss of chromatin-remodeling proteins and/or CDKN2A associates with metastasis of pancreatic neuroendocrine tumors and reduced patient survival times. Gastroenterology. 2018;154:2060–2063.e8.
21. Yuan F, et al. KRAS and DAXX/ATRX gene mutations are correlated with the clinicopathological features, advanced diseases, and poor prognosis in Chinese patients with pancreatic neuroendocrine tumors. Int J Biol Sci. 2014;10:957–65.
22. Hong X, et al. Whole-genome sequencing reveals distinct genetic bases for insulinomas and non-functional pancreatic neuroendocrine tumours: leading to a new classification system. Gut. 2020;69:877–87.
23. Chan CS, et al. ATRX, DAXX or MEN1 mutant pancreatic neuroendocrine tumors are a distinct alpha-cell signature subgroup. Nat Commun. 2018;9:4158.
24. Raj N, et al. Real-time genomic characterization of metastatic pancreatic neuroendocrine tumors has prognostic implications and identifies potential germline actionability. JCO Precis Oncol. 2018;2:1–18.
25. Mestre-Alagarda C, et al. Genetic and epigenetic prognosticators of neuroendocrine tumours of the GI tract, liver, biliary tract and pancreas: a systematic review and meta-analysis. Histopathology. 2024;84:255–65.
26. Mori JO, Keegan J, Flynn RL, Heaphy CM. Alternative lengthening of telomeres: mechanism and the pathogenesis of cancer. J Clin Pathol. 2024;77:82–6.
27. Luchini C, et al. Alternative Lengthening of Telomeres (ALT) in pancreatic neuroendocrine tumors: ready for prime-time in clinical practice? Curr Oncol Rep. 2021;23:106.
28. Hackeng WM, et al. Non-functional pancreatic neuroendocrine tumours: ATRX/DAXX and alternative lengthening of telomeres (ALT) are prognostically independent from ARX/PDX1 expression and tumour size. Gut. 2022;71:961–73.
29. Pea A, et al. Genetic analysis of small well-differentiated pancreatic neuroendocrine tumors identifies subgroups with differing risks of liver metastases. Ann Surg. 2020;271:566–73.
30. Cives M, et al. Analysis of potential response predictors to capecitabine/temozolomide in metastatic pancreatic neuroendocrine tumors. Endocr Relat Cancer. 2016;23:759–67.
31. Pipinikas CP, et al. Epigenetic dysregulation and poorer prognosis in DAXX-deficient pancreatic neuroendocrine tumours. Endocr Relat Cancer. 2015;22:L13–8.
32. Cros J, et al. MGMT expression predicts response to temozolomide in pancreatic neuroendocrine tumors. Endocr Relat Cancer. 2016;23:625–33.
33. Klieser E, et al. HDAC-linked 'proliferative' miRNA expression pattern in pancreatic neuroendocrine tumors. Int J Mol Sci. 2018;19:2781.
34. Andersson E, et al. Expression profiling of small intestinal neuroendocrine tumors identifies subgroups with clinical relevance, prognostic markers and therapeutic targets. Mod Pathol. 2016;29:616–29.
35. Andersson E, Swärd C, Stenman G, Ahlman H, Nilsson O. High-resolution genomic profiling reveals gain of chromosome 14 as a predictor of poor outcome in ileal carcinoids. Endocr Relat Cancer. 2009;16:953–66.
36. Simbolo M, et al. Mutational and copy number asset of primary sporadic neuroendocrine tumors of the small intestine. Virchows Arch. 2018;473:709–17.
37. Karpathakis A, et al. Prognostic impact of novel molecular subtypes of small intestinal neuroendocrine tumor. Clin Cancer Res. 2016;22:250–8.
38. Hieronymus H, et al. Deletion of 3p13–14 locus spanning FOXP1 to SHQ1 cooperates with PTEN loss in prostate oncogenesis. Nat Commun. 2017;8:1081.
39. Arvidsson Y, et al. miRNA profiling of small intestinal neuroendocrine tumors defines novel molecular subtypes and identifies miR-375 as a biomarker of patient survival. Mod Pathol. 2018;31:1302–17.

40. Banck MS, et al. The genomic landscape of small intestine neuroendocrine tumors. J Clin Invest. 2013;123:2502–8.
41. Fotouhi O, et al. Global hypomethylation and promoter methylation in small intestinal neuroendocrine tumors: an in vivo and in vitro study. Epigenetics. 2014;9:987–97.
42. Arnold CN, et al. Molecular characteristics and predictors of survival in patients with malignant neuroendocrine tumors. Int J Cancer. 2008;123:1556–64.
43. Yang P, et al. SET domain containing 1B gene is mutated in primary hepatic neuroendocrine tumors. Int J Cancer. 2019;145:2986–95.
44. Yachida S, et al. Comprehensive genomic profiling of neuroendocrine carcinomas of the gastrointestinal system. Cancer Discov. 2022;12:692–711.
45. van Riet J, et al. The genomic landscape of 85 advanced neuroendocrine neoplasms reveals subtype-heterogeneity and potential therapeutic targets. Nat Commun. 2021;12:4612.
46. Frilling A, et al. Treatment of liver metastases from neuroendocrine tumours in relation to the extent of hepatic disease. Br J Surg. 2009;96:175–84.
47. Deppen SA, et al. 68Ga-DOTATATE compared with 111In-DTPA-octreotide and conventional imaging for pulmonary and gastroenteropancreatic neuroendocrine tumors: a systematic review and meta-analysis. J Nucl Med. 2016;57:872–8.
48. Naraev BG, Ramirez RA, Kendi AT, Halfdanarson TR. Peptide receptor radionuclide therapy for patients with advanced lung carcinoids. Clin Lung Cancer. 2019;20:e376–92.
49. Baudin E, et al. Treatment of advanced BP-NETS with lanreotide autogel/depot vs placebo: the phase III SPINET study. Endocr Relat Cancer. 2024;31:e230337.
50. Caplin ME, et al. Lanreotide in metastatic enteropancreatic neuroendocrine tumors. N Engl J Med. 2014;371:224–33.
51. Rinke A, et al. Placebo-controlled, double-blind, prospective, randomized study on the effect of octreotide LAR in the control of tumor growth in patients with metastatic neuroendocrine midgut tumors (PROMID): results of long-term survival. Neuroendocrinology. 2017;104:26–32.
52. Singh S, et al. [177Lu]Lu-DOTA-TATE plus long-acting octreotide versus high-dose long-acting octreotide for the treatment of newly diagnosed, advanced grade 2–3, well-differentiated, gastroenteropancreatic neuroendocrine tumours (NETTER-2): an open-label, randomised, phase 3 study. Lancet. 2024;403:2807–17.
53. Strosberg J, et al. Phase 3 trial of ^{177} Lu-Dotatate for midgut neuroendocrine tumors. N Engl J Med. 2017;376:125–35.
54. Yao JC, et al. Everolimus for advanced pancreatic neuroendocrine tumors. N Engl J Med. 2011;364:514–23.
55. Yao JC, et al. Everolimus for the treatment of advanced, non-functional neuroendocrine tumours of the lung or gastrointestinal tract (RADIANT-4): a randomised, placebo-controlled, phase 3 study. Lancet. 2016;387:968–77.
56. Raymond E, et al. Sunitinib malate for the treatment of pancreatic neuroendocrine tumors. N Engl J Med. 2011;364:501–13.
57. Chan JA, et al. Phase 3 trial of cabozantinib to treat advanced neuroendocrine tumors. N Engl J Med. 2025;392:653–65.
58. Faiss S, et al. Prospective, randomized, multicenter trial on the antiproliferative effect of lanreotide, interferon alfa, and their combination for therapy of metastatic neuroendocrine gastroenteropancreatic tumors--the International Lanreotide and Interferon Alfa Study Group. J Clin Oncol. 2003;21:2689–96.
59. Nieser M, et al. Loss of chromosome 18 in neuroendocrine tumors of the small intestine: the enigma remains. Neuroendocrinology. 2017;104:302–12.
60. Pelosi G, Travis WD. Head-to-head: should Ki67 proliferation index be included in the formal classification of pulmonary neuroendocrine neoplasms? Histopathology. 2024;85:535–48.
61. Schmitt M, et al. DLL3 expression in neuroendocrine carcinomas and neuroendocrine tumours: insights from a multicentric cohort of 1294 pulmonary and extrapulmonary neuroendocrine neoplasms. Endocr Pathol. 2025;36:9.
62. Horak P, et al. Comprehensive genomic and transcriptomic analysis for guiding therapeutic decisions in patients with rare cancers. Cancer Discov. 2021;11:2780–95.
63. Bayle A, et al. ESMO study on the availability and accessibility of biomolecular technologies in oncology in Europe. Ann Oncol. 2023;34:934–45.
64. Vijayvergia N, Astsaturov IA, et al. Molecular profiling of neuroendocrine malignancies to identify prognostic and therapeutic markers: a Fox Chase Cancer Center Pilot Study. Br J Cancer. 2016. PMID: 27482655
65. Olave MC, Graham RP. Mismatch repair deficiency: the what, how and why it is important. Genes Chromosom Cancer. 2022;61:314–21.
66. Peltomäki P, Nyström M, Mecklin J-P, Seppälä TT. Lynch syndrome genetics and clinical implications. Gastroenterology. 2023;164:783–99.
67. Wang C, Zhang L, Vakiani E, Shia J. Detecting mismatch repair deficiency in solid neoplasms: immunohistochemistry, microsatellite instability, or both? Mod Pathol. 2022;35:1515–28.
68. Sha D, et al. Tumor mutational burden as a predictive biomarker in solid tumors. Cancer Discov. 2020;10:1808–25.
69. Crisafulli G, et al. Temozolomide treatment alters mismatch repair and boosts mutational burden in tumor and blood of colorectal cancer patients. Cancer Discov. 2022;12:1656–75.
70. Rizvi NA, et al. Mutational landscape determines sensitivity to PD-1 blockade in non–small cell lung cancer. Science. 2015;348:124–8.

71. Le DT, et al. PD-1 blockade in tumors with mismatch-repair deficiency. N Engl J Med. 2015;372:2509–20.
72. Le DT, et al. Mismatch repair deficiency predicts response of solid tumors to PD-1 blockade. Science. 2017;357:409–13.
73. Marabelle A, et al. Efficacy of pembrolizumab in patients with noncolorectal high microsatellite instability/mismatch repair-deficient cancer: results from the phase II KEYNOTE-158 study. J Clin Oncol. 2020;38:1–10.
74. Vijayvergia N, et al. Pembrolizumab monotherapy in patients with previously treated metastatic high-grade neuroendocrine neoplasms: joint analysis of two prospective, non-randomised trials. Br J Cancer. 2020;122:1309–14.
75. Capdevila J, et al. Durvalumab plus tremelimumab for the treatment of advanced neuroendocrine neoplasms of gastroenteropancreatic and lung origin. Nat Commun. 2023;14:2973.
76. Boilève A, et al. Molecular profiling and target actionability for precision medicine in neuroendocrine neoplasms: real-world data. Eur J Cancer. 2023;186:122–32.
77. Klempner SJ, et al. Exploiting temozolomide-induced hypermutation with pembrolizumab in a refractory high-grade neuroendocrine neoplasm: a proof-of-concept case. JCO Precis Oncol. 2020;4:614–9.
78. Owen DH, et al. A phase II clinical trial of nivolumab and temozolomide for neuroendocrine neoplasms. Clin Cancer Res. 2023;29:731–41.
79. Yu Y, et al. Temozolomide-induced hypermutation is associated with distant recurrence and reduced survival after high-grade transformation of low-grade IDH-mutant gliomas. Neuro Oncol. 2021;23:1872–84.
80. Adib E, et al. Phase II clinical trial of everolimus in a pan-cancer cohort of patients with mTOR pathway alterations. Clin Cancer Res. 2021;27:3845–53.
81. Wagle N, et al. Activating mTOR mutations in a patient with an extraordinary response on a phase I trial of everolimus and pazopanib. Cancer Discov. 2014;4:546–53.
82. Yao J, et al. Genomic profiling of NETs: a comprehensive analysis of the RADIANT trials. Endocr Relat Cancer. 2019;26:391–403.
83. Subbiah V, et al. Dabrafenib plus trametinib in BRAFV600E-mutated rare cancers: the phase 2 ROAR trial. Nat Med. 2023;29:1103–12.
84. Robert C, et al. Improved overall survival in melanoma with combined dabrafenib and trametinib. N Engl J Med. 2015;372:30–9.
85. Klempner SJ, et al. *BRAF* V600E mutations in high-grade colorectal neuroendocrine tumors may predict responsiveness to BRAF–MEK combination therapy. Cancer Discov. 2016;6:594–600.
86. Sakamoto T, Arai K, Makishima K, Yamasaki A. *BRAF* V600E-mutated combined large cell neuroendocrine carcinoma and adenocarcinoma responding to targeted therapy. BMJ Case Rep. 2021;14:e243295.
87. Ueberroth BE, Lieu CH, Lentz RW. Prolonged response to dabrafenib/trametinib in grade 3 metastatic pancreatic neuroendocrine tumor (NET G3) with BRAF V600E mutation. J Gastrointest Cancer. 2024;55:1448–52.
88. Saiki M, et al. The first case report of effective treatment with sotorasib for metastatic atypical lung carcinoid harboring KRAS G12C mutation and aggressive disseminated lung metastasis: a case report. JTO Clin Res Rep. 2024;5:100620.
89. Punekar SR, Velcheti V, Neel BG, Wong K-K. The current state of the art and future trends in RAS-targeted cancer therapies. Nat Rev Clin Oncol. 2022;19:637–55.
90. Robson M, et al. Olaparib for metastatic breast cancer in patients with a germline *BRCA* mutation. N Engl J Med. 2017;377:523–33.
91. González-Martín A, et al. Niraparib in patients with newly diagnosed advanced ovarian cancer. N Engl J Med. 2019;381:2391–402.
92. de Bono J, et al. Olaparib for metastatic castration-resistant prostate cancer. N Engl J Med. 2020;382:2091–102.
93. Kröcher A, et al. Successful combination of olaparib and ^{225}Ac-Dotatate in a patient with neuroendocrine tumor G3 and BRCA mutation. Case Rep Oncol. 2023;16:1166–71.
94. Samsom KG, et al. Driver mutations occur frequently in metastases of well-differentiated small intestine neuroendocrine tumours. Histopathology. 2021;78:556–66.
95. Du S, Liang Q, Shi J. Progress of ATM inhibitors: opportunities and challenges. Eur J Med Chem. 2024;277:116781.
96. Wilson Z, et al. ATR inhibitor AZD6738 (ceralasertib) exerts antitumor activity as a monotherapy and in combination with chemotherapy and the PARP inhibitor olaparib. Cancer Res. 2022;82:1140–52.
97. Subhi AL, et al. Loss of methylthioadenosine phosphorylase and elevated ornithine decarboxylase is common in pancreatic cancer. Clin Cancer Res. 2004;10:7290–6.
98. Rodon J, et al. First-in-human study of AMG 193, an MTA-cooperative PRMT5 inhibitor, in patients with MTAP-deleted solid tumors: results from phase I dose exploration. Ann Oncol. 2024;35:1138–47.
99. Engstrom LD, et al. MRTX1719 is an MTA-cooperative PRMT5 inhibitor that exhibits synthetic lethality in preclinical models and patients with MTAP-deleted cancer. Cancer Discov. 2023;13:2412–31.
100. Deschler-Baier B, et al. Rapid response to selpercatinib in RET fusion positive pancreatic neuroendocrine carcinoma confirmed by smartwatch. NPJ Precis Oncol. 2024;8:167.
101. Sigal DS, et al. Comprehensive genomic profiling identifies novel NTRK fusions in neuroendocrine tumors. Oncotarget. 2018;9:35809–12.

Part III

Emerging Technologies and Innovations

Emerging Technologies and Innovations

18

Donatella Lucchetti, Filomena Colella, Federica Toma, Beatrice Cellini, and Alessandro Sgambato

Advances in Sequencing Technologies

Recent advances in next-generation sequencing (NGS) technologies have enabled the comprehensive study of the transcriptome through RNA sequencing. RNA-seq is a bulk technique that quantifies RNA molecules and provides a global view of gene expression patterns. It is widely used due to its cost-effectiveness and efficiency in profiling gene expression across large cell populations. However, bulk RNA-seq cannot resolve differences among individual cells within complex tissues, which has motivated the development of single-cell RNA sequencing (scRNA-seq) approaches. Although scRNA-seq studies have generated detailed catalogues of tumour microenvironment (TME) cell types and states, they provide only limited insights into how these cells interact [1]. To address this, spatial transcriptomic technologies have emerged, revealing that the cells constituting the cancer ecosystem self-organise into microanatomical neighbourhoods. These methods allow the mapping of cellular interactions in situ, providing deeper insights into the frequency, nature, and functional consequences of cell–cell communication within tissues. In the following sections, we will first discuss the principles and applications of single-cell RNA sequencing approaches, and finally spatial transcriptomics and the integration of multimodal data to understand tissue organization and cellular interactions.

D. Lucchetti (✉) · A. Sgambato (✉)
Università Cattolica del Sacro Cuore, Rome, Italy

Multiplex Spatial Imaging Facility, Fondazione Policlinico Universitario A. Gemelli IRCCS, Rome, Italy
e-mail: donatella.lucchetti@unicatt.it; alessandro.sgambato@unicatt.it

F. Colella
Multiplex Spatial Imaging Facility, Fondazione Policlinico Universitario A. Gemelli IRCCS, Rome, Italy
e-mail: Filomena.colella@policlinicogemelli.it

F. Toma · B. Cellini
Università Cattolica del Sacro Cuore, Rome, Italy
e-mail: federica.toma@unicatt.it; Beatrice.cellini@unicatt.it

Single-Cell Transcriptomics Overview

scRNA-seq technology provides precise information on the unique characteristics of individual cells, including their gene expression profiles, mutations, and chromatin accessibility. In 2009, Tang et al. introduced the first scRNA-seq method, which provided markedly higher sensitivity and resolution compared to traditional microarray approaches, enabling detailed transcriptomic analysis of individual mouse blastomeres [2]. The scRNA-seq process involves isolating and profiling the RNA of intact individual cells. The most important step is sample prep-

© The Author(s), under exclusive license to Springer Nature Switzerland AG 2026

S. Sioletic, L. Coppola (eds.), *Next-Generation Sequencing in Solid Tumor Histopathology*, Current Clinical Pathology, https://doi.org/10.1007/978-3-032-18790-1_18

aration; obtaining high-quality single-cell suspensions is essential for successful analysis. Multiplex scRNA-seq protocols were first introduced in 2011, and by 2014, automated library preparation systems such as the Fluidigm C1 became available [3–5]. Currently, high-throughput platforms including BD Rhapsody and 10x Genomics Chromium allow single-cell transcriptomic analysis at large scale. In addition to analyzing RNA from intact cells, it is also possible to study single-nucleus RNA using single-nucleus RNA sequencing (snRNA-seq), which profiles RNA isolated from nuclei. These two approaches differ in the RNA content they capture: scRNA-seq primarily detects cytoplasmic mature mRNA ready for translation, whereas snRNA-seq examines nuclear RNA, including transcripts at various stages of processing. The choice between scRNA-seq and snRNA-seq depends on the research objectives as well as the characteristics and feasibility of the sample [6]. For instance, snRNA-seq is particularly useful for complex or hard-to-dissociate tissues as well as for archived frozen specimens. Studies of nuclear RNA in brain tissue have shown that this approach can effectively characterise neuronal cell types with a resolution comparable to that obtained from whole cells [7].

Current Platforms and Approaches for scRNA-Seq

A number of commercially available single-cell RNA sequencing technologies offer unique advantages in terms of throughput, cost, coverage, and sensitivity. These technologies can be classified by the method used for cell separation: (a) droplet-based, (b) microwell-based, (c) plate based, and (d) hydrogel based [1].

Droplet-Based Method

The droplet-based method relies on a droplet microfluidics system to encapsulate individual cells into oil droplets containing barcoded beads, allowing RNA to be captured from the lysed cells (Fig. 18.1a). Drop-seq and inDrops are open-source platform, while 10x Genomics Chromium is a commercial system. One of the main differences between these platforms lies in the type of barcoded beads used. Drop-seq and DroNc-seq employ solid beads, inDrop uses hydrogel beads with photo-cleavable oligonucleotides, and chromium uses gel beads with chemically releasable barcoded primers [8, 9]. This choice influences how RNA molecules are captured and subsequently amplified during library preparation, with Drop-seq, DroNc-seq, and chromium using a PCR-based template switching (TSO) approach, while inDrop employs in vitro transcription (IVT) for amplification [9].

Microwell-Based Method

Microwell-based methods rely on loading cells into nanoliter- or picoliter-scale microwell arrays containing barcoded beads, with cells and beads paired based on their similar density (Fig. 18.1b). This approach allows high-throughput single-cell capture while minimizing cross-contamination. Platforms include Seq-Well and Seq-Well S3 (PDMS arrays with poly (dT) mRNA beads trapped under a semipermeable polycarbonate membrane, 10 nm pores), Microwell-seq (agarose microarrays adjustable for various sample sizes), and BD Rhapsody (microfabricated plastic cartridge with a high-density microwell array for integrative transcriptome and proteome analyses) [10]. Seq-Well and Seq-Well S3 platforms differ in technical details: Seq-Well S3 incorporates a second-strand synthesis step after reverse transcription to introduce an additional PCR priming site [11]. Microwell-seq is highly accessible and low cost, and its first application enabled the production of a mammalian single-cell atlas [12]. BD Rhapsody performs second-strand synthesis to generate double-stranded cDNA, whereas Seq-Well and Microwell-seq use template switching during reverse transcription.

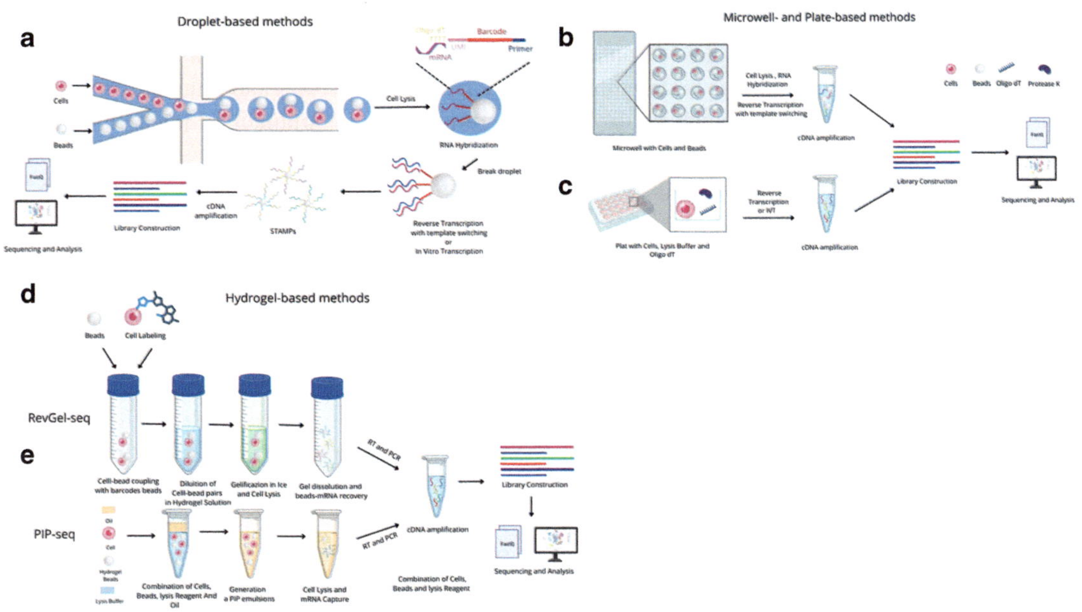

Fig. 18.1 Overview of single-cell RNA sequencing (scRNA-seq) technologies classified by cell separation method. (**a**) Droplet-based platforms (e.g. Drop-seq, inDrop, 10x Genomics Chromium) use droplet microfluidics to encapsulate individual cells with barcoded beads for RNA capture and amplification. (**b**) Microwell-based platforms (e.g. Seq-well, Seq-well S3, microwell-seq, BD rhapsody) rely on microwell arrays to co-localize cells and barcoded beads, enabling scalable capture with reduced cross-contamination. (**c**) Plate-based platforms (e.g. SMART-seq, CEL-Seq2) isolate single cells in multi-well plates, providing full-length or IVT-based transcriptome coverage depending on the amplification strategy. (**d–e**) Hydrogel-based platforms (e.g. PIP-seq, RevGel-seq) encapsulate single cells in hydrogel compartments together with barcoded beads, preserving RNA integrity and supporting efficient capture without specialized microfluidics

Plate-Based Method

Plate-based methods involve plating individual cells either into tubes or into each well of a multi-well plate (e.g. 96- or 384-well plates) (Fig. 18.1c). Common platforms include SMART-seq and CEL-Seq2, which differ in their amplification strategies. In the SMART-seq method, single cells are manually isolated in lysis buffer, and their polyadenylated RNA is reverse-transcribed into full-length cDNA using oligo (dT) primers in combination with SMART (Switching Mechanism at the 5′ End of the RNA Template) technology, enabling PCR amplification of full-length transcripts [13]. In contrast, CEL-Seq2 employs linear amplification via in vitro transcription (IVT), producing amplified RNA (cRNA) before converting it back to cDNA for sequencing [14].

Hydrogel-Based Method

Particle-templated instant partition sequencing (PIP-seq) and Reversible Hydrogel sequencing (RevGel-seq) are innovative microfluidics-free methods for single-cell RNA sequencing (scRNA-seq) sample preparation (Fig. 18.1d–e). In PIP-seq, cells, barcoded hydrogel templates, and lysis reagents are combined with oil and vortexed to generate monodisperse droplets. This simple, rapid, and scalable workflow can be performed in any laboratory equipped with standard molecular biology instruments [15]. RevGel-seq processes fresh samples without the need for freezing, fixation, or mechanical stress. First, cell-barcoding bead complexes are prepared using a bifunctional chemical linker and then diluted in a hydrogel solution that gels on ice. Cells are lysed within the gel, and the released mRNA is recovered for library preparation. This method has been successfully applied to pancreatic islet cells, peripheral blood mononuclear cells (PBMCs), and large cells such as cardiomyocytes, demonstrating its utility in clinical and translational research [16]. These hydrogel-based approaches maintain single-cell integrity by encapsulating individual cells within discrete hydrogel compartments, where each cell interacts with uniquely barcoded beads. This minimizes cross-contamination, protects RNA during handling, and allows high-efficiency capture and amplification for downstream sequencing.

Application of scRNA-Seq in Complex Disease

Single-cell RNA sequencing (scRNA-seq) is a powerful and versatile technology with broad applications across biomedical research, including developmental biology, disease pathogenesis, and stem cell studies. One key application is the dissection of the cellular composition of complex tissues, such as tumours, allowing researchers to assess how distinct cell populations respond to pharmacological treatments [17]. This approach has also been successfully applied to characterize the cellular and molecular mechanisms underlying cancer [18, 19]. In the context of autoimmune diseases, such as systemic lupus erythematosus (SLE) and rheumatoid arthritis, scRNA-seq has been instrumental in identifying cell-type-specific transcriptomic signatures, mapping the cellular landscape, and annotating disease-associated genetic variants [20, 21]. It is particularly valuable for studying the diversity, function, and interactions of immune cells within complex tissues, providing critical insights into the formation and origin of tertiary lymphoid structures (TLS) and enabling the identification of novel immune cell subsets. A major application in immunology is the analysis of T-cell and B-cell receptors (TCR-seq and BCR-seq), which is essential for understanding immune responses to infections [22, 23]. scRNA-seq is also widely used to investigate the etiopathogenesis of neurological and neurodegenerative diseases, including multiple sclerosis, Alzheimer's disease, Parkinson's disease, and various neuroinfections, by elucidating the roles and interactions of different immune cell populations [24]. In developmental biology, scRNA-seq enables detailed investigation of human embryogenesis, from the zygote stage through gastrulation. These studies not only enhance our understanding of early human development but also provide critical insights into the causes of infertility, early miscarriages, and congenital disorders [25].

Spatial Transcriptomics Overview

Life is intrinsically linked to its spatial organization at the molecular, cellular, and tissue levels. In health, tissues maintain stability through the coordinated efforts of various cells, each playing specific roles. However, disease disrupts this harmony across different cell types, leading to changes in tissue composition, structure, and organization. Understanding how the arrangement of cells and molecules at various scales relates to their overall function is fundamental to both tissue biology and pathology. Histological patterns reflect the collaborative functionality of cells and molecules, making the study of structure-function relationships crucial in this field. Understanding this organization is crucial for deciphering complex biological processes, from cellular differentiation to disease pathogenesis [26, 27]. Although single-cell sequencing techniques (scRNA-seq) have revolutionized the identification of cell subpopulations, including rare cell type, they require dissociation of tissues, resulting in the loss of fundamental spatial context and may introduce technical artifacts [28–30]. To overcome this limitation, early strategies attempted to infer spatial information indirectly. Techniques such as tomo-seq [31–33] used transcriptomic data from serial tissue sections to reconstruct spatial axes, while methods like microdissection [34, 35] and the Nanostring GeoMX DSP platform enabled region-specific transcript profiling [36–38]. Other creative approaches, including ProximID [39], PIC-seq [40, 41], and ClumpSeq [42], relied on partial dissociation to preserve physical proximity between cells or on computational inference of spatial position using gene expression signatures from scRNA-seq data. Despite these efforts, the field lacked a comprehensive method for capturing gene expression directly in intact tissues while preserving spatial architecture. The concept of ST was introduced by Ståhl et al. in 2016 [43], quickly gained recognition, so much so that it was named "Method of the Year 2020" by Nature Methods [44]. Although the term "spatial transcriptomics" only gained widespread attention in recent years, the conceptual foundation dates back several decades. As early as the 1970s, techniques such as radioactive in situ hybridization (ISH) and laser capture microdissection (LCM) were developed to explore spatial patterns of gene expression [45, 46]. These approaches reflect two distinct strategies for acquiring spatial information: either by detecting RNA molecules directly in their native tissue context and aligning them with histological features or by isolating specific regions of interest (ROIs) based on spatial location for downstream transcriptomic analysis.

Current Platforms and Approaches in Spatial Transcriptomics

Spatial transcriptomics technologies can be classified into main categories based on methodology, each defined by how spatial information is captured and how gene expression is measured in: (I) Sequencing-based methods, also known as ex situ methods, involve capturing RNA transcripts from spatially defined regions of a tissue section, tagging them with spatial barcodes, and then sequencing them externally using NGS technologies; (II) imaging-based or in situ techniques directly visualize RNA molecules within the intact tissue through repeated cycles of hybridization and fluorescence microscopy, enabling high-resolution maps of gene expression at the single-cell or even subcellular level; (III) probe-based methods use barcoded gene-specific probes to target and quantify known transcripts, combining spatial resolution with high sensitivity and compatibility with archived material; and (IV) image-guided spatially resolved single-cell RNA sequencing methods leverage microscopy to identify and isolate specific cells or regions of interest, which are then subjected to single-cell sequencing, allowing detailed molecular profiling linked directly to spatial localization within the tissue [1, 47]. Methods classification is summarized in Fig. 18.2.

Sequencing-Based Methods

Sequencing-based spatial transcriptomics methods utilize surfaces such as microarrays or bead arrays coated with spatially barcoded oligonucleotides to capture RNA from tissue sections. Released RNA binds to these oligonucleotides, is reverse transcribed, and is sequenced, enabling the mapping of each transcript to its original spatial location. These techniques are broadly categorized into array-based capture and bead-based capture methods, differing mainly in the capture substrate and spatial resolution achieved.

Array-Based Capture

Platforms in array-based capture include 10X Genomics Visium, HDST, Pixel-seq, Seq-Scope, and Stereo-seq, each with unique features in terms of spatial resolution, transcript capture efficiency, and field of view.

10X Genomics Visium

Among array-based spatial transcriptomics platforms, 10X Genomics Visium is a widely used technology that allows the acquisition of whole transcriptomes directly from tissue sections. By permeabilizing the tissue, polyadenylated RNAs are released and hybridize to spatially encoded oligonucleotides arranged on a microarray slide. These captured RNAs are then reverse transcribed and sequenced, with each sequencing read assigned to its spatial coordinates via the unique spatial barcodes. Early versions of Visium used a hexagonal array with ~5000 spots per capture area, each 55 μm in diameter and 100 μm apart, providing multicellular resolution, typically capturing transcriptomes from clusters of

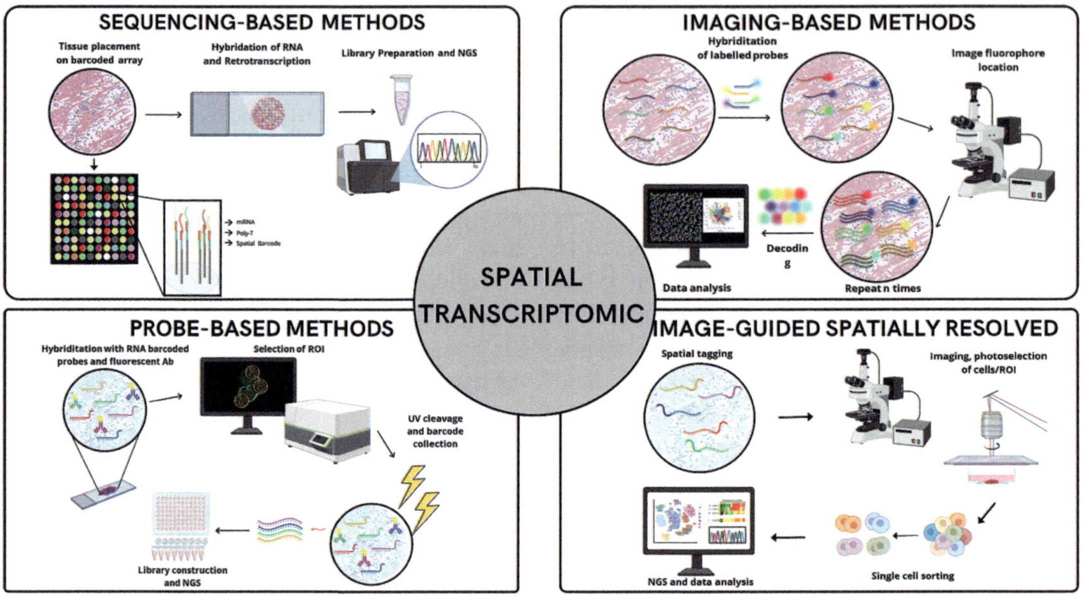

Fig. 18.2 Classification of spatial transcriptomics technologies based on methodological approach. (1) Sequencing-based (ex situ) methods capture RNA transcripts from spatially defined tissue regions, tag them with spatial barcodes, and sequence them using NGS. (2) Imaging-based (in situ) methods directly visualize RNA molecules within intact tissue by iterative hybridization and fluorescence microscopy, enabling high-resolution gene expression maps at single-cell or subcellular level. (3) Probe-based methods employ barcoded gene-specific probes to detect and quantify predefined transcripts with high sensitivity, including in archived material. (4) Image-guided spatially resolved scRNA-seq methods integrate microscopy with single-cell sequencing by isolating specific cells or regions of interest, linking spatial context to detailed molecular profiles

1–10 cells per spot. The latest version, Visium HD, further improves spatial resolution by employing a continuous array of 2 × 2 μm barcoded capture areas with no gaps, enabling near single-cell resolution within intact tissue sections. A technical limitation of the standard workflow is the need for precise alignment of the tissue section onto the small 6.5 mm × 6.5 mm capture area. To overcome this problem, 10X Genomics has introduced the Visium CytAssist instrument, which simplifies sample handling by enabling the transfer from standard glass slides to Visium arrays. Despite its strengths, the spatial resolution, even in HD mode, is not fully subcellular. Furthermore, because the platform relies on poly (A) based RNAs capture, it does not detect cleavage variants or non-polyadenylated transcripts without specialized protocols. Visium has been successfully applied in many fields, such as immune-oncology [48–51] and neuroscience [52]. Overall, 10X Genomics Visium represents a robust and scalable platform for spatial transcriptomics. As such, Visium works as a powerful discovery tool that has already contributed significantly to the understanding of tissue architecture, cellular heterogeneity, and disease-related gene expression in situ.

HDST (High-Definition Spatial Transcriptomics)

Another prominent array-based platform is HDST (high-definition spatial transcriptomics), an advanced method that enables high-resolution mapping of gene expression within tissue sections. HDST uses a dense array of barcoded microspheres placed in 2 μm wells on a slide, with positions precisely decoded by sequential hybridization. Upon tissue permeabilization, released RNAs bind to the bead-bound oligonucleotides and are subsequently sequenced. This strategy achieves near-subcellular spatial resolution, capturing hundreds of thousands of barcodes across large tissue areas. Although each spot detects relatively few transcripts, HDST provides highly specific spatial expression patterns and can be integrated with single-cell RNA-seq data to assign cell types and correlate them with histological features. The method has been successfully applied to both healthy and diseased tissues, including mouse brain and human breast cancer, offering unprecedented insights into cellular organization and molecular signatures [53].

Pixel-Seq

Pixel-seq is an advanced spatial transcriptomics method based on a modified polony approach, in which cross-linked polyacrylamide gels are used to generate amplifiable, barcoded DNA clusters (polonies) with submicron resolution. A polony ("polymerase colony") is a localized cluster of DNA copies generated from a single DNA molecule through in situ amplification on a solid support, allowing the maintenance of the spatial position of each molecule. While similar approaches using polonies or DNA clusters have previously been applied, Pixel-seq introduces a novel gel-to-gel stamping system that enables efficient, enzymatic replication of DNA barcodes without requiring sequencing of each array [54]. This drastically reduces the cost and time of array production. The technique was applied to the mouse parabrachial nucleus (PBN), a brain region involved in pain processing, to generate a single-cell atlas and uncover gene expression changes associated with chronic pain. The high resolution and RNA capture efficiency of Pixel-seq enabled spatially precise analysis of neuron and glial cell types, revealing heterogeneous responses to neuropathic pain and advancing the understanding of pain-related neural circuitry [55].

Seq-Scope

Among array-based spatial transcriptomics platforms, Seq-Scope is a technology that achieves submicrometric resolution (0.5–0.8 μm), comparable to light microscopy. It uses a two-step sequencing process: the first sequencing cycle (first-Seq) creates a high-density array of spatially barcoded RNA capture oligonucleotides on a solid surface, decoding their precise positions. The second sequencing cycle (second-Seq) captures mRNA released from tissue sections placed on this array, linking the transcript sequences to their spatial barcodes. This method makes it possible to generate detailed spatial gene expression maps with a resolution close to that of a single cell or sub-cell. Seq-Scope offers high transcriptome capture efficiency, with up to ~4700 unique molecular identifiers per cell, comparable to conventional single-cell RNA sequencing. It can distinguish cellular compartments by detecting mitochondrial transcriptomes and intronic RNA, revealing unsplit nuclear transcriptomes. The ability to visualize microscopic cellular and subcellular structures has been demonstrated in tissues such as the liver and colon, making Seq-Scope a powerful tool for high-resolution spatial transcriptomic studies that bridge the gap between histology and genomics [56, 57].

Stereo-Seq

Spatially enhanced resolution omics-sequencing is a spatial transcriptomics technology developed by BGI Genomics within the STOmics platform. It combines nanometric resolution (up to 220 nm) with a field of view (up to 13.2 × 13.2). The technology is based on the use of chips with DNA nanoballs (DNBs) containing spatial barcodes (Coordinate IDs, CIDs), arranged on high-density lithographic patterned arrays. After an initial sequencing step to map the CIDs, oligonucleotides with UMI and polyT tails are ligated to the DNBs to capture tissue RNA (frozen or FFPE). The RNA is then retro-transcribed and amplified for sequencing on the DNBSEQ platform. Notably, Stereo-seq also integrates fluorescence imaging to detect nuclear positions, allowing algorithms to reconstruct spatial gene expression maps at an approximate single-cell resolution. Successfully applied to tissues such as the murine embryo [58] and *Arabidopsis thaliana* [59], Stereo-seq enables detailed spatial maps of gene expression, facilitating the study of cellular organization and interactions with the microenvironment.

Bead-Based Capture

Bead-based capture methods represent a class of spatial transcriptomics techniques in which RNA molecules from tissue sections are captured on beads or microspheres preloaded with spatially encoded barcodes. Each bead acts as a spatially defined capture site, preserving the positional information of the transcripts. This strategy enables high-resolution mapping of gene expression while being compatible with larger tissue areas and flexible sample handling. Compared to array-based methods, bead-based approaches often allow better adaptation to irregular tissue surfaces and offer scalable capture densities, although trade-offs in sensitivity and complexity may exist depending on the platform. Key examples of bead-based capture technologies include Slide-seq/Slide-seqV2, Light-seq, and Slide-tags, each providing unique advantages in resolution, throughput, and multimodal integration.

Slide-Seq/Slide-SeqV2

These spatial transcriptomics technologies are based on NSG that enable genome-wide transcriptome profiling with high spatial resolution using region-specific RNA capture strategies. Slide-seq [60] and its improved version Slide-seqV2 [61, 62] use arrays composed of DNA-barcoded polystyrene microsphere (10 μm diameter) assembled in a monolayer on a rubber-coated coverslip. Each bead has a unique barcode sequence encoding its spatial position, and the barcode array is indexed in advance using sequencing by ligation (SOLiD or, in V2, a single-base coding strategy). Fresh and frozen tissue sections are cryosectioned directly onto the disc and the mRNA released from the tissue hybridizes with the barcoded oligonucleotides on the surface of the microsphere. After reverse transcription and amplification of the cDNA, the spatial origin of each transcript is deduced from the microsphere barcode during sequencing. Slide-seqV2 significantly improved capture sensitivity approximately tenfold through optimization of microsphere synthesis, array indexing and cDNA processing, enabling better detection of low-abundance transcripts and allowing analysis of spatially localized gene expression and developmental processes. Although these methods are cost-effective and compatible with standard laboratory equipment, they require precise array indexing and have lower sensitivity than other approaches.

Light-Seq

This technique enables light-directed barcoding of selected regions of interest (ROIs) in fixed tissue samples without damaging them. It uses barcode DNA strands containing a fast-reacting photoreactive nucleoside (CNVK), which forms covalent cross-links upon brief UV illumination. A digital micromirror device (DMD) integrated with a standard microscope precisely targets the UV light, achieving spatial resolution below 2 μm. After photolinking, a cross-junction synthesis reaction transfers both the cDNA and barcode sequences onto a new single DNA strand, compatible with standard NGS pipelines. Light-Seq has been applied, to mouse retina sections to identify transcripts from rare cell types such as dopaminergic amacrine cells, using as few as four to eight cells per section. Compared to other spatial methods, Light-Seq is low cost, and it preserves tissue morphology, requires no dissociation, and is compatible with widely available lab equipment. It also decouples imaging from sequencing, allowing flexible ROI selection. However, it currently supports fewer multiplexed regions than some other platforms, and its sensitivity could be further enhanced with protocol optimization. Still, Light-Seq's modular, scalable, and nondestructive workflow makes it a powerful tool for spatial transcriptomics, especially for studies requiring high specificity, rare cell analysis, and post-sequencing sample reuse [63].

Slide-Tags

This method captures high-resolution spatial information by tagging nuclei in situ within fresh frozen tissue sections. This is achieved by photocleaving and diffusing DNA-barcoded oligonucleotides from arrays of beads with known spatial coordinates into the tissue, where they bind nuclei at their original locations. Each nucleus thus acquires a unique spatial barcode before dissociation. After tagging, nuclei are isolated and processed using standard single-nucleus workflows such as snRNA-seq, snATAC-seq, TCR-seq, and copy-number variation (CNV) inference, preserving spatial context via the barcode. Slide-tags has been applied successfully across various tissues, including adult and embryonic mouse brain, human cortex, tonsil, and melanoma, allowing simultaneous multimodal profiling with spatial resolution of approximately 3 μm. Compared to other spatial transcriptomics methods, slide-tags offers the unique ability to integrate multimodal data (transcriptome, epigenome, immune repertoire) at true single-nucleus resolution without requiring pixel deconvolution. Limitations include the loss of nuclei during dissociation and barcoding (~75%) and current restriction to nuclei rather than whole cells, which limits applications like mitochondrial lineage tracing [64].

Imaging-Based Methods

Imaging-based spatial transcriptomics methods enable the direct visualization of RNA molecules within intact tissues, preserving spatial context. These approaches can be broadly divided into two main categories: (I) probe-based methods, which use nucleic acid probes to detect known transcripts, and (II) in situ sequencing (ISS) methods, which perform sequencing directly in tissue sections.

Probe-Based Methods

Probe-based methods are a class of techniques that use short synthetic nucleic acid sequences to detect specific DNA or RNA targets within cells or tissues. These probes are designed to be complementary to a particular sequence of interest and are typically labeled with fluorescent dyes, allowing them to be visualized by fluorescence microscopy. This fundamental approach provides the basis for several strong techniques, including FISH (Fluorescence In Situ Hybridization) which has evolved over time, providing different levels of resolution, scalability, and multiplexing capabilities [65].

smFISH/smiFISH/HT-smFISH

The concept of FISH was first introduced in 1969 by Gall and Pardue [66], who demonstrated that labeled nucleic acid probes could hybridize with specific sequences within fixed cells, preserving the spatial context and laying the foundation for in situ hybridization (ISH). Over the following decades, FISH evolved significantly, becoming a key method for visualizing gene expression and chromosomal organization. However, a major milestone in the field came in 1998, when Femino et al. reported the detection of single RNA molecules using fluorescent ISH, now known as single-molecule FISH (smFISH) [67]. SmFISH is a technique that relies on the hybridization of multiple fluorescent oligonucleotide probes to a single RNA target. By using sets of 10 to 50 probes for each transcript, an intense and highly specific signal is obtained with a low noise floor. This allows individual RNA molecules to be visualized as bright, diffraction-limited dots under a fluorescence microscope. However, a significant limitation of classical smFISH lies in its high cost, since each individual probe must be chemically labeled with a fluorophore. This becomes particularly challenging in large-scale experiments or when a higher number of probes are required to enhance signal-to-noise ratio and detection accuracy. To overcome this limitation, a cheaper and more efficient variant was developpment, single-molecule inexpensive FISH (smiFISH) [68]. In this version, the primary probes are not fluorescent but have an additional sequence called a readout, to which a labeled secondary probe is bound. This approach offers greater flexibility and reduces probe synthesis costs. However, when the complexity of experiments increases, a further technological breakthrough becomes necessary: This is where high-throughput smFISH (HT-smFISH) arises [69]. This technique automates sample preparation, hybridization and image acquisition, making systematic, high-throughput, high-precision analysis possible. HT-smFISH is therefore ideal for spatial transcriptomic studies where simultaneous mapping of the expression and localization of large numbers of RNAs at the single-cell level is required.

However, unlike sequential barcoded FISH methods, HT-smFISH multiplexing is limited by the number of spectrally distinct dyes. Furthermore, it requires stringent RNase-free conditions and careful quality control during probe preparation. Despite these limitations, HT-smFISH offers a practical and accessible approach for large-scale spatial transcriptomics in diverse cell types and tissues, making it particularly suitable for medium-throughput functional genomics studies. FISH is commonly applied in rapid prenatal screening for chromosomal abnormalities and in cancer diagnostics to detect chromosomal changes critical for tumour classification and treatment monitoring [70, 71].

MERFISH (Multiplexed Error-Robust FISH)
Merfish is a technique originally developed by Chen et al. [72] that uses combinatorial labeling and error-proof barcoding schemes to detect hundreds or thousands of RNA species in situ. Each RNA species is assigned a binary barcode, where fluorescence signals [1] or their absence (0) in multiple hybridization-imaging cycles are decoded to identify specific RNA types. Error correction is achieved by designing barcodes with large hamming distances, significantly reducing misidentification caused by imaging or hybridization errors. The technique is based on coding probes, which hybridize with target RNAs and carry sequence domains for fluorescent reading probes and is typically performed in a flow chamber through sequential cycles of hybridization, imaging, and dye removal. Recent integration with expansion microscopy (ExM) has further improved the spatial resolution and coverage of the transcriptome, enabling the profiling of over 10,000 genes in a single experiment [73]. Furthermore, MERFISH enables co-localization studies by labeling subcellular structures such as the nucleus or endoplasmic reticulum, improving spatial context in transcriptomic analysis.

seqFISH/seqFISH+
This technique was first introduced by Lubeck et al. in 2014 as an evolution of smFISH to overcome the limitations of multiplexing due to the small number of fluorophores available [74]. By applying sequential cycles of hybridization and imaging, it was possible to assign each RNA molecule a unique time barcode, allowing the detection of many RNA species in the same sample. This method was further improved by Shah et al. in 2016 [75], who demonstrated its applicability in complex tissues like the mouse hippocampus and introduced signal amplification to increase detection sensitivity. To address challenges such as optical crowding and limited resolution, Eng et al. developed seqFISH+ in 2019 [76]. This improved version expanded the color palette using 60 pseudocolors, drastically increasing the multiplexing capacity to allow the detection of up to 10,000 genes per cell. While the original seqFISH focused on targeted detection based on known gene sets, seqFISH+ supports genome-wide, discovery-based approaches, making it a more powerful tool for spatial transcriptomics in diverse biological systems.

RNAscope
RNAscope employs pairs of "double Z" probes, each containing a target-complementary region, spacer, and amplifier tail. The signal is only generated if both Z-probes hybridize correctly and near the target, triggering a highly specific amplification cascade. This approach enables the detection of single RNA molecules even in degraded FFPE samples, thanks to the use of multiple probes per target and efficient sequential amplification that can achieve up to 8000-fold signal amplification. RNAscope is compatible with both fluorescence and bright-field microscopes and can be used for multiplex analysis, making it a powerful tool for studying gene expression in situ and for the clinical application of RNA biomarkers [77, 78].

HCR/V3HCR/CycleHCR
Hybridization chain reaction (HCR) is an enzyme-free, isothermal amplification method based on metastable DNA hairpins polymerizing upon target recognition. In HCR, the presence of a short single-stranded DNA initiator triggers a chain reaction between two metastable DNA hairpins (H1 and H2), which polymerize into long chains of nicked double-stranded DNA,

amplifying the signal locally without enzymatic steps. The third-generation HCR (V3HCR) [79], introduced in 2018, was specifically optimized for mRNA detection in frozen mouse and human tissue sections, and it was designed to validate scRNA-seq data while maintaining spatial information. Due to its small probe size, it offers efficient tissue penetration, increased sensitivity for low-abundance targets, and good background suppression, as hairpin polymerization occurs only at the moment of target recognition, minimizing nonspecific signal. Building on this foundation, cycleHCR [80], introduced in 2025, represents an evolution of the method, combining separate probe coding with loop iterative HCR amplification to significantly expand multiplexing capabilities. Using unique combinations of left and right barcode sequences to define each target, this new technique enables the simultaneous detection of thousands of RNA and protein species within the same tissue sample, without the need to strip or re-hybridize primary probes.

In Situ Sequencing (ISS) Methods

In situ sequencing methods enable direct sequencing of RNA molecules within intact tissues or single cells, preserving spatial organization. Unlike traditional sequencing methods, which require tissue dissociation and RNA extraction, ISS preserves spatial context by performing molecular reactions directly in the native tissue architecture. The basic principle involves converting RNA into complementary DNA (cDNA) followed by targeted or untargeted sequencing reactions in situ.

FISSEQ/ExSEQ

FISSEQ is a pioneering technology in spatial transcriptomics that enables transcriptome-wide RNA sequencing directly within fixed cells or tissue sections, preserving the spatial context of gene expression. Developed by Lee et al. in 2014 [81] was the first nontargeted method to perform high-throughput in situ RNA sequencing, offering insights not only into RNA abundance but also into sequence-level features such as splicing events and posttranscriptional modifications. The process begins with in situ reverse transcription (RT) of cellular RNA into cDNA using aminoallyl-dUTPs, which allow subsequent chemical cross-linking of the cDNA to cellular structures, preventing it from spreading. The cDNA is circularized by CircLigase and amplified by rolling circle amplification (RCA), generating dense, localized amplicons. Sequencing is then performed using SOLiD chemistry, in which four fluorescently labeled probes are bound to the amplified DNA, visualized and iteratively cleaved in multiple cycles. This approach offers high spatial resolution and allows quantitative and qualitative analysis of RNA within intact cells. However, challenges such as optical crowding and probe design complexity remain; for this reason in 2021, ExSEQ was introduced as an innovative solution [82]. By integrating Expansion Microscopy (ExM) with FISSEQ, it addresses these limitations through physical tissue expansion, which isotropically separates densely packed RNA amplicons and improves molecular accessibility. This spatial decrowding not only enhances the resolution of RNA signals, bringing them into the nanoscale range, but also facilitates more accurate tracking of individual amplicons across multiple sequencing cycles.

Xenium (10x Genomics)

Xenium launched by 10x Genomics in 2022 [83] and developed from CARTANA technology [84] is a commercial platform for high-resolution spatial transcriptomics that combines the principles of ISH and ISS [85]. It uses a highly sensitive and specific chemistry combining hybridization and in situ sequencing, based on the use of padlock probes and RCA.

The process involves the simultaneous hybridization of two arms of the padlock probe to the target RNA, followed by highly selective ligation that occurs only in the presence of perfect pairing. The circularized probes are then locally amplified by RCA, producing intense and localized signals. After amplification, detection occurs through iterative cycles of hybridization with fluorescent probes and imaging, generating a unique optical signature for each gene. This approach makes it possible to distinguish similar transcripts, detect degraded RNAs, and obtain spatial data with subcellular resolution. The analysis is completed directly on the instrument, with artificial intelligence-assisted cell segmentation, and the resulting data can be visualized via Xenium Explorer or integrated into other software. With this combination of sensitivity, precision, and flexibility in gene panels (up to 5000 targets), Xenium represents one of the most advanced solutions for the spatial study of gene expression.

CosMx SMI (NanoString)
CosMx was introduced in 2022 by NanoString and represents a significant advancement in transcriptomics and spatial proteomics, as it enables the detection of 1000 RNA targets with resolution, and, from 2025, a panel of genes covering the entire human transcriptome (<18,000 genes) was introduced, with a spatial resolution of 50 nm [86]. After permeabilization of the tissue, a pool of five gene-specific probes is added, each binding to different regions of the target transcript. Every probe has a target-binding domain of 30–50 nucleotides long, unique for each probe in the set, and a readout domain of approximately 100 nucleotides, identical within the same set of probes. The CosMx platform is characterized by high throughput (up to four slides and one million cells per run), high flexibility (supports different sample types and areas up to 375 mm^2), and good robustness even with degraded RNA (e.g. DV200 < 30%). One of the major limitations of the technology is the very long execution time of 6–12 days per experiment, in addition to which there is an increased computational load for data analysis and the need for more storage space and the handling of high-resolution images. Nevertheless, CosMx represents a powerful tool for high-plex spatial analysis in both research and clinical pathology, especially when a profile of the entire transcriptome is not required, but high sensitivity and spatial precision are essential.

STARmap (Spatially Resolved Transcript Amplicon Readout Mapping)
This technique provides 3D mapping, at single cell resolution, of gene expression. The central innovation of STARmap resides in the use of hydrogel-tissue chemistry (HTC), a concept originally pioneered by the CLARITY method [87]. CLARITY introduced the idea of embedding biological tissues within a polymer matrix to preserve spatial architecture while enabling molecular targeting. STARmap builds on this idea by anchoring cDNA amplicons, generated from intracellular mRNA through enzymatic amplification of adjacent primer-probe pairs, directly into a hydrogel scaffold. This hydrogel network, formed through copolymerization with modified acrylamide monomers, stabilizes the spatial position of transcripts, improves optical transparency, and facilitates high-resolution volumetric imaging. Another key innovation of STARmap is the SEDAL (Sequencing with Error-reduction by Dynamic Annealing and Ligation) sequencing method, which employs short, transiently binding probes for sequencing by ligation. This technique ensures high accuracy through two-base coding and error-rejection mechanisms, preserving tissue integrity during imaging. STARmap enables the simultaneous detection of over 1000 genes in 3D space through 6 imaging cycles [88].

Probe-Based Methods
Probe-based spatial transcriptomics is a targeted approach for measuring gene expression that uses synthetic oligonucleotide probes to hybridize with specific RNA sequences within conserved tissue sections. Unlike imaging-based methods such as MERFISH or seqFISH, which rely on repeated cycles of fluorescence imaging to detect individual transcripts with subcellular resolution, probe-based platforms do not directly visualize RNA molecules. Instead, it uses barcoded probes that bind to predefined RNA targets, allowing subsequent quantification by digital counting technologies, such as the NanoString nCounter. While this strategy does not achieve single-molecule or single-cell resolution, it offers several advantages: high multiplexing capacity, compatibility with formalin-fixed paraffin-embedded (FFPE) tissues, and scalability to larger cohorts. Consequently, spatial probe-based methods are particularly suitable for studies requiring robust transcript detection

across multiple samples or patient populations, even when tissue quality is suboptimal.

GeoMx DSP (Digital Spatial Profiling)
GeoMx is a platform developed by NanoString [89], designed for multiplexed profiling of RNA (and proteins) in spatially defined regions of interest (ROIs). The system utilizes in situ hybridization probes composed of target-complementary sequences linked to indexing oligonucleotides via UV-cleavable linkers. After probe hybridization and washing, ROIs are selected according to morphological markers (e.g. CD45 for immune regions or panCK for tumour segmentation) and they can be further segmented into compartments (e.g. tumour or stroma) to allow for refined spatial resolution. Once defined, ROIs, referred to as areas of illumination (AOIs), are selectively exposed to UV light to release the indexing barcodes. The cleaved oligos are collected by microcapillary aspiration and transferred onto a microplate. These barcodes are then hybridized with fluorescent optical barcodes (GeoMx Hyb codes) and digitally counted with the NanoString nCounter system or analysed by next-generation sequencing (NGS), depending on the assay configuration. This approach enables the profiling of over 18,000 human transcripts in fresh FFPE or frozen tissue sections. The main strengths of GeoMx are its compatibility with degraded samples, its high multiplexing capacity, and its ability to integrate RNA and protein measurements in the same ROI. However, its spatial resolution is limited to groups of ~20–300 cells per ROI, without precision at the single cell or subcellular level. Furthermore, throughput and ROI selection are limited by the manual nature of ROI definition and the need for specialized instrumentation. Despite these limitations, GeoMx is widely adopted in exploratory research, particularly for the study of tumour microenvironments and FFPE archive samples, where whole transcriptome breadth and spatial context are more critical than cellular resolution [90].

Future Directions of Spatial Transcriptomics
The field has been notably accelerated by next-generation sequencing (NGS), enabling high-throughput transcriptome profiling and the extension of traditional 2D approaches into 3D tissue reconstructions through tomography-based methods. This evolution has significantly enhanced the spatial resolution and scale of analysis, from entire organ sections down to sub-millimetre regions, while preserving spatial fidelity. Despite these advances, technological trade-offs persist: A common limitation is the balance between the number of genes profiled and the capture efficiency, i.e. the proportion of transcripts successfully detected, which can range from near-complete to as low as 1% (Fig. 18.3). Moving forward, future developments in spatial transcriptomics are expected to focus on improving sensitivity, resolution, and throughput, as well as integrating multimodal measurements such as protein expression and epigenetic profiling, to provide a more comprehensive understanding of tissue architecture and cellular interactions.

Data Analysis and Integration

The advent of high-throughput technologies has fundamentally altered the landscape of translational medicine projects. This shift has increasingly focused on collecting multi-omics patient samples and, consequently, necessitates their integrated analysis [91, 92]. These advanced technologies have given rise to various "omics" fields, each studying different molecular and biological levels, including genomics, transcriptomics, proteomics, metabolomics, metagenomics, epigenomics, and epitranscriptomics, among others [92, 93]. Multi-omics integration enables a range of applications in biomedical research and clinical practice. It supports subtype identification by uncovering molecular-level similarities that go beyond traditional classifications based on histopathology or clinical symptoms, allowing the discovery of disease subtypes with different progression patterns or treatment responses. It also facilitates the

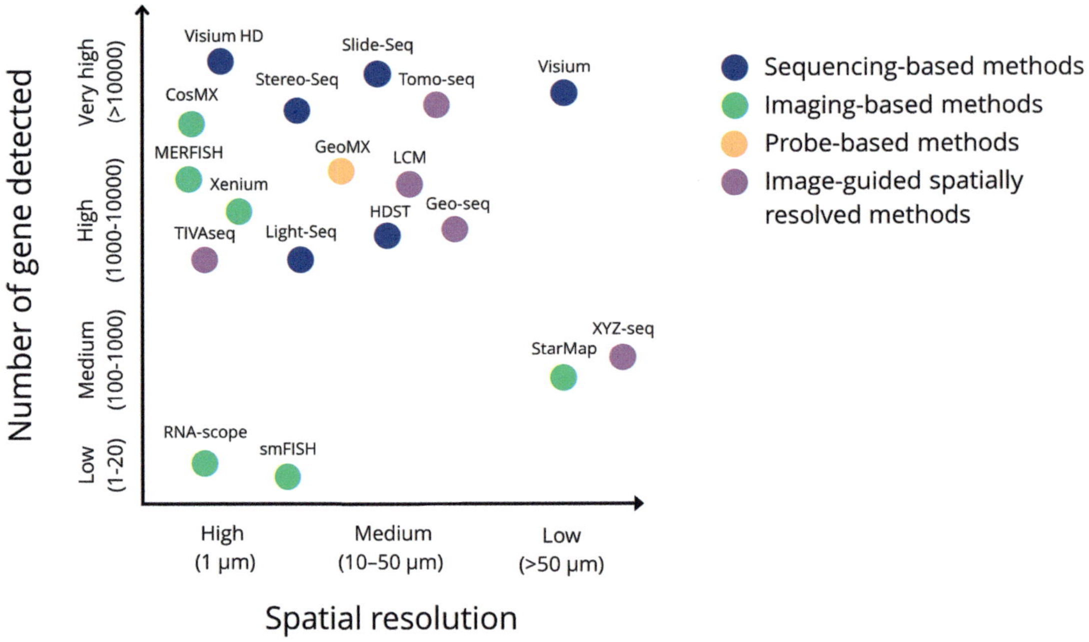

Fig. 18.3 Comparison of spatial transcriptomics (ST) methodologies in terms of resolution and transcript detection

detection of disease-associated molecular patterns, linking molecular markers with clinical traits and revealing networks or modules that serve as disease indicators. In diagnosis and prognosis, integrated molecular signatures help predict disease onset, severity, and progression, especially in complex, multifactorial diseases, improving diagnostic precision where traditional approaches fall short. For drug response prediction, multi-omics data increase the resolution of analysis, helping to explain variability in drug efficacy among patients by identifying molecular features tied to treatment outcomes. Finally, it aids in understanding regulatory processes, enabling the reconstruction of gene regulatory networks specific to diseases by combining data on gene expression and upstream molecular regulators [91].

Type of Integration

Scientific literature has identified three main categories of multi-omics data integration approaches: early, late, and intermediate integration. These distinctions are primarily based on when the combination of different datasets occurs.

Early Integration

In early integration, the different omics datasets are combined into one table or graph-based representation, which is then used as input to a machine learning (ML) model [94]. This approach refers to the concatenation of measurements obtained with different omics from the beginning, before any classification or regression analysis.

A significant advantage of early integration is the ability to observe joint effects between the different omics. However, this approach tends to disregard heterogeneity between platforms. The concatenation of data also produces very large data matrices, which generally require dimensionality reduction strategies for their analysis. While there are examples of early integration for all kinds of purposes, it has been identified that the only goal of multi-omic integration that strictly demands early integration is that of discovering multi-omic molecular mechanisms [91, 93]. Figure 18.4 provides a visual representation.

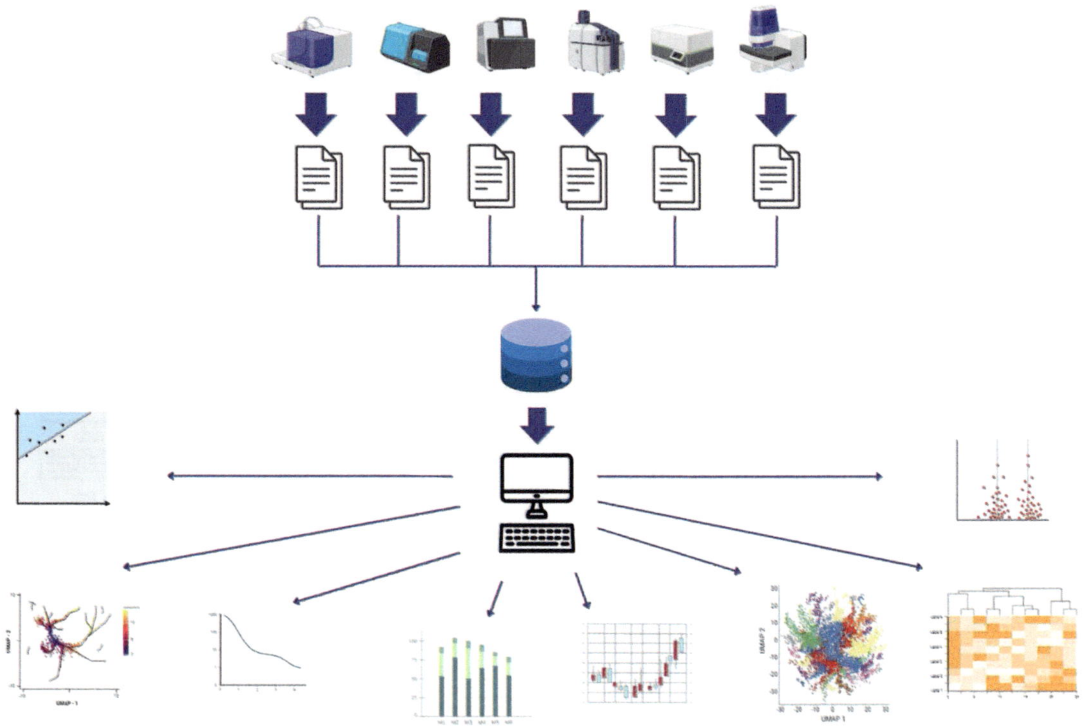

Fig. 18.4 Early integration of multi-omics data

Late Integration
Conversely, in late integration, models are applied to each omics dataset independently. Subsequently, a second model combines their predictions. This approach combines multiple predictive models, obtained separately for each omics.

Historically, late integration was the first type of multi-omics integration to emerge, and, despite providing extremely useful results, it has been progressively abandoned for other approaches. Late integration tools take independent results and do not consider relationships between omics, ignoring interactions between levels and the possibility of synergy or antagonism. Despite this, it can still satisfy classification or functional enrichment goals [91, 93, 95]. A visual representation is shown in Fig. 18.5.

Intermediate Integration
A less discussed approach is intermediate integration. In this case, a single set of data is modelled after transforming the omics through separate analysis. This approach respects the diversity of platforms but does not necessarily capture interactions between functional levels [93, 94].

Methods of Integration

Multi-omics integration tools adopt different variations and combinations of the following methods, which represent distinct computational strategies for analysing and integrating heterogeneous omics datasets. Each offers unique advantages depending on the type of data and the specific biological questions being addressed. The methods presented in the following subsections are therefore to be regarded as illustrative examples rather than a comprehensive account of all existing strategies.

Joint Dimensionality Reduction (jDR)
Joint dimensionality reduction (jDR) methods have been widely applied to address data-related

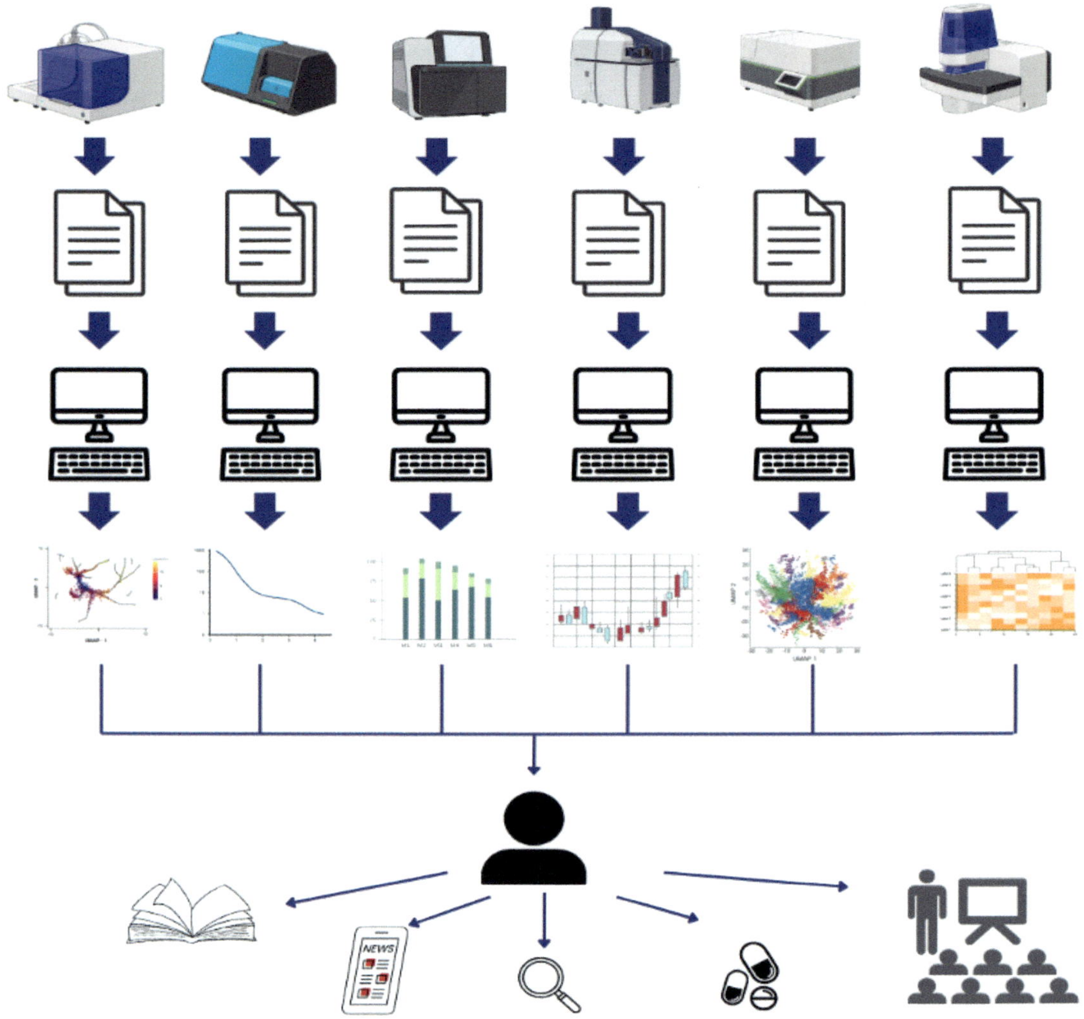

Fig. 18.5 Late integration of multi-omics data

challenges such as batch effects and outliers in both single-omics and multi-omics datasets. As such, they can serve not only as exploratory tools but also as effective pre-processing steps when used alongside subtype identification methods. jDR techniques aim to project high-dimensional omics data into a lower-dimensional space, facilitating the interpretation of complex biological signals. The rationale for using jDR in biological research lies in the fact that the state of a biological sample is influenced by multiple concurrent biological processes, ranging from general mechanisms like proliferation and inflammation to more cell-specific activities. Omics data provides a snapshot of this state, capturing a complex mixture of these underlying signals. The goal of jDR is to deconvolute this mixture, disentangling and revealing the distinct biological factors that contribute to the observed molecular profile of the sample [96].

Correlation and Covariance-Based jDR (COR)

Joint dimensionality reduction (jDR) has emerged as powerful approaches for data integration, widely used to explore and uncover complex molecular patterns. Among these, correlation- and covariance-based jDR methods play a prominent role. These techniques transform multi-view datasets by maximizing correlation or covariance within a shared lower-dimensional space. The resulting transformed representations allow for the visualization of common major patterns across different omics layers, facilitating a deeper understanding of the underlying biological structure [91]. Diablo [97] is an example of this approach.

Factor Analysis (FA)

Factor analysis methods perform dimensionality reduction by decomposing high-dimensional datasets into a smaller set of latent factors [91]. This technique is well illustrated by the tool MoCluster [98].

Probabilistic Models

Bayesian networks and Markov random fields capture the relationships between variables through probabilistic dependencies, enabling the quantification of uncertainty in predicted interactions [92, 99, 100]. This capability is particularly valuable in biological contexts, where data is frequently noisy, incomplete, and affected by multiple sources of variability [91, 101]. We can find this methodology in the tool iBAG [102].

Similarity (Kernel) Based (KB)

Compute similarity scores between pairs of patients by integrating information across multiple omics measurements [91]. This type of analysis is implemented in tools such as NEMO [103].

Network-Based Integration (NB)

Bersanelli proposed a hierarchical classification of integrative methods, distinguishing between network-based approaches and those that are network-independent [99]. While multivariate methods can produce multi-omic networks, they primarily operate at the level of the data matrix and do not require networks to perform integration. Conversely, network-based tools explicitly leverage dependency relationships between random variables, representing them as nodes and edges within a graph structure [104]. Conditional dependencies, such as partial correlations, can be estimated using Gaussian graphical models, where the network is derived from the precision matrix. Traditionally, most gene network reconstruction techniques have relied on single-omics data, particularly gene expression, to infer functional relationships among genes. However, rather than depending solely on statistical inference, multi-omic integration can also be guided by known biological networks. This approach preserves validated interactions that might otherwise be obscured by noise in complex datasets [105]. Using prior knowledge shifts the objective from discovering novel associations to utilizing existing biological insights, such as known pathways, biomarkers, or therapeutic targets, for contextual interpretation. Moreover, because this strategy does not rely entirely on statistical power, it becomes less sensitive to sample size constraints, even enabling the construction of personalized networks at the level of individual patients [93].

Regression-Based (RB)

The expression of each gene is modelled using a regression framework that incorporates measurements from other omic layers as predictors, along with their associated parameters [91]. An example of a tool that implements this approach is BMNPGRN [106].

Deep Learning (DL)

Most applications of deep learning (DL) methods in multi-omics analysis rely on an early integration strategy, where omics features are concatenated into a single input matrix. However, a new generation of tools leverage the multiple internal layers of DL architectures to learn joint representations of the input data. These deeper layers can capture complex correlations and underlying biological relationships within and across the integrated omics datasets [91, 107]. An application of this method is Subtype-GAN [108].

Portals for Visualization and Interpretation of Multi-omics Datasets

Beyond serving as repositories for multi-omics data, platforms that enable effective visualization and interpretation are critical for advancing biological discovery. Many existing tools primarily address single-omics layers, limiting the ability to capture the complex interactions across molecular domains. In recent years, however, a growing number of integrated portals have been developed to facilitate simultaneous exploration of multiple omics types. These platforms provide intuitive, multi-dimensional visualization and analysis capabilities, thereby supporting the discovery of novel relationships between molecular features and enabling deeper insights into physiological processes and disease mechanisms [92]. A summary of the main portals, including their specific features and applications, is reported in Table 18.1.

Table 18.1 Web-based portals for multi-omics data integration and visualization, summarizing supported omics types, data sources, private upload options, cancer focus, and key analytical features

Portal name	Supported omics types	Data repositories	Private data upload	Web address	Cancer focus	Highlights
cBioPortal	Mutation, CNV, gene/miRNA expression, methylation, protein abundance, clinical data	TCGA, published studies	Yes	http://www.cbioportal.org/	Yes	Multi-omics integration, network visualization, patient-centric queries, large cancer cohort data
UCSC Xena	CNV, somatic mutation, methylation, gene/exon/protein expression, phenotype	TCGA, CCLE, ICGC, GTEx, TARGET	Yes	https://xena.ucsc.edu/	Yes	Cross-study comparison, user data upload, statistical significance testing
Firebrowse	Mutation, CNV, gene/miRNA expression, methylation, protein, clinical	TCGA	No	http://firebrowse.org/	Yes	Data download, gene profiles visualization, iCoMut heatmaps
MethHC	DNA methylation, gene/miRNA expression	TCGA	No	http://methhc.mbc.nctu.edu.tw	Yes	Differential methylation, clustering, correlation, integration with UCSC genome browser and KEGG
Paintomics 3	Gene/miRNA expression, metabolite, region-specific ChIP-Seq, methyl-Seq	User data	Yes	http://www.paintomics.org/	No	Multi-omics pathway network mapping, KEGG integration, exploratory data visualization

(continued)

Table 18.1 (continued)

Portal name	Supported omics types	Data repositories	Private data upload	Web address	Cancer focus	Highlights
LinkedOmics	Clinical, CNV, mutation, gene/miRNA expression, methylation, protein, phosphoproteome, glycoproteome	TCGA, CPTAC	No	http://www.linkedomics.org/	Yes	Association and comparative analysis, pathway enrichment, pan-cancer exploration
OASIS	Mutation, CNV, gene expression	TCGA, CCLE, GTEx, published	No	http://www.oasis-genomics.org/	Yes	Pan-cancer exploratory analysis, BioMart framework
3Omics	Gene expression, protein, metabolite	User data	Yes	https://3omics.cmdm.tw/	No	Correlation, co-expression, phenotype mapping, pathway and GO enrichment
NetGestalt	Gene expression, mutation, CNV	TCGA, CPTAC, published studies	Yes	http://www.netgestalt.org/	Yes	Multi-omics on biological networks, hierarchical visualization, multi-scale data navigation

References

1. Chen T-Y, You L, Hardillo JAU, Chien M-P. Spatial transcriptomic technologies. Cells. 2023;12(16):2042. https://doi.org/10.3390/cells12162042.
2. Tang F, Barbacioru C, Wang Y, Nordman E, Lee C, Xu N, Wang X, Bodeau J, Tuch BB, Siddiqui A, Lao K, Surani MA. mRNA-Seq whole-transcriptome analysis of a single cell. Nat Methods. 2009;6(5):377–82. https://doi.org/10.1038/nmeth.1315. Epub 2009 Apr 6
3. Islam S, Kjällquist U, Moliner A, Zajac P, Fan JB, Lönnerberg P, Linnarsson S. Characterization of the single-cell transcriptional landscape by highly multiplex RNA-seq. Genome Res. 2011;21:1160–7. https://doi.org/10.1101/gr.110882.110.
4. Ke M, Elshenawy B, Sheldon H, Arora A, Buffa FM. Single cell RNA-sequencing: a powerful yet still challenging technology to study cellular heterogeneity. BioEssays. 2022;44:2200084. https://doi.org/10.1002/bies.202200084.
5. Luo G, Gao Q, Zhang S, Yan B. Probing infectious disease by single-cell RNA sequencing: progresses and perspectives. Comput Struct Biotechnol J. 2020;18:2962–71. https://doi.org/10.1016/j.csbj.2020.10.016.
6. Qu HQ, Kao C, Hakonarson H. Single-cell RNA sequencing technology landscape in 2023. Stem Cells. 2024;42(1):1–12. https://doi.org/10.1093/stmcls/sxad077. PMID: 37934608.
7. Bakken TE, Hodge RD, Miller JA, Yao Z, Nguyen TN, Aevermann B, Barkan E, Bertagnolli D, Casper T, Dee N, Garren E, Goldy J, Graybuck LT, Kroll M, Lasken RS, Lathia K, Parry S, Rimorin C, Scheuermann RH, Schork NJ, ... Tasic B. Single-nucleus and single-cell transcriptomes compared in matched cortical cell types. PloS one. 2018;13(12):e0209648. https://doi.org/10.1371/journal.pone.0209648.
8. Macosko EZ, Basu A, Satija R, Nemesh J, Shekhar K, Goldman M, Tirosh I, Bialas AR, Kamitaki N, Martersteck EM, Trombetta JJ, Weitz DA, Sanes JR, Shalek AK, Regev A, McCarroll SA. Highly parallel genome-wide expression profiling of individual cells

using Nanoliter droplets. Cell. 2015;161(5):1202–14. https://doi.org/10.1016/j.cell.2015.05.002. PMID: 26000488; PMCID: PMC4481139.
9. Salomon R, Kaczorowski D, Valdes-Mora F, Nordon RE, Neild A, Farbehi N, Bartonicek N, Gallego-Ortega D. Droplet-based single cell RNAseq tools: a practical guide. Lab Chip. 2019;19(10):1706–27. https://doi.org/10.1039/c8lc01239c. PMID: 30997473.
10. Aicher TP, Carroll S, Raddi G, Gierahn T, Wadsworth MH 2nd, Hughes TK, Love C, Shalek AK. Seq-well: a sample-efficient, portable Picowell platform for massively parallel single-cell RNA sequencing. Methods Mol Biol. 2019;1979:111–32. https://doi.org/10.1007/978-1-4939-9240-9_8. PMID: 31028635; PMCID: PMC7741456.
11. Hughes TK, Wadsworth MH, Gierahn TM, Do T, Weiss D, Andrade PR, Ma F, Silva BJdA, Shao S, Tsoi LC, et al. Second-strand synthesis-based massively parallel scRNA-seq reveals cellular states and molecular features of human inflammatory skin pathologies. Immunity. 2020;53:878–894.e7.
12. Han X, Wang R, Zhou Y, Fei L, Sun H, Lai S, Saadatpour A, Zhou Z, Chen H, Ye F, Huang D, Xu Y, Huang W, Jiang M, Jiang X, Mao J, Chen Y, Lu C, Xie J, Fang Q, Wang Y, Yue R, Li T, Huang H, Orkin SH, Yuan GC, Chen M, Guo G. Mapping the mouse cell atlas by microwell-seq. Cell. 2018;172(5):1091–1107.e17. https://doi.org/10.1016/j.cell.2018.02.001. Erratum in: Cell 2018 May 17; 173(5): 1307. https://doi.org/10.1016/j.cell.2018.05.012
13. Picelli S, Faridani OR, Björklund AK, et al. Full-length RNA-seq from single cells using smart-seq2. Nat Protoc. 2014;9(1):171–81. https://doi.org/10.1038/nprot.2014.006.
14. Hashimshony T, Senderovich N, Avital G, et al. CEL-seq2: sensitive highly-multiplexed single-cell RNA-seq. Genome Biol. 2016;17(1):77. https://doi.org/10.1186/s13059-016-0938-8.
15. Clark IC, Fontanez KM, Meltzer RH, et al. Microfluidics-free single-cell genomics with templated emulsification. Nat Biotechnol. 2023;41:1557–66. https://doi.org/10.1038/s41587-023-01685-z.
16. Komatsu J, Cico A, Poncin R, et al. RevGel-seq: instrument-free single-cell RNA sequencing using a reversible hydrogel for cell-specific barcoding. Sci Rep. 2023;13:4866. https://doi.org/10.1038/s41598-023-31915-y.
17. Zhao W, Dovas A, Spinazzi EF, et al. Deconvolution of cell type-specific drug responses in human tumor tissue with single-cell RNA-seq. Genome Med. 2021;13:82. https://doi.org/10.1186/s13073-021-00894-y.
18. Ning W, Jia W, Ning J, Zhou L, Li Z, Zhang L, Song X. Cross-cohort multi-omics analysis identifies novel clusters driven by EMT signatures in colorectal cancer. Front Immunol. 2025;16:1628005. https://doi.org/10.3389/fimmu.2025.1628005. PMID: 40574852; PMCID: PMC12198181.
19. Zhong J, Li Y, Liu Y, Qiao J, Wu Y, Kong X, Qi M, Lin Y, Yao Y, Jin Y, Bi C, Zhai A. Hepatitis B virus X protein (HBx)-mediated immune modulation and prognostic model development in hepatocellular carcinoma. PLoS One. 2025;20(6):e0325363. https://doi.org/10.1371/journal.pone.0325363.
20. Perez RK, Gordon MG, Subramaniam M, Kim MC, Hartoularos GC, Targ S, Sun Y, Ogorodnikov A, Bueno R, Lu A, Thompson M, Rappoport N, Dahl A, Lanata CM, Matloubian M, Maliskova L, Kwek SS, Li T, Slyper M, Waldman J, Dionne D, Rozenblatt-Rosen O, Fong L, Dall'Era M, Balliu B, Regev A, Yazdany J, Criswell LA, Zaitlen N, Ye CJ. Single-cell RNA-seq reveals cell type-specific molecular and genetic associations to lupus. Science. 2022;376(6589):eabf1970. https://doi.org/10.1126/science.abf1970. Epub 2022 Apr 8. Erratum in: Science. 2024 July 12; 385(6705): eadr4064. https://doi.org/10.1126/science.adr4064. PMID: 35389781; PMCID: PMC9297655.
21. Figueiredo ML. Applications of single-cell RNA sequencing in rheumatoid arthritis. Front Immunol. 2024;15:1491318. https://doi.org/10.3389/fimmu.2024.1491318. PMID: 39600707; PMCID: PMC11588722.
22. Quan K, Yang Y, Li C, Yao X. Single-cell RNA sequencing + TCR sequencing reveal the proportion and characteristics of dual TCR T cells in tertiary lymphoid structures in pemphigus. J Invest Dermatol. 2025;146:78. https://doi.org/10.1016/j.jid.2025.05.008. PMID: 40419016.
23. Iacobucci I, Zeng AGX, Gao Q, Garcia-Prat L, Baviskar P, Shah S, Murison A, Voisin V, Chan-Seng-Yue M, Cheng C, Qu C, Bailey C, Lear M, Witkowski MT, Zhou X, Zaldivar Peraza A, Gangwani K, Advani AS, Luger SM, Litzow MR, Rowe JM, Paietta EM, Stock W, Dick JE, Mullighan CG. Multipotent lineage potential in B cell acute lymphoblastic leukemia is associated with distinct cellular origins and clinical features. Nat Cancer. 2025;6:1242. https://doi.org/10.1038/s43018-025-00987-2. PMID: 40579588.
24. Ramos-Vicente D, Monterosso P, de Fàbregues O, Roch G, Vila M, Bové J. Single-cell transcriptomics for immune profiling of cerebrospinal fluid in neurological diseases. Front Immunol. 2025;16:1599303. https://doi.org/10.3389/fimmu.2025.1599303. PMID: 40510352; PMCID: PMC12158733.
25. Zhao C, Plaza Reyes A, Schell JP, et al. A comprehensive human embryo reference tool using single-cell RNA-sequencing data. Nat Methods. 2025;22:193–206. https://doi.org/10.1038/s41592-024-02493-2.
26. Palla G, Fischer DS, Regev A, Theis FJ. Spatial components of molecular tissue biology. Nat Biotechnol. 2022;40(3):308–18. https://doi.org/10.1038/s41587-021-01182-1.

27. Fomitcheva-Khartchenko A, Kashyap A, Geiger T, Kaigala GV. Space in cancer biology: its role and implications. Trends Cancer. 2022;8(12):1019–32. https://doi.org/10.1016/j.trecan.2022.07.008.
28. Van den Brink SC, Sage F, Vértesy Á, Spanjaard B, Peterson-Maduro J, Baron CS, Robin C, van Oudenaarden A. Single-cell sequencing reveals dissociation-induced gene expression in tissue subpopulations. Nat Methods. 2017;14(10):935–6. https://doi.org/10.1038/nmeth.4437.
29. Stubbington MJT, Rozenblatt-Rosen O, Regev A, Teichmann SA. Single-cell transcriptomics to explore the immune system in health and disease. Science. 2017;358(6359):58–63. https://doi.org/10.1126/science.aan6828.
30. Papalexi E, Satija R. Single-cell RNA sequencing to explore immune cell heterogeneity. Nat Rev Immunol. 2018;18(1):35–45. https://doi.org/10.1038/nri.2017.76.
31. Kruse F, Junker JP, van Oudenaarden A, Bakkers J. Tomo-seq: a method to obtain genome-wide expression data with spatial resolution. Methods Cell Biol. 2016;135:299–307. https://doi.org/10.1016/bs.mcb.2016.01.006.
32. Junker J, Noël E, Guryev V, Peterson K, Shah G, Huisken J, et al. Genome-wide RNA tomography in the zebrafish embryo. Cell. 2014;159(3):662–75. https://doi.org/10.1016/j.cell.2014.09.038.
33. Lacraz GPA, et al. Tomo-seq identifies SOX9 as a key regulator of cardiac fibrosis during ischemic injury. Circulation. 2017;136(15):1396–409. https://doi.org/10.1161/CIRCULATIONAHA.117.027790.
34. Nichterwitz S, Chen G, Aguila Benitez J, Yilmaz M, Storvall H, Cao M, Sandberg R, Deng Q, Hedlund E. Laser capture microscopy coupled with smart-seq2 for precise spatial transcriptomic profiling. Nat Commun. 2016;7:12139. https://doi.org/10.1038/ncomms12139.
35. Nichterwitz S, Benitez JA, Hoogstraaten R, Deng Q, Hedlund E. LCM-seq: a method for spatial transcriptomic profiling using laser capture microdissection coupled with PolyA-based RNA sequencing. Methods Mol Biol. 2018;1649:95–110. https://doi.org/10.1007/978-1-4939-7204-1_6.
36. Cho C, Haddadi N-S, Kidacki M, Woodard GA, Shakiba S, Yıldız-Altay Ü, Richmond JM, Vesely MD. Spatial transcriptomics in inflammatory skin diseases using GeoMx digital spatial profiling: a practical guide for applications in dermatology. JID Innov. 2025;5(1):100317. https://doi.org/10.1016/j.xjidi.2024.100317.
37. Hernandez Sharia R, Lazcano Rossana SA, Powell S, Kostousov L, Mehta J, Khan K, Lu W, Solis LM. Challenges and opportunities for immunoprofiling using a spatial high-plex technology: the NanoString GeoMx® digital spatial profiler. Front Oncol. 2022;12:890410. https://doi.org/10.3389/fonc.2022.890410.
38. Li X, Wang CY. From bulk, single-cell to spatial RNA sequencing. Int J Oral Sci. 2021;13(1):36. https://doi.org/10.1038/s41368-021-00146-0.
39. Boisset JC, Vivié J, Grün D, et al. Mapping the physical network of cellular interactions. Nat Methods. 2018;15(7):547–53. https://doi.org/10.1038/s41592-018-0009-z.
40. Giladi A, Cohen M, Medaglia C, et al. Dissecting cellular crosstalk by sequencing physically interacting cells. Nat Biotechnol. 2020;38(6):629–37. https://doi.org/10.1038/s41587-020-0442-2.
41. Koch L. Transcriptional profiling of physically interacting cells. Nat Rev Genet. 2020;21:275. https://doi.org/10.1038/s41576-020-0229-9.
42. Manco R, Averbukh I, Porat Z, et al. Clump sequencing exposes the spatial expression programs of intestinal secretory cells. Nat Commun. 2021;12:3074. https://doi.org/10.1038/s41467-021-23245-2.
43. Stahl PL, Salmén F, Vickovic S, et al. Visualization and analysis of gene expression in tissue sections by spatial transcriptomics. Science. 2016;353(6294):78–82. https://doi.org/10.1126/science.aaf2403.
44. Marx V. Method of the year: spatially resolved transcriptomics. Nat Methods. 2021;18(1):9–14. https://doi.org/10.1038/s41592-020-01033-y.
45. Emmert-Buck MR, Bonner RF, Smith PD, et al. Laser capture microdissection. Science. 1996;274(5289):998–1001. https://doi.org/10.1126/science.274.5289.998.
46. Levsky JM, Singer RH. Fluorescence in situ hybridization: past, present and future. J Cell Sci. 2003;116(14):2833–8.
47. Rao A, Barkley D, França GS, Yanai I. Exploring tissue architecture using spatial transcriptomics. Nature. 2021;596(7871):211–20. https://doi.org/10.1038/s41586-021-03634-9.
48. Oliveira MF d, Romero JP, Chung M, et al. High-definition spatial transcriptomic profiling of immune cell populations in colorectal cancer. Nat Genet. 2025;57:1512–23. https://doi.org/10.1038/s41588-025-02193-3.
49. Reyes D, Giangarra V, Williams SR, et al. Spatial whole transcriptome profiling of the tumor microenvironment in FFPE prostate carcinoma using the Visium platform. J Immunol. 2022;208(Supplement_1):179.18. https://doi.org/10.4049/jimmunol.208.Supp.179.18.
50. Nagendran M, Sapida J, Arthur J, et al. Visium HD enables spatially resolved, single-cell scale resolution mapping of FFPE human breast cancer tissue. J Immunother Cancer. 2023;11:A1620. https://doi.org/10.1136/jitc-2023-SITC2023.1457.
51. Montagne JM, Sidiropoulos DN, Mo G, et al. Spatially resolved immune receptor repertoires from Visium transcriptomic libraries. J Immunol. 2023;210(Supplement_1):251.02. https://doi.org/10.4049/jimmunol.210.Supp.251.02.

52. Maynard KR, Collado-Torres L, Weber LM, et al. Transcriptome-scale spatial gene expression in the human dorsolateral prefrontal cortex. Nat Neurosci. 2021;24:425–36. https://doi.org/10.1038/s41593-020-00787-0.
53. Vickovic S, Eraslan G, Salmén F, et al. High-definition spatial transcriptomics for in situ tissue profiling. Nat Methods. 2019;16:987–90. https://doi.org/10.1038/s41592-019-0548-y.
54. Gu L, Li C, Aach J, et al. Multiplex single-molecule interaction profiling of DNA-barcoded proteins. Nature. 2014;515:554–7. https://doi.org/10.1038/nature13761.
55. Fu X, Sun L, Dong R, et al. Polony gels enable amplifiable DNA stamping and spatial transcriptomics of chronic pain. Cell. 2022;185(24):4621–4633.e17. https://doi.org/10.1016/j.cell.2022.10.012.
56. Cho C-S, Xi J, Si Y, et al. Microscopic examination of spatial transcriptome using seq-scope. Cell. 2021;184(13):3559–3572.e22. https://doi.org/10.1016/j.cell.2021.05.040.
57. Kim Y, Cheng W, Cho CS, et al. Seq-scope: repurposing Illumina sequencing flow cells for high-resolution spatial transcriptomics. Nat Protoc. 2025;20:643–89. https://doi.org/10.1038/s41596-024-01065-0.
58. Chen A, Liao S, Cheng M, et al. Spatiotemporal transcriptomic atlas of mouse organogenesis using DNA nanoball-patterned arrays. Cell. 2022;185(10):1777–1792.e21. https://doi.org/10.1016/j.cell.2022.04.003.
59. Xia K, Sun H-X, Li J, et al. The single-cell stereo-seq reveals region-specific cell subtypes and transcriptome profiling in Arabidopsis leaves. Dev Cell. 2022;57(10):1299–1310.e4. https://doi.org/10.1016/j.devcel.2022.04.006.
60. Rodriques SG, Stickels RR, Goeva A, et al. Slide-seq: a scalable technology for measuring genome-wide expression at high spatial resolution. Science. 2019;363(6434):1463–7. https://doi.org/10.1126/science.aaw1219.
61. Stickels RR, Murray E, Kumar P, et al. Highly sensitive spatial transcriptomics at near-cellular resolution with slide-seqV2. Nat Biotechnol. 2021;39:313–9. https://doi.org/10.1038/s41587-020-0739-1.
62. Marshall JL, Noel T, Wang QS, et al. High-resolution slide-seqV2 spatial transcriptomics enables discovery of disease-specific cell neighborhoods and pathways. iScience. 2022;25(4):104097. https://doi.org/10.1016/j.isci.2022.104097.
63. Kishi JY, Liu N, West ER, et al. Light-seq: light-directed in situ barcoding of biomolecules in fixed cells and tissues for spatially indexed sequencing. Nat Methods. 2022;19:1393–402. https://doi.org/10.1038/s41592-022-01604-1.
64. Russell AJC, Weir JA, Nadaf NM, et al. Slide-tags enables single-nucleus barcoding for multimodal spatial genomics. Nature. 2024;625:101–9. https://doi.org/10.1038/s41586-023-06837-4.
65. Lawrence JB, Singer RH, Marselle LM. Highly localized tracks of specific transcripts within interphase nuclei visualized by in situ hybridization. Cell. 1989;57(3):493–502. https://doi.org/10.1016/0092-8674(89)90922-1.
66. Gall JG, Pardue ML. Formation and detection of RNA-DNA hybrid molecules in cytological preparations. Proc Natl Acad Sci. 1969;63(2):378–83. https://doi.org/10.1073/pnas.63.2.378.
67. Femino AM, Fay FS, Fogarty K, Singer RH. Visualization of single RNA transcripts in situ. Science. 1998;280(5363):585–90. https://doi.org/10.1126/science.280.5363.585.
68. Tsanov N, Samacoits A, Chouaib R, et al. smiFISH and FISH-quant—a flexible single RNA detection approach with super-resolution capability. Nucleic Acids Res. 2016;44(22):e165. https://doi.org/10.1093/nar/gkw784.
69. Safieddine A, Coleno E, Lionneton F, et al. HT-smFISH: a cost-effective and flexible workflow for high-throughput single-molecule RNA imaging. Nat Protoc. 2023;18:157–87. https://doi.org/10.1038/s41596-022-00750-2.
70. Xu F, Li P. Cytogenomic abnormalities and dosage-sensitive mechanisms for intellectual and developmental disabilities. In: Salehi A, editor. Developmental disabilities—molecules involved, diagnosis and clinical care. Rijeka: InTech; 2013. p. 1–30. https://doi.org/10.5772/54704.
71. Chrzanowska NM, Kowalewski J, Lewandowska MA. Use of fluorescence in situ hybridization (FISH) in diagnosis and tailored therapies in solid tumors. Molecules. 2020;25(8):1864. https://doi.org/10.3390/molecules25081864.
72. Chen KH, Boettiger AN, Moffitt JR, Wang S, Zhuang X. Spatially resolved, highly multiplexed RNA profiling in single cells. Science. 2015;348(6233):aaa6090. https://doi.org/10.1126/science.aaa6090.
73. Xia C, Fan J, Emanuel G, Hao J, Zhuang X. Spatial transcriptome profiling by MERFISH reveals subcellular RNA compartmentalization and cell cycle–dependent gene expression. Proc Natl Acad Sci USA. 2019;116(39):19490–9. https://doi.org/10.1073/pnas.1912459116.
74. Lubeck E, Coskun AF, Zhiyentayev T, Ahmad M, Cai L. Single-cell in situ RNA profiling by sequential hybridization. Nat Methods. 2014;11(4):360–1. https://doi.org/10.1038/nmeth.2892.
75. Shah S, Lubeck E, Zhou W, Cai L. In situ transcription profiling of single cells reveals spatial organization of cells in the mouse hippocampus. Neuron. 2016;92(2):342–57. https://doi.org/10.1016/j.neuron.2016.10.001.
76. Eng CHL, Lawson M, Zhu Q, et al. Transcriptome-scale super-resolved imaging in tissues by RNA seqFISH+. Nature. 2019;568(7751):235–9. https://doi.org/10.1038/s41586-019-1049-y.
77. Wang F, Flanagan J, Su N, et al. RNAscope: a novel in situ RNA analysis platform for formalin-

fixed, paraffin-embedded tissues. J Mol Diagn. 2012;14(1):22–9. https://doi.org/10.1016/j.jmoldx.2011.08.002.
78. Atout S, Shurrab S, Loveridge C. Evaluation of the suitability of RNAscope as a technique to measure gene expression in clinical diagnostics: a systematic review. Mol Diagn Ther. 2022;26(1):19–37. https://doi.org/10.1007/s40291-021-00570-2.
79. Choi HMT, Schwarzkopf M, Fornace ME, et al. Third-generation in situ hybridization chain reaction: multiplexed, quantitative, sensitive, versatile, robust. Development. 2018;145(12):dev165753. https://doi.org/10.1242/dev.165753.
80. Gandin V, Andronico F, Ghezzi S, et al. Deep-tissue transcriptomics and subcellular imaging at high spatial resolution. Science. 2025;388:eadq2084. https://doi.org/10.1126/science.adq2084.
81. Lee J, Daugharthy E, Scheiman J, et al. Fluorescent in situ sequencing (FISSEQ) of RNA for gene expression profiling in intact cells and tissues. Nat Protoc. 2015;10:442–58. https://doi.org/10.1038/nprot.2014.191.
82. Alon S, Goodwin DR, Sinha A, et al. Expansion sequencing: spatially precise in situ transcriptomics in intact biological systems. Science. 2021;371:eaax 2656. https://doi.org/10.1126/science.aax2656.
83. 10x Genomics. Xenium platform. Available from: https://www.10xgenomics.com/platforms/xenium.
84. Qian X, Harris KD, Hauling T, et al. Probabilistic cell typing enables fine mapping of closely related cell types in situ. Nat Methods. 2020;17:101–6. https://doi.org/10.1038/s41592-019-0631-4.
85. Ke R, Mignardi M, Pacureanu A, et al. In situ sequencing for RNA analysis in preserved tissue and cells. Nat Methods. 2013;10:857–60. https://doi.org/10.1038/nmeth.2563.
86. He S, Bhatt R, Brown C, et al. High-plex imaging of RNA and proteins at subcellular resolution in fixed tissue by spatial molecular imaging. Nat Biotechnol. 2022;40:1794–806. https://doi.org/10.1038/s41587-022-01483-z.
87. Chung K, Wallace J, Kim SY, et al. Structural and molecular interrogation of intact biological systems. Nature. 2013;497:332–7. https://doi.org/10.1038/nature12107.
88. Wang X, Allen WE, Wright MA, et al. Three-dimensional intact-tissue sequencing of single-cell transcriptional states. Science. 2018;361:eaat 5691. https://doi.org/10.1126/science.aat5691.
89. Merritt CR, Ong GT, Church SE, et al. Multiplex digital spatial profiling of proteins and RNA in fixed tissue. Nat Biotechnol. 2020;38(5):586–99. https://doi.org/10.1038/s41587-020-0472-9.
90. Vasaturo A, Fabrizio V, Vittorioso P, et al. Challenges and opportunities for immunoprofiling using a spatial high-plex technology: the NanoString GeoMx® digital spatial profiler. Front Oncol. 2022;12:890410. https://doi.org/10.3389/fonc.2022.890410.
91. Athieniti E, Spyrou GM. A guide to multi-omics data collection and integration for translational medicine. Comput Struct Biotechnol J. 2022;21:134–49. https://doi.org/10.1016/j.csbj.2022.11.050.
92. Subramanian I, Verma S, Kumar S, Jere A, Anamika K. Multi-omics data integration, interpretation, and its application. Bioinform Biol Insights. 2020;14:1177932219899051. https://doi.org/10.1177/1177932219899051.
93. Hernández-Lemus E, Ochoa S. Methods for multi-omic data integration in cancer research. Front Genet. 2024;15:1425456. https://doi.org/10.3389/fgene.2024.1425456.
94. Zitnik M, Nguyen F, Wang B, Leskovec J, Goldenberg A, Hoffman MM. Machine learning for integrating data in biology and medicine: principles, practice, and opportunities. Int J Inf fusion. 2019;50:71–91. https://doi.org/10.1016/j.inffus.2018.09.012.
95. Rohart F, Gautier B, Singh A, Lê Cao KA. mixOmics: an R package for 'omics feature selection and multiple data integration. PLoS Comput Biol. 2017;13(11):e1005752. https://doi.org/10.1371/journal.pcbi.1005752.
96. Cantini L, Zakeri P, Hernandez C, Naldi A, Thieffry D, Remy E, Baudot A. Benchmarking joint multi-omics dimensionality reduction approaches for the study of cancer. Nat Commun. 2021;12(1):124. https://doi.org/10.1038/s41467-020-20430-7.
97. Singh A, Shannon CP, Gautier B, Rohart F, Vacher M, Tebbutt SJ, Lê Cao KA. DIABLO: an integrative approach for identifying key molecular drivers from multi-omics assays. Bioinformatics (Oxford, England). 2019;35(17):3055–62. https://doi.org/10.1093/bioinformatics/bty1054.
98. Meng C, Helm D, Frejno M, Kuster B. moCluster: identifying joint patterns across multiple omics data sets. J Proteome Res. 2016;15(3):755–65. https://doi.org/10.1021/acs.jproteome.5b00824.
99. Bersanelli M, Mosca E, Remondini D, Giampieri E, Sala C, Castellani G, et al. Methods for the integration of multi-omics data: mathematical aspects. BMC Bioinformatics. 2016;17(Suppl 2):15. https://doi.org/10.1186/s12859-015-0857-9.
100. Vahabi N, Michailidis G. Unsupervised multi-omics data integration methods: a comprehensive review. Front Genet. 2022;13:854752. https://doi.org/10.3389/fgene.2022.854752.
101. Chu J, Sun NA, Hu W, Chen X, Yi N, Shen Y. The application of Bayesian methods in cancer prognosis and prediction. Cancer Genomics Proteomics. 2022;19(1):1–11. https://doi.org/10.21873/cgp.20298.
102. Wang W, Baladandayuthapani V, Morris JS, Broom BM, Manyam G, Do KA. iBAG: integrative Bayesian analysis of high-dimensional multiplatform genomics data. Bioinformatics (Oxford, England). 2013;29(2):149–59. https://doi.org/10.1093/bioinformatics/bts655.
103. Rappoport N, Shamir R. NEMO: cancer subtyping by integration of partial multi-omic data. Bioinformatics (Oxford, England). 2019;35(18):3348–56. https://doi.org/10.1093/bioinformatics/btz058.

104. Hawe JS, Theis FJ, Heinig M. Inferring interaction networks from multi-omics data. Front Genet. 2019;10:535. https://doi.org/10.3389/fgene.2019.00535.
105. Koh HWL, Fermin D, Vogel C, Choi KP, Ewing RM, Choi H. iOmicsPASS: network-based integration of multiomics data for predictive subnetwork discovery. NPJ Syst Biol Appl. 2019;5:22. https://doi.org/10.1038/s41540-019-0099-y.
106. Yuan L, Guo LH, Yuan CA, Zhang YH, Han K, Nandi A, Honig B, Huang DS. Integration of multi-omics data for gene regulatory network inference and application to breast cancer. IEEE/ACM Trans Comput Biol Bioinform. 2018; https://doi.org/10.1109/TCBB.2018.2866836. Advance online publication. https://doi.org/10.1109/TCBB.2018.2866836.
107. Guo LY, Wu AH, Wang YX, Zhang LP, Chai H, Liang XF. Deep learning-based ovarian cancer subtypes identification using multi-omics data. BioData Min. 2020;13:10. https://doi.org/10.1186/s13040-020-00222-x.
108. Yang H, Chen R, Li D, Wang Z. Subtype-GAN: a deep learning approach for integrative cancer subtyping of multi-omics data. Bioinformatics (Oxford, England). 2021;37(16):2231–7. https://doi.org/10.1093/bioinformatics/btab109.
109. Canva. Canva. https://www.canva.com (n.d.). Retrieved from 3 Sept 2025.

Liquid Biopsy and Circulating Biomarkers

19

Tancredi Didier Bazan Russo, Valerio Gristina, Francesco Pepe, Lorena Incorvaia, Antonio Galvano, Viviana Bazan, Umberto Malapelle, Antonio Giordano, and Antonio Russo

Introduction

Liquid biopsy (LB) has rapidly emerged as one of the most promising innovations in modern oncology, offering a minimally invasive approach for tumor molecular profiling [1]. Traditionally, tissue biopsy has been the cornerstone of cancer diagnosis and molecular profiling, enabling histopathological characterization and detection of genetic alterations. However, tissue sampling presents inherent limitations: It is invasive, often associated with procedural risks, and may not always provide adequate material for analysis. Furthermore, tumors are highly heterogeneous and evolve dynamically over time and across different metastatic sites, making it difficult for a single tissue specimen to capture the full molecular landscape of the disease. In this context, LB represents a complementary and, in certain clinical scenarios, alternative tool to tissue biopsy, enabling the acquisition of diagnostic, prognostic, and predictive information [2, 3].

The term LB generally refers to the analysis of tumor-derived material present in biological fluids, primarily peripheral blood plasma [1]. Among the most widely studied analytes, circulating tumor DNA (ctDNA)—a fraction of cell-free DNA (cfDNA) released into the bloodstream by tumor cells—has become the leading biomarker in clinical practice. Analysis of ctDNA allows the detection of actionable mutations, monitoring of minimal residual disease (MRD), and identification of emerging resistance mechanisms. In addition to ctDNA, other circulating components such as circulating tumor cells (CTCs), extracellular vesicles (EVs), noncoding RNAs, and tumor-educated platelets (TEPs) are gaining increasing attention for their potential

T. D. B. Russo · V. Gristina · L. Incorvaia
A. Galvano · A. Russo (✉)
Department of Precision Medicine in Medical, Surgical and Critical Care (Me.Pre.C.C.), Section of Medical Oncology, University of Palermo, Palermo, Italy
e-mail: tancredididier.bazanrusso@unipa.it; valerio.gristina@unipa.it; lorena.incorvaia@unipa.it; antonio.galvano@unipa.it; antonio.russo@unipa.it

F. Pepe · U. Malapelle
Department of Public Health, University Federico II of Naples, Naples, Italy
e-mail: francesco.pepe4@unina.it; umberto.malapelle@unina.it

V. Bazan
Department of Biomedicine, Neuroscience and Advanced Diagnostics (BIND), University of Palermo, Palermo, Italy
e-mail: viviana.bazan@unipa.it

A. Giordano
Sbarro Institute for Cancer Research and Molecular Medicine, Center for Biotechnology, College of Science and Technology, Temple University, Philadelphia, PA, USA

Department of Medical Biotechnologies, University of Siena, Siena, Italy
e-mail: antonio.giordano@temple.edu

© The Author(s), under exclusive license to Springer Nature Switzerland AG 2026

S. Sioletic, L. Coppola (eds.), *Next-Generation Sequencing in Solid Tumor Histopathology*, Current Clinical Pathology, https://doi.org/10.1007/978-3-032-18790-1_19

diagnostic and prognostic roles [4, 5]. Beyond blood, additional biological fluids such as urine, saliva, pleural effusions, and cerebrospinal fluid (CSF) may also serve as valuable sources of tumor-derived biomarkers, particularly in specific cancer contexts [6].

LB confers several advantages compared to tissue biopsy. First, it is minimally invasive, requiring only a blood draw, thus minimizing procedural risks and patient discomfort. Second, it can be performed repeatedly over time, allowing dynamic tracking of tumor evolution, which is especially relevant in advanced disease or when evaluating treatment response. Third, LB has the potential to better represent tumor spatiotemporal heterogeneity by capturing genetic material released from multiple tumor sites simultaneously [4, 7, 8]. These advantages have accelerated its translation from research into clinical practice. Notably, its application is now supported by major international guidelines, including those from the European Society for Medical Oncology (ESMO) and the American Society of Clinical Oncology (ASCO), which recommend LB in defined clinical scenarios, such as identifying actionable genomic alterations (e.g., *EGFR*, *RAS*, *BRCA*, *ESR1*) when molecular analysis on a tissue sample is found to be inconclusive for patients' clinical stratification [1, 9].

Despite its promise, LB is not without limitations. The amount of tumor-derived material in circulation is often very low, especially in early-stage cancers or in patients responding to therapy, raising challenges in sensitivity [10]. Furthermore, pre-analytical and analytical variables—including sample handling, DNA extraction methods, sequencing platforms, and bioinformatics pipelines—can significantly influence results, underscoring the need for strict standardization and quality control [11]. Current evidence supports the use of LB mainly in advanced disease settings or when tissue samples are insufficient or unavailable. However, ongoing clinical trials are expanding the role of LB to early detection, cancer screening, and MRD monitoring [1].

The importance of LB lies not only in its immediate clinical applications but also in its potential to transform cancer care in the near future. By integrating genomic, transcriptomic, and epigenomic information with advanced computational methods and artificial intelligence, LB could serve as a central tool in precision oncology, enabling personalized treatment strategies and facilitating cancer interception before overt clinical progression. In this chapter, we will provide a comprehensive overview of the main circulating biomarkers, the technologies, and methodologies for their analysis, and the current and future clinical applications of LB in solid tumors.

Definition

LB provides a minimally invasive, repeatable method for tumor molecular profiling, overcoming tissue biopsy limitations. It enables the detection of actionable mutations, monitoring of minimal residual disease (MRD), and resistance mechanisms. While promising, LB faces challenges of low analyte abundance, pre-analytical variability, and the need for standardization.

Types of Circulating Biomarkers and Biofluids

Biofluids

Peripheral blood, particularly plasma, currently represents the main source for LB in routine clinical practice. However, several biological fluids are emerging as alternative or complementary sources of tumor-derived material, especially in scenarios where analyte shedding into the bloodstream is limited or when tissue access is difficult or not repeatable. The choice of biofluid is strongly influenced by the anatomical site of the malignancy, its dissemination pattern, and the practicality of sample collection [12, 13].

Pleural effusion is among the most promising sources after blood, as it is particularly enriched in tumor-derived analytes and allows both morphological diagnosis and molecular characterization of thoracic malignancies. In patients with lung cancer, the analytical sensitivity of pleural fluid for *EGFR* mutation detection may exceed that of plasma, although collection is more invasive than venipuncture and not always feasible in frail patients [14]. Cerebrospinal fluid (CSF) is especially valuable in central nervous system tumors, such as gliomas and leptomeningeal carcinomatosis, where ctDNA release into blood is hindered by the blood–brain barrier. Nonetheless, lumbar puncture is invasive, limiting serial sampling, and tumor DNA concentrations in CSF are often low and heterogeneous, requiring highly sensitive technologies to detect subclonal alterations [15, 16].

Urine provides a completely noninvasive fluid for molecular characterization, particularly in urological cancers such as prostate and bladder cancer, where tumor-derived molecules are directly excreted. Its utility in non-urological malignancies, however, is limited by anatomical barriers and variable cfDNA content influenced by hydration, renal function, and medication use [17]. Ascitic fluid and other serous effusions, such as pericardial fluid, represent a valid alternative in peritoneal tumors, especially ovarian cancer, where high nucleic acid concentrations can increase sensitivity beyond that of plasma [18]. Similarly, saliva offers a simple and noninvasive collection method, potentially useful for head and neck cancers, though clinical application remains limited due to low tumor analyte concentrations and microbial contamination [19].

In summary, while peripheral blood remains the gold standard endorsed by international guidelines, the exploration of alternative biofluids holds promise for improving diagnostic sensitivity in anatomically confined or clinically complex cancers. Their routine use, however, requires careful evaluation of clinical feasibility, invasiveness, analytical robustness, and prospective validation before broader implementation in oncology practice.

Biofluids

Plasma represents the gold standard biological sample for LB purposes; alternatives (pleural effusion, CSF, urine, ascitic fluid, saliva) offer site-specific value but vary in feasibility and sensitivity.

Circulating Biomarkers

Circulating biomarkers analyzed through LB constitute a heterogeneous group of tumor-derived analytes detectable in peripheral blood and other biofluids (Table 19.1).

Among these, ctDNA, a fraction of cfDNA, is currently the most established in clinical practice. cfDNA is composed of short DNA fragments released into the bloodstream from apoptotic and necrotic cells, whereas ctDNA originates specifically from tumor cells and carries genetic and epigenetic alterations such as point mutations, gene rearrangements, copy number variations, and distinctive methylation profiles [20]. Despite its promise, ctDNA is present at very low concentrations (3×10^{-9} molecules/ml of blood), with a short half-life (ranging from minutes to 2,5 h), necessitating ultrasensitive methods for reliable detection [21]. Analytical approaches include digital PCR, which enables highly sensitive quantification of known mutations at allele frequencies below 0.1%, and next-generation sequencing (NGS), which allows comprehensive genomic profiling across multiple genes and variant types [22]. Beyond mutational analyses, novel approaches such as fragmentomics and methylomics have expanded ctDNA's diagnostic power. Fragmentomics investigates DNA fragment size and nucleosome positioning, revealing that ctDNA often consists of shorter fragments with altered nucleosome footprints. Methylomics focuses on aberrant DNA methylation patterns,

Table 19.1 Analytes in liquid biopsy: characteristics, isolation methods, and analysis techniques

Analyte	Characteristics	Isolation methods	Analysis techniques
cfDNA/ctDNA	Main analyte used in clinical practice; DNA fragments released from apoptotic/necrotic cells (cfDNA); ctDNA is the tumor-derived fraction	Silica columns, magnetic beads, filtration	ddPCR/dPCR, NGS, fragmentomics, methylomics
CTCs	Viable tumor cells in peripheral blood, often involved in metastasis	Positive selection (EpCAM), negative selection (CD45−), physical approaches (size, density), microfluidics	Immunological, molecular (RNA-based), functional
EVs (exosomes, microvesicles, apoptotic bodies)	"Nano-shuttle" vesicles released by cells, including tumor cells, containing miRNA, mRNA, proteins, DNA fragments	Ultracentrifugation, SEC, immunoaffinity, microfluidics	NTA, Western blot, TEM
ncRNA (miRNA, piRNA, siRNA, lncRNA)	Circulating noncoding RNAs, free or encapsulated in EVs	RNA kits specific for low molecular weight	RT-qPCR, microarray, RNA-seq
TEPs	Platelets with tumor-altered transcriptome (mRNA)	Peripheral blood collection, platelet isolation	RNA-seq, machine learning

CTCs circulating tumor cells, *ctDNA* circulating tumor DNA, *cfDNA* cell-free DNA, *EVs* extracellular vesicles, *lncRNAs* long noncoding RNAs, *miRNA* microRNA, *piRNA* piwi-interacting RNA, *SEC* size exclusion chromatography, *siRNA* small interfering RNA, *TEM* transmission electron microscopy, *TEPs* tumor-educated platelets

enabling discrimination between tumor and non-tumor DNA and even identification of the tumor tissue of origin [23, 24]. Together, these techniques provide refined tools for early cancer detection, risk stratification, and precision oncology.

CTCs represent another pivotal biomarker class. These are viable cancer cells shed from primary or metastatic lesions into the bloodstream, serving as mediators of metastatic dissemination. Their biology reflects key processes such as epithelial-to-mesenchymal transition (EMT), which enhances motility and resistance to apoptosis [25]. Although their half-life is short—approximately 25–30 minutes for single cells and even less for clusters—their presence strongly correlates with disease aggressiveness and metastatic potential [26]. CTCs exhibit marked heterogeneity, with EpCAM being the most commonly used marker for detection, although its variable expression may lead to underestimation in certain tumor types [27]. Analytical strategies for CTCs include immunological assays, RNA-based profiling, and single-cell genomic and transcriptomic analysis, which allow exploration of intratumoral heterogeneity and resistance mechanisms. Functional assays, such as EPISPOT, further assess viability and secretory activity, providing insights into therapeutic responsiveness [28]. Clinically, CTC enumeration and characterization have been associated with prognosis, prediction of therapeutic outcomes, and dynamic monitoring of treatment response [29].

Extracellular vesicles (EVs), including exosomes (30–200 nm), microvesicles (100–1000 nm), and apoptotic bodies (>1000 nm), constitute another category of circulating biomarkers. Tumor cells secrete EVs in abundance, and their cargo—comprising nucleic acids, proteins, and lipids—mirrors the molecular profile of the tumor of origin. EVs play a central role in intercellular communication, modulating processes such as immune evasion, angiogenesis, and metastatic colonization [30]. Nonetheless, technical challenges remain in EV isolation and characterization, with ultracentrifugation, chromatography, and microfluidics being among the most frequently applied approaches [31].

Noncoding RNAs (ncRNAs) further broaden the spectrum of circulating biomarkers. Small ncRNAs, including microRNAs (miRNAs), piwi-interacting RNAs, and small interfering RNAs, as well as long noncoding RNAs (lncRNAs), regulate gene expression at multiple levels and are frequently dysregulated in cancer. miRNAs, in particular, are remarkably stable in biofluids and have been extensively studied as diagnostic and prognostic markers, while lncRNAs hold significant regulatory potential but face challenges related to stability and detection. Both classes can circulate freely or within EVs, the latter enhancing their stability. Analytical methods for ncRNAs include RT-qPCR, microarrays, and small RNA sequencing, though issues such as RNase activity and low abundance necessitate optimized protocols [32, 33].

Finally, tumor-educated platelets (TEPs) represent an emerging and highly innovative biomarker. Platelets can be "reprogrammed" by tumor cells through direct interactions or secreted factors, leading to alterations in their RNA transcriptome that reflect the presence and molecular features of the tumor. Studies have demonstrated that platelet RNA signatures can discriminate cancer patients from healthy individuals, identify the tissue of origin, and detect actionable mutations such as *EGFR*, *KRAS*, or *MET*. TEPs offer practical advantages, as platelets are abundant, stable, and easily accessible from peripheral blood. However, analytical complexity, bioinformatic requirements, and potential confounders such as inflammation or thrombosis remain important limitations [34, 35].

In summary, circulating biomarkers encompass a diverse range of tumor-derived materials—cfDNA/ctDNA, CTCs, EVs, ncRNAs, and TEPs—that collectively provide a dynamic portrait of tumor biology. Their integration into clinical practice promises to enhance early detection, therapeutic stratification, and longitudinal disease monitoring.

Circulating Biomarkers

- *ctDNA*: Key tool for mutation, methylation, and fragmentomic analysis,
- *CTCs*: Reflect metastatic potential, prognostic, and predictive roles.
- *EVs*: Carry tumor-derived DNA, RNA, proteins; role in communication and resistance.
- *ncRNAs (miRNAs, lncRNAs)*: Stable, regulatory, potential diagnostic/prognostic markers,
- *TEPs*: Emerging analytes with RNA profiles mirroring tumor biology.

Phases of Sample Analysis

The analytical process of LB is not limited to the technical detection of tumor-derived analytes but rather unfolds through a sequence of interconnected steps that collectively determine the accuracy, sensitivity, and clinical reliability of the results. These can be broadly divided into three essential phases—pre-analytical, analytical, and post-analytical—each of which presents unique challenges and requires rigorous standardization to ensure reproducibility and clinical utility.

Pre-analytical Phase

The pre-analytical phase is crucial, as variability at this stage can significantly compromise downstream analyses. It encompasses all activities preceding the actual analysis, including sample collection, stabilization, storage, transport, and preparation of the biofluid. For plasma-based cfDNA/ctDNA analysis, the choice of collection tube is a critical determinant. While conventional EDTA tubes are widely used, they necessitate centrifugation within 1–2 h to prevent leukocyte lysis and subsequent contamination with genomic DNA, which may dilute the tumor-derived fraction [36, 37]. To mitigate this risk, specialized stabilizing tubes (e.g., Streck Cell-Free DNA BCT, PAXgene®, Roche cfDNA Collection Tubes) containing agents that inhibit cell lysis are increasingly employed, extending processing times to 48–72 h [38]. However, their higher cost remains a limitation for routine use. Following separation, plasma should be stored at −80 °C to maintain cfDNA integrity, with repeated freeze–thaw cycles strictly avoided [39]. RNA-based analytes, such as miRNAs or lncRNAs, are even more fragile due to RNase activity, requiring meticulous handling and rapid stabilization [32]. Centrifugation protocols also play a decisive role, with a double-spin strategy—initially at low speed to remove blood cells, followed by high-speed centrifugation to eliminate platelets and cellular debris—being the standard to minimize contamination with non-tumor nucleic acids [40]. Similar principles apply to other biofluids such as urine, pleural effusion, or cerebrospinal fluid, although standardized protocols are less well established. The lack of harmonization across laboratories remains one of the main barriers to widespread implementation, prompting international consortia and societies such as ESMO to promote initiatives for pre-analytical standardization [1].

Analytical Phase

The analytical phase encompasses the technical methodologies used to identify and quantify circulating biomarkers. The choice of platform is dictated by the analyte, the clinical question, and the required sensitivity. For ctDNA, analytical approaches can be broadly categorized into targeted assays of high sensitivity, such as droplet digital PCR (ddPCR), suitable for detecting specific known hotspot mutations at allele frequencies as low as 0.1%, and broad genomic assays such as NGS, capable of interrogating multiple genes or even the entire exome [41, 42]. Amplicon-based NGS is rapid and sensitive for defined targets, whereas hybrid-capture strategies enable wider coverage, including detection of novel or complex variants such as fusions and copy number alterations [43, 44]. The incorporation of unique molecular identifiers (UMIs) and error-suppression algorithms has become standard practice to distinguish true low-frequency variants from sequencing artifacts [45]. For ctDNA, analytical approaches can be broadly categorized into targeted assays of high sensitivity, such as droplet digital PCR (ddPCR), suitable for detecting specific known hotspot mutations at allele frequencies as low as 0.1%, and broad genomic assays such as NGS, capable of interrogating multiple genes or even the entire exome [41, 42]. dPCR represents an evolution of conventional PCR, relying on the binary detection of amplification signals within thousands of micro-reactors according to the Poisson distribution. This compartmentalization allows for the absolute quantification of mutant alleles even in the presence of a large wild-type background, enabling the reliable detection of variants at a VAF below 1.0%. Results can be expressed as absolute copy number, allelic fraction, or fractional abundance, though interpretation often requires expert evaluation, particularly for borderline findings [46, 47]. Its main limitation lies in the restricted number of loci interrogated, which makes it most useful for highly sensitive monitoring of known alterations rather than broad discovery. NGS, by contrast, enables the simultaneous analysis of multiple genomic targets, ranging from targeted panels to whole-exome or even whole-genome sequencing. It not only detects SNVs, indels, CNVs, and structural variants but also identifies novel alterations and complex fusions that cannot be captured by dPCR. Advanced methods—such as tagged-amplicon sequencing (TAm-Seq and eTAm-Seq™), Safe-SeqS, CAPP-Seq, and AmpliSeq—have achieved sensitivities down to 0.02–0.25% VAF, depending on the context, with improved accuracy through the incorporation of unique molecular identifiers (UMIs) and robust bioinformatics pipelines. Despite its breadth, the sensitivity of NGS may vary by alteration type, and false positives remain a challenge without stringent error-suppression strategies [43–45]. The complementary use of dPCR and NGS thus enables tailoring of the analytical approach to the clinical scenario: dPCR for precise, cost-effective detection of low-frequency known mutations, and NGS for comprehensive genomic profiling and discovery of resistance mechanisms. For other biomarkers, diverse techniques are required: CTCs are typically enriched using immunomagnetic or microfluidic platforms (e.g., CellSearch®, Parsortix®) and subsequently characterized through immunophenotyping or single-cell sequencing [48]; EVs are studied through nanoparticle tracking analysis, ELISA, RT-qPCR, or RNA sequencing [49]; noncoding RNAs are analyzed with RT-qPCR, microarray, or small RNA-seq platforms [32]; and TEPs require transcriptome profiling with advanced RNA-seq and bioinformatics pipelines [34]. The overarching challenge in this phase is the low abundance of tumor-derived material against a background of non-neoplastic nucleic acids and vesicles, demanding both ultrasensitive detection technologies and rigorous quality controls. Internal standards, reference materials, and validated bioinformatics workflows are indispensable for ensuring analytical accuracy and reproducibility [50].

Post-analytical Phase

The post-analytical phase transforms raw data into clinically actionable insights, encompassing interpretation, validation, and reporting. Interpretation requires careful consideration of variant allele frequency, sample quality, type of molecular alteration (point mutation, indel, rearrangement, or methylation pattern), and the patient's clinical context. A major challenge is distinguishing tumor-derived alterations from clonal hematopoiesis of indeterminate potential (CHIP) or other benign conditions, which may give rise to false positives, particularly in genes such as *DNMT3A*, *TET2*, and *ASXL1* [51]. Defining appropriate thresholds for allele frequency is critical to avoid overinterpretation of low-level or subclonal variants. Bioinformatic parameters—including sequencing depth, UMI concordance, and quality filters—must also be standardized and transparently reported. The clinical report should be concise yet comprehensive, including detected alterations, analytical method, assay sensitivity, and clinical implications, such as links to approved targeted therapies, eligibility for clinical trials, or prognostic significance. Ideally, interpretation should be undertaken by molecular pathology or precision oncology experts, as the implications often extend to treatment decision-making. Importantly, results should be discussed within a multidisciplinary framework, such as a molecular tumor board, where integration with histopathology, radiology, and clinical data maximizes the clinical value of LB findings [52, 53].

In summary, the analytical process of LB is a multistep continuum where each phase—from sample collection to final reporting—can profoundly influence clinical reliability. Ensuring standardization, minimizing variability, and integrating results within a multidisciplinary context are essential prerequisites for the successful translation of LB into routine oncology practice.

Phases of sample analysis

- *Pre-analytical:* Sample collection/processing critical; lack of harmonization is a barrier.
- *Analytical*: dPCR (high sensitivity, limited scope) vs. NGS (comprehensive profiling). Other analytes require specific methods (CTCs, EVs, ncRNAs, TEPs).
- *Post-analytical*: Interpretation, reporting, and integration into multidisciplinary tumor boards; CHIP remains a confounding factor.

Clinical Applications

LB has rapidly transitioned from a primarily research-focused technology to a clinically relevant tool that complements and, in selected contexts, substitutes tissue biopsy. By enabling minimally invasive, real-time access to the molecular landscape of cancer, it supports decision-making across multiple disease stages—from targeted therapy selection in metastatic settings to the detection of MRD and recurrence and even to early detection [5] (Fig. 19.1) (Table 19.2).

Metastatic Setting: Targeted Therapy Selection

In the metastatic setting, through ctDNA and other circulating biomarkers, clinicians can identify actionable mutations to guide targeted therapy selection, monitor the emergence of resistance mechanisms, and evaluate treatment response dynamically. This capacity makes LB a crucial tool for optimizing therapeutic strategies across multiple tumor types, in line with international guidelines such as ESMO, ASCO, NCCN, and AIOM [1, 9].

Non-small Cell Lung Cancer (NSCLC)

In advanced NSCLC, LB has gained a central role in clinical practice and is now recommended as part of the standard diagnostic algorithm, especially when tissue is insufficient or inaccessible. ctDNA analysis reliably detects clinically relevant alterations, including *EGFR*, *ALK*, *ROS1*, *KRAS p.G12C*, *BRAF p.V600*, and *TP53*, aligning with ESMO's precision medicine recommendations [1]. ctDNA testing is endorsed for all non-squamous NSCLC and selected squamous cases when tissue is not feasible or is non-

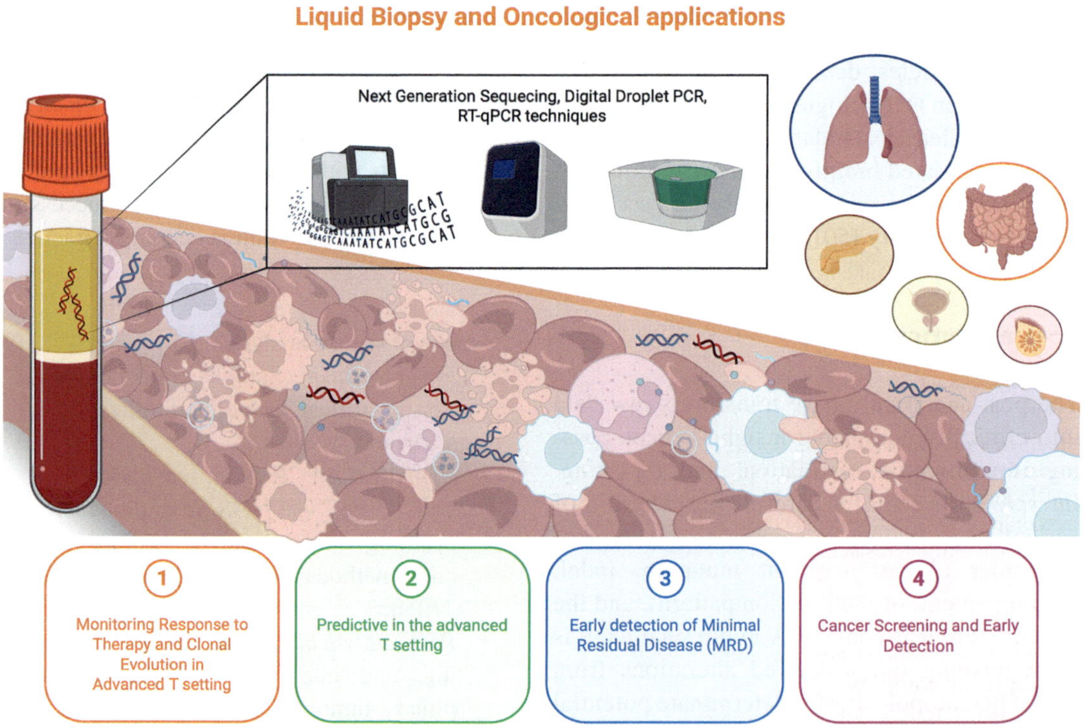

Fig. 19.1 Clinical applications of liquid biopsy across the cancer continuum: Liquid biopsy provides minimally invasive, real-time access to tumor-derived biomarkers, supporting clinical decision-making in different contexts: (i) targeted therapy selection in metastatic disease, (ii) detection of minimal residual disease (MRD) and recurrence monitoring, and (iii) early cancer detection and screening in high-risk populations. Integration of circulating tumor DNA (ctDNA), circulating tumor cells (CTCs), extracellular vesicles (EVs), and other analytes enables a comprehensive approach to precision oncology

Table 19.2 Recommendations for the use of liquid biopsy in clinical practice: genes to analyze and associated tumor types

Tumor	Gene (type of alteration)	Recommendation for ctDNA analysis
NSCLC	*EGFR* (mutations) *ALK* (fusions and acquired tyrosine kinase domain mutations) *MET* (mutations) *ROS1* (fusions and acquired resistance mutations) *KRAS p.G12C* *BRAF p.V600*	Recommended in treatment-naïve patients or in progression after TKI, only if tissue is not available or a rapid therapeutic decision is required
BC	*PIK3CA* (mutations) *ESR1* (mutations)	Recommended for second-line therapeutic choice in patients progressing after CDK4/6 inhibitors + endocrine therapy
CRC	*BRAF p.V600* (mutations) *KRAS/NRAS* (exon 2/3/4 mutations)	*KRAS/NRAS/BRAFV600E* in chemo-naïve patients only if tissue is not available or a rapid therapeutic decision is required *KRAS/NRAS/BRAF* in pretreated patients if considering anti-EGFR rechallenge
Cholangiocarcinoma	*IDH1* (mutations) *FGFR2* (fusions) *BRAF p.V600* (mutations)	Recommended only if tissue is not available or a rapid therapeutic decision is required
Urothelial carcinoma	*FGFR* (mutations) *FGFR3* (*FGFR3-TACC3*, mutations)	Recommended only if tissue is not available or not assessable
Thyroid carcinoma	*BRAF* (mutations) *RET* (mutations)	Recommended only if tissue is not available or not assessable
Tumors with MSI alterations (BC, GC, OC, PanC, PrC, CRC, cholangiocarcinoma, endometrium)	MSI (instability)	Recommended only if tissue is not available or not assessable
Tumors with *BRCA1/2* alterations (PrC, BC, OC, PanC)	*BRCA1-2* (mutations)	Recommended only if tissue is not available or not assessable
Tumors with *ERBB2* alterations (NSCLC, BC, GC)	*ERBB2* (mutations and amplifications)	Recommended only if tissue is not available or not assessable
Tumors with *NTRK* alterations (NSCLC, BC, GC, PanC, cholangiocarcinoma, urothelial, soft tissue sarcoma, thyroid)	*NTRK1-2-3* (mutations)	Recommended only if tissue is not available or a rapid therapeutic decision is required

Modified from "ESMO recommendations on the use of circulating tumour DNA assays for patients with cancer: a report from the ESMO Precision Medicine Working Group" [1]
ctDNA circulating tumor DNA, *NSCLC* non-small cell lung cancer, *BC* breast cancer, *CRC* colorectal cancer, *CT* chemotherapy, *PrC* prostate cancer, *OC* ovarian cancer, *PanC* pancreatic cancer, *GC* gastric cancer, *HCC* hepatocellular carcinoma, *MSI* microsatellite instability

diagnostic; while tissue remains the reference standard for complex events (e.g., MET exon 14 skipping). LB is a robust alternative or complement, with studies showing comparable sensitivity when the circulating tumor fraction is ≥1% [54]. Beyond static genotyping, dynamic ctDNA metrics carry prognostic and predictive weight: In FLAURA2, baseline ctDNA detectability correlated with poorer outcomes, whereas early ctDNA clearance (within ~3 weeks) associated with better responses and longer PFS, supporting ctDNA as a tool to triage patients toward intensified first-line regimens [55]. MARIPOSA reinforced this concept: Patients with high-risk biology (such as positive baseline ctDNA and/or *TP53* co-mutations) seemed to derive greater benefit from amivantamab plus lazertinib versus osimertinib alone, positioning LB to inform up-front treatment selection between standard and "boosted" strategies [56]. Additional layers are emerging from other analytes. CTC kinetics and phenotypes predict outcomes (e.g., CTONG1202 linked post-cycle CTC clearance to longer survival, whereas persistent CTCs or CTC–WBC clusters signaled resistance) [57]. EVs contribute both DNA and RNA cargo: *EGFR* alterations in EV-DNA from bronchoalveolar lavage concord with tissue, and dynamic EV-protein changes (e.g., in LEXOVE) track treatment response; and EV-borne miRNAs/lncRNAs also participate in acquired resistance to EGFR-TKIs [58, 59]. In immunotherapy-eligible, non-oncogene-addicted NSCLC, early ctDNA declines predict improved survival, blood-based TMB (bTMB) has shown predictive value in trials such as POPLAR and OAK, and PD-L1 expression on CTCs or EV-associated signatures may refine risk stratification [59, 60].

Colorectal Cancer (CRC)

In metastatic CRC, ctDNA testing for *RAS*, *BRAF*, and *EGFR* mutations is essential to guide rechallenge with anti-EGFR therapy. AIOM and ESMO guidelines recommend LB in cases where tissue is unavailable or inadequate, with tissue confirmation required in ctDNA-negative cases to avoid false negatives [1]. Importantly, LB enables dynamic monitoring of clonal evolution and supports rechallenge strategies. The CRICKET study linked RAS wild-type status in plasma at rechallenge to superior PFS with cetuximab–irinotecan [61]. CAPRI-2 GOIM further showed that, in RAS/BRAF wild-type patients receiving FOLFIRI plus cetuximab, a resistance-mutation–negative ctDNA baseline aligned with >75% ORR and prolonged PFS; notably, 80% retained wild-type status at progression, supporting reexposure to anti-EGFR with an alternative chemotherapy backbone [62]. PLATFORM-B introduced tumor-agnostic ctDNA monitoring to classify early molecular responders versus progressors, enabling adaptive escalation or de-escalation [63]. Beyond *RAS/BRAF*, ctDNA is being validated for MSI detection, guiding immunotherapy in MSI-high tumors and offering insight into hereditary syndromes such as Lynch, despite challenges in low-shedding cases [64].

Cholangiocarcinoma (CCA)

For cholangiocarcinoma, LB has emerged as an important complement to tissue testing, especially in patients where invasive biopsy is not feasible. ctDNA enables detection of actionable alterations such as *FGFR2* fusions and *IDH1* mutations, with high concordance to tissue (reported up to ~92%). In FOENIX-CCA2, ctDNA detected *FGFR2* fusions in about 85% of cases and supported futibatinib selection; longitudinal profiling uncovered on-target resistance (e.g., *FGFR2 V565F*, *N550K*) predating radiographic progression [65]. Baseline ctDNA burden associates with poorer PFS/OS, and *KRAS G12/13* positivity—especially with elevated CA19-9—portends worse outcomes. EV-derived protein panels (e.g., CRP/FIBRINOGEN/FRIL) have also correlated with survival, while serial VAF tracking in *IDH1/2*-mutant iCCA helps gauge response and emergent resistance (e.g., *ARID1A, TP53*) [66, 67].

Prostate Cancer (PC)

In metastatic prostate cancer, particularly mCRPC, LB plays a crucial role in identifying homologous recombination repair (HRR) gene mutations, especially *BRCA1/2*, when tissue is often associated with biopsy failure rates up to ~31% [68]. PROfound study validated FoundationOne Liquid CDx, showing ~80% concordance with tissue for *BRCA1/2* and *ATM* and comparable clinical outcomes; nonetheless, analytical failure remains notable (~20%) in low-shedding patients [69]. ctDNA also reveals resistance biology: TALAPRO-1 identified *BRCA2* reversion mutations and PARP1 involvement under talazoparib; higher ctDNA fractions predict faster progression on hormonal therapy; and AR copy-number gains and mutations emerge in >50% under AR-pathway inhibitors, heralding resistance [70]. CTC enumeration is prognostic for OS and response, and AR splice variants detected on CTCs provide real-time insight into endocrine escape [71, 72].

Breast Cancer

In metastatic breast cancer, LB efficiently captures subclonal heterogeneity and therapy-induced evolution. Plasma testing for *ESR1* and *PIK3CA* is guideline-supported after CDK4/6 inhibitor plus endocrine therapy: EMERALD validated ctDNA-based ESR1 detection to select elacestrant, and SOLAR-1 established ctDNA *PIK3CA* testing to identify candidates for alpelisib, even at low tumor fractions [73, 74]. Parallelly, the CAPItello-291 trial established capivasertib plus fulvestrant as a standard option after progression on ET, with significant PFS benefit in patients with tumors harboring *PIK3CA*, *AKT1*, or *PTEN* alterations (7.2 vs 3.6 mo, HR = 0.60; 95% CI, 0.51–0.71; $P < 0.001$) [75]. A large retrospective study of paired tissue and plasma samples confirmed that blood-based NGS reliably detects *PIK3CA/AKT1/PTEN* short variants when the ctDNA tumor fraction is ≥1%, with positive percent agreement above 90%; however, tissue testing remains advisable in cases of low ctDNA shedding (<1%) or for CNVs such as PTEN homozygous deletions [76]. The phase III INAVO120 trial shifted first-line management: Inavolisib plus palbociclib and fulvestrant significantly improved PFS (~17.2 vs 7.3 months) and OS (~34 vs 27 months), leading to EMA approval; first-line ctDNA *PIK3CA* testing is now recommended to triage patients to inavolisib-containing regimens [77]. Serial ctDNA monitoring detects emergent *ESR1* mutations before imaging, enabling pre-emptive endocrine switches (PADA-1, SERENA-6) with marked PFS gains (11,9 vs 5,7 mo; HR = 0,61; p = 0,004 and 16,0 vs 9,2 mo; HR = 0,44; p < 0,0001, respectively) [78, 79]. In HER2-positive disease, ctDNA correlates strongly with tissue (concordance ~86.5%), and persistent high HER2 levels predict worse PFS [80]; CTC-based ERBB2 assays (sensitivity ~85%, specificity ~94%) support noninvasive surveillance [81]. cfDNA can also reveal somatic *BRCA1/2* alterations (~13.5% in metastatic BC), enriched among younger and TNBC patients, while *BRCA1*-mutant CTC functional assays indicate PARP-inhibitor sensitivity [82].

Ovarian Cancer

In metastatic or recurrent ovarian cancer, ctDNA is particularly useful for detecting somatic *BRCA1/2* variants in the absence of available tissue as well as for identifying *BRCA1/2* reversion mutations linked to platinum or PARP inhibitor resistance [1]. Importantly, ctDNA detects *BRCA1/2* reversion mutations— ~18% in platinum-refractory and ~13% in platinum-resistant high-grade disease—with high specificity, flagging on-treatment restoration of homologous recombination and impending resistance to PARP inhibitors or platinum [67].

Minimal Residual Disease (MRD) and Recurrence Monitoring: Adjuvant, Neoadjuvant/Perioperative

LB is rapidly emerging as a transformative tool for the detection of MRD, defined as the persistence of residual tumor cells after radical treatment, undetectable with conventional imaging. By enabling the identification of ctDNA after surgery or systemic therapy, LB provides an opportunity to anticipate recurrence, refine prognostic stratification, and guide therapeutic escalation/de-escalation in a personalized manner. Two major strategies are used for MRD detection: the tumor-informed approach, which tailors monitoring to specific genomic alterations identified in the primary tumor, and the tumor-agnostic approach, which uses predefined panels to detect ctDNA without prior tumor profiling [83]. The tumor-informed method offers superior sensitivity and specificity but requires an adequate tissue sample and longer turnaround times, while the tumor-agnostic approach is more broadly applicable but carries a higher risk of false negatives [84].

Adjuvant Setting

In the adjuvant setting, ctDNA has proven highly prognostic, identifying patients at risk of relapse earlier than radiological methods. The landmark DYNAMIC trial in stage II colorectal cancer showed that a ctDNA-guided de-escalation strategy safely reduced adjuvant chemotherapy use by 28% without compromising recurrence-free survival (RFS), which remained at 93.5% at 2 years among ctDNA-negative patients [85]. Conversely, in stage III disease, DYNAMIC-III tested escalation strategies for ctDNA-positive patients, randomizing over 960 participants. Although intensification (e.g., FOLFOXIRI) did not significantly improve 2-year RFS compared to standard care, ctDNA burden strongly correlated with prognosis: Patients with high mutational load had only 22% 3-year RFS, compared to 78% in those with low burden. These results underscore the quantitative as well as qualitative value of ctDNA in risk stratification [86]. Beyond colorectal cancer, adjuvant studies in NSCLC have highlighted the utility of MRD monitoring. In ADAURA, ctDNA positivity post-surgery in *EGFR*-mutated stage IB–IIIa NSCLC was linked to a markedly higher recurrence risk, and osimertinib improved DFS, especially in ctDNA-positive patients. Molecular recurrence typically preceded radiological relapse by 4.7 months, suggesting a window for early therapeutic intervention [87]. Similarly, in high-risk early breast cancer, *monarchE* showed that persistent ctDNA during abemaciclib plus endocrine therapy predicted early relapse, whereas ctDNA clearance aligned with improved PFS [88]. In urothelial cancer, IMvigor010 found that ctDNA positivity after cystectomy identified patients most likely to benefit from adjuvant atezolizumab, while ctDNA-negative patients did not derive significant benefit [89]. Finally, in pancreatic cancer, meta-analyses confirm that ctDNA positivity post-surgery correlates with shortened RFS, supporting its potential to guide adjuvant treatment intensification in high-risk patients [90].

Neoadjuvant and Perioperative Setting

In the neoadjuvant and perioperative settings, LB offers a dynamic means to assess treatment response and guide preemptive strategies. In CheckMate 816, platinum-based chemotherapy achieved higher ctDNA clearance before surgery compared to nivolumab–ipilimumab (33% vs. 11%), suggesting a dominant cytotoxic effect on circulating tumor clones. Nonetheless, immunotherapy provided superior long-term outcomes, with significantly improved event-free survival (54.8 vs 20.9 months) and higher pCR rates (20.4% vs 4.6%) [91]. Likewise, in breast cancer, exploratory analyses of the I-SPY2 trial showed that ctDNA clearance during neoadjuvant chemotherapy predicted higher pCR rates and improved recurrence-free survival, particularly in triple-negative disease. These findings underscore the potential of ctDNA as an early surrogate for treatment efficacy. Perioperative trials have further validated this approach. CheckMate 77 T and NADIM demonstrated that perioperative nivolumab plus chemotherapy in resectable NSCLC significantly increased ctDNA clearance compared with chemotherapy alone, translating into durable PFS and OS gains: In NADIM, 5-year PFS and OS were 85% and 92% among patients with ctDNA clearance, compared with 61% and 59% in those with persistent ctDNA [92, 93]. The AEGEAN trial with durvalumab plus chemotherapy further confirmed that presurgical ctDNA clearance predicted prolonged EFS, with early clearance (by cycle 2) showing a $\geq$ 89% negative predictive value for recurrence [94].

Collectively, these studies demonstrate that ctDNA analysis not only refines prognostic assessment but also enables MRD-directed escalation and de-escalation strategies in both adjuvant and perioperative contexts.

Early Detection

Currently, only a limited number of solid tumors—such as lung, breast, colorectal, cervical, and prostate cancer—have evidence-based, guideline-recommended screening programs. Conversely, many of the cancers associated with the poorest prognosis, including pancreatic, ovarian, and liver cancer, lack established strategies for early detection. In this context, LB represents a promising opportunity to overcome the limitations of current approaches, allowing the identification of malignancies at preclinical stages through a simple blood draw. The rationale is clear: Long-term survival is strongly linked to stage at diagnosis, and detecting a tumor in its localized phase—before metastatic dissemination—enables curative treatment in a much larger proportion of patients [23, 95–99].

An area of rapid development is represented by multi-cancer early detection (MCED) tests, designed to simultaneously identify multiple tumor types from a single blood sample. CancerSEEK [100] was one of the first assays to combine ctDNA mutational analysis with plasma protein measurement, achieving very high specificity (>99%) and stage-dependent sensitivity across several tumor types, including ovary and liver, which currently lack standard screening. The Galleri test by GRAIL, based on cfDNA methylation signatures across more than 100,000 loci, can also infer the tissue of origin. Preliminary data reported sensitivity of 16.8% at stage I and 40.4% at stage II, with specificity of 99.5% [101]. In the PATHFINDER study, 1.4% of >6600 individuals ≥50 years tested positive, but only 38% had a confirmed cancer, raising concerns about false positives, downstream anxiety, and unnecessary investigations [102]. These challenges highlight the balance between sensitivity, specificity, and clinical utility in population-based screening.

Alongside MCEDs, organ-specific assays are also advancing. In colorectal cancer, Epi proColon®, a PCR-based test detecting Sept9 methylation, has been FDA-approved for average-risk individuals unwilling to undergo conventional screening. While its sensitivity is similar to fecal immunochemical testing (70–75%) and specificity lower, it may improve adherence among historically noncompliant populations [103]. The Shield™ test, validated in the large ECLIPSE study, combines cfDNA mutation, methylation, and fragmentation profiling, reaching 83.1% sensitivity for CRC (87.5% in stage I–III) and 89.6% specificity for advanced neoplasia, though sensitivity for precancerous lesions remained modest (13.2%) [104].

In ovarian cancer, integrating fragmentomics with established biomarkers has shown promise. DELFI-Pro combined cfDNA fragmentation features with CA-125 and HE4, yielding sensitivities of 72% and 69% for stage I and II tumors, respectively, while maintaining specificity >99%. Importantly, it distinguished malignant from benign ovarian masses with an AUC of 0.88, suggesting utility for both early detection and preoperative risk stratification [105].

In lung cancer, fragmentomic approaches are emerging as powerful complements to low-dose CT screening. In a prospective study of 296 symptomatic individuals referred for suspected lung cancer, median DELFI scores were significantly higher in patients with confirmed cancer compared to those without (0.94 vs 0.19; $p < 0.001$), improving diagnostic accuracy when combined with age, smoking history, and symptoms (AUC rising from 0.74 to 0.94) [106].

Despite encouraging results, integration of LB into population screening requires further prospective validation, robust cost-effectiveness analyses, and clearly defined clinical pathways for individuals with positive tests but no radiologic or clinical confirmation. LB thus represents a frontier with potential to revolutionize early detection, but careful implementation will be critical to maximize benefit and minimize harm.

Clinical Applications

- *Metastatic setting*: LB informs targeted therapy selection across cancers (NSCLC, CRC, CCA, prostate, breast, ovarian). It guides treatment, resistance detection, and dynamic monitoring.
- *MRD and recurrence*: ctDNA predicts relapse earlier than imaging and enables escalation/de-escalation of adjuvant/neoadjuvant therapy.
- *Early detection*: Multicancer early detection (MCED) tests (e.g., CancerSEEK, Galleri) and organ-specific assays show promise, though challenges remain in sensitivity, specificity, and cost-effectiveness.

From Single to Multiplex: Current Challenges and Future Perspectives

The detection of ctDNA in LB presents unique technical challenges, since tumor-derived DNA often represents <1% of total circulating DNA. This necessitates the use of highly sensitive methodologies, which can broadly be divided into single-plex assays, such as dPCR, and multiplex sequencing approaches, primarily NGS. Each technology offers distinct advantages and limitations, and in clinical practice, they are best regarded as complementary rather than mutually exclusive [107, 108].

Single-plex assays like ddPCR and BEAMing partition DNA into thousands of individual reactions, allowing absolute quantification based on Poisson statistics [109, 110]. Their main strength is sensitivity, reliably detecting mutant allele frequencies as low as 0.01–0.1% [54]. This makes them ideal for longitudinal monitoring of known alterations, MRD detection, and the identification of well-characterized hotspot mutations such as *EGFR T790M* in NSCLC, *KRAS* mutations in colorectal cancer, or *ESR1* mutations in breast cancer [111–113]. They are also cost-effective, rapid, and require minimal bioinformatics support, features that make them suitable for routine implementation in smaller referral centers with limited infrastructure. However, the major limitation of dPCR is its narrow scope: It can only interrogate mutations for which primers are designed, making it unsuitable for comprehensive profiling or the discovery of novel alterations. Multiplexing capacity is limited, and expanding coverage requires multiple assays, which increases cost and complexity [111].

In contrast, multiplex sequencing approaches based on NGS allow for broad genomic profiling across many genes simultaneously. FDA-approved assays such as Guardant360 CDx (74 genes) and FoundationOne Liquid CDx (324 genes) exemplify this strategy [114]. NGS detects a wide range of variant types, including single-nucleotide variants, indels, copy number changes, and fusions while also enabling more sophisticated analyses such as tumor mutational burden (TMB) and homologous recombination deficiency (HRD) scores [115, 116]. Advances such as UMIs, error-correction algorithms, and hybrid-capture technologies have markedly improved analytical sensitivity, allowing detection of low-frequency variants at VAFs approaching 0.01% [117]. However, broad-panel NGS is resource-intensive, with higher costs, longer turnaround times, and increased complexity of data interpretation [118]. Beyond targeted panels, whole-exome sequencing (WES) and whole-genome sequencing (WGS) represent the most comprehensive multiplex strategies. WES enables capture of mutations across all coding regions, while WGS extends coverage to noncoding regions, structural variants, and genome-wide mutational signatures, providing unparalleled breadth for discovery research and biomarker development, such as fragmentomics and methylation, which are emerging as powerful tools for early detection [119]. In real-world settings, broad panels may identify alterations with uncertain clinical utility, raising questions about cost-effectiveness. Consequently, international guidelines such as those from IASLC recommend validated, tumor-specific targeted NGS panels—covering key actionable alterations—over indiscriminate use of large panels in routine practice [54].

Clinically, a pragmatic strategy should be adopted: Single-gene PCR-based testing may be used initially in high-prevalence settings or when NGS is unavailable, but negative results should prompt reflex testing with NGS to avoid missing actionable targets. Similarly, dPCR is increasingly used as an orthogonal technology to validate NGS findings near the detection threshold. In summary, dPCR excels in sensitivity and speed for known alterations, while NGS enables comprehensive profiling and translational research.

Looking ahead, the integration of LB with artificial intelligence (AI) and machine learning (ML) has the potential to markedly enhance sensitivity, specificity, and clinical interpretability. Advanced algorithms can extract subtle and clinically meaningful signals from circulating analytes—including cfDNA, cfRNA, miRNAs, and extracellular vesicles—even in low-abundance contexts, thereby improving early diagnostic accuracy and patient risk stratification [120]. At the same time, automation of workflows, miniaturization of NGS platforms, and decentralized testing models promise to expand access, particularly in resource-limited settings where equitable implementation remains a key challenge [121]. A particularly transformative development is represented by the multi-omic approach, which integrates genomic, epigenomic, transcriptomic, and fragmentomic information into a unified framework. This strategy offers superior diagnostic power compared with single-analyte assays, especially in early-stage disease where circulating tumor material is scarce. Multi-omic LB tests are already demonstrating encouraging results in cancer screening and MRD detection while also providing a more comprehensive view of tumor heterogeneity and dynamic evolution under therapeutic pressure [100, 122].

Finally, the application of LB to cancer interception—the identification and intervention on premalignant lesions in high-risk individuals—opens entirely new perspectives for oncology prevention, enabling proactive and personalized strategies well before clinical manifestation of disease [123].

In conclusion, LB is evolving from a complementary test to a dynamic, versatile platform central to precision oncology. To unlock its full potential, large-scale prospective studies, regulatory harmonization, and sustainable reimbursement frameworks will be essential, ensuring that its benefits can be realized across diverse healthcare systems worldwide.

From Single- to Multiplex: Current Challenges and Future Perspectives

- dPCR and NGS are complementary: dPCR for known mutations, NGS for broad profiling,
- Integration of AI/ML, automation, and decentralized testing will expand clinical use.
- Multi-omic LB approaches (genomic, epigenomic, transcriptomic, fragmentomic) are emerging for screening, MRD, and cancer interception.
- Large-scale validation, regulatory harmonization, and reimbursement models are required for full clinical integration.

Declaration of Competing Interest The authors declare that they have no known competing financial interests or personal relationships that could have appeared to influence the work reported in this paper.

References

1. Pascual J, Attard G, Bidard FC, Curigliano G, De Mattos-Arruda L, Diehn M, et al. ESMO recommendations on the use of circulating tumour DNA assays for patients with cancer: a report from the ESMO precision medicine working group. Ann Oncol. 2022;33(8):750–68.
2. Lone SN, Nisar S, Masoodi T, Singh M, Rizwan A, Hashem S, et al. Liquid biopsy: a step closer to transform diagnosis, prognosis and future of cancer treatments. Mol Cancer. 2022;21(1):79.
3. Russano M, Napolitano A, Ribelli G, Iuliani M, Simonetti S, Citarella F, et al. Liquid biopsy and tumor heterogeneity in metastatic solid tumors: the potentiality of blood samples. J Exp Clin Cancer Res. 2020;39(1):95.
4. Sánchez-Herrero E, Serna-Blasco R, Robado de Lope L, González-Rumayor V, Romero A, Provencio M. Circulating tumor DNA as a cancer biomarker: an overview of biological features and factors that may impact on ctDNA analysis. Front Oncol. 2022;12:943253.
5. Ma L, Guo H, Zhao Y, Liu Z, Wang C, Bu J, et al. Liquid biopsy in cancer current: status, challenges

and future prospects. Signal Transduct Target Ther. 2024;9(1):336.

6. Santos V, Freitas C, Fernandes MG, Sousa C, Reboredo C, Cruz-Martins N, et al. Liquid biopsy: the value of different bodily fluids. Biomark Med. 2022;16(2):127–45.
7. Gilson P, Merlin JL, Harlé A. Deciphering tumour heterogeneity: from tissue to liquid biopsy. Cancers (Basel). 2022;14(6):1384.
8. Pantel K, Alix-Panabières C. Minimal residual disease as a target for liquid biopsy in patients with solid tumours. Nat Rev Clin Oncol. 2025;22(1):65–77.
9. Aredo JV, Jamali A, Zhu J, Heater N, Wakelee HA, Vaklavas C, et al. Liquid biopsy approaches for cancer characterization, residual disease detection, and therapy monitoring. Am Soc Clin Oncol Educ Book. 2025;45(3):e481114.
10. Sassorossi C, Evangelista J, Stefani A, Chiappetta M, Martino A, Campanella A, et al. The role of ctDNA for diagnosis and histological prediction in early stage non-small-cell lung cancer: a narrative review. Diagnostics (Basel). 2025;15(7):904.
11. Maass KK, Schad PS, Finster AME, Puranachot P, Rosing F, Wedig T, et al. From sampling to sequencing: a liquid biopsy pre-analytic workflow to maximize multi-layer genomic information from a single tube. Cancers (Basel). 2021;13(12):3002.
12. Martella S, Wekking D, Lai E, Lambertini M, Pettinato A, Parrino A, et al. Liquid biopsy: an innovative tool in oncology. Where do we stand? Semin Oncol. 2025;52(2):152343.
13. Batool SM, Yekula A, Khanna P, Hsia T, Gamblin AS, Ekanayake E, et al. The liquid biopsy consortium: challenges and opportunities for early cancer detection and monitoring. Cell Rep Med. 2023;4(10):101198.
14. Baburaj G, Damerla RR, Udupa KS, Parida P, Munisamy M, Kolesar J, et al. Liquid biopsy approaches for pleural effusion in lung cancer patients. Mol Biol Rep. 2020;47(10):8179–87.
15. Escudero L, Martínez-Ricarte F, Seoane J. ctDNA-based liquid biopsy of cerebrospinal fluid in brain cancer. Cancers (Basel). 2021;13(9):1989.
16. Izhar M, Ahmad Z, Moazzam M, Jader A. Targeted liquid biopsy for brain tumors. J Liq Biopsy. 2024;6:100170.
17. Oshi M, Murthy V, Takahashi H, Huyser M, Okano M, Tokumaru Y, et al. Urine as a source of liquid biopsy for cancer. Cancers (Basel). 2021;13(11):2652.
18. Werner B, Yuwono N, Duggan J, Liu D, David C, Srirangan S, et al. Cell-free DNA is abundant in ascites and represents a liquid biopsy of ovarian cancer. Gynecol Oncol. 2021;162(3):720–7.
19. Kumar P, Gupta S, Das BC. Saliva as a potential non-invasive liquid biopsy for early and easy diagnosis/prognosis of head and neck cancer. Transl Oncol. 2024;40:101827.
20. Alcaide M, Cheung M, Hillman J, Rassekh SR, Deyell RJ, Batist G, et al. Evaluating the quantity, quality and size distribution of cell-free DNA by multiplex droplet digital PCR. Sci Rep. 2020;10(1):12564.
21. Kim H, Park KU. Clinical circulating tumor DNA testing for precision oncology. Cancer Res Treat. 2023;55(2):351–66.
22. Crucitta S, Ruglioni M, Novi C, Manganiello M, Arici R, Petrini I, et al. Comparison of digital PCR systems for the analysis of liquid biopsy samples of patients affected by lung and colorectal cancer. Clin Chim Acta. 2023;541:117239.
23. Bruhm DC, Vulpescu NA, Foda ZH, Phallen J, Scharpf RB, Velculescu VE. Genomic and fragmentomic landscapes of cell-free DNA for early cancer detection. Nat Rev Cancer. 2025;25(5):341–58.
24. Crosby D, Bhatia S, Brindle KM, Coussens LM, Dive C, Emberton M, et al. Early detection of cancer. Science. 2022;375(6586):eaay9040.
25. Gu X, Wei S, Lv X. Circulating tumor cells: from new biological insights to clinical practice. Signal Transduct Target Ther. 2024;9(1):226.
26. Ring A, Nguyen-Sträuli BD, Wicki A, Aceto N. Biology, vulnerabilities and clinical applications of circulating tumour cells. Nat Rev Cancer. 2023;23(2):95–111.
27. Eslami-S Z, Cortés-Hernández LE, Alix-Panabières C. Epithelial cell adhesion molecule: an anchor to isolate clinically relevant circulating tumor cells. Cells. 2020;9(8):1836.
28. Eslami-S Z, Cortés-Hernández LE, Thomas F, Pantel K, Alix-Panabières C. Functional analysis of circulating tumour cells: the KEY to understand the biology of the metastatic cascade. Br J Cancer. 2022;127(5):800–10.
29. Capuozzo M, Ferrara F, Santorsola M, Zovi A, Ottaiano A. Circulating tumor cells as predictive and prognostic biomarkers in solid tumors. Cells. 2023;12(22):2590.
30. Kumar MA, Baba SK, Sadida HQ, Marzooqi SA, Jerobin J, Altemani FH, et al. Extracellular vesicles as tools and targets in therapy for diseases. Signal Transduct Target Ther. 2024;9(1):27.
31. Zeng Y, Qiu Y, Jiang W, Shen J, Yao X, He X, et al. Biological features of extracellular vesicles and challenges. Front Cell Dev Biol. 2022;10:816698.
32. Toden S, Goel A. Non-coding RNAs as liquid biopsy biomarkers in cancer. Br J Cancer. 2022;126(3):351–60.
33. Ghani MU, Du L, Moqbel AQ, Zhao E, Cui H, Yang L, et al. Exosomal ncRNAs in liquid biopsy: a new paradigm for early cancer diagnosis and monitoring. Front Oncol. 2025;15:1615433.
34. Gottardo A, Gristina V, Perez A, Di Giovanni E, Contino S, Barraco N, et al. Roles of tumor-educated platelets (TEPs) in the biology of non-small cell lung cancer (NSCLC): a systematic review. "Re-discovering the neglected biosources of the liquid biopsy family". J Liq Biopsy. 2024;3:100136.
35. Best MG, Sol N, Kooi I, Tannous J, Westerman BA, Rustenburg F, et al. RNA-Seq of tumor-educated

platelets enables blood-based pan-cancer, multi-class, and molecular pathway cancer diagnostics. Cancer Cell. 2015;28(5):666–76.
36. Kuligina ES, Yanus GA, Imyanitov EN. Improvement of the sensitivity of circulating tumor DNA-based liquid biopsy: current approaches and future perspectives. Explor Target Antitumor Ther. 2025;6:1002333.
37. Gerber T, Taschner-Mandl S, Saloberger-Sindhöringer L, Popitsch N, Heitzer E, Witt V, et al. Assessment of pre-analytical sample handling conditions for comprehensive liquid biopsy analysis. J Mol Diagn. 2020;22(8):1070–86.
38. Sorber L, Zwaenepoel K, Jacobs J, De Winne K, Van Casteren K, Augustus E, et al. Specialized blood collection tubes for liquid biopsy: improving the pre-analytical conditions. Mol Diagn Ther. 2020;24(1):113–24.
39. Malapelle U, Pisapia P, Addeo A, Arrieta O, Bellosillo B, Cardona AF, et al. Liquid biopsy from research to clinical practice: focus on non-small cell lung cancer. Expert Rev Mol Diagn. 2021;21(11):1165–78.
40. Ungerer V, Bronkhorst AJ, Holdenrieder S. Preanalytical variables that affect the outcome of cell-free DNA measurements. Crit Rev Clin Lab Sci. 2020;57(7):484–507.
41. Elazezy M, Joosse SA. Techniques of using circulating tumor DNA as a liquid biopsy component in cancer management. Comput Struct Biotechnol J. 2018;16:370–8.
42. Lin C, Liu X, Zheng B, Ke R, Tzeng CM. Liquid biopsy, ctDNA diagnosis through NGS. Life (Basel). 2021;11(9):890.
43. Gristina V, Russo TDB, Barraco N, Gottardo A, Pepe F, Russo G, et al. Clinical utility of ctDNA by amplicon based next generation sequencing in first line non small cell lung cancer patients. Sci Rep. 2024;14(1):22141.
44. Ryoo SB, Heo S, Lim Y, Lee W, Cho SH, Ahn J, et al. Personalised circulating tumour DNA assay with large-scale mutation coverage for sensitive minimal residual disease detection in colorectal cancer. Br J Cancer. 2023;129(2):374–81.
45. Heidrich I, Ačkar L, Mossahebi Mohammadi P, Pantel K. Liquid biopsies: potential and challenges. Int J Cancer. 2021;148(3):528–45.
46. Diehl JJ, Bennetto L, Young EC. Story recall and narrative coherence of high-functioning children with autism spectrum disorders. J Abnorm Child Psychol. 2006;34(1):87–102.
47. Chen H, An Y, Wang C, Zhou J. Circulating tumor DNA in colorectal cancer: biology, methods and applications. Discov Oncol. 2025;16(1):439.
48. Chen H, Li Y, Zhang Z, Wang S. Immunomagnetic separation of circulating tumor cells with microfluidic chips and their clinical applications. Biomicrofluidics. 2020;14(4):041502.
49. De Sousa KP, Rossi I, Abdullahi M, Ramirez MI, Stratton D, Inal JM. Isolation and characterization of extracellular vesicles and future directions in diagnosis and therapy. Wiley Interdiscip Rev Nanomed Nanobiotechnol. 2023;15(1):e1835.
50. Rolfo CD, Madison RW, Pasquina LW, Brown DW, Huang Y, Hughes JD, et al. Measurement of ctDNA tumor fraction identifies informative negative liquid biopsy results and informs value of tissue confirmation. Clin Cancer Res. 2024;30(11):2452–60.
51. Chan HT, Chin YM, Nakamura Y, Low SK. Clonal hematopoiesis in liquid biopsy: from biological noise to valuable clinical implications. Cancers (Basel). 2020;12(8):2277.
52. Malapelle U, Donne AD, Pagni F, Fraggetta F, Rocco EG, Pasello G, et al. Standardized and simplified reporting of next-generation sequencing results in advanced non-small-cell lung cancer: practical indications from an Italian multidisciplinary group. Crit Rev Oncol Hematol. 2024;193:104217.
53. Underhill HR. Leveraging the fragment length of circulating tumour DNA to improve molecular profiling of solid tumour malignancies with next-generation sequencing: a pathway to advanced non-invasive diagnostics in precision oncology? Mol Diagn Ther. 2021;25(4):389–408.
54. Rolfo C, Mack P, Scagliotti GV, Aggarwal C, Arcila ME, Barlesi F, et al. Liquid biopsy for advanced NSCLC: a consensus statement from the International Association for the Study of Lung Cancer. J Thorac Oncol. 2021;16(10):1647–62.
55. Jänne PA, Kobayashi K, Robichaux J, Lee CK, Sugawara S, Yang T-Y, et al. Abstract CT017: FLAURA2: exploratory analysis of baseline (BL) and on-treatment plasma EGFRm dynamics in patients (pts) with EGFRm advanced NSCLC treated with first-line (1L) osimertinib (osi) ± platinum-pemetrexed. Cancer Res. 2024;84(7_Supplement):CT017-CT.
56. Lee SH, Lu S, Hayashi H, Felip E, Spira AI, Girard N, et al. Lazertinib versus Osimertinib in previously untreated EGFR-mutant advanced NSCLC: a randomized, double-blind, Exploratory Analysis From MARIPOSA. J Thorac Oncol. 2025;20:1655.
57. Wang Z, Zhang XC, Feng WN, Zhang L, Liu XQ, Guo WB, et al. Circulating tumor cells dynamics during chemotherapy predict survival and response in advanced non-small-cell lung cancer patients. Ther Adv Med Oncol. 2023;15:17588359231167818.
58. Gristina V, Bazan V, Barraco N, Taverna S, Manno M, Raccosta S, et al. On-treatment dynamics of circulating extracellular vesicles in the first-line setting of patients with advanced non-small cell lung cancer: the LEXOVE prospective study. Mol Oncol. 2025;19(5):1422–35.
59. Peng XX, Yu R, Wu X, Wu SY, Pi C, Chen ZH, et al. Correlation of plasma exosomal microRNAs with the efficacy of immunotherapy in. J Immunother Cancer. 2020;8(1):e000376.
60. Kong D, Zhang W, Yang Z, Li G, Cheng S, Zhang K, et al. Correlation between PD-L1 expression ON CTCs and prognosis of patients with cancer: a

systematic review and meta-analysis. Onco Targets Ther. 2021;10(1):1938476.

61. Cremolini C, Rossini D, Dell'Aquila E, Lonardi S, Conca E, Del Re M, et al. Rechallenge for patients with RAS and BRAF wild-type metastatic colorectal cancer with acquired resistance to first-line cetuximab and irinotecan: a phase 2 single-arm clinical trial. JAMA Oncol. 2019;5(3):343–50.
62. Ciardiello D, Boscolo Bielo L, Napolitano S, Latiano TP, De Stefano A, Tamburini E, et al. Comprehensive genomic profiling by liquid biopsy portrays metastatic colorectal cancer mutational landscape to predict antitumor efficacy of FOLFIRI plus cetuximab in the CAPRI-2 GOIM trial. ESMO Open. 2025;10(4):104511.
63. Vidal J, Fernández-Rodríguez MC, Casadevall D, García-Alfonso P, Páez D, Guix M, et al. Liquid biopsy detects early molecular response and predicts benefit to first-line chemotherapy plus Cetuximab in metastatic colorectal cancer: PLATFORM-B study. Clin Cancer Res. 2023;29(2):379–88.
64. Tieng FYF, Abu N, Lee LH, Ab Mutalib NS. Microsatellite instability in colorectal cancer liquid biopsy-current updates on its potential in non-invasive detection, prognosis and as a predictive marker. Diagnostics (Basel). 2021;11(3):544.
65. Goyal L, DiToro D, Hollebecque A, Bridgewater JA, Shimura M, Kano A, et al. Genomic correlates of response and resistance to the irreversible FGFR1-4 inhibitor futibatinib based on biopsy and circulating tumor DNA profiling. Ann Oncol. 2025;36(4):414–25.
66. Thongyoo P, Chindaprasirt J, Aphivatanasiri C, Intarawichian P, Kunprom W, Kongpetch S, et al. Mutations in cholangiocarcinoma: prevalence, prognostic value, and. Cancer Genomics Proteomics. 2025;22(1):112–26.
67. Lin KK, Harrell MI, Oza AM, Oaknin A, Ray-Coquard I, Tinker AV, et al. Reversion mutations in circulating tumor DNA predict primary and acquired resistance to the PARP inhibitor Rucaparib in high-grade ovarian carcinoma. Cancer Discov. 2019;9(2):210–9.
68. Jeong SH, Kyung D, Yuk HD, Jeong CW, Lee W, Yoon JK, et al. Practical utility of liquid biopsies for evaluating genomic alterations in castration-resistant prostate cancer. Cancers (Basel). 2023;15(10):2847.
69. Matsubara N, de Bono J, Olmos D, Procopio G, Kawakami S, Ürün Y, et al. Olaparib efficacy in patients with metastatic castration-resistant prostate cancer and BRCA1, BRCA2, or ATM alterations identified by testing circulating tumor DNA. Clin Cancer Res. 2023;29(1):92–9.
70. Castro E, Laird D, Dorff T, Zhao S, van Oort IM, Gasparro D, et al. 1815P emergent circulating tumor DNA (ctDNA) variants and ctDNA burden dynamics with potential associations with talazoparib antitumor activity in TALAPRO-1. Ann Oncol. 2023;34:S983–S4.
71. Goldkorn A, Tangen C, Plets M, Bsteh D, Xu T, Pinski JK, et al. Circulating tumor cell count and overall survival in patients with metastatic hormone-sensitive prostate cancer. JAMA Netw Open. 2024;7(10):e2437871.
72. Miyamoto DT, Zheng Y, Wittner BS, Lee RJ, Zhu H, Broderick KT, et al. RNA-Seq of single prostate CTCs implicates noncanonical Wnt signaling in antiandrogen resistance. Science. 2015;349(6254):1351–6.
73. Bardia A, Aftimos P, Bihani T, Anderson-Villaluz AT, Jung J, Conlan MG, et al. EMERALD: phase III trial of elacestrant (RAD1901) vs endocrine therapy for previously treated ER+ advanced breast cancer. Future Oncol. 2019;15(28):3209–18.
74. Andre F, Ciruelos EM, Juric D, Loibl S, Campone M, Mayer IA, et al. Alpelisib plus fulvestrant for PIK3CA-mutated, hormone receptor-positive, human epidermal growth factor receptor-2-negative advanced breast cancer: final overall survival results from SOLAR-1. Ann Oncol. 2021;32(2):208–17.
75. Trapani D, Martins-Branco D, Curigliano G, Gennari A, Pentheroudakis G, Harbeck N. Updated treatment recommendations for systemic treatment: from the ESMO metastatic breast cancer living guideline†. Ann Oncol. 2025;36(11):1414–8.
76. Chaki M, Benrashid M, Puri S, Sivakumar S, Sokol ES, Briceno JM, et al. Retrospective comparison between breast cancer tissue- and blood-based next-generation sequencing results in detection of PIK3CA, AKT1, and PTEN alterations. Breast Cancer Res. 2025;27(1):122.
77. Turner NC, Im S-A, Saura C, Juric D, Loibl S, Kalinsky K, et al. INAVO120: phase III trial final overall survival (OS) analysis of first-line inavolisib (INAVO)/placebo (PBO) + palbociclib (PALBO) + fulvestrant (FULV) in patients (pts) with PIK3CA-mutated, hormone receptor-positive (HR+), HER2-negative (HER2–), endocrine-resistant advanced breast cancer (aBC). J Clin Oncol. 2025;43(16_suppl):1003.
78. Bidard FC, Hardy-Bessard AC, Dalenc F, Bachelot T, Pierga JY, de la Motte Rouge T, et al. Switch to fulvestrant and palbociclib versus no switch in advanced breast cancer with rising ESR1 mutation during aromatase inhibitor and palbociclib therapy (PADA-1): a randomised, open-label, multicentre, phase 3 trial. Lancet Oncol. 2022;23(11):1367–77.
79. Bidard FC, Mayer EL, Park YH, Janni W, Ma C, Cristofanilli M, et al. First-line Camizestrant for emerging. N Engl J Med. 2025;393(6):569–80.
80. Guan X, Liu B, Niu Y, Dong X, Zhu X, Li C, et al. Longitudinal HER2 amplification tracked in circulating tumor DNA for therapeutic effect monitoring and prognostic evaluation in patients with breast cancer. Breast. 2020;49:261–6.
81. Caro GD, Lam ET, Bourdon D, Blankfard M, Dharajiya N, Slade M, et al. A novel liquid biopsy assay for detection of *ERBB2* (HER2) amplification

in circulating tumor cells (CTCs). J Circ Biomark. 2024;13:27–35.
82. Vidula N, Dubash T, Lawrence MS, Simoneau A, Niemierko A, Blouch E, et al. Identification of somatically acquired *BRCA1/2* Mutations by cfDNA Analysis in Patients with Metastatic Breast Cancer. Clin Cancer Res. 2020;26(18):4852–62.
83. Gristina V, La Mantia M, Peri M, Iacono F, Barraco N, Perez A, et al. Navigating the liquid biopsy minimal residual disease (MRD) in non-small cell lung cancer: making the invisible visible. Crit Rev Oncol Hematol. 2023;182:103899.
84. Martínez-Castedo B, Camblor DG, Martín-Arana J, Carbonell-Asins JA, García-Micó B, Gambardella V, et al. Minimal residual disease in colorectal cancer. Tumor-informed versus tumor-agnostic approaches: unraveling the optimal strategy. Ann Oncol. 2025;36(3):263–76.
85. Tie J, Cohen JD, Lahouel K, Lo SN, Wang Y, Kosmider S, et al. Circulating tumor DNA analysis guiding adjuvant therapy in stage II colon cancer. N Engl J Med. 2022;386(24):2261–72.
86. Tie J, Wang Y, Loree JM, Cohen JD, Espinosa D, Wong R, et al. ctDNA-guided adjuvant chemotherapy escalation in stage III colon cancer: primary analysis of the ctDNA-positive cohort from the randomized AGITG dynamic-III trial (intergroup study of AGITG and CCTG). J Clin Oncol. 2025;43(16_suppl):3503.
87. Herbst RS, John T, Grohé C, Goldman JW, Kato T, Laktionov K, et al. Molecular residual disease analysis of adjuvant osimertinib in resected EGFR-mutated stage IB-IIIA non-small-cell lung cancer. Nat Med. 2025;31(6):1958–68.
88. Loi S, Johnston SRD, Arteaga CL, Graff SL, Chandarlapaty S, Goetz MP, et al. Prognostic utility of ctDNA detection in the monarchE trial of adjuvant abemaciclib plus endocrine therapy (ET) in HR+, HER2-, node-positive, high-risk early breast cancer (EBC). J Clin Oncol. 2024;42(17_suppl):LBA507–LBA.
89. Powles T, Assaf ZJ, Degaonkar V, Grivas P, Hussain M, Oudard S, et al. Updated overall survival by circulating tumor DNA status from the phase 3 IMvigor010 trial: adjuvant Atezolizumab versus observation in muscle-invasive urothelial carcinoma. Eur Urol. 2024;85(2):114–22.
90. Yanala UR, Martos MP, Dickey EM, Corona AM, Ezenwajiaku N, Pizzolato JF, et al. Utility of circulating tumor DNA (ctDNA) for the detection of minimal residual disease (MRD) after curative-intent therapy for patients with localized pancreatic adenocarcinoma (PDAC): a single institution series and meta-analysis. J Clin Oncol. 2024;42(3_suppl):695.
91. Awad MM, Forde PM, Girard N, Spicer J, Wang C, Lu S, et al. Neoadjuvant Nivolumab plus Ipilimumab versus chemotherapy in Resectable lung cancer. J Clin Oncol. 2025;43(12):1453–62.
92. Provencio M, Nadal E, Insa A, García Campelo R, Casal J, Dómine M, et al. Perioperative chemotherapy and nivolumab in non-small-cell lung cancer (NADIM): 5-year clinical outcomes from a multicentre, single-arm, phase 2 trial. Lancet Oncol. 2024;25(11):1453–64.
93. Provencio Pulla M, Awad M, Cascone T, Spicer JD, He J, Lu S, et al. LBA50 perioperative nivolumab (NIVO) v placebo (PBO) in patients (pts) with resectable NSCLC: clinical update from the phase III CheckMate 77T study. Ann Oncol. 2024;35:S1239–S40.
94. Reck M, Gale D, Zhu Z, Harpole D, Taube J, Mitsudomi T, et al. LBA49 associations of ctDNA clearance (CL) during neoadjuvant Tx with pathological response and event-free survival (EFS) in pts with resectable NSCLC (R-NSCLC): expanded analyses from AEGEAN. Ann Oncol. 2024;35:S1239.
95. Gradishar WJ, Moran MS, Abraham J, Abramson V, Aft R, Agnese D, et al. Breast cancer, version 3.2024, NCCN clinical practice guidelines in oncology. J Natl Compr Cancer Netw. 2024;22(5):331–57.
96. Wood DE, Kazerooni EA, Aberle DR, Argento C, Baines J, Boer B, et al. NCCN guidelines® insights: lung cancer screening, version 1.2025. J Natl Compr Canc Netw. 2025;23(1):e250002.
97. Ness RM, Llor X, Abbass MA, Bishu S, Chen CT, Cooper G, et al. NCCN guidelines® insights: colorectal cancer screening, version 1.2024. J Natl Compr Cancer Netw. 2024;22(7):438–46.
98. Moses KA, Sprenkle PC, Bahler C, Box G, Carlsson SV, Catalona WJ, et al. NCCN guidelines® insights: prostate cancer early detection, version 1.2023. J Natl Compr Cancer Netw. 2023;21(3):236–46.
99. Voelker RA. Cervical cancer screening. JAMA. 2023;330(20):2030.
100. Cohen JD, Li L, Wang Y, Thoburn C, Afsari B, Danilova L, et al. Detection and localization of surgically resectable cancers with a multi-analyte blood test. Science. 2018;359(6378):926–30.
101. Klein EA, Richards D, Cohn A, Tummala M, Lapham R, Cosgrove D, et al. Clinical validation of a targeted methylation-based multi-cancer early detection test using an independent validation set. Ann Oncol. 2021;32(9):1167–77.
102. Schrag D, Beer TM, McDonnell CH, Nadauld L, Dilaveri CA, Reid R, et al. Blood-based tests for multicancer early detection (PATHFINDER): a prospective cohort study. Lancet. 2023;402(10409):1251–60.
103. Loomans-Kropp HA, Song Y, Gala M, Parikh AR, Van Seventer EE, Alvarez R, et al. Methylated Septin9 (m SEPT9): a promising blood-based biomarker for the detection and screening of early-onset colorectal cancer. Cancer Res Commun. 2022;2(2):90–8.
104. Chung DC, Gray DM, Singh H, Issaka RB, Raymond VM, Eagle C, et al. A cell-free DNA blood-based

test for colorectal cancer screening. N Engl J Med. 2024;390(11):973–83.
105. Medina JE, Annapragada AV, Lof P, Short S, Bartolomucci AL, Mathios D, et al. Early detection of ovarian cancer using cell-free DNA fragmentomes and protein biomarkers. Cancer Discov. 2025;15(1):105–18.
106. Leal AIC, Mathios D, Jakubowski D, Johansen JS, Lau A, Wu T, et al. Cell-free DNA Fragmentomes in the diagnostic evaluation of patients with symptoms suggestive of lung cancer. Chest. 2023;164(4):1019–27.
107. Malapelle U, Mayo de-Las-Casas C, Rocco D, Garzon M, Pisapia P, Jordana-Ariza N, et al. Development of a gene panel for next-generation sequencing of clinically relevant mutations in cell-free DNA from cancer patients. Br J Cancer. 2017;116(6):802–10.
108. Alexandrou G, Mantikas KT, Allsopp R, Yapeter CA, Jahin M, Melnick T, et al. The evolution of affordable technologies in liquid biopsy diagnostics: the key to clinical implementation. Cancers (Basel). 2023;15(22):5434.
109. Dube S, Qin J, Ramakrishnan R. Mathematical analysis of copy number variation in a DNA sample using digital PCR on a nanofluidic device. PLoS One. 2008;3(8):e2876.
110. García-Foncillas J, Alba E, Aranda E, Díaz-Rubio E, López-López R, Tabernero J, et al. Incorporating BEAMing technology as a liquid biopsy into clinical practice for the management of colorectal cancer patients: an expert taskforce review. Ann Oncol. 2017;28(12):2943–9.
111. Scimone C, Pepe F, Russo G, Palumbo L, Ball G, Morel P, et al. Technical evaluation of a novel digital PCR platform for detecting. J Liq Biopsy. 2024;3:100133.
112. Liao Y, Chen Y, Kou X, Xiao Y, Ye J, Wu A. Diagnostic test accuracy of droplet digital PCR for the detection of EGFR mutation (T790M) in plasma: systematic review and meta-analysis. Clin Chim Acta. 2020;503:190–6.
113. Venetis K, Pepe F, Pescia C, Cursano G, Criscitiello C, Frascarelli C, et al. ESR1 mutations in HR+/HER2-metastatic breast cancer: enhancing the accuracy of ctDNA testing. Cancer Treat Rev. 2023;121:102642.
114. Febbo PG, Allo M, Alme EB, Cuyun Carter G, Dumanois R, Essig A, et al. Recommendations for the equitable and widespread implementation of liquid biopsy for cancer care. JCO Precis Oncol. 2024;8:e2300382.
115. Restrepo JC, Martínez Guevara D, Pareja López A, Montenegro Palacios JF, Liscano Y. Identification and application of emerging biomarkers in treatment of non-small-cell lung cancer: systematic review. Cancers (Basel). 2024;16(13):2338.
116. Kim H, Ahn S, Hong JY, Lee J, Park SH, Park JO, et al. The prevalence of homologous recombination deficiency (HRD) in various solid tumors and the role of HRD as a single biomarker to immune checkpoint inhibitors. J Cancer Res Clin Oncol. 2022;148(9):2427–35.
117. Passaro A, Al Bakir M, Hamilton EG, Diehn M, André F, Roy-Chowdhuri S, et al. Cancer biomarkers: emerging trends and clinical implications for personalized treatment. Cell. 2024;187(7):1617–35.
118. Moreno-Manuel A, Calabuig-Fariñas S, Obrador-Hevia A, Blasco A, Fernández-Díaz A, Sirera R, et al. dPCR application in liquid biopsies: divide and conquer. Expert Rev Mol Diagn. 2021;21(1):3–15.
119. Imperial R, Nazer M, Ahmed Z, Kam AE, Pluard TJ, Bahaj W, et al. Matched whole-genome sequencing (WGS) and whole-exome sequencing (WES) of tumor tissue with circulating tumor DNA (ctDNA) analysis: complementary modalities in clinical practice. Cancers (Basel). 2019;11(9):1399.
120. Albitar M, Charifa A, Agersborg S, Pecora A, Ip A, Goy A. Expanding the clinical utility of liquid biopsy by using liquid transcriptome and artificial intelligence. J Liq Biopsy. 2024;6:100270.
121. Abad A, Vidal J, Layos L, Morcillo C, Achaerandio I, Viteri S. Liquid biopsy, big data and artificial intelligence as a new global clinical trial model in targeted therapy. J Liq Biopsy. 2023;1:100008.
122. Athieniti E, Spyrou GM. A guide to multi-omics data collection and integration for translational medicine. Comput Struct Biotechnol J. 2023;21:134–49.
123. Serrano MJ, Garrido-Navas MC, Diaz Mochon JJ, Cristofanilli M, Gil-Bazo I, Pauwels P, et al. Precision prevention and cancer interception: the new challenges of liquid biopsy. Cancer Discov. 2020;10(11):1635–44.

Part IV

Future Directions and Research Opportunities

20 Future Directions and Research Opportunities

Giannicola Genovese and Luigi Perelli

Introduction

Over the last decade, next-generation sequencing (NGS) has transformed the clinical and laboratory workflow used for solid tumor diagnostic, enabling detection of somatic mutations, structural variants, fusions, and gene expression profile, thus providing critical information for meaningful clinical decisions aimed to explore the molecular features of solid tumors [1]. In the years to come, NGS platforms are trending to be a critical component of routine diagnostic for the detections of clonal mutational processes that could be used for patients' stratification, and the detection of actionable targets to be exploited with new classes of biological compounds [2]. Nevertheless, the full potential of NGS has yet to be unleashed: Current trends indicate that a "second wave" of NGS technologies is gradually replacing the "first generation," which consisted mostly of narrow targeted panels or bulk sequencing approaches that often overlook the full biological complexity of solid tumors. The "Second-Next-Generation" sequencing technologies will be based on three critical aspects: (i) integrating multiomic technology in the spatial context of the tumor ecosystem; (ii) longitudinal single cell resolution multiomic analysis; and (iii) long-read sequencing for the detection of structural variants that are inaccessible to the short read sequencing technology [3–5]. This broad spectrum of novel technologies that are being testing in preclinical and clinical settings holds the promise to detect the extreme heterogeneity of the tumor ecosystem at unprecedent resolution, contributing to an improved classification of several tumor types. Furthermore, the rapid "evolution" of artificial intelligence (AI) systems and large language models (LLM) in the context of health care will disrupt the traditional workflow of data handling and processing [6]. It is easy to anticipate that multiomic profiling from a single biopsy or surgical collection will be processed through multiple second-NGS platforms and interpreted by high-level analytical machines. Here we discuss the most promising NGS technologies and the future impact on the diagnostic of solid tumors and translational research.

G. Genovese (✉)
Department of Genitourinary Medical Oncology, Houston, TX, USA

TRACTION Platform, Houston, TX, USA

Department of Genomic Medicine, Houston, TX, USA
e-mail: GGenovese@mdanderson.org

L. Perelli
Department of Cancer Biology, Houston, TX, USA
e-mail: LPerelli@mdanderson.org

© The Author(s), under exclusive license to Springer Nature Switzerland AG 2026

S. Sioletic, L. Coppola (eds.), *Next-Generation Sequencing in Solid Tumor Histopathology*, Current Clinical Pathology, https://doi.org/10.1007/978-3-032-18790-1_20

Spatial Multiomic NGS

Traditional histopathology provides a uniquely spatial view of tumor biology, revealing architecture, margins, and stromal composition; at the same time, NGS technologies have been so far instrumental in detecting the molecular features of solid tumors (genomics, epigenomics, transcriptomics, proteomics, metabolomics), thus revealing the essential drivers of tumor progression. Spatial multiomic sequencing combines the state of the art of NGS preserving the spatial information that is unique of traditional histopathology, as described in detail in previous chapters. In the recent 5 years, there has been an explosion of research work focused on the development of spatially resolved genomics and transcriptomics, which allows researchers to directly map genetic and transcriptional heterogeneity onto tissue architecture [7, 8]. Co-registration of tumor samples processed with traditional histopathology methods coupled with spatial barcoded platforms offer the opportunity to identify how specific subpopulations of tumor cells localize within invasive fronts, immune niches, or perivascular regions [9, 10]. This co-localization is particularly important in understanding how tumor microenvironments support or suppress tumor progression and how clonal expansion of specific cell types may align with distinct histological features. Furthermore, spatial multiomics enables researchers to investigate not only the cancer cells themselves but also the role of stromal, endothelial, and immune cells in shaping tumor evolution and therapy resistance [11]. The application of spatial multiomic technology to surgical material has been invaluable for a complete characterization of intra- and interpatient heterogeneity. So far, studies have been conducted on pancreatic cancer, gastric cancer, colorectal cancer, lung cancer, glioblastoma, just to mention a few [10, 12–15]. These studies highlight the ability of spatial approaches to reveal hidden layers of tumor complexity—for example, spatial segregation of clones with specific mutational signatures or gene expression programs that drive metastatic potential [7]. The integration of the traditional with the NGS platform is addressing long-standing questions about the evolutionary trajectories of solid tumor cells during the metastatization process or under the influence of therapies. By linking histological features to genomic and transcriptomic profiles, researchers are beginning to reconstruct spatial evolutionary maps of tumors, providing insights into how resistance emerges under treatment pressure. The current research efforts are now focusing on developing robust pipelines that begin with pathologist-assisted selection of the region of interest, processing of spatially barcoded regions and/or nuclei within the region of interest and culminate in integrated maps of tumor-immune interactions [16]. These workflows increasingly involve machine learning and artificial intelligence approaches to align histological imaging data with high-dimensional molecular readouts, thereby generating highly detailed atlases of tumor ecosystems [17–19]. Importantly, these integrated pipelines may one day allow for real-time spatial profiling in clinical settings, complementing traditional diagnostic approaches. The application of spatial sequencing technology to the diagnosis, classification, and characterization of solid tumor is an expanding area of interest for the study of the pathology of solid tumors. However, several limitations do exist that limit its use in routinary diagnostic settings: (1) The generation of spatially barcoded slides is extremely expansive, limiting the amount of sample that can be processed through this platform; (2) the resolution of genomic material is usually low, thus limiting a deep analysis of the molecular features at single-cell resolution. In addition, challenges include sample preservation, data integration across platforms, and the computational burden of analyzing terabytes of highly complex data. In the next decade, spatial technologies will be potentiated to bypass these important limitations. Advances in chemistry and sequencing sensitivity are expected to lower costs and increase resolution, making single-cell spatial profiling more accessible for larger patient cohorts [20]. Moreover, several consortia are at work to generate guidelines and shared resources to be publicly available, as, for example, cell atlases or spatial maps of tumors. These collaborative efforts, such as the Human Tumor Atlas Network, will standardize protocols, promote reproducibility, and accelerate the adoption of spatial multiomic platforms into both research and clinical practice [21]. The implementation of spatial technologies will provide an extraordinary platform for a detailed, single-cell resolved analysis of the histopathological features of solid tumors. Ultimately, the integration of histology, spatial genomics, and computational modeling has the potential to transform the practice of pathology, bridging the gap between morphological assessment and molecular precision. Such a paradigm shift will not only improve diagnostic accuracy but also pave the way for spatially informed therapeutic interventions, where treatment strategies are guided by the spatial arrangement of tumor and immune cell populations within the tumor microenvironment.

Long-Read Sequencing NGS

The mutational processes that are observed in solid tumors are extremely complex and heterogeneous [22]. Moreover, mutational processes are dynamic and can change during the natural history of tumor progression. They are shaped by intrinsic genomic instability, extrinsic mutagenic exposures, and the selective pressures imposed by therapy [23]. For instance, while a tumor may initially be driven by a canonical mutational signature, such as UV-light-induced DNA damage in melanoma or tobacco exposure in lung cancer, additional processes such as APOBEC-mediated mutagenesis or therapy-induced DNA damage may emerge later in the disease course [24–26]. This dynamic interplay complicates both diagnosis and therapeutic targeting, as tumors evolve temporally and spatially. The application of short-read sequencing has been paradigm shifting in advancing our understanding of the somatic mutational processes in cancer; however, it remains limited in resolving complex structural alterations, repetitive regions, and isoforms. Short-read sequencing excels at profiling point mutations and small insertions or deletions but falls short in untangling larger rearrangements and highly repetitive DNA regions, which are central to the biology of many aggressive tumors. These limitations underscore the need for complementary technologies capable of providing a more comprehensive view of the cancer genome. On the other hand, long-read sequencing technologies, including nanopore and single-molecule real-time platforms, provide direct access to structural variants; gene fusions; alternative isoforms; complex chromosomal events, such as chromotripsis and chromoplexy; and extrachromosomal DNA, all of which are increasingly recognized as drivers of tumor progression and influencing patients' prognosis [27]. Unlike short-read approaches that rely on assembly and inference, long-read sequencing reads span thousands to millions of bases, allowing direct characterization of rearrangements in their native genomic context [28]. This ability is particularly relevant in cancers where structural variations, rather than point mutations, dominate the oncogenic landscape [29]. By capturing rearrangements in their entirety, long-read methods open new windows into tumor biology, allowing researchers to directly observe events that were previously hidden in fragmented sequencing data. While applying these methods to traditional histopathological methods remains challenging, this is a rapid evolving area of research. One major hurdle has been the quality of DNA and RNA obtained from formalin-fixed, paraffin-embedded (FFPE) samples, which are the mainstay of clinical pathology. Nevertheless, protocols for extracting high-molecular-weight nucleic acids from archival specimens are improving, raising the prospect that long-read sequencing could be integrated into routine diagnostic workflows [30, 31]. Furthermore, advances in sequencing throughput and cost reduction are steadily moving the field closer to clinical applicability. Long-read fusion panels may improve sensitivity of detection, classification, and prediction of therapy response in sarcomas, thyroid cancers, and gliomas, where cryptic fusions often influence tumor progression [32–34]. In many of these tumor types, the presence of a fusion not only serves as a diagnostic hallmark but also guides therapy. For example, NTRK, ALK, and RET fusions confer sensitivity to targeted inhibitors yet are often missed by conventional methods due to complex breakpoints [35]. By fully spanning the fusion junctions, long-read panels offer the potential to increase diagnostic accuracy and therapeutic matching in these contexts [36]. Beyond fusions, long-read sequencing enables to map extrachromosomal DNA and enhancer hijacking events which have been connected to disease progression in high-grade glioma and esophageal cancers, where oncogenes are usually selected within an amplification region by complex structural chromosomal events [37–39]. These circular DNA elements can carry amplified oncogenes and regulatory elements, providing tumors with rapid evolutionary adaptability [37]. Their detection and characterization require sequencing reads that capture large structural units intact—something uniquely possible with long-read approaches [40, 41]. The ability to resolve enhancer hijacking further expands the clinical utility of long-read sequencing, as it highlights not only which genes are altered but also how their regulation is rewired to drive oncogenesis. It is worth to note that long-read technologies can be applied to different types of multiomic sequencing, including single cell, spatial, transcriptomic, genomic, and epigenomic sequencing [5, 6, 27, 28, 35]. This versatility opens unprecedented opportunities to connect structural alterations to functional consequences across multiple biological layers. For example, single-cell long-read sequencing can disentangle clonal architectures and track the evolution of structural variants within individual tumors, while spatial applications can map these events in the histological context of tumor microenvironments [40]. By integrating with transcriptomic and epigenomic readouts, researchers can move beyond cataloging alterations to understanding their functional impact on transcriptional regulation, chromatin states, and cellular phenotypes [42]. This new type of technology has an unparalleled sensitivity, and it can detect very repetitive regions of the genome, such as the centromere, which have only recently been fully sequenced [43, 44]. The capacity to explore previously inaccessible "dark regions" of the genome has major implications for cancer biology, as these regions harbor structural instabilities and potential regulatory elements [45]. With complete assemblies now within reach, long-read sequencing may redefine our understanding of genome architecture and its contribution to tumor evolution. The main limitation of this new technology is the complex bioinformatic pipelines required to analyze the data and the denoising of variant calling from long-read sequencing. Error profiles remain higher compared to short-read sequencing, demanding sophisticated computational approaches to distinguish true variants from technical noise [46]. Moreover, the vast amount of data generated requires significant storage, computational infrastructure, and specialized expertise, all of which limit current adoption in clinical laboratories. Also in this case, new guidelines are being published to help navigate the complexity of the analysis of this NGS data [47]; when a consensus will be reached, it is highly likely that long-read sequencing will be a routine diagnostic technology to be exploited for some specific tumor types. As with short-read sequencing a decade ago, widespread clinical implementation will depend on the establishment of standardized best practices, regulatory approval, and demonstration of clear clinical utility. Given its rapidly expanding applications, long-read sequencing is poised to transition from research laboratories into pathology suites, transforming the molecular diagnosis and management of solid tumors.

Epigenomic and Proteogenomic NGS

In the last decade, the first NGS technologies have provided critical information on the analysis of DNA and RNA from solid tumors. These platforms have transformed the molecular characterization of cancer, allowing researchers and clinicians to systematically identify mutations, fusions, copy number alterations, and expression changes that were previously undetectable with conventional methods. However, DNA mutations alone rarely capture the full functional state of tumor cells, since many oncogenic processes are driven not only by genetic alterations but also by layers of regulation that shape how genes are expressed, and proteins are modified in the cellular context [48, 49]. Epigenomic signatures, for example, DNA methylation patterns, nucleosome footprints, and chromatin accessibility, are being investigated as diagnostic classifiers that can stratify histologically ambiguous tumors [50, 51]. These features represent a stable and highly specific molecular "fingerprint" of tumor types, reflecting developmental origins and differentiation states [52, 53]. Methylation-based classifiers have already demonstrated utility in central nervous system tumors, where they have enabled more accurate tumor subtyping and prognostication compared to morphology alone, and are posed for broader adoption in routine pathology [54]. Ongoing research is extending these approaches to other solid tumors such as sarcomas and gastrointestinal cancers, where molecular subtyping remains challenging [55]. In the future, methylation profiling may be integrated into standard workflows, both to confirm diagnoses and to provide predictive information for therapy selection. Parallel advances in RNA sequencing for FFPE tissue (please, see Spatial multiomic NGS paragraph) enable the detection of clinically actionable fusions (e.g., NTRK, ALK, RET) and splice variants, as well as immune and stromal deconvolution from bulk RNA data. This transcript-level information enriches our understanding of tumor biology by revealing aberrant signaling pathways, lineage-specific programs, and the cellular composition of the tumor microenvironment [56, 57]. In addition, RNA sequencing provides insight into dynamic processes such as immune activation, stromal remodeling, and therapy-induced plasticity, which are not captured by DNA-based analysis alone [7, 8, 42]. The incorporation of transcriptomics into clinical pathology thus represents a critical step toward functional characterization of tumors beyond static mutation profiles. The second NGS of epigenomic will be imprinted on detecting isoform-level and RNA editing biomarkers, which may predict immune escape or targeted therapy resistance more accurately than DNA alterations alone [58]. Isoform-specific signatures are increasingly recognized as important modulators of oncogenic signaling and therapeutic response—for example, splice variants of receptor tyrosine kinases or androgen receptor isoforms that confer resistance to targeted inhibitors [59]. Similarly, RNA editing events may alter antigen presentation or disrupt immune recognition, contributing to tumor evasion from immunotherapy. Research in this area is expected to generate novel biomarkers that provide more precise stratification of patients for targeted and immune-based therapies. At the same time, modification at DNA and RNA level only acquire clinical significance if they translate into altered proteins or immunogenic peptides. Proteogenomics, the integration of NGS with mass spectrometry, can confirm which mutations lead to expressed proteins, thus identifying candidate neo-antigens presented by the MHC complex [60]. By directly linking the genomic and transcriptomic layers to the proteome, proteogenomics addresses one of the central limitations of sequencing alone: the inability to determine whether mutations are functionally expressed. This approach improves the predictive value of tumor mutational burden as a biomarker of response to immunotherapies by filtering for expressed and presented variants [61]. In doing so, it moves the field from descriptive catalogs of mutations toward biologically and clinically actionable molecular features. One intense area of research in the field of proteogenomic includes mapping kinase activation states in relation to genomic drivers to build proteogenomic resistance atlases pre- and posttreatment [62, 63]. Such atlases are designed to capture how signaling pathways are rewired under therapeutic pressure, revealing adaptive resistance mechanisms that cannot be inferred from DNA or RNA sequencing alone. For instance, tumors treated with kinase inhibitors often activate bypass pathways or exploit posttranslational modifications that restore signaling flux [64]. By integrating phosphoproteomic data with genomic alterations, researchers can identify rational combination strategies aimed at preventing or overcoming these adaptive mechanisms [65]. Such integrative approaches will be key to inform to immunotherapy response and will provide insightful information for precision medicine, instructing on potential combination therapies. Importantly, their success will depend not only on the ability of sequencing to generate multi-omic data but also on basic and translational research that validates the functional role of the molecular features uncovered by NGS. Establishing mechanistic causality—for example, demonstrating how a specific splice isoform confers drug resistance, or how a neoantigen is processed and presented to the immune system—is essential to move beyond correlation and to translate sequencing discoveries into therapeutic interventions [66]. As the field advances, the integration of epigenomic, transcriptomic, and proteogenomic profiling will redefine the role of histopathology, linking morphology with molecular function and enabling a truly holistic view of tumor biology in clinical practice.

Microbiome and Virome NGS

The role of the microbiome and virome in cancer is rapidly emerging as a frontier for discovery in solid tumor histopathology, considering that key histopathological findings of gastric cancer can be traced back to the study of *H. pilori* [67]. In pancreatic ductal adenocarcinoma, for example, intratumoral bacteria have been shown to metabolize chemotherapy drugs, conferring resistance [68]. In colorectal cancer, specific taxa, such as *F. nucleatum*, are enriched within tumor tissue and have been linked to immune suppression and poor outcomes [69]. The second NGS technologies will use metagenomic sequencing, 16S rRNA amplicon sequencing, or RNA-based dual host microbe transcriptomic to identify directly the microbiome or the virome on FFPE samples [70]. At the same time, the emergence of long-read sequencing technologies is expected to provide insightful basic discovery of the tumor virome [71]. The full landscape of viral contributions to solid tumors remains incompletely mapped. The second wave of NGS technologies offers the ability to detect both viral sequences and viral integration sites with high resolution. The most exciting frontier lies in combining microbiome and virome profiling with host genomic, transcriptomic, and immune data to build a holistic view of the tumor ecosystem [72]. For example, dual RNA sequencing approaches allow simultaneous characterization of the host and microbial gene expression within the same tissue section, connecting microbial activity to immune infiltration, stromal remodeling, and cancer cell adaptation phenomena [73]. Despite the promise, significant challenges remain, particularly considering contamination from reagents and laboratory environments that can confound microbial sequencing [74]. This is a major limitation for routinely diagnostic as the processing of these samples requires rigorous negative controls and computational decontamination strategies. Clinically, it will be necessary to demonstrate that microbiome and virome profiles add actionable value beyond existing histopathologic and other NGS strategies.

Validating NGS Data

It is obvious that the second NGS technologies will provide an unprecedent depth in the profiling of solid tumors, therefore implementing diagnostic through the generation of multiomic data detailing the tumor ecosystem at an unprecedent resolution. However, a critical future direction for the field lies in establishing functional causalities between associations calculated through the analysis of molecular profiles and clinical outcomes. This topic will be a major area of research in the next decade. The enormous amount of data flowing through NGS sequencing provide strong associative correlation between molecular features and clinical parameters, but it is not yet clear if some of these molecular events are only epiphenomena of other biological processes. For example, there has been an active debate in the cancer research community about the role of sarcomatoid transformation and acquisition of mesenchymal features in epithelial tumors and its impact on tumor progression and response to therapy [75–77]. Only recent advances in preclinical modeling and genetic engineering technologies have been able to attenuate the debate with sophisticated in vivo functional experiments [7, 78]. As another example, there is increase clinical evidence showing that different point mutation events on the same gene may diverge in their way of affecting tumorigenesis and tumor progression, particularly for lung and pancreatic cancer [79, 80]. The development of NGS technologies enabling the visualization of extrachromosomal DNA in solid tumors has shown that this phenomenon is extremely prevalent in aggressive cancers; however, there are only few rigorous studies addressing an oncogenic role of extrachromosomal DNA in advanced cancers [81]. Basic research must move beyond descriptive associations to mechanistic studies that prove how specific genomic, transcriptomic, or epigenomic alterations actively shape tumor biology. This requires two essential starting points: (1) Basic research needs to move in parallel with the emergence of second NGS technologies, and it must be able to keep the pace of their application into preclinical and clinical settings; (2) basic research needs to converge toward a more translational approach, where the foundational discoveries of the biology of cancer align with unmet diagnostic and clinical needs [82]. Therefore, basic research must build a "next-generation" of technologies enabling this kind of studies. This requires the generation of preclinical models that mirror the progression of the disease observed in patients, including somatic mosaic genetically engineered mouse models, patient-derived xenotransplants and organoids, new animal models to study more complex and systemic phenomena, and novel three-dimensional culture technologies to recapitulate the microenvironment of the tumor ecosystem. For example, the implementation of CRISPR/Cas9 genome editing technologies has completely revolutionized how researchers are able to manipulate preclinical systems to recapitulate the evolution of solid tumors [78, 83]. Coupling these powerful technologies with NGS will provide critical insights for the discovery of molecular patterns that will be in future used as diagnostic tools. Without such mechanistic anchoring, many of the features identified through second NGS technologies risk to remain correlative biomarkers rather than actionable targets. Bridging this gap between profiling and functional validation will be essential for translating NGS discoveries into meaningful diagnostic tools and therapeutic strategies.

References

1. Krupina K, Goginashvili A, Cleveland DW. Scrambling the genome in cancer: causes and consequences of complex chromosome rearrangements. Nat Rev Genet. 2024;25:196–210.
2. Zehir A, et al. Mutational landscape of metastatic cancer revealed from prospective clinical sequencing of 10,000 patients. Nat Med. 2017;23:703–13.
3. Seferbekova Z, Lomakin A, Yates LR, Gerstung M. Spatial biology of cancer evolution. Nat Rev Genet. 2023;24:295–313.
4. Chakravarty D, Solit DB. Clinical cancer genomic profiling. Nat Rev Genet. 2021;22:483–501.
5. Marx V. Method of the year: long-read sequencing. Nat Methods. 2023;20:6–11.
6. Athanasopoulou K, Michalopoulou VI, Scorilas A, Adamopoulos PG. Integrating artificial intelligence in next-generation sequencing: advances, challenges, and future directions. Curr Issues Mol Biol. 2025;47(6):470.
7. Perelli L, et al. Evolutionary fingerprints of epithelial-to-mesenchymal transition. Nature. 2025;640:1083–92.
8. Russell AJC, et al. Slide-tags enables single-nucleus barcoding for multimodal spatial genomics. Nature. 2024;625:101–9.
9. Dai Y, et al. PPP2R1A mutations portend improved survival after cancer immunotherapy. Nature. 2025;644:537–46.
10. Pei G, et al. Spatial mapping of transcriptomic plasticity in metastatic pancreatic cancer. Nature. 2025;642:212–21.
11. Liu Y, et al. Conserved spatial subtypes and cellular neighborhoods of cancer-associated fibroblasts revealed by single-cell spatial multi-omics. Cancer Cell. 2025;43(5):905–924.e906.
12. Cheng X, et al. Atlas of metastatic gastric cancer links ferroptosis to disease progression and immunotherapy response. Gastroenterology. 2024;167:1345–57.
13. Han G, et al. An atlas of epithelial cell states and plasticity in lung adenocarcinoma. Nature. 2024;627:656–63.
14. Avraham-Davidi I, et al. Spatially defined multicellular functional units in colorectal cancer revealed from single cell and spatial transcriptomics. Elife. 2025;14:RP104815.

15. Miller TE, et al. Programs, origins and immunomodulatory functions of myeloid cells in glioma. Nature. 2025;640:1072–82.
16. Chen W, et al. A visual–omics foundation model to bridge histopathology with spatial transcriptomics. Nat Methods. 2025;22:1568–82.
17. Chen RJ, et al. Towards a general-purpose foundation model for computational pathology. Nat Med. 2024;30:850–62.
18. Chen RJ, et al. Pan-cancer integrative histology-genomic analysis via multimodal deep learning. Cancer Cell. 2022;40(8):865–878.e866.
19. Lu MY, et al. AI-based pathology predicts origins for cancers of unknown primary. Nature. 2021;594:106–10.
20. Juwayria, et al. Microarray integrated spatial transcriptomics (MIST) for affordable and robust digital pathology. NPJ Syst Biol Appl. 2024;10(1):142.
21. Rozenblatt-Rosen O, et al. The human tumor atlas network: charting tumor transitions across space and time at single-cell resolution. Cell. 2020;181:236–49.
22. Gerstung M, et al. The evolutionary history of 2,658 cancers. Nature. 2020;578:122–8.
23. Baker TM, Waise S, Tarabichi M, Van Loo P. Aneuploidy and complex genomic rearrangements in cancer evolution. Nat Cancer. 2024;5:228–39.
24. Alexandrov LB, et al. The repertoire of mutational signatures in human cancer. Nature. 2020;578:94–101.
25. Steele CD, et al. Signatures of copy number alterations in human cancer. Nature. 2022;606:984–91.
26. Li Y, et al. Patterns of somatic structural variation in human cancer genomes. Nature. 2020;578:112–21.
27. Logsdon GA, Vollger MR, Eichler EE. Long-read human genome sequencing and its applications. Nat Rev Genet. 2020;21:597–614.
28. Monzó C, Liu T, Conesa A. Transcriptomics in the era of long-read sequencing. Nat Rev Genet. 2025;26:681–701.
29. Cortés-Ciriano I, et al. Comprehensive analysis of chromothripsis in 2,658 human cancers using whole-genome sequencing. Nat Genet. 2020;52:331–41.
30. Afflerbach AK, et al. Nanopore sequencing from formalin-fixed paraffin-embedded specimens for copy-number profiling and methylation-based CNS tumor classification. Acta Neuropathol. 2024;147:74.
31. Bai Z, et al. Spatially exploring RNA biology in archival formalin-fixed paraffin-embedded tissues. Cell. 2024;187:6760–6779.e6724.
32. Shelton WJ, et al. Long-read sequencing for brain tumors. Front Oncol. 2024;14:1395985.
33. Wang Y, et al. Comprehensive long-read sequencing analysis discloses the transcriptome features of papillary thyroid microcarcinoma. J Clin Endocrinol Metab. 2024;109:1263–74.
34. Watkins JA, et al. Introduction and impact of routine whole genome sequencing in the diagnosis and management of sarcoma. Br J Cancer. 2024;131:860–9.
35. Sinha S, et al. Long read sequencing enhances pathogenic and novel variation discovery in patients with rare diseases. Nat Commun. 2025;16:2500.
36. Elrick H, et al. SAVANA: reliable analysis of somatic structural variants and copy number aberrations using long-read sequencing. Nat Methods. 2025;22:1436–46.
37. Bailey C, et al. Origins and impact of extrachromosomal DNA. Nature. 2024;635:193–200.
38. Luebeck J, et al. Extrachromosomal DNA in the cancerous transformation of Barrett's oesophagus. Nature. 2023;616:798–805.
39. Kim H, et al. Mapping extrachromosomal DNA amplifications during cancer progression. Nat Genet. 2024;56:2447–54.
40. Chamorro González R, et al. Parallel sequencing of extrachromosomal circular DNAs and transcriptomes in single cancer cells. Nat Genet. 2023;55:880–90.
41. Giurgiu M, et al. Reconstructing extrachromosomal DNA structural heterogeneity from long-read sequencing data using Decoil. Genome Res. 2024;34:1355–64.
42. Cittaro D, Lazarević D, Tonon G, Giannese F. Analyzing genomic and epigenetic profiles in single cells by hybrid transposase (scGET-seq). STAR Protoc. 2023;4:102176.
43. Altemose N, et al. Complete genomic and epigenetic maps of human centromeres. Science. 2022;376:eabl4178.
44. Logsdon GA, et al. The variation and evolution of complete human centromeres. Nature. 2024;629:136–45.
45. Alexander RP, Fang G, Rozowsky J, Snyder M, Gerstein MB. Annotating non-coding regions of the genome. Nat Rev Genet. 2010;11:559–71.
46. Amarasinghe SL, et al. Opportunities and challenges in long-read sequencing data analysis. Genome Biol. 2020;21:30.
47. Guo Y, et al. A detailed guide to assessing genome assembly based on long-read sequencing data using Inspector. Nat Protoc. 2025;20:2845.
48. Esteller M, et al. The epigenetic hallmarks of cancer. Cancer Discov. 2024;14:1783–809.
49. Flavahan WA, Gaskell E, Bernstein BE. Epigenetic plasticity and the hallmarks of cancer. Science. 2017;357:eaal2380.
50. Benfatto S, et al. Explainable artificial intelligence of DNA methylation-based brain tumor diagnostics. Nat Commun. 2025;16:1787.
51. Corces MR, et al. The chromatin accessibility landscape of primary human cancers. Science. 2018;362:eaav1898.
52. Yost KE, et al. Three-dimensional genome landscape of primary human cancers. Nat Genet. 2025;57:1189–200.
53. Akdemir KC, et al. Somatic mutation distributions in cancer genomes vary with three-dimensional chromatin structure. Nat Genet. 2020;52:1178–88.
54. Tran QT, et al. Comparison of DNA methylation based classification models for precision diagnostics of central nervous system tumors. NPJ Precis Oncol. 2024;8:218.
55. Koelsche C, et al. Sarcoma classification by DNA methylation profiling. Nat Commun. 2021;12:498.

56. Zhang D, et al. Spatial epigenome–transcriptome co-profiling of mammalian tissues. Nature. 2023;616:113–22.
57. Huang Y-H, et al. Unified molecular approach for spatial epigenome, transcriptome, and cell lineages. Proc Natl Acad Sci U S A. 2025;122:e2424070122.
58. Al'Khafaji AM, et al. High-throughput RNA isoform sequencing using programmed cDNA concatenation. Nat Biotechnol. 2024;42:582–6.
59. Zhang Y, Qian J, Gu C, Yang Y. Alternative splicing and cancer: a systematic review. Signal Transduct Target Ther. 2021;6:78.
60. Nesvizhskii AI. Proteogenomics: concepts, applications and computational strategies. Nat Methods. 2014;11:1114–25.
61. Huber F, et al. A comprehensive proteogenomic pipeline for neoantigen discovery to advance personalized cancer immunotherapy. Nat Biotechnol. 2025;43:1360–72.
62. Elmas A, et al. Pan-cancer proteogenomic investigations identify post-transcriptional kinase targets. Commun Biol. 2021;4:1112.
63. Li Y, et al. Pan-cancer proteogenomics connects oncogenic drivers to functional states. Cell. 2023;186:3921–3944.e3925.
64. Miao C, et al. Post-translational modifications in drug resistance. Drug Resist Updat. 2025;78:101173.
65. Müller-Dott S, et al. Comprehensive evaluation of phosphoproteomic-based kinase activity inference. Nat Commun. 2025;16:4771.
66. Zhang K, Schölkopf B, Spirtes P, Glymour C. Learning causality and causality-related learning: some recent progress. Natl Sci Rev. 2018;5:26–9.
67. Warren JR, Marshall B. Unidentified curved bacilli on gastric epithelium in active chronic gastritis. Lancet. 1983;1:1273–5.
68. Riquelme E, et al. Tumor microbiome diversity and composition influence pancreatic cancer outcomes. Cell. 2019;178:795–806.e712.
69. Zepeda-Rivera M, et al. A distinct fusobacterium nucleatum clade dominates the colorectal cancer niche. Nature. 2024;628:424–32.
70. Khan MAW, Ologun G, Arora R, McQuade JL, Wargo JA. Gut microbiome modulates response to cancer immunotherapy. Dig Dis Sci. 2020;65:885–96.
71. Elbasir A, et al. A deep learning approach reveals unexplored landscape of viral expression in cancer. Nat Commun. 2023;14:785.
72. Hermida LC, Gertz EM, Ruppin E. Predicting cancer prognosis and drug response from the tumor microbiome. Nat Commun. 2022;13:2896.
73. Macho Rendón J, Lang B, Ramos Llorens M, Gaetano Tartaglia G, Torrent Burgas M. DualSeqDB: the host-pathogen dual RNA sequencing database for infection processes. Nucleic Acids Res. 2021;49:D687–d693.
74. Austin GI, et al. Contamination source modeling with SCRuB improves cancer phenotype prediction from microbiome data. Nat Biotechnol. 2023;41:1820–8.
75. Kalluri R. EMT: when epithelial cells decide to become mesenchymal-like cells. J Clin Invest. 2009;119:1417–9.
76. Kalluri R, Weinberg RA. The basics of epithelial-mesenchymal transition. J Clin Invest. 2009;119:1420–8.
77. Zheng X, et al. Epithelial-to-mesenchymal transition is dispensable for metastasis but induces chemoresistance in pancreatic cancer. Nature. 2015;527:525–30.
78. Perelli L, et al. Interferon signaling promotes tolerance to chromosomal instability during metastatic evolution in renal cancer. Nat Cancer. 2023;4:984–1000.
79. Alonso S, et al. Concurrent genetic and non-genetic resistance mechanisms to KRAS inhibition in CRC. bioRxiv. 2025
80. McIntyre CA, et al. Distinct clinical outcomes and biological features of specific KRAS mutants in human pancreatic cancer. Cancer Cell. 2024;42:1614–1629.e1615.
81. Pradella D, et al. Engineered extrachromosomal oncogene amplifications promote tumorigenesis. Nature. 2025;637:955–64.
82. Lorsch JR, Tabak LA, Bertagnolli MM. Applied research won't flourish without basic science. elife. 2024;13:e102368.
83. Ely ZA, et al. A prime editor mouse to model a broad spectrum of somatic mutations in vivo. Nat Biotechnol. 2024;42:424–36.

Index

© The Editor(s) (if applicable) and The Author(s), under exclusive license to Springer Nature Switzerland AG 2026
S. Sioletic, L. Coppola (eds.), *Next-Generation Sequencing in Solid Tumor Histopathology*, Current Clinical Pathology, https://doi.org/10.1007/978-3-032-18790-1

Q

R

T